HARRISON'S
Manual of
Medicine

EDITORS

Dennis L. Kasper, MD, MA(HON)
William Ellery Channing Professor of Medicine,
Professor of Microbiology and Molecular Genetics,
Harvard Medical School;
Director, Channing Laboratory,
Department of Medicine,
Brigham and Women's Hospital, Boston

Eugene Braunwald, MD, MA(HON), MD(HON), ScD(HON)
Distinguished Hersey Professor of Medicine,
Harvard Medical School;
Chairman, TIMI Study Group,
Brigham and Women's Hospital, Boston

Anthony S. Fauci, MD, ScD(HON)
Chief, Laboratory of Immunoregulation; Director,
National Institute of Allergy and Infectious Diseases,
National Institutes of Health, Bethesda

Stephen L. Hauser, MD
Robert A. Fishman Distinguished Professor and Chairman,
Department of Neurology, University of
California–San Francisco,
San Francisco

Dan L. Longo, MD
Scientific Director, National Institute on Aging,
National Institutes of Health,
Bethesda and Baltimore

J. Larry Jameson, MD, PhD
Irving S. Cutter Professor and Chairman,
Department of Medicine,
Northwestern University Feinberg School of Medicine;
Physician-in-Chief, Northwestern
Memorial Hospital, Chicago

HARRISON'S Manual of Medicine

EDITORS

Dennis L. Kasper, MD

Eugene Braunwald, MD

Anthony S. Fauci, MD

Stephen L. Hauser, MD

Dan L. Longo, MD

J. Larry Jameson, MD, PhD

McGraw-Hill
Medical Publishing Division

New York   Chicago   San Francisco   Lisbon   London
Madrid   Mexico City   Milan   New Delhi   San Juan
Seoul   Singapore   Sydney   Toronto

Harrison's
PRINCIPLES OF INTERNAL MEDICINE
Sixteenth Edition
MANUAL OF MEDICINE

3 4 5 6 7 8 9 0   DOCDOC   0 9 8 7 6
ISBN 0-07-144441-6

This book was set in Times New Roman by Progressive Information Technologies. The editors were James Shanahan and Mariapaz Ramos Englis; the production supervisor was Catherine H. Saggese; the designer was Marsha Cohen. The index was prepared by Barbara Littlewood.
RR Donnelley was printer and binder.
Cover illustrations courtesy of Raymond J. Gibbons, MD;
George V. Kelvin; and Marilu Gorno-Tempini, MD.

Library of Congress Cataloging-in-Publication Data
Harrison's manual of medicine / editors, Dennis L. Kasper . . . [et al.].
    p. ; cm.
A distillation of clinical material from Harrison's principles of internal medicine, 16th ed.
Includes bibliographical references and index.
ISBN 0-07-144441-6
    1. Internal medicine—Handbooks, manuals, etc. I. Title: Manual of medicine. II. Kasper, Dennis L. III. Harrison, Tinsley Randolph, 1900–
IV. Harrison's principles of internal medicine.
    [DNLM: 1. Clinical Medicine—Handbooks. 2. Internal Medicine—Handbooks.]
RC46.H333 2005 Suppl.
616—dc22
                                                        2004065625
INTERNATIONAL EDITION ISBN 0-07-111930-2
Copyright © 2005. Exclusive rights by The McGraw-Hill Companies, Inc., for manufacture and export. This book cannot be re-exported from the country to which it is consigned by McGraw-Hill. The International Edition is not available in North America.

CONTENTS

Contributors   *xiii*

Preface   *xv*

SECTION 1
CARE OF THE HOSPITALIZED PATIENT

1 Initial Evaluation and Admission Orders for the General Medicine Patient 1

2 Assessment of Nutritional Status 2

3 Electrolytes/Acid-Base Balance 5

4 Enteral and Parenteral Nutrition 14

5 Transfusion and Pheresis Therapy 17

6 Principles of Critical Care Medicine 19

7 Respiratory Failure 22

8 Pain and Its Management 23

9 Procedures Commonly Performed by Internists 28

10 Diagnostic Imaging in Internal Medicine 32

11 Gastrointestinal Diseases 34

SECTION 2
MEDICAL EMERGENCIES

12 Acute Respiratory Distress Syndrome (ARDS) 39

13 Cardiovascular Collapse and Sudden Death 41

14 Shock 44

15 Sepsis and Septic Shock 49

16 Acute Pulmonary Edema 53

17 Confusion, Stupor, and Coma 54

18 Stroke 58

19 Subarachnoid Hemorrhage 66

20 Increased Intracranial Pressure and Head Trauma 67

21 Hypoxic-Ischemic Encephalopathy 69

22 Status Epilepticus 72

23 Poisoning and Drug Overdose 74

24 Diabetic Ketoacidosis and Hyperosmolar Coma 89

25 Hypoglycemia 91

26 Infectious Disease Emergencies 94

27 Oncologic Emergencies 101

28 Anaphylaxis 105

29 Bites, Venoms, Stings, and Marine Poisonings 106

30 Hypothermia and Frostbite 115

31 Bioterrorism 118

SECTION 3
COMMON PATIENT PRESENTATIONS

32 Chest Pain 133

33 Abdominal Pain 136

34 Headache 139

35 Back and Neck Pain 147

36 Fever, Hyperthermia, Chills, and Rash 156

37 Pain or Swelling of Joints 161

38 Syncope and Faintness 164

39 Dizziness and Vertigo 168

40 Acute Visual Loss and Double Vision 171

41 Paralysis and Movement
Disorders 175
42 Aphasias and Related
Disorders 179
43 Sleep Disorders 181
44 Dyspnea 185
45 Cough and Hemoptysis 187
46 Cyanosis 192
47 Edema 194
48 Nausea, Vomiting, and
Indigestion 197
49 Weight Loss 201
50 Dysphagia 203

51 Acute Abdomen 206
52 Diarrhea, Constipation, and
Malabsorption 208
53 Gastrointestinal Bleeding 214
54 Jaundice and Evaluation of
Liver Function 218
55 Ascites 224
56 Azotemia and Urinary
Abnormalities 227
57 Anemia and Polycythemia 232
58 Lymphadenopathy and
Splenomegaly 235

SECTION 4

DISORDERS OF THE EYE, EAR, NOSE, AND THROAT

59 Common Disorders of
Vision and Hearing 241

60 Infections of the Upper
Respiratory Tract 248

SECTION 5

DERMATOLOGY

61 General Examination of
the Skin 255

62 Common Skin Conditions 259

SECTION 6

HEMATOLOGY AND ONCOLOGY

63 Examination of Blood
Smears and Bone Marrow 265
64 Red Blood Cell Disorders 267
65 Leukocytosis and
Leukopenia 272
66 Bleeding and Thrombotic
Disorders 275
67 Prevention and Early
Detection of Cancer 280
68 Cancer Chemotherapy 284
69 Myeloid Leukemias,
Myelodysplasia, and
Myeloproliferative
Syndrome 290
70 Lymphoid Malignancies 296
71 Skin Cancer 307

72 Head and Neck Cancer 309
73 Lung Cancer 310
74 Breast Cancer 316
75 Tumors of the
Gastrointestinal Tract 320
76 Genitourinary Tract Cancer 331
77 Gynecologic Cancer 334
78 Prostate Hyperplasia and
Carcinoma 338
79 Cancer of Unknown
Primary Site 341
80 Paraneoplastic Endocrine
Syndromes 344
81 Neurologic Paraneoplastic
Syndromes 346

SECTION 7
INFECTIOUS DISEASES

82 Diagnosis of Infectious
   Diseases   351
83 Antibacterial Therapy   360
84 Immunization and Advice
   to Travelers   365
85 Infective Endocarditis   372
86 Intraabdominal Infections   380
87 Infectious Diarrheas   383
88 Sexually Transmitted
   Diseases and Reproductive
   Tract Infections   393
89 Infections of the Skin, Soft
   Tissues, Joints, and Bones   408
90 Infections in the
   Immunocompromised Host   417
91 HIV Infection and AIDS   424
92 Hospital-Acquired Infections   442
93 Pneumococcal Infections   445
94 Staphylococcal Infections   448
95 Streptococcal/Enterococcal
   Infections, Diphtheria, and
   Other Corynebacterial
   Infections   455
96 Meningococcal and Listerial
   Infections   462
97 Infections Caused by
   Haemophilus, Bordetella,
   Moraxella, and HACEK
   Group Organisms   466
98 Diseases Caused by Gram-
   Negative Enteric Bacteria,
   Pseudomonas, and
   Legionella   471

99 Infections Caused by Other
   Gram-Negative Bacilli   479
100 Anaerobic Infections   485
101 Nocardiosis and
    Actinomycosis   492
102 Tuberculosis and Other
    Mycobacterial Infections   495
103 Lyme Disease and Other
    Nonsyphilitic Spirochetal
    Infections   506
104 Rickettsial Diseases   510
105 *Mycoplasma* Infections   516
106 Chlamydial Infections   517
107 Herpesvirus Infections   520
108 Cytomegalovirus and
    Epstein-Barr Virus
    Infections   529
109 Influenza and Other Viral
    Respiratory Diseases   533
110 Rubeola, Rubella, Mumps,
    and Parvovirus Infections   539
111 Enteroviral Infections   544
112 Insect- and Animal-Borne
    Viral Infections   547
113 Fungal Infections   555
114 *Pneumocystis* Infection   565
115 Protozoal Infections   569
116 Helminthic Infections   580

SECTION 8
CARDIOVASCULAR DISEASES

117 Physical Examination of the
    Heart   593
118 Electrocardiography and
    Echocardiography   596
119 Valvular Heart Disease   603
120 Cardiomyopathies and
    Myocarditis   609
121 Pericardial Disease   612

122 Hypertension   616
123 ST-Segment Elevation
    Myocardial Infarction
    (STEMI)   621
124 Chronic Stable Angina,
    Unstable Angina, and Non-
    ST-Elevation Myocardial
    Infarction   631

125 Arrhythmias   638
126 Congestive Heart Failure
    and Cor Pulmonale   648

127 Diseases of the Aorta   653
128 Peripheral Vascular Disease   655
129 Pulmonary Hypertension   658

SECTION 9
RESPIRATORY DISEASES

130 Respiratory Function and
    Pulmonary Diagnostic
    Procedures   663
131 Asthma and Hypersensitivity
    Pneumonitis   668
132 Environmental Lung
    Diseases   673
133 Chronic Bronchitis,
    Emphysema, and Acute
    or Chronic Respiratory
    Failure   675

134 Pneumonia and Lung
    Abscess   679
135 Pulmonary
    Thromboembolism   685
136 Interstitial Lung Disease
    (ILD)   687
137 Diseases of the Pleura,
    Mediastinum, and
    Diaphragm   691
138 Disorders of Ventilation,
    Including Sleep Apnea   695

SECTION 10
RENAL DISEASES

139 Approach to the Patient with
    Renal Disease   699
140 Acute Renal Failure   702
141 Chronic Kidney Disease
    (CKD) and Uremia   707
142 Dialysis   709
143 Renal Transplantation   711

144 Glomerular Diseases   713
145 Renal Tubular Disease   720
146 Urinary Tract Infections   724
147 Renovascular Disease   728
148 Nephrolithiasis   731
149 Urinary Tract Obstruction   734

SECTION 11
GASTROINTESTINAL DISEASES

150 Peptic Ulcer and Related
    Disorders   737
151 Inflammatory Bowel
    Diseases   742
152 Colonic and Anorectal
    Diseases   746
153 Cholelithiasis, Cholecystitis,
    and Cholangitis   749

154 Pancreatitis   753
155 Acute Hepatitis   757
156 Chronic Hepatitis   762
157 Cirrhosis and Alcoholic
    Liver Disease   766
158 Portal Hypertension   769

SECTION 12
ALLERGY, CLINICAL IMMUNOLOGY, AND RHEUMATOLOGY

159 Diseases of Immediate
Type Hypersensitivity   773
160 Primary Immunodeficiency
Diseases   776
161 SLE, RA, and Other
Connective Tissue
Diseases   779
162 Vasculitis   785
163 Ankylosing Spondylitis   788

164 Psoriatic Arthritis   791
165 Reactive Arthritis and
Reiter's Syndrome   792
166 Osteoarthritis   794
167 Gout, Pseudogout, and
Related Diseases   796
168 Other Arthritides   799
169 Sarcoidosis   802
170 Amyloidosis   804

SECTION 13
ENDOCRINOLOGY AND METABOLISM

171 Disorders of the Anterior
Pituitary and Hypothalamus   807
172 Disorders of the Posterior
Pituitary   813
173 Disorders of the Thyroid   815
174 Disorders of the Adrenal
Gland   823
175 Obesity   828
176 Diabetes Mellitus   830
177 Disorders of the Male
Reproductive System   835

178 Disorders of the Female
Reproductive System   839
179 Hypercalcemic and
Hypocalcemic Disorders   847
180 Osteoporosis and
Osteomalacia   852
181 Disorders of Lipid
Metabolism   855
182 Hemochromatosis,
Porphyrias, and Wilson's
Disease   861

SECTION 14
NEUROLOGY

183 The Neurologic
Examination   867
184 Neuroimaging   873
185 Seizures and Epilepsy   875
186 Tumors of the Nervous
System   883
187 Acute Meningitis and
Encephalitis   886
188 Chronic Meningitis   896
189 Multiple Sclerosis (MS)   899
190 Alzheimer's Disease and
Other Dementias   904
191 Parkinson's Disease   910
192 Ataxic Disorders   914

193 ALS and Other Motor
Neuron Diseases   917
194 Trigeminal Neuralgia,
Bell's Palsy, and Other
Cranial Nerve Disorders   920
195 Autonomic Nervous
System Disorders   925
196 Spinal Cord Diseases   932
197 Peripheral Neuropathies,
Including Guillain-Barré
Syndrome   936
198 Myasthenia Gravis (MG)   942
199 Muscle Diseases   944
200 Chronic Fatigue Syndrome   952

SECTION 15
PSYCHIATRIC DISORDERS AND PSYCHOACTIVE SUBSTANCE USE

201 Psychiatric Disorders   955   204 Alcoholism   972
202 Psychiatric Medications   962   205 Narcotic Abuse   975
203 Eating Disorders   969

SECTION 16
ADVERSE DRUG REACTIONS

206 Adverse Drug Reactions   979

SECTION 17
WOMEN'S HEALTH

207 Women's Health   989

SECTION 18
SCREENING AND DISEASE PREVENTION

208 Health Maintenance and
    Disease Prevention   991

SECTION 19
LABORATORY VALUES

209 Appendix: Laboratory
    Values of Clinical
    Importance   995

Index   1011

NOTICE

Medicine is an ever-changing science. As new research and clinical experience broaden our knowledge, changes in treatment and drug therapy are required. The editors and the publisher of this work have checked with sources believed to be reliable in their efforts to provide information that is complete and generally in accord with the standards accepted at the time of publication. However, in view of the possibility of human error or changes in medical sciences, neither the editors nor the publisher nor any other party who has been involved in the preparation or publication of this work warrants that the information contained herein is in every respect accurate or complete, and they are not responsible for any errors or omissions or the results obtained from the use of such information. Readers are encouraged to confirm the information contained herein with other sources. For example and in particular, readers are advised to check the product information sheet included in the package of each drug they plan to administer to be certain that the information contained in this book is accurate and that changes have not been made in the recommended dose or in the contraindications for administration. This recommendation is particularly important in connection with new or infrequently used drugs.

CONTRIBUTORS

Numbers in parentheses refer to contributed chapters in the *Manual*.

TAMAR F. BARLAM, MD
Associate Professor of Medicine
Boston University School of Medicine
Boston (15, 26, 29, 36, 60, 82–116, 134, 146)

EUGENE BRAUNWALD, MD, MA(HON), MD(HON), SCD(HON)
Distinguished Hersey Professor of Medicine
Harvard Medical School
Chairman, TIMI Study Group
Brigham and Women's Hospital
Boston (11, 14, 16, 44–46, 129, 206)

ANNE CAPPOLA, MD, SCM
Assistant Professor of Medicine and Epidemiology
Division of Endocrinology, Diabetes, and Metabolism
Center for Clinical Epidemiology and Biostatistics
University of Pennsylvania School of Medicine
Philadelphia (4, 24, 25, 30, 49, 171–182, 203, 207)

PUNIT CHADHA, MD
Fellow in Medicine, Division of Hematology-Oncology
Department of Medicine
Northwestern University Feinberg School of Medicine
Northwestern Memorial Hospital
Chicago (9, 10)

GLENN CHERTOW, MD
Director of Clinical Services
Division of Nephrology
Moffitt-Long Hospitals and UCSF-Mt. Zion Medical Center
Assistant Professor of Medicine in Residence
University of California–San Francisco
San Francisco (3, 47, 56, 139–145, 147–149)

DANIEL B. EVANS, MD
Instructor in Medicine
Department of Medicine
Northwestern University Feinberg School of Medicine
Northwestern Memorial Hospital
Chicago (1, 208)

ANTHONY S. FAUCI, MD,
Chief, Laboratory of Immunoregulation
Director, NIAID, NIH
Bethesda (28, 31, 37, 54, 55, 61, 62, 91, 153–170)

STEPHEN L. HAUSER, MD
Robert A. Fishman Distinguished Professor and Chairman
Department of Neurology
University of California–San Francisco
San Francisco (8, 17–22, 34, 35, 38–43, 59, 81, 183–205)

J. LARRY JAMESON, MD, PhD
Irving S. Cutter Professor and Chairman
Department of Medicine
Northwestern University Feinberg School of Medicine
Physician-in-Chief
Northwestern Memorial Hospital
Chicago (4, 23–25, 30, 49, 172–182, 203, 207, 209)

DENNIS L. KASPER, MD, MA(HON)
William Ellery Channing Professor of Medicine
Professor of Microbiology and Molecular Genetics
Harvard Medical School
Director, Channing Laboratory
Department of Medicine
Brigham and Women's Hospital
Boston (15, 26, 29, 36, 60, 82–116, 134, 146)

CAROL A. LANGFORD, MD
Associate Professor of Medicine,
Department of Rheumatic and Immunologic Diseases,
Cleveland Clinic Foundation
Cleveland (37, 54, 55, 61, 62, 153, 154, 161–170)

LEONARD S. LILLY, MD
Associate Professor of Medicine
Harvard Medical School
Chief, Brigham and Women's/Faulkner Cardiology
Boston (13, 32, 117–128)

DAN L. LONGO, MD
Scientific Director, National Institute on Aging
NIH
Bethesda and Baltimore (5, 27, 33, 48, 50–53, 57, 58, 63–80, 150–152)

MICHAEL C. SNELLER, MD
Chief of Immunologic Diseases Section
Laboratory of Immunoregulation
NIAID, NIH
Bethesda (28, 31, 91, 155–160)

J. WOODROW WEISS, MD
Associate Professor of Medicine
Harvard Medical School, Chief, Division of Pulmonary, Critical Care and
Sleep Medicine
Beth Israel Deaconess Medical Center
Boston (6, 7, 12, 130–133, 135–138)

PREFACE

Harrison's Principles of Internal Medicine (HPIM) has always been a premier resource for clinicians and students, who require a detailed understanding of the biological and clinical aspects of quality patient care. As demands increase, especially given the expanding medical knowledge base and the increased patient-care responsibilities typical of modern health care settings, it is not always possible to read a full account of a disease or presentation before encountering the patient. It is for this reason, among others, that the Editors have condensed the clinical portions of *HPIM* into this pocket-sized *Harrison's Manual of Medicine*. Like previous editions, this new edition presents key features of the diagnosis and treatment of major diseases that are likely to be encountered on a medical service.

The purpose of the *Manual* is to provide on-the-spot summaries in preparation for a more in-depth analysis of the clinical problem. The value of the *Manual* lies in its abbreviated format, which is useful for initial diagnosis and management in time-restricted clinical situations. The *Manual* has been written for easy reference to the full text of *HPIM*, and the Editors recommend that the full textbook—or *Harrison's On Line*—be consulted as soon as time permits.

This new edition of the *Manual* includes a number of timely revisions. The first section, focusing on *care of the hospitalized patient*, is completely new and reflects the growing importance of in-patient-specific approaches. Within this section are practical and valuable chapters on *admitting orders*, *common clinical procedures,* and *approach to the patient in critical care*. A brand new chapter on key concepts in *radiographic imaging* is also included. Section 2 addresses the assessment and initial management of common medical emergencies, including the distillation of three important new chapters in *HPIM* on the likely *biological*, *chemical*, and *radiologic agents of terrorism*. Chapters on cardinal disease manifestations and on the management of common medical diseases have been completely revised and updated to reflect important developments.

The increasing time demands on clinicians are being partially offset by wider use of digital information delivery. The last edition of the *Manual* was the first to be made available in PDA format. This new edition of the *Manual* is also available digitally for PDA, and the PDA version now includes the full complement of tables and diagrams found in the print version of the *Manual*. In addition, *Harrison's On Line* includes the full text of *HPIM* and a number of other valuable features. Taken as a portfolio, *Harrison's* is now available in a variety of formats suitable for all levels of medical training and for all varieties of health care settings.

We have developed this edition of the *Manual* with the able assistance of selected contributors. The Editors also wish to acknowledge contributors to past editions of this companion handbook, whose work formed the basis for many of the chapters herein: Joseph B. Martin, MD, PhD; Daryl R. Gress, MD; John W. Engstrom, MD; Kenneth L. Tyler, MD; Sophia Vinogradov, MD. We thank Elizabeth Robbins, MD, for her editorial assistance.

1

INITIAL EVALUATION AND ADMISSION ORDERS FOR THE GENERAL MEDICINE PATIENT

Patients are admitted to the hospital when (1) they present the physician with a complex diagnostic challenge that cannot be safely or efficiently performed in the outpatient setting; or (2) they are acutely ill and require inpatient diagnostic tests, interventions, and treatments. The decision to admit a patient includes identifying the optimal clinical service (i.e., medicine, urology, neurology), the level of care (observation, general floor, telemetry, ICU), and necessary consultants. Admission should always be accompanied by clear communication with the patient, family, and other caregivers, both to procure relevant information and to outline the anticipated events in the hospital.

The scope of illnesses cared for by internists is enormous. During a single day on a typical general medical service, it is not unusual for physicians, especially residents in training, to admit ten patients with ten different diagnoses affecting ten different organ systems. Given this diversity of disease, it is important to be systematic and consistent in the approach to any new admission.

Physicians are often concerned about making errors of commission. Examples would include prescribing an improper antibiotic for a patient with pneumonia or miscalculating the dose of heparin for a patient with new deep venous thrombosis. However, errors of omission are also common and can result in patients being denied life-saving interventions. Simple examples include: not checking a lipid panel for a patient with coronary heart disease, not prescribing an angiotensin-converting enzyme (ACE) inhibitor to a diabetic with documented albuminuria, or forgetting to give a patient with an osteoporotic hip fracture calcium, vitamin D, and an oral bisphosphonate.

Inpatient medicine typically focuses on the diagnosis and treatment of acute medical problems. However, most patients have multiple medical problems, and it is equally important to prevent nosocomial complications. Prevention of common hospital complications, such as deep venous thromboses (DVT), peptic ulcers, line infections, and pressure ulcers, are important aspects of the care of all general medicine patients.

A consistent approach to the admission process helps to ensure comprehensive and clear orders that can be written and implemented in a timely manner. Several mnemonics serve as useful reminders when writing admission orders. A suggested checklist for admission orders is shown below and it includes several interventions targeted to prevent common nosocomial complications. Computerized order entry systems are also useful when designed to prompt structured sets of admission orders.

Checklist mnemonic: ADMIT VITALS AND PHYSICAL EXAM

- *A*dmit to: service (Medicine, Oncology, ICU); provide status (acute or observation).
- *D*iagnosis: state the working diagnosis prompting this particular hospitalization.
- *M*D: name the attending, resident, intern, student, primary care MD, and consultants.
- *I*solation requirements: state respiratory or contact isolation and reason for order.

- *T*elemetry: state indications for telemetry and specify monitor parameters.
- *V*ital signs (VS): frequency of VS; also specify need for pulse oximetry and orthostatic VS.
- *I*V access and IV fluid or TPN orders (see Chap. 3).
- *T*herapists: respiratory, speech, physical, and/or occupational therapy needs.
- *A*llergies: also specify type of adverse reaction.
- *L*abs: blood count, chemistries, coagulation tests, type & screen, UA, special tests.
- *S*tudies: CT scans (also order contrast), ultrasounds, angiograms, endoscopies, etc.
- *A*ctivity: weight bear/ambulating instructions, fall/seizure precautions and restraints.
- *N*ursing Orders: call intern if (*x/y/z*), also order I/Os, daily weights, and blood glucose.
- *D*iet: include NPO orders and tube feeding. State whether to resume diet after tests.
- *P*eptic ulcer prevention: proton-pump inhibitor or misoprostil for high-risk patients.
- *H*eparin or other modality (warfarin, compression boots, support hose) for DVT prophylaxis.
- *Y*ank all Foley catheters and nonessential central lines to prevent iatrogenic infections.
- *S*kin care: prevent pressure sores with heel guards, air mattresses, and RN wound care.
- *I*ncentive spirometry: prevent atelectasis and hospital-acquired pneumonia.
- *C*alcium, vitamin D, and bisphosphonates if steroid use, bone fracture, or osteoporosis.
- *A*CE inhibitor and aspirin: use for nearly all patients with coronary disease or diabetes.
- *L*ipid panel: assess and treat all cardiac and vascular patients for hyperlipidemia.
- *E*CG: for nearly every patient >50 years at the time of admission.
- *X*-rays: chest x-ray, abdominal series; evaluate central lines and endotracheal tubes.
- *A*dvanced directives: Full code or DNR; specify whether to rescind for any procedures.
- *M*edications: be specific with your medication orders.

It may be helpful to remember the medication mnemonic "Stat DRIP" for different routes of administration (*stat*, *d*aily, *r*ound-the-clock, *I*V, and *p*rn medications). For the sake of cross-covering colleagues, provide relevant prn orders for acetaminophen, diphenhydramine, calcium carbonate, and sleeping pills. Specify any stat medications since routine medication orders entered as "once daily" may not be dispensed until the following day unless ordered as stat or "first dose now."

2

ASSESSMENT OF NUTRITIONAL STATUS

Stability of body weight requires that energy intake and expenditures are balanced over time. The major categories of energy output are resting energy expenditure (REE) and physical activity; minor sources include the energy cost of metabolizing food (thermic effect of food or specific dynamic action) and shivering thermogenesis. The average energy intake is about 2800 kcal/d for men and about 1800 kcal/d for women, though these estimates vary with age, body size, and activity level. Dietary reference intakes (DRI) and recommended dietary allowances (RDA) have been defined for many nutrients, including 9 essential amino acids, 4 fat-soluble and 10 water-soluble vitamins, several minerals, fatty acids, choline, and water (Tables 60-1 and 60-2, pp. 400 and 401, in HPIM-16). The usual water requirements are 1.0–1.5 mL/kcal energy expenditure in adults, with adjustments for excessive losses. The RDA for protein is 0.6 g/kg body weight. Fat should comprise ≤30% of calories, and saturated fat should be <10% of calories. At least 55% of calories should be derived from carbohydrates.

Malnutrition

Malnutrition results from inadequate intake or abnormal gastrointestinal assimilation of dietary calories, excessive energy expenditure, or altered metabolism of energy supplies by an intrinsic disease process.

Both outpatients and inpatients are at risk for malnutrition if they meet one or more of the following criteria:

- Unintentional loss of >10% of usual body weight in the preceding 3 months
- Body weight <90% of ideal for height (Table 2-1)
- Body mass index (BMI: weight/height^2 in kg/m^2) < 18.5

Table 2-1

Ideal Weight for Height

	Men				Women		
Height[a]	Weight[a]	Height	Weight	Height	Weight	Height	Weight
145	51.9	166	64.0	140	44.9	161	56.9
146	52.4	167	64.6	141	45.4	162	57.6
147	52.9	168	65.2	142	45.9	163	58.3
148	53.5	169	65.9	143	46.4	164	58.9
149	54.0	170	66.6	144	47.0	165	59.5
150	54.5	171	67.3	145	47.5	166	60.1
151	55.0	172	68.0	146	48.0	167	60.7
152	55.6	173	68.7	147	48.6	168	61.4
153	56.1	174	69.4	148	49.2	169	62.1
154	56.6	175	70.1	149	49.8		
155	57.2	176	70.8	150	50.4		
156	57.9	177	71.6	151	51.0		
157	58.6	178	72.4	152	51.5		
158	59.3	179	73.3	153	52.0		
159	59.9	180	74.2	154	52.5		
160	60.5	181	75.0	155	53.1		
161	61.1	182	75.8	156	53.7		
162	61.7	183	76.5	157	54.3		
163	62.3	184	77.3	158	54.9		
164	62.9	185	78.1	159	55.5		
165	63.5	186	78.9	160	56.2		

[a] Values are expressed in cm for height and kg for weight. To obtain height in inches, divide by 2.54. To obtain weight in pounds, multiply by 2.2.
Source: Adapted from GL Blackburn et al.: Nutritional and metabolic assessment of the hospitalized patient. J Parenter Enteral Nutr 1:11, 1977; with permission.

A body weight <90% of ideal for height represents *risk of malnutrition*, body weight <85% of ideal constitutes *malnutrition*, <70% of ideal represents *severe malnutrition*, and <60% of ideal is usually incompatible with survival. In underdeveloped countries, two forms of severe malnutrition can be seen: *marasmus*, which refers to generalized starvation with loss of body fat and protein, and *kwashiorkor*, which refers to selective protein malnutrition with edema and fatty liver. In more developed societies, features of combined *protein-calorie malnutrition* (PCM) are more commonly seen in the context of a variety of acute and chronic illnesses.

ETIOLOGY   The major etiologies of malnutrition are starvation, stress from surgery or severe illness, and mixed mechanisms. Starvation results from decreased dietary intake (from poverty, chronic alcoholism, anorexia nervosa, fad diets, severe depression, neurodegenerative disorders, dementia, or strict vegetarianism; abdominal pain from intestinal ischemia or pancreatitis; or anorexia associated with AIDS, disseminated cancer, or renal failure) or decreased assimilation of the diet (from pancreatic insufficiency; short bowel syndrome; celiac disease; or esophageal, gastric, or intestinal obstruction). Contributors to physical stress include fever, acute trauma, major surgery, burns, acute sepsis, hyperthyroidism, and inflammation as occurs in pancreatitis, collagen vascular diseases, and chronic infectious diseases such as tuberculosis or AIDS opportunistic infections. Mixed mechanisms occur in AIDS, disseminated cancer, COPD, chronic liver disease, Crohn's disease, ulcerative colitis, and renal failure.

CLINICAL FEATURES

- *General*—weight loss, temporal and proximal muscle wasting, decreased skin-fold thickness
- *Skin, hair, nails*—easily plucked hair, easy bruising, petechiae, and perifollicular hemorrhages (vit. C), "flaky paint" rash of lower extremities (zinc), hyperpigmentation of skin in exposed areas (niacin, tryptophan); spooning of nails (iron)
- *Eyes*—conjunctival pallor (anemia), night blindness, dryness and Bitot spots (vit. A), ophthalmoplegia (thiamine)
- *Mouth and mucous membranes*—glossitis and/or cheilosis (riboflavin, niacin, vit. B_{12}, pyridoxine, folate), diminished taste (zinc); inflamed and bleeding gums (vit. C)
- *Neurologic*—disorientation (niacin, phosphorus), confabulation, cerebellar gait, or past pointing (thiamine), peripheral neuropathy (thiamine, pyridoxine, vit. E), lost vibratory and position sense (vit. B_{12})

Laboratory findings include a low serum albumin, elevated PT, and decreased cell-mediated immunity manifest as anergy to skin testing. Specific vitamin deficiencies may also be present.

For a more detailed discussion, see Dwyer J: Nutritional Requirements and Dietary Assessment, Chap. 60, p. 399; Halsted CH: Malnutrition and Nutritional Assessment, Chap. 62, p. 411; and Russell RM: Vitamin and Trace Mineral Deficiency and Excess, Chap. 61, p. 403, in HPIM-16.

3

ELECTROLYTES/ACID-BASE BALANCE

SODIUM

In most cases, disturbances of sodium concentration [Na^+] result from abnormalities of water homeostasis. Disorders of Na^+ balance usually lead to hypo- or hypervolemia. Attention to the dysregulation of volume (Na^+ balance) and osmolality (water balance) must be considered separately for each pt (see below).

HYPONATREMIA   This is defined as a serum [Na^+] < 135 mmol/L and is among the most common electrolyte abnormalities encountered in hospitalized pts. Symptoms include confusion, lethargy, and disorientation; if severe (<120 mmol/L) and abrupt, seizures or coma may develop. Hyponatremia is often iatrogenic and almost always the result of an abnormality in the action of antidiuretic hormone (ADH), deemed either "appropriate" or "inappropriate," depending on the associated clinical conditions. The serum [Na^+] by itself does not yield diagnostic information regarding the total-body Na^+ content. Therefore, a useful way to categorize pts with hyponatremia is to place them into three groups, depending on the volume status (i.e., hypovolemic, euvolemic, and hypervolemic hyponatremia).

Hypovolemic Hyponatremia   Mild to moderate degrees of hyponatremia ([Na^+] = 125–135 mmol/L) complicate GI fluid or blood loss for two reasons. First, there is activation of the three major "systems" responsive to reduced organ perfusion: the renin-angiotensin-aldosterone axis, the sympathetic nervous system, and ADH. This sets the stage for enhanced renal absorption of solutes and water. Second, replacement fluid before hospitalization or other intervention is usually hypotonic (e.g., water, fruit juices). The optimal treatment of hypovolemic hyponatremia is volume administration, either in the form of colloid or isotonic crystalloid (e.g., 0.9% NaCl or lactated Ringer's solution).

Hypervolemic Hyponatremia   The edematous disorders (CHF, hepatic cirrhosis, and nephrotic syndrome) are often associated with mild to moderate degrees of hyponatremia ([Na^+] = 125–135 mmol/L); occasionally, pts with severe CHF or cirrhosis may present with serum [Na^+] <120 mmol/L. The pathophysiology is similar to that in hypovolemic hyponatremia, except that perfusion is decreased due to (1) reduced cardiac output, (2) arteriovenous shunting, and (3) severe hypoproteinemia, respectively, rather than true volume depletion. The scenario is sometimes referred to as reduced "effective circulating arterial volume." The evolution of hyponatremia is the same: increased water reabsorption due to ADH, complicated by hypotonic fluid replacement. This problem may be compounded by increased thirst. Pts with a variety of causes of chronic kidney disease may also develop hypervolemic hyponatremia, due principally to salt and water retention due to reduced GFR, and to the diseased kidneys' inability to osmoregulate.

Management consists of treatment of the underlying disorder (e.g., afterload reduction in heart failure, large-volume paracentesis in cirrhosis, glucocorticoid therapy in some forms of nephrotic syndrome), Na^+ restriction, diuretic therapy, and, in some pts, H_2O restriction. This approach is quite distinct from that applied to hypovolemic hyponatremia.

Euvolemic Hyponatremia   The syndrome of inappropriate ADH secretion (SIADH) characterizes most cases of euvolemic hyponatremia. Common causes of the syndrome are pulmonary (e.g., pneumonia, tuberculosis, pleural effusion) and CNS diseases (e.g., tumor, subarachnoid hemorrhage, meningitis); SIADH also occurs with malignancies (e.g., small cell carcinoma of the lung) and drugs (e.g., chlorpropamide, carbamazepine, narcotic analgesics, cyclophosphamide). Optimal treatment of euvolemic hyponatremia is H_2O restriction to <1 L/d, depending on the severity of the syndrome.

 TREATMENT

The rate of correction should be relatively slow (0.5 mmol/L per h of Na^+). A useful "rule of thumb" is to limit the change in mmol/L of Na^+ to half of the total difference within the first 24 h. More rapid correction has been associated with central pontine myelinolysis, especially if the hyponatremia has been of long standing. More rapid correction (with the potential addition of hypertonic saline to the above-recommended regimens) should be reserved for pts with very severe degrees of hyponatremia and ongoing neurologic compromise (e.g., a pt with Na^+ <105 mmol/L in status epilepticus).

HYPERNATREMIA   This is rarely associated with hypervolemia, and this association is always iatrogenic, e.g., administration of hypertonic sodium bicarbonate. Rather, hypernatremia is almost always the result of a combined water and volume deficit, with losses of H_2O in excess of Na^+. The most common causes are osmotic diuresis secondary to hyperglycemia, azotemia, or drugs (radiocontrast, mannitol, etc.) or central or nephrogenic diabetes insipidus (DI) (see "Urinary Abnormalities," Chap. 56). Elderly individuals with reduced thirst and/or diminished access to fluids are at highest risk.

 TREATMENT

The approach to correction of hypernatremia is outlined in Table 3-1. As with hyponatremia, it is advisable to correct the water deficit slowly to avoid neurologic compromise. In addition to the water-replacement formula provided, other forms of therapy may be helpful in selected cases of hypernatremia. Pts with central DI may respond well to the administration of intranasal desmo-

Table 3-1

Correction of Hypernatremia

WATER DEFICIT

1. Estimate total-body water (TBW): 50–60% body weight (kg) depending on body composition
2. Calculate free-water deficit: $[(Na^+ - 140)/140] \times TBW$
3. Administer deficit over 48–72 h

ONGOING WATER LOSSES

4. Calculate free-water clearance from urinary flow rate (V) and urine (U) Na^+ and K^+ concentrations $V - V \times (U_{Na} + U_K)/140$

INSENSIBLE LOSSES

5. ~10 mL/kg per day: less if ventilated, more if febrile

TOTAL

6. Add components to determine water of D_5W administration rate (typically ~50–250 mL/h)

pressin. Pts with nephrogenic DI due to lithium may reduce their polyuria with amiloride (2.5–10 mg/d) or hydrochlorothiazide (12.5–50 mg/d) or both in combination. Paradoxically, the use of diuretics may decrease distal nephron filtrate delivery, thereby reducing free-water losses and polyuria. Occasionally, NSAIDs have also been used to treat polyuria associated with nephrogenic DI; however, their nephrotoxic potential makes them a less attractive therapeutic option.

POTASSIUM

Since potassium (K^+) is the major intracellular cation, discussion of disorders of K^+ balance must take into consideration changes in the exchange of intra- and extracellular K^+ stores (extracellular K^+ constitutes <2% of total-body K^+ content). Insulin, β_2-adrenergic agonists, and alkalosis tend to promote K^+ uptake by cells; acidosis promotes shifting of K^+.

Table 3-2

Causes of Hypokalemia

I. Decreased intake
  A. Starvation
  B. Clay ingestion
II. Redistribution into cells
  A. Acid-base
    1. Metabolic alkalosis
  B. Hormonal
    1. Insulin
    2. β_2-Adrenergic agonists (endogenous or exogenous)
    3. α-Adrenergic antagonists
  C. Anabolic state
    1. Vitamin B_{12} or folic acid (red blood cell production)
    2. Granulocyte-macrophage colony stimulating factor (white blood cell production)
    3. Total parenteral nutrition
  D. Other
    1. Pseudohypokalemia
    2. Hypothermia
    3. Hypokalemic periodic paralysis
    4. Barium toxicity
III. Increased loss
  A. Nonrenal
    1. Gastrointestinal loss (diarrhea)
    2. Integumentary loss (sweat)
  B. Renal
    1. Increased distal flow: diuretics, osmotic diuresis, salt-wasting nephropathies
    2. Increased secretion of potassium
      a. Mineralocorticoid excess: primary hyperaldosteronism, secondary hyperaldosteronism (malignant hypertension, renin-secreting tumors, renal artery stenosis, hypovolemia), apparent mineralocorticoid excess (licorice, chewing tobacco, carbenoxolone), congenital adrenal hyperplasia, Cushing's syndrome, Bartter's syndrome
      b. Distal delivery of non-reabsorbed anions: vomiting, nasogastric suction, proximal (type 2) renal tubular acidosis, diabetic ketoacidosis, glue-sniffing (toluene abuse), penicillin derivatives
      c. Other: amphotericin B, Liddle's syndrome, hypomagnesemia

HYPOKALEMIA   Major causes of hypokalemia are outlined in Table 3-2. Atrial and ventricular arrhythmias are the major health consequences of hypokalemia. Pts with concurrent magnesium deficit (e.g., after diuretic therapy) and/or digoxin therapy are at particularly increased risk. Other clinical manifestations include muscle weakness, which may be profound at serum [K$^+$] < 2.5 mmol/L, and, if prolonged, ileus and polyuria. Clinical history and urinary [K$^+$] are most helpful in distinguishing causes of hypokalemia.

℞ TREATMENT

Hypokalemia is most often managed by correction of the acute underlying disease process (e.g., diarrhea) or withdrawal of an offending medication (e.g., loop or thiazide diuretic), along with oral K$^+$ supplementation with KCl, or, in rare cases, KHCO$_3$ or K-acetate. Hypokalemia may be refractory to correction in the presence of magnesium deficiency; both cations may need to be supplemented in selected cases (e.g., cisplatin nephrotoxicity). If loop or thiazide diuretic therapy cannot be discontinued, a distal tubular K-sparing agent, such as amiloride or spironolactone, can be added to the regimen. ACE inhibition in pts with CHF attenuates diuretic-induced hypokalemia and protects against cardiac arrhythmia. If hypokalemia is severe (<2.5 mmol/L) and/or if oral supplementation is not tolerated, intravenous KCl can be administered through a central vein at rates which must not exceed 20 mmol/h, with telemetry and skilled monitoring.

HYPERKALEMIA   Causes are outlined in Table 3-3. In most cases, hyperkalemia is due to decreased K$^+$ excretion. Drugs can be implicated in many cases. Where the diagnosis is uncertain, calculation of the transtubular K gra-

Table 3-3

Major Causes of Hyperkalemia

   I. "Pseudo"-hyperkalemia
      A. Thrombocytosis, leukocytosis, in vitro hemolysis
  II. Intra- to extracellular shift
      A. Acidosis
      B. Hyperosmolality; radiocontrast, hypertonic dextrose, mannitol
      C. Beta$_2$-adrenergic antagonists (noncardioselective agents)
      D. Digoxin or ouabain poisoning
      E. Hyperkalemic periodic paralysis
 III. Inadequate excretion
      A. Distal K-sparing diuretic agents and analogues
         1. Amiloride, spironolactone, triamterene, trimethoprim
      B. Decreased distal delivery
         1. Congestive heart failure, volume depletion, NSAIDs, cyclosporine
      C. Renal tubular acidosis, type IV
         1. Tubulointerstitial diseases
            a. Reflux nephropathy, pyelonephritis, interstitial nephritis, heavy metal (e.g., Pb) nephropathy
         2. Diabetic glomerulosclerosis
      D. Advanced renal insufficiency with low GFR
      E. Decreased mineralocorticoid effects
         1. Addison's disease, congenital adrenal enzyme deficiency, other forms of adrenal insufficiency (e.g., adrenalitis), heparin, ACE inhibitors, AII antagonists

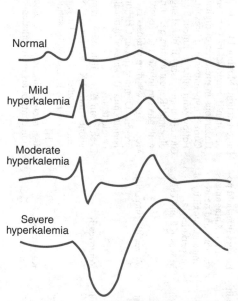

FIGURE 3-1 Diagrammatic ECGs at normal and high serum K. Peaked T waves (precordial leads) are followed by diminished R wave, wide QRS, prolonged P-R, loss of P wave, and ultimately a sine wave.

dient (TTKG) can be helpful. TTKG $= U_K P_{OSM}/P_K U_{OSM}$ (U, urine; P, plasma). TTKG < 10 suggests decreased K^+ excretion due to (1) hypoaldosteronism, or (2) renal resistance to the effects of mineralocorticoid. These can be differentiated by the administration of fludrocortisone (Florinef) 0.2 mg, with the former increasing K^+ excretion (and decreasing TTKG).

The most important consequence of hyperkalemia is altered cardiac conduction, leading to bradycardic cardiac arrest in severe cases. Hypocalcemia and acidosis accentuate the cardiac effects of hyperkalemia. Figure 3-1 shows serial ECG patterns of hyperkalemia. Stepwise treatment of hyperkalemia is summarized in Table 3-4.

ACID-BASE DISORDERS (See Fig. 3-2)

Regulation of normal pH (7.35–7.45) depends on both the lungs and kidneys. By the Henderson-Hasselbalch equation, pH is a function of the ratio of HCO_3^- (regulated by the kidney) to P_{CO_2} (regulated by the lungs). The HCO_3/P_{CO_2} relationship is useful in classifying disorders of acid-base balance. Acidosis is due to gain of acid or loss of alkali; causes may be metabolic (fall in serum HCO_3^-) or respiratory (rise in P_{CO_2}). Alkalosis is due to loss of acid or addition of base and is either metabolic ($\uparrow$ serum HCO_3) or respiratory ($\downarrow P_{CO_2}$).

To limit the change in pH, metabolic disorders evoke an immediate compensatory response in ventilation; compensation to respiratory disorders by the kidneys takes days. Simple acid-base disorders consist of one primary disturbance and its compensatory response. In mixed disorders, a combination of primary disturbances is present. Mixed disorders should be suspected when the change in anion gap is significantly higher or lower than the change in serum HCO_3 (see below).

Table 3-4

Management of Hyperkalemia

Treatment	Indication	Dose	Onset	Duration	Mechanism	Note
Calcium gluconate[a]	$K^+ > 6.5$ mmol/L with advanced ECG changes	10 mL of 10% solution IV over 2–3 min	1–5 min	30 min	Lowers threshold potential. Antagonizes cardiac and neuromuscular toxicity of hyperkalemia.	Fastest action. Monitor ECG. Repeat in 5 min if abnormal ECG persists. Hazardous in presence of digitalis. Correct hyponatremia if present. Follow with other treatment for K^+.
Insulin + glucose	Moderate hyperkalemia, peaked T waves only	10 U reg, IV + 50 mL, 50% IV	15–45 min	4–6 h	Moves K^+ into cells.	Glucose unnecessary if blood sugar elevated. Repeat insulin q15min with glucose infusion if needed.
$NaHCO_3$	Moderate hyperkalemia	90 mmol (2 ampules, IV push over 5 min)	Immediate	Short	Moves K^+ into cells.	Most effective when acidosis is present. Of more risk in CHF or hypernatremia. Beware of hypocalcemic tetany.
Kayexalate + sorbitol	Moderate hyperkalemia	Oral: 30 g, with 50 mL 20% sorbitol; rectal: 50 g in 200 mL 20% sorbitol enema, retain 45 min	1 h	4–6 h	Removes K^+.	Each gram Kayexalate orally removes about 1 mmol K^+ and about 0.5 mmol K^+ when given rectally. Repeat every 4 h. Use with caution in CHF.
Furosemide	Moderate hyperkalemia, serum creatinine <265 mmol/L (<3 mg%)	20–40 mg IV push	15 min	4 h	Kaliuresis.	Most useful if inadequate K^+ excretion contributes to hyperkalemia.
Dialysis	Hyperkalemia with renal failure		Immediate after start-up	Variable	Removes K^+.	Hemodialysis most effective. Also improves acidosis.

[a] Calcium chloride may be preferable in presence of circulatory instability or impairment.

10

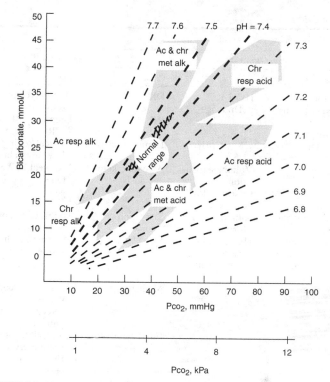

FIGURE 3-2 Nomogram, showing bands for uncomplicated respiratory or metabolic acid-base disturbances in intact subjects. Each "confidence" band represents the mean ±2 SD for the compensatory response of normal subjects or patients to a given primary disorder. Ac, acute; chr, chronic; resp, respiratory; met, metabolic; acid, acidosis; alk, alkalosis. (*From Levinsky NG: HPIM-12, p. 290; modified from Arbus GS: Can Med Assoc J 109:291, 1973.*)

METABOLIC ACIDOSIS The low HCO_3^- results from the addition of acids (organic or inorganic) or loss of HCO_3^-. The causes of metabolic acidosis are categorized by the anion gap, which equals $Na^+ - (Cl^- + HCO_3^-)$ (Table 3-5). Increased anion gap acidosis (>12 mmol/L) is due to addition of acid (other than HCl) and unmeasured anions to the body. Causes include ketoacidosis (diabetes mellitus, starvation, alcohol), lactic acidosis, poisoning (salicylates, ethylene glycol, and ethanol), and renal failure.

Diagnosis may be made by measuring BUN, creatinine, glucose, lactate, serum ketones, and serum osmolality and obtaining a toxic screen. Certain commonly prescribed drugs (e.g., metformin, antiretroviral agents) are occasionally associated with lactic acidosis.

Normal anion gap acidoses result from HCO_3^- loss from the GI tract or from the kidney, e.g., renal tubular acidosis, urinary obstruction, rapid volume expansion with saline-containing solutions, and administration of NH_4Cl, lysine HCl. Calculation of urinary anion gap may be helpful in evaluation of hyperchloremic metabolic acidosis. A negative anion gap suggests GI losses; a positive anion gap suggests altered urinary acidification.

Clinical features of acidosis include hyperventilation, cardiovascular collapse, and nonspecific symptoms ranging from anorexia to coma.

Table 3-5

Metabolic Acidosis

Non-Anion Gap Acidosis		Anion Gap Acidosis	
Cause	Clue	Cause	Clue
Diarrhea	Hx; ↑ K⁺	DKA	Hyperglycemia, ketones
Enterostomy	Drainage		
RTA		RF	Uremia, ↑ BUN, ↑ CR
Proximal	↓ K⁺		
Distal	↓ K⁺; UpH > 5.5	Lactic acidosis	Clinical setting + ↑ serum lactate
Dilutional	Volume expansion	Alcoholic keto-acidosis	Hx; weak + ketones; + osm gap
Ureterosig-moidostomy	Obstructed ileal loop		
Hyperalimentation	Amino acid infusion	Starvation	Hx; mild acidosis; + ketones
Acetazolamide, NH₄Cl, lysine HCl, arginine HCl	Hx of administration of these agents	Salicylates	Hx; tinnitus; high serum level; + ketones
		Methanol	Large AG; retinitis; + toxic screen; + osm gap
		Ethylene glycol	RF, CNS; + toxic screen; crystalluria; + osm gap

Note: RTA, renal tubular acidosis; UpH, urinary pH; DKA, diabetic ketoacidosis; RF, renal failure; AG, anion gap; osm gap, osmolar gap

℞ TREATMENT

Depends on cause and severity. Always correct the underlying disturbance. Administration of alkali is controversial. It may be reasonable to treat lactic acidosis with intravenous HCO_3^- at a rate sufficient to maintain a plasma HCO_3^- of 8–10 mmol/L and pH > 7.10. Lactic acidosis associated with cardiogenic shock may be worsened by bicarbonate administration.

Chronic acidosis should be treated when HCO_3^- < 18–20 mmol/L or symptoms of anorexia or fatigue are present. In pts with renal failure, there is some evidence that acidosis promotes protein catabolism and may worsen bone disease. Na citrate may be more palatable than oral $NaHCO_3$, although the former should be avoided in pts with advanced renal insufficiency, as it augments aluminum absorption. Oral therapy with $NaHCO_3$ usually begins with 650 mg tid and is titrated upward to maintain desired serum $[HCO_3^-]$. Other therapies for lactic acidosis remain unproven.

METABOLIC ALKALOSIS   A primary increase in serum $[HCO_3^-]$. Most cases originate with volume concentration and loss of acid from the stomach or kidney. Less commonly, HCO_3^- administered or derived from endogenous lactate is the cause and is perpetuated when renal HCO_3^- reabsorption continues. In vomiting, Cl^- loss reduces its availability for renal reabsorption with Na^+. Enhanced Na^+ avidity due to volume depletion then accelerates

Table 3-6

Metabolic Alkalosis

Cl⁻ Responsive (Low U_α)	Cl⁻ Resistant (High U_α)
Gastrointestinal causes:	Adrenal disorders:
Vomiting	Hyperaldosteronism
Nasogastric suction	Cushing's syndrome (1°, 2°, ectopic)
Chloride-wasting diarrhea	Exogenous steroids:
Villus adenoma of colon	Gluco- or mineralocorticoid
Diuretic therapy	Licorice ingestion
Posthypercapnia	Carbenoxolone
Carbenicillin or penicillin	Bartter's syndrome
	Refeeding alkalosis
	Alkali ingestion

HCO_3^- reabsorption and sustains the alkalosis. Urine Cl⁻ is typically low (<10 mmol/L) (Table 3-6). Alkalosis may also be maintained by hyperaldosteronism, due to enhancement of H⁺ secretion and HCO_3^- reabsorption. Severe K⁺ depletion also causes metabolic alkalosis by increasing HCO_3^- reabsorption; urine Cl⁻ > 20 mmol/L.

Vomiting and nasogastric drainage cause HCl and volume loss, kaliuresis, and alkalosis. Diuretics are a common cause of alkalosis due to volume contraction, Cl⁻ depletion, and hypokalemia. Pts with chronic pulmonary disease and high P_{CO_2} and serum HCO_3^- levels whose ventilation is acutely improved may develop alkalosis.

Excessive mineralocorticoid activity due to Cushing's syndrome (worse in ectopic ACTH or primary hyperaldosteronism) causes metabolic alkalosis not associated with volume or Cl⁻ depletion and not responsive to NaCl.

Severe K⁺ depletion also causes metabolic alkalosis.

Diagnosis   The [Cl⁻] from a random urine sample is useful unless diuretics have been administered. Determining the fractional excretion of Cl⁻, rather than the fractional excretion of Na⁺, is the best way to identify an alkalosis responsive to volume expansion.

℞ TREATMENT

Correct the underlying cause. In cases of Cl⁻ depletion, administer NaCl; with hypokalemia, add KCl. Pts with adrenal hyperfunction require treatment of the underlying disorder. Severe alkalosis may require, in addition, treatment with acidifying agents such as NaCl, HCl, or acetazolamide. The initial amount of H⁺ needed (in mmol) should be calculated from 0.5 × (body wt in kg) × (serum HCO_3^- − 24).

RESPIRATORY ACIDOSIS   Characterized by CO_2 retention due to ventilatory failure. Causes include sedatives, stroke, chronic pulmonary disease, airway obstruction, severe pulmonary edema, neuromuscular disorders, and cardiopulmonary arrest. Symptoms include confusion, asterixis, and obtundation.

℞ TREATMENT

The goal is to improve ventilation through pulmonary toilet and reversal of bronchospasm. Intubation may be required in severe acute cases. Acidosis due to hypercapnia is usually mild. Respiratory acidosis may accompany low tidal volume ventilation in ICU patients and may require metabolic "over-correction" to maintain a neutral pH.

RESPIRATORY ALKALOSIS   Excessive ventilation causes a primary reduction in CO_2 and ↑ pH in pneumonia, pulmonary edema, interstitial lung disease, asthma. Pain and psychogenic causes are common; other etiologies include fever, hypoxemia, sepsis, delirium tremens, salicylates, hepatic failure, mechanical overventilation, and CNS lesions. Pregnancy is associated with a mild respiratory alkalosis. Severe respiratory alkalosis may cause seizures, tetany, cardiac arrhythmias, or loss of consciousness.

Rx TREATMENT

Should be directed at the underlying disorders. In psychogenic cases, sedation or a rebreathing bag may be required.

"MIXED" DISORDERS   In many circumstances, more than a single acid-base disturbance exists. Examples include combined metabolic and respiratory acidosis with cardiogenic shock; metabolic alkalosis and acidosis in pts with vomiting and diabetic ketoacidosis; metabolic acidosis with respiratory alkalosis in pts with sepsis. The diagnosis may be clinically evident or suggested by relationships between the P_{CO_2} and HCO_3^- that are markedly different from those found in simple disorders.

In simple anion-gap acidosis, anion gap increases in proportion to fall in $[HCO_3^-]$. When increase in anion gap occurs despite a normal $[HCO_3^-]$, simultaneous anion-gap acidosis and metabolic alkalosis are suggested. When fall in $[HCO_3^-]$ due to metabolic acidosis is proportionately larger than increase in anion gap, mixed anion-gap and non-anion-gap metabolic acidosis is suggested.

For a more detailed discussion, see Singer GG, Brenner BM: Fluid and Electrolyte Disturbances, Chap. 41, p. 252; and DuBose TD Jr: Acidosis and Alkalosis, Chap. 42, p. 263, in HPIM-16.

4

ENTERAL AND PARENTERAL NUTRITION

Nutritional support should be initiated in pts with malnutrition or in those at risk for malnutrition (e.g., conditions that preclude adequate oral feeding or pts in catabolic states, such as sepsis, burns, or trauma). An approach for deciding when to use various types of specialized nutrition support (SNS) is summarized in Fig. 4-1.

Enteral therapy refers to feeding via the gut, using oral supplements or infusion of formulas via various feeding tubes (nasogastric, nasojejunal, gastrostomy, jejunostomy, or combined gastrojejunostomy). *Parenteral therapy* re-

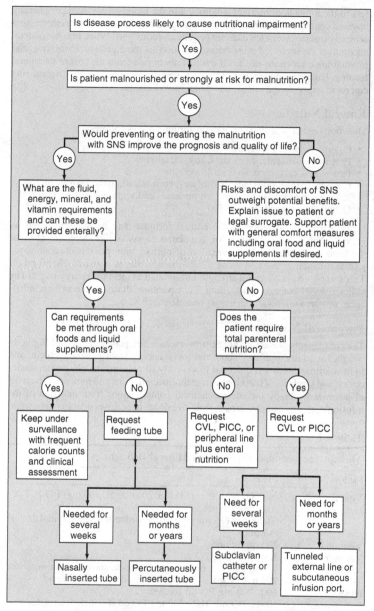

FIGURE 4-1 Decision tree for initiating specialized nutrition support (SNS). CVL, Central venous line; PICC, peripherally inserted central catheter.

fers to the infusion of nutrient solutions into the bloodstream via a peripherally inserted central catheter (PICC), a centrally inserted externalized catheter, or a centrally inserted tunneled catheter or subcutaneous port. When feasible, enteral nutrition is the preferred route because it sustains the digestive, absorptive, and immunologic functions of the GI tract, at about one-tenth the cost of parenteral feeding. Parenteral nutrition is often indicated in severe pancreatitis, necrotizing enterocolitis, prolonged ileus, and distal bowel obstruction.

Enteral Nutrition

The components of a standard enteral formula are as follows:

- Caloric density: 1 kcal/mL
- Protein: ~14% cals; caseinates, soy, lactalbumin
- Fat: ~30% cals; corn, soy, safflower oils
- Carbohydrate: ~60% cals; hydrolysed corn starch, maltodextrin, sucrose
- Recommended daily intake of all minerals and vitamins in ≥1500 kcal/d
- Osmolality (mosmol/kg): ~300

However, modification of the enteral formula may be required based on various clinical indications and/or associated disease states. After elevation of the head of the bed and confirmation of correct tube placement, continuous gastric infusion is initiated using a half-strength diet at a rate of 25–50 mL/h. This can be advanced to full strength as tolerated to meet the energy target. The major risks of enteral tube feeding are aspiration, diarrhea, electrolyte imbalance, warfarin resistance, sinusitis, and esophagitis.

Parenteral Nutrition

The components of parenteral nutrition include adequate fluid (35 mL/kg body weight for adults, plus any abnormal loss); energy from glucose, protein, and lipid solutions; nutrients essential in severely ill pts, such as glutamine, nucleotides, and products of methionine metabolism; vitamins and minerals. The risks of parenteral therapy include mechanical complications from insertion of the infusion catheter, catheter sepsis, fluid overload, hyperglycemia, hypophospha-

Table 4-1

Therapy for Common Vitamin and Mineral Deficiencies

Nutrient	Therapy
Vitamin A[a,b,c]	100,000 IU (30 mg) IM or 200,000 IU (60 mg) PO × 1 if ocular changes 50,000 IU (15 mg) PO qd × 1 month if chronic malabsorption
Vitamin C	200 mg PO qd
Vitamin E[a]	800–1200 mg PO qd
Vitamin K[a]	10 mg IV × 1, or 1–2 mg PO qd in chronic malabsorption
Thiamine[b]	100 mg IV qd × 7 days, followed by 10 mg PO qd
Niacin	100–200 mg PO tid for 5 days
Pyridoxine	50 mg PO qd, 100–200 mg PO qd if deficiency related to medication
Zinc[b,c]	60 mg PO bid

[a] Associated with fat malabsorption, along with vitamin D deficiency.
[b] Associated with chronic alcoholism; always replete thiamine before carbohydrates in alcoholics to avoid precipitation of acute thiamine deficiency.
[c] Associated with protein-calorie malnutrition.

temia, hypokalemia, acid-base and electrolyte imbalance, cholestasis, metabolic bone disease, and micronutrient deficiencies.

The following parameters should be monitored in all patients receiving supplemental nutrition, whether enteral or parenteral:

- Fluid balance (weight, intake vs. output)
- Glucose, electrolytes, BUN (daily until stable, then 2× per week)
- Serum creatinine, albumin, phosphorus, calcium, magnesium, Hb/Hct, WBC (baseline, then 2× per week)
- INR (baseline, then weekly)
- Micronutrient tests as indicated

Specific Micronutrient Deficiency

Appropriate therapies for micronutrient deficiencies are outlined in Table 4-1.

For a more detailed discussion, see Russell RM: Vitamin and Trace Mineral Deficiency and Excess, Chap. 61, p. 403; and Howard L: Enteral and Parenteral Nutrition Therapy, Chap. 63, p. 415, HPIM-16.

5

TRANSFUSION AND PHERESIS THERAPY

TRANSFUSIONS
Whole Blood Transfusion

Indicated when acute blood loss is sufficient to produce hypovolemia, whole blood provides both oxygen-carrying capacity and volume expansion. In acute blood loss, hematocrit may not accurately reflect degree of blood loss for 48 h until fluid shifts occur.

Red Blood Cell Transfusion

Indicated for symptomatic anemia unresponsive to specific therapy or requiring urgent correction. Packed RBC transfusions may be indicated in pts who are symptomatic from cardiovascular or pulmonary disease when Hb is between 70 and 90 g/L (7 and 9 g/dL). Transfusion is usually necessary when Hb < 70 g/L (<7 g/dL). One unit of packed RBCs raises the Hb by approximately 10 g/L (1 g/dL). If used instead of whole blood in the setting of acute hemorrhage, packed RBCs, fresh-frozen plasma (FFP), and platelets in an approximate ratio of 3:1:10 units are an adequate replacement for whole blood. Removal of leukocytes reduces risk of alloimmunization and transmission of CMV. Washing to remove donor plasma reduces risk of allergic reactions. Irradiation prevents graft-versus-host disease in immunocompromised recipients by killing alloreactive donor lymphocytes. Avoid related donors.

Other Indications (1) *Hypertransfusion therapy* to block production of defective cells, e.g., thalassemia, sickle cell anemia; (2) *exchange transfusion—*

hemolytic disease of newborn, sickle cell crisis; (3) *transplant recipients*— decreases rejection of cadaveric kidney transplants.

Complications   (See Table 5-1) (1) *Transfusion reaction*—immediate or delayed, seen in 1–4% of transfusions; IgA-deficient pts at particular risk for severe reaction; (2) *infection*—bacterial (rare); hepatitis C, 1 in 1,600,000 transfusions; HIV transmission, 1 in 1,960,000; (3) *circulatory overload*; (4) *iron overload*—each unit contains 200–250 mg iron; hemachromatosis may develop after 100 U of RBCs (less in children), in absence of blood loss; iron chelation therapy with deferoxamine indicated; (5) *graft-versus-host disease*; (6) *alloimmunization*.

Autologous Transfusion

Use of pt's own stored blood avoids hazards of donor blood; also useful in pts with multiple RBC antibodies. Pace of autologous donation may be accelerated using erythropoietin (50–150 U/kg SC three times a week) in the setting of normal iron stores.

Platelet Transfusion

Prophylactic transfusions usually reserved for platelet count < 10,000/μL (<20,000/μL in acute leukemia). One unit elevates the count by about 10,000/ μL if no platelet antibodies are present as a result of prior transfusions. Efficacy assessed by 1-h and 24-h posttransfusion platelet counts. HLA-matched single-donor platelets may be required in pts with platelet alloantibodies.

Table 5-1

Risks of Transfusion Complications

	Frequency, Episodes:Unit
Reactions	
Febrile (FNHTR)	1–4:100
Allergic	1–4:100
Delayed hemolytic	1:1,000
TRALI	1:5,000
Acute hemolytic	1:12,000
Fatal hemolytic	1:100,000
Anaphylactic	1:150,000
Infections[a]	
Hepatitis B	1:63,000
Hepatitis C	1:1,600,000
HIV-1	1:1,960,000
HIV-2	None reported
HTLV-I and -II	1:641,000
Malaria	1:4,000,000
Other complications	
RBC allosensitization	1:100
HLA allosensitization	1:10
Graft-versus-host disease	Rare

[a] Infectious agents rarely associated with transfusion, theoretically possible or of unknown risk include: Hepatitis A virus, parvovirus B-19, *Babesia microti* (babesiosis), *Borrelia burgdorferi* (Lyme disease), *Trypanosoma cruzi* (Chagas disease), and *Treponema pallidum*, human herpesvirus-8 and hepatitis G virus.
Note: FNHTR, febrile nonhemolytic transfusion reaction; TRALI, transfusion-related acute lung injury; HTLV, human T lymphotropic virus; RBC, red blood cell

Transfusion of Plasma Components

FFP is a source of coagulation factors, fibrinogen, antithrombin, and proteins C and S. It is used to correct coagulation factor deficiencies, rapidly reverse warfarin effects, and treat thrombotic thrombocytopenic purpura (TTP). Cryoprecipitate is a source of fibrinogen, factor VIII, and von Willebrand factor; it may be used when recombinant factor VIII or factor VIII concentrates are not available.

THERAPEUTIC HEMAPHERESIS

Hemapheresis is removal of a cellular or plasma constituent of blood; specific procedure referred to by the blood fraction removed.

Leukapheresis

Removal of WBCs; most often used in acute leukemia, esp. acute myeloid leukemia (AML) in cases complicated by marked elevation ($>100,000/\mu L$) of the peripheral blast count, to lower risk of leukostasis (blast-mediated vasoocclusive events resulting in CNS or pulmonary infarction, hemorrhage). Leukapheresis is increasingly being used to harvest hematopoietic stem cells from the peripheral blood of cancer pts; such cells are then used to promote hematopoietic reconstitution after high-dose myeloablative therapy.

Plateletpheresis

Used in some pts with thrombocytosis associated with myeloproliferative disorders with bleeding and/or thrombotic complications. Other treatments are generally used first. Also used to enhance platelet yield from blood donors.

Plasmapheresis

Indications   (1) *Hyperviscosity states*—e.g., Waldenström's macroglobulinemia; (2) *TTP*; (3) *immune-complex* and *autoantibody disorders*—e.g., Goodpasture's syndrome, rapidly progressive glomerulonephritis, myasthenia gravis; possibly Guillain-Barré, SLE, idiopathic thrombocytopenic purpura; (4) cold agglutinin disease, cryoglobulinemia.

For a more detailed discussion, see Dzieczkowski JS and Anderson KC: Transfusion Biology and Therapy, Chap. 99, p. 662, in HPIM-16.

6

PRINCIPLES OF CRITICAL CARE MEDICINE

Approach to the Critically Ill Patient

Initial care often involves resuscitation of patients at the extremes of physiologic deterioration using invasive techniques (mechanical ventilation, renal replacement therapy) to support organs on the verge of failure. Successful outcomes often depend on an aggressive approach to treatment, with a sense of urgency about intervention. Resource management and quality-of-care assessments can be facilitated by the use of illness-severity scales. APACHE II is the most common such scale in use in North America. The score is derived from determination of the type of ICU admission (elective postoperative care, nonsurgical, emergent surgical), a chronic health score, and the worst values recorded for 12 physiologic variables in the first 24 h of intensive care. APACHE should not be used to drive clinical decision-making for individual patients.

Shock (See Chap. 14)

Defined not by blood pressure measurement but by the presence of multisystem end-organ hypoperfusion. The approach to the patient in shock is outlined in Fig. 14-1.

Mechanical Ventilatory Support

Principles of advanced cardiac life support should be adhered to during initial resuscitative efforts. Any compromise of respiration should prompt consideration of endotracheal intubation and mechanical ventilatory support. Mechanical ventilation may decrease respiratory work, improve arterial oxygenation with improved tissue oxygen delivery, and reduce acidosis. Reduction in arterial pressure after institution of mechanical ventilation is common due to reduced venous return from positive thoracic pressure, reduced endogenous catecholamine output, and concurrent administration of sedative agents. This hypotension often responds in part to volume administration.

Respiratory Failure

Four common types of respiratory failure are observed, reflecting different pathophysiologic derangements.

Type I or Acute Hypoxemic Respiratory Failure Occurs due to alveolar flooding with edema (cardiac or noncardiac), pneumonia, or hemorrhage. Acute respiratory distress syndrome (ARDS) (see Chap. 12) describes diffuse lung injury with airspace edema, severe hypoxemia (ratio of arterial P_{O_2} to inspired oxygen concentration—$Pa_{O_2}/FI_{O_2} < 200$). Causes include sepsis, pancreatitis, gastric aspiration, multiple transfusions. Current ventilator strategy requires the use of low tidal volumes (4–6 mL/kg ideal body weight) to avoid ventilator-induced lung injury.

Type II Respiratory Failure This pattern reflects alveolar hypoventilation and inability to eliminate CO_2 due to:

- Impaired central respiratory drive (e.g., drug ingestion, brainstem injury, hypothyroidism)
- Impaired respiratory muscle strength (e.g., myasthenia gravis, Guillain-Barré syndrome, myopathy)
- Increased load on the respiratory system (e.g., resistive loads such as bronchospasm or upper airway obstruction, reduced chest wall compliance due to pneumothorax or pleural effusion, or increased ventilation requirements with increased dead space due to pulmonary embolism or acidosis).

Treat the underlying cause and provide mechanical support with mask or endotracheal ventilation.

Type III Respiratory Failure Occurs as a result of atelectasis—commonly occurs postoperatively. Treatment requires deep breathing and sometimes mask ventilation.

Type IV Respiratory Failure Seen as a consequence of hypoperfusion of respiratory muscles in shock or with cardiogenic pulmonary edema. Mechanical ventilatory support is required.

 TREATMENT

Care of the Mechanically Ventilated Patient Many patients receiving mechanical ventilation will require pain relief and anxiolytics. Less commonly, neuromuscular blocking agents are required to facilitate ventilation when there is extreme dyssynchrony that cannot be corrected with manipulation of the ventilator settings.

Weaning from Mechanical Ventilation Daily screening of patients who are stable while receiving mechanical support facilitates recognition of patients ready to be liberated from the ventilator. The *rapid shallow breathing index* (RSBI, or f/V_T—respiratory rate in breaths/min divided by tidal volume in liters during a brief period of spontaneous breathing)—may predict weanability. A f/V_T < 105 should prompt a spontaneous breathing trial of up to 2 h with no or minimal [5 cmH$_2$O positive end-expiratory pressure (PEEP)] support. If there is no tachypnea, tachycardia, hypotension, or hypoxia, a trial of extubation is commonly performed.

Multiorgan System Failure

Defined as dysfunction or failure of two or more organs in patients with critical illness. A common consequence of systemic inflammatory response (e.g., sepsis, pancreatitis). May cause hepatic, renal, pulmonary, or hematologic abnormalities.

Monitoring in the ICU

With critical illness, close and often continuous monitoring of vital functions is required. In addition to pulse oximetry, frequent arterial blood-gas analysis can reveal evolving acid-base disturbances. Modern ventilators have sophisticated alarms that reveal excessive pressure requirements, insufficient ventilation, or overbreathing. Intraarterial pressure monitoring and, at times, pulmonary artery pressure measurement can reveal changes in cardiac output or oxygen delivery.

Prevention of Complications

Critically ill patients are prone to a number of complications, including the following:

- Anemia—usually due to inflammation and often iatrogenic blood loss
- Venous thrombosis—may occur despite standard prophylaxis with heparin and may occur at the site of central venous catheters
- Gastrointestinal bleeding—most often in patients with bleeding diatheses or respiratory failure, necessitating acid neutralization in such patients
- Renal failure—a tendency exacerbated by nephrotoxic medications and dye studies.

Evidence suggests that strict glucose control [glucose < 6.1 mmol/L (<110 mg/dL)] improves mortality in critically ill patients.

Limitation or Withdrawal of Care

Technological advances have created a situation in which many patients can be maintained in the ICU with little or no chance of recovery. Increasingly, patients, families, and caregivers have acknowledged the ethical validity of withdrawal of care when the patient or surrogate decision maker determines that the patient's goals for care are no longer achievable with the clinical situation, as determined by the caregivers.

For a more detailed discussion, see Kress JP, Hall JB: Principles of Critical Care Medicine, Chap. 249, p. 1581, in HPIM-16.

7

RESPIRATORY FAILURE

Definition and Classification

- Defined as failure of gas exchange due to inadequate function of one or more of the essential components of the respiratory system.
- Classified as hypoxemic (Pa_{O_2} < 60 mmHg), hypercarbic (Pa_{CO_2} > 45 mmHg), or combined.
- Also classified in terms of acuity—*acute respiratory failure* reflects a sudden catastrophic deterioration, *chronic respiratory failure* reflects long-standing respiratory insufficiency, and *acute or chronic respiratory failure* is an acute deterioration in a patient with chronic respiratory failure, usually due to chronic obstructive lung disease.

Pathophysiology

Respiratory failure occurs when one or more components of the respiratory system fails.

- Disorders due to failure of the central control system can be thought of as *controller dysfunction*, or central apnea.
- Failure of the respiratory pump—the diaphragm and intercostal muscles that move the chest wall—is termed *pump dysfunction*.
- Respiratory insufficiency attributable to narrowing, collapse, spasm, or plugging of the large or small airways can be termed *airway system dysfunction*.
- Respiratory failure due to collapse or flooding of or injury to the alveolar network can be considered *alveolar network dysfunction*.
- Disease resulting from obstruction, inflammation, or hypertrophy of the pulmonary capillary vessels can be termed *pulmonary vascular dysfunction*.

Many processes will involve more than one of these components of the respiratory system, but assessment of each compartment can provide a basis for differential diagnosis.

Clinical Evaluation

Initial inspection should assess upper airway patency and signs of distress such as nasal flaring, intercostal retractions, diaphoresis, level of consciousness. Use of sternocleidomastoid muscles and pulsus paradoxus in a patient who is wheezing suggest severe asthma. Asymmetric breath sounds may indicate pneumothorax, atelectasis, or pneumonia. Oximetry permits rapid assessment of oxygenation. An arterial blood-gas measurement is required, however, to determine CO_2 level and acid-base status. Because of the potential for rapid, possibly fatal, deterioration, therapy may need to be initiated without a definite diagnosis.

• Controller dysfunction is suggested by medication history, the absence of tachypnea (respiratory rate < 12 breaths/min) in a patient with hypercarbia, altered level of consciousness.
• Pump dysfunction is suggested by supine abdominal paradox (diaphragmatic paralysis), peripheral muscle weakness, reduced maximal inspiratory pressure generation.
• Upper airway dysfunction is suggested by stridor, and lower airways dysfunction by wheezing. In ventilated patients obstruction can be deduced by inspection of the flow:time curve as displayed on most current ventilators. AutoPEEP (positive end-expiratory pressure), a sign of delayed emptying of the lungs in ventilated patients, is another sign of obstruction.
• Alveolar compartment dysfunction is evident when there are signs of consolidation on auscultation, with tubular breath sounds and dullness. Since alveolar flooding effectively increases the stiffness of the lung, respiratory compliance, as measured on the ventilator [V_T/(end-inspiratory plateau pressure − PEEP)], is reduced to <30 mL/cmH$_2$O.
• Pulmonary vascular dysfunction is reflected indirectly by signs of right heart failure on exam ($\uparrow P_2$, $\uparrow JVP$, right-sided heave).

℞ TREATMENT

• First priority is always to establish adequate oxygenation. If hypercarbia and acidosis coexist, mechanical ventilation should be strongly considered.
• Attention must always be paid to establishing airway patency, even if another cause of respiratory failure is present. This may mean removal of a foreign body, suctioning, or simply a jaw lift.
• With respiratory failure due to alveolar dysfunction, increasing end-expiratory lung volume with extrinsic PEEP may substantially improve arterial oxygenation.

For a more detailed discussion, see Lilly C, Ingenito EP, Shapiro SD: Respiratory Failure, Chap. 250, p. 1588, in HPIM-16.

8

PAIN AND ITS MANAGEMENT

Pain is the most common symptom of disease. Management depends on determining its cause, alleviating triggering and potentiating factors, and providing rapid relief whenever possible.

Organization of Pain Pathways   (See HPIM-16, Figs. 11-1 and 11-4.)

Pain-producing (nociceptive) sensory stimuli in skin and viscera activate peripheral nerve endings of primary afferent neurons, which synapse on second-order neurons in cord or medulla. These second-order neurons form crossed ascending pathways that reach the thalamus and are projected to somatosensory cortex. Parallel ascending neurons connect with brainstem nuclei and ventrocaudal and medial thalamic nuclei. These parallel pathways project to the limbic system and underlie the emotional aspect of pain. Pain transmission is regulated at the dorsal horn level by descending bulbospinal pathways that contain serotonin, norepinephrine, and several neuropeptides.

Agents that modify pain perception may act to reduce tissue inflammation (NSAIDs, prostaglandin synthesis inhibitors), to interfere with pain transmission (narcotics), or to enhance descending modulation (narcotics and antidepressants). Anticonvulsants (gabapentin, carbamazepine) may be effective for aberrant pain sensations arising from peripheral nerve injury.

Evaluation

Pain may be of somatic (skin, joints, muscles), visceral, or neuropathic (injury to nerves, spinal cord pathways, or thalamus) origin. Characteristics of each are summarized in Table 8-1.

Neuropathic pain definitions: *neuralgia*: pain in the distribution of a single nerve, as in trigeminal neuralgia; *dysesthesia*: spontaneous, unpleasant, abnormal sensations; *hyperalgesia* and *hyperesthesia*: exaggerated responses to nociceptive or touch stimulus, respectively; *allodynia*: perception of light mechanical stimuli as painful, as when vibration evokes painful sensation. Reduced pain perception is called *hypalgesia* or, when absent, *analgesia*. *Causalgia* is continuous severe burning pain with indistinct boundaries and accompanying sympathetic nervous system dysfunction (sweating; vascular, skin, and hair changes—sympathetic dystrophy) that occurs after injury to a peripheral nerve.

Sensitization (see HPIM-16, Fig. 11-2) refers to a lowered threshold for activating primary nociceptors following repeated stimulation in damaged or inflamed tissues; inflammatory mediators play a role. Sensitization contributes to tenderness, soreness, and hyperalgesia (as in sunburn).

Table 8-1

Characteristics of Somatic and Neuropathic Pain

Somatic pain
   Nociceptive stimulus usually evident
   Usually well localized
   Similar to other somatic pains in pt's experience
   Relieved by anti-inflammatory or narcotic analgesics
Visceral pain
   Most commonly activated by inflammation
   Pain poorly localized and usually referred
   Associated with diffuse discomfort, e.g., nausea, bloating
   Relieved by narcotic analgesics
Neuropathic pain
   No obvious nociceptive stimulus
   Associated evidence of nerve damage, e.g., sensory impairment, weakness
   Unusual, dissimilar from somatic pain, often shooting or electrical quality
   Only partially relieved by narcotic analgesics, may respond to antidepressants or anticonvulsants

---

Referred pain (see HPIM-16, Fig. 11-3) results from the convergence of sensory inputs from skin and viscera on single spinal neurons that transmit pain signals to the brain. Because of this convergence, input from deep structures is mislocalized to a region of skin innervated by the same spinal segment.

 TREATMENT

    Acute Somatic Pain If moderate, it can usually be treated effectively with nonnarcotic analgesics, e.g., aspirin, acetaminophen, and NSAIDs (Table 8-2). All inhibit cyclooxygenase (COX) and, except for acetaminophen, all have anti-inflammatory actions, especially at high dosages. For subacute musculoskeletal pain and arthritis, selective COX-2 inhibitors such as celecoxib are useful, especially if the pt is at risk for upper gastrointestinal ulceration or bleeding. Narcotic analgesics are usually required for relief of severe pain; the dose should be titrated to produce effective analgesia.

Chronic Pain

The problem is often difficult to diagnose, and pts may appear emotionally distraught. Psychological evaluation and behaviorally based treatment paradigms are frequently helpful, particularly in a multidisciplinary pain management center.

    Several factors can cause, perpetuate, or exacerbate chronic pain: (1) painful disease for which there is no cure (e.g., arthritis, cancer, migraine headaches, diabetic neuropathy); (2) neural factors initiated by a bodily disease that persist after the disease has resolved (e.g., damaged sensory or sympathetic nerves); (3) psychological conditions.

    Pay special attention to the medical history and to depression. Major depression is common, treatable, and potentially fatal (suicide).

 TREATMENT

    After evaluation, an explicit treatment plan should be developed, including specific and realistic goals for therapy, e.g., getting a good night's sleep, being able to go shopping, or returning to work. A multidisciplinary approach that utilizes medications, counseling, physical therapy, nerve blocks, and even surgery may be required to improve the pt's quality of life. Some pts may require referral to a pain clinic; for others, pharmacologic management alone can provide significant help. The tricyclic antidepressants are useful in management of chronic pain from many causes, including headache, diabetic neuropathy, postherpetic neuralgia, atypical facial pain, chronic low back pain, and post-stroke pain. Anticonvulsants or antiarrhythmics benefit pts with neuropathic pain and little or no evidence of sympathetic dysfunction (e.g., diabetic neuropathy, trigeminal neuralgia). The combination of the anticonvulsant gabapentin and an antidepressant such as nortriptyline may be effective for chronic neuropathic pain.

    The long-term use of opioids is accepted for pain due to malignant disease but is controversial for chronic pain of nonmalignant origin. When other approaches fail, long-acting opioid compounds such as levorphanol, methadone, sustained-release morphine, or transdermal fentanyl may be considered for these pts (Table 8-2).

Table 8-2

Drugs for Relief of Pain

NONNARCOTIC ANALGESICS: USUAL DOSES AND INTERVALS

Generic Name	Dose, mg	Interval	Comments
Acetylsalicylic acid	650 PO	q 4 h	Enteric-coated preparations available
Acetaminophen	650 PO	q 4 h	Side effects uncommon
Ibuprofen	400 PO	q 4–6 h	Available without prescription
Naproxen	250–500 PO	q 12 h	Delayed effects may be due to long half-life
Fenoprofen	200 PO	q 4–6 h	Contraindicated in renal disease
Indomethacin	25–50 PO	q 8 h	Gastrointestinal side effects common
Ketorolac	15–60 IM	q 4–6 h	Available for parenteral use (IM)
Celecoxib	100–200 PO	q 12–24 h	Useful for arthritis

NARCOTIC ANALGESICS: USUAL DOSES AND INTERVALS

Generic Name	Parenteral Dose, mg	PO Dose, mg	Comments
Codeine	30–60 q 4 h	30–60 q 4 h	Nausea common
Oxycodone	—	5–10 q 4–6 h	Usually available with acetaminophen or aspirin
Morphine	10 q 4 h	60 q 4 h	
Morphine sustained release	—	30–200 bid to tid	Oral slow-release preparation
Hydromorphone	1–2 q 4 h	2–4 q 4 h	Shorter acting than morphine sulfate
Levorphanol	2 q 6–8 h	4 q 6–8 h	Longer acting than morphine sulfate; absorbed well PO
Methadone	10 q 6–8 h	20 q 6–8 h	Delayed sedation due to long half-life

Generic Name			Comments
Meperidine	75–100 q 3–4 h	300 q 4 h	Poorly absorbed PO; normeperidine a toxic metabolite
Butorphanol	—	1–2 q 4 h	Intranasal spray
Fentanyl	25–100 µg/h	—	72 h Transdermal patch
Tramadol	—	50–100 q 4–6 h	Mixed opioid/adrenergic action

ANTIDEPRESSANTS[a]

Generic Name	Uptake Blockade 5-HT	NE	Sedative Potency	Anticholinergic Potency	Orthostatic Hypotension	Cardiac Arrhythmia	Ave. Dose, mg/d	Range, mg/d
Doxepin	++	+	High	Moderate	Moderate	Less	200	75–400
Amitriptyline	++++	++	High	Highest	Moderate	Yes	150	25–300
Imipramine	++++	++	Moderate	Moderate	High	Yes	200	75–400
Nortriptyline	+++	++	Moderate	Moderate	Low	Yes	100	40–150
Desipramine	+++	++++	Low	Low	Low	Yes	150	50–300
Venlafaxine	+++	++	Low	None	None	No	150	75–400

ANTICONVULSANTS AND ANTIARRHYTHMICS[a]

Generic Name	PO Dose, mg	Interval
Phenytoin	300	daily/qhs
Carbamazepine	200–300	q 6 h
Oxcarbazine	300	bid

Generic Name	PO Dose, mg	Interval
Clonazepam	1	q 6 h
Mexiletine	150–300	q 6–12 h
Gabapentin[b]	600–1200	q 8 h

[a] Antidepressants, anticonvulsants, and antiarrhythmics have not been approved by the U.S. Food and Drug Administration (FDA) for the treatment of pain.

[b] Gabapentin in doses up to 1800 mg/d is FDA approved for postherpetic neuralgia.

Note: 5-HT, serotonin; NE, norepinephrine.

For a more detailed discussion, see Fields HL, Martin JB: Pain: Pathophysiology and Management, Chap. 11, p. 71, in HPIM-16.

9

PROCEDURES COMMONLY PERFORMED BY INTERNISTS

Internists perform a wide range of medical procedures, although practices vary widely among institutions and by specialty. Internists, nurses, or other ancillary health care professionals perform venipuncture for blood testing, arterial puncture for blood gases, endotracheal intubation, and flexible sigmoidoscopy, and insert IV Lines, nasogastric (NG) tubes, and urinary catheters. These procedures are not covered here but require skill and practice to minimize patient discomfort and potential complications. Here, we review more invasive diagnostic and therapeutic procedures performed by internists—thoracentesis, lumbar puncture, and paracentesis. Many additional procedures are performed by specialists and require additional training and credentialing, including the following:

- Allergy—skin testing, rhinoscopy
- Cardiology—stress testing, echocardiograms, coronary catheterization, angioplasty, stent insertion, pacemakers, electrophysiology testing and ablation, implantable defibrillators, cardioversion
- Endocrinology—thyroid biopsy, dynamic hormone testing, bone densitometry
- Gastroenterology—upper and lower endoscopy, esophageal manometry, endoscopic retrograde cholangiopancreatography, stent insertion, endoscopic ultrasound, liver biopsy
- Hematology/Oncology—bone marrow biopsy, stem cell transplant, lymph node biopsy, plasmapheresis
- Pulmonary—intubation and ventilator management, bronchoscopy
- Renal—kidney biopsy, dialysis
- Rheumatology—joint aspiration

Increasingly, ultrasound, CT, and MRI are being used to guide invasive procedures, and flexible fiberoptic instruments are extending the reach into the body. For most invasive medical procedures, including those reviewed below, informed consent should be obtained in writing before beginning the procedure.

THORACENTESIS
Drainage of the pleural space can be performed at the bedside. Indications for this procedure include diagnostic evaluation of pleural fluid, removal of pleural fluid for symptomatic relief, and instillation of sclerosing agents in pts with recurrent, usually malignant pleural effusions.

PREPARATORY WORK   Familiarity with the components of a thoracentesis tray is a prerequisite to performing a thoracentesis successfully. Current PA and lateral chest radiographs with bilateral decubitus views should be obtained to document the free-flowing nature of the pleural effusion. Loculated pleural effusions should be localized by ultrasound or CT prior to drainage.

TECHNIQUE   A posterior approach is the preferred means of accessing pleural fluid. Comfortable positioning is a key to success for both pt and physician. The pt should sit on the edge of the bed, leaning forward with the arms abducted onto a pillow on a bedside stand. Pts undergoing thoracentesis frequently have severe dyspnea, and it is important to assess if they can maintain this positioning for at least 10 min. The entry site for the thoracentesis is based on the physical exam and radiographic findings. Percussion of dullness is utilized to ascertain the extent of the pleural effusion with the site of entry being the first or second highest interspace in this area. The entry site for the thoracentesis is at the superior aspect of the rib, thus avoiding the intercostal nerve, artery, and vein, which run along the inferior aspect of the rib.

The site of entry should be marked with a pen to guide the thoracentesis. The skin is then prepped and draped in a sterile fashion with the operator observing sterile technique at all times. A small-gauge needle is used to anesthetize the skin and a larger-gauge needle is used to anesthetize down to the superior aspect of the rib. The needle should then be directed over the upper margin of the rib to anesthetize down to the parietal pleura. The pleural space should be entered with the anesthetizing needle, all the while using liberal amounts of lidocaine.

A dedicated thoracentesis needle with an attached syringe should next be utilized to penetrate the skin. This needle should be advanced to the superior aspect of the rib. While maintaining gentle negative pressure, the needle should be slowly advanced into the pleural space. If a diagnostic tap is being performed, aspiration of only 30–50 mL of fluid is necessary before termination of the procedure. If a therapeutic thoracentesis is being performed, a three-way stopcock is utilized to direct the aspirated pleural fluid into collection bottles or bags. No more than 1 L of pleural fluid should be withdrawn at any given time as quantities >1–1.5 L can result in reexpansion pulmonary edema.

After all specimens have been collected, the thoracentesis needle should be withdrawn and the needle site occluded for at least 1 min.

SPECIMEN COLLECTION   The diagnostic evaluation of pleural fluid depends on the clinical situation. All pleural fluid samples should be sent for cell count and differential, Gram stain, and bacterial cultures. LDH and protein determinations should also be made to differentiate between exudative and transudative pleural effusions. The pH should be determined if empyema is a diagnostic consideration. Other studies on pleural fluid include mycobacterial and fungal cultures, glucose, triglyceride level, amylase, and cytologic determination.

POST-PROCEDURE   A post-procedural chest radiograph should be obtained to evaluate for a pneumothorax, and the pt should be instructed to notify the physician if new shortness of breath develops.

LUMBAR PUNCTURE

Evaluation of CSF is essential for the diagnosis of suspected meningeal infection, subarachnoid hemorrhage, leptomeningeal neoplastic disease, and noninfectious meningitis. Relative contraindications to LP include local skin infection in the lumbar area, suspected spinal cord mass lesion, and a suspected intracranial mass lesion. Any bleeding diathesis should also be corrected prior to performing LP to prevent the possible occurrence of an epidural hematoma. A functional platelet count $> 50,000/\mu L$ and an INR < 1.5 are advisable to perform LP safely.

PREPARATORY WORK   Familiarity with the components of a lumbar puncture tray is a prerequisite to performing LP successfully. In pts with focal neurologic deficits or with evidence of papilledema on physical exam, a CT scan of the head should be obtained prior to performing LP.

TECHNIQUE Proper positioning of the pt is important to ensure a successful LP. Two different pt positions can be used: the lateral decubitus position and the sitting position. Most routine LPs should be performed using the lateral decubitus position. The sitting position may be preferable in obese pts. With either position, the pt should be instructed to flex the spine as much as possible. In the lateral decubitus position, the pt is instructed to assume the fetal position with the knees flexed toward the abdomen. In the sitting position, the pt should bend over a bedside table with the head resting on folded arms.

The entry site for a LP is below the level of the conus medullaris, which extends to L1-L2 in most adults. Thus, either the L3-L4 or L4-L5 interspace can be utilized as the entry site. The posterior superior iliac crest should be identified and the spine palpated at this level. This represents the L3-L4 interspace, with the other interspaces referenced from this landmark. The midpoint of the interspace between the spinous processes represents the entry point for the thoracentesis needle. This entry site should be marked with a pen to guide the LP. The skin is then prepped and draped in a sterile fashion with the operator observing sterile technique at all times. A small-gauge needle is then used to anesthetize the skin and subcutaneous tissue. The spinal needle should be introduced perpendicular to the skin in the midline and should be advanced slowly. The needle stylette should be withdrawn frequently as the spinal needle is advanced. As the needle enters the subarachnoid space, a "popping" sensation can sometimes be felt. If bone is encountered, the needle should be withdrawn to just below the skin and then redirected more caudally. Once CSF begins to flow, the opening pressure can be measured. This should be measured in the lateral decubitus position with the pt shifted to this position if the procedure was begun with the pt in the sitting position. After the opening pressure is measured, the CSF should be collected in a series of specimen tubes for various tests. At a minimum, a total of 10–15 mL of CSF should be collected in the different specimen tubes.

Once the required spinal fluid is collected, the stylette should be replaced and the spinal needle removed.

SPECIMEN COLLECTION Diagnostic evaluation of CSF is based on the clinical scenario. In general, spinal fluid should always be sent for cell count with differential, protein, glucose, and bacterial cultures. Other specialized studies that can be obtained on CSF include viral cultures, fungal and mycobacterial cultures, VDRL, cryptococcal antigen, oligoclonal bands, and cytology.

POST-PROCEDURE To reduce the chance of a post-LP headache, the pt should be instructed to lie prone for at least 3 h. If a headache does develop; bedrest, hydration, and oral analgesics are often helpful. If an intractable post-LP headache ensues, the pt may have a persistent CSF leak. In this case, consultation of an anesthesiologist should be considered for the placement of a blood patch.

PARACENTESIS
Removal and analysis of peritoneal fluid is invaluable in evaluating pts with new-onset ascites or ascites of unknown etiology. It is also requisite in pts with known ascites who have a decompensation in their clinical status. Relative contraindications include bleeding diathesis, prior abdominal surgery, distended bowel, or known loculated ascites.

PREPARATORY WORK   Prior to performing a paracentesis, any severe bleeding diathesis should be corrected. Bowel distention should also be relieved by placement of a nasogastric tube, and the bladder should also be emptied before beginning the procedure. If a large-volume paracentesis is being performed, large vacuum bottles with the appropriate connecting tubing should be obtained.

TECHNIQUE   Proper pt positioning greatly improves the ease with which a paracentesis can be performed. The pt should be instructed to lie supine with the head of the bed elevated to 45°. This position should be maintained for ~15 min to allow ascitic fluid to accumulate in the dependent portion of the abdomen.

The preferred entry site for paracentesis is a midline puncture halfway between the pubic symphysis and the umbilicus; this correlates with the location of the relatively avascular linea alba. The midline puncture should be avoided if there is a previous midline surgical scar, as neovascularization may have occurred. Alternative sites of entry include the lower quadrants, lateral to the rectus abdominus, but caution should be used to avoid collateral blood vessels that may have formed in patients with portal hypertension.

The skin is prepped and draped in a sterile fashion. The skin, subcutaneous tissue, and the abdominal wall down to the peritoneum should be infiltrated with an anesthetic agent. The paracentesis needle with an attached syringe is then introduced in the midline perpendicular to the skin. To prevent leaking of ascitic fluid, "Z-tracking" can sometimes be helpful: after penetrating the skin, the needle is inserted 1–2 cm before advancing further. The needle is then advanced slowly while continuous aspiration is performed. As the peritoneum is pierced, the needle will give noticeably. Fluid should flow freely into the syringe soon thereafter. For a diagnostic paracentesis, removal of 50 mL of ascitic fluid is adequate. For a large-volume paracentesis, direct drainage into large vacuum containers using connecting tubing is a commonly utilized option.

After all samples have been collected, the paracentesis needle should be removed and firm pressure applied to the puncture site.

SPECIMEN COLLECTION   Peritoneal fluid should be sent for cell count with differential, Gram stain, and bacterial cultures. Albumin measurement of ascitic fluid is also necessary for calculating the serum–ascitic albumin gradient. Depending on the clinical scenario, other studies that can be obtained include mycobacterial cultures, amylase, adenosine deaminase, triglycerides, and cytology.

POST-PROCEDURE   The pt should be monitored carefully post-procedure and should be instructed to lie supine in bed for several hours. If persistent fluid leakage occurs, continued bedrest with pressure dressings at the puncture site can be helpful. For pts with hepatic dysfunction undergoing large-volume paracentesis, the sudden reduction in intravascular volume can precipitate hepatorenal syndrome. Administration of 25 g IV albumin following large-volume paracentesis has been shown to decrease the incidence of renal failure post-procedure. Finally, if the ascites fluid analysis shows evidence of spontaneous bacterial peritonitis, then antibiotics (directed toward gram-negative gut bacteria) and IV albumin should be administered as soon as possible.

10

DIAGNOSTIC IMAGING IN INTERNAL MEDICINE

Clinicians have a wide array of radiologic modalities at their disposal to aid them in noninvasive diagnosis. Despite the introduction of highly specialized imaging modalities, radiologic tests such as chest radiographs and ultrasound continue to serve a vital role in the diagnostic approach to patient care. At most institutions, computed tomography (CT) is available on an emergent basis and is invaluable for initial evaluation of patients with trauma, stroke, suspected CNS hemorrhage, or ischemic stroke. Magnetic resonance imaging (MRI) and related techniques (MR angiography, functional MRI, MR spectroscopy) are providing remarkable resolution of many tissues including the brain, vascular system, joints, and most large organs.

This chapter will review the indications and utility of the most commonly utilized radiologic studies used by internists.

Chest Radiography

- Can be obtained quickly and should be part of the standard evaluation for patients with cardiopulmonary complaints.
- Is able to identify life-threatening conditions such as pneumothorax, intraperitoneal air, pulmonary edema, and aortic dissection.
- Is most often normal in a patient with an acute pulmonary embolus.
- Should be repeated in 4–6 weeks in a patient with an acute pneumonic process to document resolution of the radiographic infiltrate.
- Is used in conjunction with the physical exam to support the diagnosis of congestive heart failure. Radiographic findings supporting the diagnosis of heart failure include cardiomegaly, cephalization, Kerley B lines, and pleural effusions.
- Should be obtained daily in intubated patients to examine endotracheal tube position and the possibility of barotrauma.
- Helps to identify alveolar or airspace disease. Radiographic features of such diseases include inhomogeneous, patchy opacities and air-bronchograms.
- Helps to document the free-flowing nature of pleural effusions. Decubitus views should be obtained to exclude loculated pleural fluid prior to attempts to extract such fluid.

Abdominal Radiography

- Should be the initial imaging modality in a patient with suspected bowel obstruction. Signs of small-bowel obstruction on plain radiographs include multiple air-fluid levels, absence of colonic distention, and a "stepladder" appearance of small-bowel loops.
- Should not be performed with barium enhancement when perforated bowel, portal venous gas, or toxic megacolon is suspected.
- Is used to evaluate the size of bowel:
  1. Normal small bowel is <3 cm in diameter.
  2. Normal caliber of the cecum is up to 9 cm, with the rest of the large bowel up to 6 cm in diameter.

Ultrasound

- Is more sensitive and specific than CT scanning in evaluating for the presence of gallstone disease.

• Can readily identify the size of the kidneys in a patient with renal insufficiency and can exclude the presence of hydronephrosis.
• Can expeditiously evaluate for the presence of peritoneal fluid in a patient with blunt abdominal trauma.
• Is used in conjunction with doppler studies to evaluate for the presence of arterial atherosclerotic disease.
• Is used to evaluate cardiac valves and wall motion.
• Should be used to localize loculated pleural and peritoneal fluid prior to draining such fluid.
• Can determine the size of thyroid nodules and guide fine-needle aspiration biopsy.
• Is the modality of choice for assessing known or suspected scrotal pathology.
• Should be the first imaging modality utilized when evaluating the ovaries.

Computed Tomography

• CT of the brain should be initial radiographic modality in evaluating a patient with a potential stroke.
• Is highly sensitive for diagnosing an acute subarachnoid hemorrhage and in the acute setting is more sensitive than MRI.
• CT of the brain is an essential test in evaluating a patient with mental status changes to exclude entities such as intracranial bleeding, mass effect, subdural or epidural hematomas, and hydrocephalus.
• Is better than MRI for evaluating osseous lesions of the skull and spine.
• CT of the chest should be considered in the evaluation of a patient with chest pain to rule out entities such as pulmonary embolus or aortic dissection.
• CT of the chest is essential for evaluating lung nodules to assess for the presence of thoracic lymphadenopathy.
• CT with high-resolution cuts through the lungs is the imaging modality of choice for evaluating the lung interstitium in a patient with interstitial lung disease.
• Can be used to evaluate for presence of pleural and pericardial fluid and to localize loculated effusions.
• Is an essential test in a patient with unexplained abdominal pain to evaluate for conditions such as appendicitis, mesenteric ischemia or infarction, diverticulitis, or pancreatitis.
• CT of the abdomen is also the test of choice for evaluating for nephrolithiasis in a patient with renal colic.
• Is the test of choice for evaluating for the presence of an abscess in the chest or abdomen.
• In conjunction with abdominal radiography, CT is part of the evaluation of a patient with a bowel obstruction and can help identify the cause of such an obstruction.
• Can identify abdominal conditions such as intussusception and volvulus in a patient with abdominal pain.
• Is the imaging modality of choice for evaluating the retroperitoneum.
• Should be obtained expeditiously in a patient with abdominal trauma to evaluate for the presence of intraabdominal hemorrhage and to assess injury to abdominal organs.

Magnetic Resonance Imaging

• Is more useful than CT in the evaluation of ischemic infarction, dementia, mass lesions, demyelinating diseases, and most nonosseous spinal disorders.
• Provides excellent imaging of large joints including the knee, hip, and shoulder.
• Can be used, often with CT or angiography, to assess possible dissecting aortic aneurysms and congenital anomalies of the cardiovascular system.

• Cardiac MRI is proving useful to evaluate cardiac wall motion and for assessing cardiac muscle viability in ischemic heart disease.
• Is preferable to CT for evaluating adrenal masses such as pheochromocytoma and for helping to distinguish benign and malignant adrenal masses.

MEDICAL EVALUATION OF THE SURGICAL PATIENT

GOAL

• Determine presence of comorbid disease that increases surgical morbidity and mortality.
• Reduce risk and optimize pt's condition.

The Healthy Patient Should have screening history and physical exam.

• Simple preoperative questionnaires are useful
• Determine exercise tolerance and reason for intolerance
• Routine laboratory tests in healthy pts are of little value

CARDIAC RISK ASSESSMENT

Cardiac complications are most important cause of perioperative morbidity and mortality. Risk can be estimated by adding up the number of risk factors (Table 11-1). Class II pts should receive noninvasive cardiac testing (e.g., dipyridamole-thallium testing or dobutamine stress echocardiography; see Chap. 118) for vascular surgery. Class III or IV pts should receive treatment to reduce risk prior to elective surgery.

Table 11-1

The Revised Cardiac Risk Index

Factor	Adjusted Odds Ratio for Cardiac Complications
1. High-risk surgery	2.8
2. Ischemic heart disease	2.4
3. History of congestive heart failure	1.9
4. History of cerebrovascular disease	3.2
5. Insulin therapy for diabetes mellitus	3.0
6. Preoperative serum creatinine > 2.0 mg/dL	3.0

Class	Number of Factors	Cardiac Complication Rates, %
I	0	0.5
II	1	1.0
III	2	5.0
IV	3–6	10.0

Source: Adapted from TH Lee et al: Circulation 100:1043, 1999, with permission.

Physical Examination   Evaluate for uncontrolled hypertension, signs of CHF (jugular venous distention, rales, S_3), previously unknown heart murmurs, carotid bruits. Inspect for pallor, cyanosis, poor nutritional state.

Laboratory   Examine ECG for evidence of previous MI (Q waves) or arrhythmias. Inspect CXR for signs of CHF (e.g., cardiomegaly, vascular redistribution, Kerley B lines). Additional testing is dictated by specific underlying cardiovascular disease and nature of the planned operation. See Fig. 11-1 for

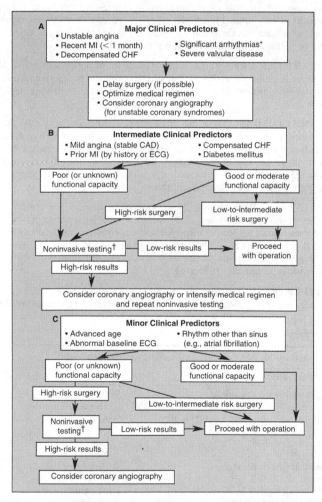

FIGURE 11-1   Approach to preoperative cardiac evaluation. *Significant arrhythmias include (1) high-grade AV block, (2) symptomatic ventricular arrhythmias, and (3) supraventricular arrhythmias with uncontrolled ventricular rate. †Exercise testing is preferred (treadmill, bicycle, arm ergometry). Perform with echo or nuclear scintigraphy if baseline ST-T waves preclude ECG interpretation. If unable to exercise, consider pharmacologic (e.g., dobutamine or adenosine) test with echo or nuclear imaging, or ambulatory ECG monitoring, if baseline ST-T waves normal. (*Modified from KA Eagle et al: Circulation 93:1278, 1996, with permission.*)

clinical predictors of increased perioperative risk of MI, CHF, or death and approaches to preoperative evaluation.

Specific Cardiac Conditions

CORONARY ARTERY DISEASE (CAD) Consider postponing purely elective operations for 6 months following an MI. Pts with stable CAD can be evaluated per algorithm in Fig. 11-1. Surgical risk is generally acceptable in pts with class I–II symptoms (e.g., able to climb one flight carrying grocery bags) and in those with low risk results from noninvasive testing. For those with high-risk results or very limited functional capacity, consider coronary angiography. Perioperative beta-blocker therapy reduces incidence of coronary events and should be included in medical regimen if no contraindications.

HEART FAILURE This is a major predictor of perioperative risk. Regimen of ACE inhibitor and diuretics should be optimized preoperatively to minimize risk of either pulmonary congestion or intravascular volume depletion postoperatively.

ARRHYTHMIAS These are often markers for underlying CHF, CAD, drug toxicities (e.g., digitalis), or metabolic abnormalities (e.g., hypokalemia, hypomagnesemia), which should be identified and corrected. Indications for antiarrhythmic therapy or pacemakers are same as in nonsurgical situations (Chap. 125). Notably, asymptomatic ventricular premature beats generally do not require suppressive therapy preoperatively.

VALVULAR DISEASES Those portending surgical risk are advanced aortic or mitral stenosis (Chap. 119), which should be repaired, if severe or symptomatic, prior to elective surgery. Ensure adequate ventricular rate control in mitral stenosis with atrial fibrillation (using beta blocker, digoxin, verapamil, or diltiazem). Endocarditis prophylaxis is indicated for operations associated with transient bacteremias (Chap. 85).

HYPERTENSION Control elevated pressure preoperatively (Chap. 122), especially using beta blocker if possible, which should be continued perioper-

Table 11-2

Risk Factors for Postoperative Pulmonary Complications

Patient-Related Risk Factors	Procedure-Related Risk Factors
Chronic obstructive pulmonary disease	Surgical site:
	Thoracic surgery
Cigarette use < 8 weeks before surgery	Abdominal aortic aneurysm
ASA class > 2	surgery
Goldman class 2–4[a]	Upper abdominal surgery
Age > 60	Neurosurgery
Dependent functional status	Peripheral vascular surgery
Albumin < 3.0 g/dL	General anesthesia
Blood urea nitrogen > 30 mg/dL	Pancuronium use
Abnormal chest radiograph	Emergency surgery
	Surgery lasting > 3 h

[a] Goldman Cardiac Risk Index. Of four classes possible; class 4 represents the highest risk.
Note: ASA, American Society of Anesthesiologists.
Source: Reprinted from GW Smetana: Clin Geriatr Med 19:35, 2003, with permission from Elsevier Science.

atively. If pheochromocytoma is a possibility, surgery should be delayed for evaluation because of high anesthetic risk.

Perioperative beta blockers reduce risk of cardiac complications in pts with two or more of the following risk factors: age ≥ 65 yrs, hypertension, current cigarette use, diabetes mellitus, and total cholesterol ≥ 240 mg/dL.

PREOPERATIVE PULMONARY EVALUATION

Table 11-2 shows risk factors for postoperative pulmonary complications. Chronic obstructive pulmonary disease (Chap. 133) increases risk fourfold. Risk increases with thoracic operations. Laparoscopic abdominal surgery is low risk.

Preoperative pulmonary function testing (Chap. 130), especially simple spirometry with FEV_1, is indicated prior to lung resection surgery.

Cigarette smoking should be stopped 8 weeks before elective surgery. Chronic obstructive pulmonary disease and asthma should be vigorously treated. Postoperative lung expansion, deep breathing exercises, and pain control reduce complications in pts with chronic pulmonary disease.

For a more detailed discussion, see Smetana GW: Medical Evaluation of the Surgical Patient, Chap. 7, p. 38, in HPIM-16.

12

ACUTE RESPIRATORY DISTRESS SYNDROME (ARDS)

Definition and Etiology

Syndrome of rapid-onset hypoxemic respiratory failure with:

1. Diffuse pulmonary infiltrates on chest radiograph
2. Arterial Pa_{O_2} (mmHg)/FI_{O_2} (inspired oxygen fraction) < 200
3. No contribution of pulmonary congestion (pulmonary capillary wedge pressure < 18 mmHg).

Acute lung injury (ALI) is a similar syndrome, with Pa_{O_2}/FI_{O_2} < 300. Caused by many medical and surgical disorders (Table 12-1), but >80% of cases caused by sepsis, bacterial pneumonia, trauma, multiple transfusions, gastric acid aspiration, and drug overdose. Risk factors include older age, chronic alcohol abuse, metabolic acidosis, and severity of critical illness.

Clinical Course and Pathophysiology

Natural history marked by three phases:

1. *Exudative phase*—Marked by disruption of normally tight alveolar-capillary membrane with consequent collection of protein-rich alveolar wall and airspace edema with collection of cytokines in edema fluid. Exudative phase duration is typically ~7 days, marked by dyspnea, tachypnea, and severe hypoxemia; differential includes cardiogenic pulmonary edema, diffuse pneumonia, alveolar hemorrhage.

2. *Proliferative phase*—If recovery does not occur, some pts will develop progressive lung injury and evidence of pulmonary interstitial inflammation and fibrosis. Duration approximately days 7–21.

3. *Fibrotic phase*—Although the majority of patients recover within 3–4 weeks of the initial insult, some experience progressive fibrosis, necessitating prolonged ventilatory support predisposing to complications of long-term intensive care. Many investigators believe the incidence of this final phase of

Table 12-1

Clinical Disorders Commonly Associated with ARDS

Direct Lung Injury	Indirect Lung Injury
Pneumonia	Sepsis
Aspiration of gastric contents	Severe trauma
Pulmonary contusion	Multiple bone fractures
Near-drowning	Flail chest
Toxic inhalation injury	Head trauma
	Burns
	Multiple transfusions
	Drug overdose
	Pancreatitis
	Post-cardiopulmonary bypass

Source: Levy BD, Shapiro SD: Chap. 251, HPIM-16.

ARDS was in part a reaction to now-abandoned ventilator strategies that employed large tidal volumes and high lung inflation pressures.

℞ TREATMENT

Progress in recent therapy has emphasized the importance of general critical care of patients with ARDS in addition to new ventilator strategies. General care requires:

- Treatment of underlying cause of lung injury
- Minimizing procedural complications
- Avoidance of preventable complications such as venous thromboembolism and GI hemorrhage with appropriate prophylactic regimes
- Recognition and treatment of nosocomial infections
- Adequate nutritional support.

Mechanical Ventilatory Support   A substantial improvement in outcome of ARDS has occurred with recognition that overdistention of normal lung units with positive pressure can produce or exacerbate lung injury, causing or worsening ARDS. This finding has prompted the introduction of ventilator strategies aimed at limiting alveolar distention while still ensuring adequate tissue oxygenation.

Current practice is to use low tidal volumes ($\leq$ 6 mL/kg predicted body weight); see http://www.ardsnet.org/. Low tidal volumes are combined with the use of positive end-expiratory pressure (PEEP) at levels that strive to achieve adequate oxygenation with the lowest $F_{I_{O_2}}$. Other techniques that may improve oxygenation while limiting alveolar distention include extending the time of inspiration on the ventilator and placing the patient in the prone position.

Ancillary Therapies   In general, patients with ARDS should receive intravenous fluids only sufficient to achieve an adequate cardiac output and tissue oxygen delivery. There is no survival advantage to increasing oxygen delivery by overresuscitation, and fluids should be given only in sufficient volumes to maintain adequate organ function as assessed by urine output, acid-base statues, arterial pressure. There is no current evidence to support the use of glucocorticoids or other pharmacologic therapies in ARDS, except as needed to treat the underlying cause of the condition.

Outcomes

Mortality from ARDS has declined steadily over the past 15 years with improvements in general care and then the introduction of low tidal volume ventilation. Current mortality is 41–65%, with most deaths due to nonpulmonary causes.

For a more detailed discussion, see Levy BD, Shapiro SD: Acute Respiratory Distress Syndrome, Chap. 251, p. 1592, in HPIM-16.

13

CARDIOVASCULAR COLLAPSE AND SUDDEN DEATH

Unexpected cardiovascular collapse and death most often result from ventricular fibrillation in pts with underlying coronary artery disease, with or without acute MI. Other common causes are listed in Table 13-1. The arrhythmic causes may be provoked by electrolyte disorders (primarily hypokalemia), hypoxemia, acidosis, or massive sympathetic discharge, as may occur in CNS injury. Immediate institution of cardiopulmonary resuscitation (CPR) followed by advanced life support measures (see below) are mandatory. Ventricular fibrillation, or asystole, without institution of CPR within 4–6 min usually causes death.

Management of Cardiac Arrest

Basic life support (BLS) must commence immediately (Fig. 13-1):

- Open mouth of patient and remove visible debris or dentures. If there is respiratory stridor, consider aspiration of a foreign body and perform Heimlich maneuver.
- Tilt head backward, lift chin, and begin mouth-to-mouth respiration if rescue equipment is not available (pocket mask is preferable to prevent transmission of infection). The lungs should be inflated twice in rapid succession for every 15 chest compressions.
- If carotid pulse is absent, perform chest compressions (depressing sternum 3–5 cm) at rate of 80–100 per min. For one rescuer, 15 compressions are performed before returning to ventilating twice.
- As soon as resuscitation equipment is available, begin advanced life support with continued chest compressions and ventilation.
- Although performed as simultaneously as possible, defibrillation takes highest priority (Fig. 13-2A), followed by placement of intravenous access and in-

Table 13-1

Differential Diagnosis of Cardiovascular Collapse and Sudden Death

1. Ventricular fibrillation due to:
   Myocardial ischemia (severe coronary artery disease, acute MI)
   Congestive heart failure
   Dilated or hypertrophic cardiomyopathy
   Myocarditis
   Right ventricular dysplasia
   Valvular disease [aortic stenosis, mitral valve prolapse (rare)]
   Preexcitation syndromes (Wolff-Parkinson-White)
   Prolonged QT syndromes (congenital, drug-induced)
   Brugada syndrome
2. Asystole or severe bradycardia
3. Sudden marked decrease in LV stroke volume from:
   Massive pulmonary embolism
   Cardiac tamponade
   Severe aortic stenosis
4. Sudden marked decrease in intravascular volume, e.g.:
   Ruptured aortic aneurysm
   Aortic dissection

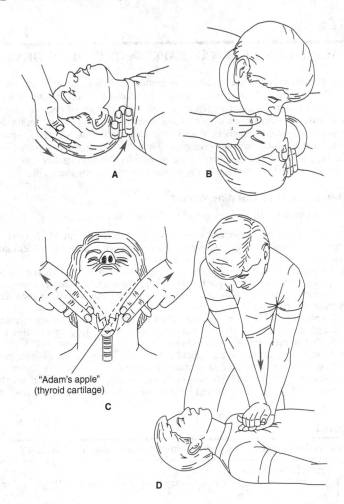

FIGURE 13-1   Major steps in cardiopulmonary resuscitation. *A*. Make certain the victim has an open airway. *B*. Start respiratory resuscitation immediately. *C*. Feel for the carotid pulse in the groove alongside the "Adam's apple" or thyroid cartilage. *D*. If pulse is absent, begin cardiac massage. Use 80–100 compressions/min with two lung inflations in rapid succession for every 15 compressions. (*From J Henderson, Emergency Medical Guide, 4th ed, New York, McGraw-Hill, 1978.*)

tubation. 100% O_2 should be administered by endotracheal tube or, if rapid intubation cannot be accomplished, by bag-valve-mask device; respirations should not be interrupted for more than 30 s while attempting to intubate.

• Initial intravenous access should be through the antecubital vein, but if drug administration is ineffective, a central line (internal jugular or subclavian) should be placed. Intravenous $NaHCO_3$ should be administered only if there is persistent severe acidosis (pH < 7.15) despite adequate ventilation. Calcium is *not* routinely administered but should be given to pts with known hypocalcemia,

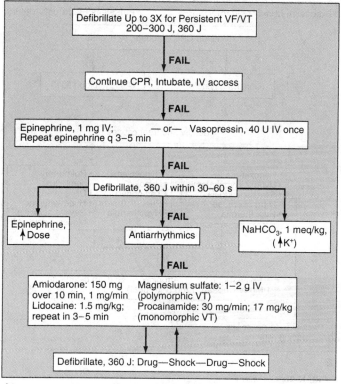

A

FIGURE 13-2A Management of cardiac arrest. *A*. The algorithm of ventricular fibrillation or hypotensive ventricular techycardia begins with defibrillation attempts. If that fails, it is followed by epinephrine and then antiarrhythmic drugs. *B*. The algorithms for bradyarrhythmia/asystole (left) or pulseless electrical activity (right) is dominated first by continued life support and a search for reversible causes. Subsequent therapy is nonspecific and accompanied by a low success rate. CPR, cardiopulmonary resuscitation; MI, myocardial infarction. (*From Myerburg RJ and Castellanos A, Chap. 256, HPIM-16.*)

those who have received toxic doses of calcium channel antagonists, or if acute hyperkalemia is thought to be the triggering event for resistant ventricular fibrillation.

• The approach to cardiovascular collapse caused by bradyarrhythmias, asystole, or pulseless electrical activity is shown in Fig. 13-2*B*.

Follow-up

If cardiac arrest was due to ventricular fibrillation in initial hours of an acute MI, follow-up is standard post-MI care (Chap. 123). For other survivors of a ventricular fibrillation arrest, extensive assessment, including evaluation of coronary anatomy, left ventricular function, and invasive electrophysiologic testing, is often recommended. In absence of a transient or reversible cause, ICD placement usually indicated.

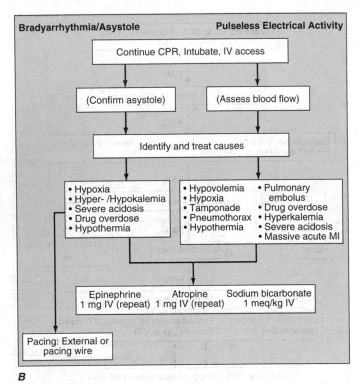

FIGURE 13-2B *(Continued)*

For a more detailed discussion, see Myerburg RJ, Castellanos A: Cardio-vascular Collapse, Cardiac Arrest, and Sudden Cardiac Death, Chap. 256, p. 1618, in HPIM-16.

14

SHOCK

Definition

Condition of severe impairment of tissue perfusion leading to cellular injury and dysfunction. Cell membrane dysfunction is a common end stage for various forms of shock. Rapid recognition and treatment are essential to prevent irreversible organ damage. Common causes are listed in Table 14-1.

Clinical Manifestations

• Hypotension (systolic bp < 90, mean bp < 60), tachycardia, tachypnea, pallor, restlessness, and altered sensorium.

Table 14-1

Common Forms of Shock

Oligemic shock
  Hemorrhage
  Volume depletion (e.g., vomiting, diarrhea, diuretic over-usage,
    ketoacidosis)
  Internal sequestration (ascites, pancreatitis, intestinal obstruction)
Cardiogenic shock
  Myopathic (acute MI, dilated cardiomyopathy)
  Mechanical (acute mitral regurgitation, ventricular septal defect, severe
    aortic stenosis)
  Arrhythmic
Extracardiac obstructive shock
  Pericardial tamponade
  Massive pulmonary embolism
  Tension pneumothorax
Distributive shock (profound decrease in systemic vascular tone)
  Sepsis
  Toxic overdoses
  Anaphylaxis
  Neurogenic (e.g., spinal cord injury)
  Endocrinologic (Addison's disease, myxedema)

* Signs of intense peripheral vasoconstriction, weak pulses, cold clammy extremities [in distributive (e.g., septic) shock, vasodilatation predominates and extremities are warm].
* Oliguria (<20 mL/h) and metabolic acidosis common.

_____ *Approach to the Patient* _____

Tissue perfusion must be restored immediately (see below); also obtain history for underlying cause, including

* Known cardiac disease (coronary disease, CHF, pericarditis)
* Recent fever or infection (leading to sepsis)
* Drugs, i.e., excess diuretics or antihypertensives
* Conditions predisposing for pulmonary embolism (Chap. 135)
* Possible bleeding from any site, particularly GI tract.

Physical Examination

* Jugular veins are flat in oligemic or distributive shock; jugular venous distention (JVD) suggests cardiogenic shock; JVD in presence of paradoxical pulse (Chap. 117) may reflect cardiac tamponade (Chap. 121).
* Look for evidence of CHF (Chap. 126), murmurs of aortic stenosis, acute regurgitation (mitral or aortic), ventricular septal defect.
* Check for asymmetry of pulses (aortic dissection) (Chap. 127).
* Tenderness or rebound in abdomen may indicate peritonitis or pancreatitis; high-pitched bowel sounds suggest intestinal obstruction. Perform stool guaiac to rule out GI bleeding.
* Fever and chills usually accompany septic shock. Sepsis may not cause fever in elderly, uremic, or alcoholic patients.
* Skin lesion may suggest specific pathogens in septic shock: petechiae or purpura (*Neisseria meningitidis*), erythyma gangrenosum (*Pseudomonas aeru-*

Table 14-2

Hemodynamic Profiles in Shock States

Diagnosis	PCW Pressure	Cardiac Output (CO)	Systemic Vascular Resistance	Comments
Cardiogenic shock	↑	↓	↑	PCW is normal or ↓ in RV infarction
Extracardiac obstructive shock				
Cardiac tamponade	↑	↓	↑	Equalization of intracardiac diastolic pressures
Massive pulmonary embolus	Normal or ↓	↓	↑	Right-sided cardiac pressures may be elevated
Oligemic shock	↓	↓	↑	
Distributive shock	↓	↑	↓	CO may ↓ later if sepsis results in LV dysfunction or if intravascular volume is inadequate

ginosa), generalized erythroderma (toxic shock due to *Staphylococcus aureus* or *Streptococcus pyogenes*).

Laboratory

• Obtain hematocrit, WBC, electrolytes. If actively bleeding, check platelet count, PT, PTT, DIC screen.

• Arterial blood gas usually shows metabolic acidosis (in septic shock, respiratory alkalosis precedes metabolic acidosis). If sepsis suspected, draw blood cultures, perform urinalysis, and obtain Gram stain and cultures of sputum, urine, and other suspected sites.

• Obtain ECG (myocardial ischemia or acute arrhythmia), chest x-ray (CHF, tension pneumothorax, aortic dissection, pneumonia). Echocardiogram may be helpful (cardiac tamponade, CHF).

• Central venous pressure or pulmonary capillary wedge (PCW) pressure measurements may be necessary to distinguish between different categories of shock (Table 14-2): Mean PCW < 6 mmHg suggests oligemic or distributive shock; PCW > 20 mmHg suggests left ventricular failure. Cardiac output (thermodilution) is decreased in cardiogenic and oligemic shock, and usually increased initially in septic shock.

℞ TREATMENT

See Fig. 14-1.

Aimed at rapid improvement of tissue hypoperfusion and respiratory impairment:

• Serial measurements of bp (intraarterial line preferred), heart rate, continuous ECG monitor, urine output, pulse oximetry, blood studies: Hct, electrolytes, creatinine, BUN, ABGs, calcium, phosphate, lactate, urine Na concentration (<20 mmol/L suggests volume depletion). Continuous monitoring of CVP and/or pulmonary artery pressure, with serial PCW pressures.

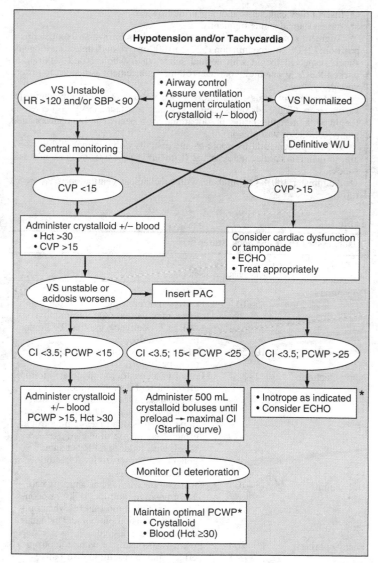

FIGURE 14-1 An algorithm for the resuscitation of the patient in shock. VS, vital signs; HR, heart rate; SBP, systolic blood pressure; W/U, work up; CVP, central venous pressure; Hct, hematocrit; ECHO, echocardiogram; PAC, pulmonary artery catheter; CI, cardiac index in (L/min)/m²; PCWP, pulmonary capillary wedge pressure in mmHg.

*Monitor SV_{O_2}, SVRI, and RVEDVI as additional markers of correction for perfusion and hypovolemia. Consider age-adjusted CI. SV_{O_2}, saturation of hemoglobin with O_2 in venous blood; SVRI, systemic vascular resistance index; RVEDVI, right-ventricular end-diastolic volume index.

- Insert Foley catheter to monitor urine flow.
- Assess mental status frequently.
- Augment systolic bp to >100 mmHg: (1) place in reverse Trendelenburg position; (2) IV volume infusion (500- to 1000-mL bolus), unless cardiogenic shock suspected (begin with normal saline, then whole blood, dextran, or packed RBCs, if anemic); continue volume replacement as needed to restore vascular volume.
- Add vasoactive drugs after intravascular volume is optimized; administer vasopressors (Table 14-3) if systemic vascular resistance (SVR) is decreased (begin with norepinephrine or dopamine; for persistent hypotension add phenylephrine or vasopressin).
- If CHF present, add inotropic agents (usually dobutamine) (Table 14-3); aim to maintain cardiac index > 2.2 (L/m^2)/min [>4.0 (L/m^2)/min in septic shock].
- Administer 100% O_2; intubate with mechanical ventilation if P_{O_2} < 70 mmHg.

Table 14-3

Vasopressors Used in Shock States [a]

Drug	Dose, (μg/kg)/min	Notes
Dopamine	1–5	Facilitates diuresis
	5–10	Positive inotropic and chronotropic effects; may increase O_2 consumption as well as O_2 delivery; use may be limited by tachycardia
	10–20	Generalized vasoconstriction (decrease renal perfusion)
Norepinephrine	2–8	Potent vasoconstrictor; moderate inotropic effect; in septic shock is thought to increase tissue O_2 consumption as well as O_2 delivery; may be chosen over dopamine in sepsis due to less chronotropic effect; may be useful in cardiogenic shock with reduced SVR but should generally be reserved for refractory hypotension
Dobutamine	1–10	Primarily for cardiogenic shock (Chap. 123): positive inotrope; lacks vasoconstrictor activity; most useful when only mild hypotension present and avoidance of tachycardia desired
Phenylephrine	20–200	Potent vasoconstrictor without inotropic effect; may be useful in distributive (septive) shock
Vasopressin	0.01–0.04 U/min[b]	Occasionally used in refractory septic (distributive) shock; restores vascular tone in vasopressin-deficient states (e.g., sepsis)

[a] Isoproterenol not recommended in shock states because of potential hypotension and arrhythmogenic effects.
[b] Dose not based on weight.
Note: SVR, systemic vascular resistance.

- If severe metabolic acidosis present (pH < 7.15), administer $NaHCO_3$ (44.6–89.2 mmol).
- Identify and treat underlying cause of shock. Cardiogenic shock in acute MI is discussed in Chap. 123. Emergent coronary revascularization may be lifesaving if persistent ischemia is present. Consider cardiac tamponade (see Chap. 121).

SEPTIC SHOCK   (See Chap. 15)

For a more detailed discussion, see Maier RV: Approach to the Patient with Shock, Chap. 253, p. 1600, in HPIM-16.

15

SEPSIS AND SEPTIC SHOCK

Definitions

Systemic inflammatory response syndrome (SIRS)— Two or more of the following, due to either an infectious or a noninfectious etiology:
- Temperature >38°C or <36°C
- Respiratory rate >24 breaths/ min
- Heart rate >90 beats/ min
- WBC count >12,000/μL or <4000/μL, or >10% bands

Sepsis—SIRS with a proven or suspected microbial etiology
Severe sepsis—Sepsis with one or more signs of organ dysfunction
Septic shock—Sepsis with arterial blood pressure <90 mmHg or 40 mmHg below pt's normal blood pressure for at least 1 h despite fluid resuscitation

Etiology

- Blood cultures are positive in 20–40% of sepsis cases and in 40–70% of septic shock cases. Of cases with positive blood cultures, ~40% are due to gram-positive bacteria, 35% to gram-negative bacteria, and 7% to fungi.
- Any class of microorganism can cause severe sepsis.
- A significant proportion of cases have negative microbiologic data.

Epidemiology and Risk Factors

The incidence of severe sepsis and septic shock is increasing in the United States, with >300,000 cases each year. Two-thirds of cases occur in pts hospitalized for other reasons. Sepsis is a contributing factor in >200,000 deaths each year in the United States.

The higher incidence of sepsis is due to the aging of the population, longer survival of pts with chronic diseases, medical treatments (e.g., with steroids or antibiotics), and invasive procedures (e.g., catheter placement). Gram-negative sepsis is associated with underlying diabetes mellitus, lymphoproliferative disorders, cirrhosis of the liver, burns, neutropenia, and indwelling urinary catheters. Gram-positive sepsis is associated with indwelling mechanical devices and intravascular catheters, IV drug use, and burns. Fungal sepsis is associated with neutropenia and broad-spectrum antimicrobial therapy.

Pathogenesis and Pathology

Local and Systemic Host Responses

• Recognition of microbial molecules by tissue phagocytes triggers production and release of cytokines and other mediators that increase blood flow to the infected site, enhance the permeability of local blood vessels, attract neutrophils to the infected site, and elicit pain.
• Through intravascular thrombosis (the hallmark of the local immune response), the body attempts to wall off invading microbes and prevent the spread of infection and inflammation. Key features of the systemic immune response include intravascular fibrin deposition, thrombosis, and DIC; the underlying mechanisms are the activation of intrinsic and extrinsic clotting pathways, impaired function of the protein C–protein S inhibitory pathway, depletion of antithrombin and protein C, and prevention of fibrinolysis by increased plasma levels of plasminogen activator inhibitor 1.

Organ Dysfunction and Shock

• Endothelial injury: Widespread endothelial injury is believed to be the major mechanism for multiorgan dysfunction.
• Septic shock: The hallmark is a decrease in peripheral vascular resistance despite increased levels of vasopressor catecholamines. Cardiac output and blood flow to peripheral tissues increase, and oxygen utilization by these tissues is greatly impaired.

Clinical Features

• Hyperventilation
• Encephalopathy (disorientation, confusion)
• Hypotension
• DIC, acrocyanosis, ischemic necrosis of peripheral tissues (e.g., digits)
• Skin: hemorrhagic lesions, bullae, cellulitis. Skin lesions may suggest specific pathogens—e.g., petechiae and purpura with *Neisseria meningitidis*, ecthyma gangrenosum in neutropenic pts with *Pseudomonas aeruginosa*.
• Gastrointestinal: nausea, vomiting, diarrhea, ileus, cholestatic jaundice
• Hypoxemia: ventilation-perfusion mismatch and increased alveolar capillary permeability with increased pulmonary water content

Major Complications

• *Cardiopulmonary manifestations*:
    Acute respiratory distress syndrome (progressive diffuse pulmonary infiltrates and arterial hypoxemia) develops in ~50% of pts with severe sepsis or septic shock.
    Hypotension: Normal or increased cardiac output and decreased systemic vascular resistance distinguish septic shock from cardiogenic or hypovolemic shock.
    Myocardial function is depressed with decreased ejection fraction.
• *Renal manifestations*: oliguria, azotemia, proteinuria, renal failure due to acute tubular necrosis
• *Coagulation*: thrombocytopenia in 10–30% of pts. With DIC, platelet counts usually fall below 50,000/μL.
• *Neurologic manifestations*: polyneuropathy with distal motor weakness in prolonged sepsis

Laboratory Findings

• Leukocytosis with a left shift, thrombocytopenia
• Prolonged thrombin time, decreased fibrinogen, presence of D-dimers, suggestive of DIC
• Hyperbilirubinemia, increase in hepatic aminotransferases, azotemia, proteinuria
• Metabolic acidosis, elevated anion gap, elevated lactate levels, hypoxemia

Diagnosis

Definitive diagnosis requires isolation of the microorganism from blood or a local site of infection. Culture of infected cutaneous lesions may help establish the diagnosis. Lacking a microbiologic diagnosis, the diagnosis is made on clinical grounds.

℞ TREATMENT

1. Antibiotic treatment: See Table 15-1.
2. Removal or drainage of a focal source of infection
   a. Remove indwelling intravascular catheters and send tips for quantitative culture; replace Foley and other drainage catheters.
   b. Rule out sinusitis in pts with nasal intubation.
   c. Perform CT or MRI to rule out occult disease or abscess.
3. Hemodynamic, respiratory, and metabolic support
   a. Maintain intravascular volume with IV fluids. Initiate treatment with 1–2 L of normal saline administered over 1–2 h, keeping pulmonary capillary wedge pressure at 12–16 mmHg or central venous pressure at 8–12 cmH$_2$O, urine output at >0.5 mL/kg per hour, mean arterial blood pressure at >65 mmHg, and cardiac index at ≥4 (L/min)/m^2. Add inotropic and vasopressor therapy if needed. Maintain central venous O$_2$ saturation at >70%, using dobutamine if necessary.
   b. Maintain oxygenation with ventilator support as indicated.
   c. Monitor for adrenal insufficiency or reduced adrenal reserve. Pts with a plasma cortisol response of ≤9 μg/dL to an ACTH challenge may have improved survival if hydrocortisone (50 mg q6h IV) and 9-α-fludrocortisone (50 μg/d via nasogastric tube) are administered for 7 days.
4. Other treatments (investigational): Antiendotoxin, anti-inflammatory, and anticoagulant drugs are being studied in severe sepsis treatment. The anticoagulant recombinant activated protein C (aPC), given as a constant infusion of 24 μg/kg per hour for 96 h, has been approved for treatment of severe sepsis or septic shock in pts with APACHE II scores of ≥25 preceding aPC infusion and low risk of hemorrhagic complications. The long-term impact of aPC is uncertain, and long-term survival data are not yet available. Other agents have not improved outcome in clinical trials.

Prognosis

In all, 20–35% of pts with severe sepsis and 40–60% of pts with septic shock die within 30 days, and further deaths occur within the first 6 months. The severity of underlying disease most strongly influences the risk of dying.

Prevention

In the United States, most episodes of severe sepsis and septic shock are complications of nosocomial infections. Thus the incidence of sepsis would be affected by measures to reduce those infections (e.g., limiting the use and duration

Table 15-1

Initial Antimicrobial Therapy for Severe Sepsis with No Obvious Source in Adults with Normal Renal Function

Clinical Condition	Antimicrobial Regimens (Intravenous Therapy)
Immunocompetent adult	The many acceptable regimens include (1) ceftriaxone (2 g q24h) *or* ticarcillin-clavulanate (3.1 g q4–6h) *or* piperacillin-tazobactam (3.375 g q4–6h); (2) imipenem-cilastatin (0.5 g q6h) *or* meropenem (1 g q8h) *or* cefepime (2 g q12h). Gentamicin *or* tobramycin (5–7 mg/kg q24h) may be *added* to either regimen. If the pt is allergic to β-lactam agents, use ciprofloxacin (400 mg q12h) *or* levofloxacin (500–750 mg q12h) *plus* clindamycin (600 mg q8h). If the institution has a high incidence of MRSA infections, add vancomycin (15 mg/kg q12h) to each of the above regimens.
Neutropenia[a] (<500 neutrophils/μL)	Regimens include (1) imipenem-cilastatin (0.5 g q6h) *or* meropenem (1 g q8h) *or* cefepime (2 g q8h); (2) ticarcillin-clavulanate (3.1 g q4h) *or* piperacillin-tazobactam (3.375 g q4h) *plus* tobramycin (5–7 mg/kg q24h). Vancomycin (15 mg/kg q12h) and cefepime should be used if the pt has an infected vascular catheter, if staphylococci are suspected, if the pt has received quinolone prophylaxis, if the pt has received intensive chemotherapy that produces mucosal damage, or if the institution has a high incidence of MRSA infections.
Splenectomy	Cefotaxime (2 g q6–8h) *or* ceftriaxone (2 g q12h) should be used. If the local prevalence of cephalosporin-resistant pneumococci is high, *add* vancomycin. If the pt is allergic to β-lactam drugs, vancomycin (15 mg/kg q12h) *plus* ciprofloxacin (400 mg q12h) *or* levofloxacin (750 mg q12h) *or* aztreonam (2 g q8h) should be used.
IV drug user	Nafcillin or oxacillin (2 g q8h) *plus* gentamicin (5–7 mg/kg q24h). If the local prevalence of MRSA is high or if the pt is allergic to β-lactam drugs, vancomycin (15 mg/kg q12h) with gentamicin should be used.
AIDS	Cefepime (2 g q8h), ticarcillin-clavulanate (3.1 g q4h), *or* piperacillin-tazobactam (3.375 g q4h) *plus* tobramycin (5–7 mg/kg q24h) should be used. If the pt is allergic to β-lactam drugs, ciprofloxacin (400 mg q12h) *or* levofloxacin (750 mg q12h) *plus* vancomycin (15 mg/kg q12h) *plus* tobramycin should be used.

[a] Adapted in part from WT Hughes et al: Clin Infect Dis 25:551, 1997.
Note: MRSA, methicillin-resistant *Staphylococcus aureus*.

of indwelling vascular and bladder catheters, aggressively treating localized infection, avoiding indiscriminate antimicrobial or glucocorticoid use, and instituting optimal infection control measures).

For a more detailed discussion, see Munford RS: Severe Sepsis and Septic Shock, Chap. 254, p. 1606, in HPIM-16.

16

ACUTE PULMONARY EDEMA

Life-threatening, acute development of alveolar lung edema often due to:

- Elevation of hydrostatic pressure in the pulmonary capillaries (left heart failure, mitral stenosis)
- Specific precipitants (Table 16-1), resulting in cardiogenic pulmonary edema in pts with previously compensated CHF or without previous cardiac history
- Increased permeability of pulmonary alveolar-capillary membrane

Physical Findings

Patient appears severely ill, sitting bolt upright, tachypneic, dyspneic, with marked perspiration; cyanosis may be present. Bilateral pulmonary rales; third heart sound may be present. Frothy and blood-tinged sputum.

Laboratory

Early ABGs show reductions of both Pa_{O_2}; and Pa_{CO_2}

- Later, with progressive respiratory failure, hypercapnia develops with progressive acidemia.
- CXR shows pulmonary vascular redistribution, diffuse haziness in lung fields with perihilar "butterfly" appearance.

Table 16-1

Precipitants of Acute Pulmonary Edema

Acute tachy- or bradyarrhythmia
Infection, fever
Acute MI
Severe hypertension
Acute mitral or aortic regurgitation
Increased circulating volume (Na ingestion, blood transfusion, pregnancy)
Increased metabolic demands (exercise, hyperthyroidism)
Pulmonary embolism
Noncompliance (sudden discontinuation) of chronic CHF medications

℞ TREATMENT

Immediate, aggressive therapy is mandatory for survival. The following measures should be instituted nearly simultaneously:

- Seat pt upright to reduce venous return.
- Administer 100% O_2 by mask to achieve $Pa_{O_2} > 60$ mmHg; in pts who can tolerate it, continuous positive airway pressure (10 cmH$_2$O pressure) by mask improves outcome. Assisted ventilation by mask or endotracheal tube is frequently necessary.
- Intravenous loop diuretic (furosemide, 40–100 mg, or bumetanide, 1 mg); use lower dose if pt does not take diuretics chronically.
- Morphine 2–4 mg IV (repetitively); assess frequently for hypotension or respiratory depression; naloxone should be available to reverse effects of morphine if necessary.

Additional therapy may be required if rapid improvement does not ensue:

- The precipitating cause of pulmonary edema (Table 16-1) should be sought and treated, particularly acute arrhythmias or infection.
- Several noncardiogenic conditions may result in pulmonary edema in the absence of left heart dysfunction; therapy is directed toward the primary condition.
- Inotropic agents, e.g., dobutamine (Chap. 14), in cardiogenic pulmonary edema with shock.
- Reduce intravascular volume by phlebotomy (removal of ~250 mL through antecubital vein) if rapid diuresis does not follow diuretic administration.
- Nitroglycerin (sublingual 0.4 mg × 3 q5min) followed by 5 to 10 μg/min IV. Alternatively, nesiritide [2-μg/kg bolus IV followed by 0.01 (μg/kg)/min] may be used.
- For refractory pulmonary edema associated with persistent cardiac ischemia, early coronary revascularization may be life-saving.

For a more detailed discussion, see Ingram RH Jr, Braunwald E: **Dyspnea and Pulmonary Edema, Chap. 29, p. 201;** and Hochman JS, Ingbar D: **Cardiogenic Shock and Pulmonary Edema, Chap. 255, p. 1612, in HPIM-16.**

17

CONFUSION, STUPOR, AND COMA

Disorders of consciousness are common; these always signify a disorder of the nervous system. Assessment should determine whether there is a change in level of consciousness (drowsy, stuporous, comatose) and/or content of consciousness (confusion, perseveration, hallucinations). *Confusion* is a lack of clarity in thinking with inattentiveness; *stupor*, a state in which vigorous stimuli are needed to elicit a response; *coma*, a condition of unresponsiveness. Patients in such states are usually seriously ill, and etiologic factors must be assessed (Table 17-1).

Table 17-1

Differential Diagnosis of Coma

1. Diseases that cause no focal or lateralizing neurologic signs, usually with normal brainstem functions; CT scan and cellular content of the CSF are normal
   a. Intoxications: alcohol, sedative drugs, opiates, etc.
   b. Metabolic disturbances: anoxia, hyponatremia, hypernatremia, hypercalcemia, diabetic acidosis, nonketotic hyperosmolar hyperglycemia, hypoglycemia, uremia, hepatic coma, hypercarbia, addisonian crisis, hypo- and hyperthyroid states, profound nutritional deficiency
   c. Severe systemic infections: pneumonia, septicemia, typhoid fever, malaria, Waterhouse-Friderichsen syndrome
   d. Shock from any cause
   e. Postseizure states, status epilepticus, subclinical epilepsy
   f. Hypertensive encephalopathy, eclampsia
   g. Severe hyperthermia, hypothermia
   h. Concussion
   i. Acute hydrocephalus
2. Diseases that cause meningeal irritation with or without fever, and with an excess of WBCs or RBCs in the CSF, usually without focal or lateralizing cerebral or brainstem signs; CT or MRI shows no mass lesion
   a. Subarachnoid hemorrhage from ruptured aneurysm, arteriovenous malformation, trauma
   b. Acute bacterial meningitis
   c. Viral encephalitis
   d. Miscellaneous: Fat embolism, cholesterol embolism, carcinomatous and lymphomatous meningitis, etc.
3. Diseases that cause focal brainstem or lateralizing cerebral signs, with or without changes in the CSF; CT and MRI are abnormal
   a. Hemispheral hemorrhage (basal ganglionic, thalamic) or infarction (large middle cerebral artery territory) with secondary brainstem compression
   b. Brainstem infarction due to basilar artery thrombosis or embolism
   c. Brain abscess, subdural empyema
   d. Epidural and subdural hemorrhage, brain contusion
   e. Brain tumor with surrounding edema
   f. Cerebellar and pontine hemorrhage and infarction
   g. Widespread traumatic brain injury
   h. Metabolic coma (see above) with preexisting focal damage
   i. Miscellaneous: cortical vein thrombosis, herpes simplex encephalitis, multiple cerebral emboli due to bacterial endocarditis, acute hemorrhagic leukoencephalitis, acute disseminated (postinfectious) encephalomyelitis, thrombotic thrombocytopenic purpura, cerebral vasculitis, gliomatosis cerebri, pituitary apoplexy, intravascular lymphoma, etc.

Note: CT, computed tomography; CSF, cerebrospinal fluid; WBCs, white blood cells; RBCs, red blood cells; MRI, magnetic resonance imaging.

_____ *Approach to the Patient* _____

1. Support vital functions.
2. Administer glucose, thiamine, and naloxone if etiology is not clear.
3. Utilize history, examination, and laboratory and radiologic information to rapidly establish the cause of the disorder.

4. Urgent lumbar puncture indicated if meningitis suspected (fever, headache, meningismus).
5. Provide appropriate medical and surgical treatment.

History

The pt should be aroused, if possible, and questioned regarding use of insulin, narcotics, anticoagulants, other prescription drugs, suicidal intent, recent trauma, headache, epilepsy, significant medical problems, and preceding symptoms. Witnesses and family members should be interviewed, often by phone. History of sudden headache followed by loss of consciousness suggests intracranial hemorrhage; preceding vertigo, nausea, diplopia, ataxia, hemisensory disorder suggest basilar insufficiency; chest pain, palpitations, and faintness suggest cardiovascular cause.

Immediate Assessment

Vital signs should be evaluated, and appropriate support initiated. Blood should be drawn for glucose, electrolytes, calcium, and renal (BUN) and hepatic (ammonia, transaminases) function; also screen for presence of alcohol and other toxins if these are possibilities. Arterial blood-gas analysis is helpful in pts with lung disease and acid-base disorders. Fever, especially with petechial rash, suggests meningitis. Examination of CSF is essential in diagnosis of meningitis and encephalitis; lumbar puncture should not be deferred if meningitis is a possibility. Fever with dry skin suggests heat shock or intoxication with anticholinergics. Hypothermia suggests myxedema, intoxication, sepsis, exposure, or hypoglycemia. Marked hypertension occurs with increased intracranial pressure (ICP) and hypertensive encephalopathy.

Neurologic Evaluation

Focus on establishing pt's best level of function and uncovering signs that enable a specific diagnosis. Although confused states may occur with unilateral cerebral lesions, stupor and coma are signs of bihemispheral dysfunction or damage to midbrain-tegmentum (reticular activating system). Lack of movement on one side suggests hemiplegia; multifocal myoclonus indicates that a metabolic disorder is likely; intermittent twitching may be the only sign of a seizure.

Responsiveness Stimuli of increasing intensity are applied to gauge the degree of unresponsiveness and any asymmetry in sensory or motor function. Motor responses may be purposeful or reflexive. Spontaneous flexion of elbows with leg extension, termed *decortication*, accompanies severe damage to contralateral hemisphere above midbrain. Internal rotation of the arms with extension of elbows, wrists, and legs, termed *decerebration*, suggests damage to midbrain or diencephalon. These postural reflexes occur in profound encephalopathic states.

Pupils In comatose pts, equal, round, reactive pupils exclude midbrain damage as cause and suggest a metabolic abnormality. Pinpoint pupils occur in narcotic overdose (except meperidine, which causes midsize pupils), with pontine damage, hydrocephalus, or thalamic hemorrhage; the response to naloxone and presence of reflex eye movements can distinguish these. A unilateral, enlarged, often oval, poorly reactive pupil is caused by midbrain lesions or compression of third cranial nerve, as occurs in transtentorial herniation. Bilaterally dilated, unreactive pupils indicate severe bilateral midbrain damage, anticholinergic overdose, or ocular trauma.

Eye Movements   Examine spontaneous and reflex eye movements. Intermittent horizontal divergence is common in drowsiness. Slow, to-and-fro horizontal movements suggest bihemispheric dysfunction. Conjugate eye deviation to one side indicates damage to the pons on the opposite side or a lesion in the frontal lobe on the same side (*"The eyes look toward a hemispheral lesion and away from a brainstem lesion"*). An adducted eye at rest with impaired ability to turn eye laterally indicates an abducens (VI) nerve palsy, common in raised ICP or pontine damage. The eye with a dilated, unreactive pupil is often abducted at rest and cannot adduct fully due to third nerve dysfunction, as occurs with transtentorial herniation. Vertical separation of ocular axes (skew deviation) occurs in pontine or cerebellar lesions. Doll's head maneuver (oculocephalic reflex) and cold caloric–induced eye movements allow diagnosis of gaze or cranial nerve palsies in pts who do not move their eyes purposefully. Doll's head maneuver is tested by observing eye movements in response to lateral rotation of head (neck injury is a contraindication); full movement of eyes occurs in bihemispheric dysfunction. In comatose pts with intact brainstem function, raising head to 60° above the horizontal and irrigating external auditory canal with cool water causes tonic deviation of gaze to side of irrigated ear. In conscious pts, it causes nystagmus, vertigo, and emesis.

Respirations   Respiratory pattern may suggest site of neurologic damage. Cheyne-Stokes (periodic) breathing occurs in bihemispheric dysfunction and is common in metabolic encephalopathies. Respiratory patterns composed of gasps or other irregular breathing patterns are indicative of lower brainstem damage; such pts usually require intubation and ventilatory assistance.

Other   Comatose pt's best motor and sensory function should be assessed by testing reflex responses to noxious stimuli; carefully note any asymmetric responses, which suggest a focal lesion. If possible, pts with disordered consciousness should have gait examined. Ataxia may be the prominent neurologic finding in a stuporous pt with a cerebellar mass.

Radiologic Examination

Lesions causing raised ICP commonly cause impaired consciousness. CT or MRI scan of the brain is often abnormal in coma but may not be diagnostic; appropriate therapy should not be postponed while awaiting a CT or MRI scan. Pts with disordered consciousness due to high ICP can deteriorate rapidly; emergent CT study is necessary to confirm presence of mass effect and to guide surgical decompression. CT scan is normal in some pts with subarachnoid hemorrhage; the diagnosis then rests on clinical history combined with RBCs in spinal fluid. MR angiography or cerebral angiography may be necessary to establish basilar artery stroke as cause of coma in pts with brainstem signs. The EEG is useful in metabolic or drug-induced states but is rarely diagnostic; exceptions are coma due to seizures, herpesvirus encephalitis, or prion disease.

Brain Death

This results from total cessation of cerebral function and blood flow at a time when cardiopulmonary function continues but is dependent on ventilatory assistance. The pt is unresponsive to all forms of stimulation, brainstem reflexes are absent, and there is complete apnea. Demonstration of apnea requires that the P_{CO_2} be high enough to stimulate respiration, while P_{O_2} and bp are maintained. EEG is isoelectric at high gain. The absence of deep tendon reflexes is not required because the spinal cord may remain functional. Special care must be taken to exclude drug toxicity and hypothermia prior to making a diagnosis of brain death. Diagnosis should be made only if the state persists for some agreed-upon period, usually 6–24 h.

For a more detailed discussion, see Ropper AH: Acute Confusional States and Coma, Chap. 257, p. 1624, in HPIM-16.

18

STROKE

Sudden onset of a neurologic deficit from a vascular mechanism: 85% are ischemic; 15% are primary hemorrhages [subarachnoid (Chap. 19) and intraparenchymal]. An ischemic deficit that resolves rapidly is termed a *transient ischemic attack* (TIA); 24 h is a useful boundary between TIA and stroke, although most TIAs last between 5 and 15 min. Stroke is the leading cause of neurologic disability in adults; 200,000 deaths annually in the United States. Much can be done to limit morbidity and mortality through prevention and acute intervention.

Ischemic stroke is most often due to embolic occlusion of large cerebral vessels; source of emboli may be heart, aortic arch, or a more proximal arterial lesion. Primary involvement of intracerebral vessels with atherosclerosis is less common than in coronary vessels. Small, deep ischemic lesions are most often related to intrinsic small-vessel disease (lacunar strokes). Low-flow strokes are seen with severe proximal stenosis and inadequate collaterals challenged by systemic hypotensive episodes. Hemorrhage most frequently results from rupture of aneurysms or small vessels within brain tissue.

Clinical Presentation

Ischemic Stroke   Abrupt and dramatic onset of focal neurologic symptoms is typical of ischemic stroke; with hemmorhage, deficits typically evolve more slowly and drowsiness is common. Pts may not seek assistance on their own because they are rarely in pain and may lose appreciation that something is wrong (*anosagnosia*). Symptoms reflect the vascular territory involved (Table 18-1). Transient monocular blindness (amaurosis fugax) is a particular form of TIA due to retinal ischemia; pts describe a shade descending over the visual field. Rapid resolution of symptoms excludes hemorrhage as cause. Variability in stroke recovery is influenced by collateral vessels, blood pressure, and specific site and mechanism of vessel occlusion.

Lacunar Syndromes   Most common are (1) pure motor hemiparesis of face, arm, and leg (internal capsule or pons); (2) pure sensory stroke (ventro-

Table 18-1

Anatomic Localization in Stroke

Signs and Symptoms

CEREBRAL HEMISPHERE, LATERAL ASPECT (MIDDLE CEREBRAL A.)

Hemiparesis
Hemisensory deficit
Motor aphasia (Broca's)—hesitant speech with word-finding difficulty and
  preserved comprehension
Central aphasia (Wernicke's)—anomia, poor comprehension, jargon speech
Unilateral neglect, apraxias
Homonymous hemianopia or quadrantanopia
Gaze preference with eyes deviated to side of lesion

CEREBRAL HEMISPHERE, MEDIAL ASPECT (ANTERIOR CEREBRAL A.)

Paralysis of foot and leg with or without paresis of arm
Cortical sensory loss over leg
Grasp and sucking reflexes
Urinary incontinence
Gait apraxia

CEREBRAL HEMISPHERE, POSTERIOR ASPECT (POSTERIOR CEREBRAL A.)

Homonymous hemianopia
Cortical blindness
Memory deficit
Dense sensory loss, spontaneous pain, dysesthesias, choreoathetosis

BRAINSTEM, MIDBRAIN (POSTERIOR CEREBRAL A.)

Third nerve palsy and contralateral hemiplegia
Paralysis/paresis of vertical eye movement
Convergence nystagmus, disorientation

BRAINSTEM, PONTOMEDULLARY JUNCTION (BASILAR A.)

Facial paralysis
Paresis of abduction of eye
Paresis of conjugate gaze
Hemifacial sensory deficit
Horner's syndrome
Diminished pain and thermal sense over half body (with or without face)
Ataxia

BRAINSTEM, LATERAL MEDULLA (VERTEBRAL A.)

Vertigo, nystagmus
Horner's syndrome (miosis, ptosis, decreased sweating)
Ataxia, falling toward side of lesion
Impaired pain and thermal sense over half body with or without face

---

lateral thalamus); (3) ataxic hemiparesis (pons); (4) dysarthria–clumsy hand
(pons or genu of internal capsule); and (5) pure motor hemiparesis with motor
(Broca's) aphasia (internal capsule and adjacent corona radiata).

Intracranial Hemorrhage   Vomiting occurs in most cases, and headache
in about one-half. Signs and symptoms not usually confined to a single vascular
territory. Hypertensive hemorrhage typically occurs in (1) the putamen, adjacent
internal capsule, and central white matter; (2) thalamus; (3) pons; and (4) cere-

bellum. A neurologic deficit that evolves relentlessly over 5–30 min strongly suggests intracerebral bleeding. Ocular signs are important in localization: (1) putaminal—eyes deviated to side opposite paralysis (toward lesion); (2) thalamic—eyes deviated downward, sometimes with unreactive pupils; (3) pontine—reflex lateral eye movements impaired and small (1–2 mm), reactive pupils; (4) cerebellar—eyes initially deviated to side opposite lesion.

 TREATMENT

Principles of management are outlined in Table 18-2. Stroke needs to be distinguished from potential mimics, including seizure, tumor, migraine, and metabolic derangements. After initial stabilization, an emergency noncontrast head CT scan is necessary to differentiate ischemic from hemorrhagic stroke.

Table 18-2

Clinical Management of Acute Stroke

New onset of neuro-logic deficit: Stroke or TIA?	Differential diagnosis of new focal deficit
	 Stroke or TIA
	 Seizure with postictal Todd's paresis
	 Tumor
	 Migraine
	 Metabolic encephalopathy
	  Fever/infection and old stroke
	  Hyperglycemia
	  Hypercalcemia
	  Hepatic encephalopathy

Initial assessment and management	ABCs, serum glucose
	 Noncontrast head CT
	  Hemorrhage
	   Medical and surgical management
	  Tumor or other CNS process
	   Treat as indicated
	  Normal or hypodense area consistent with acute ischemic stroke
	   Consider thrombolysis, aspirin
	   Maintain blood pressure and hydrate
	   Admit patient to appropriate level of care depending on concomitant medical problems and airway

Subsequent hospital management	Establish cause of stroke and risk factors Plan for secondary prophylaxis (drugs, risk factor modifications) Obtain physical, occupational, and speech therapy consultation and social work as appropriate Provide nutrition Plan for discharge, including prescriptions for risk factor reduction, including when to institute antihypertensive treatment, and antithrombotic medication prophylaxis

Note: ABCs, airway management, breathing, cardiac status; CNS, central nervous system; CT, computed tomography; TIA, transient ischemic attack.

With large ischemic strokes, CT abnormalities usually evident within the first few hours, but small infarcts can be difficult to visualize by CT.

Acute Ischemic Stroke

Treatments designed to reverse or lessen tissue infarction include: (1) medical support, (2) thrombolysis, (3) antiplatelet agents, (4) anticoagulation, and (5) neuroprotection.

Medical Support   Immediate goal is to optimize perfusion in ischemic penumbra surrounding the infarct. Blood pressure should never be lowered precipitously (exacerbates the underlying ischemia), and only in the most extreme situations should gradual lowering be undertaken (e.g., malignant hypertension or, if thrombolysis planned, bp > 185/110 mmHg). Intravascular volume should be maintained with isotonic fluids as volume restriction is rarely helpful. Osmotic therapy with mannitol may be necessary to control edema in large infarcts, but isotonic volume must be replaced to avoid hypovolemia. In cerebellar infarction (or hemorrhage), rapid deterioration can occur from brainstem compression and hydrocephalus, requiring neurosurgical intervention.

Thrombolysis   Ischemic deficits of <3 h duration, with no hemorrhage by CT criteria, may benefit from thrombolytic therapy with IV recombinant tissue plasminogen activator (Table 18-3). Only a small percentage of stroke pts are seen early enough to receive treatment with this agent.

Antiplatelet Agents   Aspirin (up to 325 mg/d) is safe and has a small but definite benefit in acute stroke.

Anticoagulation   Role uncertain; clinical trials show no clear benefit of low molecular-weight heparin or SC heparin over aspirin. Heparin is often used for crescendo TIAs (TIAs that increase in frequency) and for progressive stroke worsening over hours or days (20% of pts), despite absence of data.

Neuroprotection   Hypothermia is effective in coma following cardiac arrest but has not been adequately studied in pts with stroke.

Acute Intracerebral Hemorrhage

Noncontrast head CT will confirm diagnosis. Rapidly identify and correct any coagulopathy. Nearly 50% of pts die; prognosis is determined by volume and location of hematoma. Neurosurgical consultation should be sought for possible urgent evacuation of cerebellar hematoma; in other locations, evacuation is usually not helpful. Treatment for edema and mass effect with osmotic agents and induced hyperventilation may be necessary; glucocorticoids not helpful.

Determining the Cause of Stroke

Although initial management of acute ischemic stroke or TIA does not depend on the etiology, establishing a cause is essential to reduce risk of recurrence (Table 18-4). Nearly 30% of strokes remain unexplained despite extensive evaluation, however. Clinical examination should be focused on the peripheral and cervical vascular system. Routine studies include CXR and ECG, CBC/platelets, electrolytes, glucose, ESR, lipid profile, PT, PTT, and serologic tests for syphilis. If a hypercoagulable state is suspected, further studies of coagulation are indicated. Imaging evaluation may include brain MRI (compared with CT, increased sensitivity for small infarcts of cortex and brainstem); MR angiography (evaluate patency of intracranial vessels and extracranial carotid and vertebral vessels); noninvasive carotid tests ("duplex" studies, combine ultrasound imaging of the vessel with Doppler evaluation of blood flow characteristics); or cerebral angiography ("gold standard" for evaluation of intracranial and extra-

Table 18-3

Administration of Intravenous Recombinant Tissue Plasminogen Activator (rtPA) for Acute Ischemic Stroke[a]

Indication	Contraindication
Clinical diagnosis of stroke	Sustained BP > 185/110 despite treatment
Onset of symptoms to time of drug administration ≤3 h	Platelets < 100,000; HCT < 25%; glucose < 50 or > 400 mg/dL
CT scan showing no hemorrhage or edema of >⅓ of the MCA territory	Use of heparin within 48 h and prolonged PTT, or elevated INR
Age ≥18 years	Rapidly improving symptoms
Consent by patient or surrogate	Prior stroke or head injury within 3 months; prior intracranial hemorrhage
	Major surgery in preceding 14 days
	Minor stroke symptoms
	Gastrointestinal bleeding in preceding 21 days
	Recent myocardial infarction
	Coma or stupor

Administration of rtPA

Intravenous access with two peripheral IV lines (avoid arterial or central line placement)

Review eligibility for rtPA

Administer 0.9 mg/kg intravenously (maximum 90 mg) IV as 10% of total dose by bolus, followed by remainder of total dose over 1 h

Frequent cuff blood pressure monitoring

No other antithrombotic treatment for 24 h

For decline in neurologic status or uncontrolled blood pressure, stop infusion, give cryoprecipitate, and reimage brain emergently

Avoid urethral catheterization for ≥2 h

[a] See Activase (tissue plasminogen activator) package insert for complete list of contraindications and dosing.
Note: BP, blood pressure; CT, computed tomography; HCT, hematocrit; INR, international normalized ratio; MCA, middle cerebral artery; PTT, partial thromboplastin time.

cranial vascular disease). For suspected cardiogenic source, cardiac ultrasound with attention to right-to-left shunts, and 24-h Holter monitoring indicated.

Primary and Secondary Prevention of Stroke

Risk Factors   Atherosclerosis is a systemic disease affecting arteries throughout the body. Multiple factors including hypertension, diabetes, hyperlipidemia, and family history influence stroke and TIA risk (Table 18-5). Cardioembolic risk factors include atrial fibrillation, MI, valvular heart disease, and cardiomyopathy. Hypertension and diabetes are also specific risk factors for lacunar stroke and intraparenchymal hemorrhage. Smoking is a potent risk factor for all vascular mechanisms of stroke. *Identification of modifiable risk factors and prophylactic interventions to lower risk is probably the best approach to stroke overall.*

Table 18-4

Causes of Ischemic Stroke

Common Causes	Uncommon Causes
Thrombosis	Hypercoagulable disorders
Lacunar stroke (small	Protein C deficiency
vessel)	Protein S deficiency
Large vessel thrombosis	Antithrombin III deficiency
Dehydration	Antiphospholipid syndrome
Embolic occlusion	Factor V Leiden mutation[a]
Artery-to-artery	Prothrombin G20210 mutation[a]
Carotid bifurcation	Systemic malignancy
Aortic arch	Sickle cell anemia
Arterial dissection	β-Thalassemia
Cardioembolic	Polycythemia vera
Atrial fibrillation	Systemic lupus erythematosus
Mural thrombus	Homocysteinemia
Myocardial infarction	Thrombotic thrombocytopenic
Dilated cardiomyopathy	purpura
Valvular lesions	Disseminated intravascular
Mitral stenosis	coagulation
Mechanical valve	Dysproteinemias
Bacterial endocarditis	Nephrotic syndrome
Paradoxical embolus	Inflammatory bowel disease
Atrial septal defect	Oral contraceptives
Patent foramen ovale	Venous sinus thrombosis[b]
Atrial septal aneurysm	Fibromuscular dysplasia
Spontaneous echo	Vasculitis
contrast	Systemic vasculitis (PAN, Wegner's,
	Takayasu's, giant cell arteritis)
	Primary CNS vasculitis
	Meningitis (syphilis, tuberculosis,
	fungal, bacterial, zoster)
	Cardiogenic
	Mitral valve calcification
	Atrial myxoma
	Intracardiac tumor
	Marantic endocarditis
	Libman-Sacks endocarditis
	Subarachnoid hemorrhage vasospasm
	Drugs: cocaine, amphetamine
	Moyamoya disease
	Eclampsia

[a] Chiefly cause venous sinus thrombosis.
[b] May be associated with any hypercoagulable disorder.
Note: CNS, central nervous system; PAN, polyarteritis nodosa.

Antiplatelet Agents   Platelet antiaggregation agents can prevent athero-thrombotic events, including TIA and stroke, by inhibiting the formation of intraarterial platelet aggregates. Aspirin (50–325 mg/d) inhibits thromboxane A_2, a platelet aggregating and vasoconstricting prostaglandin. Aspirin, clopidogril (blocks the platelet ADP receptor), and the combination of aspirin plus extended-release dipyrimadole (inhibits platelet uptake of adenosine) are the

Table 18-5

Risk Factors for Stroke

Risk Factor	Relative Risk	Relative Risk Reduction with Treatment	Number Needed to Treat[a]	
			Primary Prevention	Secondary Prevention
Hypertension	2–5	38%	100–300	50–100
Atrial fibrillation	1.8–2.9	68% warfarin, 21% aspirin	20–83	13
Diabetes	1.8–6	No proven effect		
Smoking	1.8	50% at 1 year, baseline risk at 5 years post cessation		
Hyperlipidemia	1.8–2.6	10–29%		
Asymptomatic carotid stenosis	2.0	53%	85	N/A
Symptomatic carotid stenosis (70–99%)		65% at 2 years	N/A	12
Symptomatic carotid stenosis (50–69%)		29% at 5 years	N/A	77

[a] Number needed to treat to prevent one stroke annually. Prevention of other cardiovascular outcomes is not considered here.

Note: N/A, not applicable.

Table 18-6

Consensus Recommendation for Antithrombotic Prophylaxis
in Atrial Fibrillation

Age	Risk Factors[a]	Recommendation
Age ≤65	≥1	Warfarin INR 2–3
	0	Aspirin or no treatment
Age 65–75	≥1	Warfarin INR 2–3
	0	Warfarin INR 2–3 or aspirin
Age >75		Warfarin INR 2–3

[a] Risk factors include previous transient ischemic attack or stroke, hypertension, heart failure, diabetes, clinical coronary artery disease, mitral stenosis, prosthetic heart valves, or thyrotoxicosis.

Source: Modified from GW Albers et al: Chest 119:194S, 2001; with permission.

antiplatelet agents most commonly used. In general, antiplatelet agents reduce new stroke events by 25–30%. Every patient who has experienced an atherothrombotic stroke or TIA and has no contraindication should take an antiplatelet agent regularly because the average annual risk of another stroke is 8–10%.

Embolic Stroke In pts with atrial fibrillation, the choice between warfarin or aspirin prophylaxis is determined by age and risk factors (Table 18-6). Anticoagulation reduces the risk of embolism in acute MI; most clinicians recommend a 3-month course of therapy when there is anterior Q-wave infarction or other complications; warfarin is recommended long term if atrial fibrillation persists. For prosthetic heart valve pts, a combination of aspirin and warfarin (INR, 3–4) is recommended. If an embolic source cannot be eliminated, anticoagulation is usually continued indefinitely. For patients who "fail" one form of therapy, many neurologists recommend combining antiplatelet agents with anticoagulation.

Anticoagulation Therapy for Noncardiogenic Stroke In contrast to cardiogenic stroke, there are few data to support long-term warfarin for preventing atherothrombotic stroke. Secondary prophylaxis for ischemic stroke of unknown origin is controversial; some physicians prescribe anticoagulation for 3–6 months, followed by antiplatelet treatment.

Surgical Therapy Carotid endarterectomy benefits many pts with *symptomatic* severe (>70%) *carotid stenosis*; the relative risk reduction is ~65%. However, if the perioperative stroke rate is >6% for any surgeon, the benefit is lost. Surgical results in pts with *asymptomatic carotid stenosis* are less robust, and medical therapy for reduction of atherosclerosis risk factors plus aspirin is generally recommended in this group.

For a more detailed discussion, see Smith WS, Johnston SC, Easton JD: Cerebrovascular Diseases, Chap. 349, p. 2372, in HPIM-16.

19

SUBARACHNOID HEMORRHAGE

Excluding head trauma, most common cause of subarachnoid hemorrhage (SAH) is rupture of an intracranial (saccular) aneurysm; other etiologies include mycotic aneurysms in subacute bacterial endocarditis, vascular anomalies, bleeding dyscrasias, and rarely infections or tumors. Approximately 2% of the population harbor aneurysms; rupture risk for aneurysms ≥10 mm in size is 0.5–1% per year.

CLINICAL PRESENTATION   Sudden, severe headache, often with transient loss of consciousness at onset; vomiting is common. Bleeding may injure adjacent brain tissue and produce focal neurologic deficits. A progressive third nerve palsy with severe headache suggests posterior communicating artery aneurysm. In addition to dramatic presentations, aneurysms can undergo small ruptures with leaks of blood into the subarachnoid space (sentinel bleeds).

LABORATORY EVALUATION   Noncontrast CT is the initial study of choice and usually demonstrates the hemorrhage. On occasion, LP is required for diagnosis of suspected SAH if CT is nondiagnostic. Cerebral angiography is necessary to define anatomy, location, and type of vascular malformation, such as aneurysm or arteriovenous malformation; also assesses vasospasm. Usually performed as soon as possible after diagnosis of SAH is made. ECG may reveal ST-segment changes, prolonged QRS complex, increased QT interval, and prominent or inverted T waves; some changes reflect SAH, others indicate associated myocardial ischemic injury.

 TREATMENT

Standard management includes bed rest in a quiet darkened room, analgesics, and stool softeners. Closely follow serum electrolytes and osmolality; hyponatremia frequently develops several days after SAH. Cerebral salt wasting is common, and supplemental oral salt plus IV normal saline may be used to overcome renal losses; some pts require hypertonic saline. Anticonvulsants are begun at diagnosis and continued at least until the aneurysm is treated. Risk of early *rebleeding* is high (20–30% over 2 weeks), thus early treatment (within 1–3 days) is advocated to avoid rerupture and allow aggressive treatment of *vasospasm*. Endovascular coiling of aneurysms in accessible locations (via a catheter passed from the femoral artery) or neurosurgical clipping of the aneurysm neck are the definitive treatments. Severe *hydrocephalus* may require urgent placement of a ventricular catheter for external CSF drainage. Blood pressure is carefully monitored and regulated to assure adequate cerebral perfusion while avoiding excessive elevations. Symptomatic *vasospasm* may occur by day 4 and continue through day 14, leading to focal ischemia and possible stroke. Medical treatment, including nimodipine, may reduce sequelae of vasospasm. Cerebral perfusion can be improved in vasospasm by increasing mean arterial pressure with vasopressor agents such as phenylephrine or dopamine. Intravascular volume can be expanded with crystalloid. Angioplasty of the cerebral vessels can be effective in severe vasospasm when ischemic symptoms persist despite maximal medical therapy.

For a more detailed discussion, see Smith WS, Johnston SC, Easton JD: Cerebrovascular Diseases, Chap. 349, p. 2372, in HPIM-16.

20

INCREASED INTRACRANIAL PRESSURE AND HEAD TRAUMA

Increased Intracranial Pressure

A limited volume of extra tissue, blood, CSF, or edema fluid can be added to the intracranial contents without raising the intracranial pressure (ICP). Clinical deterioration or death may follow increases in ICP that shift intracranial contents, distort vital brainstem centers, or compromise cerebral perfusion. Cerebral perfusion pressure (CPP), defined as the mean systemic bp minus the ICP, is the driving force for circulation across capillary beds of the brain.

CLINICAL MANIFESTATIONS   Symptoms of high ICP include headache (especially a constant ache that is worse upon awakening), nausea, emesis, drowsiness, diplopia, and blurred vision. Papilledema and sixth nerve palsies are common. If not controlled, then cerebral hypoperfusion, pupillary dilation, coma, decerebrate posturing, abnormal respirations, systemic hypertension, and bradycardia may result.

A posterior fossa mass, which may initially cause ataxia, stiff neck, and nausea, is especially dangerous because it can compress vital brainstem structures and cause obstructive hydrocephalus. Masses that cause raised ICP also distort midbrain and diencephalic anatomy, leading to stupor and coma. Brain tissue is pushed away from the mass against fixed intracranial structures and into spaces not normally occupied. Herniation syndromes include (1) medial cortex displaced under the midline falx → anterior or posterior cerebral artery occlusion and stroke; (2) uncus displaced through the tentorium, compressing the third cranial nerve and pushing the cerebral peduncle against the tentorium → ipsilateral pupillary dilation, contralateral hemiparesis, and posterior cerebral artery occlusion; (3) cerebellar tonsils displaced into the foramen magnum, causing medullary compression → cardiorespiratory collapse; and (4) downward displacement of the diencephalon through the tentorium.

℞ TREATMENT

Elevated ICP may occur in a wide range of disorders including head trauma, intracerebral hemorrhage, subarachnoid hemorrhage (SAH) with hydrocephalus, and fulminant hepatic failure. A number of different interventions may lower ICP, and ideally the selection of treatment will be based on the underlying mechanism responsible for the elevated ICP (Table 20-1). For example, in hydrocephalus from SAH, the principal cause of elevated ICP is impaired CSF drainage; in this setting, ventricular drainage of CSF is likely to be sufficient. In head trauma and stroke, cytotoxic edema may be most responsible, and the use of osmotic diuretics such as mannitol becomes an appropriate early step. As noted above, elevated ICP may cause tissue ischemia. This can lead to reflex cerebral vasodilatation that further worsens ischemia;

Table 20-1

Stepwise Approach to Treatment of Elevated Intracranial Pressure[a]

Insert ICP monitor—ventriculostomy versus parenchymal device
General goals: maintain ICP < 20 mmHg and CPP > 70 mmHg

For ICP > 20–25 mmHg for >5 min:
1. Drain CSF via ventriculostomy (if in place)
2. Elevate head of the bed
3. Osmotherapy—mannitol 25–100 g q4h as needed (maintain serum osmolality <320 mosmol)
4. Glucocorticoids—dexamethasone 4 mg q6h for vasogenic edema from tumor, abscess (avoid glucocorticoids in head trauma, ischemic and hemorrhagic stroke)
5. Sedation (e.g., morphine, propofol, or midazolam); add neuromuscular paralysis if necessary (patient will require endotracheal intubation and mechanical ventilation at this point, if not before)
6. Hyperventilation—to Pa_{CO_2} 30–35 mmHg
7. Pressor therapy—phenylephrine, dopamine, or norepinephrine to maintain adequate MAP to ensure CPP > 70 mmHg (maintain euvolemia to minimize deleterious systemic effects of pressors)
8. Consider second-tier therapies for refractory elevated ICP
   a. High-dose barbiturate therapy ("pentobarb coma")
   b. Aggressive hyperventilation to Pa_{CO_2} < 30 mmHg
   c. Hemicraniectomy

---

[a] Throughout ICP treatment algorithm, consider repeat head CT to identify mass lesions amenable to surgical evacuation.
Note: CPP, cerebral perfusion pressure; MAP, mean arterial pressure; Pa_{CO_2}, arterial partial pressure of carbon dioxide.

paradoxically, administration of vasopressor agents to increase mean arterial pressure may actually lower ICP by increasing perfusion. ICP monitoring can guide medical and surgical decisions in pts with cerebral edema. Hypertension should be treated carefully, if at all. Free H_2O should be restricted, and fever treated aggressively. Hyperventilation is best used for short periods of time until a more definitive treatment can be instituted. After stabilization and initiation of the above therapies, a CT scan (or MRI, if feasible) is performed to delineate the cause of the elevated ICP. Emergency surgical intervention is sometimes necessary to decompress the intracranial contents. Hydrocephalus, cerebellar stroke with edema, surgically accessible cerebral hemorrhage or tumor, and subdural or epidural hemorrhage often require lifesaving neurosurgery.

Head Trauma

Head trauma can cause immediate loss of consciousness. If transient and unaccompanied by other serious brain pathology, it is called *concussion*. Prolonged alterations in consciousness may be due to parenchymal, subdural, or epidural hematoma or to diffuse shearing of axons in the white matter. Skull fracture should be suspected in pts with CSF rhinorrhea, hemotympanum, and periorbital or mastoid ecchymoses. Spinal cord trauma can cause transient loss of function or a permanent loss of motor, sensory, and autonomic function below the damaged spinal level.

   Minor Concussive Injury   The pt with minor head injury who is alert and attentive after a short period of unconsciousness (<1 min) may have headache, a brief amnestic period, difficulty with concentration, a single episode of emesis, or mild vertigo; vasovagal syncope may also occur. After several hours of observation, pts with this category of injury can be accompanied home and observed by family or friends. Most pts do not have a skull fracture on x-ray or hemorrhage on CT. Constant headache is common in the days following trauma; persistent severe headache and repeated vomiting are usually benign if the neurologic exam remains normal, but in such situations radiologic studies should be obtained and hospitalization is justified.

Injury of Intermediate Severity   Pts who are not comatose but who have persistent confusion, behavioral changes, subnormal alertness, extreme dizziness, or focal neurologic signs such as hemiparesis should be admitted to the hospital and soon thereafter have a CT scan. Usually a contusion or subdural hematoma is found. CT scan may be normal in comatose pts with axonal shearing lesions in cerebral white matter. Pts with intermediate head injury require medical observation to detect increasing drowsiness, respiratory dysfunction, and pupillary enlargement, as well as to ensure fluid restriction (unless there is diabetes insipidus). Abnormalities of attention, intellect, spontaneity, and memory tend to return to normal weeks or months after the injury.

Severe Injury   Patients who are comatose from onset require immediate neurologic attention and often resuscitation. After intubation, with care taken to avoid deforming the cervical spine, the depth of coma, pupillary size and reactivity, limb movements, and Babinski responses are assessed. As soon as vital functions permit and cervical spine x-rays and a CT scan have been obtained, the pt should be transported to a critical care unit. The finding of an epidural or subdural hematoma or large intracerebral hemorrhage requires prompt decompressive surgery in otherwise salvageable pts. Subsequent treatment is probably best guided by direct measurement of ICP. All potentially exacerbating factors should be eliminated. Hypoxia, hyperthermia, hypercarbia, awkward head positions, and high mean airway pressures from mechanical ventilation all increase cerebral blood volume and ICP. Persistently raised ICP after institution of this therapy generally indicates a poor outcome.

For a more detailed discussion, see Hemphill JC: Critical Care Neurology, Chap. 258, p. 1631; and Ropper AH: Concussion and Other Head Injuries, Chap. 357, p. 2447, in HPIM-16.

21

HYPOXIC-ISCHEMIC ENCEPHALOPATHY

Results from lack of delivery of oxygen to the brain because of hypotension or respiratory failure. Most common causes are MI, cardiac arrest, shock, asphyxiation, paralysis of respiration, and carbon monoxide or cyanide poisoning. In some circumstances, hypoxia may predominate. Carbon monoxide and cyanide poisoning are termed *histotoxic hypoxia* since they cause a direct impairment of the respiratory chain.

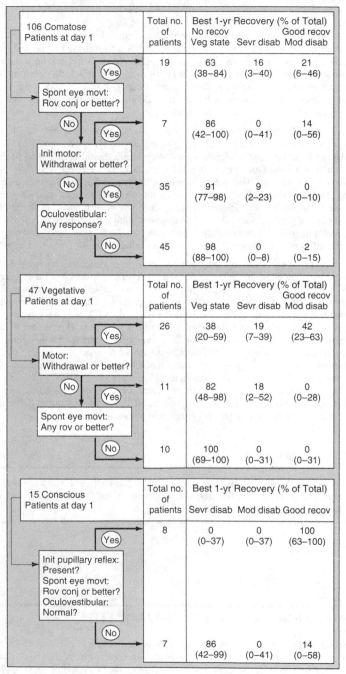

FIGURE 21-1 Clinical examination at day 1 provides useful prognostic information in hypoxic-ischemic encephalopathy. Numbers in parentheses represent 95% confidence intervals. Recov, recovery; veg, vegetative; sevr, severe; mod, moderate; spont eye movt, spontaneous eye movement; rov conj, roving conjugate. (*From DE Levy et al: Predicting outcome for hypoxic-ischemic coma. JAMA 253:1420, 1985.*)

Clinical Manifestations

Mild degrees of pure hypoxia (e.g., high altitude) cause impaired judgment, inattentiveness, motor incoordination, and, at times, euphoria. However, with hypoxia-ischemia, such as occurs with circulatory arrest, consciousness is lost within seconds. If circulation is restored within 3–5 min, full recovery may occur, but with longer periods permanent cerebral damage is the rule. It may be difficult to judge the precise degree of hypoxia-ischemia, and some pts make a relatively full recovery even after 8–10 min of global ischemia. The distinction between pure hypoxia and hypoxia-ischemia is important, since a Pa_{O_2} as low as 2.7 kPa (20 mmHg) can be well tolerated if it develops gradually and normal blood pressure is maintained, but short periods of very low or absent cerebral circulation may result in permanent impairment.

Clinical examination at different time points after an insult (especially cardiac arrest) helps to assess prognosis (Fig. 21-1). The prognosis is better for pts with intact brainstem function, as indicated by normal pupillary light responses, intact oculocephalic (doll's eyes) reflexes, and oculovestibular (caloric) and corneal reflexes (Chap. 17). Absence of these reflexes and the presence of persistently dilated pupils that do not react to light are grave prognostic signs. A uniformly dismal prognosis is conveyed by the absence of pupillary light reflex or absence of a motor response to pain on day 3 following the injury. Bilateral absence of the cortical somatosensory evoked response also conveys a poor prognosis. Long-term consequences include persistent coma or vegetative state, dementia, visual agnosia, parkinsonism, choreoathetosis, ataxia, myoclonus, seizures, and an amnestic state.

 TREATMENT

Initial treatment is directed at restoring normal cardiorespiratory function. This includes securing a clear airway, ensuring adequate oxygenation and ventilation, and restoring cerebral perfusion, whether by cardiopulmonary resuscitation, fluids, pressors, or cardiac pacing. Mild hypothermia (33°C), initiated as early as possible and continued for 12–24 h, may improve outcome in pts who remain comatose after cardiac arrest. Severe carbon monoxide intoxication may be treated with hyperbaric oxygen. Anticonvulsants are not usually given prophylactically but may be used to control seizures. Posthypoxic myoclonus can be controlled with clonazepam (1.5–10 mg/d) or sodium valproate (300–1200 mg/d) in divided doses. Myoclonic status epilepticus after a hypoxic-ischemic insult portends a universally poor prognosis.

For a more detailed discussion, see Hemphill JC, Critical Care Neurology, Chap. 258, p. 1631, in HPIM-16.

22

STATUS EPILEPTICUS

Defined as continuous seizures (>15–30 min) or repetitive, discrete seizures with impaired consciousness in the interictal period. May occur with all kinds of seizures: grand mal (tonic-clonic) status, myoclonic status, petit mal status, and temporal lobe (complex partial) status. Generalized, tonic-clonic seizures are most common and are usually clinically obvious early in the course. After 30–45 min, the signs may become increasingly subtle and include only mild clonic movements of the fingers or fine, rapid movements of the eyes. In some situations, EEG may be the only method of diagnosis. Generalized status is life-threatening when accompanied by hyperpyrexia, acidosis (from prolonged muscle activity), respiratory or cardiovascular compromise. Irreversible neuronal injury may occur from persistent seizures, even when pt is paralyzed from neuromuscular blockade.

Etiology

Principal causes of tonic-clonic status are antiepileptic drug withdrawal or noncompliance, metabolic disturbances, alcohol or drug related, CNS infections, CNS tumors, refractory epilepsy, cerebrovascular disease, and head trauma.

℞ TREATMENT

Generalized tonic-clonic status epilepticus is a medical emergency. Pts must be evaluated promptly and appropriate therapy instituted without delay (Fig. 22-1). In parallel, it is essential to determine the cause of the seizures to prevent recurrence and treat any underlying abnormalities.

1. Assess carefully for evidence of respiratory or cardiovascular insufficiency. With careful monitoring and standard airway protection, pts usually do not require intubation (if intubation is necessary, use short-acting paralytics). Treat hyperthermia. Establish IV and administer 50 mL 50% dextrose in water, 100 mg thiamine, and 0.4 mg naloxone.
2. Perform a brief medical and neurologic examination; send samples for laboratory studies aimed at identifying metabolic abnormalities (CBC with differential, serum electrolytes including calcium, glucose, liver and renal function tests, toxicology if indicated).
3. Administer lorazepam, 0.1 mg/kg (4–8 mg) at 2 mg/min.
4. Immediately after lorazepam, administer phenytoin, 20 mg/kg (1000–1500 mg) IV slowly over 20 min (50 mg/min) or fosphenytoin, 20 mg/kg (150 mg/min). Monitor bp, ECG, and, if possible, EEG during infusion. Phenytoin can cause precipitous fall in bp if given too quickly, especially in elderly pts. (Do not administer phenytoin with 5% dextrose in water—phenytoin precipitates at low pH. This is not a problem with fosphenytoin.) If seizures are not controlled, a repeat bolus of phenytoin (5–10 mg/kg) or fosphenytoin (5–10 mg/kg) may be given.
5. If seizures persist, administer phenobarbital 20 mg/kg (1000–1500 mg) slowly over 30 min. Endotracheal intubation will often be required by this stage. If seizures continue, give additional dose of phenobarbital (5–10 mg/kg).
6. If seizures remain refractory after 60–90 min, consider placing pt in midazolam, propofol, or pentobarbital coma. Consultation with a neurologist and anesthesiologist is advised.

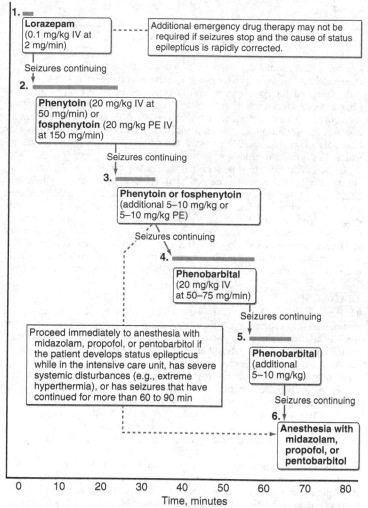

FIGURE 22-1 Pharmacologic treatment of generalized tonic-clonic status epilepticus in adults. IV, intravenous; PE, phenytoin equivalents. The horizontal bars indicate the approximate duration of drug infusions.

Prognosis

The mortality rate is 20% in tonic-clonic status, and the incidence of permanent neurologic sequelae is 10–30%.

For a more detailed discussion, see Lowenstein DH: Seizures and Epilepsy, Chap. 348, p. 2357, in HPIM-16.

23

POISONING AND DRUG OVERDOSE

Poisoning refers to the development of harmful effects following exposure to chemicals. *Overdosage* is exposure to excessive amounts of a substance normally intended for consumption and does not necessarily imply poisoning. Chemical exposures result in an estimated 5 million requests in the United States for medical advice or treatment each year, and about 5% of victims of chemical exposure require hospitalization. Suicide attempts account for most serious or fatal poisonings. Up to 30% of psychiatric admissions are prompted by attempted suicide via overdosage.

Carbon monoxide (CO) poisoning is the leading cause of death. Acetaminophen toxicity is the most common pharmaceutical agent causing fatalities. Other drug-related fatalities are commonly due to analgesics, antidepressants, sedative-hypnotics, neuroleptics, stimulants and street drugs, cardiovascular drugs, anticonvulsants, antihistamines, and asthma therapies. Nonpharmaceutical agents implicated in fatal poisoning include alcohols and glycols, gases and fumes, chemicals, cleaning substances, pesticides, and automotive products. The diagnosis of poisoning or drug overdose must be considered in any pt who presents with coma, seizure, or acute renal, hepatic, or bone marrow failure.

DIAGNOSIS

The correct diagnosis can usually be reached by history, physical exam, and routine and toxicologic laboratory evaluation. All available sources should be used to determine the exact nature of the ingestion or exposure. The *history* should include the time, route, duration, and circumstances (location, surrounding events, and intent) of exposure; time of onset, nature, and severity of symptoms; relevant past medical and psychiatric history. The Physicians Desk Reference, regional poison control centers, and local/hospital pharmacies may be useful for identification of ingredients and potential effects of toxins.

The *physical exam* should focus initially on the vital signs, cardiopulmonary system, and neurologic status including assessment of mental status and documentation of neuromuscular abnormalities. Focal neurologic signs are uncommon in poisoning.

Examination of the eyes (for nystagmus, pupil size, and reactivity), abdomen (for bowel activity and bladder size), and skin (for burns, bullae, color, warmth, moisture, pressure sores, and puncture marks) may narrow the diagnosis to a particular disorder. The pt should also be examined for evidence of trauma and underlying illnesses. When the history is unclear, all orifices should be examined for the presence of chemical burns and drug packets. The odor of breath or vomitus and the color of nails, skin, or urine may provide diagnostic clues.

Initial laboratory studies should include glucose, serum electrolytes, serum osmolality, BUN/Cr, LFTs, PT/PTT, and ABGs. An increased anion-gap metabolic acidosis is characteristic of advanced methanol, ethylene glycol, and salicylate intoxication but can occur with other agents and in any poisoning that results in hepatic, renal, or respiratory failure; seizures; or shock. An increased osmolal gap—the difference between the serum osmolality (measured by freezing point depression) and that calculated from the serum sodium, glucose, and BUN of >10 mmol/L—suggests the presence of a low-molecular-weight solute such as an alcohol, glycol, or ketone or an unmeasured electrolyte or sugar. Ketosis suggests acetone, isopropyl alcohol, or salicylate poisoning. Hypoglycemia may be due to poisoning with β-adrenergic blockers, ethanol, insulin, oral hypoglycemic agents, quinine, and salicylates, whereas hyperglycemia can occur in poisoning with acetone, β-adrenergic agonists, calcium channel blockers, iron, theophylline, or Vacor.

Radiologic studies should include a chest x-ray to exclude aspiration or ARDS. Radiopaque densities may be visible on abdominal x-rays. Head CT or MRI is indicated in stuporous or comatose pts to exclude structural lesions or subarachnoid hemorrhage, and LP should be performed when CNS infection is suspected. The *ECG* can be useful to assist with the differential diagnosis and to guide treatment. *Toxicologic analysis* of urine and blood (and occasionally of gastric contents and chemical samples) may be useful to confirm or rule out suspected poisoning. Although rapid screening tests for a limited number of drugs of abuse are available, comprehensive screening tests require 2 to 6 h for completion, and immediate management must be based on the history, physical exam, and routine ancillary tests. Quantitative analysis is useful for poisoning with acetaminophen, acetone, alcohol (including ethylene glycol), antiarrhythmics, anticonvulsants, barbiturates, digoxin, heavy metals, lithium, paraquat, salicylate, and theophylline, as well as for carboxyhemoglobin and methemoglobin. Results can often be available within an hour.

The response to antidotes may be useful for diagnostic purposes. Resolution of altered mental status and abnormal vital signs within minutes of intravenous administration of dextrose, naloxone, or flumazenil is virtually diagnostic of hypoglycemia, narcotic poisoning, and benzodiazepine intoxication, respectively. The prompt reversal of acute dystonic (extrapyramidal) reactions following an intravenous dose of benztropine or diphenhydramine confirms a drug etiology. Although physostigmine reversal of both central and peripheral manifestations of anticholinergic poisoning is diagnostic, it may cause arousal in patients with CNS depression of any etiology.

℞ TREATMENT

Goals of therapy include support of vital signs, prevention of further absorption, enhancement of elimination, administration of specific antidotes, and prevention of reexposure. Fundamentals of poisoning management are listed in Table 23-1. Treatment is usually initiated before routine and toxicologic data are known. All symptomatic pts need large-bore IV access, supplemental O_2, cardiac monitoring, continuous observation, and, if mental status is altered, 100 mg thiamine (IM or IV), 1 ampule of 50% dextrose in water, and 4 mg of naloxone along with specific antidotes as indicated. Unconscious pts should be intubated. Activated charcoal may be given PO or via a large-bore gastric tube; gastric lavage requires an orogastric tube. Severity of poisoning determines the management. Admission to an ICU is indicated for pts with severe poisoning (coma, respiratory depression, hypotension, cardiac conduction abnormalities, arrhythmias, hypothermia or hyperthermia, seizures); those needing close monitoring; antidotes; enhanced elimination therapy; progressive clinical deterioration; significant underlying medical problems. Suicidal pts require constant observation by qualified personnel.

Supportive Care Airway protection is mandatory. Gag reflex alone is not a reliable indicator of the need for intubation. Need for O_2 supplementation and ventilatory support can be assessed by measurement of ABGs. Drug-induced pulmonary edema is usually secondary to hypoxia, but myocardial depression may contribute. Measurement of pulmonary artery pressure may be necessary to establish etiology. Electrolyte imbalances should be corrected as soon as possible.

Supraventricular tachycardia (SVT) with hypertension and CNS excitation is almost always due to sympathetic, anticholinergic, or hallucinogenic stim-

Table 23-1

Fundamentals of Poisoning Management

SUPPORTIVE CARE

Airway protection	Treatment of seizures
Oxygenation/ventilation	Correction of temperature abnormalities
Treatment of arrhythmias	Correction of metabolic derangements
Hemodynamic support	Prevention of secondary complications

PREVENTION OF FURTHER POISON ABSORPTION

GI decontamination	Decontamination of other sites
Syrup of ipecac–induced	Eye decontamination
emesis	Skin decontamination
Gastric lavage	Body cavity evacuation
Activated charcoal	
Whole-bowel irrigation	
Catharsis	
Dilution	
Endoscopic/surgical removal	

ENHANCEMENT OF POISON ELIMINATION

Multiple-dose activated charcoal	Extracorporeal removal
Forced diuresis	Peritoneal dialysis
Alteration of urinary pH	Hemodialysis
Chelation	Hemoperfusion
Hyperbaric oxygenation	Hemofiltration
	Plasmapheresis
	Exchange transfusion

ADMINISTRATION OF ANTIDOTES

Neutralization by antibodies	Metabolic antagonism
Neutralization by chemical binding	Physiologic antagonism

PREVENTION OF REEXPOSURE

Adult education	Notification of regulatory agencies
Child-proofing	Psychiatric referral

Source: Modified from CH Linden, MJ Burns: Table 377-3, p. 2582 in HPIM-16.

ulation or to drug withdrawal. Treatment is indicated if associated with hemodynamic instability, chest pain, or ischemia on ECG. Treatment with combined alpha and beta blockers or combinations of beta blocker and vasodilator is indicated in severe sympathetic hyperactivity. Physostigmine is useful for anticholinergic hyperactivity. SVT without hypertension usually responds to fluid administration.

Ventricular tachycardia (VT) can be caused by sympathetic stimulation, myocardial membrane destabilization, or metabolic derangements. Lidocaine and phenytoin are generally safe. Drugs that prolong the QT interval (quinidine, procainamide) should not be used in VT due to tricyclic antidepressant overdose. Magnesium sulfate and overdrive pacing (by isoproterenol or a pacemaker) may be useful for torsades de pointes. Arrhythmias may be resistant to therapy until underlying acid-base and electrolyte derangements, hypoxia, and hypothermia are corrected. It is acceptable to observe hemodynamically stable pts without pharmacologic intervention.

Seizures are best treated with γ-aminobutyric acid agonists such as benzodiazepines or barbiturates. Barbiturates should only be given after intubation. Seizures caused by isoniazid overdose may respond only to large doses of pyridoxine IV. Seizures from beta blockers or tricyclic antidepressants may require phenytoin and benzodiazepines.

Prevention of Poison Absorption   Whether or not to perform GI decontamination, and which procedure to use, depends on the time since ingestion; the existing and predicted toxicity of the ingestant; the availability, efficacy, and contraindications of the procedure; and the nature, severity, and risk of complications. The efficacy of activated charcoal, gastric lavage, and syrup of ipecac decreases with time, and there are insufficient data to support or exclude a beneficial effect when they are used >1 h after ingestion. Activated charcoal has comparable or greater efficacy, fewer contraindications and complications, and is less invasive than ipecac or gastric lavage and is the preferred method of GI decontamination in most situations.

Activated charcoal is prepared as a suspension in water, either alone or with a cathartic. It is given orally via a nippled bottle (for infants), or via a cup, straw, or small-bore nasogastric tube. The recommended dose is 1 g/kg body weight, using 8 mL of diluent per gram of charcoal if a pre-mixed formulation is not available. Charcoal may inhibit absorption of other orally administered agents and is contraindicated in pts with corrosive ingestion.

When indicated, gastric lavage is performed using a 28F orogastric tube in children and a 40F orogastric tube in adults. Saline or tap water may be used in adults or children (use saline in infants). Place pt in Trendelenburg and left lateral decubitus position to minimize aspiration (occurs in 10% of pts). Lavage is contraindicated with corrosives and petroleum distillate hydrocarbons because of risk of aspiration-induced pneumonia and gastroesophageal perforation.

Whole-bowel irrigation may be useful with ingestions of foreign bodies, drug packets, and slow-release medications. Golytely is given orally or by gastric tube up to a rate of 2 L/h. Cathartic salts (magnesium citrate) and saccharides (sorbitol, mannitol) promote evacuation of the rectum. Dilution of corrosive acids and alkali is accomplished by having pt drink 5 mL water/kg. Endoscopy or surgical intervention may be required in large foreign-body ingestion, heavy metal ingestion, and when ingested drug packets leak or rupture.

Syrup of ipecac is administered orally in doses of 30 mL for adults, 15 mL for children, and 10 mL for infants. Vomiting should occur within 20 min. Ipecac is contraindicated with marginal airway patency, CNS depression, recent GI surgery, seizures, corrosive (lye) ingestion, petroleum hydrocarbon ingestion, and rapidly acting CNS poisons (camphor, cyanide, tricyclic antidepressants, propoxyphene, strychnine). Ipecac is particularly useful in the field.

Skin and eyes are decontaminated by washing with copious amounts of water or saline.

Enhancement of Elimination   Activated charcoal in repeated doses of 1 g/kg q2–4h is useful for ingestions of drugs with enteral circulation such as carbamazepine, dapsone, diazepam, digoxin, glutethimide, meprobamate, methotrexate, phenobarbital, phenytoin, salicylate, theophylline, and valproic acid.

Forced alkaline diuresis enhances the elimination of chlorphenoxyacetic acid herbicides, chlorpropamide, diflunisal, fluoride, methotrexate, phenobarbital, sulfonamides, and salicylates. Sodium bicarbonate, 1–2 ampules per liter of 0.45% NaCl, is given at a rate sufficient to maintain urine pH $\geq$ 7.5 and urine output at 3–6 mL/kg per h. Acid diuresis is no longer recommended. Saline diuresis may enhance elimination of bromide, calcium, fluoride, lithium, meprobamate, potassium, and isoniazid; contraindications include CHF, renal failure, and cerebral edema.

Peritoneal dialysis or hemodialysis may be useful in severe poisoning due to barbiturates, bromide, chloral hydrate, ethanol, ethylene glycol, isopropyl alcohol, lithium, heavy metals, methanol, procainamide, and salicylate. Hemoperfusion may be indicated for chloramphenicol, disopyramide, and hypnotic-sedative overdose. Exchange transfusion removes poisons affecting red blood cells.

SPECIFIC POISONS

ACETAMINOPHEN   A dose of $\geq$140 mg/kg of acetaminophen saturates metabolism to sulfate and glucuronide metabolites, resulting in increased metabolism of acetaminophen to mercapturic acid. Nonspecific toxic manifestations (and not predictive of hepatic toxicity) include nausea, vomiting, diaphoresis, and pallor 2–4 h after ingestion. Laboratory evidence of hepatotoxicity includes elevation of AST, ALT, and, in severe cases, PT and bilirubin, with ultimate hyperammonemia. A serum acetaminophen level drawn 4–24 h after ingestion is useful for purposes of predicting risk.

Initial therapy consists of activated charcoal (particularly within 30 min of ingestion), then *N*-acetylcysteine therapy, which is indicated up to 24 h after ingestion. Loading dose is 140 mg/kg PO, followed by 70 mg/kg PO q4h for 17 doses. Therapy should be started immediately and may be discontinued when serum level is below toxic range.

ALKALI AND ACID   Alkalis include industrial-strength bleach, drain cleaners (sodium hydroxide), surface cleaners (ammonia, phosphates), laundry and dishwashing detergents (phosphates, carbonates), disk batteries, denture cleaners (borates, phosphates, carbonates), and Clinitest tablets (sodium hydroxide). Common acids include toilet bowl cleaners (hydrofluoric, phosphoric, and sulfuric acids), soldering fluxes (hydrochloric acid), anti-rust compounds (hydrofluoric and oxalic acids), automobile battery fluid (sulfuric acid), and stone cleaners (hydrofluoric and nitric acids). Clinical signs include burns, pain, drooling, vomiting of blood or mucus, and ulceration. Lack of oral manifestations does not rule out esophageal involvement. The esophagus and stomach can perforate, and aspiration can cause fulminant tracheitis.

Endoscopy is safe within 48 h of ingestion to document site and severity of injury.

Immediate treatment consists of dilution with milk or water. Glucocorticoids should be given within 48 h to pts with alkali (not acid) burns of the esophagus and continued for at least 2 weeks. Antacids may be useful for stomach burns. Prophylactic broad-spectrum antibiotics are recommended.

ANTIARRHYTHMIC DRUGS   Acute ingestion of >2× the usual daily dose is potentially toxic and causes symptoms within 1 h. Manifestations include nausea, vomiting, diarrhea, lethargy, confusion, ataxia, bradycardia, hypotension, and cardiovascular collapse. Anticholinergic effects are seen with disopyramide ingestion. Quinidine and class IB agents (lidocaine, mexiletine, phenytoin, tocainide) can cause agitation, dysphoria, and seizures. Ventricular fibrillation (including torsades de pointes) and QT prolongation are characteristic of class IA (disopyramide, procainamide, quinidine) and IC (encainide, moricizine, propafenone, flecainide) poisonings. Myocardial depression may precipitate pulmonary edema.

Activated charcoal is the treatment of choice for GI decontamination. Persistent hypotension and bradycardia may require monitoring of pulmonary artery pressure, cardiac pacing, intraaortic balloon pump counterpulsation, and cardiopulmonary bypass. Ventricular tachyarrhythmias are treated with lidocaine. Sodium bicarbonate or lactate may be useful in class IA or IC overdoses.

Torsades de pointes is treated with magnesium sulfate (4 g or 40 mL of 10% solution IV over 10–20 min) or overdrive pacing (with isoproterenol or pacemaker).

ANTICHOLINERGIC AGENTS Antimuscarinic agents inhibit acetylcholine in the CNS and parasympathetic postganglionic muscarinic neuroreceptors and include antihistamines (H_1-receptor blockers and over-the-counter hypnotics), belladonna alkaloids (atropine, homatropine, scopolamine), Parkinsonian drugs (benztropine, biperiden, trihexyphenidyl), mydriatics (cyclopentolate, tropicamide), phenothizaines, skeletal muscle relaxants (cyclobenzaprine, orphenadrine), smooth-muscle relaxants (clinidinium, dicyclomine), tricyclic antidepressants, and a variety of plants (stramonium, jimsonweed) and mushrooms. Manifestations begin 1 h to 3 d after ingestion; agitation, ataxia, confusion, delirium, hallucinations, and choreoathetosis can lead to lethargy, respiratory depression, and coma; dry skin and mucous membranes.

Treatment involves GI decontamination with activated charcoal, supportive measures, and, in severe cases, the acetylcholinesterase inhibitor physostigmine; 1 to 2 mg is given IV over 2 min, and the dose may be repeated for incomplete response or recurrent toxicity. Physostigmine is contraindicated in the presence of cardiac conduction defects or ventricular arrhythmias.

ANTICONVULSANTS These drugs include carbamazepine, lamotrigine, phenytoin and other hydantoins, topiramate, valproate, barbiturates, ethosuximide, methsuximide, felbamate, gabapentin, and benzodiazepines (see below). Anticonvulsants are well absorbed after oral administration and primarily cause CNS depression. Cerebellar and vestibular function are affected first, with cerebral depression occurring later. Ataxia, blurred vision, diplopia, dizziness, nystagmus, slurred speech, tremors, and nausea and vomiting are common initial manifestations. Coma with respiratory depression usually occurs at serum carbamazepine concentrations >20 µg/mL, serum phenytoin levels >60 µg/mL, and serum valproate levels of >180 µg/mL. Anticholinergic effects (see above) may be present in carbamazepine poisoning, and tricyclic antidepressant–like cardiotoxicity (see below) can occur at drug levels >30 µg/mL. Hypotension and arrhythmias (e.g., bradycardia, conduction disturbances, ventricular tachyarrhythmias) can occur during the rapid infusion of phenytoin. Cardiovascular toxicity after oral phenytoin overdose, however, is essentially nonexistent. Extravasation of phenytoin can result in local tissue necrosis due to the high pH of this formulation. Intravenous phenytoin may also cause the "purple glove syndrome" (limb edema, discoloration, and pain). Multiple metabolic abnormalites, including anion-gap metabolic acidosis, hyperosmolality, hypocalcemia, hypoglycemia, hypophosphatemia, hypernatremia, and hyperammonemia (with or without other evidence of hepatotoxicity) can occur in valproate poisoning. Three or more days may be required for resolution of toxicity in severe carbamazepine, phenytoin, and valproate poisoning.

The diagnosis of carbamazepine, phenytoin, and valproate poisoning can be confirmed by measuring serum drug concentrations. Serial drug levels should be obtained until a peak is observed following acute overdose. Quantitative serum levels of other agents are not generally available. Most anticonvulsants can be detected by comprehensive urine screening tests.

Activated charcoal is the method of choice for GI decontamination. Multiple-dose charcoal therapy can enhance the elimination of carbamezpine, phenytoin, valproate, and perhaps other agents. Airway protection and support of respirations with endotracheal intubation and mechanical ventilation, if necessary, are the mainstays of treatment. Seizures should be treated with benzodiazepines or barbiturates. Flumazenil can be used for benzodiazepine or zolpidem poisoning. Physostigmine (see "Anticholinergic Agents," above) should be considered for anticholinergic poisoning due to carbamazepine. Occasionally, CNS depression due to valproate will respond to naloxone (2 mg IV). Hemodialysis and hemoperfusion should be reserved for patients with persistently high drug levels (e.g., carbamazepine $\geq$ 40 μg/mL and valproate $\geq$ 1000 μg/mL) who do not respond to supportive care.

ARSENIC Poisoning can occur from natural sources (contamination of deep-water wells); from occupational exposure (a byproduct of the smelting of ores and use in the microelectronic industry); commercial use of arsenic in wood preservatives, pesticides, herbicides, fungicides, and paints; and through foods and tobacco treated with arsenic-containing pesticides. Acute poisoning causes hemorrhagic gastroenteritis, fluid loss, and hypotension followed by delayed cardiomyopathy, delirium, coma, and seizures. Acute tubular necrosis and hemolysis may develop. Arsine gas causes severe hemolysis. Chronic exposure causes skin and nail changes (hyperkeratosis, hyperpigmentation, exfoliative dermatitis, and transverse white striae of the fingernails), sensory and motor polyneuritis that may lead to paralysis, and inflammation of the respiratory mucosa. Chronic exposure is associated with increased risk of skin cancer and possibly of systemic cancers and with vasospasm and peripheral vascular insufficiency.

Treatment of acute ingestion includes ipecac-induced vomiting, gastric lavage, activated charcoal with a cathartic, aggressive administration of IV fluids and electrolyte correction, and dimercaprol IM at an initial dose of 3–5 mg/kg every q4h for 2 days, q6h on day 3, and q12h for 7 days. Succimer is an alternative agent if adverse reactions develop to dimercaprol. With renal failure doses should be adjusted carefully. Other than avoidance of additional exposure, specific therapy is not of proven benefit for chronic arsenic toxicity.

BARBITURATES Overdose may result in confusion, lethargy, coma, hypotension, hypothermia, pulmonary edema, and death.

Treatment consists of GI decontamination and repetitive charcoal administration for long-acting barbiturates. Renal excretion of phenobarbital is enhanced by alkalinization of urine to a pH of 8 and by saline diuresis. Hemoperfusion and hemodialysis can be used in severe poisoning with short- or long-acting barbiturates.

BENZODIAZEPINES Long-acting agents include chlordiazepoxide, clonazepam, clorazepate, diazepam, flurazepam, prazepam, and quazepam; short-acting drugs include alprazolam, flunitrazepam, lorazepam, and oxazepam; and ultrashort-acting agents include estazolam, midazolam, temazepam, and triazolam. Effects may begin within 30 min of overdosage and include weakness, ataxia, drowsiness, coma, and respiratory depression. Pupils are constricted and do not respond to naloxone.

Treatment includes GI decontamination and support of vital signs. Flumazenil, a competitive benzodiazepine-receptor antagonist, can reverse CNS and respiratory depression and is given IV in incremental doses of 0.2, 0.3, and 0.5 mg at 1-min intervals until the desired effect is achieved or a total dose of 3 to 5 mg is given; flumazenil must be used with caution in pts who have benzodiazepine dependency or have coingested stimulants and benzodiazepines.

BETA-ADRENERGIC BLOCKING AGENTS Some beta blockers are cardioselective (acebutolol, atenolol, betaxolol, bisoprolol, esmolol, metoprolol), some have sympathomimetic activity (acebutolol, cartelol, pindolol, timolol, possibly penbutolol), and some have quinidine-like effects (acebutolol, metoprolol, pindolol, propranolol, sotalol, possibly betaxolol). Toxicity is usually manifest within 30 min of ingestion. Symptoms include nausea, vomiting, diarrhea, bradycardia, hypotension, and CNS depression. Agents with intrinsic sympathomimetic activity can cause hypertension and tachycardia. Bronchospasm and pulmonary edema may occur. Hyperkalemia, hypoglycemia, metabolic acidosis, all degrees of AV block, bundle branch block, QRS prolongation, ventricular tachyarrhythmias, torsades de pointes, and asystole may occur.

Treatment includes GI decontamination, supportive measures, and administration of calcium (10% chloride or gluconate salt solution, IV 0.2 mL/kg, up to 10 mL) and glucagon (5–10 mg IV, then infusion of 1–5 mg/L). Bradycardia and hypotension sometimes respond to atropine, isoproterenol, and vasopressors. Cardiac pacing or an intraaortic balloon pump may be required. Bronchospasm is treated with inhaled β agonists.

CADMIUM Foods can be contaminated with cadmium from sewage, polluted ground water, or mining effluents. Airborne cadmium can be released from smelting or incineration of wastes containing plastics and batteries, and occupational exposure occurs in the metal-plating, pigment, battery, and plastics industries. Acute inhalation can cause pleuritic chest pain, dyspnea, cyanosis, fever, tachycardia, nausea, and pulmonary edema. Ingestion can cause severe nausea, vomiting, salivation, abdominal cramps, and diarrhea. Chronic exposure causes anosmia, microcytic hypochromic anemia, renal tubular dysfunction with proteinuria, and osteomalacia with pseudofractures.

Treatment involves avoidance of further exposure and supportive therapy. Chelation therapy is not useful, and dimercaprol may worsen nephrotoxicity and is contraindicated.

CALCIUM CHANNEL BLOCKERS These agents include amlodipine, bepridil, diltiazem, felodipine, flunarizine, isradipine, lacidipine, nicardipine, nifedipine, nimodipine, nisoldipine, nitrendipine, and verapamil. Toxicity usually develops within 30–60 min following ingestion of 5–10 $\times$ usual dose. Manifestations include confusion, drowsiness, coma, seizure, hypotension, bradycardia, cyanosis, and pulmonary edema. ECG findings include all degrees of AV block, prolonged QRS and QT intervals, ischemia or infarction, and asystole. Metabolic acidosis and hyperglycemia may result.

Treatment consists of GI decontamination with activated charcoal, supportive care, calcium, and glucagon (as above). Electrical pacing or intraaortic balloon pump may be required, and persistent hypotension may require vasopressors.

CARBON MONOXIDE CO binds to hemoglobin (forming carboxyhemoglobin) with an affinity 200 times that of O_2 and hence causes cellular anoxia. An elevated carboxyhemoglobin fraction confirms exposure but must be interpreted relative to the time elapsed from exposure. Once exposure is discontinued, CO is excreted via the lungs with a half-life of 4–6 h. The half-life decreases to 40–80 min with 100% O_2 therapy and to 15–30 min with hyperbaric O_2. Manifestations include shortness of breath, dyspnea, tachypnea, headache, nausea, vomiting, emotional lability, confusion, impaired judgment, and clumsiness. Pulmonary edema, aspiration pneumonia, arrhythmias, and hypotension may occur. The "cherry red" color of skin and mucous membranes is rare; cyanosis is usual.

Treatment consists of giving 100% O_2 via a tightly fitting mask until CO levels are <10% and all symptoms have resolved. Hyperbaric O_2 is recommended for comatose pts with CO levels $\geq$ 40%, for pts with CO levels $\geq$ 25% who also have seizures or intractable arrhythmias, and for pts with delayed onset of sequelae. Pts with loss of consciousness are at risk for neuropsychiatric sequelae 1 to 3 weeks later.

CARDIAC GLYCOSIDES, INCLUDING DIGOXIN   Poisoning with digitalis occurs with therapeutic or suicidal use of digoxin and with plant (foxglove, oleander, squill) ingestion. Symptoms include vomiting, confusion, delirium, hallucinations, blurred vision, disturbed color perception (yellow vision), photophobia, all types of arrhythmias, and all degrees of AV block. The combination of SVT and AV block suggests digitalis toxicity. Hypokalemia is common with chronic intoxication, while hyperkalemia occurs with acute overdosage. Diagnosis is confirmed by measuring the serum digoxin level.

GI decontamination is done carefully to avoid vagal stimulation, repeated doses of activated charcoal are given, and hyperkalemia is treated with Kayexalate, insulin, and glucose. Atropine and electrical pacing may be required. In severe poisoning digoxin-specific Fab antibodies are given; dosage (in 40-mg vials) is calculated by dividing ingested dose of digoxin (mg) by 0.6 mg/vial. If dose and serum levels are unknown, give 5–10 vials to an adult.

CYANIDE   Cyanide blocks electron transport, resulting in decreased oxidative metabolism and oxidative utilization, decreased ATP production, and lactic acidosis. Lethal dose is 200–300 mg of sodium cyanide and 500 mg of hydrocyanic acid. Early effects include headache, vertigo, excitement, anxiety, burning of mouth and throat, dyspnea, tachycardia, hypertension, nausea, vomiting, and diaphoresis. Breath may have a bitter almond odor. Later effects include coma, seizures, opisthotonos, trismus, paralysis, respiratory depression, arrhythmias, hypotension, and death.

Treatment should begin immediately based on history. Supportive measures, 100% O_2, and GI decontamination are begun concurrently with specific therapy. Amyl nitrite is inhaled for 30 s each min, and a new ampule is broken q3min. (Nitrite produces methemoglobinemia, which has a higher affinity for cyanide and promotes release from peripheral sites.) Sodium nitrite is then given as a 3% solution IV at a rate of 2.5–5.0 mL/min up to a total dose of 10–15 mL. Then, 50 mL of 25% sodium thiosulfate is given IV over 1–2 min, producing sodium thiocyanate, which is excreted in urine. (Children should be given 0.33 mL/kg sodium nitrite and 1.65 mL/kg sodium thiosulfate.) If symptoms persist, repeat half the dose of sodium nitrite and sodium thiosulfate.

CYCLIC ANTIDEPRESSANTS   These agents include amitriptyline, imipramine, nortriptyline, desipramine, chlomipramine, doxepin, protriptyline, trimipramine, amoxapine, bupropion, maprotiline, mirtazepine, and trazadone. Depending on the agent, they block reuptake of synaptic transmitters (norepinephrine, dopamine) and have central and peripheral anticholinergic activity. Manifestations include anticholinergic symptoms (fever, mydriasis, flushing of skin, urinary retention, decreased bowel motility). CNS manifestations include excitation, restlessness, myoclonus, hyperreflexia, disorientation, confusion, hallucinations, coma, and seizures. Cardiac effects include prolongation of the QRS complex, other AV blocks, and arrhythmias. QRS duration ≥ 0.10 ms is correlated with seizures and life-threatening cardiac arrhythmias. Serum levels ≥ 3300 nmol/L (≥ 1000 ng/mL) indicate serious poisoning.

Treatment with ipecac is contraindicated. Activated charcoal is the preferred method of GI decontamination and may require repeated treatments. Metabolic acidosis is treated with sodium bicarbonate; hypotension with volume expansion, norepinephrine, or high-dose dopamine; seizures with benzodiazepines and barbiturates; arrhythmias with sodium bicarbonate (0.5–1 mmol/kg) and lidocaine. β-Adrenergic blockers and class 1A antiarrhythmics should be avoided. The efficacy of phenytoin is not established. Physostigmine reverses anticholinergic signs and may be given in mild poisoning.

ETHYLENE GLYCOL   Ethylene glycol is used as a solvent for paints, plastics, and pharmaceuticals and in the manufacture of explosives, fire extinguishers, foams, hydraulic fluids, windshield cleaners, radiator antifreeze, and de-icer preparations. As little as 120 mg or 0.1 mL/kg can be hazardous. Manifestations include nausea, vomiting, slurred speech, ataxia, nystagmus, lethargy, sweet breath odor, coma, seizures, cardiovascular collapse, and death. Hypocalcemia occurs in half of pts. Anion-gap metabolic acidosis, elevated serum osmolality, and oxalate crystalluria suggest the diagnosis. Renal failure may result from glycolic acid production.

GI lavage should be followed by activated charcoal, and airway protection should be initiated immediately. Calcium salts should be given IV at a rate of 1 mL/min for a total dose of 7–14 mL (10% solution diluted 10:1). Metabolic acidosis should be treated with sodium bicarbonate. Phenytoin and benzodiazepines are given for seizures. Ethanol and fomepizole bind to alcohol dehydrogenase with higher affinity than ethylene glycol and block the production of toxic metabolites. Ethanol is administered when ethylene glycol level is >3 mmol/L (>20 mg/dL) and acidosis is present; ethanol is given as follows: the loading dose is 10 mL/kg of 10% ethanol IV or 1 mL/kg of 95% ethanol PO; the maintenance dose is 1.5 (mL/kg)/h of 10% ethanol IV and 3 (mL/kg)/h of 10% ethanol during dialysis. A serum ethanol level ≥ 20 mmol/L (≥100 mg/dL) is required to inhibit alcohol dehydrogenase, and levels must be monitored closely. Fomepizole is diluted in 100 mL of IV fluid and administered over 30 min in a loading dose of 15 mg/kg followed by 10 mg/kg every 12 h for four doses and 15 mg/kg thereafter until the ethylene glycol level falls below 1.5 mmol/L (10 mg/dL). Hemodialysis is indicated in cases not responding to above therapy, when serum levels are ≥ 8 mmol/L (≥50 mg/dL), and for renal failure. Give thiamine and pyridoxine supplements.

HALLUCINOGENS   Mescaline, lysergic acid (LSD), and psilocybin cause disorders of mood, thought, and perception lasting 4–6 h. Psilocybin can cause fever, hypotension, and seizures. Symptoms include mydriasis, conjunctival injection, piloerection, hypertension, tachycardia, tachypnea, anorexia, tremors, and hyperreflexia.

Treatment is nonspecific: a calm environment, benzodiazepines for acute panic reactions, and haloperidol for psychotic reactions.

IRON   Ferrous iron injures mitochondria, causes lipid peroxidation, and results in renal, tubular, and hepatic necrosis and occasionally in myocardial and pulmonary injury. Ingestion of 20 mg/kg causes GI symptoms, and 60 mg/kg causes fever, hyperglycemia, leukocytosis, lethargy, hypotension, metabolic acidosis, seizures, coma, vascular collapse, jaundice, elevated liver enzymes, prolongation of PT, and hyperammonemia. X-ray may identify iron tablets in stomach. Serum iron levels greater than iron-binding capacity indicate serious toxicity. A positive urine deferoxamine provocative test (50 mg/kg IV or IM up to 1 g) produces a vin rosé color that indicates presence of ferrioxamine.

Gastric lavage and whole-bowel irrigation should be administered, followed by x-ray to check adequacy of decontamination. Charcoal is ineffective. Endoscopic removal of tablets may be necessary. Volume depletion should be corrected, and sodium bicarbonate is used to correct metabolic acidosis. Deferoxamine is infused at 10–15 (mg/kg)/h (up to 1–2 g) if iron exceeds binding capacity. If iron level > 180 μmol/L (>1000 μg/dL), larger doses of deferoxamine can be given, followed by exchange transfusion or plasmapheresis to remove deferoxamine complex.

ISONIAZID   Acute overdose decreases synthesis of γ-aminobutyric acid and causes CNS stimulation. Symptoms begin within 30 min of ingestion and include nausea, vomiting, dizziness, slurred speech, coma, seizures, and metabolic acidosis.

Activated charcoal is the preferred method of GI decontamination. Pyridoxine (vitamin B_6) should be given slowly IV in weight equivalency to ingested dose of isoniazid. If dose is not known, give 5 g pyridoxine IV over 30 min as a 5–10% solution.

ISOPROPYL ALCOHOL Isopropyl alcohol is present in rubbing alcohol, solvents, aftershave lotions, antifreeze, and window cleaners. Its metabolite, acetone, is found in cleaners, solvents, and nail polish removers. Manifestations begin promptly and include vomiting, abdominal pain, hematemesis, myopathy, headache, dizziness, confusion, coma, respiratory depression, hypothermia, and hypotension. Hypoglycemia, anion-gap (small) metabolic acidosis, elevated serum osmolality, false elevations of serum creatinine, and hemolytic anemia may be present.

Treatment consists of GI decontamination by gastric aspiration and supportive measures. Activated charcoal is not effective. Dialysis may be needed in severe cases.

LEAD Exposure to lead occurs through paints, cans, plumbing fixtures, leaded gasolines, vegetables grown in lead-contaminated soils, improperly glazed ceramics, lead-containing glass, and industrial sources such as battery manufacturing, demolition of lead-contaminated buildings, and the ceramics industry. Manifestations in childhood include abdominal pain followed by lethargy, anorexia, anemia, ataxia, and slurred speech. Severe manifestations include convulsions, coma, generalized cerebral edema, and renal failure. Impairment of cognition is dose-dependent. In adults symptoms of chronic exposure include abdominal pain, headache, irritability, joint pain, fatigue, anemia, motor neuropathy, and deficits in memory. Encephalopathy is rare. A "lead line" may appear at the gingiva-tooth border. Chronic, low-level exposure can cause interstitial nephritis, tubular damage, hyperuricemia, and decreased glomerular filtration. Elevation of bone lead level is a risk for anemia and hypertension.

Treatment first involves prevention of further exposure and the use of chelating agents such as oral succimer or IM edetate calcium disodium. Chelation may not improve subclinical manifestations such as impaired cognition.

LITHIUM Manifestations begin within 2–4 h of ingestion and include nausea, vomiting, diarrhea, weakness, fasciculations, twitching, ataxia, tremor, myoclonus, choreoathetosis, seizures, confusion, coma, and cardiovascular collapse. Laboratory abnormalities include leukocytosis, hyperglycemia, albuminuria, glycosuria, nephrogenic diabetes insipidus, ECG changes (AV block, prolonged QT), and ventricular arrhythmias.

Within 2–4 h of ingestion, gastric lavage and bowel irrigation should be performed. Charcoal is not effective. Endoscopy should be considered if concretions are suspected. Serial serum lithium levels should be measured until trend is downward. Supportive care includes saline diuresis and alkalinization of the urine for levels > 2–3 mmol/L. Hemodialysis is indicated for acute or chronic intoxication with symptoms and/or a serum level > 3 mmol/L.

MERCURY Mercury is used in thermometers, dental amalgams, and some batteries and is combined with other chemicals to form inorganic or organic mercury compounds. Fish can concentrate mercury at high levels, and occupational exposure continues in some chemical, metal-processing, electrical, and automotive manufacturing; building industries; and medical and dental services (e.g., ordinary dental amalgam). Inhalation of mercury vapor causes diffuse infiltrates or a pneumonitis, respiratory distress, pulmonary edema, fibrosis, and desquamation of the bronchiolar epithelium. Neurologic manifestations include tremors, emotional lability, and polyneuropathy. Chronic exposure to metallic mercury produces intention tremor and erethism (excitability, memory loss, insomnia, timidity, and sometimes delirium); acute high-dose ingestion of metallic mercury may lead to hematemesis and abdominal pain, acute renal failure, and cardiovascular collapse. Organic mercury compounds can cause a neurotoxicity characterized by paresthesia; impaired vision, hearing, taste, and smell; unsteadiness of gait; weakness; memory loss; and depression. Exposed mothers give birth to infants with mental retardation and multiple neurologic derangements.

Treatment acutely involves emesis or gastric lavage followed by the oral administration of polythiol resins to bind mercury in the GI tract. Chelating agents include dimercaprol, succimer, and penicillamine. Acute poisoning is treated with dimercaprol in divided doses IM, not exceeding 24 mg/kg per day; 5-day courses are usually separated by rest periods. Peritoneal dialysis, hemodialysis, and extracorporeal hemodialysis with succimer have been used for renal failure. Chronic inorganic mercury poisoning is best treated with acetyl penicillamine.

METHANOL   Methanol is a component of shellacs, varnishes, paint removers, Sterno, windshield-washer solutions, copy machine fluid, and denaturants for ethanol. It is metabolized to formic acid, which causes metabolic acidosis. Manifestations begin within $1-2$ h of ingestion and include nausea, vomiting, abdominal pain, headache, vertigo, confusion, obtundation, and ethanol-like intoxication. Late manifestations are due to formic acid and include an anion-gap metabolic acidosis, coma, seizures, and death. Ophthalmic manifestations $15-19$ h after ingestion include clouding, diminished acuity, dancing and flashing spots, dilated or fixed pupils, hyperemia of the disc, retinal edema, and blindness. An osmol gap is often present.

Gastric aspiration should be undertaken. Activated charcoal is not effective. Acidosis is corrected with sodium bicarbonate. Seizures respond to diazepam and phenytoin. Ethanol or fomepizole therapy (as described for ethylene glycol) is indicated in pts with visual symptoms or a methanol level > 6 mmol/L (>20 mg/dL). Therapy with ethanol is continued until the methanol level falls to <6 mmol/L. Hemodialysis is indicated when visual signs are present or when metabolic acidosis is unresponsive to sodium bicarbonate.

METHEMOGLOBINEMIA   Chemicals that oxidize ferrous hemoglobin (Fe^{2+}) to its ferric (Fe^{3+}) state include aniline, aminophenols, aminophenones, chlorates, dapsone, local anesthetics, nitrates, nitrites, nitroglycerine, naphthalene, nitrobenzene, nitrogen oxides, phenazopyridine, primiquine, and sulfonamides. Cyanosis occurs with methemoglobin levels $> 15\%$. When levels exceed $20-30\%$, symptoms include fatigue, headache, dizziness, tachycardia, and weakness. At levels $> 45\%$, dyspnea, bradycardia, hypoxia, acidosis, seizures, coma, and arrhythmias occur. Death usually occurs with levels $> 70\%$. Hemolytic anemia may lead to hyperkalemia and renal failure $1-3$ days after exposure. Cyanosis in conjunction with a normal O_2 and decreased O_2 saturation (measured by oximeter) and "chocolate brown" blood suggest the diagnosis. The chocolate color does not redden with exposure to O_2 but fades when exposed to 10% potassium cyanide.

Ingested toxins should be removed by treatment with activated charcoal. Methylene blue is indicated for methemoglobin level > 30 g/L or methemoglobinemia with hypoxia. Dosage is $1-2$ mg/kg as a 1% solution over 5 min. Additional doses may be needed. Methylene blue is contraindicated in G6PD deficiency. Administration of 100% O_2 and packed red blood cell transfusion to a hemoglobin level of 150 g/L can enhance O_2-carrying capacity of the blood. Exchange transfusions may be indicated in G6PD-deficient pts.

MUSCLE RELAXANTS   Manifestations of poisoning by carisoprodol, chlorphenesin, chlorzoxazone, and methocarbamol include nausea, vomiting, dizziness, headache, nystagmus, hypotonia, and CNS depression. Cyclobenzaprine and orphenadrine cause agitation, hallucinations, seizures, stupor, coma, and hypotension. Orphenadrine can also cause ventricular tachyarrhythmias. Baclofen causes CNS depression, hypothermia, excitability, delirium, myoclonus, seizures, conduction abnormalities, arrhythmias, and hypotension.

Prompt GI decontamination, single-dose activated charcoal (repeated for baclofen overdose), and cathartics are indicated. Physostigmine (1–2 mg IV over 2–5 min) is useful for anticholinergic effects.

NEUROLEPTICS   The phenothiazines chlorpromazine, fluphenazine, mesoridazine, perphenazine, prochlorperazine, promazine, promethazine, and thioridazine and pharmacologically similar agents such as haloperidol, loxapine, pimozide, and thiothixene are CNS depressants and can cause lethargy, obtundation, respiratory depression, and coma. Pupils are often constricted. Hypothermia, hypotension, SVT, AV block, arrhythmias (including torsades de pointes), prolongation of PR, QRS, and QT intervals, and T-wave abnormalities are seen. Malignant neuroleptic syndrome occurs rarely. Acute dystonic reaction symptoms include rigidity, opisthotonos, stiff neck, hyperreflexia, irritability, dystonia, fixed speech, torticollis, tremors, trismus, and oculogyric crisis.

Treatment of overdose includes GI decontamination with activated charcoal. Seizures should be treated with benzodiazepines; hypotension responds to volume expansion and α agonists. Sodium bicarbonate is given for metabolic acidosis. Avoid the use of procainamide, quinidine, or any agent that prolongs cardiac repolarization. Acute dystonic reactions respond to diphenhydramine (1–2 mg/kg IV) or benztropine (1–2 mg). Doses may be repeated in 20 min if necessary.

ORGANOPHOSPHATE AND CARBAMATE INSECTICIDES   Organophosphates (chlorpyrifos, phosphorothioic acid, dichlorvos, fenthion, malathion, parathion, sarin, and numerous others) irreversibly inhibit acetylcholinesterase and cause accumulation of acetylcholine at muscarinic and nicotinic synapses. Carbamates (carbaryl, aldicarb, propoxur, and bendicarb) reversibly inhibit acetylcholinesterase; therapeutic carbonates include ambenonium, neostigmine, physostigmine, and pyridostigmine. Both types are absorbed through the skin, lungs, and GI tract and produce nausea, vomiting, abdominal cramps, urinary and fecal incontinence, increased bronchial secretions, coughing, sweating, salivation, lacrimation, and miosis; carbamates are shorter acting. Bradycardia, conduction blocks, hypotension, twitching, fasciculations, weakness, respiratory depression, seizures, confusion, and coma may result. A decrease in cholinesterase activity $\geq$50% in plasma or red cells is diagnostic.

Treatment begins with washing exposed surfaces with soap and water and, in cases of ingestion, GI decontamination, then activated charcoal. Atropine, 0.5–2 mg is given IV q15min until complete atropinization is achieved (dry mouth). Pralidoxime (2-PAM), 1–2 g IV over several minutes, can be repeated q8h until nicotinic symptoms resolve. Use of 2-PAM in carbamate poisoning is controversial. Seizures should be treated with benzodiazepines.

SALICYLATES   Poisoning with salicylates causes vomiting, tachycardia, hyperpnea, fever, tinnitus, lethargy, and confusion. Severe poisoning can result in seizures, coma, respiratory and cardiovascular failure, cerebral edema, and renal failure. Respiratory alkalosis is commonly coupled with metabolic acidosis (40–50%), but respiratory alkalosis (20%) and metabolic acidosis (20%) can occur separately. Lactic and other organic acids are responsible for the increased anion gap. PT may be prolonged. Salicylates in blood or urine can be detected by ferric chloride test. Levels > 2.2 mmol/L (30 mg/dL) are associated with toxicity.

Treatment includes repeated administration of activated charcoal for up to 24 h. Forced alkaline diuresis (urine pH > 8.0) increases excretion and decreases serum half-life. Seizures can be controlled with diazepam or phenobarbital. Hemodialysis should be considered in pts who fail conventional therapy or have cerebral edema or hepatic or renal failure.

SEROTONIN SYNDROME   This syndrome is due to excessive CNS and peripheral serotonergic (5HT-1a and possibly 5HT-2) activity and results from the concomitant use of agents that promote the release of serotonin from presynaptic neurons [e.g., amphetamines, cocaine, codeine, methylenedioxy-methamphetamine, or MDMA (Ecstasy), reserpine, some MAO inhibitors], inhibit its reuptake (e.g., cyclic antidepressants, particularly the SSRIs, ergot derivatives, dextromethorphan, meperidine, pentacozine, sumatriptan and related agents, tramadol, some MAO inhibitors) or metabolism (e.g., cocaine, MAO inhibitors), or stimulate postsynaptic serotonin receptors (e.g., bromocryptine, bupropion, buspirone, levodopa, lithium, L-tryptophan, LSD, mescaline, trazodone). Less often, it results from the use or overdose of a single serotonergic agent or when one agent is taken soon after another has been discontinued (up to 2 weeks for some agents).

Manifestations include altered mental status (agitation, confusion, delirium, mutism, coma, and seizures), neuromuscular hyperactivity (restlessness, incoordination, hyperreflexia, myoclonus, rigidity, and tremors), and autonomic dysfunction (abdominal pain, diarrhea, diaphoresis, fever, elevated and fluctuating blood pressure, flushed skin, mydriasis, tearing, salivation, shivering, and tachycardia). Complications include hyperthermia, lactic acidosis, rhabdomyolysis, kidney and liver failure, ARDS, and DIC.

Gastrointestinal decontamination may be indicated for acute overdose. Supportive measures include hydration with intravenous fluids, airway protection and mechanical ventilation, benzodiazepines (and paralytics, if necessary) for neuromuscular hyperactivity, and mechanical cooling measures for hyperthermia. Cyproheptadine (Periactin), an antihistamine with 5HT-1a and 5HT-2 receptor blocking activity, and chlorpromazine (Thorazine), a nonspecific serotonin receptor antagonist, have been used with success. Cyproheptadine is given orally or by gastric tube in an initial dose of 4 to 8 mg and repeated as necessary every 2 to 4 h up to a maximum of 32 mg in 24 h. Chlorpromazine can be given parenterally (intramuscularly or by slow IV injection in doses of 50 to 100 mg).

SYMPATHOMIMETICS   Amphetamines; bronchodilators such as albuterol and metaproterenol; decongestants such as ephedrine, pseudoephedrine, phenylephrine, and phenylpropanolamines; and cocaine can cause nausea, vomiting, diarrhea, abdominal cramps, irritability, confusion, delirium, euphoria, auditory and visual hallucinations, tremors, hyperreflexia, seizures, palpitations, tachycardia, hypertension, arrhythmias, and cardiovascular collapse. Sympathomimetic symptoms include dilated pupils, dry mouth, pallor, flushing of skin, and tachypnea. Severe manifestations include hyperpyrexia, seizures, rhabdomyolysis, hypertensive crisis, intracranial hemorrhage, cardiac arrhythmias, and cardiovascular collapse. Rhabdomyolysis and intracranial hemorrhage can occur.

Activated charcoal is preferred for GI decontamination. Seizures are treated with benzodiazepines; hypertension with a nonselective beta blocker or the α-adrenergic antagonist phentolamine (1 to 5 mg IV q5min); fever with salicylates; and agitation with sedatives and, if necessary, paralyzing agents. Propranolol is useful for tachycardia.

THALLIUM Thallium is used as insecticide, in fireworks, in manufacturing, as an alloy, and in cardiac imaging, and epidemic poisoning has occurred with ingestion of grain contaminated with thallium. Acute manifestations include nausea and vomiting, abdominal pain, bloody diarrhea, and hematemesis. Subsequent manifestations include confusion, psychosis, choreoathetosis, organic brain syndrome, convulsions, coma, and sensory and motor neuropathy; autonomic nervous system effects include tachycardia, hypertension, and salivation. Optic neuritis, ophthalmoplegia, ptosis, strabismus, and cranial nerve palsies may occur. Late effects include diffuse hair loss, memory defects, ataxia, tremor, and foot drop.

Treatment includes GI decontamination by lavage or ipecac syrup and cathartics, forced diuresis with furosemide and KCl supplements, and either peritoneal dialysis, hemodialysis, or charcoal hemoperfusion. Prussian blue (250 g/kg) prevents absorption.

THEOPHYLLINE Theophylline, caffeine, and other methylxanthines are phosphodiesterase inhibitors that reduce the degradation of cyclic AMP, thereby enhancing the actions of endogenous catecholamines. Vomiting, restlessness, irritability, agitation, tachypnea, tachycardia, and tremors are common. Coma and respiratory depression, generalized tonic-clonic and partial seizures, atrial arrhythmias, ventricular arrhythmias, and fibrillation can occur. Rhabdomyolysis with acute renal failure develops occasionally. Laboratory abnormalities include ketosis, metabolic acidosis, elevated amylase, hyperglycemia, and decreased potassium, calcium, and phosphorus.

Treatment requires prompt administration of activated charcoal every 2–4 h for 12–24 h after ingestion. Tachyarrhythmias are treated with propranolol; hypotension requires volume expansion. Seizures are treated with benzodiazepines and barbiturates; phenytoin is ineffective. Indications for hemodialysis and hemoperfusion with acute ingestion include a serum level > 500 μmol/L (>100 mg/L) and with chronic ingestion a serum level > 200–300 μmol/L (>40–60 mg/L). Dialysis is also indicated in pts with lower serum levels who have refractory seizures or arrhythmias.

For a more detailed discussion, see Linden CH, Burns MJ: Poisoning and Drug Overdosage, Chap. 377, p. 2580; and Hu H: Heavy Metal Poisoning, Chap. 376, p. 2577, in HPIM-16.

24

DIABETIC KETOACIDOSIS AND HYPEROSMOLAR COMA

Diabetic ketoacidosis (DKA) and hyperglycemic hyperosmolar state (HHS) are acute complications of diabetes mellitus (DM). DKA is seen primarily in individuals with type 1 DM and HHS in individuals with type 2 DM. Both disorders are associated with absolute or relative insulin deficiency, volume depletion, and altered mental status. The metabolic similarities and differences in DKA and HHS are summarized in Table 24-1.

DIABETIC KETOACIDOSIS

ETIOLOGY   DKA results from insulin deficiency with a relative or absolute increase in glucagon and may be caused by inadequate insulin administration, infection (pneumonia, UTI, gastroenteritis, sepsis), infarction (cerebral, coronary, mesenteric, peripheral), surgery, drugs (cocaine), or pregnancy.

CLINICAL FEATURES   The initial symptoms of DKA include anorexia, nausea, vomiting, polyuria, and thirst. Abdominal pain, altered mental function, or frank coma may ensue. Classic signs of DKA include Kussmaul respirations and an acetone odor on the pt's breath. Volume depletion can lead to dry mucous membranes, tachycardia, and hypotension. Fever and abdominal tenderness may also be present. Laboratory evaluation reveals hyperglycemia, ketosis (β-hydroxybutyrate > acetoacetate), and metabolic acidosis (arterial pH 6.8–7.3) with an increased anion gap (Table 24-1). The fluid deficit is often 3–5 L. Despite a total-body potassium deficit, the serum potassium at presentation may

Table 24-1

Laboratory Values in Diabetic Ketoacidosis (DKA) and Hyperglycemic Hyperosmolar State (HHS) (Representative Ranges at Presentation)

	DKA	HHS
Glucose,[a] mmol/L (mg/dL)	13.9–33.3 (250–600)	33.3–66.6 (600–1200)
Sodium, meq/L	125–135	135–145
Potassium,[a] meq/L	Normal to ↑[b]	Normal
Magnesium[a]	Normal[b]	Normal
Chloride[a]	Normal	Normal
Phosphate[a]	↓	Normal
Creatinine, μmol/L (mg/dL)	Slightly ↑	Moderately ↑
Osmolality (mOsm/mL)	300–320	330–380
Plasma ketones[a]	++++	+/−
Serum bicarbonate,[a] meq/L	<15 meq/L	Normal to slightly ↓
Arterial pH	6.8–7.3	>7.3
Arterial P_{CO_2},[a] mmHg	20–30	Normal
Anion gap[a] [Na − (Cl + HCO₃)], meq/L	↑	Normal to slightly ↑

[a] Large changes occur during treatment of DKA.
[b] Although plasma levels may be normal or high at presentation, total-body stores are usually depleted.

be normal or mildly high as a result of acidosis. Leukocytosis, hypertriglycer-idemia, and hyperlipoproteinemia are common. Hyperamylasemia is usually of salivary origin but may suggest a diagnosis of pancreatitis. The measured serum sodium is reduced as a consequence of hyperglycemia (1.6-meq reduction for each 100-mg/dL rise in the serum glucose).

 TREATMENT

The management of DKA is outlined in Table 24-2.

HYPERGLYCEMIC HYPEROSMOLAR STATE

ETIOLOGY   Relative insulin deficiency and inadequate fluid intake are the underlying causes of HHS. Hyperglycemia induces an osmotic diuresis that

Table 24-2

Management of Diabetic Ketoacidosis

1. Confirm diagnosis (↑ plasma glucose, positive serum ketones, metabolic acidosis).
2. Admit to hospital; intensive-care setting may be necessary for frequent monitoring or if pH < 7.00 or unconscious.
3. Assess: Serum electrolytes (K^+, Na^+, Mg^{2+}, Cl^-, bicarbonate, phosphate)
   Acid-base status—pH, HCO_3^-, P_{CO_2}, β-hydroxybutyrate
   Renal function (creatinine, urine output)
4. Replace fluids: 2–3 L of 0.9% saline over first 1–3 h (5–10 mL/kg per hour); subsequently, 0.45% saline at 150–300 mL/h; change to 5% glucose and 0.45% saline at 100–200 mL/h when plasma glucose reaches 14 mmol/L, (250 mg/dL).
5. Administer regular insulin: IV (0.1 units/kg) or IM (0.4 units/kg), then 0.1 units/kg per hour by continuous IV infusion; increase 2- to 10-fold if no response by 2–4 h. If initial serum potassium is < 3.3 mmol/L (3.3 meq/L), do not administer insulin until the potassium is corrected to > 3.3 mmol/L (3.3.meq/L).
6. Assess patient: What precipitated the episode (noncompliance, infection, trauma, infarction, cocaine)? Initiate appropriate workup for precipitating event (cultures, CXR, ECG).
7. Measure capillary glucose every 1–2 h; measure electrolytes (especially K^+, bicarbonate, phosphate) and anion gap every 4 h for first 24 h.
8. Monitor blood pressure, pulse, respirations, mental status, fluid intake and output every 1–4 h.
9. Replace K^+: 10 meq/h when plasma K^+ < 5.5 meq/L, ECG normal, urine flow and normal creatinine documented; administer 40–80 meq/h when plasma K^+ <3.5 meq/L or if bicarbonate is given.
10. Continue above until patient is stable, glucose goal is 150–250 mg/dL, and acidosis is resolved. Insulin infusion may be decreased to 0.05–0.1 units/kg per hour.
11. Administer intermediate or long-acting insulin as soon as patient is eating. Allow for overlap in insulin infusion and subcutaneous insulin injection.

Note: CXR, chest x-ray; ECG, electrocardiogram.
Source: Adapted from M Sperling, in *Therapy for Diabetes Mellitus and Related Disorders*, American Diabetes Association, Alexandria, VA, 1998; and AE Kitabchi et al: Diabetes Care 24:131, 2001.

leads to profound intravascular volume depletion. HHS is often precipitated by a serious, concurrent illness such as myocardial infarction or sepsis and compounded by conditions that impede access to water.

CLINICAL FEATURES Presenting symptoms include polyuria, thirst, and altered mental state, ranging from lethargy to coma. Notably absent are symptoms of nausea, vomiting, and abdominal pain and the Kussmaul respirations characteristic of DKA. The prototypical pt is an elderly individual with a several week history of polyuria, weight loss, and diminished oral intake. The laboratory features are summarized in Table 24-1. In contrast to DKA, acidosis and ketonemia are usually not found; however, a small anion gap may be due to lactic acidosis, and moderate ketonuria may occur from starvation. Though the measured serum sodium may be normal or slightly low, the corrected serum sodium is usually increased (add 1.6 meq to measured sodium for each 100-mg/dL rise in the serum glucose).

℞ TREATMENT

The precipitating problem should be sought and treated. Sufficient IV fluids (1–3 L of 0.9% normal saline over the first 2–3 h) must be given to stabilize the hemodynamic status. The calculated free water deficit (usually 8–10 L) should be reversed over the next 1–2 days, using 0.45% saline initially then 5% dextrose in water. Potassium repletion is usually necessary. The plasma glucose may drop precipitously with hydration alone, though insulin therapy with an intravenous bolus of 5–10 units followed by a constant infusion rate (3–7 units/h) is usually required. Glucose should be added to intravenous fluid when the plasma glucose falls to 13.9 mmol/L (250 mg/dL). The insulin infusion should be continued until the patient has resumed eating and can be transitioned to a subcutaneous insulin regimen.

For a more detailed discussion, see Powers AC: Diabetes Mellitus, Chap. 323, p. 2152, in HPIM-16.

25

HYPOGLYCEMIA

Glucose is an obligate metabolic fuel for the brain. Hypoglycemia should be considered in any patient with confusion, altered level of consciousness, or seizures. Counterregulatory responses to hypoglycemia include insulin suppression and the release of catecholamines, glucagon, growth hormone, and cortisol.

The laboratory diagnosis of hypoglycemia is usually defined as a plasma glucose level <2.5–2.8 mmol/L (<45–50 mg/dL), although the absolute glucose level at which symptoms occur varies among individuals. For this reason,

Whipple's triad should be present: (1) symptoms consistent with hypoglycemia, (2) a low plasma glucose concentration, and (3) relief of symptoms after the plasma glucose level is raised.

Etiology

Hypoglycemia occurs most commonly as a result of treating patients with diabetes mellitus. However, a number of other disorders are also associated with hypoglycemia, and it is useful to divide these into those associated with fasting or the postprandial state.

1. Fasting:
   a. *Underproduction of glucose*: hormone deficiencies (hypopituitarism and adrenal insufficiency), inherited enzyme defects, hepatic failure, renal failure, hypothermia, and drugs (ethanol, beta blockers, and rarely salicylates).
   b. *Overutilization of glucose*: hyperinsulinism (exogenous insulin, sulfonylureas, insulin or insulin receptor antibodies, insulinoma, endotoxic shock, renal failure, and use of pentamidine, quinine, or disopyramide) and with appropriate insulin levels but increased levels of insulin-like growth factors such as IGF-II (mesenchymal or other extrapancreatic tumors and prolonged starvation).
2. Postprandial (reactive): after gastric surgery and in children with rare enzymatic defects.

Clinical Features

Symptoms of hypoglycemia can be divided into autonomic (adrenergic: palpitations, tremor, and anxiety; and cholinergic: sweating, hunger, and paresthesia) and neuroglycopenic (behavioral changes, confusion, fatigue, seizure, loss of consciousness, and, if hypoglycemia is severe and prolonged, death). Tachycardia, elevated systolic blood pressure, pallor, and diaphoresis may be present on physical examination.

Recurrent hypoglycemia shifts thresholds for the autonomic symptoms and counterregulatory responses to lower glucose levels, leading to hypoglycemic unawareness. Under these circumstances, the first manifestation of hypoglycemia is neuroglycopenia, placing patients at risk of being unable treat themselves.

Diagnosis

Diagnosis of the hypoglycemic mechanism is critical for choosing a treatment that prevents recurrent hypoglycemia (Fig. 25-1). Urgent treatment is often necessary in patients with suspected hypoglycemia. Nevertheless, blood should be drawn at the time of symptoms, whenever possible before the administration of glucose, to allow documentation of the glucose level. If the glucose level is low and the cause of hypoglycemia is unknown, additional assays should be performed on blood obtained at the time of a low plasma glucose. These should include insulin, C-peptide, sulfonylurea levels, cortisol, and ethanol. In the absence of documented spontaneous hypoglycemia, overnight fasting or food deprivation during observation in the outpatient setting will sometimes elicit hypoglycemia and allow diagnostic evaluation. An extended (up to 72 h) fast under careful supervision in the hospital may otherwise be required—the test should be terminated if plasma glucose drops below 2.5 mmol/L (45 mg/dL) and the patient has symptoms.

Interpretation of fasting test results is shown in Table 25-1.

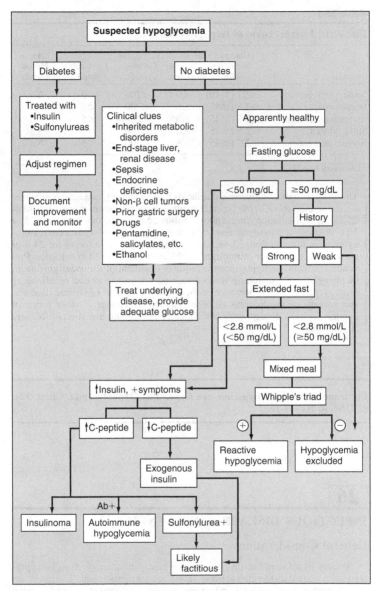

FIGURE 25-1 Diagnostic approach to a patient with suspected hypoglycemia based on a history of symptoms, a low plasma glucose concentration, or both.

Rx **TREATMENT**

The syndrome of hypoglycemic unawareness in patients with diabetes mellitus is reversible after as little as 2 weeks of scrupulous avoidance of hypoglycemia.

Table 25-1

Diagnostic Interpretation of Hypoglycemia

Diagnosis	Glucose, mmol/L (mg/dL)	Insulin, μU/mL	C-Peptide, pmol/L	Proinsulin, pmol/L	Urine or Plasma Sulfonylurea
Nonhypoglycemic	≥2.2 (≥40)	<6	<200	<5	No
Insulinoma	≤2.5 (≤45)	≥6	≥200	≥5	No
Exogenous insulin	≤2.5 (≤45)	≥6[a]	<200	<5	No
Sulfonylurea	≤2.5 (≤45)	≥6	≥200	≥5	Yes
Non-insulin mediated	≤2.5 (≤45)	<6	<200	<5	No

[a] Often very high.

This involves a shift of glycemic thresholds back to higher glucose concentrations.

Acute therapy of hypoglycemia requires administration of oral glucose or 25 g of a 50% solution intravenously followed by a constant infusion of 5 or 10% dextrose if parenteral therapy is necessary. Hypoglycemia from sulfonylureas is often prolonged, requiring treatment and monitoring for 24 h or more. Subcutaneous or intramuscular glucagon can be used in diabetics. Prevention of recurrent hypoglycemia requires treatment of the underlying cause of hypoglycemia, including discontinuation or dose reduction of offending drugs, replacement of hormonal deficiencies, treatment of critical illnesses, and surgery of insulinomas or other tumors. Treatment of other forms of hypoglycemia is dietary, with avoidance of fasting and ingestion of frequent small meals.

For a more detailed discussion, see Cryer PE: Hypoglycemia, Chap. 324, p. 2180, in HPIM-16.

26

INFECTIOUS DISEASE EMERGENCIES

General Considerations

• Acutely ill infected febrile pts requiring emergent attention must be appropriately evaluated and treated at presentation to improve outcome. The physician should quickly assess general appearance to gain a subjective sense of whether the pt is septic or toxic.
• *History*: The physician should assess:
   Onset and duration of symptoms, changes in severity or rate of progression over time
   Host factors (e.g., alcoholism, IV drug use) and comorbid conditions (e.g., asplenia, diabetes)
   Potential nidus for invasive infection (e.g., URI or influenza, trauma, burn, foreign body)

Exposure history (e.g., travel, pets, diet, medication use, sick contacts, menstruation history, sexual contacts)

- *Physical examination*
  General appearance (e.g., agitation or lethargy, vital signs)
  Special attention to skin and soft tissue examination, neurologic examination, assessment of mental status
- *Diagnostic workup*
  Bloodwork: cultures, CBC with differential, electrolytes, renal function tests, LFTs, blood smear examination, buffy coat
  CSF cultures if meningitis is possible. With focal neurologic signs, papilledema, or abnormal mental status, obtain blood cultures, begin antibiotics, perform brain imaging, and then consider LP.
  CT or MRI to evaluate focal abscesses; cultures of wounds or scraping of skin lesions as indicated. No diagnostic procedure should delay treatment for more than minutes.
- *Treatment*
  See Table 26-1. Urgent surgical attention may be indicated.

Specific Presentations (Table 26-1)

Sepsis without an Obvious Focus of Primary Infection Nonspecific symptoms and signs progressing rapidly to hypotension, tachycardia, tachypnea, altered mental status, and/or DIC

1. Septic shock: primary site not initially identified, bacteremia and shock evident
2. Overwhelming infection in asplenic pts
   a. The risk of severe sepsis remains increased throughout life, but 50–70% of cases occur in the first 2 years after splenectomy.
   b. *Streptococcus pneumoniae* is the most common etiologic agent, with mortality rates up to 80%.
3. Babesiosis: history of travel to endemic areas, tick bite 1–4 weeks previously
   a. Asplenia and age >60 years are risk factors for severe disease.
   b. *Babesia microti* is transmitted by *Ixodes scapularis*, the tick that also transmits *Borrelia burgdorferi* (Lyme disease) and ehrlichiae. Co-infections can result in more severe disease.
   c. European strain, *B. divergens*, causes more fulminant disease.
   d. Symptoms are nonspecific fever, chills, anorexia, headache, myalgias that can progress to hemolysis, jaundice, and renal and respiratory failure.
4. Other sepsis syndromes
   a. Tularemia (associated with wild rabbit, tick, and tabanid fly contact) and plague (associated with contact with squirrels, prairie dogs, chipmunks); also category A agents of bioterrorism
   b. Mortality rates for typhoidal or septic forms of these infections are ~30%.

Sepsis with Skin Manifestations

1. Maculopapular rashes: usually not emergent but seen in early meningococcemia and rickettsial disease. Primary HIV infection can present with rash; early recognition and treatment can improve prognosis.
2. Petechiae
   a. Meningococcemia: young children at greatest risk; outbreaks in schools and army barracks
      Headache, nausea, myalgias, altered mental status, meningismus
      Petechiae begin at ankles, wrists, axillae, and mucosal surfaces and progress to purpura and DIC.

Table 26-1

Common Infectious Disease Emergencies

Clinical Syndrome	Possible Etiologies	Treatment	Comments	Reference Chapter(s) in HPIM-16
SEPSIS WITHOUT A CLEAR FOCUS				
Gram-negative sepsis	*Pseudomonas* spp., gram-negative enteric bacilli	Piperacillin/tazobactam (3.75 g q4h) **plus** Tobramycin (5 mg/kg per day)	See Chap. 254, HPIM-16.	136, 254
Gram-positive sepsis	*Staphylococcus* spp., *Streptococcus* spp.	*or* Ceftazidime (2 g q8h) **plus** Vancomycin (1 g q12h) **plus** Gentamicin (5 mg/kg per day)	If a β-lactam-sensitive strain is identified, antibiotics should be altered.	120, 121, 254
Overwhelming post-splenectomy sepsis	*Streptococcus pneumoniae, Haemophilus influenzae, Neisseria meningitidis*	Ceftriaxone (2 g q12h)[a]	If the isolate is penicillin-sensitive, penicillin is the drug of choice.	254
Babesiosis	*Babesia microti* (U.S.), *B. divergens* (Europe)	*Either:* Clindamycin (600 mg tid) **plus** Quinine (650 mg tid) *or* Atovaquone (750 mg q12h) **plus** Azithromycin (500-mg loading dose, then 250 mg/d)	Atovaquone and azithromycin have been shown to be as effective as clindamycin and quinine and are associated with fewer side effects. Treatment with doxycycline (100 mg bid) for potential coinfection with *Borrelia burgdorferi* or *Ehrlichia* spp. may be prudent.	193, 195

SEPSIS WITH SKIN FINDINGS

Petechiae: Meningococcemia	*N. meningitidis*	Penicillin (4 mU q4h) *or* Ceftriaxone (2 g q12h)	Consider protein C replacement in fulminant meningococcemia.	127, 158
Rocky Mountain spotted fever	*Rickettsia rickettsii*	Doxycycline (100 mg bid)	If both meningococcemia and Rocky Mountain spotted fever are being considered, use chloramphenicol (50–75 mg/kg per day in four divided doses). *Do not add doxycycline to a regimen including a β-lactam agent.* If Rocky Mountain spotted fever is diagnosed, doxycycline is the proven superior agent.	
Purpura fulminans	*S. pneumoniae, H. influenzae, N. meningitidis*	Ceftriaxone (2 g q12h)[a]	If the isolate is penicillin-sensitive, penicillin is the drug of choice.	127, 254
Erythroderma: toxic shock syndrome	Group A *Streptococcus*, *Staphylococcus aureus*	Penicillin (2 mU q4h) *or* Oxacillin (2 g q4h) *plus* Clindamycin (600 mg q8h)	Site of toxigenic bacteria should be debrided; if necessary, intravenous immunoglobulin can be used in severe cases. The optimal dose of IVIg has not been determined, but the median dose in observational studies is 2 g/kg (total dose administered over 1–5 days).	120, 121

(continued)

Table 26-1 (*Continued*)

Common Infectious Disease Emergencies

Clinical Syndrome	Possible Etiologies	Treatment	Comments	Reference Chapter(s) in HPIM-16
SEPSIS WITH SOFT TISSUE FINDINGS				
Necrotizing fasciitis	Group A *Streptococcus*, mixed aerobic/anaerobic flora	Penicillin (2 mU q4h) *plus* Clindamycin (600 mg q8h) *plus* Gentamicin (5 mg/kg per day)	Urgent surgical evaluation is critical.	110, 121
Clostridial myonecrosis	*Clostridium perfringens*	Penicillin (2 mU q4h) *plus* Clindamycin (600 mg q8h)	Urgent surgical evaluation is critical.	126
NEUROLOGIC INFECTIONS				
Bacterial meningitis	*S. pneumoniae, N. meningitidis*	Ceftriaxone (2 g q12h)[a]	If the isolate is penicillin-sensitive, penicillin is the drug of choice. If the pt is >50 years old, add ampicillin for *Listeria* coverage. Dexamethasone (10 mg q6h × 4 days) improves outcome in adult pts with meningitis (especially that due to *S. pneumoniae*) and cloudy CSF, positive CSF Gram's stain, or CSF leukocyte count >1000/μL.	360
Suppurative intracranial infections	*Staphylococcus* spp., *Streptococcus* spp., anaerobes, gram-negative bacilli	Oxacillin (2 g q4h)[b] *plus* Metronidazole (500 mg tid) *plus* Ceftriaxone (2 g q12h)	Urgent surgical evaluation is critical.	360

98

Brain abscess	Streptococcus spp., anaerobes, Staphylococcus spp.	Penicillin (4 mU q4h) **or** Oxacillin (2 g q4h)[b] **plus** Metronidazole (500 mg tid)	Surgical evaluation is essential.	360
Cerebral malaria	Plasmodium falciparum	Quinine (650 mg tid for 3 days) **plus** Tetracycline (250 mg tid for 7 days)	Do not use glucocorticoids.	193, 195
Spinal epidural abscess	Staphylococcus spp.	Oxacillin (2 g q4h)[c]	Surgical evaluation is essential.	356

FOCAL INFECTIONS

Acute bacterial endocarditis	S. aureus, β-hemolytic streptococci, HACEK group,[d] Neisseria spp., S. pneumoniae	Ceftriaxone (2 g q12h) **plus** Vancomycin (1 g q12h)	Adjust treatment when culture data become available. Surgical evaluation is essential.	109

[a] If resistant pneumococci are prevalent, add vancomycin (1 g q12h).

[b] Vancomycin (1 g q12h) should replace oxacillin if methicillin-resistant strains are highly prevalent.

[c] In HIV-infected IV drug users with suspected spinal epidural abscess, empirical therapy must cover gram-negative rods and methicillin-resistant S. aureus.

[d] Haemophilus aphrophilus, H. paraphrophilus, H. parainfluenzae, Actinobacillus actinomycetemcomitans, Cardiobacterium hominis, Eikenella corrodens, and Kingella kingae.

Mortality rates exceed 90% among pts without meningitis, with rash, hypotension, and normal/low WBC count and ESR.
   b. Rocky Mountain spotted fever: history of tick bite and/or travel or outdoor activity
      Headache, malaise, myalgias, nausea, vomiting, anorexia
      By day 3, blanching macules that become hemorrhagic, starting at wrists and ankles and spreading to legs and trunk, then palms and soles
      Hypotension, noncardiogenic pulmonary edema, confusion, lethargy, encephalitis, coma in progressive disease
   c. Purpura fulminans: cutaneous manifestation of DIC; large ecchymotic areas and hemorrhagic bullae; associated with CHF, septic shock, acute renal failure, acidosis
3. Ecthyma gangrenosum: hemorrhagic vesicles with central necrosis and ulceration in septic shock with *Pseudomonas aeruginosa* or *Aeromonas hydrophila*
4. Other emergent infections associated with rash
   a. *Vibrio vulnificus* and other noncholera vibrios: bacteremic infections and sepsis after contaminated shellfish ingestion, typically in hosts with liver disease. Skin findings: lower-extremity bullous or hemorrhagic lesions
   b. *Capnocytophaga canimorsus*: septic shock in asplenic pts, typically after dog bite. Skin manifestations: exanthem, erythema multiforme, peripheral cyanosis, petechiae
5. Erythroderma: diffuse sunburn-like rash that desquamates after 1–2 weeks; hypotension; multiorgan failure; renal failure (may precede hypotension)
   a. *Staphylococcus aureus* toxic shock syndrome (TSS): usually no primary focal infection, colonization of vagina or postoperative wound, 5–15% mortality
   b. Streptococcal TSS: less frequent desquamation, 30–70% mortality

Sepsis with a Soft Tissue/Muscle Primary Focus

1. Necrotizing fasciitis
   a. Can arise at site of minimal trauma, postoperative incision, varicella
   b. Risk factors: diabetes, peripheral vascular disease, IV drug use, NSAID use in setting of soft tissue infection
   c. Bacteremia, hypotension, physical findings minimal compared to degree of pain, fever, toxicity; infected area red, hot, shiny, exquisitely tender
   d. Progression to bullae, necrosis; decrease in pain due to peripheral nerve destruction an ominous sign
   e. Mortality: 100% without surgery, 70% in setting of TSS, 30% overall
2. Clostridial myonecrosis
   a. Either secondary to trauma or surgery or spontaneous (associated with *Clostridium septicum* infection and underlying malignancy)
   b. Massive necrotizing gangrene, toxicity, shock, death within hours
   c. Pain and toxicity out of proportion to physical findings. Pts are apathetic, tachycardic, and tachypneic, with a sense of impending doom.
   d. Mottled, bronze-colored overlying skin or bullous lesions; drainage with mousy or sweet odor; crepitus
   e. Mortality: 12% (extremity myonecrosis) to 63–65% (trunk or spontaneous myonecrosis)

Neurologic Infections with or without Septic Shock

1. Bacterial meningitis
   a. Classic triad of headache, meningismus, and fever in one-half to two-thirds of pts

   b. Blood cultures positive in 50–60% of pts
   c. Mortality associated with coma, respiratory distress, shock, CSF protein >2.5 g/L, peripheral WBC count <5000/μL, serum Na level <135 mmol/L
2. Brain abscess
   a. Often without systemic signs, can present as space-occupying lesion
   b. Headache, focal neurologic signs, papilledema
   c. From contiguous foci or hematogenous infection (e.g., endocarditis)
3. Spinal epidural abscesses
   a. Risk factors: diabetes, IV drug use, chronic alcohol use, spinal trauma or surgery, epidural anesthesia
   b. Thoracic or lumbar spine most common sites
   c. Back pain, neurologic deficits, fever, elevated ESR and WBC counts

Focal Syndromes with a Fulminant Course

1. Rhinocerebral mucormycosis
   a. Risk factors: diabetes, malignancy
   b. Low-grade fever, dull sinus pain, diplopia, decreased mental status, chemosis, proptosis, hard-palate lesions that respect the midline
2. Acute bacterial endocarditis
   a. Risk factors: malignancy, diabetes, IV drug use, alcoholism
   b. Rapid onset, changing murmur, CHF
   c. Rapid valvular destruction, pulmonary edema, hypotension, myocardial abscesses, conduction abnormalities and arrhythmias, large friable vegetations, major arterial emboli with tissue infarction
3. Inhalational anthrax: *Bacillus anthracis*, category A agent of bioterrorism
   a. Malaise, fever, cough, nausea, sweats, shortness of breath, headache
   b. CXR: mediastinal widening, pulmonary infiltrates, pleural effusions

---

For a more detailed discussion, see Barlam TF, Kasper DL: Approach to the Acutely Ill Infected Febrile Patient, Chap. 106, p. 706, in HPIM-16.

27

ONCOLOGIC EMERGENCIES

Emergencies in the cancer pt may be classified into three categories: effects from tumor expansion, metabolic or hormonal effects mediated by tumor products, and treatment complications.

STRUCTURAL/OBSTRUCTIVE ONCOLOGIC EMERGENCIES

The most common problems are: superior vena cava syndrome; pericardial effusion/tamponade, spinal cord compression; seizures (Chap. 185) and/or increased intracranial pressure; and intestinal, urinary, or biliary obstruction. The last three conditions are discussed in Chap. 88 in HPIM-16.

SUPERIOR VENA CAVA SYNDROME Obstruction of the superior vena cava reduces venous return from the head, neck, and upper extremities.

About 85% of cases are due to lung cancer; lymphoma and thrombosis of central venous catheters are also causes. Pts often present with facial swelling, dyspnea, and cough. In severe cases, the mediastinal mass lesion may cause tracheal obstruction. Dilated neck veins and increased collateral veins on anterior chest wall are noted on physical exam. CXR documents widening of the superior mediastinum; 25% of pts have a right-sided pleural effusion.

 TREATMENT

Radiation therapy is the treatment of choice for non-small cell lung cancer; addition of chemotherapy to radiation therapy is effective in small cell lung cancer and lymphoma. Symptoms recur in 10–30% and can be palliated by venous stenting. Clotted central catheters producing this syndrome should be withdrawn, and anticoagulation therapy initiated. Catheter clots may be prevented with warfarin, 1 mg/d.

PERICARDIAL EFFUSION/TAMPONADE Accumulation of fluid in the pericardium impairs filling of the heart and decreases cardiac output. Most commonly seen in pts with lung or breast cancers, leukemias, or lymphomas; pericardial tamponade may also develop as a late complication of mediastinal radiation therapy. Common symptoms are dyspnea, cough, chest pain, orthopnea, and weakness. Pleural effusion, sinus tachycardia, jugular venous distention, hepatomegaly, and cyanosis are frequent physical findings. Paradoxical pulse, decreased heart sounds, pulsus alternans, and friction rub are less common with malignant than nonmalignant pericardial disease. Echocardiography is diagnostic; pericardiocentesis may show serous or bloody exudate, and cytology usually shows malignant cells.

 TREATMENT

Drainage of fluid from the pericardial sac may be lifesaving until a definitive surgical procedure can be performed.

SPINAL CORD COMPRESSION Primary spinal cord tumors occur rarely, and cord compression is most commonly due to epidural metastases from vertebral bodies involved with tumor, especially from prostate, lung, breast, lymphoma, and myeloma primaries. Pts present with back pain, worse when recumbent, with local tenderness. Loss of bowel and bladder control may occur. On physical exam, pts have a loss of sensation below a horizontal line on the trunk, called a *sensory level*, that usually corresponds to one or two vertebrae below the site of compression. Weakness and spasticity of the legs and hyperactive reflexes with upgoing toes on Babinski testing are often noted. Spine radiographs may reveal erosion of the pedicles (winking owl sign), lytic or sclerotic vertebral body lesions, and vertebral collapse. Collapse alone is not a reliable indicator of tumor; it is a common manifestation of a more common disease, osteoporosis. MRI can visualize the cord throughout its length and define the extent of tumor involvement.

 TREATMENT

Radiation therapy plus dexamethasone, 4 mg IV or PO q4h, is successful in arresting and reversing symptoms in about 75% of pts who are diagnosed while still ambulatory. Only 10% of pts made paraplegic by the tumor recover the ability to ambulate.

EMERGENT PARANEOPLASTIC SYNDROMES

Most paraneoplastic syndromes have an insidious onset (Chap. 80). Hypercalcemia, syndrome of inappropriate antidiuretic hormone (SIADH), and adrenal insufficiency may present as emergencies.

HYPERCALCEMIA   The most common paraneoplastic syndrome, it occurs in about 10% of cancer pts, particularly those with lung, breast, head and neck, and kidney cancer and myeloma. Bone resorption mediated by parathormone-related protein is the most common mechanism; IL-1, IL-6, TNF, and transforming growth factor-β may act locally in tumor-involved bone. Pts usually present with nonspecific symptoms: fatigue, anorexia, constipation, weakness. Hypoalbuminemia associated with malignancy may make symptoms worse for any given serum calcium level because more calcium will be free rather than protein bound.

 TREATMENT

Saline hydration, antiresorptive agents (e.g., pamidronate, 60–90 mg IV over 4 h, or zoledronate, 4–8 mg IV) and glucocorticoids usually lower calcium levels significantly within 1–3 days. Treatment effects usually last several weeks. Treatment of the underlying malignancy is also important.

SIADH   Induced by the action of arginine vasopressin produced by certain tumors (especially small cell cancer of the lung), SIADH is characterized by hyponatremia, inappropriately concentrated urine, and high urine sodium excretion in the absence of volume depletion. Most pts with SIADH are asymptomatic. When serum sodium falls to <115 meq/L, pts may experience anorexia, depression, lethargy, irritability, confusion, weakness, and personality changes.

 TREATMENT

Water restriction controls mild forms. Demeclocycline (150–300 mg PO tid or qid) inhibits the effects of vasopressin on the renal tubule but has a slow onset of action (1 week). Treatment of the underlying malignancy is also important. If the patient has mental status changes with sodium levels <115 meq/L, normal saline infusion plus furosemide to increase free water clearance may provide more rapid improvement. Rate of correction should not exceed 0.5–1 meq/L per hour.

ADRENAL INSUFFICIENCY   The infiltration of the adrenals by tumor and their destruction by hemorrhage are the two most common causes. Symptoms such as nausea, vomiting, anorexia, and orthostatic hypotension may be attributed to progressive cancer or to treatment side effects. Certain treatments (e.g., ketoconazole, aminoglutethimide) may directly interfere with steroid synthesis in the adrenal.

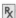 **TREATMENT**

In emergencies, a bolus of 100 mg IV hydrocortisone is followed by a continuous infusion of 10 mg/h. In nonemergent but stressful circumstances, 100–200 mg/d oral hydrocortisone is the beginning dose, tapered to maintenance of 15–37.5 mg/d. Fludrocortisone (0.1 mg/d) may be required in the presence of hyperkalemia.

TREATMENT COMPLICATIONS

Complications from treatment may occur acutely or emerge only many years after treatment. Toxicity may be related either to the agents used to treat the cancer or from the response of the cancer to the treatment (e.g., leaving a perforation in a hollow viscus or causing metabolic complications such as the tumor lysis syndrome). Several treatment complications present as emergencies. Fever and neutropenia and tumor lysis syndrome will be discussed here; others are discussed in Chap. 88 in HPIM-16.

FEVER AND NEUTROPENIA   Many cancer pts are treated with myelotoxic agents. When peripheral blood granulocyte counts are <1000/μL, the risk of infection is substantially increased (48 infections/100 pts). A neutropenic pt who develops a fever (>38°C) should undergo physical exam with special attention to skin lesions, mucous membranes, IV catheter sites, and perirectal area. Two sets of blood cultures from different sites should be drawn, and a CXR performed, and any additional tests should be guided by findings from the history and physical exam. Any fluid collections should be tapped, and urine and/or fluids should be examined under the microscope for evidence of infection.

 TREATMENT

After cultures are obtained, all pts should receive IV broad-spectrum antibiotics (e.g., ceftazidime, 1 g q8h). If an obvious infectious site is found, the antibiotic regimen is designed to cover organisms that may cause the infection. Usually therapy should be started with an agent or agents that cover both gram-positive and -negative organisms. If the fever resolves, treatment should continue until neutropenia resolves. If the pt remains febrile and neutropenic after 7 days, amphotericin B should be added to the antibiotic regimen.

TUMOR LYSIS SYNDROME   When rapidly growing tumors are treated with effective chemotherapy regimens, the rapid destruction of tumor cells can lead to the release of large amounts of nucleic acid breakdown products (chiefly uric acid), potassium, phosphate, and lactic acid. The phosphate elevations can lead to hypocalcemia. The increased uric acid, especially in the setting of acidosis, can precipitate in the renal tubules and lead to renal failure. The renal failure can exacerbate the hyperkalemia.

 TREATMENT

Prevention is the best approach. Maintain hydration with 3 L/d of saline, keep urine pH > 7.0 with bicarbonate administration, and start allopurinol, 300 mg/m^2 per day, 24 h before starting chemotherapy. Once chemotherapy is given, monitor serum electrolytes every 6 h. If after 24 h, uric acid (>8 mg/dL) and serum creatinine (>1.6 mg/dL) are elevated, rasburicase (recombinant urate oxidase), 0.2 mg/kg IV daily, may lower uric acid levels. If serum potassium > 6.0 meq/L and renal failure ensues, hemodialysis may be required. Maintain normal calcium levels.

For a more detailed discussion, see Finberg R: Infections in Patients with Cancer, Chap. 72, p. 489; and Gucalp R, Dutcher J: Oncologic Emergencies, Chap. 88, p. 575, in HPIM-16.

28

ANAPHYLAXIS

Definition

A life-threatening systemic hypersensitivity reaction to contact with an allergen; it may appear within minutes of exposure to the offending substance. Manifestations include respiratory distress, pruritus, urticaria, mucous membrane swelling, gastrointestinal disturbances (including nausea, vomiting, pain, and diarrhea), and vascular collapse. Virtually any allergen may incite an anaphylactic reaction, but among the more common agents are proteins such as antisera, hormones, pollen extracts, Hymenoptera venom, foods; drugs (especially antibiotics); and diagnostic agents. Atopy does not seem to predispose to anaphylaxis from penicillin or venom exposures. Anaphylactic transfusion reactions are covered in Chap. 5.

Clinical Presentation

Time to onset is variable, but symptoms usually occur within seconds to minutes of exposure to the offending antigen:

- Respiratory: mucous membrane swelling, hoarseness, stridor, wheezing
- Cardiovascular: tachycardia, hypotension
- Cutaneous: pruritus, urticaria, angioedema

Diagnosis

Made by obtaining history of exposure to offending substance with subsequent development of characteristic complex of symptoms.

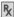 TREATMENT

Mild symptoms such as pruritus and urticaria can be controlled by administration of 0.2 to 0.5 mL of 1:1000 epinephrine solution SC, repeated at 20-min intervals as necessary.

An IV infusion should be initiated. Hypotension should be treated by IV administration of 2.5 mL of 1:10,000 epinephrine solution at 5- to 10-min intervals, volume expanders, e.g., as normal saline, and vasopressor agents, e.g., dopamine, if intractable hypotension occurs.

Epinephrine provides both α- and β-adrenergic effects, resulting in vasoconstriction and bronchial smooth-muscle relaxation. Beta blockers are relatively contraindicated in persons at risk for anaphylactic reactions.

The following should also be used as necessary:

- Antihistamines such as diphenhydramine 50 to 100 mg IM or IV
- Aminophylline 0.25 to 0.5 g IV for bronchospasm
- Oxygen
- Glucocorticoids—IV; not useful for acute manifestations but may help control persistent hypotension or bronchospasm

Prevention

Avoidance of offending antigen, where possible; skin testing and desensitization to materials such as penicillin and Hymenoptera venom, if necessary. Individuals should wear an informational bracelet and have immediate access to an unexpired epinephrine kit.

For a more detailed discussion, see Austen KF: Allergies, Anaphylaxis, and Systemic Mastocytosis, Chap. 298, p. 1947, HPIM-16.

29

BITES, VENOMS, STINGS, AND MARINE POISONINGS

MAMMALIAN BITES

More than 4 million animal bite wounds are sustained in the United States each year.

Dog Bites

Epidemiology Of all mammalian bite wounds, 80% are inflicted by dogs, and 15–20% of these wounds become infected.

Etiology (See Table 29-1.) In addition to bacterial infections, dog bites may transmit rabies (Chap. 112) and may lead to tetanus (Chap. 100) or tularemia (Chap. 99).

Clinical Features

• Pain, cellulitis, and a purulent, sometimes foul-smelling discharge may develop 8–24 h after the bite.
• Infection is usually localized, but systemic spread (e.g., bacteremia, endocarditis, brain abscess) can occur.
• *Capnocytophaga canimorsus* infection can present as sepsis syndrome, DIC, and renal failure, particularly in pts who are splenectomized, have hepatic dysfunction, or are otherwise immunosuppressed.

Cat Bites

Epidemiology In >50% of cases, infection occurs as a result of deep tissue penetration of narrow, sharp feline incisors. Cat bites are more likely than dog bites to cause septic arthritis or osteomyelitis.

Etiology The microflora is usually mixed, although *Pasteurella multocida* is the most important pathogen. Cat bites may transmit rabies or may lead to tetanus. Cat bites and scratches may also transmit *Bartonella henselae*, the agent of cat-scratch disease, as well as *Francisella tularensis*, the agent of tularemia (Chap. 99).

Clinical Features *P. multocida* can cause rapidly advancing, painful inflammation that may manifest only a few hours after the bite as well as purulent or serosanguineous discharge. Dissemination may occur.

Other Nonhuman Mammalian Bites

• Bite infections reflect oral flora. Bites from Old World monkeys (*Macaca* spp.) may transmit herpes B virus (*Herpesvirus simiae*), which can cause CNS infections with high mortality.
• Small rodents and the animals that prey on them may transmit *rat-bite fever*, caused by *Streptobacillus moniliformis* (in the United States) or *Spirillum minor* (in Asia). Infection with *S. moniliformis* manifests 3–10 days after the bite as fever, chills, myalgias, headache, and migratory arthralgias; these manifesta-

Table 29-1

Management of Wound Infections Following Animal Bites

Biting Species	Commonly Isolated Pathogens	Preferred Antibiotic(s)[a]	Alternative Agent(s) for Penicillin-Allergic Patients	Recommendation for Prophylaxis in Patients with Recent Uninfected Wounds[b]	Other Considerations
Dog	*Staphylococcus aureus, Streptococcus* spp., *Pasteurella* spp., anaerobes, *Capnocytophaga canimorsus*	Amoxicillin/clavulanic acid (250–500 mg PO tid); or ampicillin/sulbactam (1.5–3.0 g IV q6h)	Clindamycin (150–300 mg PO qid) plus either TMP-SMX (1 double-strength tablet bid) or ciprofloxacin (500 mg PO bid)	Sometimes[c]	Consider rabies prophylaxis.
Cat	*Pasteurella multocida, S. aureus, Streptococcus* spp., anaerobes	Amoxicillin/clavulanic acid or ampicillin/sulbactam, as for dog bite	Clindamycin plus either TMP-SMX or a fluoroquinolone	Usually	Consider rabies prophylaxis; carefully evaluate for joint/bone penetration.
Human: occlusional bite	Viridans streptococci, *S. aureus, Haemophilus influenzae*, anaerobes	Amoxicillin/clavulanic acid or ampicillin/sulbactam, as for dog bite	Erythromycin, fluoroquinolone	Always	—
Human: clenched-fist injury	As for occlusional bite plus *Eikenella corrodens*	Ampicillin/sulbactam, as for dog bite, or imipenem	Cefoxitin[d] (1.5 g IV q6h)	Always	Examine for tendon/nerve/joint involvement.

(continued)

107

Table 29-1 *(Continued)*

Management of Wound Infections Following Animal Bites

Biting Species	Commonly Isolated Pathogens	Preferred Antibiotic(s)[a]	Alternative Agent(s) for Penicillin-Allergic Patients	Recommendation for Prophylaxis in Patients with Recent Uninfected Wounds[b]	Other Considerations
Monkey	As for human bite	As for human bite	As for human bite	Always	For macaque monkeys, consider B virus prophylaxis with acyclovir.
Snake[e]	*Pseudomonas aeruginosa, Proteus* spp., *Bacteroides fragilis, Clostridium* spp.	Ceftriaxone (1–2 g IV q12–24h); or ampicillin/sulbactam, as for dog bite	Clindamycin plus either TMP-SMX or a fluoroquinolone	Sometimes, especially for venomous snakebite	Use antivenin for venomous snakebite.
Rodent	*Streptobacillus moniliformis, Leptospira* spp., *P. multocida*	Penicillin VK (500 mg PO bid)	Doxycycline (100 mg PO qd)	Sometimes[c]	—

[a] Antibiotic choices should be based on culture data, when available. Duration of therapy must be guided by response, but normally a minimum course of 10 to 14 days is required for established soft tissue infection. Osteomyelitis and septic arthritis require longer treatment. These suggestions for empirical therapy need to be tailored to individual circumstances and local conditions. IV regimens should be used for hospitalized pts. When the pt is to be discharged after initial management, a single IV dose of antibiotic may be followed by oral therapy.

[b] Prophylactic antibiotics are usually given for 3 to 5 days.

[c] Prophylactic antibiotics are suggested for severe or extensive wounds, facial wounds, or crush injuries; when bone or joint may be involved; or when comorbidity exists.

[d] Cefoxitin may be hazardous to pts with immediate-type hypersensitivity to penicillin.

[e] See Chap. 378.

Note: TMP-SMX, trimethoprim-sulfamethoxazole.

tions are followed by a maculopapular rash. Complications can include meta-static abscesses, endocarditis, meningitis, or pneumonia. Diagnosis can be made by culture on enriched media and serologic testing. Infection with *S. minor* causes local inflammation, pain, and regional lymphadenopathy 1–4 weeks after the bite, with evolution into a systemic illness. Diagnosis can be made by detection of spirochetes on microscopic examination.

Human Bites

Human bites become infected more frequently than bite wounds from other animals. *Occlusional* injuries are inflicted by actual biting. *Clenched-fist* injuries result when the fist of one individual strikes the teeth of another. These injuries are particularly prone to serious infection.

Etiology   See Table 29-1.

 TREATMENT

- *Wound management*: Wound closure is controversial in bite injuries. After thorough cleansing, facial wounds are usually sutured for cosmetic reasons and because the abundant facial blood supply lessens the risk of infection. For wounds elsewhere on the body, many authorities do not attempt primary closure, preferring instead to irrigate the wound copiously, debride devitalized tissue, remove foreign bodies, and approximate the margins. Delayed primary closure may be undertaken after the risk of infection has passed.
- *Antibiotic therapy*: See Table 29-1.
- *Tetanus*: A booster for pts immunized previously but not boosted within 5 years should be considered, as should primary immunization and tetanus immune globulin administration for pts not previously immunized.

VENOMOUS SNAKEBITES

Etiology and Epidemiology   Worldwide, at least 30,000 to 40,000 people die each year from venomous snakebite injuries, most often in temperate and tropical regions. The overall mortality rate for venomous snakebite is <1% among U.S. victims who receive antivenom. Eastern and western diamondback rattlesnakes are responsible for most deaths from snakebite in the United States. Snake venoms are complex mixtures of enzymes and other substances that promote vascular leaking and bleeding, tissue necrosis, and neurotoxicity and affect the coagulation cascade.

 TREATMENT

Field Management

- Get the victim to definitive care as soon as possible.
- Keep the victim inactive to minimize systemic spread of venom.
- If the victim is >60 min from medical care, a proximal lymphatic-occlusive constriction band may limit the spread of venom but should be applied so as not to interfere with arterial flow.
- Splint a bitten extremity and keep it at heart level.
- *Avoid* incisions into the bite wound, cooling, consumption of alcoholic beverages by the victim, and electric shock.

Hospital Management

- Monitor vital signs, cardiac rhythm, and O_2 saturation closely.
- Note the level of erythema and swelling and the limb circumference every 15 min until swelling has stabilized.

- Treat shock initially with crystalloid fluid resuscitation (normal saline or Ringer's lactate). If hypotension persists, try 5% albumin and vasopressors.
- Begin the search for appropriate, specific antivenom early in all cases of known venomous snakebite, regardless of symptoms. In the United States, round-the-clock assistance is available from the University of Arizona Poison and Drug Information Center (520-626-6016).

1. Rapidly progressive and severe local findings or manifestations of systemic toxicity (signs and symptoms or laboratory abnormalities) are indications for IV antivenom.
2. Most antivenoms are of equine origin and carry risks of anaphylactic, anaphylactoid, or delayed-hypersensitivity reactions. The newest antivenom available in the United States for pit viper bites reduces this risk.
3. Pts should be premedicated with IV antihistamines (e.g., diphenhydramine, 1 mg/kg up to a maximum dose of 100 mg; plus cimetidine, 5–10 mg/kg up to a maximum dose of 300 mg) and given IV crystalloids to expand intravascular volume. Epinephrine should be immediately available. The antivenom should be administered slowly in dilute solution with a physician present in case of an acute reaction.

- Elevate the bitten extremity only when antivenom is available.
- Update tetanus immunization.
- Observe pts with signs of envenomation in the hospital for at least 24 h. Pts with "dry" bites should be watched for at least 8 h because symptoms are commonly delayed.

MARINE ENVENOMATIONS
Invertebrates
Injuries from nematocysts (stinging cells) of hydroids, fire coral, jellyfish, Portuguese man-of-war, and sea anemones cause similar clinical symptoms that differ in severity.

Clinical Features   Pain (prickling, burning, and throbbing), pruritus, and paresthesia develop immediately at the site of the bite. Neurologic, GI, renal, cardiovascular, respiratory, rheumatologic, and ocular symptoms have been described.

℞ TREATMENT

- Decontaminate the skin immediately with vinegar (5% acetic acid) or rubbing alcohol (40–70% isopropanol). Baking soda, unseasoned meat tenderizer (papain), or lemon or lime juice may be effective.
- Shaving the skin may help remove nematocysts.
- After decontamination, topical anesthetics, antihistamines, or steroid lotions may be helpful.
- Narcotics may be necessary for persistent pain.
- Muscle spasms may respond to IV 10% calcium gluconate (5–10 mL) or diazepam (2–5 mg titrated upward as needed).

Vertebrates
Marine vertebrates, including stingrays, scorpionfish, and catfish, are capable of envenomating humans.

Clinical Features
- Immediate and intense pain at the site can last up to 48 h.

- Systemic symptoms include weakness, diaphoresis, nausea, vomiting, diarrhea, dysrhythmia, syncope, hypotension, muscle cramps, muscle fasciculations, and paralysis. Fatal cases are rare.
- Stingray wounds can become ischemic and heal poorly.
- The sting of a stonefish is the most serious marine vertebrate envenomation and can be life-threatening.

 TREATMENT

- Immerse the affected part immediately in nonscalding hot water (113°F/45°C) for 30–90 min.
- Explore, debride, and vigorously irrigate the wound.
- Antivenom is available for stonefish and scorpionfish envenomations.
- Leave wounds to heal by secondary intention or to be treated by delayed primary closure.
- Update tetanus immunization.
- Consider empirical antibiotics to cover *Staphylococcus* and *Streptococcus* spp. for serious wounds or envenomations in immunocompromised hosts.

Sources of Antivenoms and Other Assistance

Antivenom for stonefish and severe scorpionfish envenomation is available in the United States through the pharmacies of Sharp Cabrillo Hospital Emergency Department, San Diego, CA (619-221-3429) and Community Hospital of Monterey Peninsula (CHOMP) Emergency Department, Monterey, CA (408-625-4900). Divers Alert Network is a source of helpful information (round-the-clock at 919-684-8111 or http://www.diversalertnetwork.org).

MARINE POISONINGS
Ciguatera

Ciguatera poisoning is the most common nonbacterial food poisoning associated with fish in the United States. Tropical and semitropical marine coral reef fish are usually the source; 75% of cases involve barracuda, snapper, jack, or grouper. Toxins may not affect the appearance or taste of the fish and are resistant to heat, cold, freeze-drying, and gastric acid.

Clinical Features Most victims experience diarrhea, vomiting, and abdominal pain 3–6 h after ingestion of contaminated fish and develop myriad symptoms within 12 h, including neurologic signs (e.g., paresthesia, weakness, fasciculations, ataxia), maculopapular or vesicular rash, and hemodynamic instability. A pathognomonic symptom—reversal of hot and cold perception—develops within 3–5 days and can last for months. Death is rare. A diagnosis is made on clinical grounds.

 TREATMENT

Therapy is supportive and based on symptoms. Cool showers, hydroxyzine (25 mg PO q6–8h), or amitriptyline (25 mg PO bid) may ameliorate pruritus and dysesthesias. During recovery, the pt should avoid ingestion of fish, shellfish, fish oils, fish or shellfish sauces, alcohol, nuts, and nut oils.

Paralytic Shellfish Poisoning (PSP)

PSP is induced by ingestion of contaminated clams, oysters, scallops, mussels, and other species that concentrate water-soluble, heat- and acid-stable chemical toxins. Pts develop oral paresthesias that progress to the neck and extremities and that change to numbness within minutes to hours after ingestion of contaminated shellfish. Flaccid paralysis and respiratory insufficiency may follow 2–12 h later. Treatment is supportive. If pts present within hours of ingestion, gastric lavage and stomach irrigation with 2 L of a 2% sodium bicarbonate solution may help. The pt should be monitored for respiratory paralysis for at least 24 h.

Scombroid

Etiology and Clinical Features   Scombroid poisoning is a histamine intoxication due to inadequately preserved or refrigerated scombroid fish (e.g., tuna, mackerel, saury, needlefish, wahoo, skipjack, and bonito); it can also occur with exposure to nonscombroid fish, including sardines and herring. Within 15–90 min of ingestion, victims present with flushing, pruritus or urticaria, bronchospasm, GI symptoms, tachycardia, and hypotension. Symptoms generally resolve within 8–12 h.

 TREATMENT

Treatment consists of antihistamine (H_1 or H_2) administration.

Pfiesteria Poisoning

Etiology and Clinical Features   *Pfiesteria*, a dinoflagellate identified in Maryland waters, releases a neurotoxin that kills fish within minutes. In people, exposure to *Pfiesteria* can cause a syndrome defined by the CDC as either of two groups of signs or symptoms: (1) memory loss/confusion or acute skin burning on contact with infested water; or (2) at least three of the following: headache, rash, eye irritation, upper respiratory irritation, muscle cramps, and GI symptoms. Neurocognitive defects improve within 3–6 months after cessation of exposure.

 TREATMENT

Milk of magnesia (1 tsp qd) followed by cholestyramine (1 scoop in 8 oz water qid) for 2 weeks has been a successful remedy in some cases.

ARTHROPOD BITES AND STINGS
Spider Bites

RECLUSE SPIDER BITES   Severe necrosis of skin and SC tissue follows a bite by the brown recluse spider. The spider is 7–15 mm in body length, has a 2- to 4-cm leg span, and has a dark violin-shaped spot on its dorsal surface. Spiders seek dark, undisturbed spots and bite only if threatened or pressed against the skin. The venoms contain enzymes that produce necrosis and hemolysis.

Clinical Features

• Initially the bite is painless or stings, but within hours the site becomes painful, pruritic, and indurated, with zones of ischemia and erythema.
• Fever and other nonspecific systemic symptoms may develop within 3 days of the bite.
• Lesions typically resolve within 2–3 days, but severe cases can leave a large ulcer and a depressed scar that take months to years to heal. Deaths are rare and are due to hemolysis and renal failure.

℞ TREATMENT

> • Wound care, cold compress application, elevation and loose immobilization of the affected limb, and administration of analgesics, antihistamines, antibiotics, and tetanus prophylaxis should be undertaken as indicated.
> • Dapsone administration within 48–72 h (50–100 mg PO bid after G6PD deficiency has been ruled out) may halt progression of necrotic lesions.

WIDOW SPIDER BITES   *Etiology and Clinical Features*   The black widow spider is found in every U.S. state except Alaska but is most abundant in the Southeast. It measures up to 1 cm in body length and 5 cm in leg span, is shiny black, and has a red hourglass marking on the ventral abdomen. Female widow spiders produce a potent neurotoxin that binds irreversibly to nerves and causes release and depletion of acetylcholine and other neurotransmitters from presynaptic terminals. Within 30–60 min, painful cramps spread from the bite site to large muscles of the extremities and trunk. Extreme abdominal muscular rigidity and pain may mimic peritonitis, but the abdomen is nontender. Other features include salivation, diaphoresis, vomiting, hypertension, tachycardia, and myriad neurologic signs. Respiratory arrest, cerebral hemorrhage, or cardiac failure may occur.

℞ TREATMENT

> Treatment consists of local cleansing of the wound, application of ice packs to slow the spread of the venom, and tetanus prophylaxis. Analgesics, antispasmodics, and other supportive care should be given. Equine antivenom is available; rapid IV administration of 1 or 2 vials relieves pain and can be lifesaving. However, antivenom use should be reserved for severe cases involving respiratory arrest, refractory hypertension, seizures, or pregnancy because of anaphylaxis risk and serum sickness.

Scorpion Stings

Etiology and Clinical Features   Among the venoms of scorpions in the United States, only the venom of the bark scorpion (*Centruroides sculpturatus* or *C. exilicauda*) is potentially lethal. The bark scorpion is yellow-brown and 7 cm long and is found in the southwestern United States and northern Mexico. Its neurotoxin opens sodium channels, and neurons fire repetitively. The sting causes little swelling, but pain, paresthesia, and hyperesthesia are prominent. Cranial nerve dysfunction and skeletal muscle hyperexcitability develop within hours. Symptoms include restlessness, blurred vision, abnormal eye movements, profuse salivation, slurred speech, diaphoresis, nausea, and vomiting. Complications include tachycardia, arrhythmias, hypertension, hyperthermia, rhabdomyolysis, and acidosis. Manifestations peak at 5 h and subside within a day or two, although paresthesias can last for weeks.

℞ TREATMENT

> Aggressive supportive care should include pressure dressings and cold packs to decrease the absorption of venom. Continuous IV administration of midazolam to decrease agitation and involuntary muscle movements may be needed. The benefit of scorpion antivenom has not been established in controlled trials.

Hymenoptera Stings

The hymenoptera include apids (bees and bumblebees), vespids (wasps, hornets, and yellow jackets), and ants. About 50 deaths from hymenoptera stings occur annually in the United States, nearly all due to allergic reactions to venoms.

Clinical Features

• Honeybees can sting only once; other bees, vespids, and ants can sting many times in succession.
• Uncomplicated stings cause pain, a wheal-and-flare reaction, and local edema that subsides within hours.
• Multiple stings can lead to vomiting, diarrhea, generalized edema, dyspnea, hypotension, rhabdomyolysis, renal failure, and death.
• Large (>10-cm) local reactions progressing over 1–2 days are not uncommon and resemble cellulitis but are hypersensitivity reactions.
• About 0.4–4% of the U.S. population exhibits immediate-type hypersensitivity to insect stings. Serious reactions occur within 10 min of the sting and include upper airway edema, bronchospasm, hypotension, shock, and death.

TREATMENT

• Stingers embedded in skin should be removed promptly by any method.
• The site should be cleansed and ice packs applied. Elevation of the bite site and administration of analgesics, oral antihistamines, and topical calamine lotion may ease symptoms.
• Oral glucocorticoids are indicated for large local reactions.
• Anaphylaxis is treated with epinephrine hydrochloride (0.3–0.5 mL of a 1:1000 solution, given SC q20–30min as needed). For profound shock, epinephrine (2–5 mL of a 1:10,000 solution by slow IV push) is indicated. Pts should be observed for 24 h because of the risk of recurrence.
• Pts with a history of allergy to insect stings should carry a sting kit and seek medical attention immediately after the kit is used. Adults with a history of anaphylaxis should undergo desensitization.

Tick Bites and Tick Paralysis

Etiology and Clinical Features

• Ticks are important carriers of vector-borne diseases in the United States.
• Ticks attach and feed painlessly on blood from their hosts, but tick secretions may produce local reactions. Tick bites may cause a small area of induration and erythema. A necrotic ulcer occasionally develops; chronic nodules or tick granulomata may require surgical excision. Tick-induced fever and malaise resolve 24–36 h after tick removal.
• Tick paralysis is an ascending flaccid paralysis due to a toxin in tick saliva that causes neuromuscular block and decreased nerve conduction. Paralysis begins in the lower extremities 5–6 days after the tick's attachment and ascends symmetrically, causing complete paralysis of the extremities and cranial nerves. Deep tendon reflexes are decreased or absent, but sensory examination and LP yield normal findings. Tick removal results in improvement within hours. Failure to remove the tick may lead ultimately to respiratory paralysis and death. The tick is usually found on the scalp.

TREATMENT

Ticks should be removed with forceps applied close to the point of attachment, and the site of attachment should then be disinfected. Removal within 48 h of attachment usually prevents transmission of the agents of Lyme disease, babesiosis, and ehrlichiosis. Protective clothing and DEET application are protective measures that can be effective against ticks.

For a more detailed discussion, see Madoff LC: Infectious Complications of Bites and Burns, Chap. 109A in *Harrison's Online*; Auerbach PS, Norris RL: Disorders Caused by Reptile Bites and Marine Animal Exposures, Chap. 378, p. 2593; and Maguire JH et al: Ectoparasite Infestations and Arthropod Bites and Stings, Chap. 379, p. 2600, in HPIM-16.

30

HYPOTHERMIA AND FROSTBITE

HYPOTHERMIA

Hypothermia is defined as a core body temperature of ≤35°C and is classified as mild (32.2°–35°C), moderate (28°–32.2°C), or severe (<28°C).

   ETIOLOGY   Most cases occur during the winter in cold climates, but hypothermia may occur in mild climates and is usually multifactorial. Heat is generated in most tissues of the body and is lost by radiation, conduction, convection, evaporation, and respiration. Factors that impede heat generation and/or increase heat loss lead to hypothermia (Table 30-1).

Table 30-1

Risks Factors for Hypothermia

Age extremes	Endocrine-related
Elderly	Hypoglycemia
Neonates	Hypothyroidism
Outdoor exposure	Adrenal insufficiency
Occupational	Hypopituitarism
Sports-related	Neurologic-related
Inadequate clothing	Stroke
Drugs and intoxicants	Hypothalamic disorders
Ethanol	Parkinson's disease
Phenothiazines	Spinal cord injury
Barbiturates	Multisystem
Anesthetics	Malnutrition
Neuromuscular blockers	Sepsis
Others	Shock
	Hepatic or renal failure
	Burns and exfoliative dermato-logic disorders
	Immobility or debilitation

CLINICAL FEATURES Acute cold exposure causes tachycardia, increased cardiac output, peripheral vasoconstriction, and increased peripheral vascular resistance. As body temperature drops below 32°C, cardiac conduction becomes impaired, the heart rate slows, and cardiac output decreases. Atrial fibrillation with slow ventricular response is common. Other ECG changes include Osborn (J) waves. Additional manifestations of hypothermia include volume depletion, hypotension, increased blood viscosity (which can lead to thrombosis), coagulopathy, thrombocytopenia, DIC, acid-base disturbances, and bronchospasm. CNS abnormalities are diverse and can include ataxia, amnesia, hallucinations, delayed deep tendon reflexes, and (in severe hypothermia) an isoelectric EEG.

DIAGNOSIS Hypothermia is confirmed by measuring the core body temperature, preferably at two sites. Since oral thermometers are usually calibrated only as low as 34.4°C, the exact temperature of a patient whose initial reading is <35°C should be determined with a thermometer reading down to 15°C or, ideally, with a rectal thermocouple probe inserted to ≥15 cm. Simultaneously, an esophageal probe should be placed 24 cm below the larynx.

 TREATMENT

Cardiac monitoring should be instituted, along with attempts to limit further heat loss. Mild hypothermia is managed by passive external rewarming and insulation. The pt should be placed in a warm environment and covered with blankets to allow endogenous heat production to restore normal body temperature. Active rewarming is necessary for moderate to severe hypothermia, cardiovascular instability, age extremes, CNS dysfunction, endocrine insufficiency, or hypothermia due to complications from systemic disorders. Active rewarming may be external (forced-air heating blankets, radiant heat sources, and hot packs) or internal (by inspiration of heated, humidified oxygen warmed to 40°–45°C; by administration of IV fluids warmed to 40°–42°C; or by peritoneal or pleural lavage with dialysate or saline warmed to 40°–45°C). The most efficient active internal rewarming techniques are extracorporeal rewarming by hemodialysis and cardiopulmonary bypass. External rewarming may cause a fall in blood pressure by relieving peripheral vasoconstriction. Volume should be repleted with warmed isotonic solutions; lactated Ringer's solution should be avoided because of impaired lactate metabolism in hypothermia. If sepsis is a possibility, empirical broad-spectrum antibiotics should be administered after sending blood cultures. Atrial arrhythmias usually require no specific treatment. Ventricular fibrillation is often refractory. Only a single sequence of 3 defibrillation attempts (2 J/kg) should be attempted when the temperature is <30°C. Since it is sometimes difficult to distinguish profound hypothermia from death, cardiopulmonary resuscitation efforts and active internal rewarming should continue until the core temperature is >32°C or cardiovascular status has been stabilized.

FROSTBITE

Frostbite occurs when the tissue temperature drops below 0°C. Clinically, it is most practical to classify frostbite as superficial (without tissue loss) or deep (with tissue loss). Classically, frostbite is retrospectively graded like a burn (first- to fourth-degree) once the resultant pathology is demarcated over time.

CLINICAL FEATURES The initial presentation of frostbite can be deceptively benign. The symptoms always include a sensory deficit affecting light touch, pain, and temperature perception. Deep frostbitten tissue can appear

Table 30-2

Treatment for Frostbite

Before Thawing	During Thawing	After Thawing
Remove from environment	Consider parenteral analgesia and ketorolac	Gently dry and protect part; elevate; pledgets between toes, if macerated
Prevent partial thawing and refreezing	Administer ibuprofen, 400 mg PO	If clear vesicles are intact, the fluid will reabsorb in days; if broken, debride and dress with antibiotic or sterile aloe vera ointment
Stabilize core temperature and treat hypothermia	Immerse part in 37°–40°C (thermometer-monitored) circulating water containing an antiseptic soap until distal flush (10–45 min)	Leave hemorrhagic vesicles intact to prevent infection
Protect frozen part—no friction or massage	Encourage patient to gently move part	Continue ibuprofen 400 mg PO (12 mg/kg per day) q8–12h
Address medical or surgical conditions	If pain is refractory, reduce water temperature to 33°–37°C	Consider tetanus and streptococcal prophylaxis; elevate part Hydrotherapy at 37°C

waxy, mottled, yellow, or violaceous-white. Favorable presenting signs include some warmth or sensation with normal color.

Rx TREATMENT

A treatment protocol for frostbite is summarized in Table 30-2. Frozen tissue should be rapidly and completely thawed by immersion in circulating water at 37°–40°C. Thawing should not be terminated prematurely due to pain from reperfusion; ibuprofen, 400 mg, should be given, and parenteral narcotics are often required. If cyanosis persists after rewarming, the tissue compartment pressures should be monitored carefully.

For a more detailed discussion, see Danzl DF: Hypothermia and Frostbite, Chap. 19, p. 121, in HPIM-16.

31

BIOTERRORISM

MICROBIAL BIOTERRORISM

Microbial bioterrorism refers to the use of microbial pathogens as weapons of terror that target civilian populations. A primary goal of bioterrorism is not necessarily to produce mass casualties but to destroy the morale of a society through creating fear and uncertainty. The events of September 11, 2001, followed by the anthrax attacks through the U.S. Postal Service illustrate the vulnerability of the American public to terrorist attacks, including those that use microbes. The key to combating bioterrorist attacks is a highly functioning system of public health surveillance and education that rapidly identifies and effectively contains the attack.

Agents of microbial bioterrorism may be used in their natural form or may be deliberately modified to maximize their deleterious effect. Modifications that increase the deleterious effect of a biologic agent include genetic alteration of microbes to produce antimicrobial resistance, creation of fine-particle aerosols, chemical treatment to stabilize and prolong infectivity, and alteration of the host range through changes in surface protein receptors. Certain of these approaches fall under the category of *weaponization*, a term that describes the processing of microbes or toxins in a manner that enhances their deleterious effect after release. The key features that characterize an effective biologic weapon are summarized in Table 31-1.

The U.S. Centers for Disease Control and Prevention (CDC) has classified microbial agents that could potentially be used in bioterrorism attacks into three categories: A, B, and C (Table 31-2). Category A agents are the highest-priority pathogens. They pose the greatest risk to national security because they (1) can be easily disseminated or transmitted from person to person, (2) are associated with high case fatality rates, (3) have potential to cause significant public panic and social disruption, and (4) require special action and public health preparedness.

Category A Agents

ANTHRAX (*BACILLUS ANTHRACIS*) *Anthrax as a Bioweapon*
Anthrax in many ways is the prototypic bioweapon. Although it is only rarely spread by person-to-person contact, it has many of the other features of an ideal

Table 31-1

Key Features of Biologic Agents Used as Bioweapons

1. High morbidity and mortality
2. Potential for person-to-person spread
3. Low infective dose and highly infectious by aerosol
4. Lack of rapid diagnostic capability
5. Lack of universally available effective vaccine
6. Potential to cause anxiety
7. Availability of pathogen and feasibility of production
8. Environmental stability
9. Database of prior research and development
10. Potential to be "weaponized"

Source: From L Borio et al: JAMA 287:2391, 2002; with permission.

Table 31-2

CDC Category A, B, and C Agents

Category A
  Anthrax (*Bacillus anthracis*)
  Botulism (*Clostridium botulinum* toxin)
  Plague (*Yersinia pestis*)
  Smallpox (Variola major)
  Tularemia (*Francisella tularensis*)
  Viral hemorrhagic fevers
    Arenaviruses: Lassa, New World (Machupo, Junin, Guanarito, and Sabia)
    Bunyaviridae: Crimean Congo, Rift Valley
    Filoviridae: Ebola, Marburg
    Flaviviridae: Yellow fever; Omsk fever; Kyasanur Forest
Category B
  Brucellosis (*Brucella* spp.)
  Epsilon toxin of *Clostridium perfringens*
  Food safety threats (e.g., *Salmonella* spp., *Escherichia coli* 0157:H7, *Shigella*)
  Glanders (*Burkholderia mallei*)
  Melioidosis (*B. pseudomallei*)
  Psittacosis (*Chlamydia psittaci*)
  Q fever (*Coxiella burnetii*)
  Ricin toxin from *Ricinus communis* (castor beans)
  Staphylococcal enterotoxin B
  Typhus fever (*Rickettsia prowazekii*)
  Viral encephalitis [alphaviruses (e.g., Venezuelan, eastern, and western equine encephalitis)]
  Water safety threats (e.g., *Vibrio cholerae*, *Cryptosporidium parvum*)
Category C
  Emerging infectious diseases threats such as Nipah, hantavirus, and SARS coronavirus.

Source: Centers for Disease Control and Prevention and the National Institute of Allergy and Infectious Diseases.

biologic weapon listed in Table 31-1. The potential impact of anthrax as a bioweapon is illustrated by the apparent accidental release in 1979 of anthrax spores from a Soviet bioweapons facility in Sverdlosk, Russia. As a result of this atmospheric release of anthrax spores, at least 77 cases of anthrax (of which 66 were fatal) occurred in individuals within an area 4 km downwind of the facility. Deaths were noted in livestock up to 50 km from the facility. The interval between probable exposure and onset of symptoms ranged from 2 to 43 days, with the majority of cases occurring within 2 weeks. In September of 2001 the American public was exposed to anthrax spores delivered through the U.S. Postal Service. There were 22 confirmed cases: 11 cases of inhaled anthrax (5 died) and 11 cases of cutaneous anthrax (no deaths). Cases occurred in individuals who opened contaminated letters as well as in postal workers involved in processing the mail.

Microbiology and Clinical Features   (See also Chap. 205, HPIM-16)

• Anthrax is caused by infections with *B. anthracis*, a gram-positive, non-motile, spore-forming rod that is found in soil and predominantly causes disease in cattle, goats, and sheep.

Table 31-3

Treatment Strategies for Diseases Caused by Category A Agents

Agent	Diagnosis	Treatment	Prophylaxis
Bacillus anthracis (anthrax)	Culture, Gram stain, PCR, Wright stain of peripheral smear	*Postexposure:* Ciprofloxacin, 500 mg, PO bid × 60 d *or* Doxycycline, 100 mg PO bid ×60 d Amoxicillin, 500 mg PO q8h, likely to be effective if strain penicillin sensitive *Active disease:* Ciprofloxacin, 400 mg IV q12h *or* Doxycycline, 100 mg IV q12 *plus* Clindamycin, 900 mg IV q8h and/or rifampin, 300 mg IV q12h; switch to PO when stable ×60 d total *Antitoxin strategies:* Neutralizing monoclonal antibodies are under study	Anthrax vaccine adsorbed Recombinant protective antigen vaccines are under study
Yersinia pestis (pneumonic plague)	Culture, Gram stain, direct fluorescent antibody, PCR	Gentamicin, 2.0 mg/kg IV loading then 1.7 mg/kg q8h IV *or* Streptomycin, 1.0 g q12h IM or IV Alternatives include doxycycline, 100 mg bid PO or IV; chloramphenicol 500 mg bid PO or IV	Doxycycline, 100 mg PO bid (ciprofloxacin may also be active) Formalin-fixed vaccine (FDA licensed; not available)

120

Agent	Diagnosis	Treatment	Prophylaxis
Variola major (smallpox)	Culture, PCR, electron microscopy	Supportive measures; consideration for cidofovir, antivaccinia immunoglobulin	Vaccinia immunization
Francisella tularensis (tularemia)	Gram stain, culture, immunohistochemistry, PCR	Streptomycin, 1 g IM bid *or* Gentamicin, 5 mg/kg per day div q8h IV for 14 days *or* Doxycycline, 100 mg IV bid *or* Chlorphenid, 15 mg/kg IV qid *or* Ciprofloxacin, 400 mg IV bid	Doxycycline, 100 mg PO bid × 14 days *or* Ciprofloxacin, 500 mg PO bid × 14 days
Viral hemorrhagic fevers	RT-PCR, serologic testing for antigen or antibody; Viral isolation by CDC or U.S. Army Medical Institute of Infectious Diseases (USAMRIID)	Supportive measures; Ribavirin 30 mg/kg up to 2 g × 1, followed by 16 mg/kg IV up to 1 g q6h for 4 days, followed by 8 mg/kg IV up to 0.5 g q8h × 6 days	No known chemoprophylaxis; Consideration for ribavirin in high-risk situations; Vaccine exists for yellow fever
Botulinum toxin (*Clostridium botulinum*)	Mouse bioassay, toxin immunoassay	Supportive measures including ventilation; 5000–9000 IU equine antitoxin	Administration of antitoxin

Note: CDC, U.S. Centers for Disease Control and Prevention; FDA, U.S. Food and Drug Administration; PCR, polymerase chain reaction; RT-PCR, reverse transcriptase PCR.

- Spores can remain viable for decades in the environment and be difficult to destroy with standard decontamination procedures. These properties make anthrax an ideal bioweapon.
- Naturally occurring human infection generally results from exposure to infected animals or contaminated animal products.

There are three major clinical forms of anthrax:

1. *Gastrointestinal anthrax* is rare and is unlikely to result from a bioterrorism event.
2. *Cutaneous anthrax* follows introduction of spores through an opening in the skin. The lesion begins as a papule followed by the development of a black eschar. Prior to the availability of antibiotics, about 20% of cutaneous anthrax cases were fatal.
3. *Inhalation anthrax* is the form most likely to result in serious illness and death in a bioterrorism attack. It occurs following inhalation of spores that become deposited in the alveolar spaces. The spores are phagocytosed by alveolar macrophages and are transported to regional lymph nodes where they germinate. Following germination, rapid bacterial growth and toxin production occur. Subsequent hematologic dissemination leads to cardiovascular collapse and death. The earliest symptoms are typically those of a viral-like prodrome with fever, malaise, and abdominal/chest symptoms that rapidly progress to a septic shock picture. Widening of the mediastinum and pleural effusions are typical findings on chest radiography. Once considered 100% fatal, experience from the Sverdlosk and U.S. Postal outbreaks indicate that with prompt initiation of appropriate antibiotic therapy, survival may be >50%.

Rx **TREATMENT**   (See Table 31-3)

Anthrax can be successfully treated if the disease is promptly recognized and appropriate antibiotic therapy is initiated.

- Penicillin, ciprofloxacin, and doxycycline are currently licensed for the treatment of anthrax.
- Clindamycin and rifampin have in vitro activity against the organism and may be used as part of the treatment regimen.
- Patients with inhalation anthrax are not contagious and do not require special isolation procedures.

Vaccination and Prevention

- Currently there is a single vaccine licensed for use; produced from a cell-free culture supernatant of an attenuated strain of *B. anthracis* (Stern strain).
- Since the efficacy of this vaccine in the postexposure setting has not been established, current recommendation for postexposure prophylaxis is 60 days of antibiotics (see Table 31-1)

PLAGUE (*YERSINIA PESTIS*)   (See also Chap. 99)   ***Plague as a Bioweapon***   Although plague lacks the environmental stability of anthrax, the highly contagious nature of the infection and the high mortality rate make it a potentially important agent of bioterrorism. As a bioweapon, plague would likely be delivered via an aerosol leading to primary pneumonic plague. In such an attack, person-to-person transmission of plague via respiratory aerosol could lead to large numbers of secondary cases.

Microbiology and Clinical Features   See Chap. 99, p. 482.

℞ TREATMENT   See Table 31-3 and Chap. 99, p. 482.

SMALLPOX (*VARIOLA MAJOR* AND *V. MINOR*)   (See also Chap. 167, HPIM-16)   *Smallpox as a Bioweapon*   Smallpox as a disease was globally eradicated by 1980 through a worldwide vaccination program. However, with the cessation of smallpox immunization programs in the United States in 1972 (and worldwide in 1980), close to half the U.S. population is fully susceptible to smallpox today. Given the infectious nature and the 10–30% mortality of smallpox in unimmunized individuals, the deliberate release of virus could have devastating effects on the population. In the absence of effective containment measures, an initial infection of 50–100 persons in a first generation of cases could expand by a factor of 10 to 20 with each succeeding generation. These considerations make smallpox a formidable bioweapon.

Microbiology and Clinical Features   The disease smallpox is caused by one of two closely related double-strand DNA viruses, *V. major* and *V. minor*. Both viruses are members of the Orthopoxvirus genus of the Poxviridae family. Infection with *V. minor* is generally less severe, with low mortality rates; thus, *V. major* is the only one considered as a potential bioweapon. Infection with *V. major* typically occurs following contact with an infected person from the time that a maculopapular rash appears through scabbing of the pustular lesions. Infection is thought to occur from inhalation of virus-containing saliva droplets from oropharyngeal lesions. Contaminated clothing or linen can also spread infection. About 12–14 days following initial exposure the patient develops high fever, malaise, vomiting, headache, back pain, and a maculopapular rash that begins on the face and extremities and spreads to the trunk. The skin lesions evolve into vesicles that eventually become pustular with scabs. The oral mucosa also develops macular lesions that progress to ulcers. Smallpox is associated with a 10–30% mortality. Historically, about 5–10% of naturally occurring cases manifest as highly virulent atypical forms, classified as *hemorrhagic* and *malignant*. These are difficult to recognize due to their atypical manifestations. Both forms have similar onset of a severe prostrating illness characterized by high fever, severe headache, and abdominal and back pain. In the hemorrhagic form, cutaneous erythema develops followed by petechiae and hemorrhage into the skin and mucous membranes. In the malignant form, confluent skin lesions develop but never progress to the pustular stage. Both of these forms are often fatal, with death occurring in 5–6 days.

℞ **TREATMENT**

Treatment is supportive. There is no licensed specific antiviral therapy for smallpox. While certain antiviral agents, such as cidofovir, have in vitro activity against *V. major*, these agents have not been tested clinically. Smallpox is highly infectious to close contacts; patients who are suspected cases should be handled with strict isolation procedures.

Vaccination and Prevention   Smallpox is a preventable disease following immunization with vaccinia. Past and current experience indicates that the smallpox vaccine is associated with a very low incidence of severe complications (see Table 205-5, p. 1285, HPIM-16). The current dilemma facing our society regarding assessment of the risk/benefit of smallpox vaccination is that, while the risks of vaccination are known, the risk of someone deliberately and effectively releasing smallpox into the general population is unknown.

TULAREMIA (*FRANCISELLA TULARENSIS*)   (See also Chap. 99) *Tularemia as a Bioweapon*   Tularemia has been studied as a biologic agent since the mid-twentieth century. Reportedly, both the United States and the former Soviet Union had active programs investigating this organism as a possible bioweapon. It has been suggested that the Soviet program extended into the era of molecular biology and that some strains of *F. tularensis* may have been genetically engineered to be resistant to commonly used antibiotics. *F. tularensis* is extremely infectious and can cause significant morbidity and mortality. These facts make it reasonable to consider this organism as a possible bioweapon that could be disseminated by either aerosol or contamination of food or drinking water.

Microbiology and Clinical Features   See Chap. 99, p. 481.

 TREATMENT   See Table 31-3 and Chap. 99, p. 481.

VIRAL HEMORRHAGIC FEVERS   (See also Chap. 112.)   *Hemorrhagic Fever Viruses as Bioweapons*   Several of the hemorrhagic fever viruses have been reported to have been weaponized by the former Soviet Union and the United States. Nonhuman primate studies indicate that infection can be established with very few virions and that infectious aerosol preparations can be produced.

Microbiology and Clinical Features   See Chap. 112, p. 554.

 TREATMENT   See Table 31-3 and Chap. 112, p. 555.

BOTULINUM TOXIN (*CLOSTRIDIUM BOTULINUM*)   (See also Chap. 100)   *Botulinum Toxin as a Bioweapon*   In a bioterrorism attack, botulinum toxin would likely be dispersed as an aerosol or used to contaminate food. Contamination of the water supply is possible, but the toxin would likely be degraded by chlorine used to purify drinking water. The toxin can also be inactivated by heating food to >85° C for >5 min. The United States, the former Soviet Union, and Iraq have all acknowledged studying botulinum toxin as a potential bioweapon. Unique among the Category A agents for not being a live organism, botulinum toxin is one of the most potent and lethal toxins known to man. It has been estimated that 1 g of toxin is sufficient to kill 1 million people if adequately dispersed.

Microbiology and Clinical Features   See Chap. 100, p. 487.

 TREATMENT   See Table 31-3 and Chap. 100, p. 487.

Category B and C Agents   (See Table 31-2)

Category B agents are the next highest priority and include agents that are moderately easy to disseminate, produce moderate morbidity and low mortality, and require enhanced diagnostic capacity.

Category C agents are the third highest priority agents in the biodefense agenda. These agents include emerging pathogens, such as SARS (severe acute respiratory syndrome) coronavirus, to which the general population lacks immunity. Category C agents could be engineered for mass dissemination in the future. It is important to note that these categories are empirical, and, depending on future circumstances, the priority ratings for a given microbial agent may change.

Prevention and Preparedness

As indicated above, a diverse array of agents have the potential to be used against a civilian population in a bioterrorism attack. The medical profession must maintain a high index of suspicion that unusual clinical presentations or clustering of rare diseases may not be a chance occurrence, but rather the first sign of a bioterrorism attack. Possible early indicators of a bioterrorism attack could include:

- The occurrence of rare diseases in healthy populations
- The occurrence of unexpectedly large numbers of a rare infection
- The appearance in an urban population of an infectious disease that is usually confined to rural settings

Given the importance of rapid diagnosis and early treatment for many of these diseases, it is important that the medical care team report any suspected cases of bioterrorism immediately to local and state health authorities and/or the CDC (888-246-2675).

CHEMICAL BIOTERRORISM

The use of chemical warfare agents (CWAs) as weapons of terror against civilian populations is a potential threat that must be addressed by public health officials and the medical profession. The use of both nerve agents and sulfur mustard by Iraq against Iranian military and Kurdish civilians and the sarin attacks in 1994–1995 in Japan underscore this threat.

A detailed description of the various CWAs can be found in Chap. 206, HPIM-16, and on the CDC website at *www.bt.cdc.gov/agent/agentlistchem.asp*. In this section only vesicants and nerve agents will be discussed as these are considered the most likely agents to be used in a terrorist attack.

Vesicants (Sulfur Mustard, Nitrogen Mustard, Lewisite)

Sulfur mustard is the prototype for this group of CWAs and was first used on the battlefields of Europe in World War I. This agent constitutes both a vapor and liquid threat to exposed epithelial surfaces. The organs most commonly affected are the skin, eyes, and airways. Exposure to large quantities of sulfur mustard can result in bone marrow toxicity. Sulfur mustard dissolves slowly in aqueous media such as sweat or tears, but once dissolved it forms reactive compounds that react with cellular proteins, membranes, and importantly DNA. Much of the biologic damage from this agent appears to result from DNA alkylation and cross-linking in rapidly dividing cells in the corneal epithelium, skin, bronchial mucosal epithelium, GI epithelium, and bone marrow. Sulfur mustard reacts with tissue within minutes of entering the body.

Clinical Features   The topical effects of sulfur mustard occur in the skin, airways, and eyes. Absorption of the agent may produce effects in the bone marrow and GI tract (direct injury to the GI tract may occur if sulfur mustard is ingested in contaminated food or water).

- Skin: erythema is the mildest and earliest manifestation; involved areas of skin then develop vesicles that coalesce to form bullae; high-dose exposure may lead to coagulation necrosis within bullae.
- Airways: initial and, with mild exposures, the only airway manifestations are burning of the nares, epistaxis, sinus pain, and pharyngeal pain. With ex-

posure to higher concentrations, damage to the trachea and lower airways may occur, producing laryngitis, cough, and dyspnea. With large exposures, necrosis of the airway mucosa occurs leading to pseudomembrane formation and airway obstruction. Secondary infection may occur due to bacterial invasion of denuded respiratory mucosa.

• Eyes: the eyes are the most sensitive organ to injury by sulfur mustard. Exposure to low concentrations may produce only erythema and irritation. Exposure to higher concentrations produces progressively more severe conjunctivitis, photophobia, blepharospasm pain, and corneal damage.

• GI tract manifestations include nausea and vomiting, lasting up to 24 h.

• Bone marrow suppression with peaks at 7–14 days following exposure may result in sepsis due to leukopenia.

 TREATMENT

Immediate decontamination is essential to minimize damage. Immediately remove clothing and gently wash skin with soap and water. Eyes should be flushed with copious amounts of water or saline. Subsequent medical care is supportive. Cutaneous vesicles should be left intact. Larger bullae should be debrided and treated with topical antibiotic preparations. Intensive care similar to that given to severe burn patients is required for pts with severe exposure. Oxygen may be required for mild/moderate respiratory exposure. Intubation and mechanical ventilation may be necessary for laryngeal spasm and severe lower airway damage. Pseudomembranes should be removed by suctioning; bronchodilators are of benefit for bronchospasm. The use of granulocyte colony-stimulating factor and/or stem cell transplantation may be effective for severe bone marrow suppression.

Nerve Agents

The organophosphorus nerve agents are the deadliest of the CWAs and work by inhibiting synaptic acetylcholinesterase, creating an acute cholinergic crisis. The "classic" organophosphorus nerve agents are tabun, sarin, soman, cyclosarin, and VX. All agents are liquid at standard temperature and pressure. With the exception of VX, all these agents are highly volatile, and the spilling of even a small amount of liquid agent represents a serious vapor hazard.

Mechanism Inhibition of acetylcholinesterase accounts for the major life-threatening effects of these agents. At the cholinergic synapse, the enzyme acetylcholinesterase functions as a "turn off" switch to regulate cholinergic synaptic transmission. Inhibition of this enzyme allows released acetylcholine to accumulate, resulting in end-organ overstimulation and leading to what is clinically referred to as *cholinergic crisis*.

Clinical Features The clinical manifestations of nerve agent exposure are identical for vapor and liquid exposure routes. Initial manifestations include miosis, blurred vision, headache, and copious oropharyngeal secretions. Once the agent enters the bloodstream (usually via inhalation of vapors) manifestations of cholinergic overload include nausea, vomiting, abdominal cramping, muscle twitching, difficulty breathing, cardiovascular instability, loss of consciousness, seizures, and central apnea. The onset of symptoms following vapor exposure is rapid (seconds to minutes). Liquid exposure to nerve agents results in differences in speed of onset and order of symptoms. Contact of a nerve agent with intact skin produces localized sweating followed by localized muscle fasciculations. Once in the muscle, the agent enters the circulation and causes the symptoms described above.

℞ TREATMENT

Since nerve agents have a short circulating half-life, improvement should be rapid if exposure is terminated and supportive care and appropriate antidotes are given. Thus, the treatment of acute nerve agent poisoning involves decontamination, respiratory support, antidotes.

1. *Decontamination*: Procedures are the same as those described above for sulfur mustard.
2. *Respiratory support*: Death from nerve agent exposure is usually due to respiratory failure. Ventilation will be complicated by increased airway resistance and secretions. Atropine should be given before mechanical ventilation is instituted.
3. *Antidotal therapy* (see Table 31-4):
   a. *Atropine*: Generally the preferred anticholinergic agent of choice for treating acute nerve agent poisoning. Atropine rapidly reverses cholinergic overload at muscarinic synapses but has little effect at nicotinic synapses. Thus, atropine can rapidly treat the life-threatening respiratory effects of nerve agents but will probably not help neuromuscular effects. The field loading dose is 2–6 mg IM, with repeat doses given every 5–10 min until breathing and secretions improve. In the mildly affected pt with miosis and no systemic symptoms, atropine or homoatropine eye drops may suffice.
   b. *Oxime therapy*: Oximes are nucleophiles that help restore normal enzyme function by reactivating the cholinesterase whose active site has been occupied and bound by the nerve agent. The oxime available in the United States is 2-pralidoxime chloride (2-PAM Cl). Treatment with 2-PAM may cause blood pressure elevation.
   c. *Anticonvulsant*: Seizures caused by nerve agents do not respond to the usual anticonvulsants such as phenytoin, phenobarbital, carbamazepine, valproate, and lamotrigine. The only class of drugs known to have efficacy in treating nerve agent–induced seizures are the benzodiazepines. Diazepam is the only benzodiazepine approved by the U.S. Food and Drug Administration for the treatment of seizures (although other benzodiazepines have been shown to work well in animal models of nerve agent–induced seizures).

RADIATION BIOTERRORISM

Nuclear or radiation-related devices represent a third category of weapon that could be used in a terrorism attack. There are two major types of attacks that could occur. The first is the use of radiologic dispersal devices that cause the dispersal of radioactive material without detonation of a nuclear explosion. Such devices could use conventional explosives to disperse radionuclides. The second, and less probable, scenario would be the use of actual nuclear weapons by terrorists against a civilian target.

Types of Radiation

Alpha radiation consists of heavy, positively charged particles containing two protons and two neutrons. Due to their large size, alpha particles have limited penetrating power. Cloth and human skin can usually prevent alpha particles from penetrating into the body. If alpha particles are internalized, they can cause significant cellular damage.

Beta radiation consists of electrons and can travel only short distances in tissue. Plastic layers and clothing can stop most beta particles. Higher energy beta particles can cause injury to the basal stratum of skin similar to a thermal burn.

Table 31-4

Antidote Recommendations Following Exposure to Nerve Agents

Patient Age	Antidotes		Other Treatment
	Mild/Moderate Effects[a]	Severe Effects[b]	
Infants (0–2 yrs)	Atropine: 0.05 mg/kg IM, or 0.02 mg/kg IV; and 2-PAM chloride: 15 mg/kg IM or IV slowly	Atropine: 0.1 mg/kg IM, or 0.02 mg/kg IV; and 2-PAM chloride: 25 mg/kg IM, or 15 mg/kg IV slowly	Assisted ventilation after antidotes for severe exposure. Repeat atropine (2 mg IM, or 1 mg IM for infants) at 5- to 10-min intervals until secretions have diminished and breathing is comfortable or airway resistance has returned to near normal. Phentolamine for 2-PAM-induced hypertension: (5 mg IV for adults; 1 mg IV for children). Diazepam for convulsions: (0.2 to 0.5 mg IV for infants <5 years: 1 mg IV for children >5 years; 5 mg IV for adults).
Child (2 to 10 yrs)	Atropine: 1 mg IM, or 0.02 mg/kg IV; and 2-PAM chloride[c]: 15 mg/kg IM or IV slowly	Atropine: 2 mg IM, or 0.02 mg/kg IV; and 2-PAM chloride[c]: 25 mg/kg IM, or 15 mg/kg IV slowly	
Adolescent (>10 yrs)	Atropine: 2 mg IM, or 0.02 mg/kg IV; and 2-PAM chloride[c]: 15 mg/kg IM or IV slowly	Atropine: 4 mg IM, or 0.02 mg/kg IV; and 2-PAM chloride[c]: 25 mg/kg IM, or 15 mg/kg IV slowly	
Adult	Atropine: 2 to 4 mg IM or IV; and 2-PAM chloride: 600 mg IM, or 15 mg/kg IV slowly	Atropine: 6 mg IM; and 2-PAM chloride: 1800 mg IM, or 15 mg/kg IV slowly	
Elderly, frail	Atropine: 1 mg IM; and 2-PAM chloride: 10 mg/kg IM, or 5 to 10 mg/kg IV slowly	Atropine: 2 to 4 mg IM; and 2-PAM chloride: 25 mg/kg IM, or 5 to 10 mg/kg IV slowly	

[a] Mild/moderate effects include localized sweating, muscle fasciculations, nausea, vomiting, weakness, dyspnea.

[b] Severe effects include unconsciousness, convulsions, apnea, flaccid paralysis.

[c] If calculated dose exceeds the adult IM dose, adjust accordingly.

Note: 2-PAM chloride is pralidoxime chloride or protopam chloride.

Source: State of New York, Department of Health.

Gamma radiation and *x-rays* are forms of electromagnetic radiation discharged from the atomic nucleus. Sometimes referred to as *penetrating radiation*, both gamma and x-rays easily penetrate matter and are the principle type of radiation to cause whole-body exposure (see below).

Neutron particles are heavy and uncharged; often emitted during a nuclear detonation. Their ability to penetrate tissues is variable, depending upon their energy. They are less likely to be generated in various scenarios of radiation bioterrorism.

The commonly used units of radiation are the *rad* and the *gray*. The rad is the energy deposited within living matter and is equal to 100 ergs/g of tissue. The rad has been replaced by the SI unit of the gray (Gy). 100 rad = 1 Gy.

Types of Exposure

Whole-body exposure represents deposition of radiation energy over the entire body. Alpha and beta particles have limited penetration power and do not cause significant whole-body exposure unless they are internalized in large amounts. Whole-body exposure from gamma rays, x-rays, or high-energy neutron particles can penetrate the body, causing damage to multiple tissues and organs.

External contamination results from fallout of radioactive particles landing on the body surface, clothing, and hair. This is the dominant form of contamination likely to occur in a terrorist strike that utilizes a dispersal device. The most likely contaminants would emit alpha and beta radiation. Alpha particles do not penetrate the skin and thus would produce minimal systemic damage. Beta emitters can cause significant cutaneous burns. Gamma emitters cannot only cause cutaneous burns but can also cause significant internal damage.

Internal contamination will occur when radioactive material is inhaled, ingested, or is able to enter the body via a disruption in the skin. The respiratory tract is the main portal of entrance for internal contamination, and the lung is the organ at greatest risk. Radioactive material entering the GI tract will be absorbed according to its chemical structure and solubility. Penetration through the skin usually occurs when wounds or burns have disrupted the cutaneous barrier. Absorbed radioactive materials will travel throughout the body. Liver, kidney, adipose tissue, and bone tend to bind and retain radioactive material more than do other tissues.

Localized exposure results from close contact between highly radioactive material and a part of the body, resulting in discrete damage to the skin and deeper structures.

Acute Radiation Sickness

Radiation interactions with atoms can result in ionization and free radical formation that damages tissue by disrupting chemical bonds and molecular structures in the cell, including DNA. Radiation can lead to cell death; cells that recover may have DNA mutations that pose a higher risk for malignant transformation. Cell sensitivity to radiation damage increases as replication rate increases. Bone marrow and mucosal surfaces in the GI tract have high mitotic activity and thus are significantly more prone to radiation damage than slowly dividing tissues such as bone and muscle. Acute radiation sickness (ARS) can develop following exposure of all or most of the human body to ionizing radiation. The clinical manifestation of ARS reflect the dose and type of radiation as well as the parts of the body that are exposed.

Clinical Features ARS produces signs and symptoms related to damage of three major organ systems: GI tract, bone marrow, and neurovascular. The type and dose of radiation and the part of the body exposed will determine the dominant clinical picture.

- There are four major stages of ARS:
  1. *Prodrome* occurs between hours to 4 days after exposure and lasts from hours to days. Manifestations include: nausea, vomiting, anorexia, and diarrhea.
  2. The *latent stage* follows the prodrome and is associated with minimal or no symptoms. It most commonly lasts up to 2 weeks but can last as long as 6 weeks.
  3. *Illness* follows the latent stage.
  4. *Death or recovery* is the final stage of ARS.
- The higher the radiation dose, the shorter and more severe the stage.
- At low radiation doses (0.7 to 4 Gy), bone marrow suppression occurs and constitutes the main illness. The pt may develop bleeding or infection secondary to thrombocytopenia and leukopenia. The bone marrow will generally recover in most pts. Care is supportive (transfusion, antibiotics, colony-stimulating factors).
- With exposure to 6–8 Gy, the clinical picture is more complicated; the bone marrow may not recover and death will ensue. Damage to the GI mucosa producing diarrhea, hemorrhage, sepsis, fluid and electrolyte imbalance may occur and complicate the clinical picture.
- Whole-body exposure to >10 Gy is usually fatal. In addition to severe bone marrow and GI tract damage, a neurovascular syndrome characterized by vascular collapse, seizures, and death may occur (especially at doses >20 Gy).

℞ TREATMENT

Treatment of ARS is largely supportive (Fig. 31-1).

1. Persons contaminated either externally or internally should be decontaminated as soon as possible. Contaminated clothes should be removed; showering or washing the entire skin and hair is very important. A radiation detector should be used to check for residual contamination. Decontamination of medical personnel should occur following emergency treatment and decontamination of the pt.
2. Treatment for the hematopoietic system includes appropriate therapy for neutropenia and infection, transfusion of blood products as needed, and hematopoietic growth factors. The value of bone marrow transplantation in this situation is unknown.
3. Partial or total parenteral nutrition is appropriate supportive therapy for pts with significant injury to the GI mucosa.
4. Treatment of internal radionuclide contamination is aimed at reducing absorption and enhancing elimination of the ingested material (Table 207-2, HPIM-16).
   a. Clearance of the GI tract may be achieved by gastric lavage, emetics, or purgatives, laxatives, ion exchange resins, and aluminum-containing antacids.
   b. Administration of *blocking agents* is aimed at preventing the entrance of radioactive materials into tissues (e.g., potassium iodide, which blocks the uptake of radioactive iodine by the thyroid).
   c. *Diluting agents* decrease the absorption of the radionuclide (e.g., water in the treatment of tritium contamination).
   d. *Mobilizing agents* are most effective when given immediately; however, they may still be effective for up to 2 weeks following exposure. Examples include antithyroid drugs, glucocorticoids, ammo-

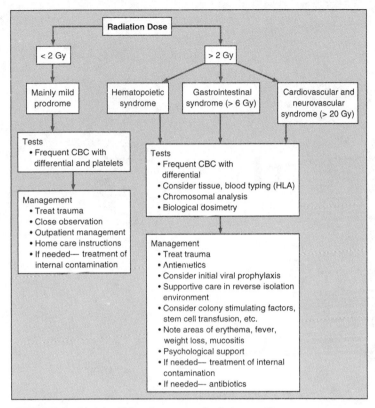

FIGURE 31-1 General guidelines for treatment of radiation casualties.

nium chloride, diuretics, expectorants, and inhalants. All of these should induce the release of radionuclides from tissues.
  e. *Chelating agents* bind many radioactive materials, after which the complexes are excreted from the body.

For a more detailed discussion, see Lane HC, Fauci AS: Microbial Bioterrorism, Chap. 205, p. 1279; Hurst CG, Newmark J, Romano JA: Chemical Bioterrorism, Chap. 206, p. 1288; Tochner ZA, Lehavi O, Glatstein E: Radiation Bioterrorism, Chap. 207, p. 1294; in HPIM-16.

COMMON PATIENT PRESENTATIONS

32

CHEST PAIN

There is little correlation between the severity of chest pain and the seriousness of its cause.

POTENTIALLY SERIOUS CAUSES

The differential diagnosis of chest pain is shown in Fig. 32-1. It is useful to characterize the chest pain as (1) new, acute, and ongoing; (2) recurrent, episodic; and (3) persistent, sometimes for days (Table 32-1).

MYOCARDIAL ISCHEMIA *Angina Pectoris* Substernal pressure, squeezing, constriction, with radiation typically to left arm; usually on exertion, especially after meals or with emotional arousal. Characteristically relieved by rest and nitroglycerin.

Acute Myocardial Infarction (Chap. 123) Similar to angina but usually more severe, of longer duration (≥ 30 min), and not immediately relieved by rest or nitroglycerin. S_3 and S_4 common.

PULMONARY EMBOLISM (Chap. 135) May be substernal or lateral, pleuritic in nature, and associated with hemoptysis, tachycardia, and hypoxemia.

AORTIC DISSECTION (Chap. 127) Very severe, in center of chest, a "ripping" quality, radiates to back, not affected by changes in position. May be associated with weak or absent peripheral pulses.

MEDIASTINAL EMPHYSEMA Sharp, intense, localized to substernal region; often associated with audible crepitus.

ACUTE PERICARDITIS (Chap. 121) Usually steady, crushing, substernal; often has pleuritic component aggravated by cough, deep inspiration, supine position, and relieved by sitting upright; one-, two-, or three-component pericardial friction rub often audible.

PLEURISY Due to inflammation; less commonly tumor and pneumothorax. Usually unilateral, knifelike, superficial, aggravated by cough and respiration.

LESS SERIOUS CAUSES

COSTOCHONDRAL PAIN In anterior chest, usually sharply localized, may be brief and darting or a persistent dull ache. Can be reproduced by pressure on costochondral and/or chondrosternal junctions. In Tietze's syndrome (costochondritis), joints are swollen, red, and tender.

CHEST WALL PAIN Due to strain of muscles or ligaments from excessive exercise or rib fracture from trauma; accompanied by local tenderness.

ESOPHAGEAL PAIN Deep thoracic discomfort; may be accompanied by dysphagia and regurgitation.

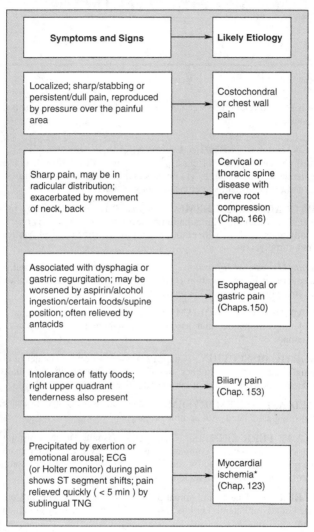

FIGURE 32-1 Differential diagnosis of recurrent chest pain. *If myocardial ischemia suspected, also consider aortic valve disease (Chap. 119) and hypertrophic obstructive cardiomyopathy (Chap. 120) if systolic murmur present.

EMOTIONAL DISORDERS Prolonged ache or dartlike, brief, flashing pain; associated with fatigue, emotional strain.

OTHER CAUSES
(1) Cervical disk; (2) osteoarthritis of cervical or thoracic spine; (3) abdominal disorders: peptic ulcer, hiatus hernia, pancreatitis, biliary colic; (4) tracheo-bronchitis, pneumonia; (5) diseases of the breast (inflammation, tumor); (6) intercostal neuritis (herpes zoster).

FIGURE 32-2 Differential diagnosis of acute chest pain.

	Acute myocardial infarction (Chap. 123)	Aortic dissection (Chap. 127)	Acute pericarditis (Chap. 121)	Pulmonary embolism (Chap. 135)	Acute pneumothorax (Chap. 137)	Rupture of esophagus
Description of pain	Oppressive, constrictive, or squeezing; may radiate to arm(s), neck, back	"Tearing" or "ripping"; may travel from anterior chest to mid-back	Crushing, sharp, pleuritic; relieved by sitting forward	Pleuritic, sharp; possibly accompanied by cough/hemoptysis	Very sharp, pleuritic	Intense substernal and epigastric; accompanied by vomiting ± hematemesis
Background history	Less severe, similar pain on exertion; + coronary risk factors (Chap. 122)	Hypertension or Marfan syndrome (Chap. 161)	Recent upper respiratory tract infection, or other conditions which predispose to pericarditis (Chap. 121)	Recent surgery or other immobilization	Recent chest trauma, or history of chronic obstructive lung disease	Recent recurrent vomiting/retching
Key Physical findings	Diaphoresis, pallor; S4 common; S3 less common	Weak, asymmetric peripheral pulses; possible diastolic murmur or aortic insufficiency (Chap. 117)	Pericardial friction rub (usually 3 components, best heard by sitting patient forward)	Tachypnea; possible pleural friction rub	Tachypnea; breath sounds & hyperresonance over affected lung field	Subcutaneous emphysema; audible crepitus adjacent to the sternum
Consider						
Confirmatory tests	• Serial ECGs • Serial cardiac markers (esp. troponins, CK)	• CXR – widened mediastinal silhouette • MRI, CT, or transesophageal echogram: intimal flap visualized • Aortic angiogram: definitive diagnosis	• ECG: diffuse ST elevation and PR segment depression • Echogram: pericardial effusion often visualized	• Arterial blood gas: hypoxemia & respiratory alkalosis • Lung scan: V/Q mismatch • Pulmonary angiogram: arterial luminal filling defects	• CXR: radiolucency within pleural space; poss. collapse of adjacent lung segment; if tension pneumothorax, mediastinum is shifted to opp. side	• CXR: pneumo-mediastinum • Esophageal endoscopy is diagnostic

Table 32-1

Differential Diagnoses of Patients Admitted to Hospital with Acute Chest Pain Ruled Not Myocardial Infarction

Diagnosis	Percent
Gastroesophageal disease[a]	42
Gastroesophageal reflux	
Esophageal motility disorders	
Peptic ulcer	
Gallstones	
Ischemic heart disease	31
Chest wall syndromes	28
Pericarditis	4
Pleuritis/pneumonia	2
Pulmonary embolism	2
Lung cancer	1.5
Aortic aneurysm	1
Aortic stenosis	1
Herpes zoster	1

[a] In order of frequency.
Source: Fruergaard P et al: Eur Heart J 17:1028, 1996.

————————————— *Approach to the Patient* —————————————

A meticulous history of the behavior of pain, what precipitates it and what relieves it, aids diagnosis of recurrent chest pain. Figure 32-2 presents clues to diagnosis and workup of acute, life-threatening chest pain.

For a more detailed discussion, see Lee TH: Chest Discomfort and Palpitations, Chap. 12, p. 76, in HPIM-16.

33

ABDOMINAL PAIN

Numerous causes, ranging from acute, life-threatening emergencies to chronic functional disease and disorders of several organ systems, can generate abdominal pain. Evaluation of acute pain requires rapid assessment of likely causes and early initiation of appropriate therapy (see Chap. 51). A more detailed and time-consuming approach to diagnosis may be followed in less acute situations. Table 33-1 lists the common causes of abdominal pain.

Table 33-1

Common Etiologies of Abdominal Pain

Mucosal or muscle inflammation in hollow viscera: Peptic disease (ulcers, erosions, inflammation), hemorrhagic gastritis, gastroesophageal reflux, appendicitis, diverticulitis, cholecystitis, cholangitis, inflammatory bowel diseases (Crohn's, ulcerative colitis), infectious gastroenteritis, mesenteric lymphadenitis, colitis, cystitis, or pyelonephritis

Visceral spasm or distention: Intestinal obstruction (adhesions, tumor, intussusception), appendiceal obstruction with appendicitis, strangulation of hernia, irritable bowel syndrome (muscle hypertrophy and spasm), acute biliary obstruction, pancreatic ductal obstruction (chronic pancreatitis, stone), ureteral obstruction (kidney stone, blood clot), fallopian tubes (tubal pregnancy)

Vascular disorders: Mesenteric thromboembolic disease (arterial or venous), arterial dissection or rupture (e.g., aortic aneurysm), occlusion from external pressure or torsion (e.g., volvulus, hernia, tumor, adhesions, intussusception), hemoglobinopathy (esp. sickle cell disease)

Distention or inflammation of visceral surfaces: Hepatic capsule (hepatitis, hemorrhage, tumor, Budd-Chiari syndrome, Fitz-Hugh-Curtis syndrome), renal capsule (tumor, infection, infarction, venous occlusion), splenic capsule (hemorrhage, abscess, infarction), pancreas (pancreatitis, pseudocyst, abscess, tumor), ovary (hemorrhage into cyst, ectopic pregnancy, abscess)

Peritoneal inflammation: Bacterial infection (perforated viscus, pelvic inflammatory disease, infected ascites), intestinal infarction, chemical irritation, pancreatitis, perforated viscus (esp. stomach and duodenum), reactive inflammation (neighboring abscess, incl. diverticulitis, pleuropulmonary infection or inflammation), serositis (collagen-vascular diseases, familial Mediterranean fever), ovulation (mittelschmerz).

Abdominal wall disorders: Trauma, hernias, muscle inflammation or infection, hematoma (trauma, anticoagulant therapy), traction from mesentery (e.g., adhesions)

Toxins: Lead poisoning, black widow spider bite

Metabolic disorders: Uremia, ketoacidosis (diabetic, alcoholic), Addisonian crisis, porphyria, angioedema (C1 esterase deficiency), narcotic withdrawal

Neurologic disorders: Herpes zoster, tabes dorsalis, causalgia, compression or inflammation of spinal roots, (e.g., arthritis, herniated disk, tumor, abscess), psychogenic

Referred pain: From heart, lungs, esophagus, genitalia (e.g., cardiac ischemia, pneumonia, pneumothorax, pulmonary embolism, esophagitis, esophageal spasm, esophageal rupture)

_____ *Approach to the Patient* _____

History

History is of critical diagnostic importance. Physical exam may be unrevealing or misleading, and laboratory and radiologic exams delayed or unhelpful.

Characteristic Features of Abdominal Pain

Duration and Pattern These provide clues to nature and severity, although acute abdominal crisis may occasionally present insidiously or on a background of chronic pain.

Type and location provide a rough guide to nature of disease. *Visceral pain* (due to distention of a hollow viscus) localizes poorly and is often perceived in the midline. Intestinal pain tends to be crampy; when originating proximal to the ileocecal valve, it usually localizes above and around the umbilicus. Pain of colonic origin is perceived in the hypogastrium and lower quadrants. Pain from biliary or ureteral obstruction often causes pts to writhe in discomfort. *Somatic pain* (due to peritoneal inflammation) is usually sharper and more precisely localized to the diseased region (e.g., acute appendicitis; capsular distention of liver, kidney, or spleen), exacerbated by movement, causing pts to remain still. Pattern of radiation may be helpful: right shoulder (hepatobiliary origin), left shoulder (splenic), midback (pancreatic), flank (proximal urinary tract), groin (genital or distal urinary tract).

Factors that Precipitate or Relieve Pain Ask about its relationship to eating (e.g., upper GI, biliary, pancreatic, ischemic bowel disease), defecation (colorectal), urination (genitourinary or colorectal), respiratory (pleuropulmonary, hepatobiliary), position (pancreatic, gastroesophageal reflux, musculoskeletal), menstrual cycle/menarche (tuboovarian, endometrial, including endometriosis), exertion (coronary/intestinal ischemia, musculoskeletal), medication/specific foods (motility disorders, food intolerance, gastroesophageal reflux, porphyria, adrenal insufficiency, ketoacidosis, toxins), and stress (motility disorders, nonulcer dyspepsia, irritable bowel syndrome).

Associated Symptoms Look for fevers/chills (infection, inflammatory disease, infarction), weight loss (tumor, inflammatory diseases, malabsorption, ischemia), nausea/vomiting (obstruction, infection, inflammatory disease, metabolic disease), dysphagia/odynophagia (esophageal), early satiety (gastric), hematemesis (esophageal, gastric, duodenal), constipation (colorectal, perianal, genitourinary), jaundice (hepatobiliary, hemolytic), diarrhea (inflammatory disease, infection, malabsorption, secretory tumors, ischemia, genitourinary), dysuria/hematuria/vaginal or penile discharge (genitourinary), hematochezia (colorectal or, rarely, urinary), skin/joint/eye disorders (inflammatory disease, bacterial or viral infection).

Predisposing Factors Inquire about family history (inflammatory disease, tumors, pancreatitis), hypertension and atherosclerotic disease (ischemia), diabetes mellitus (motility disorders, ketoacidosis), connective tissue disease (motility disorders, serositis), depression (motility disorders, tumors), smoking (ischemia), recent smoking cessation (inflammatory disease), ethanol use (motility disorders, hepatobiliary, pancreatic, gastritis, peptic ulcer disease).

Physical Examination

Evaluate abdomen for prior trauma or surgery, current trauma; abdominal distention, fluid, or air; direct, rebound, and referred tenderness; liver and spleen size; masses, bruits, altered bowel sounds, hernias, arterial masses. Rectal examination for presence and location of tenderness, masses, blood (gross or occult). Pelvic examination in women is essential. *General examination*: evaluate for evidence of hemodynamic instability, acid-base disturbances, nutritional deficiency, coagulopathy, arterial occlusive disease, stigmata of liver disease, cardiac dysfunction, lymphadenopathy, and skin lesions.

Routine Laboratory and Radiologic Studies

Choices depend on clinical setting (esp. severity of pain, rapidity of onset): may include CBC, serum electrolytes, coagulation parameters, serum glucose, and biochemical tests of liver, kidney, and pancreatic function; CXR to determine the presence of diseases involving heart, lung, mediastinum, and pleura; ECG is helpful to exclude referred pain from cardiac disease; plain abdominal radiographs to evaluate bowel displacement, intestinal distention, fluid and gas pattern, free peritoneal air, liver size, and abdominal calcifications (e.g., gallstones, renal stones, chronic pancreatitis).

Special Studies

These include abdominal ultrasonography (to visualize biliary ducts, gallbladder, liver, pancreas, and kidneys); CT to identify masses, abscesses, evidence of inflammation (bowel wall thickening, mesenteric "stranding," lymphadenopathy), aortic aneurysm; barium contrast radiographs (barium swallow, upper GI series, small-bowel follow-through, barium enema); upper GI endoscopy, sigmoidoscopy, or colonoscopy; cholangiography (endoscopic, percutaneous, or via MRI), angiography (direct or via CT or MRI), and radionuclide scanning. In selected cases, percutaneous biopsy, laparoscopy, and exploratory laparotomy may be required.

ACUTE, CATASTROPHIC ABDOMINAL PAIN
See Chap. 51, Acute Abdomen, page 206.

For a more detailed discussion, see Silen W: Abdominal Pain, Chap. 13, p. 82, in HPIM-16.

34

HEADACHE

Causes of headache are summarized in Table 34-1. First step—distinguish serious from benign etiologies. Symptoms that raise the suspicion for a serious cause are listed in Table 34-2; serious causes are summarized in Table 34-3. Intensity of head pain rarely has diagnostic value; most pts who present to emergency ward with worst headache of their lives have migraine. Headache location can suggest involvement of local structures (temporal pain in giant cell arteritis, facial pain in sinusitis). Ruptured aneurysm (instant onset), cluster headache (peak over 3–5 min), and migraine (onset over minutes to hours) differ in time to peak intensity. Provocation by environmental factors suggests a benign cause.

Evaluation

Complete neurologic exam is essential first step. If exam is abnormal or if serious underlying cause is suspected for any reason, an imaging study (CT or MRI) is indicated. Lumbar puncture is required when meningitis (stiff neck, fever) is a possibility.

Migraine

Classic Migraine   Onset usually in childhood, adolescence, or early adulthood; however, initial attack may occur at any age. Family history often posi-

Table 34-1
_____
International Headache Society Classification of Headache
_____
1. **Migraine**
   Migraine without aura
   Migraine with aura
   Ophthalmoplegic migraine
   Retinal migraine
   Childhood periodic syndromes that may be precursors to or
      associated with migraine
   Migrainous disorder not fulfilling above criteria
2. **Tension-type headache**
   Episodic tension-type headache
   Chronic tension-type headache
3. **Cluster headache and chronic paroxysmal hemicrania**
   Cluster headache
   Chronic paroxysmal hemicrania
4. **Miscellaneous headaches not associated with structural
   lesion**
   Idiopathic stabbing headache
   External compression headache
   Cold stimulus headache
   Benign cough headache
   Benign exertional headache
   Headache associated with sexual activity
5. **Headache associated with head trauma**
   Acute posttraumatic headache
   Chronic posttraumatic headache
6. **Headache associated with vascular disorders**
   Acute ischemic cerebrovascular disorder
   Intracranial hematoma
   Subarachnoid hemorrhage
   Unruptured vascular malformation
   Arteritis
   Carotid or vertebral artery pain
   Venous thrombosis
   Arterial hypertension
   Other vascular disorder
7. **Headache associated with nonvascular intracranial
   disorder**
   High CSF pressure
   Low CSF pressure
   Intracranial infection
_____
Source: After J Olesen: Cephalalgia 8(Suppl 7):1, 1988.

tive. More frequent in women. Classic triad: premonitory visual (scotoma or scintillations) sensory or motor symptoms, unilateral throbbing headache, nausea and vomiting. Photo- and phonophobia common. Vertigo may occur. Focal neurologic disturbances without headache or vomiting (migraine equivalents) may also occur. An attack lasting 2–6 h is typical, as is relief after sleep. Attacks may be triggered by wine, cheese, chocolate, contraceptives, stress, exercise, or travel.

   Common Migraine   Unilateral or bilateral headache with nausea, but no focal neurologic symptoms. Moderate-to-severe head pain, pulsating quality,

7. **Headache associated with nonvascular intracranial disorder** (*cont.*)
   Sarcoidosis and other noninfectious inflammatory diseases
   Related to intrathecal injections
   Intracranial neoplasm
   Associated with other intracranial disorder
8. **Headache associated with substances or their withdrawal**
   Headache induced by acute substance use or exposure
   Headache induced by chronic substance use or exposure
   Headache from substance withdrawal (acute use)
   Headache from substance withdrawal (chronic use)
9. **Headache associated with noncephalic infection**
   Viral infection
   Bacterial infection
   Other infection
10. **Headache associated with metabolic disorder**
    Hypoxia
    Hypercapnia
    Mixed hypoxia and hypercapnia
    Hypoglycemia
    Dialysis
    Other metabolic abnormality
11. **Headache or facial pain associated with disorder of facial or cranial structures**
    Cranial bone
    Eyes
    Ears
    Nose and sinuses
    Teeth, jaws, and related structures
    Temporomandibular joint disease
12. **Cranial neuralgias, nerve trunk pain, and deafferentation pain**
    Persistent (in contrast to ticlike) pain of cranial nerve origin
    Trigeminal neuralgia
    Glossopharyngeal neuralgia
    Nervus intermedius neuralgia
    Superior laryngeal neuralgia
    Occipital neuralgia
    Central causes of head and facial pain other than tic douloureux
13. **Headache not classifiable**

unilateral, worse with activity; associated with photophobia, phonophobia, multiple attacks. More common in women. Onset more gradual than in classic migraine; duration 4–72 h.

 TREATMENT

Three approaches to migraine treatment: nonpharmacologic (Table 34-4), drug treatment of acute attacks (Table 34-5), and prophylaxis (Table 34-6). Drug treatment necessary for most migraine pts, but avoidance or manage-

Table 34-2

Headache Symptoms that Suggest a Serious Underlying Disorder

"Worst" headache ever
First severe headache
Subacute worsening over days or weeks
Abnormal neurologic examination
Fever or unexplained systemic signs
Vomiting precedes headache
Induced by bending, lifting, cough
Disturbs sleep or presents immediately upon awakening
Known systemic illness
Onset after age 55

ment of environmental triggers is sufficient for some. General principles of pharmacologic treatment: (1) response rates vary from 60–90%; (2) initial drug choice is empirical—influenced by patient age, coexisting illnesses, and side effect profile; (3) efficacy of prophylactic treatment may take several months to assess with each drug; (4) when an acute attack requires additional medication 60 min after the first dose, then the initial drug dose should be increased for subsequent attacks. A staged approach to treatment is outlined in Table 34-7. Mild-to-moderate acute migraine attacks often respond to over-the-counter (OTC) NSAIDs when taken early in the attack. Triptans are widely used also, but recurrence of head pain after the first dose (40–78%) is a major limitation. There is less frequent headache recurrence when using ergots, but more frequent side effects. For prophylaxis, amitriptyline is a good first choice for young people with difficulty falling asleep; verapamil is often a first choice for prophylaxis in the elderly.

Table 34-3

Symptoms of Serious Underlying Causes of Headache

Cause	Symptoms
Meningitis	Nuchal rigidity, headache, photophobia, and prostration; may not be febrile. Lumbar puncture is diagnostic.
Intracranial hemorrhage	Nuchal rigidity and headache; may not have clouded consciousness or seizures. Hemorrhage may not be seen on CT scan. Lumbar puncture shows "bloody tap" that does not clear by the last tube. A fresh hemorrhage may not be xanthochromic.
Brain tumor	May present with prostrating pounding headaches that are associated with nausea and vomiting. Should be suspected in progressively severe new "migraine" that is invariably unilateral.
Temporal arteritis	May present with a unilateral pounding headache. Onset generally in older patients (>50 years) and frequently associated with visual changes. The erythrocyte sedimentation rate is the best screening test and is usually markedly elevated (i.e., >50). Definitive diagnosis can be made by arterial biopsy.
Glaucoma	Usually consists of severe eye pain. May have nausea and vomiting. The eye is usually painful and red. The pupil may be partially dilated.

Table 34-4

Nonpharmacologic Approaches to Migraine

Identify and then avoid trigger factors such as:
Alcohol (e.g., red wine)
Foods (e.g., chocolate, certain cheeses, monosodium glutamate, nitrate-
  containing foods)
Hunger (avoid missing meals)
Irregular sleep patterns (both lack of sleep and excessive sleep)
Organic odors
Sustained exertion
Acute changes in stress levels
Miscellaneous (glare, flashing lights)
Attempt to manage environmental shifts such as:
Time zone shifts
High altitude
Barometric pressure changes
Weather changes
Assess menstrual cycle relationship

Table 34-5

Treatment of Acute Migraine

Drug	Trade Name	Dosage
NSAIDs		
Acetaminophen, aspirin, caffeine	Excedrin Migraine	Two tablets or caplets q6h (max 8 per day)
5-HT$_1$ AGONISTS		
Oral		
Ergotamine	Ergomar	One 2 mg sublingual tablet at onset and q1/2h (max 3 per day, 5 per week)
Ergotamine 1 mg, caffeine 100 mg	Ercaf, Wigraine	One or two tablets at onset, then one tablet q1/2h (max 6 per day, 10 per week)
Naratriptan	Amerge	2.5 mg tablet at onset; may repeat once after 4 h
Rizatriptan	Maxalt Maxalt-MLT	5 to 10 mg tablet at onset; may repeat after 2 h (max 30 mg/d)
Sumatriptan	Imitrex	50 to 100 mg tablet at onset; may repeat after 2 h (max 200 mg/d)
Zolmitriptan	Zomig Zomig Rapimelt	2.5 mg tablet at onset; may repeat after 2 h (max 10 mg/d)
Nasal		
Dihydroergotamine	Migranal Nasal Spray	Prior to nasal spray, the pump must be primed 4 times; one spray (0.5 mg) is administered followed, in 15 min, by a second spray

(continued)

Table 34-5 *(Continued)*

Treatment of Acute Migraine

Sumatriptan	Imitrex Nasal Spray	5 to 20 mg intranasal spray as 4 sprays of 5 mg or a single 20 mg spray (may repeat once after 2 h, not to exceed a dose of 40 mg/d)
Parenteral		
Dihydroergotamine	DHE-45	1 mg IV, IM, or SC at onset and q1h (max 3 mg/d, 6 mg per week)
Sumatriptan	Imitrex Injection	6 mg SC at onset (may repeat once after 1 h for max of two doses in 24 h)

DOPAMINE ANTAGONISTS

Oral		
Metoclopramide	Reglan,[a] generic[a]	5–10 mg/d
Prochlorperazine	Compazine,[a] generic[a]	1–25 mg/d
Parenteral		
Chlorpromazine	Generic[a]	0.1 mg/kg IV at 2 mg/min; max 35 mg/d
Metoclopramide	Reglan,[a] generic	10 mg IV
Prochlorperazine	Compazine,[a] generic[a]	10 mg IV

OTHER

Oral		
Acetaminophen, 325 mg, *plus* dichloralphenazone, 100 mg, *plus* isometheptene, 65 mg	Midrin, Duradrin, generic	Two capsules at onset followed by 1 capsule q1h (max 5 capsules)
Nasal		
Butorphanol	Stadol[a]	1 mg (1 spray in 1 nostril), may repeat if necessary in 1–2 h
Parenteral		
Narcotics	Generic[a]	Multiple preparations and dosages; see Table 8-2.

[a] Not specifically indicated by the U.S. Food and Drug Administration for migraine.
Note: 5-HT, 5-hydroxytryptamine.

Tension Headache Common in all age groups. Pain is holocephalic, described as pressure or a tight band. May persist for hours or days. Often related to stress; responds to relaxation and OTC analgesics (Table 34-8). Amitriptyline may be helpful for prophylaxis. Distinction from common migraine may be difficult.

Cluster Headache Characterized by episodes of recurrent, nocturnal, unilateral, retroorbital searing pain. Typically, a young male (90%) awakens 2–4 h after sleep onset with severe pain, unilateral lacrimation, and nasal and conjunctival congestion. Visual complaints, nausea, or vomiting are rare. Pain

Table 34-6

Drugs Effective in the Prophylactic Treatment of Migraine

Drug	Trade Name	Dosage
β-Adrenergic agents		
Propranolol	Inderal	80–320 mg qd
	Inderal LA	
Timolol	Blocadren	20–60 mg qd
Anticonvulsants		
Sodium valproate	Depakote	250 mg bid (max 1000 mg/d)
Tricyclic antidepressants		
Amitriptyline	Elavil,[a] generic	10–50 mg qhs
Nortriptyline	Pamelor,[a] generic	25–75 mg qhs
Monoamine oxidase inhibitors		
Phenelzine	Nardil[a]	15 mg tid
Serotonergic drugs		
Methysergide	Sansert	4–8 mg qd
Cyproheptadine	Periactin[a]	4–16 mg qd
Other		
Verapamil	Calan[a]	80–480 mg qd
	Isoptin[a]	

[a] Not specifically indicated for migraine by the U.S. Food and Drug Administration.

lasts 30–120 min but tends to recur at the same time of night or several times each 24 h over 4–8 weeks (a cluster). Diurnal periodicity (recurrent pain during the same hour each day of the cluster) occurs in 85%. A pain-free period of months or years may be followed by another cluster of headaches. Alcohol provokes attacks in 70%. Prophylaxis with lithium (600–900 mg qd) or prednisone (60 mg for 7 days followed by a rapid taper). Ergotamine, 1-mg sup-

Table 34-7

A Staged Approach to Migraine Pharmacotherapy

Stage	Diagnosis	Therapies
Mild migraine	Occasional throbbing headaches	NSAIDs
		Combination analgesics
	No major impairment of functioning	Oral 5-HT$_1$ agonists
Moderate migraine	Moderate or severe headaches	Oral, nasal, or SC 5-HT$_1$ agonists
	Nausea common	Oral dopamine antagonists
	Some impairment of functioning	
Severe migraine	Severe headaches >3 times per month	SC, IM, or IV 5-HT$_1$ agonists
	Significant functional impairment	IM or IV dopamine antagonists
	Marked nausea and/or vomiting	Prophylactic medications

Note: 5-HT, 5-hydroxytryptamine.

Table 34-8

Drugs Effective in the Treatment of Tension-Type Headache

Drug	Trade Name	Dosage
NONSTEROIDAL ANTI-INFLAMMATORY AGENTS		
Acetaminophen	Tylenol, generic	650 mg PO q4–6h
Aspirin	Generic	650 mg PO q4–6h
Diclofenac	Cataflam, generic	50–100 mg q4–6h (max 200 mg/d)
Ibuprofen	Advil, Motrin, Nuprin, generic	400 mg PO q3–4h
Naproxen sodium	Aleve, Anaprox, generic	220–550 mg bid
COMBINATION ANALGESICS		
Acetaminophen, 325 mg, *plus* butalbital, 50 mg	Phrenilin, generic	1–2 tablets; max 6 per day
Acetaminophen, 650 mg, *plus* butalbital, 50 mg	Phrenilin Forte	1 tablet; max 6 per day
Acetaminophen, 325 mg, *plus* butalbital, 50 mg, *plus* caffeine, 40 mg	Fioricet; Esgic, generic	1–2 tablets; max 6 per day
Acetaminophen, 500 mg, *plus* butalbital, 50 mg, *plus* caffeine, 40 mg	Esgicplus	1–2 tablets; max 6 per day
Aspirin, 325 mg, *plus* butalbital, 50 mg, *plus* caffeine, 40 mg	Fiorinal	1–2 tablets; max 6 per day
Aspirin, 650 mg, *plus* butalbital, 50 mg	Axotal	1 tablet q4h; max 6 per day
PROPHYLACTIC MEDICATIONS		
Amitriptyline	Elavil, generic	10–50 mg at bedtime
Doxepin	Sinequan, generic	10–75 mg at bedtime
Nortriptyline	Pamelor, generic	25–75 mg at bedtime

pository 1–2 h before expected attack, may prevent daily episode. High-flow oxygen (9 L/min) or sumatriptan (6 mg SC) is useful for the acute attack.

Other Headaches

Post-Concussion Headache   Common following motor vehicle collisions, other head trauma; severe injury or loss of consciousness often not present. Symptoms of headache, dizziness, vertigo, impaired memory, poor concentration, irritability; typically remits after several weeks to months. Neurologic examination and neuroimaging studies normal. Not a functional disorder; cause unknown.

Lumbar Puncture Headache   Typical onset 24–48 h after LP; follows 10–30% of LPs. Positional: onset when pt sits or stands, relief by lying flat. Most cases remit spontaneously in ≤1 week. Intravenous caffeine (500 mg IV, repeat in 1 h if dose ineffective) successful in 85%; epidural blood patch effective immediately in refractory cases.

Cough Headache Transient severe head pain with coughing, bending, lifting, sneezing, or stooping; lasts from seconds to several minutes; men > women. Usually benign, but posterior fossa mass lesion in ~25%. Consider brain MRI.

Facial Pain

Most common cause of facial pain is dental; triggered by hot, cold, or sweet foods. Exposure to cold repeatedly induces dental pain. Trigeminal neuralgia consists of paroxysmal, electric shock–like episodes of pain in the distribution of trigeminal nerve; occipital neuralgia presents as lancinating occipital pain. These disorders are discussed in Chap. 194.

For a more detailed discussion, see Raskin NH: Headache, Chap. 14, p. 85, in HPIM-16.

35

BACK AND NECK PAIN

LOW BACK PAIN

FIVE TYPES OF LOW BACK PAIN (LBP)

• *Local pain*—caused by activation of pain-sensitive nerve endings near affected part of the spine (i.e., tears, stretching).

• *Pain referred to the back*—abdominal or pelvic origin; back pain unaffected by spine movement.

• *Pain of spine origin*—restricted to the back or referred to lower limbs. Diseases of upper lumbar spine refer pain to upper lumbar region, groin, or anterior thighs. Diseases of lower lumbar spine refer pain to buttocks or posterior thighs.

• *Radicular pain*—radiates from spine to leg in specific nerve root territory. Coughing, sneezing, lifting heavy objects, or straining may elicit pain.

• *Pain associated with muscle spasm*—diverse causes; accompanied by taut paraspinal muscles.

EXAMINATION Include abdomen, pelvis, and rectum to search for visceral sources of pain. Inspection may reveal scoliosis or muscle spasm. Palpation may elicit pain over a diseased spine segment. Pain from hip may be confused with spine pain; manual internal/external rotation of leg at hip (knee and hip in flexion) reproduces the hip pain. Straight-leg raising (SLR) sign—elicited by passive flexion of extended leg at the hip with pt in supine position; maneuver stretches L5/S1 nerve roots and sciatic nerve passing posterior to the hip; SLR is positive if maneuver reproduces the pain. Crossed SLR sign—positive when SLR on one leg reproduces symptoms in opposite leg or buttocks; nerve/nerve root lesion is on the painful side. Reverse SLR sign—passive extension of leg backwards with pt standing; maneuver stretches L2–L4 nerve roots and femoral nerve passing anterior to the hip. Neurologic exam—search for focal atrophy, weakness, reflex loss, diminished sensation in a dermatomal distribution. Findings with radiculopathy are summarized in Table 35-1.

LABORATORY STUDIES "Routine" laboratory studies and lumbar spine x-rays—rarely needed for acute LBP but indicated when risk factors for serious underlying disease are present (Table 35-2). MRI and CT-myelography are tests of choice for anatomic definition of spine disease. Electromyography (EMG) and nerve conduction studies useful for functional assessment of peripheral nervous system.

ETIOLOGY *Lumbar Disk Disease* Common cause of low back and leg pain; usually at L4-L5 or L5-S1 levels. Dermatomal sensory loss, reduction or loss of deep tendon reflexes, or myotomal pattern of weakness more informative than pain pattern for localization. Usually unilateral; bilateral with large central disk herniations compressing multiple nerve roots—may cause cauda equina syndrome. Indications for lumbar disk surgery: (1) progressive motor weakness from nerve root injury, (2) progressive motor impairment by EMG, (3) abnormal bowel or bladder function, (4) incapacitating nerve root pain despite conservative treatment for at least 4 weeks, and (5) recurrent incapacitating pain despite conservative treatment. The latter two criteria are controversial.

Spinal Stenosis A narrowed spinal canal producing neurogenic claudication, i.e., back, buttock, and/or leg pain induced by walking or standing and relieved by sitting. Symptoms are usually bilateral. Unlike vascular claudication, symptoms are provoked by standing without walking. Unlike lumbar disk disease, symptoms are relieved by sitting. Focal neurologic deficits common; severe neurologic deficits (paralysis, incontinence) rare. Stenosis results from acquired (75%), congenital, or mixed acquired/congenital factors. Symptomatic treatment adequate for mild disease; surgery indicated when pain interferes with activities of daily living or focal neurologic signs present. Surgery successful in 65–80%; 25% develop recurrent stenosis within 5 years.

Trauma *Low back strain* or *sprain* used to describe minor, self-limited injuries associated with LBP. *Vertebral fractures* from trauma result in wedging or compression of vertebral bodies; burst fractures involving anterior and posterior spine elements can occur. Neurologic impairment common with vertebral fractures; early surgical intervention indicated. Most common cause of *nontraumatic fracture* is osteoporosis; others are osteomalacia, hyperparathyroidism, hyperthyroidism, multiple myeloma, or metastatic carcinoma; glucocorticoid use may predispose vertebral body to fracture. Clinical context, exam findings, and spine x-rays establish diagnosis.

Spondylolisthesis Slippage of anterior spine forward, leaving posterior elements behind; L4-L5 > L5-S1 levels; can produce LBP or radiculopathy/cauda equina syndrome (see Chap. 196).

Osteoarthritis Back pain induced by spine movement. Increases with age; radiologic findings do not correlate with severity of pain. Facet syndrome—radicular symptoms and signs, nerve root compression by unilateral facet hypertrophy. Foraminotomy and facetectomy—long-term pain relief in 80–90%. Loss of intervertebral disk height reduces vertical dimensions of intervertebral foramen; descending pedicle can compress the exiting nerve root.

Vertebral Metastases Back pain most common neurologic symptom in patients with systemic cancer. Metastatic carcinoma, multiple myeloma, and lymphomas frequently involve spine. Back pain may be presenting symptom of

Table 35-1

Lumbosacral Radiculopathy—Neurologic Findings

Lubosacral Nerve Roots	Reflex	Sensory	Motor	Pain Distribution
L2[a]	—	Upper anterior thigh	Psoas[b] (hip flexion)	Anterior thigh
L3[a]	—	Lower anterior thigh Anterior knee	Psoas[b] (hip flexion) Quadriceps (knee extension) Thigh adduction	Anterior thigh, knee
L4[a]	Quadriceps (knee)	Medial calf	Quadriceps[b] (knee extension) Thigh adduction Tibialis anterior (foot dorsiflexion)	Knee, medial calf, anterolateral thigh
L5[c]	—	Dorsal surface—foot Lateral calf	Peroneii[b] (foot eversion) Tibialis anterior (foot dorsiflexion) Gluteus medius (hip abduction) Toe dorsiflexors	Lateral calf, dorsal foot, posterolateral thigh, buttocks
S1[a]	Gastrocnemius/soleus (ankle)	Plantar surface—foot Lateral aspect—foot	Gastrocnemius/soleus[b] (foot plantar flexion) Abductor hallucis (toe flexors) Gluteus maximus (hip extension)	Bottom foot, posterior calf, posterior thigh, buttocks

[a] Reverse straight-leg raising sign present—see "Examination."

[b] These muscles receive the majority of innervation from the root in the same horizontal row.

[c] Straight-leg raising sign present—see "Examination."

Table 35-2

Risk Factors for Possible Serious Causes of Acute LBP

HISTORY

Pain worse at rest or at night   Age >50 years
Prior history of cancer   Intravenous drug use
History of chronic infection (esp. Glucocorticoid use
  pulmonary, urinary tract, or skin) Rapidly progressive neurologic deficit
History of trauma

EXAMINATION

Unexplained fever
Unexplained weight loss
Straight-leg raising sign
Percussion tenderness—low spine or costovertebral angle
Abdominal, rectal, or pelvic mass
Rapidly progressive focal neurologic deficit (e.g., sensory loss, leg weakness,
  asymmetric or absent leg reflexes, abnormal bladder function)

---

cancer; pain typically unrelieved by rest. MRI or CT-myelography demonstrates vertebral body metastasis; disk space is spared.

Vertebral Osteomyelitis   Back pain unrelieved by rest; focal spine tenderness, elevated ESR. Primary source of infection (lung, urinary tract, or skin) found in 40%; IV drug abuse a risk factor. Destruction of the vertebral bodies and disk space common. Lumbar spinal epidural abscess presents as back pain and fever; exam may be normal or show radicular findings, spinal cord involvement, or cauda equina syndrome; abscess extent best defined by MRI.

Lumbar Arachnoiditis   May follow inflammatory response to local tissue injury within subarachnoid space; fibrosis results in clumping of nerve roots, best seen by MRI; treatment is unsatisfactory.

Immune Disorders   Ankylosing spondylitis, rheumatoid arthritis, Reiter's syndrome, psoriatic arthritis, and chronic inflammatory bowel disease. Ankylosing spondylitis—typically male <40 years with nocturnal back pain; pain unrelieved by rest but improves with exercise.

Osteoporosis   Loss of bone substance resulting from hyperparathyroidism, chronic glucocorticoid use, immobilization, or other medical disorders. Sole manifestation may be back pain exacerbated by movement.

Visceral Diseases   (Table 35-3)   Pelvis refers pain to sacral region, lower abdomen to lumbar region, upper abdomen to lower thoracic or upper lumbar region. Local signs are absent; normal movements of the spine are painless. A contained rupture of abdominal aortic aneurysm may produce isolated back pain.

Other   Chronic LBP with no clear cause; psychiatric disorders, substance abuse may be associated.

 TREATMENT

Acute Low Back Pain (ALBP)

Pain of <3 months' duration; full recovery occurs in 85%. Management controversial; few well-controlled clinical trials exist. Algorithms presented in

Table 35-3

Visceral Causes of Low Back Pain

Stomach (posterior wall)—Gallbladder—gallstones
Pancreas—tumor, cyst, pancreatitis
Retroperitoneal—hemorrhage, tumor, pyelonephritis
Vascular—abdominal aortic aneurysm, renal artery and vein thrombosis
Colon—colitis, diverticulitis, neoplasm
Uterosacral ligaments—endometriosis, carcinoma
Uterine malposition
Menstrual pain
Neoplastic infiltration of nerves
Radiation neurosis of tumors/nerves
Prostate—carcinoma, prostatitis
Kidney—renal stones, inflammatory disease, neoplasm, infection

Fig. 35-1. If "risk factors" (Table 35-2) are absent, initial treatment is symptomatic and no diagnostic tests necessary. Spine infections, fractures, tumors, or rapidly progressive neurologic deficits require urgent diagnostic evaluation. Patients with no risk factors and no improvement over 4 weeks are subdivided by the presence/absence of leg symptoms and managed accordingly.

Clinical trials do not show benefit from bed rest >2 days. Possible benefits of early activity—cardiovascular conditioning, disk and cartilage nutrition, bone and muscle strength, increased endorphin levels. Studies of traction or posture modification fail to show benefit. Proof lacking to support acupuncture, ultrasound, diathermy, transcutaneous electrical nerve stimulation, massage, biofeedback, or electrical stimulation. Self-application of ice or heat or use of shoe insoles is optional given low cost and risk; benefit of exercises uncertain. A short course of spinal manipulation or physical therapy may lessen pain and improve function. Temporary suspension of activities known to increase mechanical stress on the spine (heavy lifting, straining at stool, prolonged sitting/bending/twisting) may relieve symptoms. Value of education ("back school") in long-term prevention is unclear.

Pharmacologic treatment of ALBP includes NSAIDs and acetaminophen. Muscle relaxants (cyclobenzaprine, methocarbanol) provide short-term benefit (4–7 days), but drowsiness limits use. Opioids are not superior to NSAIDs or acetaminophen for ALBP. Epidural anesthetics, glucocorticoids, opioids, or tricyclic antidepressants are not indicated as initial treatment.

Chronic Low Back Pain (CLBP)

Pain lasting >3 months; differential diagnosis includes most conditions described above. CLBP causes can be clarified by neuroimaging and EMG/nerve conduction studies; diagnosis of radiculopathy secure when results concordant with findings on neurologic exam. Management is complex and not amenable to a simple algorithmic approach. Treatment based upon identification of underlying cause; when specific cause not found, conservative management necessary. Pharmacologic and comfort measures similar to those described for ALBP. Exercise ("work hardening") regimens effective in returning some pts to work, diminishing pain, and improving walking distances. Hydrotherapy may be useful, and some pts experience short-term pain relief with percutaneous electrical nerve stimulation.Surgical intervention based upon neuroimaging alone not recommended: up to one-third of asymptomatic young adults have a herniated lumbar disk by CT or MRI.

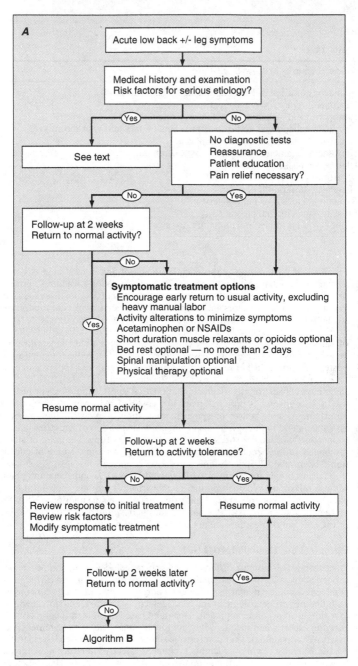

FIGURE 35-1A Algorithms for management of acute low back pain, age ≥ 18 years. *A.* Symptoms <3 months, first 4 weeks. *B.* Management weeks 4–12. ①, entry point from Algorithm *C* postoperatively or if patient declines surgery. *C.* Surgical options. (NCV, nerve conduction velocity studies.)

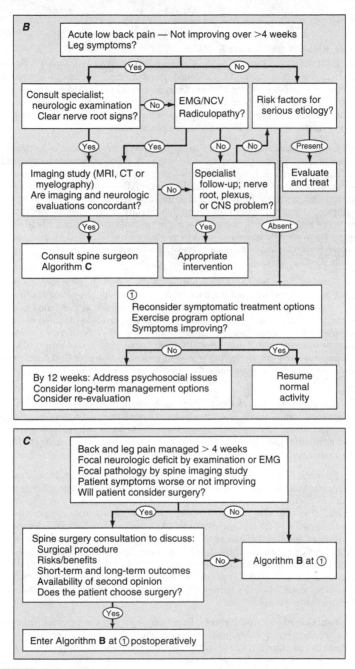

FIGURE 35-1B and C

NECK AND SHOULDER PAIN

ETIOLOGY *Trauma to the Cervical Spine* *Whiplash injury* is due to trauma (usually automobile accidents) causing cervical musculoligamental sprain or strain due to hyperflexion or hyperextension. This diagnosis should not be applied to pts with fractures, disk herniation, head injury, or altered consciousness. In one study, 18% of pts with whiplash injury had persistent injury-related symptoms 2 years after the car accident.

Cervical Disk Disease Herniation of a lower cervical disk is a common cause of neck, shoulder, arm, or hand pain. Neck pain (worse with movement), stiffness, and limited range of neck motion are common. With nerve root compression, pain may radiate into a shoulder or arm. Extension and lateral rotation of the neck narrows the intervertebral foramen and may reproduce radicular symptoms (Spurling's sign). In young individuals, acute radiculopathy from a ruptured disk is often traumatic. *Subacute radiculopathy* is less likely to be related to a specific traumatic incident and may involve both disk disease and spondylosis. Clinical features of cervical nerve root lesions are summarized in Table 35-4.

Cervical Spondylosis Osteoarthritis of the cervical spine may produce neck pain that radiates into the back of the head, shoulders, or arms; can also be source of headaches in the posterior occipital region. A combined radiculopathy and myelopathy may occur. An electrical sensation elicited by neck flexion and radiating down the spine from the neck (Lhermitte's symptom) usually indicates cervical or upper thoracic spinal cord involvement. MRI or CT-myelography can define the anatomic abnormalities, and EMG and nerve conduction studies can quantify the severity and localize the levels of nerve root injury.

Other Causes of Neck Pain Includes *rheumatoid arthritis* of the cervical apophyseal joints, ankylosing spondylitis, *herpes zoster* (shingles), *neoplasms* metastatic to the cervical spine, *infections* (osteomyelitis and epidural abscess), and *metabolic bone diseases*. Neck pain may also be referred from the heart with coronary artery ischemia (cervical angina syndrome).

Thoracic Outlet An anatomic region containing the first rib, the subclavian artery and vein, the brachial plexus, the clavicle, and the lung apex. Injury may result in posture- or task-related pain around the shoulder and supraclavicular region. *True neurogenic thoracic outlet syndrome* results from compression of the lower trunk of the brachial plexus by an anomalous band of tissue; treatment consists of surgical division of the band. *Arterial thoracic outlet syndrome* results from compression of the subclavian artery by a cervical rib; treatment is with thrombolyis or anticoagulation, and surgical excision of the cervical rib. *Disputed thoracic outlet syndrome* includes a large number of patients with chronic arm and shoulder pain of unclear cause; surgery is controversial, and treatment often unsuccessful.

Brachial Plexus and Nerves Pain from injury to the brachial plexus or arm peripheral nerves can mimic pain of cervical spine origin. *Neoplastic infiltration* can produce this syndrome, as can *postradiation fibrosis* (pain less often present). *Acute brachial neuritis* consists of acute onset of severe shoulder or scapular pain followed over days by weakness of proximal arm and shoulder girdle muscles innervated by the upper brachial plexus; onset often preceded by an infection or immunization. Complete recovery occurs in 75% of pts after 2 years and in 89% after 3 years.

Table 35-4

Cervical Radiculopathy—Neurologic Features

Cervical Nerve Roots	Examination Findings				
	Sensory	Reflex	Motor		Pain Distribution
C5	Over lateral deltoid	Biceps	Supraspinatus[a] (initial arm abduction) Infraspinatus[a] (arm external rotation) Deltoid[a] (arm abduction) Biceps (arm flexion)		Lateral arm, medial scapula
C6	Thumb, index fingers Radial hand/forearm	Biceps	Biceps (arm flexion) Pronator teres (internal forearm rotation)		Lateral forearm, thumb, index finger
C7	Middle fingers Dorsum forearm	Triceps	Triceps[a] (arm extension) Wrist extensors[a] Extensor digitorum[a] (finger extension)		Posterior arm, dorsal forearm, lateral hand
C8	Little finger Medial hand and forearm	Finger flexors	Abductor pollicis brevis (abduction D1) First dorsal interosseous (abduction D2) Abductor digiti minimi (abduction D5)		4th and 5th fingers, medial forearm
T1	Axilla and medial arm	Finger flexors	Abductor pollicis brevis (abduction D1) First dorsal interosseous (abduction D2) Abductor digiti minimi (abduction D5)		Medial arm, axilla

[a] These muscles receive the majority of innervation from this root.

Shoulder   If signs of radiculopathy are absent, differential diagnosis includes mechanical shoulder pain (tendonitis, bursitis, rotator cuff tear, dislocation, adhesive capsulitis, and cuff impingement under the acromion) and referred pain (subdiaphragmatic irritation, angina, Pancoast tumor). Mechanical pain is often worse at night, associated with shoulder tenderness, and aggravated by abduction, internal rotation, or extension of the arm.

TREATMENT

Symptomatic treatment of neck pain includes analgesic medications and/or a soft cervical collar. Indications for cervical disk and lumbar disk surgery are similar; however, with cervical disease an aggressive approach is indicated if spinal cord injury is threatened. Surgery of *cervical herniated disks* consists of an anterior approach with diskectomy followed by anterior interbody fusion; a simple posterior partial laminectomy with diskectomy is an acceptable alternative. The cumulative risk of subsequent radiculopathy or myelopathy at cervical segments adjacent to the fusion is 3% per year and 26% per decade. *Nonprogressive cervical radiculopathy* (associated with a focal neurologic deficit) due to a herniated cervical disk may be treated conservatively with a high rate of success. *Cervical spondylosis* with bony, compressive cervical radiculopathy is generally treated with surgical decompression to interrupt the progression of neurologic signs; *spondylotic myelopathy* is managed with anterior decompression and fusion or laminectomy.

For more detailed discussion, see Engstrom JW: Back and Neck Pain, Chap. 15, p. 94, in HPIM-16.

36

FEVER, HYPERTHERMIA, CHILLS, AND RASH

FEVER

DEFINITIONS   *Temperature*: Normal body temperature is maintained (≤37.2°C/98.9°F in the morning and ≤37.7°C/99.9°F in the evening) because the hypothalamic thermoregulatory center balances excess heat production from metabolic activity in muscle and liver with heat dissipation from the skin and lungs.

Fever: An elevation of normal body temperature in conjunction with an increase in the hypothalamic set point. Infectious causes are common.

Fever of unknown origin (FUO):

1. *Classic FUO*: Three outpt visits or 3 days in the hospital without elucidation of a cause of fever; *or* 1 week of unproductive intelligent and invasive ambulatory investigation, temperatures >38.3°C (101°F) on several occasions, and duration of fever for >3 weeks
2. *Nosocomial FUO*: At least 3 days of investigation and 2 days of culture incubation failing to elucidate a cause of fever in a hospitalized pt with

temperatures >38.3°C (101°F) on several occasions and no infection on admission
3. *Neutropenic FUO*: At least 3 days of investigation and 2 days of culture incubation failing to elucidate a cause of fever in a pt with temperatures >38.3°C (101°F) on several occasions whose neutrophil count is <500 μL or is expected to fall to that level within 1–2 days
4. *HIV-associated FUO*: Failure of appropriate investigation to reveal a cause of fever in an HIV-infected pt with temperatures >38.3°C (101°F) on several occasions over a period of >4 weeks for outpatients and >3 days for hospitalized pts.

Hyperpyrexia: Temperatures >41.5°C (106.7°F) that can occur with severe infections but more commonly occur with CNS hemorrhages

ETIOLOGY Most fevers are associated with self-limited infections (usually viral) and have causes that are easily identified.

• *Classic FUO*: As the duration of fever increases, the likelihood of an infectious etiology decreases. Etiologies to consider include:
1. Infection—e.g., extrapulmonary tuberculosis; EBV, CMV, or HIV infection; occult abscesses; endocarditis; fungal disease
2. Neoplasm—e.g., lymphoma and hematologic malignancies, hepatoma, renal cell carcinoma
3. Miscellaneous noninfectious inflammatory diseases
   a. Systemic rheumatologic disease or vasculitis—e.g., Still's disease, lupus erythematosus
   b. Granulomatous disease—e.g., granulomatous hepatitis, sarcoidosis, Crohn's disease
   c. Miscellaneous diseases—e.g., pulmonary embolism, hereditary fever syndromes, drug fever, factitious fevers

• *Nosocomial FUO*
   Infectious—e.g., infected foreign bodies or catheters, *Clostridium difficile* colitis, sinusitis
   Noninfectious—e.g., drug fever, pulmonary embolism
• *Neutropenic FUO*: More than 50–60% of pts infected or at risk for bacterial and certain fungal and viral infections
• *HIV-associated FUO*: More than 80% of pts infected, but drug fever and lymphoma also possible etiologies

PATHOGENESIS Hypothalamic set point increases; pt feels cold due to peripheral vasoconstriction and shivering that are needed to raise body temperature to new set point; peripheral vasodilation and sweating commence when set point is lowered again by resolution or treatment of the fever.
   Fever caused by:

Exogenous pyrogens (e.g., lipopolysaccharide endotoxin)
Endogenous pyrogens (e.g., interleukin 1, tumor necrosis factor) induced by exogenous pyrogens
Prostaglandin E_2 (in CNS, raises hypothalamic set point; in peripheral tissues, causes myalgias and arthralgias)

CLINICAL FEATURES Generalized symptoms: myalgias, arthralgias, anorexia, somnolence, chills, sweats, rigors, change in mental status, rash

History A meticulous history is essential.

Symptom chronology (in case of rash: site of onset and direction and rate of spread) in relation to medications, treatments, occupational and potential toxic exposures, pets, sick contacts, sexual contacts, travel, diet, hobbies

Tobacco, alcohol, marijuana, or IV drug use
Trauma, tick bites, other animal bites
Transfusions, immunizations, allergies

Physical Examination   Special attention to skin, lymph nodes, eyes, nail beds, cardiovascular system, chest, abdomen, musculoskeletal system, nervous system. Rectal and pelvic examinations must be included.
   Skin examination can be especially revealing in pts with fever.

1. Type of lesion (e.g., macule, papule, nodule, vesicle, pustule, purpura, ulcer)
2. Classification of rash
   a. Centrally distributed maculopapular eruptions (e.g., measles, rubella)
   b. Peripheral eruptions (e.g., Rocky Mountain spotted fever, secondary syphilis)
   c. Confluent desquamative erythemas (e.g., toxic shock syndrome)
   d. Vesiculobullous eruptions (e.g., varicella, smallpox, rickettsialpox)
   e. Urticarial eruptions: Hypersensitivity reactions are usually not associated with fever. The presence of fever suggests serum sickness, connective-tissue disease, or infection (hepatitis B, enteroviral or parasitic infection).
   f. Nodular eruptions (e.g., disseminated candidiasis, cryptococcosis, erythema nodosum, Sweet's syndrome)
   g. Purpuric eruptions (e.g., acute meningococcemia, echovirus 9 infection, disseminated gonococcemia)
   h. Eruptions with ulcers or eschars (e.g., scrub typhus or rickettsialpox)

DIAGNOSIS   In most cases, initial history, physical examination, and laboratory tests (including CBC with differential, ESR, electrolytes, LFTs, urinalysis, and CXR; CT, MRI, or nuclear scans as indicated; and appropriate smears and cultures and sampling of abnormal fluid collections) lead to a diagnosis, or the pt recovers spontaneously. If fever continues for 2–3 weeks and repeat physical examinations and laboratory tests are unrevealing, the pt is diagnosed as having FUO. The approach to diagnosis of FUO is found in Fig. 36-1.

Rx TREATMENT

The diagnosed infection should be treated appropriately. In pts with FUO, "shotgun" empirical therapy should be avoided if vital signs are stable and the pt is not neutropenic. Cirrhosis, asplenia, immunosuppressive drug use, or recent exotic travel may be appropriate settings for empirical treatment.
   Treatment of the fever with antipyretics may mask important clinical indicators; examples include a relapsing pattern seen in malaria and a reversal of the usual times of peak and trough temperatures in typhoid fever and disseminated tuberculosis. However, treatment of fever is appropriate to ameliorate symptoms and reduce oxygen demand in pts with underlying cardiovascular or pulmonary disease or to prevent seizures in children with a history of febrile seizures. Antipyretic treatment should be given on a regular schedule rather than intermittently; otherwise, it will aggravate chills and sweats.
   Aspirin, NSAIDs, and glucocorticoids are effective antipyretics, but acetaminophen is preferred because it does not mask signs of inflammation, does not impair platelet function, and is not associated with Reye's syndrome.

PROGNOSIS   Failure to identify the source of FUO for >6 months is generally associated with a good prognosis. Debilitating symptoms can be treated with antipyretics.

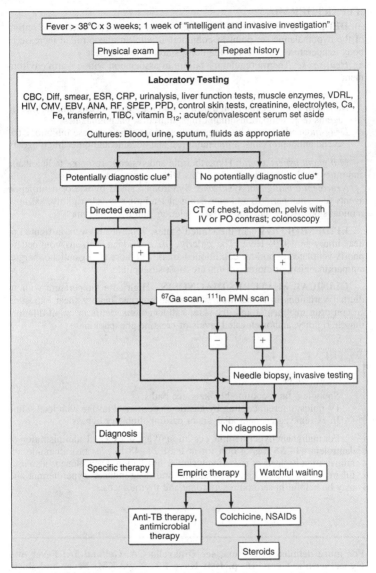

FIGURE 36-1 Approach to the pt with classic FUO. *"Potentially diagnostic clues," as outlined by EMHA DeKleijn and colleagues (Medicine 76:401, 1997), may be key findings in the history, localizing signs, or key symptoms. Abbreviations: CRP, C-reactive protein; Diff, differential; RF, rheumatoid factor; SPEP, serum protein electrophoresis; TB, tuberculosis; TIBC, total iron-binding capacity.

HYPERTHERMIA

DEFINITIONS AND ETIOLOGY   *Hyperthermia*: An unchanged setting of the hypothalamic set point in conjunction with an uncontrolled increase in body temperature that exceeds the body's ability to lose heat

Heat stroke: Thermoregulatory failure in association with a warm environment

Exertional: Caused by exercise in high heat or humidity

Nonexertional: Occurs in high heat or humidity in pts taking anticholinergic agents (e.g., antiparkinsonian drugs, diuretics, phenothiazines)

Drug-induced: Caused by drugs such as monoamine oxidase inhibitors, tricyclic antidepressants, amphetamines, and cocaine and other illicit agents

Malignant hyperthermia: Hyperthermic and systemic response to halothane and other inhalational anesthetics in pts with genetic abnormality

Neuroleptic malignant syndrome: Syndrome caused by use of neuroleptic agents (e.g., haloperidol) and consisting of lead-pipe muscle rigidity, extrapyramidal side effects, autonomic dysregulation, and hyperthermia

EPIDEMIOLOGY   In the United States, 7000 deaths were attributed to heat injury in 1979–1997. The elderly, the bedridden, persons confined to poorly ventilated or non-air-conditioned areas, and those taking anticholinergic, antiparkinsonian, or diuretic drugs are most susceptible.

CLINICAL FEATURES/DIAGNOSIS   High core temperature without diurnal variations in association with an appropriate history (heat exposure, certain drug treatments) and dry skin, hallucinations, delirium, pupil dilation, muscle rigidity, and/or elevated levels of creatine phosphokinase

 TREATMENT

Physical cooling:

Sponging, fans, cooling blankets, ice baths
IV fluids, internal cooling by gastric or peritoneal lavage with iced saline
In extreme cases, hemodialysis or cardiopulmonary bypass

For malignant hyperthermia, cessation of anesthesia and administration of dantrolene (1–2.5 mg/kg q6h for at least 24–48 h) *plus* procainamide administration because of risk of ventricular fibrillation. Dantrolene is also useful in neuroleptic malignant syndrome and drug-induced hyperthermia and may be helpful in serotonin syndrome and thyrotoxicosis.

For more detailed discussion, see Dinarello CA, Gelfand JA: Fever and Hyperthermia, Chap. 16, p. 104; Kaye ET, Kaye KM: Fever and Rash, Chap. 17, p. 108; and Gelfand JA, Callahan MV: Fever of Unknown Origin, Chap. 18, p. 116, in HPIM-16.

37

PAIN OR SWELLING OF JOINTS

Musculoskeletal complaints are extremely common in outpatient medical practice and are among the leading causes of disability and absenteeism from work. Pain in the joints must be evaluated in a uniform, thorough, and logical fashion to ensure the best chance of accurate diagnosis and to plan appropriate follow-up testing and therapy. Joint pain and swelling may be manifestations of disorders affecting primarily the musculoskeletal system or may reflect systemic disease.

Goals for the Initial Assessment of a Musculoskeletal Complaint   (See Fig. 37-1)

1. *Articular versus nonarticular*. Is the pain located in a joint or in a periarticular structure such as soft tissue or muscle?
2. *Inflammatory versus noninflammatory*. Inflammatory disease is suggested by local signs of inflammation (erythema, warmth, swelling), systemic features (morning stiffness, fatigue, fever, weight loss), or laboratory evidence of inflammation (thrombocytosis, elevated ESR or C-reactive protein).
3. *Acute (≤6 weeks) versus chronic*.
4. *Localized versus systemic*.

Historic Features

- Age, sex, race, and family history
- Symptom onset (abrupt or indolent), evolution (chronic constant, intermittent, migratory, additive), and duration (acute versus chronic)
- Number and distribution of involved structures: monarticular (one joint), oligoarticular (2–3 joints), polyarticular (>3 joints); symmetry
- Other articular features: morning stiffness, effect of movement, features that improve/worsen Sx
- Extraarticular Sx: e.g., fever, rash, weight loss, visual change, dyspnea, diarrhea, dysuria, numbness, weakness
- Recent events: e.g., trauma, drug administration, travel, other illnesses.

Physical Examination

Complete examination is essential: particular attention to skin, mucous membranes, nails (may reveal characteristic pitting in psoriasis), eyes. Careful and thorough examination of involved and uninvolved joints and periarticular structures; this should proceed in an organized fashion from head to foot or from extremities inward toward axial skeleton; special attention should be paid to identifying the presence or absence of

- Warmth and/or erythema
- Swelling
- Synovial thickening
- Subluxation, dislocation, joint deformity
- Joint instability
- Limitations to active and passive range of motion
- Crepitus
- Periarticular changes
- Muscular changes including weakness, atrophy

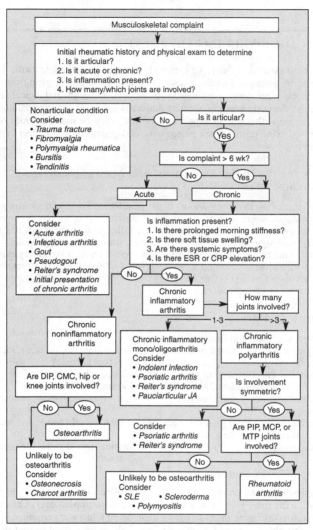

FIGURE 37-1 Algorithm for the diagnosis of musculoskeletal complaints. An approach to formulating a differential diagnosis (shown in italics). ESR, erythrocyte sedimentation rate; CRP, C-reactive protein; DIP, distal interphalangeal; CMC, carpometacarpal; PIP, proximal interphalangeal; MCP, metacarpophalangeal; MTP, metatarsophalangeal; SLE, systemic lupus erythematosus; JA, juvenile arthritis.

Laboratory Investigations

Additional evaluation usually indicated for monarticular, traumatic, inflammatory, or chronic conditions or for conditions accompanied by neurologic changes or systemic manifestations.

- For all evaluations: include CBC, ESR, or C-reactive protein

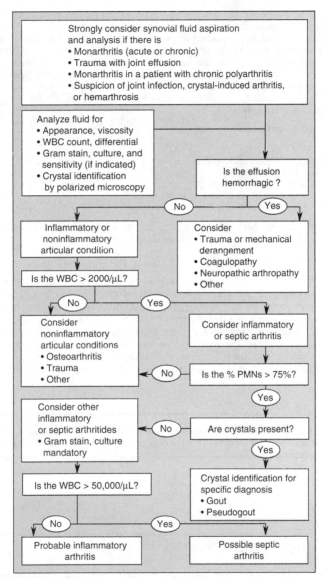

FIGURE 37-2 Algorithmic approach to the use and interpretation of synovial fluid aspiration and analysis.

• Should be performed where there are suggestive clinical features: rheumatoid factor, ANA, antineutrophilic cytoplasmic antibodies (ANCA), antistreptolysin O titer, Lyme antibodies

• Where systemic disease is present or suspected: renal/hepatic function tests, UA

- Uric acid—useful only when gout diagnosed and therapy contemplated
- CPK, aldolase—consider with muscle pain, weakness
- Synovial fluid aspiration and analysis: always indicated for acute monarthritis or when infectious or crystal-induced arthropathy is suspected. Should be examined for (1) appearance, viscosity; (2) cell count and differential (suspect septic joint if WBC count $> 50,000/\mu L$); (3) crystals using polarizing microscope; (4) Gram's stain, cultures (Fig. 37-2).

Diagnostic Imaging

Plain radiographs should be considered for

- Trauma
- Suspected chronic infection
- Progressive disability
- Monarticular involvement
- Baseline assessment of a chronic process
- When therapeutic alterations are considered

Additional imaging procedures, including ultrasound, radionuclide scintigraphy, CT, and MRI, may be helpful in selected clinical settings.

Special Considerations in the Elderly Patient

The evaluation of joint and musculoskeletal disorders in the elderly pt presents a special challenge given the frequently insidious onset and chronicity of disease in this age group, the confounding effect of other medical conditions, and the increased variability of many diagnostic tests in the geriatric population. Although virtually all musculoskeletal conditions may afflict the elderly, certain disorders are especially frequent. Special attention should be paid to identifying the potential rheumatic consequences of intercurrent medical conditions and therapies when evaluating the geriatric pt with musculoskeletal complaints.

For a more detailed discussion, see Cush JJ, Lipsky PE: Approach to Articular and Musculoskeletal Disorders, Chap. 311, p. 2029, in HPIM-16.

38

SYNCOPE AND FAINTNESS

Syncope is a transient loss of consciousness due to reduced cerebral blood flow. Syncope is associated with postural collapse and spontaneous recovery. It may occur suddenly, without warning, or may be preceded by presyncopal symptoms such as lightheadedness, weakness, nausea, dimming vision, ringing in ears, or sweating. *Faintness* refers to prodromal symptoms that precede the loss of consciousness in syncope. The syncopal pt appears pale, has a faint, rapid, or irregular pulse, and breathing may be almost imperceptible; transient myoclonic or clonic movements may occur. Recovery of consciousness is prompt if the pt is maintained in a horizontal position and cerebral perfusion is restored.

Features Distinguishing Syncope from Seizure

The differential diagnosis is often between syncope and a generalized seizure. Syncope is more likely if the event was provoked by acute pain or anxiety or occurred immediately after arising from a lying or sitting position. Seizures are typically not related to posture. Pts with syncope often describe a stereotyped transition from consciousness to unconsciousness that develops over a few seconds. Seizures occur either very abruptly without a transition or are preceded by premonitory symptoms such as an epigastric rising sensation, perception of odd odors, or racing thoughts. Pallor is seen during syncope; cyanosis is usually seen during a seizure. The duration of unconsciousness is usually very brief (i.e., seconds) in syncope and more prolonged (i.e., >5 min) in a seizure. Injury from falling and incontinence are common in seizure, rare in syncope. Headache and drowsiness, which with mental confusion are the usual sequelae of a seizure, do not follow a syncopal attack.

Etiology

Transiently decreased cerebral blood flow is usually due to one of three general mechanisms: disorders of vascular tone or blood volume including vasovagal syncope and postural hypotension, cardiovascular disorders including cardiac arrhythmias, or uncommonly cerebrovascular disease (Table 38-1). Not infrequently the cause of syncope is multifactorial.

Neurocardiogenic (Vasovagal and Vasodepressor) Syncope The common faint, experienced by normal persons and accounting for approximately half of all episodes of syncope. Frequently recurrent and may be provoked by hot or crowded environment, alcohol, fatigue, pain, hunger, prolonged standing, or stressful situations.

Postural (Orthostatic) Hypotension Cause of syncope in 30% of elderly; polypharmacy with antihypertensive or antidepressant drugs often a contributor; physical deconditioning may also play a role. Also occurs with autonomic nervous system disorders, either peripheral (diabetes, nutritional, or amyloid) or central (multiple system atrophy, Parkinson's disease). Some cases are idiopathic.

―――――――――――― *Approach to the Patient* ――――――――――――

The cause of syncope may be apparent only at the time of the event, leaving few, if any, clues when the pt is seen by the physician. First consider causes that represent serious underlying etiologies; among these are massive internal hemorrhage or myocardial infarction, which may be painless, and cardiac arrhythmias. In elderly persons, a sudden faint without obvious cause should arouse the suspicion of complete heart block or a tachyarrhythmia, even if all findings are negative when the pt is seen. Loss of consciousness in particular situations, such as during venipuncture or micturition, suggests a benign abnormality of vascular tone. The position of the pt at the time of the syncopal episode is important; syncope in the supine position is unlikely to be vasovagal and suggests an arrhythmia or a seizure. Medications must be considered, including nonprescription drugs or health store supplements, with particular attention to recent changes. Symptoms of impotence, bowel and bladder difficulties, or disturbed sweating, or an abnormal neurologic exam, suggest a primary neurogenic cause. An algorithmic approach to syncope is presented in Fig. 38-1.

Table 38-1

Causes of Syncope

I. Disorders of vascular tone or blood volume
   A. Vasovagal (vasodepressor, neurocardiogenic)
      Postural (orthostatic) hypotension
      1. Drug-induced (especially antihypertensive or vasodilator drugs)
         Peripheral neuropathy (diabetic, alcoholic, nutritional, amyloid)
         Idiopathic postural hypotension
         Multisystem atrophies
         Physical deconditioning
         Sympathectomy
         Acute dysautonomia (Guillain-Barré syndrome variant)
         Decreased blood volume (adrenal insufficiency, acute blood loss, etc.)
   B. Carotid sinus hypersensitivity
      Situational
      1. Cough
         Micturition
         Defecation
         Valsalva
         Deglutition
   C. Glossopharyngeal neuralgia
II. Cardiovascular disorders
   A. Cardiac arrhythmias
      1. Bradyarrhythmias
         a. Sinus bradycardia, sinoatrial block, sinus arrest, sick-sinus syndrome
         b. Atrioventricular block
      2. Tachyarrhythmias
         a. Supraventricular tachycardia with structural cardiac disease
         b. Atrial fibrillation associated with the Wolff-Parkinson-White syndrome
         c. Atrial flutter with 1:1 atrioventricular conduction
         d. Ventricular tachycardia
   B. Other cardiopulmonary etiologies
      1. Pulmonary embolism
         Pulmonary hypertension
         Atrial myxoma
         Myocardial disease (massive myocardial infarction)
         Left ventricular myocardial restriction or constriction
         Pericardial constriction or tamponade
         Aortic outflow tract obstruction
         Aortic valvular stenosis
         Hypertrophic obstructive cardiomyopathy
III. Cerebrovascular disease
   A. Vertebrobasilar insufficiency
      Basilar artery migraine
IV. Other disorders that may resemble syncope
   A. Metabolic
      1. Hypoxia
         Anemia
         Diminished carbon dioxide due to hyperventilation
         Hypoglycemia
   B. Psychogenic
      1. Anxiety attacks
         Hysterical fainting
   C. Seizures

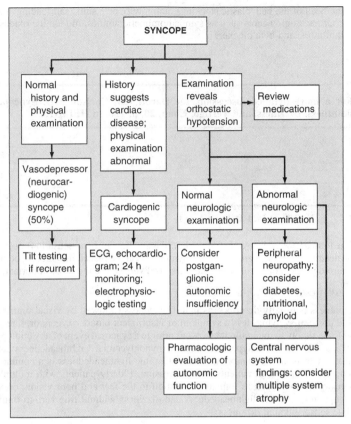

FIGURE 38-1 Approach to the patient with syncope.

℞ TREATMENT

Therapy is determined by the underlying cause. Pts with vasovagal syncope should be instructed to avoid situations or stimuli that provoke attacks. Episodes associated with intravascular volume depletion may be prevented by salt and fluid preloading. β-Adrenergic antagonists (metoprolol 25–50 mg bid; atenolol 25–50 mg qd; or nadolol 10–20 mg bid; all starting doses) are the most widely used agents; serotonin reuptake inhibitors (paroxetine 20–40 mg qd, or sertraline 25–50 mg qd) and bupropion SR (150 mg qd) are also effective. The mineralocorticoid hydrofludrocortisone (0.1–0.2 mg qd) or the α-agonist proamatine (2.5–10 mg bid or tid) may be helpful for refractory pts with recurrent vasovagal syncope but side effects, including increases in resting bp, limit their usefulness. Permanent cardiac pacing is effective for pts whose episodes of vasovagal syncope are frequent or associated with prolonged asystole.

Pts with orthostatic hypotension should be instructed to rise slowly from the bed or chair and to move legs prior to rising to facilitate venous return from the extremities. Medications that aggravate the problem should be discontinued when possible. Other useful treatments may include elevation of the head of the bed, elastic stockings, antigravity or g suits, salt loading, and pharmacologic agents such as sympathomimetic amines, monomine oxidase inhibitors, and beta blockers.

For a more detailed discussion, see Daroff RB, Carlson MD: Syncope, Faintness, Dizziness, and Vertigo, Chap. 20, p. 126, in HPIM-16.

39

DIZZINESS AND VERTIGO

The term *dizziness* is used by pts to describe a variety of head sensations or gait unsteadiness. With a careful history, symptoms can be placed into more specific neurologic categories, of which faintness and vertigo are the most important.

Faintness

Faintness is usually described as light-headedness followed by visual blurring and postural swaying. It is a symptom of insufficient blood, oxygen, or, rarely, glucose supply to the brain. It can occur prior to a syncopal event of any etiology (Chap. 38) and with hyperventilation or hypoglycemia. Lightheadedness can also occur as an aura before a seizure. Chronic lightheadedness is a common somatic complaint in patients with depression. Elderly patients with multiple sensory deficits, such as impaired sensation in the feet and poor vision, often complain of chronic lightheadedness and dizziness without true vertigo (multiple sensory-deficit dizziness).

Vertigo

An illusion of movement, most commonly a sensation of spinning. Usually due to a disturbance in the vestibular system; abnormalities in the visual or somatosensory systems may also contribute to vertigo. Frequently accompanied by nausea, postural unsteadiness, and gait ataxia, and may be provoked or worsened by head movement. *Physiologic vertigo* results from unfamiliar head movement (seasickness) or a mismatch between visual-proprioceptive-vestibular system inputs (height vertigo, visual vertigo). True vertigo almost never occurs as a presyncopal symptom.

Pathologic vertigo may be caused by a peripheral (labyrinth or eighth nerve) or central CNS lesion. Distinguishing between these causes is the essential first step in diagnosis (Table 39-1).

Peripheral Vertigo   Usually severe, accompanied by nausea and emesis. Tinnitus, a feeling of ear fullness, or hearing loss may occur. The pt may appear pale and diaphoretic. A characteristic jerk nystagmus is almost always present. The nystagmus does not change direction with a change in direction of gaze, it is horizontal with a torsional component and has its fast phase away from the side of the lesion. It is inhibited by visual fixation. The pt senses spinning motion away from the lesion and tends to fall towards the side of the lesion. No other neurologic abnormalities are present.

Table 39-1

Differentiation of Peripheral and Central Vertigo

Sign or Symptom	Peripheral (Labyrinth)	Central (Brainstem or Cerebellum)
Direction of associated nystagmus	Unidirectional; fast phase opposite lesion[a]	Bidirectional or unidirectional
Purely horizontal nystagmus without torsional component	Uncommon	Common
Vertical or purely torsional nystagmus	Never present	May be present
Visual fixation	Inhibits nystagmus and vertigo	No inhibition
Severity of vertigo	Marked	Often mild
Direction of spin	Toward fast phase	Variable
Direction of fall	Toward slow phase	Variable
Duration of symptoms	Finite (minutes, days, weeks) but recurrent	May be chronic
Tinnitus and/or deafness	Often present	Usually absent
Associated central abnormalities	None	Extremely common
Common causes	Infection (labyrinthitis), Ménière's, neuronitis, ischemia, trauma, toxin	Vascular, demyelinating, neoplasm

[a] In Ménière's disease, the direction of the fast phase is variable.

Acute unilateral labyrinthine dysfunction may be caused by infection, trauma, or ischemia. Often no specific etiology is uncovered, and the nonspecific term *acute labyrinthitis* (or *vestibular neuronitis*) is used to describe the event. The attacks are brief and leave the patient for some days with a mild positional vertigo: recurrent episodes may occur. *Acute bilateral labyrinthine dysfunction* is usually due to drugs (aminoglycoside antibiotics) or alcohol. *Recurrent labyrinthine dysfunction* with signs of cochlear disease is usually due to *Ménière's disease* (recurrent vertigo accompanied by tinnitus and deafness). Positional

Table 39-2

Benign Paroxysmal Positional Vertigo and Central Positional Vertigo

Features	BPPV	Central
Latency[a]	3–40 s	None: immediate vertigo and nystagmus
Fatigability[b]	Yes	No
Habituation[c]	Yes	No
Intensity of vertigo	Severe	Mild
Reproducibility[d]	Variable	Good

[a] Time between attaining head position and onset of symptoms.
[b] Disappearance of symptoms with maintenance of offending position.
[c] Lessening of symptoms with repeated trials.
[d] Likelihood of symptom production during any examination session.

Table 39-3

Treatment of Vertigo	
Agent[a]	Dose[b]
Antihistamines	
Meclizine	25–50 mg 3 times/day
Dimenhydrinate	50 mg 1–2 times/day
Promethazine[c]	25–50-mg suppository or IM
Benzodiazepines	
Diazepam	2.5 mg 1–3 times/day
Clonazepam	0.25 mg 1–3 times/day
Phenothiazines	
Prochlorperazine[c]	5 mg IM or 25-mg suppository
Anticholinergic[d]	
Scopolamine transdermal	Patch
Sympathomimetics[d]	
Ephedrine	25 mg/d
Combination preparations[d]	
Ephedrine and promethazine	25 mg/d of each
Exercise therapy	
Repositioning maneuvers[e]	
Vestibular rehabilitation[f]	
Other	
Diuretics or low-salt (1 g/d) diet[g]	
Antimigrainous drugs[h]	
Inner ear surgery[i]	
Glucocorticoids[c]	

[a] All listed drugs are U.S. Food and Drug Administration approved, but most are not approved for the treatment of vertigo.
[b] Usual oral (unless otherwise stated) starting dose in adults; maintenance dose can be reached by a gradual increase.
[c] For acute vertigo only.
[d] For motion sickness only.
[e] For benign paroxysmal positional vertigo.
[f] For vertigo other than Ménière's and positional.
[g] For Ménière's disease.
[h] For migraine-associated vertigo (see Chap. 34 for a listing of prophylactic antimigrainous drugs).
[i] For perilymphatic fistula and refractory cases of Ménière's disease.

vertigo is usually precipitated by a recumbent head position. *Benign paroxysmal positional vertigo* (BPPV) of the posterior semicircular canal is particularly common; the pattern of nystagmus is distinctive (Table 39-2). BPPV may follow trauma but is usually idiopathic; it generally abates spontaneously after weeks or months. Schwannomas of the eighth cranial nerve (acoustic neuroma) usually present as auditory symptoms of hearing loss and tinnitus, sometimes accompanied by facial weakness and sensory loss due to involvement of cranial nerves VII and V. *Psychogenic vertigo* should be suspected in pts with chronic incapacitating vertigo who also have agoraphobia, a normal neurologic exam, and no nystagmus.

Central Vertigo Identified by associated abnormal brainstem or cerebellar signs such as dysarthria, diplopia, paresthesia, weakness, limb ataxia; depending on the cause, headache may be present. The nystagmus can take almost any form, i.e., vertical or multidirectional, but is often purely horizontal without a torsional component. Central nystagmus is not inhibited by fixation. Central vertigo may be chronic, mild, and is often unaccompanied by tinnitus or hearing loss. It may be due to demyelinating, vascular, or neoplastic disease. Vertigo may be a manifestation of migraine or, rarely, of temporal lobe epilepsy.

_____ *Approach to the Patient* _____

The "dizzy" patient usually requires provocative tests to reproduce the symptoms. Valsalva maneuver, hyperventilation, or postural changes may reproduce faintness. Rapid rotation in a swivel chair is a simple provocative test to reproduce vertigo. Benign positional vertigo is identified by positioning the turned head of a recumbent patient in extension over the edge of the bed to elicit vertigo and the characteristic nystagmus. If a vestibular nerve or central cause for the vertigo is suspected (e.g., signs of peripheral vertigo are absent or other neurologic abnormalities are present), then prompt evaluation for central pathology is required. The initial test is usually an MRI scan of the posterior fossa, and depending upon the results evoked potentials or vertebrobasilar angiography may be indicated. Vestibular function tests, including electronystagmography (calorics), can help distinguish between central and peripheral etiologies.

℞ TREATMENT

Treatment of acute vertigo consists of bed rest and vestibular suppressant drugs (Table 39-3). If the vertigo persists more than a few days, most authorities advise ambulation in an attempt to induce central compensatory mechanisms. BPPV may respond to repositioning exercises such as the Epley procedure designed to empty particulate debris from the posterior semicircular canal (www.charite.de/ch/neuro/vertigo.html). Ménière's disease may respond to a low-salt diet (1 g/d) or to a diuretic.

For a more detailed discussion, see Daroff RB, Carlson MD: Syncope, Faintness, Dizziness, and Vertigo, Chap. 20, p. 126, in HPIM-16.

40

ACUTE VISUAL LOSS AND DOUBLE VISION

Clinical Assessment

Accurate measurement of visual acuity in each eye (with glasses) is of primary importance. Additional assessments include testing of pupils, eye movements, ocular alignment, and visual fields. Slit-lamp examination can exclude corneal infection, trauma, glaucoma, uveitis, and cataract. Ophthalmoscopic exam to inspect the optic disc and retina often requires pupillary dilation using 1% topicamide and 2.5% phenylephrine; risk of provoking an attack of narrow-angle glaucoma is remote.

Visual field mapping by finger confrontation localizes lesions in the visual pathway (Fig. 40-1); formal testing using a perimeter may be necessary. The goal is to determine whether the lesion is anterior, at, or posterior to the optic chiasm. A scotoma confined to one eye is caused by an anterior lesion affecting the optic nerve or globe; swinging flashlight test may reveal an afferent pupil defect. History and ocular exam are usually sufficient for diagnosis. If a bitemporal hemianopia is present, lesion is located at optic chiasm (e.g., pituitary adenoma, meningioma). Homonymous visual field loss signals a retrochiasmal lesion, affecting the optic tract, lateral geniculate body, optic radiations, or vi-

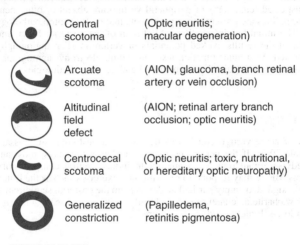

OPTIC NERVE OR RETINA

Central scotoma — (Optic neuritis; macular degeneration)

Arcuate scotoma — (AION, glaucoma, branch retinal artery or vein occlusion)

Altitudinal field defect — (AION; retinal artery branch occlusion; optic neuritis)

Centrocecal scotoma — (Optic neuritis; toxic, nutritional, or hereditary optic neuropathy)

Generalized constriction — (Papilledema, retinitis pigmentosa)

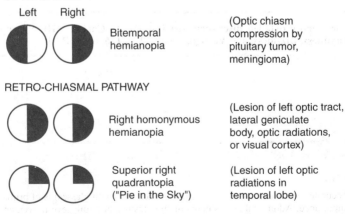

OPTIC CHIASM

Left   Right

Bitemporal hemianopia — (Optic chiasm compression by pituitary tumor, meningioma)

RETRO-CHIASMAL PATHWAY

Right homonymous hemianopia — (Lesion of left optic tract, lateral geniculate body, optic radiations, or visual cortex)

Superior right quadrantopia ("Pie in the Sky") — (Lesion of left optic radiations in temporal lobe)

Macular sparing — (Bilateral visual cortex lesions)

FIGURE 40-1 Deficits in visual fields caused by lesions affecting visual pathways.

sual cortex (e.g., stroke, tumor, abscess). Neuroimaging is recommended for any pt with a bitemporal or homonymous hemianopia.

Transient or Sudden Visual Loss

Amaurosis fugax (transient monocular blindness) usually occurs from a retinal embolus or severe ipsilateral carotid stenosis. Prolonged occlusion of the central retinal artery results in classic fundus appearance of a milky, infarcted retina with cherry-red fovea. Any pt with compromise of the retinal circulation should be evaluated promptly for stroke risk factors (e.g., carotid atheromata, heart disease, atrial fibrillation).

Vertebrobasilar insufficiency or emboli can be confused with amaurosis fugax, because many pts mistakenly ascribe symptoms to their left or right eye, when in fact they are occurring in the left or right hemifield of both eyes. Interruption of blood flow to the visual cortex causes sudden graying of vision, occasionally with flashing lights or other symptoms that mimic *migraine*. The history may be the only guide to the correct diagnosis. Pts should be questioned about the precise pattern and duration of visual loss and other neurologic symptoms such as diplopia, vertigo, numbness, or weakness, which may help decide between compromise of the anterior or posterior cerebral circulation.

Malignant hypertension can cause visual loss from exudates, hemorrhages, cotton-wool spots (focal nerve fiber layer infarcts), and optic disc edema. In central or branch *retinal vein occlusion*, the fundus exam reveals engorged, dusky veins with extensive retinal bleeding. In age-related *macular degeneration*, characterized by extensive drusen and scarring of the pigment epithelium, leakage of blood or fluid from subretinal neovascular membranes can produce sudden central visual loss. Flashing lights and floaters may indicate a fresh *vitreous detachment*. Separation of the vitreous from the retina is a frequent involutional event in the elderly. It is not harmful unless it creates sufficient traction to produce a retinal detachment. *Vitreous hemorrhage* may occur in diabetic pts from retinal neovascularization.

Papilledema refers to bilateral optic disc edema from raised intracranial pressure. Transient visual obscurations are common, but visual acuity is not affected unless the papilledema is severe, long-standing, or accompanied by macular exudates or hemorrhage. Neuroimaging should be obtained to exclude an intracranial mass. If negative, an LP is required to confirm elevation of the intracranial pressure. *Pseudotumor cerebri* (idiopathic intracranial hypertension) is a diagnosis of exclusion. Most pts are young, female, and obese; some are found to have occult cerebral venous sinus thrombosis. Treatment is with acetazolamide, repeated LPs, and weight loss; some pts require lumboperitoneal shunting or optic nerve sheath fenestration. *Optic neuritis* is a common cause of monocular optic disc swelling and visual loss, although it rarely affects both eyes. If site of inflammation is retrobulbar, fundus will appear normal on initial exam. The typical pt is female, age 15–45, with pain provoked by eye movements. Glucocorticoids, consisting of intravenous methylprednisolone (1 g daily for 3 days) followed by oral prednisone (1 mg/kg daily for 11 days), may hasten recovery in severely affected patients. If an MR scan shows multiple demyelinating lesions, treatment for multiple sclerosis should be considered. *Anterior ischemic optic neuropathy* (AION) is an infarction of the optic nerve head due to inadequate perfusion via the posterior ciliary arteries. Pts have sudden visual loss, often upon awakening, and painless swelling of the optic disc. It is important to differentiate between nonarteritic (idiopathic) AION and arteritic AION. The latter is caused by *temporal arteritis* and requires immediate glucocorticoid therapy. The ESR should be checked in any elderly pt with acute optic disc swelling or symptoms suggestive of polymyalgia rheumatica.

Double Vision (Diplopia)

If pt has diplopia while being examined, motility testing will usually reveal abnormality in ocular excursions. However, if the degree of angular separation between the double images is small, the limitation of eye movements may be subtle and difficult to detect. In this situation, the cover test is useful. While the pt is fixating upon a distant target, one eye is covered while observing the other eye for a movement of redress as it takes up fixation. If none is seen, the procedure is repeated with the other eye. With genuine diplopia, this test should reveal ocular malalignment, especially if the head is turned or tilted in the position that gives rise to the worst symptoms.

The most frequent causes of diplopia are summarized in Table 40-1. The physical findings in isolated ocular motor nerve palsies are:

- CN III: Ptosis and deviation of the eye down and outwards, causing vertical and horizontal diplopia. Pupil dilation suggests direct compression of the third nerve; if present, the possibility of an aneurysm of the posterior communicating artery must be considered urgently.
- CN IV: Vertical diplopia with cyclotorsion; the affected eye is slightly elevated, and limitation of depression is seen when the eye is held in adduction. The pt may assume a head tilt to the opposite side (e.g., left head tilt in right fourth nerve paresis).
- CN VI: Horizontal diplopia with crossed eyes; the affected eye cannot abduct.

Isolated ocular motor nerve palsies often occur in pts with hypertension or diabetes. They usually resolve spontaneously over several months. The apparent occurrence of multiple ocular motor nerve palsies, or diffuse ophthalmoplegia, raises the possibility of myasthenia gravis. In this disease, the pupils are always normal. Systemic weakness may be absent. Diplopia that cannot be explained by a single ocular motor nerve palsy may also be caused by carcinomatous or

Table 40-1

Common Causes of Diplopia

Brainstem stroke (skew deviation, nuclear or fascicular palsy)
Microvascular infarction (III, IV, VI nerve palsy)
Tumor (brainstem, cavernous sinus, superior orbital fissure, orbit)
Multiple sclerosis (internuclear ophthalmoplegia, ocular motor nerve palsy)
Aneurysm (III nerve)
Raised intracranial pressure (VI nerve)
Postviral inflammation
Meningitis (bacterial, fungal, granulomatosis, neoplastic)
Carotid-cavernous fistula or thrombosis
Herpes zoster
Tolosa-Hunt syndrome
Wernicke-Korsakoff syndrome
Botulism
Myasthenia gravis
Guillain-Barré or Fisher syndrome
Graves' disease
Orbital pseudotumor
Orbital myositis
Trauma
Orbital cellulitis

fungal meningitis, Graves' disease, Guillain-Barré syndrome, Fisher's syndrome, or Tolosa-Hunt syndrome.

For a more detailed discussion, see Horton JC: Disorders of the Eye, Chap. 25, p. 162, in HPIM-16.

41

PARALYSIS AND MOVEMENT DISORDERS

PARALYSIS OR WEAKNESS

GENERAL CONSIDERATIONS The loss of power or control of voluntary muscle is usually described by pts as "weakness" or as some difficulty that can be interpreted as "loss of dexterity." The diagnostic approach begins by determining which part of the nervous system is involved. It is important to distinguish weakness arising from disorders of upper motor neurons (i.e., motor neurons in the cerebral cortex and their axons that descend through the subcortical white matter, internal capsule, brainstem, and spinal cord) from disorders of the motor unit (i.e., lower motor neurons in the ventral horn of the spinal cord and their axons in the spinal roots and peripheral nerves, neuromuscular junction, and skeletal muscle). In general:

- *Upper motor neuron dysfunction*: increased muscle tone (spasticity), brisk deep tendon reflexes, and Babinski sign.
- *Lower motor neuron dysfunction*: reduced muscle tone, diminished reflexes, and muscle atrophy.

Table 41-1 summarizes patterns with lesions of different parts of the nervous system. Table 41-2 lists common causes of weakness by the primary site of pathology.

EVALUATION The history should focus on the tempo of development of weakness, presence of sensory and other neurologic symptoms, medication history, predisposing medical conditions, and family history. The physical exam aids in localization (Table 41-1). An algorithm for the initial workup of weakness is shown in Fig. 41-1.

MOVEMENT DISORDERS

Divided into akinetic rigid forms, with muscle rigidity and slowness of movement, and hyperkinetic forms, with involuntary movements. In both types, preservation of strength is the rule. Most movement disorders arise from disruption of basal ganglia circuits; common causes are degenerative diseases (hereditary and idiopathic), drug-induced, organ system failure, CNS infection, and ischemia. Clinical features of the various movement disorders are summarized below.

BRADYKINESIA Inability to initiate changes in activity or perform ordinary volitional movements rapidly and easily. There is a slowness of move-

Table 41-1

Clinical Differentiation of Weakness Arising from Different Areas of the Nervous System

Location of Lesion	Pattern of Weakness	Associated Signs
UPPER MOTOR NEURON		
Cerebral cortex	Hemiparesis (face and arm predominantly, or leg predominantly)	Hemisensory loss, seizures, homonymous hemianopia or quadrantanopia, aphasia, apraxias, gaze preference
Internal capsule	Hemiparesis (face, arm, leg may be equally affected)	Hemisensory deficit; homonymous hemianopia or quadrantanopia
Brainstem	Hemiparesis (arm and leg; face may not be involved at all)	Vertigo, nausea and vomiting, ataxia and dysarthria, eye movement abnormalities, cranial nerve dysfunction, altered level of consciousness, Horner's syndrome
Spinal cord	Quadriparesis if midcervical or above	Sensory level; bowel and bladder dysfunction
	Paraparesis if low cervical or thoracic	
	Hemiparesis below level of lesion (Brown-Séquard)	Contralateral pain/temperature loss below level of lesion
MOTOR UNIT		
Spinal motor neuron	Diffuse weakness, may involve control of speech and swallowing	Muscle fasciculations and atrophy; no sensory loss
Spinal root	Radicular pattern of weakness	Dermatomal sensory loss; radicular pain common with compressive lesions
Peripheral nerve		
Polyneuropathy	Distal weakness, usually feet more than hands; usually symmetric	Distal sensory loss, usually feet more than hands
Mononeuropathy	Weakness in distribution of single nerve	Sensory loss in distribution of single nerve
Neuromuscular junction	Fatigable weakness, usually with ocular involvement producing diplopia and ptosis	No sensory loss; no reflex changes
Muscle	Proximal weakness	No sensory loss; diminished reflexes only when severe; may have muscle tenderness

Table 41-2

Common Causes of Weakness

UPPER MOTOR NEURON

Cortex: ischemia; hemorrhage; intrinsic mass lesion (primary or metastatic cancer, abscess); extrinsic mass lesion (subdural hematoma); degenerative (amyotrophic lateral sclerosis)

Subcortical white matter/internal capsule: ischemia; hemorrhage; intrinsic mass lesion (primary or metastatic cancer, abscess); immunologic (multiple sclerosis); infectious (progressive multifocal leukoencephalopathy)

Brainstem: ischemia; immunologic (multiple sclerosis)

Spinal cord: extrinsic compression (cervical spondylosis, metastatic cancer, epidural abscess); immunologic (multiple sclerosis, transverse myelitis); infectious (AIDS-associated myelopathy, HTLV-1–associated myelopathy, tabes dorsalis); nutritional deficiency (subacute combined degeneration)

MOTOR UNIT

Spinal motor neuron: degenerative (amyotrophic lateral sclerosis); infectious (poliomyelitis)

Spinal root: compressive (degenerative disc disease); immunologic (Guillain-Barré syndrome); infectious (AIDS-associated polyradiculopathy, Lyme disease)

Peripheral nerve: metabolic (diabetes mellitus, uremia, porphyria); toxic (ethanol, heavy metals, many drugs, diphtheria); nutritional (B_{12} deficiency); inflammatory (polyarteritis nodosa); hereditary (Charcot-Marie-Tooth); immunologic (paraneoplastic, paraproteinemia); infectious (AIDS-associated polyneuropathies and mononeuritis multiplex); compressive (entrapment)

Neuromuscular junction: immunologic (myasthenia gravis); toxic (botulism, aminoglycosides)

Muscle: inflammatory (polymyositis, inclusion body myositis); degenerative (muscular dystrophy); toxic (glucocorticoids, ethanol, AZT); infectious (trichinosis); metabolic (hypothyroid, periodic paralyses); congenital (central core disease)

---

ment and a paucity of automatic motions such as eye blinking and arm swinging while walking. Usually due to Parkinson's disease.

TREMOR Rhythmic oscillation of a part of the body, usually involving the distal limbs and less commonly the head, tongue, and jaw. A coarse tremor at rest, 4–5 beats/s, is usually due to Parkinson's disease. A fine postural tremor of 8–10 beats/s may be an exaggeration of normal physiologic tremor or indicate familial essential tremor; the latter often responds to propranolol or primidone. An intention tremor, most pronounced during voluntary movement towards a target, is found with cerebellar pathway disease.

ASTERIXIS Brief, arrhythmic interruptions of sustained voluntary muscle contraction, usually observed as a brief lapse of posture of wrists in dorsiflexion with arms outstretched. This "liver flap" may be seen in any encephalopathy related to drug intoxication, organ system failure, or CNS infection. Therapy is correction of underlying disorder.

MYOCLONUS Rapid, brief, irregular movements that are usually multifocal. Like asterixis, often indicates a diffuse encephalopathy. Following cardiac arrest, diffuse cerebral hypoxia may produce multifocal myoclonus. Clonazepam, valproate, or baclofen may be effective.

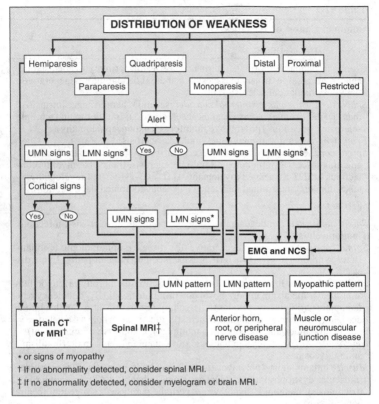

FIGURE 41-1 An algorithm for the initial workup of a patient with weakness. CT, computed tomography; EMG, electromyography; LMN, lower motor neuron; MRI, magnetic resonance imaging; NCS, nerve conduction studies; UMN, upper motor neuron.

DYSTONIA Involuntary, sustained deviation in posture about one or more joints. Postures attained are often bizarre, with forceful extensions and twisting. Dystonias may be generalized or focal (e.g., spasmodic torticollis, blepharospasm). Symptoms may respond to high doses of anticholinergics, benzodiazepines, baclofen, and anticonvulsants. Local injection of botulinum toxin is effective in certain focal dystonias.

CHOREOATHETOSIS A combination of chorea (rapid, jerky movements) and athetosis (slow writhing movements). The two usually exist together, though one may be more prominent. Choreic movements are the predominant involuntary movements in rheumatic (Sydenham's) chorea and Huntington's disease. Athetosis is prominent in some forms of cerebral palsy. Chronic neuroleptic use may lead to tardive dyskinesia, in which choreoathetotic movements are usually restricted to the buccal, lingual, and mandibular areas. Benzodiazepines, reserpine, and low-dose neuroleptics may suppress choreoathetotic movements but are often ineffective.

TICS Stereotypical, purposeless movements such as eye blinks, sniffling, and clearing of the throat. Gilles de la Tourette syndrome is a rare but severe multiple tic disorder that may involve motor tics (especially twitches of the face, neck, and shoulders), vocal tics (grunts, words), and "behavioral tics" (coprolalia, echolalia). The cause is unknown. Haloperidol usually reduces frequency and severity of the tics.

For a more detailed discussion, see Olney RK: Weakness, Disorders of Movement, and Imbalance, Chap. 21, p. 134, in HPIM-16.

42

APHASIAS AND RELATED DISORDERS

Aphasias are disturbances in the comprehension or production of spoken or written language. Clinical examination should assess naming, spontaneous speech, comprehension, repetition, reading, and writing. A classification scheme is presented in Table 42-1; the most common aphasias are summarized below.

Wernicke's Aphasia

Clinical Manifestations   Although speech sounds grammatical, melodic, and effortless ("fluent"), it is virtually incomprehensible due to errors in word usage, structure, and tense and the presence of neologisms and paraphasia ("jargon"). Comprehension of written and spoken material is severely impaired, as are reading, writing, and repetition. The pt usually seems unaware of the deficit. Associated symptoms can include parietal lobe sensory deficits and homonymous hemianopia. Motor disturbances are rare.

Etiology   Lesion located in posterior perisylvian region. Most common cause is embolic occlusion of inferior division of dominant middle cerebral artery (MCA); less commonly hemorrhage, tumor, encephalitis, or abscess is responsible.

Broca's Aphasia

Clinical Manifestations   Speech output is sparse, slow, labored, interrupted by many word-finding pauses, telegraphic, and usually dysarthric; output may be reduced to a grunt or single word. Naming and repetition also impaired. Most patients have severe writing impairment. Comprehension of written and spoken language is relatively preserved. Patient is often aware of and visibly frustrated by deficit. With large lesions, a dense hemiparesis may occur, and the eyes may deviate toward side of lesion. More commonly, lesser degrees of contralateral face and arm weakness are present. Sensory loss is rarely found, and visual fields are intact. Buccolingual apraxia is common, with difficulty imitating movements with tongue and lips or performing these movements on command.

Etiology   Lesion involves dominant inferior frontal convolution (Broca's area), although cortical and subcortical areas along superior sylvian fissure and insula are often involved. Commonly caused by vascular lesions involving the

Table 42-1

Clinical Features of Aphasias and Related Conditions

	Comprehension	Repetition of Spoken Language	Naming	Fluency
Wernicke's	Impaired	Impaired	Impaired	Preserved or increased
Broca's	Preserved (except grammar)	Impaired	Impaired	Decreased
Global	Impaired	Impaired	Impaired	Decreased
Conduction	Preserved	Impaired	Impaired	Preserved
Nonfluent (motor) transcortical	Preserved	Preserved	Impaired	Impaired
Fluent (sensory) transcortical	Impaired	Preserved	Impaired	Preserved
Isolation	Impaired	Echolalia	Impaired	No purposeful speech
Anomic	Preserved	Preserved	Impaired	Preserved except for word-finding pauses
Pure word deafness	Impaired only for spoken language	Impaired	Preserved	Preserved
Pure alexia	Impaired only for reading	Preserved	Preserved	Preserved

Source: M-M Mesulam: HPIM-16, p. 146.

superior division of the MCA; less commonly due to tumor, abscess, metastasis, subdural hematoma, encephalitis.

Global Aphasia

All aspects of speech and language are impaired. Patient cannot read, write, or repeat and has poor auditory comprehension. Speech output is minimal and nonfluent. Usually hemiplegia, hemisensory loss, and homonymous hemianopia are present. Syndrome represents the combined dysfunction of Wernicke's and Broca's areas, usually resulting from occlusion of MCA supplying dominant hemisphere (less commonly hemorrhage, trauma, or tumor).

Conduction Aphasia

Comprehension of speech and writing is largely intact, and speech output is fluent, although paraphasia is common. Repetition is severely affected. Lesion spares, but functionally disconnects, Wernicke's and Broca's areas. Most cases are embolic, involving supramarginal gyrus of dominant parietal lobe, dominant superior temporal lobe, or arcuate fasciculus.

Laboratory Studies in Aphasia

CT scan or MRI usually identifies the location and nature of the causative lesion. Angiography helps in accurate definition of specific vascular syndromes.

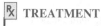 TREATMENT

Speech therapy may be helpful in treatment of certain types of aphasia.

For a more detailed discussion, see Mesulam M-M: Aphasia, Memory Loss, and Other Focal Cerebral Disorders, Chap. 23, p. 145, in HPIM-16.

43

SLEEP DISORDERS

Disorders of sleep are among the most common problems seen by clinicians. More than one-half of adults experience at least occasional insomnia, and 15–20% have a chronic sleep disturbance.

Approach to the Patient

Pts may complain of (1) difficulty in initiating and maintaining sleep (insomnia); (2) excessive daytime sleepiness, fatigue, or tiredness; (3) behavioral phenomena occurring during sleep [sleepwalking, rapid eye movement (REM) behavioral disorder, periodic leg movements of sleep, etc.]; or (4) circadian rhythm disorders associated with jet lag, shift work, and delayed sleep phase syndrome. A careful history of sleep habits and reports from the sleep partner (e.g., heavy snoring, falling asleep while driving) are a cornerstone of diagnosis. Completion of a day-by-day sleep-work-drug log for at least 2 weeks is often helpful. Work and sleep times (including daytime naps and nocturnal awakenings) as well as drug and alcohol use, including caffeine and hypnotics, should be noted each day. Objective sleep laboratory recording is necessary to evaluate sleep apnea, narcolepsy, REM behavior disorder, periodic leg movements, and other suspected disorders.

Insomnia

Insomnia, or the complaint of inadequate sleep, may be subdivided into difficulty falling asleep (*sleep-onset insomnia*), frequent or sustained awakenings (*sleep-offset insomnia*), or persistent sleepiness despite sleep of adequate duration (*nonrestorative sleep*). An insomnia complaint lasting one to several nights is termed *transient insomnia* and is typically due to situational stress or a change in sleep schedule or environment (e.g., jet lag). *Short-term insomnia* lasts from a few days up to 3 weeks; it is often associated with more protracted stress such as recovery from surgery or short-term illness. *Long-term (chronic) insomnia* lasts for months or years and, in contrast to short-term insomnia, requires a thorough evaluation for underlying causes. Chronic insomnia is often a waxing and waning disorder, with spontaneous or stressor-induced exacerbations.

EXTRINSIC INSOMNIA *Transient situational insomnia* can occur after a change in the sleeping environment (e.g., in an unfamiliar hotel or hospital bed) or before or after a significant life event or anxiety-provoking situation. Treatment is symptomatic, with intermittent use of hypnotics and resolution of the underlying stress. *Inadequate sleep hygiene* is characterized by a behavior pattern prior to sleep and/or a bedroom environment that is not conducive to sleep. In preference to hypnotic medications, the pt should attempt to avoid stressful activities before bed, reserve the bedroom environment for sleeping, and maintain regular rising times.

PSYCHOPHYSIOLOGIC INSOMNIA Pts with this behavioral disorder are preoccupied with a perceived inability to sleep adequately at night. Rigorous attention should be paid to sleep hygiene and correction of counterproductive, arousing behaviors before bedtime. Behavioral therapies are the treatment of choice.

DRUGS AND MEDICATIONS Caffeine is probably the most common pharmacologic cause of insomnia. Alcohol and nicotine can also interfere with sleep, despite the fact that many pts use these agents to relax and promote sleep. A number of prescribed medications, including antidepressants, sympathomimetics, and glucocorticoids, can produce insomnia. In addition, severe rebound insomnia can result from the acute withdrawal of hypnotics, especially following use of high doses of benzodiazepines with a short half-life. For this reason, hypnotic doses should be low to moderate, the total duration of hypnotic therapy should be limited to 2–3 weeks, and prolonged drug tapering is encouraged.

MOVEMENT DISORDERS Pts with *restless legs syndrome* complain of creeping dysesthesia deep within the calves or feet associated with an irresistible urge to move the affected limbs; symptoms are typically worse at night. Treatment is with dopaminergic drugs (pramipexole 0.25 to 1.0 mg daily at 8 P.M.. or ropinirole 0.5 to 4.0 mg daily at 8 P.M.). *Periodic limb movement disorder* consists of stereotyped extensions of the great toe and dorsiflexion of the foot recurring every 20–40 s during non-rapid eye movement sleep. This common condition is present in 1% of the population; treatment options include dopaminergic medications or benzodiazepines.

OTHER NEUROLOGIC DISORDERS A variety of neurologic disorders produce sleep disruption through both indirect, nonspecific mechanisms (e.g., neck or back pain) or by impairment of central neural structures involved in the generation and control of sleep itself. Common disorders to consider include *dementia* from any cause, *epilepsy*, *Parkinson's disease*, and *migraine*.

PSYCHIATRIC DISORDERS Approximately 80% of pts with mental disorders complain of impaired sleep. The underlying diagnosis may be depression, mania, an anxiety disorder, or schizophrenia.

MEDICAL DISORDERS In *asthma*, daily variation in airway resistance results in marked increases in asthmatic symptoms at night, especially during sleep. Treatment of asthma with theophylline-based compounds, adrenergic agonists, or glucocorticoids can independently disrupt sleep. Inhaled glucocorticoids that do not disrupt sleep may provide a useful alternative to oral drugs. *Cardiac ischemia* is also associated with sleep disruption; the ischemia itself may result from increases in sympathetic tone as a result of sleep apnea. Pts may present with complaints of nightmares or vivid dreams. *Paroxysmal nocturnal dyspnea* can also occur from cardiac ischemia that causes pulmonary congestion exacerbated by the recumbent posture. *Chronic obstructive pulmonary disease, hyperthyroidism, menopause,* and *gastroesophageal reflux* are other causes.

 TREATMENT

> ***Insomnia without Identifiable Cause*** Primary insomnia is a diagnosis of exclusion. Treatment is directed toward behavior therapies for anxiety and negative conditioning, pharmacotherapy for mood/anxiety disorders, an emphasis on good sleep hygiene, and intermittent hypnotics for exacerbations of insomnia. Cognitive therapy emphasizes understanding the nature of normal sleep, the circadian rhythm, the use of light therapy, and visual imagery to block unwanted thought intrusions. Behavioral modification involves bedtime restriction, set schedules, and careful sleep environment practices. Judicious use of benzodiazepine receptor agonists with short half-lives can be effective; options include zaleplon (5–20 mg), zolpidem (5–10 mg), or triazolam (0.125–0.25 mg). Limit use to 2–4 weeks maximum for acute insomnia or intermittent use for chronic. Some pts benefit from low-dose sedating antidepressants (e.g., trazodone, 25–100 mg).

Hypersomnias (Disorders of Excessive Daytime Sleepiness)

Differentiation of sleepiness from subjective complaints of fatigue may be difficult. Quantification of daytime sleepiness can be performed in a sleep laboratory using a multiple sleep latency test (MSLT), the repeated daytime measurement of sleep latency under standardized conditions. Common causes are summarized in Table 43-1.

SLEEP APNEA SYNDROMES Respiratory dysfunction during sleep is a common cause of excessive daytime sleepiness and/or disturbed nocturnal sleep, affecting an estimated 2 to 5 million individuals in the U.S. Episodes may be due to occlusion of the airway (obstructive sleep apnea), absence of respiratory effort (central sleep apnea), or a combination of these factors (mixed sleep apnea). Obstruction is exacerbated by obesity, supine posture, sedatives (especially alcohol), nasal obstruction, and hypothyroidism. Sleep apnea is particularly prevalent in overweight men and in the elderly and is often undiagnosed. Treatment consists of correction of the above factors, positive airway pressure devices, oral appliances, and sometimes surgery (see Chap 137).

NARCOLEPSY (Table 43-2) A disorder of excessive daytime sleepiness and intrusion of REM-related sleep phenomena into wakefulness (cataplexy, hypnagogic hallucinations, and sleep paralysis). Cataplexy, the abrupt loss of muscle tone in arms, legs, or face, is precipitated by emotional stimuli such as laughter or sadness. The excessive daytime sleepiness usually appears in adolescence, and the other phenomena, variably, later in life. The prevalence is 1 in 4000. Hypothalamic neurons containing the neuropeptide orexin (hypocretin) regulate the sleep/wake cycle and have been implicated in narcolepsy. Sleep studies confirm a short daytime sleep latency and a rapid transition to REM sleep.

 TREATMENT

> Somnolence is treated with modafinil, a novel wake-promoting agent; the usual dose is 200–400 mg/d given as a single dose. Older stimulants such as

Table 43-1

Evaluation of the Patient with the Complaint of Excessive Daytime Somnolence

Findings on History and Physical Examination	Diagnostic Evaluation	Diagnosis	Therapy
Obesity, snoring, hypertension	Polysomnography with respiratory monitoring	Obstructive sleep apnea	Continuous positive airway pressure; ENT surgery (e.g., uvulopalatopharyngoplasty); dental appliance; pharmacologic therapy (e.g., protriptyline); weight loss
Cataplexy, hypnogogic hallucinations, sleep paralysis, family history	Polysomnography with multiple sleep latency testing	Narcolepsy-cataplexy syndrome	Stimulants (e.g., modafinil, methylphenidate); REM-suppressant antidepressants (e.g., protriptyline); genetic counseling
Restless legs syndrome, disturbed sleep, predisposing medical condition (e.g., anemia or renal failure)	Polysomnography with bilateral anterior tibialis EMG monitoring	Periodic limb movements of sleep	Treatment of predisposing condition, if possible; dopamine agonists (e.g., pramipexole); benzodiazepines (e.g., clonazepam)
Disturbed sleep, predisposing medical conditions (e.g., asthma) and/or predisposing medical therapies (e.g., theophylline)	Sleep-wake diary recording	Insomnias (see text)	Treatment of predisposing condition and/or change in therapy, if possible; behavioral therapy; short-acting benzodiazepine receptor agonist (e.g., zolpidem)

Note: ENT, ears, nose, throat; REM, rapid eye movement; EMG, electromyogram.
Source: From Czeisler CA et al: HPIM-16, p. 156.

Table 43-2

Prevalence of Symptoms in Narcolepsy	
Symptom	Prevalence, %
Excessive daytime somnolence	100
Disturbed sleep	87
Cataplexy	76
Hypnagogic hallucinations	68
Sleep paralysis	64
Memory problems	50

Source: Modified from TA Roth, L Merlotti in SA Burton et al (eds), *Narcolepsy 3rd International Symposium: Selected Symposium Proceedings*, Chicago, Matrix Communications, 1989.

methylphenidate (10 mg bid–20 mg qid); pemoline, dextroamphetamine, and methamphetamine are alternatives, particularly in refractory pts. Adequate nocturnal sleep time and the use of short naps are other useful measures. Cataplexy, hypnagogic hallucinations, and sleep paralysis respond to the tricyclic antidepressants protriptyline (10–40 mg/d) and clomipramine (25–50 mg/d) and to the selective serotonin uptake inhibitor fluoxetine (10–20 mg/d).

Disorders of Circadian Rhythmicity

Insomnia or hypersomnia may occur in disorders of sleep timing rather than sleep generation. Such conditions may be (1) organic—due to a defect in the hypothalamic circadian pacemaker, or (2) environmental—due to a disruption of entraining stimuli (light/dark cycle). Examples of the latter include jet-lag syndrome and shift work. *Delayed sleep phase syndrome* is characterized by late sleep onset and awakening with otherwise normal sleep architecture. Bright-light phototherapy in the morning hours or melatonin therapy during the evening hours may be effective. *Advanced sleep phase syndrome* moves sleep onset to the early evening hours with early morning awakening. These pts may benefit from bright light phototherapy during the evening hours.

For a more detailed discussion, see Czeisler CA, Winkleman JW, Richardson GS: Sleep Disorders, Chap. 24, p. 153, in HPIM-16.

44

DYSPNEA

Definition

Abnormally uncomfortable awareness of breathing; intensity quantified by establishing the amount of physical exertion necessary to produce the sensation. Dyspnea occurs when work of breathing is excessive.

Causes

HEART DISEASE

• Dyspnea most commonly due to ↑ pulmonary capillary pressure, and sometimes fatigue of respiratory muscles. Vital capacity and lung compliance are ↓ and airway resistance ↑.

• Begins as exertional breathlessness → orthopnea → paroxysmal nocturnal dyspnea and dyspnea at rest.

• Diagnosis depends on recognition of heart disease, e.g., Hx of MI, presence of S_3, S_4, murmurs, cardiomegaly, jugular vein distention, hepatomegaly, and peripheral edema (Chap. 126). Objective quantification of ventricular function (echocardiography, radionuclide ventriculography) is often helpful.

AIRWAY OBSTRUCTION   (Chap. 133)

• May occur with obstruction anywhere from extrathoracic airways to lung periphery.

• Acute dyspnea with difficulty *inhaling* suggests *upper* airway obstruction. Physical exam may reveal inspiratory stridor and retraction of supraclavicular fossae.

• Acute intermittent dyspnea with expiratory wheezing suggests reversible intrathoracic obstruction due to asthma.

• Chronic, slowly progressive exertional dyspnea characterizes emphysema and CHF.

• Chronic cough with expectoration is typical of chronic bronchitis and bronchiectasis.

DIFFUSE PARENCHYMAL LUNG DISEASES   (Chap. 136)   Many parenchymal lung diseases, from sarcoidosis to pneumoconioses, may cause dyspnea. Dyspnea is usually related to exertion early in the course of the illness. Physical exam typically reveals tachypnea and late inspiratory rales.

PULMONARY EMBOLISM   (Chap. 135)   Dyspnea is most common symptom of pulmonary embolus. Repeated discrete episodes of dyspnea may occur with recurrent pulmonary emboli; tachypnea is frequent.

DISEASE OF THE CHEST WALL OR RESPIRATORY MUSCLES
(Chap. 137)   Severe kyphoscoliosis may produce chronic dyspnea, often with chronic cor pulmonale. Spinal deformity must be severe before respiratory function is compromised.

Pts with bilateral diaphragmatic paralysis appear normal while standing, but complain of severe orthopnea and display paradoxical abnormal respiratory movement when supine.

––––––––––––––––––– *Approach to the Patient* –––––––––––––––––––

Elicit a description of the amount of physical exertion necessary to produce the sensation and whether it varies under different conditions.

• If acute upper airway obstruction is suspected, lateral neck films or fiberoptic exam of upper airway may be helpful.

• With chronic upper airway obstruction the respiratory flow-volume curve may show inspiratory cutoff of flow, suggesting variable extrathoracic obstruction.

• Dyspnea due to emphysema is reflected in a reduction in expiratory flow rates (FEV_1), and often by a reduction in diffusing capacity for carbon monoxide (DL_{CO}).

• Pts with intermittent dyspnea due to asthma may have normal pulmonary function if tested when asymptomatic.

Table 44-1

Differentiation between Cardiac and Pulmonary Dyspnea

• *Careful history*: Dyspnea of lung disease usually more gradual in onset than that of heart disease; nocturnal exacerbations common with each.
• *Examination*: Usually obvious evidence of cardiac or pulmonary disease. Findings may be absent at rest when symptoms are present only with exertion.
• *Brain natriuretic peptide (BNP)*: Elevated in cardiac but not pulmonary dyspnea.
• *Pulmonary function tests*: Pulmonary disease rarely causes dyspnea unless tests of obstructive disease (FEV_1, FEV_1/FVC) or restrictive disease (total lung capacity) are reduced (<80% predicted).
• *Ventricular performance*: LV ejection fraction at rest and/or during exercise usually depressed in cardiac dyspnea.

• Cardiac dyspnea usually begins as breathlessness on strenuous exertion with gradual (months-to-years) progression to dyspnea at rest.
• Pts with dyspnea due to both cardiac and pulmonary diseases may report orthopnea. Paroxysmal nocturnal dyspnea occurring after awakening from sleep is characteristic of CHF.
• Dyspnea of chronic obstructive lung disease tends to develop more gradually than that of heart disease.
• PFTs should be performed when etiology is not clear. When the diagnosis remains obscure a pulmonary stress test is often useful.
• Management depends on elucidating etiology.

Differentiation between cardiac and pulmonary dyspnea is summarized in Table 44-1.

For a more detailed discussion, see Ingram RH Jr., Braunwald E: Dyspnea and Pulmonary Edema, Chap. 29, p. 201, HPIM-16.

45

COUGH AND HEMOPTYSIS

COUGH

Produced by inflammatory, mechanical, chemical, and thermal stimulation of cough receptors.

ETIOLOGY

• *Inflammatory*—edema and hyperemia of airways and alveoli due to laryngitis, tracheitis, bronchitis, bronchiolitis, pneumonitis, lung abscess.
• *Mechanical*—inhalation of particulates (dust) or compression of airways (pulmonary neoplasms, foreign bodies, granulomas, bronchospasm).

- *Chemical*—inhalation of irritant fumes, including cigarette smoke.
- *Thermal*—inhalation of cold or very hot air.

_____ *Approach to the Patient* _____

Diagnosis (Fig. 45-1)   *History* should consider:

- *Duration*—acute or chronic
- *Presence of fever or wheezing*

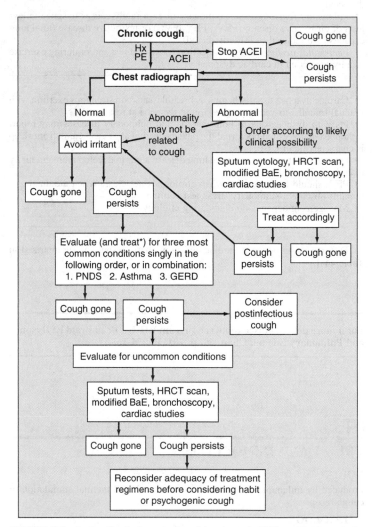

FIGURE 45-1   An algorithm for the evaluation of chronic cough. ACEI, angiotensin-converting enzyme inhibitor; BaE, barium esophagography; GERD, gastroesophageal reflux disease; HRCT, high resolution computed tomography; Hx, history; PE, physical examination; PNDS, postnasal drip syndrome. *Treatment is either targeted to a presumptive diagnosis or given empirically. [*Adapted from RS Irwin: Chest 114(Suppl):1335, 1998, with permission.*]

• *Sputum quantity and character*—change in sputum character, color, or volume in a smoker with "smoker's cough" necessitates investigation.

• *Temporal or seasonal pattern*—seasonal cough may indicate "cough asthma."

• *Risk factors for underlying disease*—environmental exposures may suggest occupational asthma or interstitial lung disease.

• *Past medical history*—past history of recurrent pneumonias may indicate bronchiectasis, particularly if associated with purulent or copious sputum production. A change in the character of chronic cigarette cough raises suspicion of bronchogenic carcinoma. Chronic CHF causes cough.

• *Drugs*—is pt. on ACE inhibitor? Causes chronic cough in 5–20%

Short duration with associated fever suggests acute viral or bacterial infection. Persistent cough after viral illness suggests postinflammatory cough. Postnasal drip is common cause of chronic cough. Nocturnal cough may indicate chronic sinus drainage or esophageal reflux.

Physical exam should assess upper and lower airways and lung parenchyma.

• Stridor suggests upper airway obstruction; wheezing suggests bronchospasm as the cause of cough.

• Midinspiratory crackles indicate airways disease (e.g., chronic bronchitis).

• Fine end-inspiratory crackles occur in interstitial fibrosis and heart failure.

• CXR may show neoplasm, infection, interstitial disease, or the hilar adenopathy of sarcoidosis.

• High-resolution computed tomography (HRCT) helpful in unexplained chronic cough.

• PFTs may reveal obstruction or restriction.

• Sputum exam can indicate malignancy or infection.

• Fiberoptic bronchoscopy helpful in defining endobronchial causes.

COMPLICATIONS   (1) Syncope, due to transient decrease in venous return; (2) rupture of an emphysematous bleb with pneumothorax; (3) rib fractures—may occur in otherwise normal individuals.

R̲x̲ TREATMENT

• When possible, therapy of cough is that of underlying disease. Eliminate ACE inhibitors and cigarette smoking.

• If no cause can be found, a trial of an inhaled anticholinergic agent (e.g., ipratropium 2–4 puffs qid), an inhaled β agonist (e.g., albuterol) or an inhaled steroid (e.g., triamcinolone) can be attempted. Inhaled steroids may take 7–10 days to be effective when used for an irritative cough.

• Cough productive of significant volumes of sputum should generally not be suppressed. Sputum clearance can be facilitated with adequate hydration, expectorants, and mechanical devices. Iodinated glycerol (30 mg qid) may be useful in asthma or chronic bronchitis.

• When symptoms from an irritative cough are severe, the cough may be suppressed with a narcotic antitussive agent such as codeine, 15–30 mg up to qid, or a nonnarcotic such as dextromethorphan (15 mg qid).

HEMOPTYSIS

Includes both streaked sputum and coughing up of gross blood.

ETIOLOGY   (Table 45-1) Bronchitis and pneumonia are common causes. Neoplasm may be the cause, particularly in smokers and when hemoptysis is persistent. Hemoptysis rare in metastatic neoplasm to lung. Pulmonary

Table 45-1

Differential Diagnosis of Hemoptysis

Source other than the lower respiratory tract
    Upper airway (nasopharyngeal) bleeding
    Gastrointestinal bleeding
Tracheobronchial source
    Neoplasm (bronchogenic carcinoma, endobronchial metastatic tumor,
      Kaposi's sarcoma, bronchial carcinoid)
    Bronchitis (acute or chronic)
    Bronchiectasis
    Broncholithiasis
    Airway trauma
    Foreign body
Pulmonary parenchymal source
    Lung abscess
    Pneumonia
    Tuberculosis
    Mycetoma ("fungus ball")
    Goodpasture's syndrome
    Idiopathic pulmonary hemosiderosis
    Wegener's granulomatosis
    Lupus pneumonitis
    Lung contusion
Primary vascular source
    Arteriovenous malformation
    Pulmonary embolism
    Elevated pulmonary venous pressure (esp. mitral stenosis)
    Pulmonary artery rupture secondary to balloon-tip pulmonary artery catheter
      manipulation
Miscellaneous/rare causes
    Pulmonary endometriosis
    Systemic coagulopathy or use of anticoagulants or thrombolytic agents

Source: Adapted from SE Weinberger, *Principles of Pulmonary Medicine*, 3d ed, Philadelphia, Saunders, 1998.

thromboembolism and infection are other causes. Diffuse hemoptysis may occur with vasculitis involving the lung. Five to 15% of cases with hemoptysis remain undiagnosed.

_____ *Approach to the Patient* _____

Diagnosis (Fig. 45-2)   Essential to determine that blood is coming from respiratory tract. Often frothy, may be preceded by a desire to cough.

• History may suggest diagnosis: chronic hemoptysis in otherwise asymptomatic young woman suggests bronchial adenoma.
• Hemoptysis, weight loss, and anorexia in a smoker suggest carcinoma.
• Hemoptysis with acute pleuritic pain suggests infarction; fever or chills with blood streaked sputum suggests pneumonia.

Physical exam may also suggest diagnosis: pleural friction rub raises possibility of pulmonary embolism or some other pleural-based lesion (lung abscess, coccidioidomycosis cavity, vasculitis); diastolic rumbling murmur suggests mitral stenosis; localized wheeze suggests bronchogenic carcinoma.

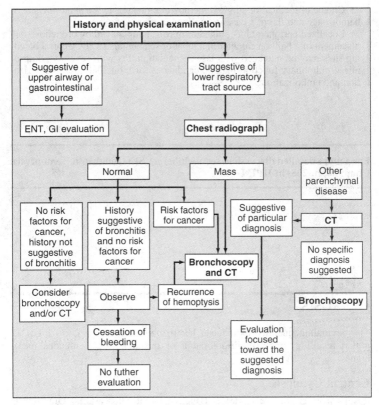

FIGURE 45-2 Diagnostic approach to hemoptysis. (From Chap. 30 in HPIM-16.)

Initial evaluation includes CXR. A normal CXR does not exclude tumor or bronchiectasis as a source of bleeding. The CXR may show an air-fluid level suggesting an abscess or atelectasis distal to an obstructing carcinoma. Follow with chest CT.

Most pts should be assessed by fiberoptic bronchoscopy. Rigid bronchoscopy helpful when bleeding is massive or from proximal airway lesion and when endotracheal intubation is contemplated.

℞ **TREATMENT**

• Treat the underlying condition
• Mainstays are bed rest and cough suppression with an opiate (codeine, 15–30 mg, or hydrocodone, 5 mg q4–6h).
• Pts with massive hemoptysis (>600 mL/d) and pts with respiratory compromise due to aspiration of blood should be monitored intensively with suction and intubation equipment close by so that selective intubation to isolate the bleeding lung can be accomplished. In massive hemoptysis, highest priority is to maintain gas exchange, and this may require intubation with double-lumen endotracheal tubes.

• Choice of medical or surgical therapy often relates to the anatomic site of hemorrhage and the pt's baseline pulmonary function.

• Localized peripheral bleeding sites may be tamponaded by bronchoscopic placement of a balloon catheter in a lobar or segmental airway. Central bleeding sites may be managed with laser coagulation. Pts with severely compromised pulmonary function may be candidates for bronchial artery catherization and embolization.

For a more detailed discussion, see Weinberger SE: Cough and Hemoptysis, Chap. 30, p. 205, in HPIM-16.

46

CYANOSIS

The circulating quantity of reduced hemoglobin is elevated [>50 g/L (>5 g/dL)] resulting in bluish discoloration of the skin and/or mucous membranes.

Central Cyanosis

Results from arterial desaturation. Usually evident when arterial saturation is ≤85%. Cyanosis may not be detected until saturation is 75% in dark-skinned individuals.

• *Impaired pulmonary function*: Poorly ventilated alveoli or impaired oxygen diffusion; most frequent in pneumonia, pulmonary edema, and chronic obstructive pulmonary disease (COPD); in COPD with cyanosis, polycythemia is often present.

• *Anatomic vascular shunting*: Shunting of desaturated venous blood into the arterial circulation may result from congenital heart disease or pulmonary AV fistula.

• *Decreased inspired O_2*: Cyanosis may develop in ascents to altitudes >2400 m (>8000 ft).

• *Abnormal hemoglobins*: Methemoglobinemia, sulfhemoglobinemia, and mutant hemoglobins with low oxygen affinity (see HPIM-16, Chap. 91).

Peripheral Cyanosis

Occurs with normal arterial O_2 saturation with increased extraction of O_2 from capillary blood caused by decreased localized blood flow. Vasoconstriction due to cold exposure, decreased cardiac output (in shock, Chap. 14), heart failure (Chap 126), and peripheral vascular disease (Chap. 128) with arterial obstruction or vasospasm (Table 46-1). Local (e.g., thrombophlebitis) or central (e.g., constrictive pericarditis) venous hypertension intensifies cyanosis.

Table 46-1

Causes of Cyanosis

CENTRAL CYANOSIS

Decreased arterial oxygen saturation
    Decreased atmospheric pressure—high altitude
    Impaired pulmonary function
        Alveolar hypoventilation
        Uneven relationships between pulmonary ventilation and perfusion
        (perfusion of hypoventilated alveoli)
        Impaired oxygen diffusion
    Anatomic shunts
        Certain types of congenital heart disease
        Pulmonary arteriovenous fistulas
        Multiple small intrapulmonary shunts
    Hemoglobin with low affinity for oxygen
Hemoglobin abnormalities
    Methemoglobinemia—hereditary, acquired
    Sulfhemoglobinemia—acquired
    Carboxyhemoglobinemia (not true cyanosis)

PERIPHERAL CYANOSIS

Reduced cardiac output
Cold exposure
Redistribution of blood flow from extremities
Arterial obstruction
Venous obstruction

_____ *Approach to the Patient* _____

• Inquire about duration (cyanosis since birth suggests congenital heart disease) and exposures (drugs or chemicals that result in abnormal hemoglobins).
• Differentiate central from peripheral cyanosis by examining nailbeds, lips, and mucous membranes. Peripheral cyanosis most intense in nailbeds and may resolve with gentle warming of extremities.
• Check for clubbing of fingers and toes; clubbing is the selective enlargement of the distal segments of fingers and toes. Clubbing may be hereditary, idiopathic, or acquired and is associated with a variety of disorders. Combination of clubbing and cyanosis is frequent in congenital heart disease and occasionally with pulmonary disease (lung abscess, pulmonary AV shunts but *not* with uncomplicated obstructive lung disease).
• Examine chest for evidence of pulmonary disease, pulmonary edema, or murmurs associated with congenital heart disease.
• If cyanosis is localized to an extremity, evaluate for peripheral vascular obstruction.
• Obtain arterial blood gas to measure systemic O_2 saturation. Repeat while pt inhales 100% O_2; if saturation fails to increase to >95%, intravascular shunting of blood bypassing the lungs is likely (e.g., right-to-left intracardiac shunts).
• Evaluate abnormal hemoglobins by hemoglobin electrophoresis, spectroscopy, and measurement of methemoglobin level.

For a more detailed discussion, see Braunwald E: Hypoxia and Cyanosis, Chap. 31, p. 209, in HPIM-16.

47

EDEMA

Definition

Soft tissue swelling due to abnormal expansion of interstitial fluid volume. Edema fluid is a plasma transudate that accumulates when movement of fluid from vascular to interstitial space is favored. Since detectable generalized edema in the adult reflects a gain of ≥3 L, renal retention of salt and water is necessary for edema to occur. Distribution of edema can be an important guide to cause.

LOCALIZED EDEMA   Limited to a particular organ or vascular bed; easily distinguished from generalized edema. Unilateral extremity edema is usually due to venous or lymphatic obstruction (e.g., deep venous thrombosis, tumor obstruction, primary lymphedema). Stasis edema of a paralyzed lower extremity may also occur. Allergic reactions ("angioedema") and superior vena caval obstruction are causes of localized facial edema. Bilateral lower extremity edema may have localized causes, e.g., inferior vena caval obstruction, compression due to ascites, abdominal mass. Ascites (fluid in peritoneal cavity) and hydrothorax (in pleural space) may also present as isolated localized edema, due to inflammation or neoplasm.

GENERALIZED EDEMA   Soft tissue swelling of most or all regions of the body. Bilateral lower extremity swelling, more pronounced after standing for several hours, and pulmonary edema are usually cardiac in origin. Periorbital edema noted on awakening often results from renal disease and impaired Na excretion. Ascites and edema of lower extremities and scrotum are frequent in cirrhosis or CHF. In *CHF*, diminished cardiac output and effective arterial blood volume result in both decreased renal perfusion and increased venous pressure with resultant renal Na retention due to renal vasoconstriction, intrarenal blood flow redistribution, direct Na-retentive effects of norepinephrine and angiotensin II, and secondary hyperaldosteronism.

In *cirrhosis*, arteriovenous shunts lower effective renal perfusion, resulting in Na retention. Ascites accumulates when increased intrahepatic vascular resistance produces portal hypertension. Reduced serum albumin and increased abdominal pressure also promote lower extremity edema.

In *nephrotic syndrome*, massive renal loss of albumin lowers plasma oncotic pressure, promoting fluid transudation into interstitium; lowering of effective blood volume stimulates renal Na retention.

In acute or chronic *renal failure*, edema occurs if Na intake exceeds kidney's ability to excrete Na secondary to marked reductions in glomerular filtration. Severe hypoalbuminemia [<25 g/L (2.5 g/dL)] of any cause (e.g., nephrosis, nutritional deficiency states, chronic liver disease) may lower plasma oncotic pressure sufficiently to cause edema, if accompanied by low levels of non-albumin proteins [total protein <54 g/L (5.4 g/dL)].

Less common causes of generalized edema: *idiopathic edema*, a syndrome of recurrent rapid weight gain and edema in women of reproductive age; *hypothyroidism*, in which myxedema is typically located in the pretibial region; *drugs* such as glucocorticoids, estrogens, thiozolidinediones, and vasodilators; pregnancy; refeeding after starvation.

℞ TREATMENT

Primary management is to identify and treat the underlying cause of edema (Fig. 47-1).

Dietary Na restriction (<500 mg/d) may prevent further edema formation. Bed rest enhances response to salt restriction in CHF and cirrhosis. Supportive stockings and elevation of edematous lower extremities will help mobilize interstitial fluid. If severe hyponatremia (<132 mmol/L) is present, water intake should also be reduced (<1500 mL/d). Diuretics (Table 47-1) are indicated for marked peripheral edema, pulmonary edema, CHF, inadequate dietary salt restriction. Complications are listed in Table 47-2. Weight loss by diuretics should

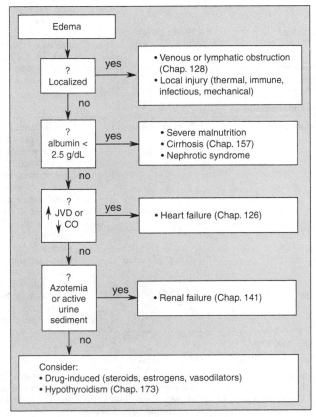

FIGURE 47-1 Diagnostic approach to edema. JVD, jugular venous distention; CO, cardiac output.

Table 47-1

Diuretics for Edema*

Drug	Usual Dose	Comments
LOOP (MAY BE ADMINISTERED PO OR IV)		
Furosemide	40–120 mg qd or bid	Short-acting; potent; effective with low GFR
Bumetanide	0.5–2 mg qd or bid	May be used if allergic to furosemide
Ethacrynic acid	50–200 mg qd	Longer-acting
DISTAL, K-LOSING		
Hydrochlorothiazide	25–200 mg qd	First choice; causes hypokalemia; need GFR > 25 mL/min
Chlorthalidone	100 mg qd or qod	Long-acting (up to 72 h); hypokalemia; need GFR > 25 mL/min
Metolazone	1–10 mg qd	Long-acting; hypokalemia; effective with low GFR, especially when combined with a loop diuretic
DISTAL, K-SPARING		
Spironolactone	25–100 mg qd to qid	Hyperkalemia; acidosis; blocks aldosterone; gynecomastia, impotence, amenorrhea; onset takes 2–3 days; avoid use in renal failure or in combination with ACE inhibitors or potassium supplements
Amiloride	5–10 mg qd or bid	Hyperkalemia; once daily; less potent than spironolactone
Triamterene	100 mg bid	Hyperkalemia; less potent than spironolactone; renal stones

* See also Table 17-2.

be limited to 1–1.5 kg/d. Distal ("potassium sparing") diuretics or metolazone may be added to loop diuretics for enhanced effect. Note that intestinal edema may impair absorption of oral diuretics and reduce effectiveness. When desired weight is achieved, diuretic doses should be reduced.

In *CHF* (Chap. 126), avoid overdiuresis because it may bring a fall in cardiac output and prerenal azotemia. Avoid diuretic-induced hypokalemia, which predisposes to digitalis toxicity.

Table 47-2

Complications of Diuretics

Common	Uncommon
Volume depletion	Interstitial nephritis (thiazides,
Prerenal azotemia	furosemide)
Potassium depletion	Pancreatitis (thiazides)
Hyponatremia (thiazides)	Loss of hearing (loop diuretics)
Metabolic alkalosis	Anemia, leukopenia, thrombocyto-
Hypercholesterolemia	penia (thiazides)
Hyperglycemia (thiazides)	
Hyperkalemia (K-sparing)	
Hypomagnesemia	
Hyperuricemia	
Hypercalcemia (thiazides)	
GI complaints	
Rash (thiazides)	

In *cirrhosis* and other hepatic causes of edema, spironolactone is the diuretic of choice but may produce acidosis and hyperkalemia. Thiazides or small doses of loop diuretics may also be added. However, renal failure may result from volume depletion. Overdiuresis may result in hyponatremia, hypokalemia, and alkalosis, which may worsen hepatic encephalopathy (Chap. 157).

For a more detailed discussion, see Braunwald E: Edema, Chap. 32, p. 212, in HPIM-16.

48

NAUSEA, VOMITING, AND INDIGESTION

NAUSEA AND VOMITING

Nausea refers to the imminent desire to vomit and often precedes or accompanies vomiting. *Vomiting* refers to the forceful expulsion of gastric contents through the mouth. *Retching* refers to labored rhythmic respiratory activity that precedes emesis. *Regurgitation* refers to the gentle expulsion of gastric contents in the absence of nausea and abdominal diaphragmatic muscular contraction. *Rumination* refers to the regurgitation, rechewing, and reswallowing of food from the stomach.

PATHOPHYSIOLOGY   Gastric contents are propelled into the esophagus when there is relaxation of the gastric fundus and gastroesophageal sphincter followed by a rapid increase in intraabdominal pressure produced by contraction of the abdominal and diaphragmatic musculature. Increased intrathoracic pressure results in further movement of the material to the mouth. Reflex elevation of the soft palate and closure of the glottis protects the nasopharynx and trachea and completes the act of vomiting. Vomiting is controlled by two brainstem areas, the vomiting center and chemoreceptor trigger zone. Activation of the chemoreceptor trigger zone results in impulses to the vomiting center, which controls the physical act of vomiting.

ETIOLOGY Nausea and vomiting are manifestations of a large number of disorders (Table 48-1).

EVALUATION The history, including a careful drug history, and the timing and character of the vomitus can be helpful. For example, vomiting that occurs predominantly in the morning is often seen in pregnancy, uremia, and alcoholic gastritis; feculent emesis implies distal intestinal obstruction or gastrocolic fistula; projectile vomiting suggests increased intracranial pressure; vomiting during or shortly after a meal may be due to psychogenic causes or peptic ulcer disease. Associated symptoms may also be helpful: vertigo and tinnitus in Ménière's disease, relief of abdominal pain with vomiting in peptic ulcer, and early satiety in gastroparesis. Plain radiographs can suggest diagnoses such as intestinal obstruction. The upper GI series assesses motility of the proximal GI tract as well as the mucosa. Other studies may be indicated such as gastric emptying scans (diabetic gastroparesis) and CT scan of the brain.

COMPLICATIONS Rupture of the esophagus (Boerhaave's syndrome), hematemesis from a mucosal tear (Mallory-Weiss syndrome), dehydration, malnutrition, dental caries and erosions, metabolic alkalosis, hypokalemia, and aspiration pneumonitis.

 TREATMENT

This should be directed toward correcting the specific cause. The effectiveness of antiemetic medications depends on etiology of symptoms, pt responsiveness, and side effects. Antihistamines such as dimenhydrinate and promethazine hydrochloride are effective for nausea due to inner ear dysfunction. Anticholinergics such as scopolamine are effective for nausea associated with motion sickness. Haloperidol and phenothiazine derivatives such as prochlorperazine are often effective in controlling mild nausea and vomiting, but sedation, hypotension, and parkinsonian symptoms are common side effects. Selective dopamine antagonists such as metoclopramide may be superior to the phenothiazines in treating severe nausea and vomiting and are particularly useful in treatment of gastroparesis. Intravenous metoclopramide may be effective as prophylaxis against nausea when given prior to chemotherapy. Cisapride, the preferred drug for gastroparesis, exerts peripheral antiemetic effects but is devoid of the CNS effects of metoclopramide. Ondansetron and palosetron, serotonin receptor blockers, and glucocorticoids are used for treating nausea and vomiting associated with cancer chemotherapy. Aprepitant, a neurokinin receptor blocker, is effective at controlling nausea from highly emetic drugs like cisplatin. Erythromycin is effective in some pts with gastroparesis.

INDIGESTION

Indigestion is a nonspecific term that encompasses a variety of upper abdominal complaints including heartburn, regurgitation, and dyspepsia (upper abdominal discomfort or pain). These symptoms are overwhelmingly due to gastroesophageal reflux disease (GERD).

PATHOPHYSIOLOGY GERD occurs as a consequence of acid reflux into the esophagus from the stomach, gastric motor dysfunction, or visceral afferent hypersensitivity. A wide variety of situations promote GERD: increased

Table 48-1

Causes of Nausea and Vomiting

Intraperitoneal	Extraperitoneal	Medications/Metabolic Disorders
Obstructing disorders	Cardiopulmonary disease	Drugs
Pyloric obstruction	Cardiomyopathy	Cancer chemotherapy
Small bowel obstruction	Myocardial infarction	Antibiotics
Colonic obstruction	Labyrinthine disease	Cardiac antiarrhythmics
Superior mesenteric artery syndrome	Motion sickness	Digoxin
Enteric infections	Labyrinthitis	Oral hypoglycemics
Viral	Malignancy	Oral contraceptives
Bacterial	Intracerebral disorders	Endocrine/metabolic disease
Inflammatory diseases	Malignancy	Pregnancy
Cholecystitis	Hemorrhage	Uremia
Pancreatitis	Abscess	Ketoacidosis
Appendicitis	Hydrocephalus	Thyroid and parathyroid disease
Hepatitis	Psychiatric illness	Adrenal insufficiency
Impaired motor function	Anorexia and bulimia nervosa	Toxins
Gastroparesis	Depression	Liver failure
Intestinal pseudoobstruction	Psychogenic vomiting	Ethanol
Functional dyspepsia	Postoperative vomiting	
Gastroesophageal reflux	Cyclic vomiting syndrome	
Biliary colic		
Abdominal irradiation		

gastric contents (from a large meal, gastric stasis, or acid hypersecretion), physical factors (lying down, bending over), increased pressure on the stomach (tight clothes, obesity, ascites, pregnancy), loss (usually intermittent) of lower esophageal sphincter tone (diseases such as scleroderma, smoking, anticholinergics, calcium antagonists). Hiatal hernia also promotes acid flow into the esophagus.

NATURAL HISTORY Heartburn is reported once monthly by 40% of Americans and daily by 7%. Functional dyspepsia is defined as >3 months of dyspepsia without an organic cause. Functional dyspepsia is the cause of symptoms in 60% of pts with dyspeptic symptoms. However, peptic ulcer disease from either *Helicobacter pylori* infection or ingestion of NSAIDs is present in 15% of cases.

In most cases, the esophagus is not damaged, but 5% of pts develop esophageal ulcers and some form strictures. 8–20% develop glandular epithelial cell metaplasia, termed *Barrett's esophagus*, which can progress to adenocarcinoma.

Extraesophageal manifestations include asthma, laryngitis, chronic cough, aspiration pneumonitis, chronic bronchitis, sleep apnea, dental caries, halitosis, and hiccups.

EVALUATION The presence of dysphagia, odynophagia, unexplained weight loss, recurrent vomiting leading to dehydration, occult or gross bleeding, or a palpable mass or adenopathy are "alarm" signals that demand directed radiographic, endoscopic, and surgical evaluation. Pts without alarm features are generally treated empirically. Individuals >45 years can be tested for the presence of *H. pylori*. Pts positive for the infection are treated to eradicate the organism. Pts who fail to respond to *H. pylori* treatment, those >45 years old, and those with alarm factors generally undergo upper GI endoscopy.

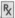 **TREATMENT**

Weight reduction; elevation of the head of the bed; and avoidance of large meals, smoking, caffeine, alcohol, chocolate, fatty food, citrus juices, and NSAIDs may prevent GERD. Antacids are widely used. Clinical trials suggest that proton pump inhibitors (omeprazole) are more effective than histamine receptor blockers (ranitidine) in patients with or without esophageal erosions. *H. pylori* eradication regimens are discussed in Chap. 150. Cisapride can stimulate gastric emptying. Omeprazole plus cisapride is a rational combination.

Surgical techniques (Nissan fundoplication, Belsey procedure) can be used in the rare pts who are refractory to medical management. Clinical trials have not documented the superiority of one over another.

For a more detailed discussion, see Hasler WL: Nausea, Vomiting, and Indigestion, Chap. 34, p. 219, in HPIM-16.

49

WEIGHT LOSS

Significant unintentional weight loss in a previously healthy individual is often a harbinger of underlying systemic disease. The routine medical history should always include inquiry about changes in weight. Rapid fluctuations of weight over days suggest loss or gain of fluid, whereas long-term changes usually involve loss of tissue mass. Loss of 5% of body weight over 6–12 months should prompt further evaluation.

Etiology

A list of possible causes of weight loss is extensive (Table 49-1). In older persons the most common causes of weight loss are depression, cancer, and benign gastrointestinal disease. In younger individuals diabetes mellitus, hyperthyroidism, anorexia nervosa, and infection, especially with HIV, should be considered.

Table 49-1

Causes of Weight Loss

Cancer

Endocrine and metabolic causes
  Hyperthyroidism
  Diabetes mellitus
  Pheochromocytoma
  Adrenal insufficiency

Gastrointestinal disorders
  Malabsorption
  Obstruction
  Pernicious anemia

Cardiac disorders
  Chronic ischemia
  Chronic congestive heart failure

Respiratory disorders
  Emphysema
  Chronic obstructive pulmonary disease

Renal insufficiency

Rheumatologic disease

Infections
  HIV
  Tuberculosis
  Parasitic infection
  Subacute bacterial endocarditis

Medications
  Antibiotics
  Nonsteroidal anti-inflammatory drugs
  Serotonin reuptake inhibitors
  Metformin
  Levodopa
  ACE inhibitors
  Other drugs

Disorders of the mouth and teeth

Age-related factors
  Physiologic changes
  Decreased taste and smell
  Functional disabilities

Neurologic causes
  Stroke
  Parkinson's disease
  Neuromuscular disorders
  Dementia

Social causes
  Isolation
  Economic hardship

Psychiatric and behavioral causes
  Depression
  Anxiety
  Bereavement
  Alcoholism
  Eating disorders
  Increased activity or exercise

Idiopathic

Table 49-2

___

Screening Tests for Evaluation of Involuntary Weight Loss
___

Initial testing	Additional testing
CBC	HIV test
Electrolytes, calcium, glucose	Upper and/or lower gastrointes-
Renal and liver function tests	tinal endoscopy
Urinalysis	Abdominal CT scan or MRI
Thyroid-stimulating hormone	Chest CT scan
Chest x-ray	
Recommended cancer screening	

___

Clinical Features

Before extensive evaluation is undertaken, it is important to confirm that weight loss has occurred. In the absence of documentation, changes in belt notch size or the fit of clothing may help to determine loss of weight.

The *history* should include questions about fever, pain, shortness of breath or cough, palpitations, and evidence of neurologic disease. A history of GI symptoms should be obtained, including difficulty eating, dysphagia, anorexia, nausea, and change in bowel habits. Travel history, use of cigarettes, alcohol, and all medications should be reviewed, and pts should be questioned about previous illness or surgery as well as diseases in family members. Risk factors for HIV should be assessed. Signs of depression, evidence of dementia, and social factors, including financial issues that might affect food intake, should be considered.

Physical examination should begin with weight determination and documentation of vital signs. The skin should be examined for pallor, jaundice, turgor, surgical scars, and stigmata of systemic disease. Evaluation for oral thrush, dental disease, thyroid gland enlargement, and adenopathy and for respiratory, cardiac, or abdominal abnormalities should be performed. All men should have a rectal examination, including the prostate; all women should have a pelvic examination; and both should have testing of the stool for occult blood. Neurologic examination should include mental status assessment and screening for depression.

Initial *laboratory evaluation* is shown in Table 49-2, with appropriate treatment based on the underlying cause of the weight loss. If an etiology of weight loss is not found, careful clinical follow-up, rather than persistent undirected testing, is reasonable.

___

For a more detailed discussion, see Reife CM: Weight Loss, Chap. 36, p. 233, in HPIM-16.
___

50

DYSPHAGIA

DYSPHAGIA

Dysphagia is difficulty moving food or liquid through the mouth, pharynx, and esophagus. The pt senses swallowed material sticking along the path. *Odynophagia* is pain on swallowing. *Globus pharyngeus* is the sensation of a lump lodged in the throat, but swallowing is unaffected.

PATHOPHYSIOLOGY   Dysphagia is caused by two main mechanisms: mechanical obstruction or motor dysfunction. Mechanical causes of dysphagia can be luminal (e.g., large food bolus, foreign body), intrinsic to the esophagus (e.g., inflammation, webs and rings, strictures, tumors), or extrinsic to the esophagus (e.g., cervical spondylitis, enlarged thyroid or mediastinal mass, vascular compression). The motor function abnormalities that cause dysphagia may be related to defects in initiating the swallowing reflex (e.g., tongue paralysis, lack of saliva, lesions affecting sensory components of cranial nerves X and XI), disorders of the pharyngeal and esophageal striated muscle (e.g., muscle disorders such as polymyositis and dermatomyositis, neurologic lesions such as myasthenia gravis, polio, or amyotrophic lateral sclerosis), and disorders of the esophageal smooth muscle (e.g., achalasia, scleroderma, myotonic dystrophy).

_____ *Approach to the Patient* _____

History can provide a presumptive diagnosis in about 80% of pts. Difficulty only with solids implies mechanical dysphagia. Difficulty with both solids and liquids may occur late in the course of mechanical dysphagia but is an early sign of motor dysphagia. Pts can sometimes pinpoint the site of food sticking. Weight loss out of proportion to the degree of dysphagia may be a sign of underlying malignancy. Hoarseness may be related to involvement of the larynx in the primary disease process (e.g., neuromuscular disorders), neoplastic disruption of the recurrent laryngeal nerve, or laryngitis from gastroesophageal reflux.

Physical exam may reveal signs of skeletal muscle, neurologic, or oropharyngeal diseases. Neck exam can reveal masses impinging on the esophagus. Skin changes might suggest the systemic nature of the underlying disease (e.g., scleroderma).

Dysphagia is nearly always a symptom of organic disease rather than a functional complaint. If oropharyngeal dysphagia is suspected, videofluoroscopy of swallowing may be diagnostic. Mechanical dysphagia can be evaluated by barium swallow and esophagogastroscopy with endoscopic biopsy. Barium swallow and esophageal motility studies can show the presence of motor dysphagia.

_____

OROPHARYNGEAL DYSPHAGIA   Pt has difficulty initiating the swallow; food sticks at the level of the suprasternal notch; nasopharyngeal regurgitation and aspiration may be present.

Causes include: for solids only, carcinoma, aberrant vessel, congenital or acquired web (Plummer-Vinson syndrome in iron deficiency), cervical osteophyte; for solids and liquids, cricopharyngeal bar (e.g., hypertensive or hypotensive upper esophageal sphincter), Zenker's diverticulum (outpouching in the posterior midline at the intersection of the pharynx and the cricopharyngeus muscle), myasthenia gravis, glucocorticoid myopathy, hyperthyroidism, hypothyroidism, myotonic dystrophy, amyotrophic lateral sclerosis, multiple sclerosis, Parkinson's disease, stroke, and bulbar and pseudobulbar palsy.

ESOPHAGEAL DYSPHAGIA   Food sticks in the mid or lower sternal area; can be associated with regurgitation, aspiration, odynophagia. Causes include: for solids only, lower esophageal ring (Schatzki's ring, symptoms are usually intermittent), peptic stricture (heartburn accompanies this), carcinoma, lye stricture; for solids and liquids, diffuse esophageal spasm (occurs with chest pain and is intermittent), scleroderma (progressive and occurs with heartburn), achalasia (progressive and occurs without heartburn).

NONCARDIAC CHEST PAIN

Thirty percent of pts presenting with chest pain have an esophageal source rather than angina. History and physical exam often cannot distinguish cardiac from noncardiac pain. Exclude cardiac disease first. Causes include: gastroesophageal reflux disease, esophageal motility disorders, peptic ulcer disease, gallstones, psychiatric disease (anxiety, panic attacks, depression).

Evaluation   Consider a trial of antireflux therapy (omeprazole); if no response, 24-h ambulatory luminal pH monitoring; if negative, esophageal manometry may show motor disorder. Trial of imipramine, 50 mg PO qhs, may be worthwhile. Consider psychiatric evaluation in selected cases.

ESOPHAGEAL MOTILITY DISORDERS

Pts may have a spectrum of manometric findings ranging from nonspecific abnormalities to defined clinical entities.

ACHALASIA   Motor obstruction caused by hypertensive lower esophageal sphincter (LES), incomplete relaxation of LES, or loss of peristalsis in smooth-muscle portion of esophagus. Causes include: primary (idiopathic) or secondary due to Chagas' disease, lymphoma, carcinoma, chronic idiopathic intestinal pseudoobstruction, ischemia, neurotropic viruses, drugs, toxins, radiation therapy, postvagotomy.

Evaluation   Chest x-ray shows absence of gastric air bubble. Barium swallow shows dilated esophagus with distal beaklike narrowing and air-fluid level. Endoscopy is done to rule out cancer, particularly in persons >50 years. Manometry shows normal or elevated LES pressure, decreased LES relaxation, absent peristalsis.

℞ TREATMENT

Pneumatic balloon dilatation is effective in 85%, 3–5% risk of perforation or bleeding. Injection of botulinum toxin at endoscopy to relax LES is safe and effective but effects last only about 12 months. Myotomy of LES (Heller procedure) is effective, but 10–30% of pts develop gastroesophageal reflux. Nifedipine, 10–20 mg, or isosorbide dinitrate, 5–10 mg SL ac, may avert need for dilatation or surgery.

SPASTIC DISORDERS   Diffuse esophageal spasm involves multiple spontaneous and swallow-induced contractions of the esophageal body that are of simultaneous onset, long duration, and recurrent. Causes include: primary (idiopathic) or secondary due to gastroesophageal reflux disease, emotional stress, diabetes, alcoholism, neuropathy, radiation therapy, ischemia, or collagen vascular disease.

An important variant is nutcracker esophagus: high-amplitude (>180 mmHg) peristaltic contractions; particularly associated with chest pain or dysphagia, but correlation between symptoms and manometry is inconsistent. Condition may resolve over time or evolve into diffuse spasm; associated with increased frequency of depression, anxiety, and somatization.

Evaluation   Barium swallow shows corkscrew esophagus, pseudodiverticula, and diffuse spasm. Manometry shows spasm with multiple simultaneous esophageal contractions of high amplitude and long duration. In nutcracker esophagus, the contractions are peristaltic and of high amplitude. If heart disease has been ruled out, edrophonium, ergonovine, or bethanecol can be used to provoke spasm.

 TREATMENT

Anticholinergics are usually of limited value; nitrates (isosorbide dinitrate, 5–10 mg PO ac) and calcium antagonists (nifedipine, 10–20 mg PO ac) are more effective. Those refractory to medical management may benefit from balloon dilatation. Rare pts require surgical intervention; longitudinal myotomy of esophageal circular muscle. Treatment of concomitant depression or other psychological disturbance may help.

SCLERODERMA   Atrophy of the esophageal smooth muscle and fibrosis can make the esophagus aperistaltic and lead to an incompetent LES with attendant reflux esophagitis and stricture. Treatment of gastroesophageal reflux disease is discussed in Chap. 48.

ESOPHAGEAL INFLAMMATION

VIRAL ESOPHAGITIS   Herpesviruses I and II, varicella-zoster virus, and CMV can all cause esophagitis; particularly common in immunocompromised pts (e.g., AIDS). Odynophagia, dysphagia, fever, and bleeding are symptoms and signs. Diagnosis is made by endoscopy with biopsy, brush cytology, and culture.

 TREATMENT

Disease is usually self-limited in the immunocompetent person; viscous lidocaine can relieve pain; in prolonged cases and in immunocompromised hosts, herpes and varicella esophagitis are treated with acyclovir, 5–10 mg/kg IV q8h for 10–14 d, then 200–400 mg PO 5 times a day. CMV is treated with ganciclovir, 5 mg/kg IV q12h, until healing occurs, which may take weeks. Oral valganciclovir (900 mg bid) is an effective alternative to parenteral treatment. In nonresponders, foscarnet, 60 mg/kg IV q12h for 21 days, may be effective.

CANDIDA ESOPHAGITIS   In immunocompromised hosts, malignancy, diabetes, hypoparathyroidism, hemoglobinopathy, SLE, corrosive esophageal injury, candidal esophageal infection may present with odynophagia, dysphagia, and oral thrush (50%). Diagnosis is made on endoscopy by identifying yellow-white plaques or nodules on friable red mucosa. Characteristic hyphae are seen on KOH stain. In patients with AIDS, the development of symptoms may prompt an empirical therapeutic trial.

TREATMENT

Oral nystatin (100,000 U/mL), 5 mL q6h, or clotrimazole, 10-mg tablet sucked q6h, is effective. In immunocompromised host, fluconazole, 100–200 mg PO daily for 1–3 weeks, is treatment of choice; alternatives include itraconazole, 200 mg PO bid, or ketoconazole, 200–400 mg PO daily; long-term maintenance therapy is often required. Poorly responsive pts may respond to higher doses of fluconazole (400 mg/d) or to amphotericin, 10–15 mg IV q6h for a total dose of 300–500 mg.

PILL-RELATED ESOPHAGITIS Doxycycline, tetracycline, aspirin, NSAIDs, KCl, quinidine, ferrous sulfate, clindamycin, alprenolol, and alendronate can induce local inflammation in the esophagus. Predisposing factors include recumbency after swallowing pills with small sips of water, anatomic factors impinging on the esophagus and slowing transit.

 TREATMENT

Withdraw offending drug, use antacids, and dilate any resulting stricture.

OTHER CAUSES OF ESOPHAGITIS IN AIDS *Mycobacteria, Cryptosporidium, Pneumocystis carinii*, idiopathic esophageal ulcers, giant ulcers (possible cytopathic effect of HIV) can occur. Ulcers may respond to systemic glucocorticoids.

For a more detailed discussion, see Goyal RK: Dysphagia, Chap. 33, p. 217; and Diseases of the Esophagus, Chap. 273, p. 1739, in HPIM-16.

51

ACUTE ABDOMEN

Acute, Catastrophic Abdominal Pain

Intense abdominal pain of acute onset or pain associated with syncope, hypotension, or toxic appearance necessitates rapid yet orderly evaluation. Consider obstruction, perforation, or rupture of hollow viscus; dissection or rupture of major blood vessels (esp. aortic aneurysm); ulceration; abdominal sepsis; ketoacidosis; and adrenal crisis.

Brief History and Physical Examination Historic features of importance include age; time of onset of the pain; activity of the pt when the pain began; location and character of the pain; radiation to other sites; presence of nausea, vomiting, or anorexia; temporal changes; changes in bowel habits; and menstrual history. Physical exam should focus on the pt's overall appearance [writhing in pain (ureteral lithiasis) vs. still (peritonitis, perforation)], position (a pt leaning forward may have pancreatitis or gastric perforation into the lesser sac), presence of fever or hypothermia, hyperventilation, cyanosis, bowel sounds, direct or rebound abdominal tenderness, pulsating abdominal mass, abdominal bruits, ascites, rectal blood, rectal or pelvic tenderness, and evidence of coagulopathy. Useful laboratory studies include hematocrit (may be normal with acute hemorrhage or misleadingly high with dehydration), WBC with differential count, arterial blood gases, serum electrolytes, BUN, creatinine, glucose, lipase or amylase, and UA. Females of reproductive age should have a pregnancy test. Radiologic studies should include supine and upright abdominal films (left lateral decubitus view if upright unobtainable) to evaluate bowel caliber and presence of free peritoneal air, cross-table lateral film to assess aortic diameter; CT (when available) to detect evidence of bowel perforation, inflammation, solid organ infarction, retroperitoneal bleeding, abscess, or tumor. Abdominal paracentesis (or peritoneal lavage in cases of trauma) can detect evidence of bleeding or peritonitis. Abdominal ultrasound (when available) reveals evidence of abscess, cholecystitis, biliary or ureteral obstruction, or hematoma and is used to determine aortic diameter.

Diagnostic Strategies   The initial decision point is based on whether the pt is hemodynamically stable. If not, one must suspect a vascular catastrophe such as a leaking abdominal aortic aneurysm. Such pts receive limited resuscitation and move immediately to surgical exploration. If the pt is hemodynamically stable, the next decision point is whether the abdomen is rigid. Rigid abdomens are most often due to perforation or obstruction. The diagnosis can generally be made by a chest and plain abdominal radiograph.

If the abdomen is not rigid, the causes may be grouped based on whether the pain is poorly localized or well localized. In the presence of poorly localized pain, one should assess whether an aortic aneurysm is possible. If so, a CT scan can make the diagnosis; if not, early appendicitis, early obstruction, mesenteric ischemia, inflammatory bowel disease, pancreatitis, and metabolic problems are all in the differential diagnosis.

Pain localized to the epigastrium may be of cardiac origin, esophageal inflammation or perforation, gastritis, peptic ulcer disease, biliary colic or cholecystitis, and pancreatitis. Pain localized to the right upper quadrant includes those same entities plus pyelonephritis or nephrolithiasis, hepatic abscess, subdiaphragmatic absess, pulmonary embolus, or pneumonia or be of musculoskeletal origin. Additional considerations with left upper quadrant localization are infarcted or ruptured spleen, splenomegaly, and gastric or peptic ulcer. Right lower quadrant pain may be from appendicitis, Meckel's diverticulum, Crohn's disease, diverticulitis, mesenteric adenitis, rectus sheath hematoma, psoas abscess, ovarian abscess or torsion, ectopic pregnancy, salpingitis, familial fever syndromes, uterolithiasis, herpes zoster. Left lower quadrant pain may be due to diverticulitis, perforated neoplasm, and other entities previously mentioned.

 TREATMENT

Intravenous fluids, correction of life-threatening acid-base disturbances, and assessment of need for emergent surgery are the first priority; careful follow-up with frequent reexamination (when possible, by the same examiner) is essential. The use of narcotic analgesia is controversial. Traditionally, narcotic analgesics were withheld pending establishment of diagnosis and therapeutic plan, since masking of diagnostic signs may delay needed intervention. However, evidence that narcotics actually mask a diagnosis is sparse.

For a more detailed discussion, see Silen W: Abdominal Pain, Chap. 13, p. 82, in HPIM-16.

52

DIARRHEA, CONSTIPATION, AND MALABSORPTION

NORMAL GASTROINTESTINAL FUNCTION

ABSORPTION OF FLUID AND ELECTROLYTES Fluid delivery to the GI tract is 8–10 L/d, including 2 L/d ingested; most is absorbed in small bowel. Colonic absorption is normally 0.05–2 L/d, with capacity for 6 L/d if required. Intestinal water absorption passively follows active transport of Na^+, Cl^-, glucose, and bile salts. Additional transport mechanisms include Cl^-/HCO_3^- exchange, Na^+/H^+ exchange, H^+, K^+, Cl^-, and HCO_3^- secretion, Na^+-glucose cotransport, and active Na^+ transport across the basolateral membrane by Na^+,K^+-ATPase.

NUTRIENT ABSORPTION

1. *Proximal small intestine*: iron, calcium, folate, fats (after hydrolysis of triglycerides to fatty acids by pancreatic lipase and colipase), proteins (after hydrolysis by pancreatic and intestinal peptidases), carbohydrates (after hydrolysis by amylases and disaccharidases); triglycerides absorbed as micelles after solubilization by bile salts; amino acids and dipeptides absorbed via specific carriers; sugars absorbed by active transport.
2. *Distal small intestine*: vitamin B_{12}, bile salts, water.
3. *Colon*: water, electrolytes.

INTESTINAL MOTILITY Allows propulsion of intestinal contents from stomach to anus and separation of components to facilitate nutrient absorption. Propulsion is controlled by neural, myogenic, and hormonal mechanisms; mediated by migrating motor complex, an organized wave of neuromuscular activity that originates in the distal stomach during fasting and migrates slowly down the small intestine. Colonic motility is mediated by local peristalsis to propel feces. Defecation is effected by relaxation of internal anal sphincter in response to rectal distention, with voluntary control by contraction of external anal sphincter.

DIARRHEA

PHYSIOLOGY Formally defined as fecal output >200 g/d on low-fiber (western) diet; also frequently used to connote loose or watery stools. Mediated by one or more of the following mechanisms:

Osmotic Diarrhea Nonabsorbed solutes increase intraluminal oncotic pressure, causing outpouring of water; usually ceases with fasting; stool osmolal gap > 40 (see below). Causes include disaccharidase (e.g., lactase) deficiencies, pancreatic insufficiency, bacterial overgrowth, lactulose or sorbitol ingestion, polyvalent laxative abuse, celiac or tropical sprue, and short bowel syndrome. Lactase deficiency can be either primary (more prevalent in blacks and Asians, usually presenting in early adulthood) or secondary (from viral, bacterial, or protozoal gastroenteritis, celiac or tropical sprue, or kwashiorkor).

Secretory Diarrhea   Active ion secretion causes obligatory water loss; diarrhea is usually watery, often profuse, unaffected by fasting; stool Na^+ and K^+ are elevated with osmolal gap < 40. Causes include viral infections (e.g., rotavirus, Norwalk virus), bacterial infections (e.g., cholera, enterotoxigenic *Escherichia coli*, *Staphylococcus aureus*), protozoa (e.g., *Giardia*, *Isospora*, *Cryptosporidium*), AIDS-associated disorders (including mycobacterial and HIV-induced), medications (e.g., theophylline, colchicine, prostaglandins, diuretics), Zollinger-Ellison syndrome (excess gastrin production), vasoactive intestinal peptide (VIP)-producing tumors, carcinoid tumors (histamine and serotonin), medullary thyroid carcinoma (prostaglandins and calcitonin), systemic mastocytosis, basophilic leukemia, distal colonic villous adenomas (direct secretion of potassium-rich fluid), collagenous and microscopic colitis, and cholerrheic diarrhea (from ileal malabsorption of bile salts).

Exudative   Inflammation, necrosis, and sloughing of colonic mucosa; may include component of secretory diarrhea due to prostaglandin release by inflammatory cells; stools usually contain PMNs as well as occult or gross blood. Causes include bacterial infections [e.g., *Campylobacter*, *Salmonella*, *Shigella*, *Yersinia*, invasive or enterotoxigenic *E. coli*, *Vibrio parahemolyticus*, *Clostridium difficile* colitis (frequently antibiotic-induced)], colonic parasites (e.g., *Entamoeba histolytica*), Crohn's disease, ulcerative proctocolitis, idiopathic inflammatory bowel disease, radiation enterocolitis, cancer chemotherapeutic agents, and intestinal ischemia.

Altered Intestinal Motility   Alteration of coordinated control of intestinal propulsion; diarrhea often intermittent or alternating with constipation. Causes include diabetes mellitus, adrenal insufficiency, hyperthyroidism, collagen-vascular diseases, parasitic infestations, gastrin and VIP hypersecretory states, amyloidosis, laxatives (esp. magnesium-containing agents), antibiotics (esp. erythromycin), cholinergic agents, primary neurologic dysfunction (e.g., Parkinson's disease, traumatic neuropathy), fecal impaction, diverticular disease, and irritable bowel syndrome. Blood in intestinal lumen is cathartic, and major upper GI bleeding leads to diarrhea from increased motility.

Decreased Absorptive Surface   Usually arises from surgical manipulation (e.g., extensive bowel resection or rearrangement) that leaves inadequate absorptive surface for fat and carbohydrate digestion and fluid and electrolyte absorption; occurs spontaneously from enteroenteric fistulas (esp. gastrocolic).

EVALUATION   *History*   Diarrhea must be distinguished from fecal incontinence, change in stool caliber, rectal bleeding, and small, frequent, but otherwise normal stools. Careful medication history is essential. Alternating diarrhea and constipation suggests fixed colonic obstruction (e.g., from carcinoma) or irritable bowel syndrome. A sudden, acute course, often with nausea, vomiting, and fever, is typical of viral and bacterial infections, diverticulitis, ischemia, radiation enterocolitis, or drug-induced diarrhea and may be the initial presentation of inflammatory bowel disease. >90% of acute diarrheal illnesses are infectious in etiology. A longer (>4 weeks), more insidious course suggests malabsorption, inflammatory bowel disease, metabolic or endocrine disturbance, pancreatic insufficiency, laxative abuse, ischemia, neoplasm (hypersecretory state or partial obstruction), or irritable bowel syndrome. Parasitic and certain forms of bacterial enteritis can also produce chronic symptoms. Particularly foul-smelling or oily stool suggests fat malabsorption. Fecal impaction may cause apparent diarrhea because only liquids pass partial obstruction. Several infectious causes of diarrhea are associated with an immunocompromised state (Table 52-1).

Table 52-1

Infectious Causes of Diarrhea in Patients with AIDS

NONOPPORTUNISTIC PATHOGENS	OPPORTUNISTIC PATHOGENS
Shigella	Protozoa
Salmonella	*Cryptosporidium*
Campylobacter	*Isospora belli*
Entamoeba histolytica	Microsporidia
Chlamydia	*Blastocystis hominis*
Neisseria gonorrhoeae	Viruses
Treponema pallidum and other	Cytomegalovirus
spirochetes	Herpes simplex
Giardia lamblia	Adenovirus
	HIV
	Bacteria
	Mycobacterium avium complex

Physical Examination   Signs of dehydration are often prominent in severe, acute diarrhea. Fever and abdominal tenderness suggest infection or inflammatory disease but are often absent in viral enteritis. Evidence of malnutrition suggests chronic course. Certain signs are frequently associated with specific deficiency states secondary to malabsorption (e.g., cheilosis with riboflavin or iron deficiency, glossitis with B_{12}, folate deficiency).

Stool Examination   Culture for bacterial pathogens, examination for leukocytes, measurement of *C. difficile* toxin, and examination for ova and parasites are important components of evaluation of pts with severe, protracted, or bloody diarrhea. Presence of blood (fecal occult blood test) or leukocytes (Wright's stain) suggests inflammation (e.g., ulcerative colitis, Crohn's disease, infection, or ischemia). Gram's stain of stool can be diagnostic of *Staphylococcus*, *Campylobacter*, or *Candida* infection. Steatorrhea (determined with Sudan III stain of stool sample or 72-h quantitative fecal fat analysis) suggests malabsorption or pancreatic insufficiency. Measurement of Na^+ and K^+ levels in fecal water helps to distinguish osmotic from other types of diarrhea; osmotic diarrhea is implied by stool osmolal gap > 40, where stool osmolal gap $= osmol_{serum} - [2 \times (Na^+ + K^+)_{stool}]$.

Laboratory Studies   CBC may indicate anemia (acute or chronic blood loss or malabsorption of iron, folate, or B_{12}), leukocytosis (inflammation), eosinophilia (parasitic, neoplastic, and inflammatory bowel diseases). Serum levels of calcium, albumin, iron, cholesterol, folate, B_{12}, vitamin D, and carotene; serum iron-binding capacity; and prothrombin time can provide evidence of intestinal malabsorption or maldigestion.

Other Studies   D-Xylose absorption test is a convenient screen for small-bowel absorptive function. Small-bowel biopsy is especially useful for evaluating intestinal malabsorption. Specialized studies include Schilling test (B_{12} malabsorption), lactose H_2 breath test (carbohydrate malabsorption), [^{14}C]xylose and lactulose H_2 breath tests (bacterial overgrowth), glycocholic breath test (ileal malabsorption), triolein breath test (fat malabsorption), and bentiromide and secretin tests (pancreatic insufficiency). Sigmoidoscopy or colonoscopy with biopsy is useful in the diagnosis of colitis (esp. pseudomembranous, ischemic, microscopic); it may not allow distinction between infectious and noninfectious (esp. idiopathic ulcerative) colitis. Barium contrast x-ray studies may suggest malabsorption (thickened bowel folds), inflammatory bowel disease (ileitis or colitis), tuberculosis (ileocecal inflammation), neoplasm, intestinal fistula, or motility disorders.

℞ TREATMENT

An approach to the management of acute diarrheal illnesses is shown in Fig. 52-1. Symptomatic therapy includes vigorous rehydration (IV or with oral glucose-electrolyte solutions), electrolyte replacement, binders of osmotically active substances (e.g., kaolin-pectin), and opiates to decrease bowel motility (e.g., loperamide, diphenoxylate); opiates may be contraindicated in infectious or inflammatory causes of diarrhea. An approach to the management of chronic diarrhea is shown in Fig. 52-2.

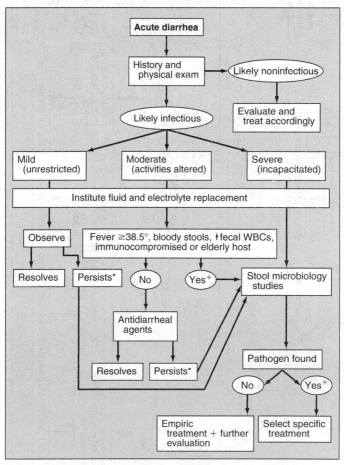

FIGURE 52-1 Algorithm for the management of acute diarrhea. Before evaluation, consider empiric Rx with (*) metronidazole and with (+) quinolone.

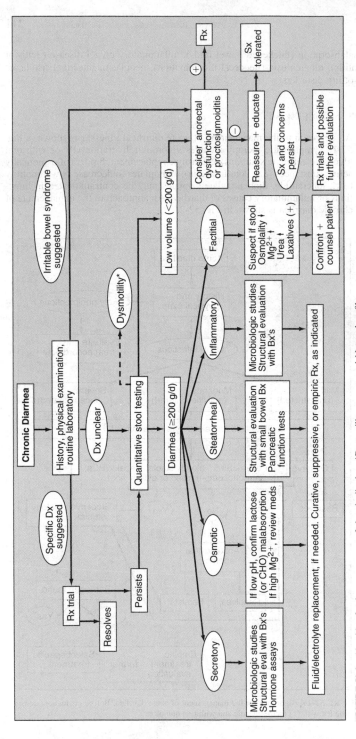

FIGURE 52-2 Algorithm for the management of chronic diarrhea. *Dysmotility presents variable stool profile.

MALABSORPTION SYNDROMES

Intestinal malabsorption of ingested nutrients may produce osmotic diarrhea, steatorrhea, or specific deficiencies (e.g., iron; folate; B_{12}; vitamins A, D, E, and K). Table 52-2 lists common causes of intestinal malabsorption. Protein-losing enteropathy may result from several causes of malabsorption; it is associated with hypoalbuminemia and can be detected by measuring stool α_1-antitrypsin or radiolabeled albumin levels. Therapy is directed at the underlying disease.

CONSTIPATION

Defined as decrease in frequency of stools to <1 per week or difficulty in defecation; may result in abdominal pain, distention, and fecal impaction, with consequent obstruction or, rarely, perforation. A frequent and often subjective complaint. Contributory factors may include inactivity, low-fiber diet, and inadequate allotment of time for defecation.

SPECIFIC CAUSES Altered colonic motility due to neurologic dysfunction (diabetes mellitus, spinal cord injury, multiple sclerosis, Chagas' disease, Hirschsprung's disease, chronic idiopathic intestinal pseudoobstruction, idiopathic megacolon), scleroderma, drugs (esp. anticholinergic agents, opiates, aluminum- or calcium-based antacids, calcium channel blockers, iron supplements, sucralfate), hypothyroidism, Cushing's syndrome, hypokalemia, hypercalcemia, dehydration, mechanical causes (colorectal tumors, diverticulitis, volvulus, hernias, intussusception), and anorectal pain (from fissures, hemorrhoids, abscesses, or proctitis) leading to retention, constipation, and fecal impaction.

 TREATMENT

In absence of identifiable cause, constipation may improve with reassurance, exercise, increased dietary fiber, bulking agents (e.g., psyllium), and increased fluid intake. Specific therapies include removal of bowel obstruction (fecolith,

Table 52-2

Common Causes of Malabsorption

Maldigestion: Chronic pancreatitis, cystic fibrosis, pancreatic carcinoma

Bile salt deficiency: Cirrhosis, cholestasis, bacterial overgrowth (blind loop syndromes, intestinal diverticula, hypomotility disorders), impaired ileal reabsorption (resection, Crohn's disease), bile salt binders (cholestyramine, calcium carbonate, neomycin)

Inadequate absorptive surface: Massive intestinal resection, gastrocolic fistula, jejunoileal bypass

Lymphatic obstruction: Lymphoma, Whipple's disease, intestinal lymphangiectasia

Vascular disease: Constrictive pericarditis, right-sided heart failure, mesenteric arterial or venous insufficiency

Mucosal disease: Infection (esp. *Giardia*, Whipple's disease, tropical sprue), inflammatory diseases (esp. Crohn's disease), radiation enteritis, eosinophilic enteritis, ulcerative jejunitis, mastocytosis, tropical sprue, infiltrative disorders (amyloidosis, scleroderma, lymphoma, collagenous sprue, microscopic colitis), biochemical abnormalities (gluten-sensitive enteropathy, disaccharidase deficiency, hypogammaglobulinemia, abetalipoproteinemia, amino acid transport deficiencies), endocrine disorders (diabetes mellitus, hypoparathyroidism, adrenal insufficiency, hyperthyroidism, Zollinger-Ellison syndrome, carcinoid syndrome)

tumor), discontinuance of nonessential hypomotility agents (esp. aluminum- or calcium-containing antacids, opiates) or substitute magnesium-based antacids for aluminum-based antacids. For symptomatic relief, magnesium-containing agents or other cathartics are occasionally needed. With severe hypo- or dysmotility or in presence of opiates, osmotically active agents (e.g., oral lactulose, intestinal polyethylene glycol–containing lavage solutions) and oral or rectal emollient laxatives (e.g., docusate salts) and mineral oil are most effective.

For a more detailed discussion, see Ahlquist DA, Camilleri M: Diarrhea and Constipation, Chap. 35, p. 224; and Binder HJ: Disorders of Absorption, Chap. 275, p. 1763, in HPIM-16.

53

GASTROINTESTINAL BLEEDING

PRESENTATION

1. *Hematemesis*: Vomiting of blood or altered blood ("coffee grounds") indicates bleeding proximal to ligament of Treitz.

2. *Melena*: Altered (black) blood per rectum (>100 mL blood required for one melenic stool) usually indicates bleeding proximal to ligament of Treitz but may be as distal as ascending colon; pseudomelena may be caused by ingestion of iron, bismuth, licorice, beets, blueberries, charcoal.

3. *Hematochezia*: Bright red or maroon rectal bleeding usually implies bleeding beyond ligament of Treitz but may be due to rapid upper GI bleeding (>1000 mL).

4. *Positive fecal occult blood test with or without iron deficiency.*

5. *Symptoms of blood loss*: e.g., light-headedness or shortness of breath.

HEMODYNAMIC CHANGES Orthostatic drop in Bp > 10 mmHg usually indicates >20% reduction in blood volume (± syncope, light-headedness, nausea, sweating, thirst).

SHOCK Bp < 100 mmHg systolic usually indicates <30% reduction in blood volume (± pallor, cool skin).

LABORATORY CHANGES Hematocrit may not reflect extent of blood loss because of delayed equilibration with extravascular fluid. Mild leukocytosis and thrombocytosis. Elevated BUN is common in upper GI bleeding.

ADVERSE PROGNOSTIC SIGNS Age >60, associated illnesses, coagulopathy, immunosuppression, presentation with shock, rebleeding, onset of bleeding in hospital, variceal bleeding, endoscopic stigmata of recent bleeding [e.g., "visible vessel" in ulcer base (see below)].

UPPER GI BLEEDING

CAUSES *Common* Peptic ulcer (accounts for ~50%), gastropathy (alcohol, aspirin, NSAIDs, stress), esophagitis, Mallory-Weiss tear (mucosal tear at gastroesophageal junction due to retching), gastroesophageal varices.

Less Common Swallowed blood (nosebleed); esophageal, gastric, or intestinal neoplasm; anticoagulant and fibrinolytic therapy; hypertrophic gastropathy (Ménétrier's disease); aortic aneurysm; aortoenteric fistula (from aortic graft); AV malformation; telangiectases (Osler-Rendu-Weber syndrome); Dieulafoy lesion (ectatic submucosal vessel); vasculitis; connective tissue disease (pseudoxanthoma elasticum, Ehlers-Danlos syndrome); blood dyscrasias; neurofibroma; amyloidosis; hemobilia (biliary origin).

EVALUATION After hemodynamic resuscitation (see below and Fig. 53-1).

• History and physical examination: Drugs (increased risk of upper and lower GI tract bleeding with aspirin and NSAIDs), prior ulcer, bleeding history, family history, features of cirrhosis or vasculitis, etc. Hyperactive bowel sounds favor upper GI source.

• Nasogastric aspirate for gross blood, if source (upper versus lower) not clear from history; may be falsely negative in up to 16% of pts if bleeding has ceased or duodenum is the source. Testing aspirate for occult blood is meaningless.

• Upper endoscopy: Accuracy >90%; allows visualization of bleeding site and possibility of therapeutic intervention; mandatory for suspected varices,

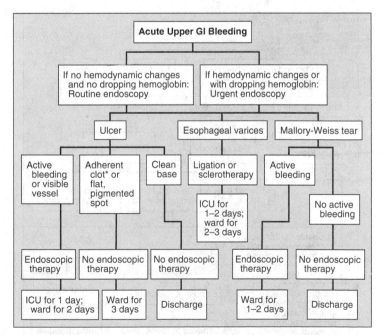

FIGURE 53-1 Suggested algorithm for patients with acute UGIB. Recommendations on level of care and time of discharge assume patient is stabilized without further bleeding or other concomitant medical problems. Upper GI endoscopy is the major diagnostic and therapeutic tool. *Some authors suggest endoscopic therapy for adherent clots.

aortoenteric fistulas; permits identification of "visible vessel" (protruding artery in ulcer crater), which connotes high (~50%) risk of rebleeding.
• Upper GI barium radiography: Accuracy ~80% in identifying a lesion, though does not confirm source of bleeding; acceptable alternative to endoscopy in resolved or chronic low-grade bleeding.
• Selective mesenteric arteriography: When brisk bleeding precludes identification of source at endoscopy.
• Radioisotope scanning (e.g., ^{99}Tc tagged to red blood cells or albumin); used primarily as screening test to confirm bleeding is rapid enough for arteriography to be of value or when bleeding is intermittent and of unclear origin.

LOWER GI BLEEDING

CAUSES   Anal lesions (hemorrhoids, fissures), rectal trauma, proctitis, colitis (ulcerative colitis, Crohn's disease, infectious colitis, ischemic colitis, radiation), colonic polyps, colonic carcinoma, angiodysplasia (vascular ectasia), diverticulosis, intussusception, solitary ulcer, blood dyscrasias, vasculitis, connective tissue disease, neurofibroma, amyloidosis, anticoagulation.

EVALUATION   See below and Fig. 53-2.

• History and physical examination.
• In the presence of hemodynamic changes, perform upper endoscopy followed by colonoscopy. In the absence of hemodynamic changes, perform anoscopy and either flexible sigmoidoscopy or colonoscopy: Exclude hemorrhoids, fissure, ulcer, proctitis, neoplasm.

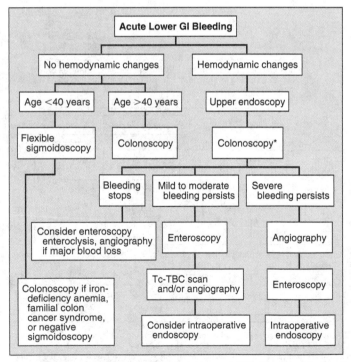

FIGURE 53-2 Suggested algorithm for patients with acute LGIB. *If massive bleeding does not allow time for colonic lavage, proceed to angiography.

- Colonoscopy: Often test of choice, but may be impossible if bleeding is massive.
- Barium enema: No role in active bleeding.
- Arteriography: When bleeding is severe (requires bleeding rate >0.5 mL/min; may require prestudy radioisotope bleeding scan as above); defines site of bleeding or abnormal vasculature.
- Surgical exploration (last resort).

BLEEDING OF OBSCURE ORIGIN   Often small-bowel source. Consider small-bowel enteroclysis x-ray (careful barium radiography via peroral intubation of small bowel), Meckel's scan, enteroscopy (small-bowel endoscopy), or exploratory laparotomy with intraoperative enteroscopy.

 TREATMENT

> ### *Upper and Lower GI Bleeding*
>
> - Venous access with large bore IV (14–18 gauge); central venous line for major bleed and pts with cardiac disease; monitor vital signs, urine output, Hct (fall may lag). Gastric lavage of unproven benefit but clears stomach before endoscopy. Iced saline may lyse clots; room-temperature tap water may be preferable. Intubation may be required to protect airway.
> - Type and cross-match blood (6 units for major bleed).
> - Surgical standby when bleeding is massive.
> - Support blood pressure with isotonic fluids (normal saline); albumin and fresh-frozen plasma in cirrhotics. Packed red blood cells when available (whole blood if massive bleeding); maintain Hct >25–30. Fresh-frozen plasma and vitamin K (10 mg SC or IV) in cirrhotics with coagulopathy.
> - IV calcium (e.g., up to 10–20 mL 10% calcium gluconate IV over 10–15 min) if serum calcium falls (due to transfusion of citrated blood). Empirical drug therapy (antacids, H_2 receptor blockers, omeprazole) of unproven benefit.
> - Specific measures: *Varices*: octreotide (50-μg bolus, 50-μg/h infusion for 2–5 days), Blakemore-Sengstaken tube tamponade, endoscopic sclerosis, or band ligation; propranolol or nadolol in doses sufficient to cause beta blockade reduces risk of recurrent or initial variceal bleeding (do not use in acute bleed) (Chap. 158); *ulcer with visible vessel or active bleeding*: endoscopic bipolar, heater-probe, or laser coagulation or injection of epinephrine; *gastritis*: embolization or vasopressin infusion of left gastric artery; *GI telangiectases*: ethinylestradiol/norethisterone (0.05/1.0 mg PO qd) may prevent recurrent bleeding, particularly in pts with chronic renal failure; *diverticulosis*: mesenteric arteriography with intraarterial vasopressin; *angiodysplasia*: colonoscopic bipolar or laser coagulation, may regress with replacement of stenotic aortic valve.
> - Indications for emergency surgery: Uncontrolled or prolonged bleeding, severe rebleeding, aortoenteric fistula. For intractable variceal bleeding, consider transjugular intrahepatic portosystemic shunt (TIPS).

For a more detailed discussion, see Laine L: Gastrointestinal Bleeding, Chap. 37, p. 235, in HPIM-16.

54

JAUNDICE AND EVALUATION OF LIVER FUNCTION

JAUNDICE

DEFINITION   Yellow skin pigmentation caused by elevation in serum bilirubin level (also termed *icterus*); often more easily discernible in sclerae. Scleral icterus becomes clinically evident at a serum bilirubin level of ≥ 51 μmol/L (≥ 3 mg/dL); yellow skin discoloration also occurs with elevated serum carotene levels but without pigmentation of the sclerae.

BILIRUBIN METABOLISM   Bilirubin is the major breakdown product of hemoglobin released from senescent erythrocytes. Initially it is bound to albumin, transported into the liver, conjugated to a water-soluble form (glucuronide) by glucuronosyl transferase, excreted into the bile, and converted to urobilinogen in the colon. Urobilinogen is mostly excreted in the stool; a small portion is reabsorbed and excreted by the kidney. Bilirubin can be filtered by the kidney only in its conjugated form (measured as the "direct" fraction); thus increased *direct* serum bilirubin level is associated with bilirubinuria. Increased bilirubin production and excretion (even without hyperbilirubinemia, as in hemolysis) produce elevated urinary urobilinogen levels.

ETIOLOGY   Hyperbilirubinemia occurs as a result of (1) overproduction; (2) impaired uptake, conjugation, or excretion of bilirubin; (3) regurgitation of unconjugated or conjugated bilirubin from damaged hepatocytes or bile ducts (Table 54-1).

EVALUATION   The initial steps in evaluating the pt with jaundice are to determine whether (1) hyperbilirubinemia is conjugated or unconjugated, and

Table 54-1

Causes of Isolated Hyperbilirubinemia

I. Indirect hyperbilirubinemia
   A. Hemolytic disorders
      1. Inherited
         a. Spherocytosis, elliptocytosis
         b. Glucose-6-phosphate dehydrogenase and pyruvate kinase deficiencies
         c. Sickle cell anemia
      2. Acquired
         a. Microangiopathic hemolytic anemias
         b. Paroxysmal nocturnal hemoglobinuria
         c. Immune hemolysis
   B. Ineffective erythropoiesis
      1. Cobalamin, folate, thalassemia, and severe iron deficiencies
   C. Drugs
      1. Rifampicin, probenecid, ribavirin
   D. Inherited conditions
      1. Crigler-Najjar types I and II
         Gilbert's syndrome
II. Direct hyperbilirubinemia
   A. Inherited conditions
      1. Dubin-Johnson syndrome
         Rotor's syndrome

(2) other biochemical liver tests are abnormal (Fig. 54-1, Tables 54-2 and 54-3). Essential clinical examination includes history (especially duration of jaundice, pruritus, associated pain, risk factors for parenterally transmitted diseases, medications, ethanol use, travel history, surgery, pregnancy, presence of any

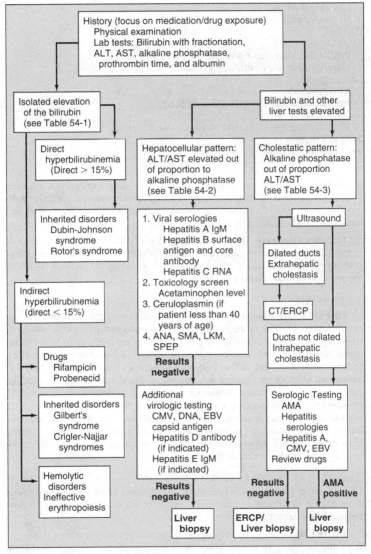

FIGURE 54-1 Evaluation of the patient with jaundice. ERCP, endoscopic retrograde cholangiopancreatography; CT, computed tomography; ALT, alanine aminotransferase; AST, aspartate aminotransferase; SMA, smooth muscle antibody; AMA, antimitochondrial antibody; LKM; liver-kidney microsomal antibody; SPEP, serum protein electrophoresis; CMV, cytomegalovirus; EBV, Epstein-Barr virus.

Table 54-2

Hepatocellular Conditions That May Produce Jaundice

Viral hepatitis
  Hepatitis A, B, C, D, and E
  Epstein-Barr virus
  Cytomegalovirus
  Herpes simplex
Alcohol
Drug toxicity
  Predictable, dose-dependent, e.g., acetaminophen
  Unpredictable, idosyncratic, e.g., isoniazid
Environmental toxins
  Vinyl chloride
  Jamaica bush tea—pyrrolizidine alkaloids
  Kava Kava
  Wild mushrooms—*Amanita phalloides* or *A. verna*
Wilson's disease
Autoimmune hepatitis

accompanying symptoms), physical examination (hepatomegaly, tenderness over liver, palpable gallbladder, splenomegaly, gynecomastia, testicular atrophy, other stigmata of chronic liver disease), blood liver tests (see below), and complete blood count.

Gilbert's Syndrome   Impaired conjugation of bilirubin due to reduced bilirubin UDP glucuronosyltransferase activity. Results in mild unconjugated hyperbilirubinemia almost always <103 μmol/L (<6 mg/dL). Affects 3–7% of the population; males/females 2–7:1.

HEPATOMEGALY

DEFINITION   Generally a span of >12 cm in the right midclavicular line or a palpable left lobe in the epigastrium. It is important to exclude low-lying liver (e.g., with chronic obstructive pulmonary disease and lung hyperinflation) and other RUQ masses (e.g., enlarged gallbladder or bowel or kidney tumor). Independent assessment of size best obtained from ultrasound (US) or CT examination. Contour and texture are important: Focal enlargement or rocklike consistency suggests tumor; tenderness suggests inflammation (e.g., hepatitis) or rapid enlargement (e.g., right-sided heart failure, Budd-Chiari syndrome, fatty infiltration). Cirrhotic livers are usually firm and nodular, often enlarged until late in course. Pulsations frequently connote tricuspid regurgitation. Arterial bruit or hepatic rub suggests tumor. Portal hypertension is occasionally associated with continuous venous hum.

BLOOD TESTS OF LIVER FUNCTION

Used to detect presence of liver disease, discriminate among different types of liver disease (Table 54-4), gauge the extent of known liver damage, follow response to treatment.

BILIRUBIN   Provides indication of hepatic uptake, metabolic (conjugation) and excretory functions; conjugated fraction (direct) distinguished from unconjugated by chemical assay (Table 54-1).

AMINOTRANSFERASES (TRANSAMINASES)   Aspartate aminotransferase (AST; SGOT) and alanine aminotransferase (ALT; SGPT); sensitive

Table 54-3

Cholestatic Conditions That May Produce Jaundice

I. Intrahepatic
   A. Viral hepatitis
      1. Fibrosing cholestatic hepatitis—hepatitis B and C
         Hepatitis A, Epstein-Barr virus, cytomegalovirus
   B. Alcoholic hepatitis
   C. Drug toxicity
      1. Pure cholestasis—anabolic and contraceptive steroids
         Cholestatic hepatitis—chlorpromazine, erythromycin estolate
         Chronic cholestasis—chlorpromazine and prochlorperazine
   D. Primary biliary cirrhosis
   E. Primary sclerosing cholangitis
   F. Vanishing bile duct syndrome
      1. Chronic rejection of liver transplants
         Sarcoidosis
         Drugs
   G. Inherited
      1. Benign recurrent cholestasis
   H. Cholestasis of pregnancy
    I. Total parenteral nutrition
    J. Nonhepatobiliary sepsis
   K. Benign postoperative cholestasis
   L. Paraneoplastic syndrome
   M. Venoocclusive disease
   N. Graft-versus-host disease
II. Extrahepatic
   A. Malignant
      1. Cholangiocarcinoma
         Pancreatic cancer
         Gallbladder cancer
         Ampullary cancer
         Malignant involvement of the porta hepatis lymph nodes
   B. Benign
      1. Choledocholithiasis
         Primary sclerosing cholangitis
         Chronic pancreatitis
         AIDS cholangiopathy

indicators of liver cell injury; greatest elevations seen in hepatocellular necrosis (e.g., viral hepatitis, toxic or ischemic liver injury, acute hepatic vein obstruction), occasionally with sudden, complete biliary obstruction (e.g., from gallstone); milder abnormalities in cholestatic, cirrhotic, and infiltrative disease; poor correlation between degree of liver cell damage and level of aminotransferases; ALT more specific measure of liver cell injury, since AST also found in striated muscle and other organs; ethanol-induced liver injury usually produces modest increases with more prominent elevation of AST than ALT.

    ALKALINE PHOSPHATASE Sensitive indicator of cholestasis, biliary obstruction (enzyme increases more quickly than serum bilirubin), and liver infiltration; mild elevations in other forms of liver disease; limited specificity because of wide tissue distribution; elevations also seen in childhood, pregnancy, and bone diseases; tissue-specific isoenzymes can be distinguished by

Table 54-4

Patterns of Liver Test Abnormalities

Test	Type of Liver Disease Hepatocellular	Obstructive	Ischemic	Infiltrative
AST, ALT[a]	↑↑↑	↑	↑–↑↑↑	N–↑
Alkaline phosphatase	↑–↑↑	↑↑↑	↑–↑↑	↑–↑↑↑
5′-Nucleotidase	↑–↑↑	↑↑↑	↑	↑–↑↑↑
Bilirubin	↑–↑↑↑	↑–↑↑↑	N–↑	N
Prothrombin time	↑–↑↑↑	N[b]	N–↑↑	N
Albumin	N–↓↓↓	N[c]	N–↓	N

[a] In *acute complete obstruction*, serum transaminases may rise rapidly and dramatically but return to near normal levels after 1–3 days even in the presence of continued obstruction.
[b] May increase with prolonged biliary obstruction and secondary biliary cirrhosis.
[c] May decrease with prolonged biliary obstruction and secondary biliary cirrhosis.
Note: N, normal; ↑, elevated; ↓, decreased.

fractionation or by differences in heat stability (liver enzyme activity stable under conditions that destroy bone enzyme activity).

5′-NUCLEOTIDASE (5′-NT)   Pattern of elevation in hepatobiliary disease similar to alkaline phosphatase; has greater specificity for liver disorders; used to determine whether liver is source of elevation in serum alkaline phosphatase, esp. in children, pregnant women, pts with possible concomitant bone disease.

γ-GLUTAMYLTRANSPEPTIDASE (GGT)   Correlates with serum alkaline phosphatase activity. Elevation is less specific for cholestasis than alkaline phosphatase or 5′-NT.

PROTHROMBIN TIME (PT)   (See also Chap. 66)   Measure of clotting factor activity; prolongation results from clotting factor deficiency or inactivity; all clotting factors except factor VIII are synthesized in the liver, and deficiency can occur rapidly from widespread liver disease as in hepatitis, toxic injury, or cirrhosis; single best acute measure of hepatic synthetic function; helpful in Dx and prognosis of acute liver disease. Clotting factors II, VII, IX, X function only in the presence of the fat-soluble vitamin K; PT prolongation from fat malabsorption distinguished from hepatic disease by rapid and complete response to vitamin K replacement.

ALBUMIN   Decreased serum levels result from decreased hepatic synthesis (chronic liver disease or prolonged malnutrition) or excessive losses in urine or stool; insensitive indicator of acute hepatic dysfunction, since serum half-life is 2 to 3 weeks; in pts with chronic liver disease, degree of hypoalbuminemia correlates with severity of liver dysfunction.

GLOBULIN   Mild polyclonal hyperglobulinemia often seen in chronic liver diseases; marked elevation frequently seen in *autoimmune* chronic active hepatitis.

AMMONIA   Elevated blood levels result from deficiency of hepatic detoxification pathways and portal-systemic shunting, as in fulminant hepatitis, hepatotoxin exposure, and severe portal hypertension (e.g., from cirrhosis); elevation of blood ammonia does not correlate well with hepatic function or the presence or degree of acute encephalopathy.

HEPATOBILIARY IMAGING PROCEDURES

ULTRASONOGRAPHY   Rapid, noninvasive examination of abdominal structures; no radiation exposure; relatively low cost, equipment portable; images and interpretation strongly dependent on expertise of examiner; particularly valuable for detecting biliary duct dilatation and gallbladder stones (>95%); much less sensitive for intraductal stones (~60%); most sensitive means of detecting ascites; moderately sensitive for detecting hepatic masses but excellent for discriminating solid from cystic structures; useful in directing percutaneous needle biopsies of suspicious lesions; Doppler US useful to determine patency and flow in portal, hepatic veins and portal-systemic shunts; imaging improved by presence of ascites but severely hindered by bowel gas; endoscopic US less affected by bowel gas and is sensitive for determination of depth of tumor invasion through bowel wall.

CT   Particularly useful for detecting, differentiating, and directing percutaneous needle biopsy of abdominal masses, cysts, and lymphadenopathy; imaging enhanced by intestinal or intravenous contrast dye and unaffected by intestinal gas; somewhat less sensitive than US for detecting stones in gallbladder but more sensitive for choledocholithiasis; may be useful in distinguishing certain forms of diffuse hepatic disease (e.g., fatty infiltration, iron overload).

MRI   Most sensitive detection of hepatic masses and cysts; allows easy differentiation of hemangiomas from other hepatic tumors; most accurate noninvasive means of assessing hepatic and portal vein patency, vascular invasion by tumor; useful for monitoring iron, copper deposition in liver (e.g., in hemochromatosis, Wilson's disease).

RADIONUCLIDE SCANNING   Using various radiolabeled compounds, different scanning methods allow sensitive assessment of biliary excretion (HIDA, PIPIDA, DISIDA scans), parenchymal changes (technetium sulfur colloid liver/spleen scan), and selected inflammatory and neoplastic processes (gallium scan); HIDA and related scans particularly useful for assessing biliary patency and excluding acute cholecystitis in situations where US is not diagnostic; CT, MRI, and colloid scans have similar sensitivity for detecting liver tumors and metastases; CT and combination of colloidal liver and lung scans sensitive for detecting right subphrenic (suprahepatic) abscesses.

CHOLANGIOGRAPHY   Most sensitive means of detecting biliary ductal calculi, biliary tumors, sclerosing cholangitis, choledochal cysts, fistulas, and bile duct leaks; may be performed via endoscopic (transampullary) or percutaneous (transhepatic) route; allows sampling of bile and ductal epithelium for cytologic analysis and culture; allows placement of biliary drainage catheter and stricture dilatation; endoscopic route (ERCP) permits manometric evaluation of sphincter of Oddi, sphincterotomy, and stone extraction.

ANGIOGRAPHY   Most accurate means of determining portal pressures and assessing patency and direction of flow in portal and hepatic veins; highly sensitive for detecting small vascular lesions and hepatic tumors (esp. primary hepatocellular carcinoma); "gold standard" for differentiating hemangiomas from solid tumors; most accurate means of studying vascular anatomy in preparation for complicated hepatobiliary surgery (e.g., portal-systemic shunting, biliary reconstruction) and determining resectability of hepatobiliary and pancreatic tumors. Similar anatomic information (but not intravascular pressures) can often be obtained noninvasively by CT- and MR-based techniques.

PERCUTANEOUS LIVER BIOPSY   Most accurate in disorders causing diffuse changes throughout the liver; subject to sampling error in focal infiltrative disorders such as metastasis; should not be the initial procedure in the Dx of cholestasis.

For a more detailed discussion, see Pratt DS, Kaplan MM: Jaundice, Chap. 38, p. 238; and Pratt DS, Kaplan MM: Evaluation of Liver Function, Chap. 283, p. 1813, in HPIM-16.

55

ASCITES

Definition

Accumulation of fluid within the peritoneal cavity. Small amounts may be asymptomatic; increasing amounts cause abdominal distention and discomfort, anorexia, nausea, early satiety, heartburn, flank pain, and respiratory distress.

Detection

PHYSICAL EXAMINATION   Bulging flanks, fluid wave, shifting dullness, "puddle sign" (dullness over dependent abdomen with pt on hands and knees). May be associated with penile or scrotal edema, umbilical or inguinal herniation, pleural effusion. Evaluation should include rectal and pelvic examination, assessment of liver and spleen. Palmar erythema and spider angiomata seen in cirrhosis. Periumbilical nodule (*Sister Mary Joseph's nodule*) suggests metastatic disease from a pelvic or GI tumor.

ULTRASONOGRAPHY/CT   Very sensitive; able to distinguish fluid from cystic masses.

Evaluation

Diagnostic paracentesis (50–100 mL) essential. Routine evaluation includes inspection, protein, albumin, glucose, cell count and differential, Gram's and acid-fast stains, culture, cytology; in selected cases check amylase, LDH, triglycerides, culture for TB. Rarely, laparoscopy or even exploratory laparotomy may be required. Ascites due to CHF (e.g., pericardial constriction) may require evaluation by right-sided heart catheterization.

DIFFERENTIAL DIAGNOSIS   More than 90% of cases due to cirrhosis, neoplasm, CHF, tuberculosis.

1. *Diseases of peritoneum*: Infections (bacterial, tuberculous, fungal, parasitic), neoplasms, connective tissue disease, miscellaneous (Whipple's disease, familial Mediterranean fever, endometriosis, starch peritonitis, etc.).
2. *Diseases not involving peritoneum*: Cirrhosis, CHF, Budd-Chiari syndrome, hepatic venocclusive disease, hypoalbuminemia (nephrotic syndrome, protein-losing enteropathy, malnutrition), miscellaneous (myxedema, ovarian diseases, pancreatic disease, chylous ascites).

PATHOPHYSIOLOGIC CLASSIFICATION USING SERUM-ASCITES ALBUMIN GRADIENT   Difference in albumin concentrations between serum and ascites as a reflection of imbalances in hydrostatic pressures:

1. *Low gradient* (serum-ascites albumin gradient <1.1): 2° bacterial peritonitis, neoplasm, pancreatitis, vasculitis, nephrotic syndrome.
2. *High gradient* (serum-ascites albumin gradient >1.1 suggests ascites is due to portal hypertension): cirrhosis, CHF, Budd-Chiari syndrome.

REPRESENTATIVE FLUID CHARACTERISTICS See Table 55-1.

CIRRHOTIC ASCITES

PATHOGENESIS Contributing factors: (1) portal hypertension, (2) hypoalbuminemia, (3) hepatic lymph, (4) renal sodium retention—secondary to hyperaldosteronism, increased sympathetic nervous activity (renin-angiotensin production). Initiating event may be peripheral arterial vasodilation triggered by endotoxin and cytokines and mediated by nitric oxide; results in decreased "effective" plasma volume and activation of compensatory mechanisms to retain renal Na and preserve intravascular volume.

R̽ TREATMENT

Maximum mobilization ~700 mL/d (peripheral edema may be mobilized faster).

1. Rigid salt restriction (400 mg Na/d).
2. Fluid restriction of 1–1.5 L only if hyponatremia.
3. Diuretics if no response to salt restriction after 1 week or if urine Na concentration <25 meq/L; spironolactone (mild, potassium-sparing, aldosterone-antagonist) 100 mg/d PO increased by 100 mg q4–5d to maximum of 400 mg/d; furosemide 40–80 mg/d PO or IV may be added if necessary (greater risk of hepatorenal syndrome, encephalopathy), can increase by 40 mg/d to maximum of 160 mg/d until effect achieved or complication occurs.
4. Monitor weight, urinary Na and K, serum electrolytes, and creatinine.
5. Repeated large-volume paracentesis (5 L) with IV infusions of albumin (10 g/L ascites removed) is preferable for initial management of massive ascites because of fewer side effects than diuretics.
6. In refractory cases, consider transjugular intrahepatic portosystemic shunt (TIPS), though 20–30% risk of encephalopathy and high rate of shunt stenosis and occlusion. Peritoneovenous (LeVeen, Denver) shunt (high complication rate—occlusion, infection, DIC) and side-to-side portacaval shunt (high mortality rate in end-stage cirrhotic pt) have fallen out of favor. Consider liver transplantation in appropriate candidates (Chap. 157).

Complications

SPONTANEOUS BACTERIAL PERITONITIS Suspect in cirrhotic pt with ascites and fever, abdominal pain, worsening ascites, ileus, hypotension, worsening jaundice, or encephalopathy; low ascitic protein concentration (low opsonic activity) is predisposing factor. Diagnosis suggested by ascitic fluid PMN cell count >250/μL and symptoms or PMN count >500/μL; confirmed by positive culture (usually Enterobacteriaceae, group D streptococci, *Streptococcus pneumoniae*, *S. viridans*). Initial treatment: Cefotaxime 2 g IV q8h; efficacy demonstrated by marked decrease in ascitic PMN count after 48 h; treat 5–10 days or until ascitic PMN count is normal. Risk of recurrence can be reduced with norfloxacin 400 mg PO qd, trimethoprim-sulfamethoxazole 1 double-strength PO bid 5 days a week, or possibly ciprofloxacin 750 mg PO once

Table 55-1

Representative Fluid Characteristics

Cause	Appearance	Protein, g/dL	Serum-Ascites Albumin Gradient	Cell Count, per µL		Other
				RBC	WBC	
Cirrhosis	Straw-colored	<2.5	>1.1	Low	<250	—
Neoplasm	Straw-colored, hemorrhagic, mucinous, or chylous	>2.5	Variable	Often high	>1000 (>50% lymphs)	+ Cytology
2° Bacterial peritonitis	Turbid or purulent	>2.5	<1.1	Low	>10,000	+ Gram's stain, culture (often multiple organisms)
Spontaneous bacterial peritonitis	Turbid or purulent	<2.5	>1.1	Low	>250 polys	+ Gram's stain, culture
Tuberculous peritonitis	Clear, hemorrhagic, or chylous	>2.5	<1.1	Occ. high	>1000 (>70% lymphs)	+ AFB stain, culture
CHF	Straw-colored, rarely chylous	>2.5	>1.1	Low	<1000 (mesothelial)	—
Pancreatitis	Turbid, hemorrhagic, or chylous	>2.5	<1.1	Variable	Variable	Increased amylase

a week. Consider prophylactic therapy (before first episode of peritonitis) in pts with cirrhotic ascites and an ascitic albumin level <10 g/L (<1 g/dL).

HEPATORENAL SYNDROME Progressive renal failure characterized by azotemia, oliguria with urinary sodium concentration <10 mmol/L, hypotension, and lack of response to volume challenge. May be spontaneous or precipitated by bleeding, sepsis, excessive diuresis or paracentesis. Thought to result from altered renal hemodynamics. Prognosis poor. Treatment: Trial of plasma expansion; TIPS of doubtful benefit; liver transplantation in selected cases.

For a more detailed discussion, see Glickman RM: Abdominal Swelling and Ascites, Chap. 39, p. 243; and Chung RT, Podolsky DK: Cirrhosis and Its Complications, Chap. 289, p. 1858, in HPIM-16.

56

AZOTEMIA AND URINARY ABNORMALITIES

ABNORMALITIES OF RENAL FUNCTION, AZOTEMIA

Azotemia is the retention of nitrogenous waste products excreted by the kidney. Increased levels of blood urea nitrogen (BUN) [>10.7 mmol/L (>30 mg/dL)] and creatinine [>133 μmol/L (>1.5 mg/dL)] are ordinarily indicative of impaired renal function. Renal function can be estimated by determining the clearance of creatinine (CL_{cr}) (normal > 100 mL/min). CL_{cr} overestimates glomerular filtration rate (GFR), particularly at lower levels. A formula that allows an estimate of creatinine clearance in men that accounts for age-related decreases in GFR, body weight, and sex has been derived by Cockcroft-Gault:

$$\text{Creatinine clearance (mL/min)} = \frac{(140 - \text{age}) \times \text{lean body weight (kg)}}{\text{plasma creatinine (mg/dL)} \times 72}$$

This value should be multiplied by 0.85 for women.

GFR may also be estimated using serum creatinine–based equations derived from the Modification of Diet in Renal Disease Study. Isotopic markers (e.g., iothalamate) provide more accurate estimates of GFR.

Manifestations of impaired renal function include: volume overload, hypertension, electrolyte abnormalities (e.g., hyperkalemia, hypocalcemia, hyperphosphatemia), metabolic acidosis, hormonal disturbances (e.g., insulin resistance, functional vitamin D deficiency, secondary hyperparathyroidism), and, when severe, "uremia" (one or more of the following: anorexia, lethargy, confusion, asterixis, pleuritis, pericarditis, enteritis, pruritus, sleep and taste disturbance, nitrogenous fetor).

An approach to the patient with azotemia is shown in Fig. 56-1.

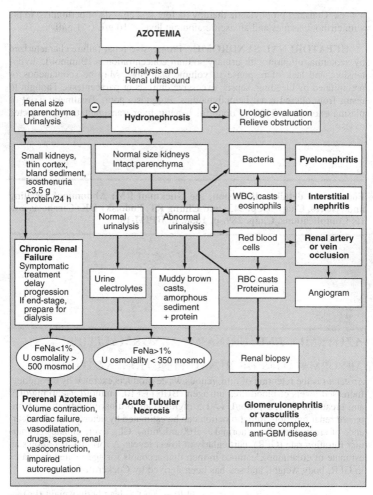

FIGURE 56-1   Approach to the patient with azotemia. WBC, white blood cell; RBC, red blood cell; GBM, glomerular basement membrane. *(From Denker BM, Brenner BM in HPIM-16.)*

ABNORMALITIES OF URINE VOLUME

OLIGURIA   This refers to sparse urine output, usually defined as <400 mL/d. Oligoanuria refers to a more marked reduction in urine output, i.e., <100 mL/d. Anuria indicates the absence of urine output. Oliguria most often occurs in the setting of volume depletion and/or renal hypoperfusion, resulting in "prerenal azotemia" and acute renal failure (Chap. 140). Anuria can be caused by complete bilateral urinary tract obstruction; a vascular catastrophe (dissection or arterial occlusion); renal vein thrombosis; and hypovolemic, cardiogenic, or septic shock. Oliguria is never normal, since at least 400 mL of maximally concentrated urine must be produced to excrete the obligate daily osmolar load.

POLYURIA   Polyuria is defined as a urine output >3 L/d. It is often accompanied by nocturia and urinary frequency and must be differentiated from

Table 56-1

Major Causes of Polyuria

Excessive fluid intake
  Primary polydipsia
  Iatrogenic (intravenous fluids)
Therapeutic
  Diuretic agents
Osmotic diuresis
  Hyperglycemia
  Azotemia
  Mannitol
  Radiocontrast

Nephrogenic diabetes insipidus
  Lithium exposure
  Urinary tract obstruction
  Papillary necrosis
  Reflux nephropathy
  Interstitial nephritis
  Hypercalcemia
Central diabetes insipidus
  Tumor
  Postoperative
  Head trauma
  Basilar meningitis
  Neurosarcoidosis

other more common conditions associated with lower urinary tract pathology and urinary urgency or frequency (e.g., cystitis, prostatism). It is often accompanied by hypernatremia (Chap. 3). Polyuria (Table 56-1) can occur as a response to a solute load (e.g., hyperglycemia) or to an abnormality in antidiuretic hormone (ADH) action. Diabetes insipidus is termed *central* if due to the insufficient hypothalmic production of ADH and *nephrogenic* if the result of renal insensitivity to the action of ADH. Excess fluid intake can lead to polyuria, but primary polydipsia rarely results in changes in plasma osmolality unless urinary diluting capacity is impaired, as with chronic renal failure. Tubulointerstitial diseases and urinary tract obstruction can be associated with nephrogenic diabetes insipidus.

The approach to the pt with polyuria is shown in Fig. 56-2.

Table 56-2

Major Causes of Hematuria

LOWER URINARY TRACT

Bacterial cystitis
Intestitial cystitis
Urethritis (infectious or inflammatory)
Passed or passing kidney stone
Transitional cell carcinoma of bladder or structures proximal to it
Squamous cell carcinoma of bladder (e.g., following schistosomiasis)

UPPER URINARY TRACT

Renal cell carcinoma
Age-related renal cysts
Other neoplasms (e.g., oncocytoma, hamartoma)
Acquired renal cystic disease
Congenital cystic disease, including autosomal dominant form
Glomerular diseases
Interstitial renal diseases
Nephrolithiasis
Pyelonephritis
Renal infarction

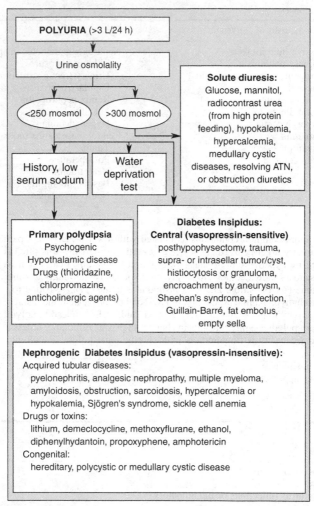

FIGURE 56-2 Approach to the patient with polyuria. (OSM, osmolality; ATN, acute tubular necrosis.) *(From Denker BM, Brenner BM in HPIM-16.)*

ABNORMALITIES OF URINE COMPOSITION

PROTEINURIA This is the hallmark of glomerular disease. Levels up to 150 mg/d are considered within normal limits. Typical measurements are semi-quantitative, using a moderately sensitive dipstick that estimates protein concentration; therefore, the degree of hydration may influence the dipstick protein determination. Most commercially available urine dipsticks detect albumin and do not detect smaller proteins, such as light chains, that require testing with sulfosalicylic acid. More sensitive assays can be used to detect microalbuminuria in diabetes mellitus. A urine albumin to creatinine ratio >30 mg/g defines the presence of micoalbuminuria.

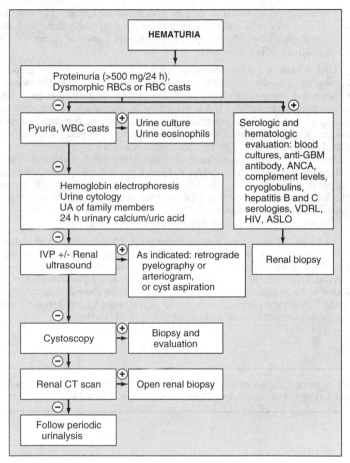

FIGURE 56-3 Approach to the patient with hematuria. RBC, red blood cell; WBC, white blood cell; GBM, glomerular basement membrane; ANCA, antineutrophil cytoplasmic antibody; VDRL, venereal disease research laboratory; ASLO, antistreptolysin O; UA, urinalysis; IVP, intravenous pyelography; CT, computed tomography.

Urinary protein excretion rates between 500 mg/d and 3 g/d are nonspecific and can be seen in a variety of renal diseases (including hypertensive nephrosclerosis, interstitial nephritis, vascular disease, and other primary renal diseases with little or no glomerular involvement). Lesser degrees of proteinuria (500 mg/d to 1.5 g/d) may be seen after vigorous exercise, changes in body position, fever, or congestive heart failure. Protein excretion rates >3 g/d are termed *nephrotic range proteinuria* and are accompanied by hypoalbuminemia, hypercholesterolemia, and edema in the nephrotic syndrome. Massive degrees of proteinuria (>10 g/d) can be seen with minimal change disease, primary focal segmental sclerosis, membranous nephropathy, collapsing glomerulopathy, and HIV-associated nephropathy and can be associated with a variety of extrarenal complications (Chap. 144).

Pharmacologic inhibition of ACE or blockade of angiotensin II or aldosterone receptors may reduce proteinuria in some pts, particularly those with diabetic nephropathy. Specific therapy for a variety of causes of nephrotic syndrome is discussed in Chap. 144.

HEMATURIA Gross hematuria refers to the presence of frank blood in the urine and is more characteristic of lower urinary tract disease and/or bleeding diatheses than intrinsic renal disease (Table 56-2). Cyst rupture in polycystic kidney disease and flares of IgA nephropathy are exceptions. Microscopic hematuria (>1–2 RBC/high powered field) accompanied by proteinuria, hypertension, and an active urinary sediment (the "nephritic syndrome") is most likely related to an inflammatory glomerulonephritis (Chap. 144).

Free hemoglobin and myoglobin are detected by dipstick; a negative urinary sediment with strongly heme-positive dipstick are characteristic of either hemolysis or rhabdomyolysis, which can be differentiated by clinical history and laboratory testing. Red blood cell casts are not commonly seen but are highly specific for glomerulonephritis.

The approach to the pt with hematuria is shown in Fig. 56-3.

PYURIA This may accompany hematuria in inflammatory glomerular diseases. Isolated pyuria is most commonly observed in association with an infection of the upper or lower urinary tract. Pyuria may also occur with allergic interstitial nephritis (often with a preponderance of eosinophils), transplant rejection, and noninfectious, nonallergic tubulointerstitial diseases. The finding of "sterile" pyuria (i.e., urinary white blood cells without bacteria) in the appropriate clinical setting should raise suspicion of renal tuberculosis.

For a more detailed discussion, see Denker BM, Brenner BM: Azotemia and Urinary Abnormalities, Chap. 40, p. 246, in HPIM-16.

57

ANEMIA AND POLYCYTHEMIA

ANEMIA

According to WHO criteria, anemia is defined as blood hemoglobin (Hb) concentration < 130 g/L (<13 g/dL) or hematocrit (Hct) < 39% in adult males; Hb < 120 g/L (<12 g/dL) or Hct < 37% in adult females.

Signs and symptoms of anemia are varied, depending on the level of anemia and the time course over which it developed. Acute anemia is nearly always due to blood loss or hemolysis. In acute blood loss, hypovolemia dominates the clinical picture; hypotension and decreased organ perfusion are the main issues. Symptoms associated with more chronic onset vary with the age of the pt and the adequacy of blood supply to critical organs. Moderate anemia is associated with fatigue, loss of stamina, breathlessness, and tachycardia. The pt's skin and mucous membranes may appear pale. If the palmar creases are lighter in color than the surrounding skin with the fingers extended, Hb level is often <80 g/L

(8 g/dL). In pts with coronary artery disease, anginal episodes may appear or increase in frequency and severity. In pts with carotid artery disease, lightheadedness or dizziness may develop.

A physiologic approach to anemia diagnosis is based on the understanding that a decrease in circulating red blood cells (RBC) can be related to either inadequate production of RBCs or increased RBC destruction or loss. Within the category of inadequate production, erythropoiesis can be either ineffective, due to an erythrocyte maturation defect (which usually results in RBCs that are too small or too large), or hypoproliferative (which usually results in RBCs of normal size, but too few of them).

Basic evaluations include: (1) reticulocyte index (RI), (2) review of blood smear and RBC indices [particularly mean corpuscular volume (MCV)] (Fig. 57-1).

The RI is a measure of RBC production. The reticulocyte count is corrected for the Hct level and for early release of marrow reticulocytes into the circulation, which leads to an increase in the life span of the circulating reticulocyte beyond the usual 1 day. Thus, RI = (% reticulocytes × pt Hct/45%) × (1/shift correction factor). The shift correction factor varies with the Hct: 1.5 for Hct =

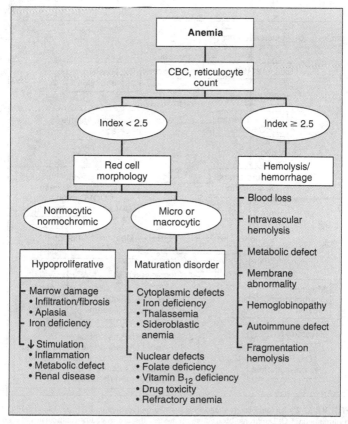

FIGURE 57-1 The physiologic classification of anemia. CBC, complete blood count.

35%, 2 for Hct = 25%, 2.5 for Hct = 15%. RI < 2–2.5% implies inadequate RBC production for the particular level of anemia; RI > 2.5% implies excessive RBC destruction or loss.

If the anemia is associated with a low RI, RBC morphology helps distinguish a maturation disorder from hypoproliferative marrow states. Cytoplasmic maturation defects such as iron deficiency or Hb synthesis problems produce smaller RBCs, MCV < 80; nuclear maturation defects such as B_{12} and folate deficiency and drug effects produce larger RBCs, MCV > 100. In hypoproliferative marrow states, RBCs are generally normal in morphology but too few are produced. Bone marrow examination is often helpful in the evaluation of anemia but is done most frequently to diagnose hypoproliferative marrow states.

Other laboratory tests indicated to evaluate particular forms of anemia depend on the initial classification based on the pathophysiology of the defect. These are discussed in more detail in Chap. 64.

POLYCYTHEMIA (ERYTHROCYTOSIS)

This is an increase above the normal range of RBCs in the circulation. Concern that the Hb level may be abnormally high should be triggered at a level of 170 g/L (17 g/dL) in men and 150 g/L (15 g/dL) in women. Polycythemia is usually

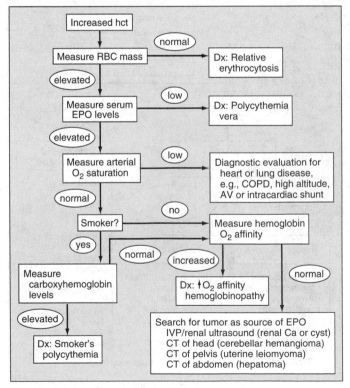

FIGURE 57-2 An approach to diagnosing pts with polycythemia. RBC, red blood cell; EPO, erythropoietin; COPD, chronic obstructive pulmonary disease; AV, atrioventricular; IVP, intravenous pyelogram; CT, computed tomography.

found incidentally at routine blood count. Relative erythrocytosis, due to plasma volume loss (e.g., severe dehydration, burns), does not represent a true increase in total RBC mass. Absolute erythrocytosis is a true increase in total RBC mass.

CAUSES Polycythemia vera (a clonal myeloproliferative disorder), erythropoietin-producing neoplasms (e.g., renal cancer, cerebellar hemangioma), chronic hypoxemia (e.g., high altitude, pulmonary disease), carboxyhemoglobin excess (e.g., smokers), high-affinity hemoglobin variants, Cushing's syndrome, androgen excess. Polycythemia vera is distinguished from secondary polycythemia by the presence of splenomegaly, leukocytosis, thrombocytosis, and elevated vitamin B_{12} levels, and by decreased erythropoietin levels. An approach to evaluate polycythemic pts is shown in Fig. 57-2.

COMPLICATIONS Hyperviscosity (with diminished O_2 delivery) with risk of ischemic organ injury and thrombosis (venous or arterial) are most common.

 TREATMENT

Phlebotomy recommended for Hct $\geq$ 55%, regardless of cause, to low-normal range.

For a more detailed discussion, see Adamson JW, Longo DL: Anemia and Polycythemia, Chap. 52, p. 329, in HPIM-16.

58

LYMPHADENOPATHY AND SPLENOMEGALY

LYMPHADENOPATHY

Exposure to antigen through a break in the skin or mucosa results in antigen being taken up by an antigen-presenting cell and carried via lymphatic channels to the nearest lymph node. Lymph channels course throughout the body except for the brain and the bones. Lymph enters the node through the afferent vessel and leaves through an efferent vessel. As antigen-presenting cells pass through lymph nodes, they present antigen to lymphocytes residing there. Lymphocytes in a node are constantly being replaced by antigen-naive lymphocytes from the blood. They are retained in the node via special homing receptors. B cells populate the lymphoid follicles in the cortex; T cells populate the paracortical regions. When a B cell encounters an antigen to which its surface immunoglobulin can bind, it stays in the follicle for a few days and forms a germinal center where the immunoglobulin gene is mutated in an effort to make an antibody with higher affinity for the antigen. The B cell then migrates to the medullary region, differentiates into a plasma cell, and secretes immunoglobulin into the efferent lymph.

When a T cell in the node encounters an antigen it recognizes, it proliferates and joins the efferent lymph. The efferent lymph laden with antibodies and T cells specific for the inciting antigen passes through several nodes on its way to the thoracic duct, which drains lymph from most of the body. From the thoracic duct, lymph enters the bloodstream at the left subclavian vein. Lymph from the head and neck and the right arm drain into the right subclavian vein. From the bloodstream, the antibody and T cells localize to the site of infection.

Lymphadenopathy may be caused by infections, immunologic diseases, malignancies, lipid storage diseases, or a number of disorders of uncertain etiology (e.g., sarcoidosis, Castleman's disease; Table 58-1). The two major mechanisms of lymphadenopathy are *hyperplasia*, in response to immunologic or infectious stimuli, and *infiltration*, by cancer cells or lipid- or glycoprotein-laden macrophages.

Approach to the Patient

History Age, occupation, animal exposures, sexual orientation, substance abuse history, medication history, and concomitant symptoms influence diagnostic workup. Adenopathy is more commonly malignant in origin in those over age 40. Farmers have an increased incidence of brucellosis and lymphoma. Male homosexuals may have AIDS-associated adenopathy. Alcohol and tobacco abuse increase risk of malignancy. Phenytoin may induce adenopathy. The concomitant presence of cervical adenopathy with sore throat or with fever, night sweats, and weight loss suggests particular diagnoses (mononucleosis in the former instance, Hodgkin's disease in the latter).

Physical Examination Location of adenopathy, size, node texture, and the presence of tenderness are important in differential diagnosis. Generalized adenopathy (three or more anatomic regions) implies systemic infection or lymphoma. Subclavian or scalene adenopathy is always abnormal and should be biopsied. Nodes > 4 cm should be biopsied immediately. Rock hard nodes fixed to surrounding soft tissue are usually a sign of metastatic carcinoma. Tender nodes are most often benign.

Laboratory Tests Usually lab tests are not required in the setting of localized adenopathy. If generalized adenopathy is noted, an excisional node biopsy should be performed for diagnosis, rather than a panoply of laboratory tests.

℞ TREATMENT

Pts over age 40, those with scalene or supraclavicular adenopathy, those with lymph nodes > 4 cm in diameter, and those with hard nontender nodes should undergo immediate excisional biopsy. In younger patients with smaller nodes that are rubbery in consistency or tender, a period of observation for 7–14 days is reasonable. Empirical antibiotics are not indicated. If the nodes shrink, no further evaluation is necessary. If they enlarge, excisional biopsy is indicated.

SPLENOMEGALY

Just as the lymph nodes are specialized to fight pathogens in the tissues, the spleen is the lymphoid organ specialized to fight bloodborne pathogens. It has no afferent lymphatics. The spleen has specialized areas like the lymph node for making antibodies (follicles) and amplifying antigen-specific T cells (periarteriolar lymphatic sheath, or PALS). In addition, it has a well-developed reticuloendothelial system for removing particles and antibody-coated bacteria. The flow of blood through the spleen permits it to filter pathogens from the blood and to maintain quality control over erythrocytes (RBCs)—those that are

Table 58-1

Diseases Associated with Lymphadenopathy

1. Infectious diseases
   a. Viral—infectious mononucleosis syndromes (EBV, CMV), infectious hepatitis, herpes simplex, herpesvirus-6, varicella-zoster virus, rubella, measles, adenovirus, HIV, epidemic keratoconjunctivitis, vaccinia, herpesvirus-8
   b. Bacterial—streptococci, staphylococci, cat-scratch disease, brucellosis, tularemia, plague, chancroid, melioidosis, glanders, tuberculosis, atypical mycobacterial infection, primary and secondary syphilis, diphtheria, leprosy
   c. Fungal—histoplasmosis, coccidioidomycosis, paracoccidioidomycosis
   d. Chlamydial—lymphogranuloma venereum, trachoma
   e. Parasitic—toxoplasmosis, leishmaniasis, trypanosomiasis, filariasis
   f. Rickettsial—scrub typhus, rickettsialpox
2. Immunologic diseases
   a. Rheumatoid arthritis
   b. Juvenile rheumatoid arthritis
   c. Mixed connective tissue disease
   d. Systemic lupus erythematosus
   e. Dermatomyositis
   f. Sjögren's syndrome
   g. Serum sickness
   h. Drug hypersensitivity—diphenylhydantoin, hydralazine, allopurinol, primidone, gold, carbamazepine, etc.
   i. Angioimmunoblastic lymphadenopathy
   j. Primary biliary cirrhosis
   k. Graft-vs.-host disease
   l. Silicone-associated
3. Malignant diseases
   a. Hematologic—Hodgkin's disease, non-Hodgkin's lymphomas, acute or chronic lymphocytic leukemia, hairy cell leukemia, malignant histiocytosis, amyloidosis
   b. Metastatic—from numerous primary sites
4. Lipid storage diseases—Gaucher's, Niemann-Pick, Fabry, Tangier
5. Endocrine diseases—hyperthyroidism
6. Other disorders
   a. Castleman's disease (giant lymph node hyperplasia)
   b. Sarcoidosis
   c. Dermatopathic lymphadenitis
   d. Lymphomatoid granulomatosis
   e. Histiocytic necrotizing lymphadenitis (Kikuchi's disease)
   f. Sinus histiocytosis with massive lymphadenopathy (Rosai-Dorfman disease)
   g. Mucocutaneous lymph node syndrome (Kawasaki's disease)
   h. Histiocytosis X
   i. Familial mediterranean fever
   j. Severe hypertriglyceridemia
   k. Vascular transformation of sinuses
   l. Inflammatory pseudotumor of lymph node

Note: EBV, Epstein-Barr virus; CMV, cytomegalovirus.

Table 58-2

Diseases Associated with Splenomegaly Grouped by Pathogenic Mechanism

---

ENLARGEMENT DUE TO INCREASED DEMAND FOR SPLENIC FUNCTION

Reticuloendothelial system hyperplasia (for removal of defective erythrocytes)
  Spherocytosis
  Early sickle cell anemia
  Ovalocytosis
  Thalassemia major
  Hemoglobinopathies
  Paroxysmal nocturnal hemoglobinuria
  Nutritional anemias
Immune hyperplasia
  Response to infection (viral, bacterial, fungal, parasitic)

Infectious mononucleosis	Splenic abscess
AIDS	Tuberculosis
Viral hepatitis	Histoplasmosis
Cytomegalovirus	Malaria
Subacute bacterial	Leishmaniasis
endocarditis	Trypanosomiasis
Bacterial septicemia	Ehrlichiosis
Congenital syphilis	

  Disordered immunoregulation

Rheumatoid arthritis	Drug reactions
(Felty's syndrome)	Angioimmunoblastic
Systemic lupus erythematosus	lymphadenopathy
Collagen vascular diseases	Sarcoidosis
Serum sickness	Thyrotoxicosis (benign
Immune hemolytic anemias	lymphoid hypertrophy)
Immune thrombocytopenias	Interleukin 2 therapy
Immune neutropenias	

Extramedullary hematopoiesis
  Myelofibrosis
  Marrow damage by toxins, radiation, strontium
  Marrow infiltration by tumors, leukemias, Gaucher's disease

---

ENLARGEMENT DUE TO ABNORMAL SPLENIC OR PORTAL BLOOD FLOW

Cirrhosis
Hepatic vein obstruction
Portal vein obstruction, intrahepatic or extrahepatic
Cavernous transformation of the portal vein
Splenic vein obstruction
Splenic artery aneurysm
Hepatic schistosomiasis
Congestive heart failure
Hepatic echinococcosis
Portal hypertension (any cause including the above): "Banti's disease"

(continued)

Table 58-2 *(Continued)*

Diseases Associated with Splenomegaly Grouped by Pathogenic Mechanism

INFILTRATION OF THE SPLEEN

Intracellular or extracellular depositions
  Amyloidosis
  Gaucher's disease
  Niemann-Pick disease
  Tangier disease
  Hurler's syndrome and other mucopolysaccharidoses
  Hyperlipidemias
Benign and malignant cellular infiltrations
  Leukemias (acute, chronic, lymphoid, myeloid, monocytic)
  Lymphomas
  Hodgkin's disease
  Myeloproliferative syndromes (e.g., polycythemia vera)
  Angiosarcomas
  Metastatic tumors (melanoma is most common)
  Eosinophilic granuloma
  Histiocytosis X
  Hamartomas
  Hemangiomas, fibromas, lymphangiomas
  Splenic cysts

UNKNOWN ETIOLOGY

Idiopathic splenomegaly
Berylliosis
Iron-deficiency anemia

old and nondeformable are destroyed, and intracellular inclusions (sometimes including pathogens such as babesia and malaria) are culled from the cells in a process called *pitting*. Under certain conditions, the spleen can generate hematopoietic cells in place of the marrow.

The normal spleen is about 12 cm in length and 7 cm in width and is not normally palpable. Dullness from the spleen can be percussed between the ninth and eleventh ribs with the pt lying on the right side. Palpation is best performed with the pt supine with knees flexed. The spleen may be felt as it descends when the pt inspires. Physical diagnosis is not sensitive. CT or ultrasound are superior tests.

Spleen enlargement occurs by three basic mechanisms: (1) hyperplasia or hypertrophy due to an increase in demand for splenic function (e.g., hereditary spherocytosis where demand for removal of defective RBCs is high or immune hyperplasia in response to systemic infection or immune diseases); (2) passive vascular congestion due to portal hypertension; and (3) infiltration with malignant cells, lipid- or glycoprotein-laden macrophages, or amyloid (Table 58-2). Massive enlargement, with spleen palpable >8 cm below the left costal margin, usually signifies a lymphoproliferative or myeloproliferative disorder.

Peripheral blood RBC count, WBC count, and platelet count may be normal, decreased, or increased depending on the underlying disorder. Decreases in one or more cell lineages could indicate hypersplenism, increased destruction. In cases with hypersplenism, the spleen is removed and the cytopenia is generally reversed. In the absence of hypersplenism, most causes of splenomegaly are diagnosed on the basis of signs and symptoms and laboratory abnormalities associated with the underlying disorder. Splenectomy is rarely performed for diagnostic purposes.

Individuals who have had splenectomy are at increased risk of sepsis from a variety of organisms including the pneumococcus and *Haemophilus influenzae*. Vaccines for these agents should be given before splenectomy is performed. Splenectomy compromises the immune response to these T-independent antigens.

For a more detailed discussion, see Henry PH, Longo DL: Enlargement of Lymph Nodes and Spleen, Chap. 54, p. 343, in HPIM-16.

59

COMMON DISORDERS OF VISION AND HEARING

DISORDERS OF THE EYE
Clinical Assessment

The history and examination permit accurate diagnosis of most eye disorders, without need for laboratory or imaging studies. The essential ocular exam includes assessment of the visual acuity, pupil reactions, eye movements, eye alignment, visual fields, and intraocular pressure. The lids, conjunctiva, cornea, anterior chamber, iris, and lens are examined with a slit lamp. The fundus is viewed with an ophthalmoscope.

Acute visual loss or double vision in a pt with quiet, uninflamed eyes often signifies a serious ocular or neurologic disorder and should be managed emergently (Chap. 40). Ironically, the occurrence of a red eye, even if painful, has less dire implications as long as the visual acuity is spared.

Specific Disorders

RED OR PAINFUL EYE   Most common causes listed in Table 59-1.

Minor Trauma   This may result in corneal abrasion, subconjunctival hemorrhage, or foreign body. The integrity of the corneal epithelium is assessed by placing a drop of fluorescein in the eye and looking with a slit lamp or a blue penlight. The conjunctival fornices should be searched carefully for foreign bodies. Topical anesthesia with a drop of 0.5% proparacaine may be necessary to perform an adequate examination.

 TREATMENT

Chemical splashes and foreign bodies are treated by copious saline irrigation. Corneal abrasions may require application of a topical antibiotic, a mydriatic agent (1% cyclopentolate), and an eye patch for 24 h.

Table 59-1

Causes of a Red or Painful Eye

Blunt or penetrating trauma	Dacrocystitis
Chemical exposure	Episcleritis
Corneal abrasion	Scleritis
Foreign body	Anterior uveitis (iritis or
Contact lens (overuse or infection)	iridocyclitis)
Corneal exposure (5th, 7th nerve	Endophthalmitis
palsy, ectropion)	Acute angle-closure glaucoma
Subconjunctival hemorrhage	Medicamentosus
Blepharitis	Pinguecula
Conjunctivitis (infectious or allergic)	Pterygium
Corneal ulcer	Proptosis (retrobulbar mass, orbital
Herpes keratitis	cellulitis, Graves' ophthalmopa-
Herpes zoster ophthalmicus	thy, orbital pseudotumor, carotid-
Keratoconjunctivitis sicca (dry eye)	cavernous fistula)

Infection   Infection of the eyelids and conjunctiva (blepharoconjunctivitis) produces redness and irritation but should not cause visual loss or pain. Adenovirus is the most common cause of "pink eye." It produces a thin, watery discharge, whereas bacterial infection causes a more mucopurulent exudate. On slit-lamp exam one should confirm that the cornea is not affected, by observing that it remains clear and lustrous. Corneal infection (keratitis) is a more serious condition than blepharoconjunctivitis because it can cause scarring and permanent visual loss. A localized abscess or ulcer within the cornea produces visual loss, pain, anterior chamber inflammation, and hypopyon. A dendritic pattern of corneal fluorescein staining is characteristic of herpes simplex keratitis.

 TREATMENT

Strict handwashing and broad-spectrum topical antibiotics for blepharoconjunctivitis (sulfacetamide 10%, polymyxin-bacitracin-neomycin, or trimethoprim-polymyxin). Keratitis requires empirical antibiotics (usually topical and subconjunctival) pending culture results. Herpes keratitis is treated with topical antiviral agents, cycloplegics, and oral acyclovir.

Inflammation   Eye inflammation, without infection, can produce episcleritis, scleritis, or uveitis (iritis or iridocyclitis). Most cases are idiopathic, but some occur in conjunction with autoimmune disease. There is no discharge. A ciliary flush results from injection of deep conjunctival and episcleral vessels near the corneal limbus. The diagnosis of iritis hinges on the slit-lamp observation of inflammatory cells floating in the aqueous of the anterior chamber (cell and flare) or deposited on the corneal endothelium (keratic precipitates).

 TREATMENT

Mydriatic agents (1% cyclopentolate), NSAIDs, and topical glucocorticoids. (Note: prolonged treatment with ocular glucocorticoids causes cataract and glaucoma.)

Acute Angle-Closure Glaucoma   This is a rare but important cause of a red, painful eye. Because the anterior chamber is shallow, aqueous outflow via the canal of Schlemm becomes blocked by the peripheral iris. Intraocular pressure rises abruptly, causing ocular pain, injection, headache, nausea, and blurred vision. The key diagnostic step is measurement of the intraocular pressure during an attack.

 TREATMENT

The acute attack is broken by constricting the pupil with a drop of 4% pilocarpine and by lowering the intraocular pressure with topical 0.5% apraclonidine, 0.5% timolol, and a single oral dose of 500 mg acetazolamide. Future attacks are prevented by performing an iridotomy with a laser.

CHRONIC VISUAL LOSS   Most common causes are listed in Table 59-2.

Cataract   A cloudy lens, due principally to aging. It is treated by surgical extraction and replacement with an artificial intraocular lens.

Table 59-2

Causes of Chronic, Progressive Visual Loss

Cataract	Intraocular tumor
Glaucoma	Retinitis pigmentosa
Macular degeneration	Epiretinal membrane
Diabetic retinopathy	Macular hole
Optic nerve or optic chiasm tumor	

Glaucoma   An optic neuropathy that leads to progressive visual loss from death of retinal ganglion cells. It is associated with elevated intraocular pressure, but many pts have normal pressure. Angle closure accounts for only a few cases; most pts have open angles and no identifiable cause for their pressure elevation. The diagnosis is made by documenting arcuate (nerve fiber bundle) scotomas on visual field exam and by observing "cupping" of the optic disc.

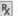 **TREATMENT**

Topical adrenergic agonists (epinephrine, dipivefrin, apraclonidine, brimonidine), cholinergic agents (pilocarpinc), beta blockers (betaxolol, carteolol, levobunolol, metipranolol, timolol), and prostaglandin analogues (latanaprost); oral carbonic anhydrase inhibitors (acetazolamide). Surgical filter to reduce pressure (trabeculectomy).

Macular Degeneration   This occurs in both a "dry" and "wet" form. In the dry form, clumps of extracellular debris, called *drusen*, are deposited beneath the retinal pigment epithelium. As they accumulate, vision is slowly lost. In the wet form, neovascular vessels proliferate beneath the retinal pigment epithelium. Bleeding from these neovascular vessels can cause sudden, central visual loss in the elderly. Macular exam shows drusen and subretinal hemorrhage.

 TREATMENT

Treatment with vitamins C and E, beta carotene, and zinc may retard dry macular degeneration. Wet macular degeneration can be treated with laser photocoagulation of the leaking vessels.

Diabetic Retinopathy   Appears in most pts 10–15 years after onset of the disease. Background diabetic retinopathy consists of intraretinal hemorrhage, exudates, nerve fiber layer infarcts (cotton-wool spots), and macular edema. Proliferative diabetic retinopathy is characterized by ingrowth of neovascular vessels on the retinal surface, causing blindness from vitreous hemorrhage and retinal detachment.

 TREATMENT

All diabetics should be examined regularly by an ophthalmologist for surveillance of diabetic retinopathy. Macular edema is treated by focal or grid laser application. Neovascularization is treated by panretinal laser photocoagulation.

Tumors   Tumors of the optic nerve or chiasm are comparatively rare but often escape detection because they produce insidious visual loss and few physical findings, except for optic disc pallor. Pituitary tumor is the most common lesion. It causes bitemporal or monocular visual loss.

 TREATMENT

Large pituitary tumors producing chiasm compression are removed transsphenoidally. In some cases, small tumors can be observed or controlled pharmacologically (e.g., bromocriptine for prolactinoma).

HEARING DISORDERS

Nearly 10% of the adult population has some hearing loss; up to 35% of individuals over the age of 65 have hearing loss of sufficient magnitude to require a hearing aid. Hearing loss can result from disorders of the auricle, external auditory canal, middle ear, inner ear, or central auditory pathways. *In general, lesions in the auricle, external auditory canal, or middle ear cause conductive hearing losses, while lesions in the inner ear or eighth nerve cause sensorineural hearing losses.*

—————————— *Approach to the Patient* ——————————

Ascertain onset (sudden vs. insidious), progression (rapid vs. slow), and whether symptoms are unilateral or bilateral. Ask about tinnitus, vertigo, imbalance, aural fullness, otorrhea, headache, and facial or other cranial nerve symptoms. Prior head trauma, exposure to ototoxins, occupational or recreational noise exposure, or family history of hearing impairment also important.

Exam should include the auricle, external ear canal, and tympanic membrane. The external ear canal of the elderly is often dry and fragile; it is preferable to clean cerumen with wall-mounted suction and cerumen loops and to avoid irrigation. Inspect the nose, nasopharynx, cranial nerves, and upper respiratory tract. Unilateral serous effusion should prompt a fiberoptic exam of the nasopharynx to exclude neoplasm.

The Weber and Rinne tuning fork tests differentiate conductive from sensorineural hearing losses. *Rinne test*: the tines of a vibrating tuning fork are held near the opening of the external auditory canal, and then the stem is placed on the mastoid process. Normally, and with sensorineural hearing loss, air conduction is louder than bone conduction; however, with conductive hearing loss, bone conduction is louder. *Weber test*: the stem of a vibrating tuning fork on the forehead in the midline. With a unilateral conductive hearing loss, the tone is perceived in the affected ear; with a unilateral sensorineural hearing loss, the tone is perceived in the unaffected ear.

Laboratory Assessment of Hearing

Audiologic Assessment   *Pure tone audiometry* assesses severity of hearing impairment on each side and the type of hearing loss. Speech recognition requires greater synchronous neural firing than necessary for appreciation of pure tones; clarity of hearing is tested in *speech audiometry. Tympanometry* measures impedance of middle ear to sound; useful in diagnosis of middle-ear effusions. *Otoacoustic emissions* (OAE), measured with microphones inserted in external auditory canal, indicate that outer hair cells of the organ of Corti are intact; useful to assess auditory thresholds and distinguish sensory from neural hearing loss. *Electrocochleography* measures earliest evoked potentials generated in cochlea and auditory nerve; useful in diagnosis of Ménière's disease. *Brainstem auditory evoked responses* (BAER) localize site of sensorineural hearing loss.

Imaging Studies   CT of temporal bone with fine 1-mm cuts can define the caliber of the external auditory canal, integrity of the ossicular chain, presence of middle ear or mastoid disease, inner ear malformations, and bone erosion (chronic otitis media and cholesteatoma). MRI superior to CT for imaging of retrocochlear structures including cerebellopontine angle (vestibular schwannoma) and brainstem.

Causes of Hearing Loss (Fig. 59-1)

CONDUCTIVE HEARING LOSS   May result from obstruction of the external auditory canal by cerumen, debris, and foreign bodies; swelling of the lining of the canal; atresia of the ear canal; neoplasms of the canal; perforations of the tympanic membrane; disruption of the ossicular chain, as occurs with necrosis of the long process of the incus in trauma or infection; otosclerosis; and fluid, scarring, or neoplasms in the middle ear. Hearing loss with otorrhea most likely due to otitis media or cholesteatoma.

Cholesteatoma, i.e., stratified squamous epithelium in the middle ear or mastoid, is a benign, slowly growing lesion that destroys bone and normal ear tissue. A chronically draining ear that fails to respond to appropriate antibiotic therapy suggests cholesteatoma; surgery is required.

Conductive hearing loss with a normal ear canal and intact tympanic membrane suggests ossicular pathology. Fixation of the stapes from *otosclerosis* is a common cause of low-frequency conductive hearing loss; onset is between the late teens to the forties. In women, the hearing loss is often first noticeable during pregnancy. A hearing aid or a surgical stapedectomy can provide auditory rehabilitation.

Eustachian tube dysfunction is common and may predispose to acute otitis media (AOM) or serous otitis media (SOM). Trauma, AOM, or chronic otitis media are the usual factors responsible for tympanic membrane perforation. While small perforations often heal spontaneously, larger defects usually require surgical tympanoplasty (>90% effective). Otoscopy is usually sufficient to diagnose AOM, SOM, chronic otitis media, cerumen impaction, tympanic membrane perforation, and eustachian tube dysfunction.

SENSORINEURAL HEARING LOSS   Damage to the hair cells of the organ of Corti may be caused by intense noise, viral infections, ototoxic drugs (e.g., salicylates, quinine and its analogues, aminoglycoside antibiotics, diuretics such as furosemide and ethacrynic acid, and cancer chemotherapeutic agents such as cisplatin), fractures of the temporal bone, meningitis, cochlear otosclerosis (see above), Ménière's disease, and aging. Sudden unilateral hearing loss may represent a viral infection of the inner ear or a cerebrovascular accident. Congenital malformations of the inner ear may cause hearing loss in some adults. Genetic predisposition alone or in concert with environmental influences may also be responsible.

Presbycusis (age-associated hearing loss) is the most common cause of sensorineural hearing loss in adults. In early stages, symmetric high frequency hearing loss is typical; with progression, the hearing loss involves all frequencies. The hearing impairment is associated with loss in clarity. Hearing aids provide limited rehabilitation; cochlear implants are treatment of choice for severe cases.

Ménière's disease is characterized by episodic vertigo, fluctuating sensorineural hearing loss, tinnitus, and aural fullness. It is caused by an increase in endolymphatic fluid pressure due to endolymphatic sac dysfunction. Low-frequency, unilateral sensorineural hearing impairment is usually present. MRI should be obtained to exclude retrocochlear pathology such as cerebellopontine angle tumors or demyelinating disorders. Therapy directed toward control of

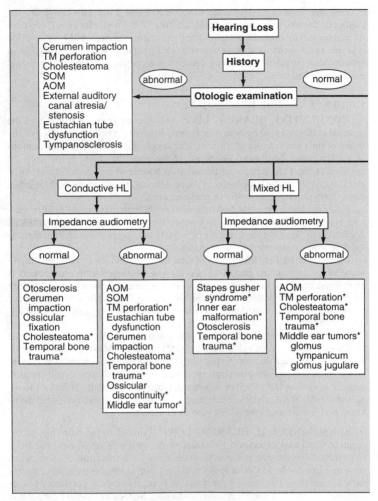

FIGURE 59-1A   An algorithm for the approach to hearing loss. HL, hearing loss; SNHL, sensorineural hearing loss; TM, tympanic membrane; SOM, serous otitis media; AOM, acute otitis media; BAER, brainstem auditory evoked response; *, CT scan of temporal bone; †, MRI scan.

vertigo; a low-salt diet, diuretics, a short course of glucocorticoids, and intra-tympanic gentamicin may be useful. For unresponsive cases, labyrinthectomy and vestibular nerve section abolish rotatory vertigo. There is no effective therapy for hearing loss, tinnitus, or aural fullness.

Vestibular schwannomas present with asymmetric hearing impairment, tinnitus, imbalance (rarely vertigo); cranial neuropathy (trigeminal or facial nerve) may accompany larger tumors.

Sensorineural hearing loss may also result from any neoplastic, vascular, demyelinating, infectious (including HIV), or degenerative disease or trauma affecting the central auditory pathways.

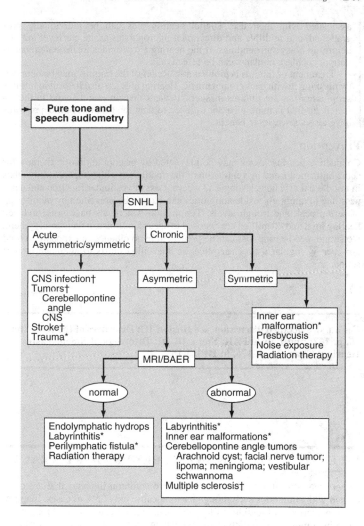

TINNITUS   Defined as the perception of a sound when there is no sound in the environment. It may have a buzzing, roaring, or ringing quality and may be pulsatile (synchronous with the heartbeat). Tinnitus is often associated with either a conductive or sensorineural hearing loss and may be the first symptom of a serious condition such as a vestibular schwannoma. Pulsatile tinnitus requires evaluation of the vascular system of the head to exclude vascular tumors such as glomus jugulare tumors, aneurysms, and stenotic arterial lesions; it may also occur with SOM.

Rx **TREATMENT**

Hearing aids have been improved to provide greater fidelity and miniaturized so that they can be placed entirely within the ear canal, reducing the stigma associated with their use. Digital hearing aids can be individually programmed, and multiple and directional microphones at the ear level may be helpful in noisy surroundings. If the hearing aid provides inadequate rehabilitation, cochlear implants can be effective.

Treatment of tinnitus is problematic. Relief of the tinnitus may be obtained by masking it with background music. Hearing aids are also helpful in tinnitus suppression, as are tinnitus maskers, devices that present a sound to the affected ear that is more pleasant to listen to than the tinnitus. Antidepressants have also shown some benefit.

Prevention

Conductive hearing losses may be prevented by prompt antibiotic therapy for acute otitis media and by ventilation of the middle ear with tympanostomy tubes in middle-ear effusions lasting ≥ 12 weeks. Loss of vestibular function and deafness due to aminoglycoside antibiotics can largely be prevented by monitoring of serum peak and trough levels. Ten million Americans have noise-induced hearing loss, and 20 million are exposed to hazardous noise in their employment. Noise-induced hearing loss can be prevented by avoidance of exposure to loud noise or by regular use of ear plugs or fluid-filled muffs to attenuate intense sound.

For a more detailed discussion, see Horton JC: Disorders of the Eye, Chap. 25, p. 162; and Lalwani AK, Snow JB Jr.: Disorders of Smell, Taste, and Hearing, Chap. 26, p. 176, in HPIM-16.

60

INFECTIONS OF THE UPPER RESPIRATORY TRACT

Upper respiratory tract infections (URIs) are common illnesses that are often treated with antibiotics even though bacteria cause only 25% of cases. Inappropriate prescribing of antibiotics for URIs is a leading cause of antibiotic resistance in common community-acquired pathogens such as *Streptococcus pneumoniae*.

NONSPECIFIC URIs

The "common cold" is an acute, mild, catarrhal syndrome that lasts ~1 week and is caused by a wide variety of viruses, including rhinoviruses, coronaviruses, parainfluenza viruses, influenza viruses, adenoviruses, and respiratory syncytial virus. Symptoms include rhinorrhea, nasal congestion, cough, sore throat, hoarseness, malaise, sneezing, and fever. Because secondary bacterial infection complicates only 0.5–2% of colds, antibiotics are not indicated. Only symptom-based treatments should be used.

SINUS INFECTIONS

Sinusitis is an inflammatory condition most commonly involving the maxillary sinus; the next most common sites are the ethmoid, frontal, and sphenoid sinuses. Sinuses become infected when sinus ostia are obstructed or when ciliary clearance is impaired.

Acute Sinusitis

Etiology and Epidemiology Acute sinusitis, defined as disease of <4 weeks' duration, is usually caused by the same viruses that cause nonspecific URIs. *S. pneumoniae*, nontypable *Haemophilus influenzae*, and (in children) *Moraxella catarrhalis* cause acute bacterial sinusitis. Nosocomial cases, which are associated with nasotracheal intubation, are commonly caused by *Staphylococcus aureus* and gram-negative bacilli and are often polymicrobial and highly resistant to antibiotics. Acute fungal sinusitis occurs in compromised hosts (e.g., rhinocerebral mucormycosis in diabetic pts or aspergillosis in neutropenic pts).

Clinical Features Common manifestations of acute sinusitis include nasal drainage, congestion, facial pain or pressure, headache, thick purulent nasal discharge, and tooth pain. Pain localizes to the involved sinus and is often worse when the pt bends over or is supine. Rarely, sphenoid or ethmoid sinusitis causes severe frontal or retroorbital pain, cavernous sinus thrombosis, and orbital cellulitis. Advanced frontal sinusitis can present as "Pott's puffy tumor": swelling and edema over the frontal bone. Life-threatening complications include meningitis, epidural abscess, and brain abscess.

Diagnosis It is difficult to distinguish viral from bacterial sinusitis clinically. Disease of <7 days' duration is considered viral. Of pts with symptoms of >7 days' duration, 40–50% have bacterial sinusitis. If fungal sinusitis is a consideration, biopsies of involved areas should be performed. Nosocomial sinusitis should be confirmed with a CT scan of the sinuses.

 TREATMENT

See Table 60-1 for recommended regimens for adults. (Regimens for children can be found in Table 27-1 in HPIM-16.)
  Most pts improve without therapy. Treatment to facilitate drainage (e.g., oral and topical decongestants) should be used. Pts without improvement or with severe disease at presentation should be given antibiotics. Lack of response may mandate surgical drainage or lavage. Surgery should be considered for pts with severe disease or intracranial complications. Extensive debridement is usually needed for invasive fungal sinusitis in immunocompromised pts. Nosocomial disease requires agents active against *S. aureus* and gram-negative bacilli, including *Pseudomonas aeruginosa*.

Chronic Sinusitis

Sinusitis of >12 weeks' duration is considered chronic.

• *Chronic bacterial sinusitis*: repeated infections due to impaired mucociliary clearance. Pts have constant nasal congestion and sinus pressure with periods of increased severity. Sinus CT scans can define the extent of disease and response to treatment. Tissue samples for histology and culture should be obtained to guide treatment. Repeated courses of antibiotics are required for 3–4 weeks at a time. Adjunctive treatments include intranasal administration of glucocorticoids, sinus irrigation, and surgical evaluation. Recurrence is common.
• *Chronic fungal sinusitis*: a noninvasive disease in immunocompetent hosts. Mild, indolent disease is usually curable without antifungal agents by endoscopic surgery. Unilateral disease with a mycetoma within the sinus (fungus

Table 60-1

Guidelines for the Diagnosis and Treatment of Selected Upper Respiratory Tract Infections in Adults[a]

Syndrome, Diagnostic Criteria	Treatment Recommendations
Acute sinusitis	

Moderate symptoms (e.g., nasal purulence/congestion or cough) for >7 d *or*	Initial therapy:
	  Amoxicillin, 875 mg PO bid for 10 d *or*
	  TMP-SMX, 1 DS tablet PO bid for 10 d

Severe symptoms (any duration), including unilateral/focal facial swelling or tooth pain	Exposure to antibiotics within 30 d:
	  Amoxicillin, 1000 mg PO bid for 10 d *or*
	  Amoxicillin/clavulanate, 875 mg PO bid for 10 d *or*
	  Antipneumococcal fluoroquinolone (e.g., levofloxacin, 500 mg PO qd) for 7 d

	Recent treatment failure:
	  Amoxicillin (1500 mg) *plus* clavulanate (125 mg) PO bid for 10 d
	  or
	  Amoxicillin (1500 mg) *plus* clindamycin (300 mg qid) PO for 10 d
	  or
	  Antipneumococcal fluoroquinolone (e.g., levofloxacin, 500 mg PO qd) for 7 d

Acute pharyngitis	
Clinical suspicion of streptococcal pharyngitis (e.g., fever, tonsillar swelling, exudate, enlarged/tender anterior cervical lymph nodes, absence of cough or coryza)[b] *with* History of rheumatic fever *or* Documented household exposure *or* Positive rapid strep screen	Penicillin V, 500 mg PO bid for 10 d *or* Cephalexin, 250 mg PO qid for 10 d *or* Erythromycin, 250 mg PO qid for 10 d *or* Benzathine penicillin G, single dose of 1.2 million units IM

Acute otitis media

Fluid in middle ear, evidenced by decreased tympanic membrane mobility, air/fluid level behind tympanic membrane, bulging tympanic membrane, purulent otorrhea *and*

Signs and symptoms of middle-ear disease, including fever, irritability, otalgia, decreased hearing, tinnitus, vertigo

Initial therapy[c]:

Amoxicillin, 90 mg/kg per day (up to 2 g) PO in divided doses (bid or tid) *or*

Amoxicillin, 90 mg/kg per day (up to 2 g), *plus* clavulanate, 6.4 mg/kg per day; both PO in divided doses (bid) *or*

Cefdinir, 14 mg/kg PO qd *or*

Clindamycin, 20 mg/kg per day PO in divided doses (tid), *plus* TMP-SMX, 10 mg/kg per day PO in divided doses (bid)

Exposure to antibiotics within 30 d or recent treatment failure:

Amoxicillin, 90 mg/kg per day (up to 2 g), *plus* clavulanate, 6.4 mg/kg per day; both PO in divided doses (bid) for 10 d *or*

Cefdinir, 14 mg/kg PO qd for 10 d *or*

Ceftriaxone, 50 mg/kg IM qd for 3 d *or*

Consider myringotomy

[a] For detailed information regarding diagnosis and treatment in children, see Table 27-1 in HPIM-16.

[b] Some organizations support treating adults with these symptoms and signs without the need for rapid streptococcal antigen testing.

[c] Duration: 5–7 d (with consideration of observation only in previously healthy individuals with mild disease).

Note: DS, double-strength; TMP-SMX, trimethoprim-sulfamethoxazole.

Source: RJ Cooper et al: Ann Intern Med 134:509, 2001; JM Hickner et al: Ann Intern Med 134:498, 2001; KL O'Brien et al: Pediatrics 101:174, 1998; SF Dowell et al: Pediatrics 101:165, 1998; B Schwartz et al: Pediatrics 101:171, 1998.

ball) is treated with surgery and—if bony erosion has occurred—antifungal agents. Allergic fungal sinusitis is seen in pts with nasal polyps and asthma.

INFECTIONS OF THE EAR AND MASTOID
External Ear Infections

• *Auricular cellulitis*: Tenderness, erythema, and swelling of the external ear, particularly the lobule, follow minor trauma. Warm compresses are applied, and antibiotics active against *S. aureus* and streptococci (e.g., dicloxacillin) are given.

• *Perichondritis*: Infection of the perichondrium of the auricular cartilage follows minor trauma (e.g., ear piercing). Treatment should be directed at the most common etiologic agents, *P. aeruginosa* and *S. aureus*, and may consist of an antipseudomonal penicillin or a penicillinase-resistant penicillin (e.g., nafcillin) plus an antipseudomonal quinolone (e.g., ciprofloxacin). Surgical drainage may be needed; resolution can take weeks.

• *Otitis externa*

1. *Acute localized otitis externa*, furunculosis in the outer third of the ear canal, is usually due to *S. aureus*.

2. *Acute diffuse otitis externa* is known as "swimmer's ear." *P. aeruginosa* or other gram-negative or gram-positive bacteria cause infection in macerated, irritated canals. Pts have severe pain, erythema and swelling of the canal, and white clumpy discharge from the ear. Treatment includes cleansing of the canal and use of topical antibiotics (e.g., preparations with neomycin and polymyxin), with or without glucocorticoids, to reduce inflammation.

3. *Chronic otitis externa* usually arises from persistent drainage from a chronic middle-ear infection, repeated irritation, or rare chronic infections such as tuberculosis or leprosy. Pts have pruritus rather than pain. Treatment is directed against the offending process; resolution is difficult.

4. *Malignant* or *necrotizing otitis externa* is an aggressive, potentially life-threatening disease occurring primarily in elderly diabetic or immunocompromised pts. The disease progresses over weeks to months. Severe otalgia and purulent otorrhea and erythema of the ear and canal are evident. On exam, granulation tissue in the posteroinferior wall of the canal, near the junction of bone and cartilage, is seen. Untreated, this condition has a high mortality rate and can involve the base of the skull, meninges, cranial nerves, and brain. *P. aeruginosa* is the most common etiologic agent, but other gram-negative bacilli, *S. aureus*, *Staphylococcus epidermidis*, and *Aspergillus* can also cause the disease. Biopsy should be performed for diagnostic purposes. IV antipseudomonal agents (e.g., piperacillin, ceftazidime) with an aminoglycoside or fluoroquinolone plus antibiotic drops active against *Pseudomonas* should be given along with glucocorticoids.

Middle Ear Infections

Eustachian tube dysfunction, often in association with URIs, causes sterile inflammation. Infection results when viral or bacterial superinfection occurs.

• *Acute otitis media*: A viral URI can cause otitis media or predispose to bacterial otitis media. *S. pneumoniae* is the most common bacterial cause; next in frequency are nontypable *H. influenzae* and *M. catarrhalis*. Pts have fluid in the middle ear. The tympanic membrane is immobile, erythematous, and bulging or retracted and can perforate spontaneously. Other findings include otalgia, otorrhea, decreased hearing, fever, and irritability. Most cases resolve within 1 week without treatment. U.S. physicians usually prescribe antibiotics at presentation. However, pts with mild to moderate disease will do well if treated with analgesia and anti-inflammatory agents initially, with antibiotics reserved for pts who do not improve in 2–3 days. Amoxicillin remains the drug of choice, despite rising antibiotic resistance. See Table 60-1 for treatment options.

• *Serous otitis media*: Otitis media with effusion can persist for months without signs of infection. Antibiotic therapy or myringotomy with tympanostomy tubes is reserved for pts with bilateral effusions that have persisted for at least 3 months and are associated with bilateral hearing loss.

• *Chronic otitis media*: persistent or recurrent purulent otorrhea with tympanic membrane perforation. Active disease may lead to erosion of bone, meningitis, and brain abscess and is treated surgically. Inactive disease is treated with repeated courses of topical antibiotic drops during periods of drainage.

• *Mastoiditis* has been uncommon in the antibiotic era. Mastoid air cells connect with the middle ear, and purulent exudates can cause erosion of surrounding bone and abscess-like cavities. Pts have pain, erythema, and mastoid process swelling along with the signs and symptoms of otitis media. Rare complications include subperiosteal abscess, deep neck abscess, and septic thrombosis of the lateral sinus. Cultures should be performed and used to direct therapy.

INFECTIONS OF THE PHARYNX AND ORAL CAVITY
Acute Pharyngitis

• *Viral*: Respiratory viruses typically cause mild disease associated with nonspecific URI symptoms, tender cervical adenopathy, and minimal fever. Influenza virus and adenovirus can cause severe exudative pharyngitis with fever. Herpes simplex virus (HSV) causes pharyngeal inflammation and exudates with vesicles and ulcers on the palate. Coxsackievirus A causes small vesicles on the soft palate and uvula that form shallow white ulcers. EBV and CMV cause exudative pharyngitis in association with other signs of infectious mononucleosis. HIV causes fever, myalgias, malaise, and sometimes a maculopapular rash.

• *Bacterial*: Group A *Streptococcus* (GAS) accounts for ~5–15% of cases of pharyngitis in adults but is primarily a disease of children 5–15 years old. Other bacterial causes include streptococci of groups C and G, *Neisseria gonorrhoeae*, *Corynebacterium diphtheriae*, and anaerobic bacteria. Streptococcal pharyngitis ranges from mild disease to profound pharyngeal pain, fever, chills, abdominal pain, and a hyperemic pharyngeal membrane with tonsillar hypertrophy and exudates. Coryzal symptoms are absent. The diagnosis is made by rapid antigen-detection testing for GAS. Most experts recommend that children have a throat culture performed if rapid testing is negative, but this course is not recommended for adults because of the low incidence of disease. For treatment options, see Table 60-1 and Chap. 95.

Oral Infections

Oral-labial herpesvirus infections and oral thrush caused by *Candida* are discussed in Chaps. 107 and 113, respectively.

INFECTIONS OF THE LARYNX AND EPIGLOTTIS

• *Laryngitis*: a common syndrome caused by nearly all the major respiratory viruses and only rarely by bacteria (e.g., GAS, *C. diphtheriae*, and *M. catarrhalis*). Pts are hoarse, exhibit reduced vocal pitch or aphonia, and have coryzal symptoms. Treatment consists of humidification, voice rest, and—if GAS is cultured—antibiotic administration.

• *Croup*: viral disease marked by swelling of the subglottic region and primarily affecting children <6 years old

• *Epiglottitis*: acute, rapidly progressive cellulitis of the epiglottis and adjacent structures. Vaccination against *H. influenzae* type b has reduced disease rates among children by >90%, but the incidence among adults is stable. Epiglottitis in adults is caused by GAS, *S. pneumoniae*, *Haemophilus parainfluenzae*, and *S. aureus*. Symptoms include fever, severe sore throat, and systemic toxicity, and pts sometimes drool while sitting forward. Signs of respiratory obstruction may develop and progress rapidly. Adolescents and adults have less acute presentations than children. Examination may reveal respiratory distress, inspiratory stridor, and chest wall retractions. Direct fiberoptic laryngoscopy in a controlled environment (e.g., an operating room) may be performed for diagnosis, procurement of specimens for culture, and placement of an endotracheal tube. Treatment focuses on protection of the airway. Blood and, in some cases, the epiglottis should be cultured; after samples are obtained, IV antibiotics active against *H. influenzae* (e.g., ampicillin/sulbactam or a second- or third-generation cephalosporin) should be given for 7–10 days.

INFECTIONS OF DEEP NECK STRUCTURES

These infections, which include Ludwig's angina, Lemierre's syndrome, and retropharyngeal abscess, are discussed in Chap. 100.

For a more detailed discussion, see Rubin MA et al: Infections of the Upper Respiratory Tract, Chap. 27, p. 185, in HPIM-16.

61

GENERAL EXAMINATION OF THE SKIN

As dermatologic evaluation relies heavily on the objective cutaneous appearance, physical examination is often performed prior to taking a complete history in pts presenting with a skin problem. A differential diagnosis can usually be generated on the basis of a thorough examination with precise descriptions of the skin lesion(s) and narrowed with pertinent facts from the history. Laboratory or diagnostic procedures are then used, when appropriate, to clarify the diagnosis.

PHYSICAL EXAMINATION

Examination of skin should take place in a well-illuminated room with pt completely disrobed. Helpful ancillary equipment includes a hand lens and a pocket flashlight to provide peripheral illumination of lesions. The examination often begins with an assessment of the entire skin viewed at a distance, which is then narrowed down to focus on the individual lesions.

DISTRIBUTION   As illustrated in Fig. 61-1, the distribution of skin lesions can provide valuable clues to the identification of the disorder: Generalized (systemic diseases); sun-exposed (SLE, photoallergic, phototoxic, polymorphous light eruption, porphyria cutanea tarda); dermatomal (herpes zoster); extensor surfaces (elbows and knees in psoriasis); flexural surfaces (antecubital and popliteal fossae in atopic dermatitis).

ARRANGEMENT AND SHAPE   Can describe individual or multiple lesions.

Linear [contact dermatitis such as poison ivy, lesions that appear at sites of local skin trauma (Koebner phenomenon)]; *annular*—"ring-shaped" lesion with an active border and central clearing (erythema chronicum migrans, erythema annulare centrificum, tinea corporis); *iris* or *target lesion*—two or three concentric circles of differing hue (erythema multiforme); *circinate*—circular lesion (urticaria, herald patch of pityriasis rosea); *nummular*—"coin-shaped" (nummular eczema); *guttate*—droplike (guttate psoriasis); *morbilliform*—"measles-like" with small confluent papules coalescing into unusual shapes (measles, drug eruption); *reticulated*—"netlike" (livedo reticularis); *herpetiform*—grouped vesicles, papules, or erosions (herpes simplex).

PRIMARY LESIONS   Cutaneous changes caused directly by disease process.

Macule—a flat circumscribed lesion of a different color, allowing for differentiation from surrounding skin; *patch*—macule >2 cm in diameter; *papule*—elevated, circumscribed lesion of any color <1 cm in diameter, with the major portion of lesion projecting above surrounding skin; *nodule*—palpable lesion similar to a papule but >1 cm in diameter; *plaque*—an elevated, flat-topped lesion >1 cm in diameter; *vesicle*—sharply marginated elevated lesion <1 cm in diameter filled with clear fluid; *bulla*—vesicular lesion >1 cm in diameter; *pustule*—a well-marginated focal accumulation of inflammatory cells within skin; *wheal*—a transient elevated lesion due to accumulation of fluid in upper dermis; *cyst*—lesion consisting of liquid or semisolid material contained within limits of cyst wall (true cyst).

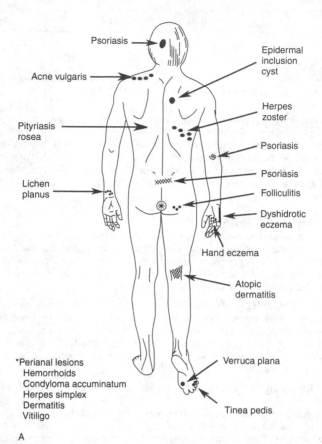

Psoriasis

Epidermal
inclusion
cyst

Acne vulgaris

Herpes
zoster

Pityriasis
rosea

Psoriasis

Psoriasis

Lichen
planus

Folliculitis

Dyshidrotic
eczema

Hand eczema

Atopic
dermatitis

*Perianal lesions
Hemorrhoids
Condyloma accuminatum
Herpes simplex
Dermatitis
Vitiligo

Verruca plana

Tinea pedis

A

FIGURE 61-1 The distribution of some common dermatologic diseases and lesions.

SECONDARY LESIONS Changes in area of primary pathology often due to secondary events, e.g., scratching, secondary infection, bleeding.

Scale—a flaky accumulation of excess keratin that is partially adherent to skin; *crust*—a circumscribed collection of inflammatory cells and dried serum on skin surface; *excoriation*—linear, angular erosions caused by scratching; *erosion*—a circumscribed, usually depressed, moist lesion resulting from loss of overlying epidermis; *ulcer*—a deeper erosion involving epidermis plus underlying papillary dermis; may leave a scar on healing; *atrophy*: (1) epidermal—thinning of skin with loss of normal skin surface markings, (2) dermal—depression of skin surface due to loss of underlying collagen or dermal ground substance; *lichenification*—thickening of skin with accentuation of normal skin surface markings most commonly due to chronic rubbing; *scar*—collection of fibrous tissue replacing normal dermal constituents.

OTHER DESCRIPTIVE TERMS Color, e.g., violaceous, erythematous; physical characteristics, e.g., warm, tender; sharpness of edge, surface contour—flat-topped, pedunculated (on a stalk), verrucous (wartlike), umbilicated (containing a central depression).

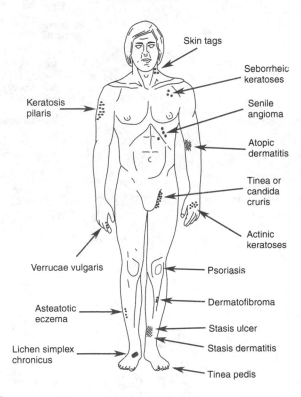

B

FIGURE 61-1 *(Continued)*

HISTORY

A complete history should be obtained, with special attention being paid to the following points:

1. Evolution of the lesion—site of onset, manner in which eruption progressed or spread, duration, periods of resolution or improvement in chronic eruptions
2. Symptoms associated with the eruption—itching, burning, pain, numbness; what has relieved symptoms; time of day when symptoms are most severe
3. Current or recent medications—both prescription and over-the-counter
4. Associated systemic symptoms (e.g., malaise, fatigue, arthralgias)
5. Ongoing or previous illnesses
6. History of allergies
7. Presence of photosensitivity
8. Review of systems

ADDITIONAL DIAGNOSTIC PROCEDURES

POTASSIUM HYDROXIDE PREPARATION Useful for detection of dermatophyte or yeast. Scale is collected from advancing edge of a scaling lesion by gently scraping with side of a microscope slide. Nail lesions are best sampled by trimming back nail and scraping subungual debris. A drop of 10–

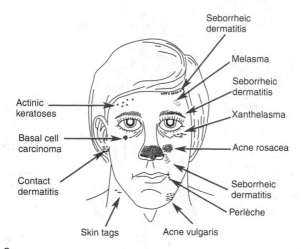

C

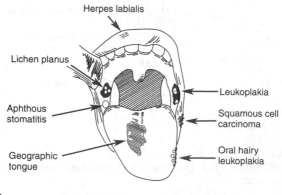

D

FIGURE 61-1 *(Continued)*

15% potassium hydroxide is added to slide, and coverslip is applied. The slide may be gently heated and examined under microscope. Positive preparations show translucent, septate branching hyphae among keratinocytes.

TZANCK PREPARATION   Useful for determining presence of herpes viruses. Optimal lesion to sample is an early vesicle. Lesion is gently unroofed with no. 15 scalpel blade, and base of vesicle is gently scraped with belly of blade (keep blade perpendicular to skin surface to prevent laceration). Scrapings are transferred to slide and stained with Wright's or Giemsa stain. A positive preparation has multinucleate giant cells.

SKIN BIOPSY   Minor surgical procedure. Choice of site very important.

DIASCOPY   Assesses whether a lesion blanches with pressure. Done by pressing a magnifying lens or microscope slide on lesion and observing changes in vascularity. For example, hemangiomas will usually blanch; purpuric lesions will not.

WOOD'S LIGHT EXAMINATION Useful for detecting bacterial or fungal infection or accentuating features of some skin lesions.

PATCH TESTS To document cutaneous sensitivity to specific antigens.

For a more detailed discussion, see Lawley TJ, Yancey KB: Approach to the Patient with a Skin Disorder, Chap. 46, p. 283, in HPIM-16.

62

COMMON SKIN CONDITIONS

PAPULOSQUAMOUS DISORDERS
Disorders exhibiting papules and scale.

PSORIASIS A chronic, recurrent disorder. Classic lesion is a well-marginated, erythematous plaque with silvery-white surface scale. Distribution includes extensor surfaces (i.e., knees, elbows, and buttocks); may also involve palms and scalp (particularly anterior scalp margin). Associated findings include psoriatic arthritis (Chap. 164) and nail changes (onycholysis, pitting or thickening of nail plate with accumulation of subungual debris).

 TREATMENT

Maintain cutaneous hydration; topical glucocorticoids; topical vitamin D analogue (calcipotriol) and retinoid (tazarotene); UV light (PUVA when UV used in combination with psoralens); for severe disease methotrexate or cyclosporine; acitretin can also be used but is teratogenic. Efalizumab (humanized monoclonal antibody directed against CD11a) or alefacept (dimeric fusion protein: LFA-3/Fc human IgG1) can be considered for chronic moderate to severe plaque psoriasis. Etanercept (dimeric fusion protein: TNF receptor/Fc human IgG1) is approved for psoriatic arthritis and is being studied in psoriasis.

PITYRIASIS ROSEA A self-limited condition lasting 3–8 weeks. Initially, there is a single 2- to 6-cm annular salmon-colored patch (herald patch) with a peripheral rim of scale, followed in days to weeks by a generalized eruption involving the trunk and proximal extremities. Individual lesions are similar to but smaller than the herald patch and are arranged in symmetric fashion with long axis of each individual lesion along skin lines of cleavage. Appearance may be similar to that of secondary syphilis.

 TREATMENT

Disorder is self-limited, so treatment is directed at symptoms; oral antihistamines for pruritus; topical glucocorticoids; UV-B phototherapy in some cases.

LICHEN PLANUS Disorder of unknown cause; can follow administration of certain drugs and in chronic graft-versus-host disease; lesions are pruritic, polygonal, flat-topped, and violaceous. Course is variable, but most pts have spontaneous remissions 6–24 months after onset of disease.

 TREATMENT

Topical glucocorticoids.

ECZEMATOUS DISORDERS

ECZEMA Eczema, or dermatitis, is a reaction pattern that presents with variable clinical and histologic findings; it is the final common expression for a number of disorders.

ATOPIC DERMATITIS One aspect of atopic triad of hayfever, asthma, and eczema. Usually an intermittent, chronic, severely pruritic, eczematous dermatitis with scaly erythematous patches, vesiculation, crusting, and fissuring. Lesions are most commonly on flexures, with prominent involvement of antecubital and popliteal fossae; generalized erythroderma in severe cases. Most pts with atopic dermatitis are chronic carriers of *Staphylococcus aureus* in anterior nares and on skin.

 TREATMENT

Avoidance of irritants; cutaneous hydration; topical glucocorticoids; treatment of infected lesions. Systemic glucocorticoids only for severe exacerbations unresponsive to topical conservative therapy.

ALLERGIC CONTACT DERMATITIS A delayed hypersensitivity reaction that occurs after cutaneous exposure to an antigenic substance. Lesions occur at site of contact and are vesicular, weeping, crusting; linear arrangement of vesicles is common. Most frequent allergens are resin from plants of the *Rhus* (or *Toxicodendron*) genus (poison ivy, oak, sumac), nickel, rubber, and cosmetics.

 TREATMENT

Avoidance of sensitizing agent; topical glucocorticoids; consideration of systemic glucocorticoids over 2–3 weeks for widespread disease.

IRRITANT CONTACT DERMATITIS Inflammation of the skin due to direct injury by an exogenous agent. The most common area of involvement is the hands, where dermatitis is initiated or aggravated by chronic exposure to water and detergents. Features may include skin dryness, cracking, erythema, edema.

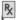 **TREATMENT**

Avoidance of irritants; barriers (use of vinyl gloves); topical glucocorticoids; treatment of secondary bacterial or dermatophyte infection.

SEBORRHEIC DERMATITIS A chronic noninfectious process characterized by erythematous patches with greasy yellowish scale. Lesions are gen-

erally on scalp, eyebrows, nasolabial folds, axillae, central chest, and posterior
auricular area.

 TREATMENT

Nonfluorinated topical glucocorticoids; shampoos containing coal tar, salicylic acid, or selenium sulfide.

INFECTIONS

IMPETIGO   A superficial infection of skin secondary to either *S. aureus*
or group A β-hemolytic streptococci. The primary lesion is a superficial pustule
that ruptures and forms a "honey-colored" crust. Tense bullae are associated
with *S. aureus* infections (bullous impetigo). Lesions may occur anywhere but
commonly involve the face.

 TREATMENT

Gentle debridement of adherent crusts with soaks and topical antibiotics; appropriate oral antibiotics depending on organism (Chap. 83).

ERYSIPELAS   Superficial cellulitis, most commonly on face, characterized by a bright red, sharply demarcated, intensely painful, warm plaque. Because of superficial location of infection and associated edema, surface of plaque
may exhibit a *peau d'orange* (orange peel) appearance. Most commonly due to
infection with group A β-hemolytic streptococci, occurring at sites of trauma
or other breaks in skin.

 TREATMENT

Appropriate antibiotics depending on organism (Chap. 83).

HERPES SIMPLEX   (See also Chap. 107)   Recurrent eruption characterized by grouped vesicles on an erythematous base that progress to erosions;
often secondarily infected with staphylococci or streptococci. Infections frequently involve mucocutaneous surfaces around the oral cavity, genitals, or
anus. Can also cause severe visceral disease including esophagitis, pneumonitis,
encephalitis, and disseminated herpes simplex virus infection. Tzanck preparation of an unroofed early vesicle reveals multinucleate giant cells.

 TREATMENT

Will differ based on disease manifestations and level of immune competence
(Chap. 107); appropriate antibiotics for secondary infections, depending on
organism.

HERPES ZOSTER   (See also Chap. 107)   Eruption of grouped vesicles
on an erythematous base usually limited to a single dermatome ("shingles");
disseminated lesions can also occur, especially in immunocompromised pts.
Tzanck preparation reveals multinucleate giant cells; indistinguishable from herpes simplex except by culture. Postherpetic neuralgia, lasting months to years,
may occur, especially in the elderly.

TREATMENT

Will differ based on disease manifestations and level of immune competence (Chap. 107).

DERMATOPHYTE INFECTION   Skin fungus, may involve any area of body; due to infection of stratum corneum, nail plate, or hair. Appearance may vary from mild scaliness to florid inflammatory dermatitis. Common sites of infection include the foot (tinea pedis), nails (tinea unguium), groin (tinea cruris), or scalp (tinea capitis). Classic lesion of tinea corporis ("ringworm") is an erythematous papulosquamous patch, often with central clearing and scale along peripheral advancing border. Hyphae are often seen on KOH preparation, although tinea capitis and tinea corporis may require culture or biopsy.

 TREATMENT

Depends on affected site and type of infection. Topical imidazoles, triazoles, and allylamines may be effective. Haloprogin, undecylenic acid, ciclopiroxolamine, and tolnaftate are also effective, but nystatin is not active against dermatophytes. Griseofulvin, 500 mg/d, if systemic therapy required. Itraconazole or terbinafine may be effective for nail infections.

CANDIDIASIS   Fungal infection caused by a related group of yeasts. Manifestations may be localized to the skin or rarely systemic and life-threatening. Predisposing factors include diabetes mellitus, cellular immune deficiencies, and HIV (Chap. 91). Frequent sites include the oral cavity, chronically wet macerated areas, around nails, intertriginous areas. Diagnosed by clinical pattern and demonstration of yeast on KOH preparation or culture.

 TREATMENT

(See also Chap. 113) Removal of predisposing factors; topical nystatin or azoles; systemic therapy reserved for immunosuppressed patients, unresponsive chronic or recurrent disease; vulvovaginal candidiasis may respond to a single dose of fluconazole, 150 mg.

WARTS   Cutaneous neoplasms caused by human papilloma viruses (HPVs). Typically dome-shaped lesions with irregular filamentous surface. Propensity for the face, arms, and legs; often spread by shaving. HPVs are also associated with genital or perianal lesions and play a role in the development of neoplasia of the uterine cervix and external genitalia in females (Chap. 88).

 TREATMENT

Cryotherapy with liquid nitrogen, keratinolytic agents (salicylic acid). For genital warts, application of podophyllin solution is effective but can be associated with marked local reactions; topical imiquinod has also been used.

ACNE

ACNE VULGARIS   Usually a self-limited disorder of teenagers and young adults. Comedones (small cyst formed in hair follicle) are clinical hallmark; often accompanied by inflammatory lesions of papules, pustules, or nodules. May scar in severe cases.

TREATMENT

Careful cleaning and removal of oils; oral tetracycline or erythromycin; topical antibacterials (e.g., benzoyl peroxide), topical retinoic acid. Systemic isotretinoin only for unresponsive severe nodulocystic acne (risk of severe adverse events including teratogenicity and possible association with depression).

ACNE ROSACEA   Inflammatory disorder affecting predominantly the central face, rarely affecting pts <30 years of age. Tendency toward exaggerated flushing, with eventual superimposition of papules, pustules, and telangiectases. May lead to rhinophyma and ocular problems.

 TREATMENT

Oral tetracycline, 250–1000 mg/d; topical metronidazole and topical non-fluorinated glucocorticoids may be useful.

VASCULAR DISORDERS

ERYTHEMA NODOSUM   Septal panniculitis characterized by erythematous, warm, tender subcutaneous nodular lesions typically over anterior tibia. Lesions are usually flush with skin surface but are indurated and have appearance of an erythematous/violaceous bruise. Lesions usually resolve spontaneously in 3–6 weeks without scarring. Commonly seen in sarcoidosis, treatment with some drugs (esp. sulfonamides, oral contraceptives, and estrogens), and a wide range of infections including streptococcal and tubercular; may be idiopathic.

 TREATMENT

Identification and treatment/removal of underlying cause. NSAID for severe or recurrent lesions; systemic glucocorticoids are effective but dangerous if underlying infection is not appreciated.

ERYTHEMA MULTIFORME   A reaction pattern of skin consisting of a variety of lesions but most commonly erythematous papules and bullae. "Target" or "iris" lesion is characteristic and consists of concentric circles of erythema and normal flesh-colored skin, often with a central vesicle or bulla.

Distribution of lesions classically acral, esp. palms and soles. Three most common causes are drug reaction (particularly penicillins and sulfonamides) or concurrent herpetic or *Mycoplasma* infection. Can rarely affect mucosal surfaces and internal organs (erythema multiforme major or Stevens-Johnson syndrome).

 TREATMENT

Provocative agent should be sought and eliminated if drug-related. In mild cases limited to skin, only symptomatic treatment is needed (antihistamines, NSAID). For Stevens-Johnson, systemic glucocorticoids are controversial; prevention of secondary infection and maintenance of nutrition and fluid/electrolyte balance are critical.

URTICARIA   A common disorder, either acute or chronic, characterized by evanescent (individual lesions lasting <24 h), pruritic, edematous, pink to erythematous plaques with a whitish halo around margin of individual lesions.

Lesions range in size from papules to giant coalescent lesions (10–20 cm in diameter). Often due to drugs, systemic infection, or foods (esp. shellfish). Food additives such as tartrazine dye (FD & C yellow no. 5), benzoate, or salicylates have also been implicated. If individual lesions last >24 h, consider diagnosis of urticarial vasculitis.

 TREATMENT   See Chap. 159.

VASCULITIS   Palpable purpura (nonblanching, elevated lesions) is the cutaneous hallmark of vasculitis. Other lesions include petechiae (esp. early lesions), necrosis with ulceration, bullae, and urticarial lesions (urticarial vasculitis). Lesions usually most prominent on lower extremities. Associations include infections, collagen-vascular disease, primary systemic vasculitides, malignancy, hepatitis B and C, drugs (esp. thiazides), and inflammatory bowel disease. May occur as an idiopathic, predominantly cutaneous vasculitis.

 TREATMENT

Will differ based on cause. Pursue identification and treatment/elimination of an exogenous cause or underlying disease. If part of a systemic vasculitis, treat based on major organ-threatening features (Chap. 162). Immunosuppressive therapy should be avoided in idiopathic predominantly cutaneous vasculitis as disease frequently does not respond and rarely causes irreversible organ system dysfunction.

CUTANEOUS DRUG REACTIONS

Cutaneous reactions are among the most frequent medication toxicities. These can have a wide range of severity and manifestations including urticaria, photosensitivity, erythema multiforme, fixed drug reactions, erythema nodosum, vasculitis, lichenoid reactions, bullous drug reactions, Stevens-Johnson syndrome, and toxic epidermal necrolysis (TEN). Diagnosis is usually made by appearance and careful medication history.

 TREATMENT

Withdrawal of the medication. Treatment based on nature and severity of cutaneous pathology.

For a more detailed discussion, see McCall CO, Lawley TJ: *Eczema, Psoriasis, Cutaneous Infections, Acne, and Other Common Skin Disorders*, Chap. 47, p. 288; Chosidow OM, Stern RS, Wintroub BU: *Cutaneous Drug Reactions*, Chap. 50, p. 318; and Bolognia JL, Braverman IM: *Skin Manifestations of Internal Disease*, Chap. 48, p. 296, in HPIM-16.

63

EXAMINATION OF BLOOD SMEARS AND BONE MARROW

BLOOD SMEARS
Erythrocyte (RBC) Morphology

- Normal: 7.5-μm diameter.
- *Reticulocytes* (Wright's stain)—large, grayish-blue, admixed with pink (polychromasia).
- *Anisocytosis*—variation in RBC size; large cells imply delay in erythroid precursor DNA synthesis caused by folate or B_{12} deficiency or drug effect; small cells imply a defect in hemoglobin synthesis caused by iron deficiency or abnormal hemoglobin genes.
- *Poikilocytosis*—abnormal RBC shapes; the following are examples:

  1. *Acanthocytes* (spur cells)—irregularly spiculated; abetalipoproteinemia, severe liver disease, rarely anorexia nervosa.
  2. *Echinocytes* (burr cells)—regularly shaped, uniformly distributed spiny projections; uremia, RBC volume loss.
  3. *Elliptocytes*—elliptical; hereditary elliptocytosis.
  4. *Schistocytes* (schizocytes)—fragmented cells of varying sizes and shapes; microangiopathic or macroangiopathic hemolytic anemia.
  5. *Sickled cells*—elongated, crescentic; sickle cell anemias.
  6. *Spherocytes*—small hyperchromic cells lacking normal central pallor; hereditary spherocytosis, extravascular hemolysis as in autoimmune hemolytic anemia, G6PD deficiency.
  7. *Target cells*—central and outer rim staining with intervening ring of pallor; liver disease, thalassemia, hemoglobin C and sickle C diseases.
  8. *Teardrop cells*—myelofibrosis, other infiltrative processes of marrow (e.g., carcinoma).
  9. *Rouleaux formation*—alignment of RBCs in stacks; may be artifactual or due to paraproteinemia (e.g., multiple myeloma, macroglobulinemia).

RBC Inclusions

- *Howell-Jolly bodies*—1-μm diameter basophilic cytoplasmic inclusion that represents a residual nuclear fragment, usually single; asplenic pts.
- *Basophilic stippling*—multiple, punctate basophilic cytoplasmic inclusions composed of precipitated mitochondria and ribosomes; lead poisoning, thalassemia, myelofibrosis.
- *Pappenheimer (iron) bodies*—iron-containing granules usually composed of mitochondria and ribosomes resemble basophilic stippling but also stain with Prussian blue; lead poisoning, other sideroblastic anemias.
- *Heinz bodies*—spherical inclusions of precipitated hemoglobin seen only with supravital stains, such as crystal violet; G6PD deficiency (after oxidant stress such as infection, certain drugs), unstable hemoglobin variants.
- *Parasites*—characteristic intracytoplasmic inclusions; malaria, babesiosis.

Leukocyte Inclusions and Nuclear Contour Abnormalities

- *Toxic granulations*—dark cytoplasmic granules; bacterial infection.
- *Döhle bodies*—1- to 2-μm blue, oval cytoplasmic inclusions; bacterial infection, Chédiak-Higashi anomaly.

• *Auer rods*—eosinophilic, rodlike cytoplasmic inclusions; acute myeloid leukemia (some cases).
• *Hypersegmentation*—neutrophil nuclei contain more than the usual 2–4 lobes; usually >5% have ≥5 lobes or a single cell with 7 lobes is adequate to make the diagnosis; folate or B_{12} deficiency, drug effects.
• *Hyposegmentation*—neutrophil nuclei contain fewer lobes than normal, either one or two: Pelger-Hüet anomaly, pseudo-Pelger-Hüet or acquired Pelger-Hüet anomaly in acute leukemia.

Platelet Abnormalities

Platelet clumping—an in vitro artifact—is often readily detectable on smear; can lead to falsely low platelet count by automated cell counters.

BONE MARROW

Aspiration assesses cell morphology. *Biopsy* assesses overall marrow architecture, including degree of cellularity. Biopsy should precede aspiration to avoid aspiration artifact (mainly hemorrhage) in the specimen.

Indications

ASPIRATION Hypoproliferative or unexplained anemia, leukopenia, or thrombocytopenia, suspected leukemia or myeloma or marrow defect, evaluation of iron stores, workup of some cases of fever of unknown origin.

Special Tests Histochemical staining (leukemias), cytogenetic studies (leukemias, lymphomas), microbiology (bacterial, mycobacterial, fungal cultures), Prussian blue (iron) stain (assess iron stores, diagnosis of sideroblastic anemias).

BIOPSY Performed in addition to aspiration for pancytopenia (aplastic anemia), metastatic tumor, granulomatous infection (e.g., mycobacteria, brucellosis, histoplasmosis), myelofibrosis, lipid storage disease (e.g., Gaucher's, Niemann-Pick), any case with "dry tap" on aspiration; evaluation of marrow cellularity.

Special Tests Histochemical staining (e.g., acid phosphatase for metastatic prostate carcinoma), immunoperoxidase staining (e.g., immunoglobulin or cell surface marker detection in multiple myeloma, leukemia, or lymphoma; lysozyme detection in monocytic leukemia), reticulin staining (increased in myelofibrosis), microbiologic staining (e.g., acid-fast staining for mycobacteria).

Interpretation

CELLULARITY Defined as percentage of space occupied by hematopoietic cells. Decreases with age after age 65 years from about 50% to 25–30% with a corresponding increase in fat.

ERYTHROID:GRANULOCYTIC (E:G) RATIO Normally about 1:2, the E:G ratio is decreased in acute and chronic infection, leukemoid reactions (e.g., chronic inflammation, metastatic tumor), acute and chronic myeloid leukemia, myelodysplastic disorders ("preleukemia"), and pure red cell aplasia; increased in agranulocytosis, anemias with erythroid hyperplasia (megaloblastic, iron-deficiency, thalassemia, hemorrhage, hemolysis, sideroblastic), and erythrocytosis (excessive RBC production); normal in aplastic anemia (though marrow hypocellular), myelofibrosis (marrow hypocellular), multiple myeloma, lymphoma, anemia of chronic disease. Some centers use the term M:E (myeloid to erythroid) ratio; normal value is 2:1 and increases with diseases that promote myeloid activity or inhibit erythroid activity and decreases with diseases that inhibit myeloid activity or promote erythroid activity.

For a more detailed discussion, see Adamson JW, Longo DL: Anemia and Polycythemia, Chap. 52, p. 329; and Holland SM, Gallin JI: Disorders of Granulocytes and Monocytes, Chap. 55, p. 349, in HPIM-16.

64

RED BLOOD CELL DISORDERS

Anemia is a common clinical problem in medicine. A physiologic approach to anemia diagnosis (outlined in Chap. 57) provides the most efficient path to diagnosis and management. Anemias arise either because RBC production is inadequate or RBC lifespan is shortened through loss from the circulation or destruction.

HYPOPROLIFERATIVE ANEMIAS

These are the most common anemias encountered in clinical practice. Usually the RBC morphology is normal and the reticulocyte index (RI) is low. Marrow damage, early iron deficiency, and decreased erythropoietin production or action may produce anemia of this type.

Marrow damage may be caused by infiltration of the marrow with tumor or fibrosis that crowds out normal erythroid precursors or by the absence of erythroid precursors (aplastic anemia) as a consequence of exposure to drugs, radiation, chemicals, viruses (e.g., hepatitis), autoimmune mechanisms, or genetic factors, either hereditary (e.g., Fanconi's anemia) or acquired (e.g., paroxysmal nocturnal hemoglobinuria). Most cases of aplasia are idiopathic. The tumor or fibrosis that infiltrates the marrow may originate in the marrow (as in leukemia or myelofibrosis) or be secondary to processes originating outside the marrow (as in metastatic cancer or myelophthisis).

Early iron-deficiency anemia (or iron-deficient erythropoiesis) is associated with a decrease in serum ferritin levels (<15 μg/L), moderately elevated total iron-binding capacity (TIBC) (>380 μg/dL), serum iron (SI) level <50 μg/dL, and an iron saturation of $<30\%$ but $>10\%$ (Fig. 64-1). RBC morphology is generally normal until iron deficiency is severe (see below).

Decreased stimulation of erythropoiesis can be a consequence of inadequate erythropoietin production [e.g., renal disease destroying the renal tubular cells that produce it or hypometabolic states (endocrine deficiency or protein starvation) in which insufficient erythropoietin is produced] or of inadequate erythropoietin action. The anemia of chronic disease is a common entity. It is multifactorial in pathogenesis: inhibition of erythropoietin production, inhibition of iron reutilization (which blocks the response to erythropoietin), and inhibition of erythroid colony proliferation by inflammatory cytokines (e.g., TNF, interferonγ). Hepcidin, a small iron-binding molecule produced by the liver during an acute-phase inflammatory response, may bind iron and prevent its reutili-

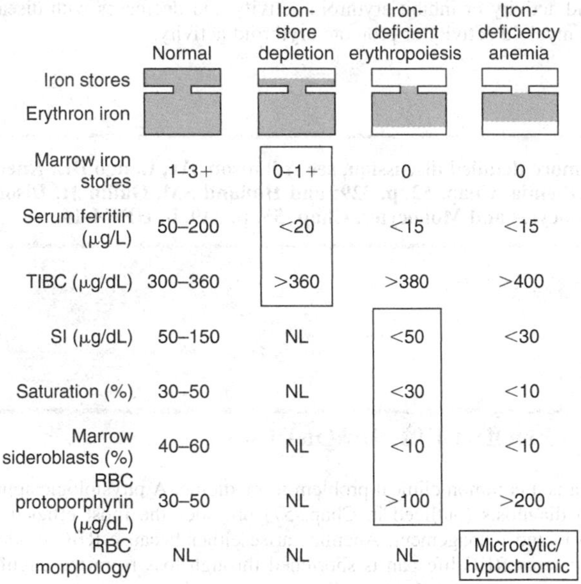

FIGURE 64-1 Laboratory studies in the evolution of iron deficiency. Measurements of marrow iron stores, serum ferritin, and TIBC are sensitive to early iron-store depletion. Iron-deficient erythropoiesis is recognized from additional abnormalities in the SI, percent saturation of transferrin, the pattern of marrow sideroblasts, and the red blood cell protoporphyrin level. Finally, patients with iron-deficiency anemia demonstrate all of these same abnormalities plus an anemia characterized by microcytic hypochromic morphology. (*From RS Hillman, CA Finch: Red Cell Manual, 7th. ed, Philadelphia, Davis, 1996, with permission.*)

Table 64-1

Diagnosis of Hypoproliferative Anemias

Tests	Iron Deficiency	Inflammation	Renal Disease	Hypo-metabolic States
Anemia	Mild to severe	Mild	Mild to severe	Mild
MCV (fL)	70–90	80–90	90	90
Morphology	Normo-microcytic	Normocytic	Normocytic	Normocytic
SI	<30	<50	Normal	Normal
TIBC	>360	>300	Normal	Normal
Saturation (%)	<10	10–20	Normal	Normal
Serum ferritin (μg/L)	<15	30–200	115–150	Normal
Iron stores	0	2–4+	1–4+	Normal

Note: MCV, mean corpuscular volume; SI, serum iron; TIBC, total iron-binding capacity.

Table 64-2

Diagnosis of Microcytic Anemia

Tests	Iron Deficiency	Thalassemia	Sideroblastic Anemia
Smear	Micro/hypo	Micro/hypo with targeting	Variable
SI	<30	Normal to high	Normal to high
TIBC	>360	Normal	Normal
Percent saturation	<10	30–80	30–80
Ferritin (μg/L)	<15	50–300	50–300
Hemoglobin pattern	Normal	Abnormal	Normal

Note: SI, serum iron; TIBC, total iron-binding capacity.

zation in hemoglobin synthesis. The laboratory tests shown in Table 64-1 may assist in the differential diagnosis of hypoproliferative anemias. Measurement of hepcidin in the urine is not yet practical or widely available.

MATURATION DISORDERS

These result from either defective hemoglobin synthesis, leading to cytoplasmic maturation defects and small relatively empty red cells, or abnormally slow DNA replication, leading to nuclear maturation defects and large full red cells. Defects in hemoglobin synthesis usually result from insufficient iron supply (iron deficiency), decreased globin production (thalassemia), or are idiopathic (sideroblastic anemia). Defects in DNA synthesis are usually due to nutritional problems (vitamin B_{12} and folate deficiency), toxic (methotrexate or other cancer chemotherapeutic agent) exposure, or intrinsic marrow maturation defects (refractory anemia, myelodysplasia).

Laboratory tests useful in the differential diagnosis of the microcytic anemias are shown in Table 64-2. Mean corpuscular volume (MCV) is generally 60 to 80 fL. Increased lactic dehydrogenase (LDH) and indirect bilirubin levels suggest an increase in RBC destruction and favor a cause other than iron deficiency. Iron status is best assessed by measuring SI, TIBC, and ferritin levels. Macrocytic MCVs are >94 fL. Folate status is best assessed by measuring red blood cell folate levels. Vitamin B_{12} status is best assessed by measuring serum

Table 64-3

Classifications of Hemolytic Anemias

Intracorpuscular	1. Abnormalities of RBC interior
	  a. Enzyme defects
	  b. Hemoglobinopathies
	2. RBC membrane abnormalities
	  a. Hereditary spherocytosis, etc.
		Hereditary

	b. Paroxysmal nocturnal hemoglobinuria c. Spur cell anemia	

Extracorpuscular	3. Extrinsic factors
	  a. Hypersplenism
	  b. Antibody: immune hemolysis
	  c. Microangiopathic hemolysis
	  d. Infections, toxins, etc.
		Acquired

Table 64-4

Drugs Causing Hemolysis in Subjects Deficient in G6PD

Antimalarials: Primaquine, pamaquine, dapsone
Sulfonamides: Sulfamethoxazole
Nitrofurantoin
Analgesics: Acetanilid
Miscellaneous: Vitamin K (water-soluble form), doxorubicin, methylene blue,
  nalidixic acid, furazolidone, niridazole, phenazopyridine

B_{12}, homocysteine, and methylmalonic acid levels. Homocysteine and methylmalonic acid levels are elevated in the setting of B_{12} deficiency.

ANEMIA DUE TO RBC DESTRUCTION OR ACUTE BLOOD LOSS

BLOOD LOSS Trauma, GI hemorrhage (may be occult) are common causes; less common are genitourinary sources (menorrhagia, gross hematuria), internal bleeding such as intraperitoneal from spleen or organ rupture, retroperitoneal, iliopsoas hemorrhage (e.g., in hip fractures). Acute bleeding is associated with manifestations of hypovolemia, reticulocytosis, macrocytosis; chronic bleeding is associated with iron deficiency, hypochromia, microcytosis.

HEMOLYSIS Causes are listed in Table 64-3.

1. *Intracellular RBC abnormalities*—most are inherited enzyme defects [glucose-6-phosphate dehydrogenase (G6PD) deficiency ≫ pyruvate kinase deficiency], hemoglobinopathies, sickle cell anemia and variants, thalassemia, unstable hemoglobin variants.

2. *G6PD deficiency*—leads to episodes of hemolysis precipitated by ingestion of drugs that induce oxidant stress on RBCs. These include antimalarials (chloroquine), sulfonamides, analgesics (phenacetin), and other miscellaneous drugs (Table 64-4).

3. *Sickle cell anemia*—is characterized by a single amino acid change in β globin (valine for glutamic acid in the 6th residue) that produces a molecule of decreased solubility, especially in the absence of O_2. Although anemia and chronic hemolysis are present, the major disease manifestations relate to vasoocclusion from misshapen sickled RBCs. Infarcts in lung, bone, spleen, retina, brain, and other organs lead to symptoms and dysfunction (Table 64-5).

Table 64-5

Clinical Manifestations of Sickle Cell Anemia

Constitutional
  Impaired growth and development
  Increased susceptibility to infection
Vasoocclusive
  Microinfarcts → Painful crisis
  Macroinfarcts
      Organ damage
Anemia
  Severe hemolysis
  Aplastic crises

Source: See Chap. 107, p. 648 in HPIM-14.

4. *Membrane abnormalities* (rare)—spur cell anemia (cirrhosis, anorexia nervosa), paroxysmal nocturnal hemoglobinuria, hereditary spherocytosis (increased RBC osmotic fragility, spherocytes), hereditary elliptocytosis (causes mild hemolytic anemia).

5. *Immunohemolytic anemia* (positive Coombs' test, spherocytes). Two types: (a) *warm antibody* (usually IgG)—idiopathic, lymphoma, chronic lymphocytic leukemia, SLE, drugs (e.g., methyldopa, penicillins, quinine, quinidine, isoniazid, sulfonamides); and (b) *cold antibody*—cold agglutinin disease (IgM) due to *Mycoplasma* infection, infectious mononucleosis, lymphoma, idiopathic; paroxysmal cold hemoglobinuria (IgG) due to syphilis, viral infections.

6. *Mechanical trauma* (macro- and microangiopathic hemolytic anemias; schistocytes)—prosthetic heart valves, vasculitis, malignant hypertension, eclampsia, renal graft rejection, giant hemangioma, scleroderma, thrombotic thrombocytopenic purpura, hemolytic-uremic syndrome, DIC, march hemoglobinuria (e.g., marathon runners, bongo drummers).

7. *Direct toxic effect*—infections (e.g., malaria, *Clostridium welchii* toxin, toxoplasmosis).

8. *Hypersplenism* (pancytopenia may be present).

LABORATORY ABNORMALITIES   Elevated reticulocyte index, polychromasia and nucleated RBCs on smear; also spherocytes, elliptocytes, schistocytes, or target, spur, or sickle cells may be present depending on disorder; elevated unconjugated serum bilirubin and LDH, elevated plasma hemoglobin, low or absent haptoglobin; urine hemosiderin present in intravascular but not extravascular hemolysis, Coombs' test (immunohemolytic anemias), osmotic fragility test (hereditary spherocytosis), hemoglobin electrophoresis (sickle cell anemia, thalassemia), G6PD assay (best performed after resolution of hemolytic episode to prevent false-negative result).

 TREATMENT

General Approaches   The acuteness and severity of the anemia determine whether transfusion therapy with packed RBCs is indicated. Rapid occurrence of severe anemia (e.g., after acute GI hemorrhage resulting in Hct < 25%, following volume repletion) is an indication for transfusion. Hct should increase 3 to 4% [Hb by 10 g/L (1 g/dL)] with each unit of packed RBCs, assuming no ongoing losses. Chronic anemia (e.g., vitamin B_{12} deficiency), even when severe, may not require transfusion therapy if the pt is compensated and specific therapy (e.g., vitamin B_{12}) is instituted.

Specific Disorders

1. *Iron deficiency*: find and treat cause of blood loss, oral iron (e.g., $FeSO_4$ 300 mg tid).
2. *Folate deficiency*: common in malnourished, alcoholics; less common now than before folate food supplementation; folic acid 1 mg PO qd (5 mg qd for pts with malabsorption).
3. *Vitamin B_{12} deficiency*: can be managed either with parenteral vitamin B_{12} 100 μg IM qd for 7 d, then 100–1000 μg IM per month or 2 mg oral crystalline vitamin B_{12} per day.
4. *Anemia of chronic disease*: treat underlying disease; in uremia use recombinant human erythropoietin, 50–150 U/kg three times a week; role of erythropoietin in other forms of anemia of chronic disease is less clear; response more likely if serum erythropoietin levels are low.
5. *Sickle cell anemia*: hydroxyurea (antisickling) 10–30 mg/kg per day PO, treat infections early, supplemental folic acid; painful crises treated with oxygen, analgesics, hydration, and hypertransfusion; consider allogeneic bone marrow transplantation in pts with increasing frequency of crises.

6. *Thalassemia*: transfusion to maintain Hb > 90 g/L (>9 g/dL), folic acid, prevention of Fe overload with deferoximine chelation; consider splenectomy and allogeneic bone marrow transplantation.
7. *Aplastic anemia*: antithymocyte globulin ± cyclosporine, bone marrow transplantation in young pts with a matched donor.
8. *Autoimmune hemolysis*: glucocorticoids, sometimes immunosuppressive agents, danazol, plasmapheresis, rituximab.
9. *G6PD deficiency*: avoid agents known to precipitate hemolysis.

For a more detailed discussion, see Adamson JW et al: Chaps. 90–94, pp. 586–626, in HPIM-16.

65

LEUKOCYTOSIS AND LEUKOPENIA

LEUKOCYTOSIS
Approach

Review smear (? abnormal cells present) and obtain differential count. The normal values for concentration of blood leukocytes are shown in Table 65-1.

Neutrophilia

Absolute neutrophil count (polys and bands) > 10,000/μL. The pathophysiology of neutrophilia involves increased production, increased marrow mobilization, or decreased margination (adherence to vessel walls).

   Causes   (1) *Exercise, stress*; (2) *infections*—esp. bacterial; smear shows increased numbers of immature neutrophils ("left shift"), toxic granulations, Döhle bodies; (3) *burns*; (4) *tissue necrosis* (e.g., myocardial, pulmonary, renal infarction); (5) *chronic inflammatory disorders* (e.g., gout, vasculitis); (6) *drugs* (e.g., glucocorticoids, epinephrine, lithium); (7) *cytokines* (e.g., G-CSF, GM-CSF); (8) *myeloproliferative disorders* (Chap. 69); (9) *metabolic* (e.g., ketoacidosis, uremia); (10) *other*—malignant neoplasms, acute hemorrhage or hemolysis, after splenectomy.

Table 65-1

Normal Values for Leukocyte Concentration in Blood

Cell Type	Mean, cells/μL	95% Confidence Limits, cells/μL	Percent Total WBC
Neutrophil	3650	1830–7250	30–60%
Lymphocyte	2500	1500–4000	20–50%
Monocyte	430	200–950	2–10%
Eosinophil	150	0–700	0.3–5%
Basophil	30	0–150	0.6–1.8%

Leukemoid Reaction

Extreme elevation of leukocyte count ($>50,000/\mu L$) composed of mature and/or immature neutrophils.

Causes   (1) *Infection* (severe, chronic, e.g., tuberculosis), esp. in children; (2) *hemolysis* (severe); (3) *malignant neoplasms* (esp. carcinoma of the breast, lung, kidney); (4) *cytokines* (e.g., G-CSF, GM-CSF). May be distinguished from chronic myeloid leukemia (CML) by measurement of the leukocyte alkaline phosphatase (LAP) level: elevated in leukemoid reactions, depressed in CML.

Leukoerythroblastic Reaction

Similar to leukemoid reaction with addition of nucleated RBCs and schistocytes on blood smear.

Causes   (1) *Myelophthisis*—invasion of the bone marrow by tumor, fibrosis, granulomatous processes; smear shows "teardrop" RBCs; (2) *myelofibrosis*—same pathophysiology as myelophthisis, but the fibrosis is a primary marrow disorder; (3) *hemorrhage* or *hemolysis* (rarely, in severe cases).

Lymphocytosis

Absolute lymphocyte count $>5000/\mu L$.

Causes   (1) *Infection*—infectious mononucleosis, hepatitis, CMV, rubella, pertussis, tuberculosis, brucellosis, syphilis; (2) *endocrine disorders*—thyrotoxicosis, adrenal insufficiency; (3) *neoplasms*—chronic lymphocytic leukemia (CLL), most common cause of lymphocyte count $> 10,000/\mu L$.

Monocytosis

Absolute monocyte count $> 800/\mu L$.

Causes   (1) *Infection*—subacute bacterial endocarditis, tuberculosis, brucellosis, rickettsial diseases (e.g., Rocky Mountain spotted fever), malaria, leishmaniasis; (2) *granulomatous diseases*—sarcoidosis, Crohn's disease; (3) *collagen vascular diseases*—rheumatoid arthritis, SLE, polyarteritis nodosa, polymyositis, temporal arteritis; (4) *hematologic diseases*—leukemias, lymphoma, myeloproliferative and myelodysplastic syndromes, hemolytic anemia, chronic idiopathic neutropenia; (5) *malignant neoplasms*.

Eosinophilia

Absolute eosinophil count $> 500/\mu L$.

Causes   (1) *Drugs*, (2) *parasitic infections*, (3) *allergic diseases*, (4) *collagen vascular diseases*, (5) *malignant neoplasms*, (6) *hypereosinophilic syndromes*.

Basophilia

Absolute basophil count $> 100/\mu L$.

Causes   (1) *Allergic diseases*, (2) *myeloproliferative disorders* (esp. CML), (3) *chronic inflammatory disorders* (rarely).

LEUKOPENIA

Total leukocyte count $< 4300/\mu L$.

Neutropenia

Absolute neutrophil count < 2000/μL (increased risk of bacterial infection with count < 1000/μL). The pathophysiology of neutropenia involves decreased production or increased peripheral destruction.

Causes (1) *Drugs*—cancer chemotherapeutic agents are most common cause, also phenytoin, carbamazepine, indomethacin, chloramphenicol, penicillins, sulfonamides, cephalosporins, propylthiouracil, phenothiazines, captopril, methyldopa, procainamide, chlorpropamide, thiazides, cimetidine, allopurinol, colchicine, ethanol, penicillamine, and immunosuppressive agents; (2) *infections*—viral (e.g., influenza, hepatitis, infectious mononucleosis, HIV), bacterial (e.g., typhoid fever, miliary tuberculosis, fulminant sepsis), malaria; (3) *nutritional*—B$_{12}$, folate deficiencies; (4) *benign*—mild cyclic neutropenia common in blacks, no associated risk of infection; (5) *hematologic diseases*—cyclic neutropenia (q21d, with recurrent infections common), leukemia, myelodysplasis (preleukemia), aplastic anemia, bone marrow infiltration (uncommon cause), Chédiak-Higashi syndrome; (6) *hypersplenism*—e.g., Felty's syndrome, congestive splenomegaly, Gaucher's disease; (7) *autoimmune diseases*—idiopathic, SLE, lymphoma (may see positive antineutrophil antibodies).

 TREATMENT

> *Of the Febrile, Neutropenic Patient* (See Chap. 26)　In addition to usual sources of infection, consider paranasal sinuses, oral cavity (including teeth and gums), anorectal region; empirical therapy with broad-spectrum antibiotics (e.g., ceftazidime) is indicated after blood and other appropriate cultures are obtained. Prolonged febrile neutropenia (>7 days) leads to increased risk of disseminated fungal infections; requires addition of antifungal chemotherapy (e.g., amphotericin B). The duration of chemotherapy-induced neutropenia may be shortened by a few days by treatment with the cytokines GM-CSF or G-CSF.

Lymphopenia

Absolute lymphocyte count < 1000/μL.

Causes (1) *Acute stressful illness*—e.g., myocardial infarction, pneumonia, sepsis; (2) *glucocorticoid therapy*; (3) *lymphoma* (esp. Hodgkin's disease); (4) *immunodeficiency syndromes*—ataxia telangiectasia and Wiskott-Aldrich and DiGeorge's syndromes; (5) *immunosuppressive therapy*—e.g., antilymphocyte globulin, cyclophosphamide; (6) *large-field radiation therapy* (esp. for lymphoma); (7) *intestinal lymphangiectasia* (increased lymphocyte loss); (8) *chronic illness*—e.g., CHF, uremia, SLE, disseminated malignancies; (9) *bone marrow failure/replacement*—e.g., aplastic anemia, miliary tuberculosis.

Monocytopenia

Absolute monocyte count < 100/μL.

Causes (1) *Acute stressful illness*, (2) *glucocorticoid therapy*, (3) *aplastic anemia*, (4) *leukemia* (certain types, e.g., hairy cell leukemia), (5) *chemotherapeutic and immunosuppressive agents*.

Eosinopenia

Absolute eosinophil count < 50/μL.

Causes (1) *Acute stressful illness*, (2) *glucocorticoid therapy*.

For a more detailed discussion, see Holland SM, Gallin JI: Disorders of Granulocytes and Monocytes, Chap. 55, p. 349; Young NS: Aplastic Anemia, Myelodysplasia, and Related Bone Marrow Failure Syndromes, Chap. 94, p. 617; Spivak JL: Polycythemia Vera and Other Myeloproliferative Diseases, Chap. 95, p. 626, in HPIM-16.

66

BLEEDING AND THROMBOTIC DISORDERS

BLEEDING DISORDERS

Bleeding may result from abnormalities of (1) platelets, (2) blood vessel walls, or (3) coagulation. Platelet disorders characteristically produce petechial and purpuric skin lesions and bleeding from mucosal surfaces. Defective coagulation results in ecchymoses, hematomas, and mucosal and, in some disorders, recurrent joint bleeding (hemarthroses).

Platelet Disorders

THROMBOCYTOPENIA Normal platelet count is 150,000–350,000/μL. Thrombocytopenia is defined as a platelet count < 100,000/μL. Bleeding time, a measurement of platelet function, is abnormally increased if platelet count < 100,000/μL; injury or surgery may provoke excess bleeding. Spontaneous bleeding is unusual unless count < 20,000/μL; platelet count < 10,000/μL is often associated with serious hemorrhage. Bone marrow examination shows increased number of megakaryocytes in disorders associated with accelerated platelet destruction; decreased number in disorders of platelet production.

Causes (1) Production defects such as marrow injury (e.g., drugs, irradiation), marrow failure (e.g., aplastic anemia), marrow invasion (e.g., carcinoma, leukemia, fibrosis); (2) sequestration due to splenomegaly; (3) accelerated destruction: causes include:

- *Drugs* such as chemotherapeutic agents, thiazides, ethanol, estrogens, sulfonamides, quinidine, quinine, methyldopa.
- *Heparin-induced thrombocytopenia* is seen in 5% of pts receiving >5 days of therapy and is due to in vivo platelet aggregation often from anti-platelet factor-4 antibodies. Arterial and occasionally venous thromboses may result.
- *Autoimmune destruction* by an antibody mechanism; may be idiopathic or associated with SLE, lymphoma, HIV.
- *Idiopathic thrombocytopenic purpura* (ITP) has two forms: an acute, self-limited disorder of childhood requiring no specific therapy, and a chronic disorder of adults (esp. women 20–40 years). Chronic ITP may be due to autoantibodies to glycoprotein IIb-IIIa or glycoprotein Ib-IX complexes.
- *Disseminated intravascular coagulation* (DIC)—platelet consumption with coagulation factor depletion (prolonged PT, PTT) and stimulation of fibrinolysis (generation of fibrin split products, FSP). Blood smear shows microangiopathic hemolysis (schistocytes). Causes include infection (esp. meningococcal, pneumococcal, gram-negative bacteremias), extensive burns, trauma, or thrombosis; giant hemangioma, retained dead fetus, heat stroke, mismatched blood transfusion, metastatic carcinoma, acute promyelocytic leukemia.

• *Thrombotic thrombocytopenic purpura* (TTP)—rare disorder characterized by microangiopathic hemolytic anemia, fever, thrombocytopenia, renal dysfunction (and/or hematuria), and neurologic dysfunction caused by failure to cleave von Willebrand factor normally.

• *Hemorrhage with extensive transfusion.*

PSEUDOTHROMBOCYTOPENIA Platelet clumping secondary to collection of blood in EDTA (0.3% of pts). Examination of blood smear establishes diagnosis.

THROMBOCYTOSIS Platelet count > 350,000/μL. Either primary (thrombocythemia; Chap. 69) or secondary (reactive); latter secondary to severe hemorrhage, iron deficiency, surgery, after splenectomy (transient), malignant neoplasms (esp. Hodgkin's disease), chronic inflammatory diseases (e.g., inflammatory bowel disease), recovery from acute infection, vitamin B_{12} deficiency, drugs (e.g., vincristine, epinephrine). Rebound thrombocytosis may occur after marrow recovery from cytotoxic agents, alcohol. Primary thrombocytosis may be complicated by bleeding and/or thrombosis; secondary rarely causes hemostatic problems.

DISORDERS OF PLATELET FUNCTION Suggested by the finding of prolonged bleeding time with normal platelet count. Defect is in platelet adhesion, aggregation, or granule release. Causes include: (1) Drugs—aspirin, other NSAIDs, dipyridamole, clopidogrel, heparin, penicillins, esp. carbenicillin, ticarcillin; (2) uremia; (3) cirrhosis; (4) dysproteinemias; (5) myeloproliferative and myelodysplastic disorders; (6) von Willebrand's disease (see below); (7) cardiopulmonary bypass.

Hemostatic Disorders Due to Blood Vessel Wall Defects

Causes include: (1) aging; (2) drugs—e.g., glucocorticoids (chronic therapy), penicillins, sulfonamides; (3) vitamin C deficiency; (4) TTP; (5) hemolytic uremic syndrome; (6) Henoch-Schönlein purpura; (7) paraproteinemias; (8) hereditary hemorrhagic telangiectasia (Osler-Rendu-Weber disease).

Disorders of Blood Coagulation

CONGENITAL DISORDERS

1. *Hemophilia A*—incidence 1:10,000; sex-linked recessive deficiency of factor VIII (low plasma factor VIII coagulant activity, but normal amount of factor VIII–related antigen—von Willebrand's factor). Laboratory features: elevated PTT, normal PT.

2. *Hemophilia B* (Christmas disease)—incidence 1:100,000, sex-linked recessive, due to factor IX deficiency. Clinical and laboratory features similar to hemophilia A.

3. *von Willebrand's disease*—most common inherited coagulation disorder (1:800–1000), usually autosomal dominant; primary defect is reduced synthesis or chemically abnormal factor VIII–related antigen produced by platelets and endothelium, resulting in abnormal platelet function.

ACQUIRED DISORDERS

1. *Vitamin K deficiency*—impairs production of factors II (prothrombin), VII, IX, and X; vitamin K is a cofactor in the carboxylation of glutamate residues on prothrombin complex proteins; major source of vitamin K is dietary (esp. green vegetables), with minor production by gut bacteria. Laboratory features: elevated PT and PTT.

2. *Liver disease*—results in deficiencies of all clotting factors except VIII. Laboratory features: elevated PT, normal or elevated PTT.

3. *Other disorders*—DIC, fibrinogen deficiency (liver disease, L-asparaginase therapy, rattlesnake bites), other factor deficiencies, circulating anticoagulants (lymphoma, SLE, idiopathic), massive transfusion (dilutional coagulopathy).

℞ TREATMENT

Thrombocytopenia Caused by Drugs Includes discontinuation of possible offending agents; expect recovery in 7–10 days. Platelet transfusions may be needed if platelet count < 10,000/µL.

Heparin-Induced Thrombocytopenia Includes prompt discontinuation of heparin. Warfarin or one of the newer direct thrombin inhibitors such as lepirudin (0.4-mg/kg bolus, 0.15-mg/kg per hour infusion; PTT target 1.5–2.5 × baseline) or argatroban (2 µg/kg per min infusion; PTT target 1.5–3 × baseline) should be used for treatment of thromboses.

Chronic ITP Prednisone, initially 1–2 (mg/kg)/d, then slow taper, to keep the platelet count > 60,000/µL. IV immunoglobulin to block phagocytic destruction may be useful. Rituximab is effective in patients refractory to glucocorticoids. Splenectomy, danazol (androgen), or other agents (e.g., vincristine, cyclophosphamide, fludarabine) are indicated for refractory pts or those requiring >5–10 mg prednisone daily.

DIC Control of underlying disease most important; platelets, fresh-frozen plasma (FFP) to correct clotting parameters. Heparin may be beneficial in pts with acute promyelocytic leukemia.

TTP Plasmapheresis and FFP infusions, possibly IV IgG; recovery in two-thirds of cases. Plasmapheresis removes inhibitors of the vWF cleavage enzyme (ADAMTS13), and FFP replaces the enzyme.

Disorders of Platelet Function Remove or reverse underlying cause. Dialysis and/or cryoprecipitate infusions (10 bags/24 h) may be helpful for platelet dysfunction associated with uremia.

Hemostatic Disorders Withdraw offending drugs, replace vitamin C, plasmapheresis, and plasma infusion for TTP.

Hemophilia A Factor VIII replacement for bleeding or before surgical procedure; degree and duration of replacement depends on severity of bleeding. Give factor VIII to obtain a 15% (for mild bleeding) to 50% (for severe bleeding) factor VIII level. The duration should range from a single dose of factor VIII to therapy bid for up to 2 weeks.

Hemophilia B FFP or factor IX concentrates (Proplex, Konyne).

von Willebrand's Disease Cryoprecipitate (plasma product rich in factor VIII) or factor VIII concentrate (Humate-P, Koate HS); up to 10 bags bid for 48–72 h, depending on the severity of bleeding. Desmopressin (vasopressin analogue) may benefit some pts.

Vitamin K Deficiency Vitamin K, 10 mg SC or slow IV.

Liver Disease Fresh-frozen plasma.

THROMBOTIC DISORDERS
Hypercoagulable State

Consider in pts with recurrent episodes of venous thrombosis (i.e., deep venous thrombosis, DVT; pulmonary embolism, PE). Causes include: (1) venous stasis (e.g., pregnancy, immobilization); (2) vasculitis; (3) myeloproliferative disorders; (4) oral contraceptives; (5) lupus anticoagulant—antibody to platelet phospholipid, stimulates coagulation; (6) heparin-induced thrombocytopenia; (7) deficiencies of endogenous anticoagulant factors—antithrombin III, protein C, protein S; (8) factor V Leiden—mutation in factor V (Arg → Glu at position 506) confers resistance to inactivation by protein C, accounts for 25% of cases of recurrent thrombosis; (9) prothrombin gene mutation—Glu → Arg at position 20210 results in increased prothrombin levels; accounts for about 6% of thromboses; (10) other—paroxysmal nocturnal hemoglobinuria, dysfibrinogenemias (abnormal fibrinogen).

℞ TREATMENT

Correct underlying disorder whenever possible; long-term warfarin therapy is otherwise indicated.

Anticoagulant Agents

1. *Heparin* (Table 66-1)—enhances activity of antithrombin III; parenteral agent of choice. Low-molecular-weight heparin is the preparation of choice (enoxaparin or dalteparin). It can be administered SC, monitoring of the PTT is unnecessary, and it is less likely to induce antibodies and thrombocytopenia. The usual dose is 100 U/kg SC bid. Unfractionated heparin should be given only if low-molecular-weight heparin is unavailable. In adults, the dose of unfractionated heparin is 25,000–40,000 U continuous IV infusion over 24 h following initial IV bolus of 5000 U; monitor by following

Table 66-1

Anticoagulant Therapy with Low-Molecular-Weight and Unfractionated Heparin

Clinical Indication	Heparin Dose and Schedule	Target PTT[a]	LMWH Dose and Schedule[b]
Venous thrombosis pulmonary embolism			
Treatment	5000 U IV bolus; 1000–1500 U/h	2–2.5	100 U/kg SC bid
Prophylaxis	5000 U SC q8–12h	<1.5	100 U/kg SC bid
Acute myocardial infarction			
With thrombo- lytic therapy	5000 U IV bolus; 1000 U/h	1.5–2.5	100 U/kg SC bid
With mural thrombus	8000 U SC q8h + warfarin	1.5–2.0	100 U /kg SC bid
Unstable angina	5000 U IV bolus; 1000 U/h	1.5–2.5	100 U/kg SC bid
Prophylaxis			
General surgery	5000 U SC bid	<1.5	100 U/kg SC before and bid
Orthopedic surgery	10000 U SC bid	1.5	100 U/kg SC before and bid
Medical patients with CHF, MI	10000 U SC bid	1.5	100 U/kg SC bid

[a] Times normal control; assumes PTT has been standardized to heparin levels so that 1.5–2.5× normal equals 0.2–0.4 U/mL; if PTT is normal (27–35 S), start with 5000 U bolus 1300 U/h infusion monitoring PTT; if PTT at recheck is <50 S, rebolus with 5000 U and increase infusion by 100 U/h; if PTT at recheck is 50–60 s, increase infusion rate by 100 U/h; if PTT at recheck is 60–85 s, no change; if PTT at recheck is 85–100 s, decrease infusion rate 100 U/h; if PTT at recheck is 100–120 s, stop infusion for 30 min and decrease rate 100 U/h at restart; if PTT at recheck is >120 s, stop infusion for 60 min and decrease rate 200 U/h at restart.
[b] LMWH does not affect PTT and PTT is not used to adjust dosage.
Note: PTT, partial thromboplastin time; LMWH, low-molecular-weight heparin; CHF, congestive heart failure; MI, myocardial infarction.

PTT; should be maintained between 1.5 and 2 times upper normal limit. Prophylactic anticoagulation to lower risk of venous thrombosis recommended in some pts (e.g., postoperative, immobilized) (Table 66-1). Major complication of unfractionated heparin therapy is hemorrhage—manage by discontinuing heparin; for severe bleeding, administer protamine (1 mg/100 U heparin); results in rapid neutralization.

    2.   *Warfarin* (Coumadin)—vitamin K antagonist, decreases levels of factors II, VII, IX, X, and anticoagulant proteins C and S. Administered over 2–3 days; initial load of 5–10 mg PO qd followed by titration of daily dose to keep PT 1.5–2 times control PT or 2–3 times if the International Normalized Ratio method is used. Complications include hemorrhage, warfarin-induced skin necrosis (rare, occurs in persons deficient in protein C), teratogenic effects. Warfarin effect reversed by administration of vitamin K; FFP infused if urgent reversal necessary. Numerous drugs potentiate or antagonize warfarin effect. Potentiating agents include chlorpromazine, chloral hydrate, sulfonamides, chloramphenicol, other broad-spectrum antibiotics, allopurinol, cimetidine, tricyclic antidepressants, disulfiram, laxatives, high-dose salicylates, thyroxine, clofibrate. Antagonizing agents include vitamin K, barbiturates, rifampin, cholestyramine, oral contraceptives, thiazides.

    3.   *Newer agents*—Fondaparinux is a pentapeptide that directly inhibits factor Xa. It is given SC and does not require monitoring. Argatroban and lepirudin are direct thrombin inhibitors. These agents are being compared to LMWH and are commonly used in patients with heparin-induced thrombocytopenia.

    In-hospital anticoagulation usually initiated with heparin, with subsequent maintenance on warfarin after an overlap of 3 days. Duration of therapy depends on underlying condition; calf DVT with clear precipitating cause, 6 wks–3 mos; proximal or idiopathic DVT, 3–6 mos; recurrent idiopathic DVT, 12 mos minimum; PE, 6 mos minimum; embolic disease with ongoing risk factor, long-term, indefinite (Fig. 66-1).

Fibrinolytic Agents

Tissue plasminogen activator (tPA, alteplase), streptokinase, and urokinase; mediate clot lysis by activating plasmin, which degrades fibrin. Indications include treatment of DVT, with lower incidence of postphlebitic syndrome (chronic venous stasis, skin ulceration) than with heparin therapy; massive PE, arterial embolic occlusion of extremity, treatment of acute MI, unstable angina pectoris. Dosages for fibrinolytic agents: (1) tPA—for acute MI and massive PE (adult > 65 kg), 10-mg IV bolus over 1–2 min, then 50 mg IV over 1 h and 40 mg IV over next 2 h (total dose = 100 mg). tPA is slightly more effective but more expensive than streptokinase for treatment of acute MI. (2) Streptokinase—for acute MI, 1.5 million IU IV over 60 min; or 20,000 IU as a bolus intracoronary (IC) infusion, followed by 2000 IU/min for 60 min IC. For PE or arterial or deep venous thrombosis, 250,000 IU over 30 min, then 100,000 IU/h for 24 h (PE) or 72 h (arterial or deep venous thrombosis). (3) Urokinase—for PE, 4400 IU/kg IV over 10 min, then 4400 (IU/kg)/h IV for 12 h.

    Fibrinolytic therapy is usually followed by period of anticoagulant therapy with heparin. Fibrinolytic agents are contraindicated in pts with: (1) active internal bleeding; (2) recent (<2–3 months) cerebrovascular accident; (3) intracranial neoplasm, aneurysm, or recent head trauma.

Antiplatelet Agents

Aspirin (160–325 mg/d) plus clopidogrel (400-mg loading dose then 75 mg/d) may be beneficial in lowering incidence of arterial thrombotic events (stroke, MI) in high-risk pts.

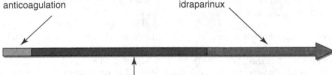

Initial-Phase Anticoagulation
4 to 14 days
Acute management usually with a parenteral agent (heparin or LMWH) intended to rapidly abrogate thrombin generation, prevent thrombus extension, and serve as a "bridge" to subacute anticoagulation

Chronic-Phase Anticoagulation
Long term
Chronic management usually with subacute-phase intensity or reduced-intensity (INR, 1.5 to 2.0) oral warfarin and perhaps in the future with oral ximelagatran or once-weekly SC idraparinux

Subacute-Phase Anticoagulation
up to 6 months
Subacute management usually with an oral agent such as warfarin (INR, 2.0 to 3.0) or SC LMWH intended to stabilize the thrombus, prevent early recurrence, and allow time for endogenous fibrinolysis-mediated recanalization

FIGURE 66-1   Phases of anticoagulation for venous thromboembolic events. Anticoagulation for a venous thromboembolic event can be divided into three distinct phases. Acute-phase anticoagulation usually consists of several days of parenteral therapy with intravenous unfractionated heparin or subcutaneous low-molecular-weight heparin (LMWH). Acute-phase therapy is usually continued for at least 4 days and until stable-dose, subacute-phase anticoagulation has been achieved. Subacute anticoagulation traditionally consists of oral warfarin for up to 6 months. Low-molecular-weight heparin therapy may offer superior and more convenient subacute anticoagulation in select populations. Long-term, chronic-phase anticoagulation consists of identical intensity therapy as is employed during subacute-phase therapy in high-risk patients and attenuated-intensity warfarin in others.

For a more detailed discussion, see Handin RI: Bleeding and Thrombosis, Chap. 53, p. 337; Disorders of the Platelet and Vessel Wall, Chap. 101, p. 673; Disorders of Coagulation and Thrombosis, Chap. 102, p. 680; and Deitcher SR: Antiplatelet, Anticoagulant, and Fibrinolytic Therapy, Chap. 103, p. 687, in HPIM-16.

67

PREVENTION AND EARLY DETECTION OF CANCER

One of the most important functions of medical care is to prevent disease or discover it early enough that treatment might be more effective. All risk factors for cancer have not yet been defined. However, a substantial number of factors that elevate risk are within a person's control. Some of these factors are listed in Table 67-1. Every physician visit is an opportunity to teach and reinforce the elements of a healthy life-style.

Cancer screening in the aymptomatic population at average risk is a complicated issue. To be of value, screening must detect disease at a stage that is more readily curable than disease that is treated after symptoms appear. For cervix cancer and colon cancer, screening has been shown to save lives. For other tumors, benefit is less clear. Screening can cause harm; complications may

Table 67-1

Life-Style Factors That Reduce Cancer Risk

Do not use any tobacco products
Maintain a healthy weight; eat a well-balanced diet[a]; maintain caloric balance
Exercise at least 3 times a week
Prevent sun exposure
Avoid excessive alcohol intake
Practice safe sex; use condoms

---

[a] Not precisely defined, but current recommendations include 5 servings of fruits and vegetables per day, 25 g fiber, and <30% of calories coming from fat.

ensue from the screening test or the tests done to validate a positive screening test or from treatments for the underlying disease. Furthermore, quality of life can be adversely affected by false-positive tests. Evaluation of screening tools can be biased and needs to rely on prospective randomized studies. *Lead-time bias* occurs when the natural history of disease is unaffected by the diagnosis, but the patient is diagnosed earlier in the course of disease than normal; thus, the patient spends more of his/her life span knowing the diagnosis. *Length bias* occurs when slow-growing cancers are detected during screening that might never have come to medical attention. *Overdiagnosis* is a form of length bias when a cancer is detected that is not growing and is not an influence on length of survival. *Selection bias* is the term for the fact that people who volunteer for screening trials may be different from the general population. Volunteers might have family history concerns that actually elevate their risk or they may be generally more health-conscious, which can affect outcome.

The various groups that evaluate and recommend screening practice guidelines have used varying criteria to make their recommendations (Table 67-2). The absence of data on survival for a number of diseases has led to a lack of consensus. In particular, four areas are worth noting.

1. *Prostate cancer*: Prostate-specific antigen (PSA) levels are elevated in prostate cancer, but a substantial number of the cancers detected appear to be non-life-threatening. PSA screening has not been shown to improve survival. Efforts are underway to develop better tests (predominantly using bound vs. free and rate of increase of PSA) to distinguish lethal and nonlethal cancers.

2. *Breast cancer*: The data on annual mammography support its use in women over age 50 years. However, the benefit for women age 40–49 years is quite small. One study shows some advantage to women who are screened starting at age 40 that appears 15 years later; however, it is unclear if this benefit would not have also been derived by starting screening at age 50 years. Women age 40–49 years have a much lower incidence of breast cancer and a higher false-positive rate on mammography. Here, too, refined methods of screening are in development.

3. *Colon cancer*: Annual fecal occult blood testing after age 50 years is felt to be useful. However, colonoscopy is the "gold standard" in colorectal cancer detection, but it is expensive and has not been shown to be cost effective in asymptomatic people.

4. *Lung cancer*: Chest radiographs and sputum cytology in smokers appear to identify more early-stage tumors, but paradoxically, the screened patients do not have improved survival. Spiral CT scanning is being evaluated, but it is known to have more false-positive tests.

CANCER PREVENTION IN HIGH-RISK GROUPS

BREAST CANCER   Risk factors include age, early menarche, nulliparity or late first pregnancy, high body-mass index, radiation exposure before age 30

Table 67-2

Screening Recommendations for Asymptomatic Normal-Risk Subjects[a]

Test or Procedure	USPSTF	ACS	CTFPHC
Sigmoidoscopy	>50, periodically <50, not recommended	≥50, every 3–5 years	Insufficient evidence
Fecal occult blood testing	≥50, every year	≥50, every year	Insufficient evidence
Digital rectal examination	No recommendation	≥40, every year	Poor evidence to include or exclude
Prostate-specific antigen	Insufficient evidence to recommend	M: ≥50, every year	Recommendation against
Pap test	F: 18–65, every 1–3 years	F with uterine cervix, beginning 3 years after first intercourse or by age 21. Yearly for standard Pap; every 2 years with liquid test.	Fair evidence to include in examination of sexually active women
Pelvic examination	Do not recommend, advise adnexal palpation during exam for other reasons	F: 18–40, every 1–3 years with Pap test; >40, every year	Not considered
Endometrial tissue sampling	Not considered	At menopause if obese or a history of unopposed estrogen use	Not considered
Breast self-examination	No recommendation	≥20, monthly	Insufficient evidence to make a recommendation
Breast clinical examination		F: 20–40, every 3 years; >40, yearly	F: >50, every year
Mammography	F: >50, every year F: 40–75, every 1–2 years	F: ≥40, every year	F: 50–69, every year
Complete skin examination	Not recommended	20–39, every 3 years	Poor evidence to include or exclude

[a] Summary of the screening procedures recommended for the general population by U.S. Preventive Services Task Force (USPSTF), the American Cancer Society (ACS), and the Canadian Task Force on Prevention Health Care (CTFPHC). These recommendations refer to asymptomatic persons who have no risk factors, other than age or gender, for the targeted condition.

Note: F, female; M, male.

years, hormone-replacement therapy (HRT), alcohol consumption, family history, presence of mutations in *BRCA1* or *BRCA2*, and prior history of breast neoplasia. Risk assessment models have been developed to predict an individual's likelihood of developing breast cancer (see *brca.nci.nih.gov/brc/*).

Diagnosis MRI scanning is a more effective screening tool than mammography in women with a familial breast cancer risk.

Interventions Women whose risk exceeds 1.66% in the next 5 years have been shown to have a 50% reduction in breast cancer from taking tamoxifen. Raloxifene also appears to reduce the risk and may have less toxicity. Aromatase inhibitors have generally been superior to tamoxifen in the adjuvant treatment of hormone-sensitive breast cancer but are still being evaluated as preventive agents. Women with strong family histories should undergo testing for mutations in *BRCA1* and *BRCA2*. Mutations in these genes carry a lifetime probability of >80% for developing breast cancer. Bilateral prophylactic mastectomy prevents at least 90% of these cancers but is a more radical prevention than the usual treatment for the disease. In addition, bilateral salpingo-oophorectomy reduces ovarian and fallopian tube cancer risk by about 96% in women with *BRCA1* or *BRCA2* mutations.

COLORECTAL CANCER Risk factors include diets high in saturated fats and low in fruits and vegetables, smoking, and alcohol consumption. Stronger but less prevalent risk factors are the presence of inflammatory bowel disease or genetic disorders such as familial polyposis (autosomal dominant germline mutation in *APC*) and hereditary nonpolyposis colorectal cancer (mutations in DNA mismatch repair genes *hMSH2* and *hMLH1*).

Interventions Pts with ulcerative colitis and familial polyposis generally undergo total colectomy. In familial polyposis, NSAIDs reduce the number and size of polyps. Celecoxib, sulindac, and even aspirin appear to be effective, and celecoxib is FDA-approved for this indication. Calcium supplementation can lead to a decrease in the recurrence of adenomas, but it is not yet clear that the risk of colorectal cancer is decreased and survival increased. The Women's Health Study noted a significant reduction in the risk of colorectal cancer in women taking HRT, but the increase in thrombotic events and breast cancers counterbalanced this benefit. Studies are underway to assess NSAIDs with and without inhibitors of the epidermal growth factor (EGF) receptor in other risk groups.

LUNG CANCER Risk factors include smoking, exposure to radiation, asbestos, radon.

Interventions Smoking cessation is the only effective prevention. NSAIDs and EGF receptor inhibitors are being evaluated. Carotenoids, selenium, retinoids, and α-tocopheral do not work.

PROSTATE CANCER Risk factors include age, family history, and possibly dietary fat intake. African Americans are at increased risk. The disease is highly prevalent, with autopsy studies finding prostate cancer in 70–80% of men over age 70.

Interventions In a group of men $\geq$55 years with normal rectal examinations and PSA levels < 3 ng/mL, daily finasteride reduced the incidence of prostate cancer by 25%. Finasteride also prevents the progression of benign prostate hyperplasia. However, some men experience decreased libido as a side effect. The Gleason grade of tumors seen in men taking finasteride prevention was somewhat higher than the controls; however, androgen deprivation alters the morphology of the cells and it is not yet clear that the Gleason grade is a reliable indicator of tumor aggressiveness in the setting of androgen deprivation. Some data suggest that selenium and α-tocopherol may lower risk of prostate cancer. In a lung cancer prevention trial, men taking vitamin E had a 34% lower incidence of prostate cancer during the 6-year study period.

CERVICAL CANCER Risk factors include early age at first intercourse, multiple sexual partners, smoking, and infection with human papillomavirus (HPV) types 16, 18, 45, and 56.

Interventions Regular Pap testing can detect nearly all cases of the premalignant lesion called *cervical intraepithelial neoplasia*. Untreated, the lesion can progress to carcinoma in situ and invasive cervical cancer. Surgical removal, cryotherapy, or laser therapy is used to treat the disease and is effective in 80%. Risk of recurrence is highest in women over age 30, those with prior HPV infection, and those who have had prior treatment for the same condition. Chemoprevention and HPV vaccine studies are ongoing, but no other intervention has been proven effective.

HEAD AND NECK CANCER Risk factors include smoking, alcohol consumption, and possibly HPV infection.

Interventions Oral leukoplakia, white lesions of the oral mucosa, occur in 1–2 persons in 1000, and 2–3% of these pts go on to develop head and neck cancer. Spontaneous regression of oral leukoplakia is seen in 30–40% of pts. Retinoid treatment (13-*cis* retinoid acid) can increase the regression rate. Vitamin A induces complete remission in ~50% of pts. The use of retinoids in pts who have been diagnosed with head and neck cancer and received definitive local therapy has not produced consistent results. Initial studies claimed that retinoids prevented the development of second primary tumors, a common feature of head and neck cancer. However, large randomized studies did not confirm this benefit. Other studies are underway combining retinoids and NSAIDs with and without EGF receptor inhibitors.

For a more detailed discussion, see Brawley OW, Kramer BS: Prevention and Early Detection of Cancer, Chap. 67, p. 441, in HPIM-16.

68

CANCER CHEMOTHERAPY

BIOLOGY OF TUMOR GROWTH

Two essential features of cancer cells are uncontrolled growth and the ability to metastasize. The malignant phenotype of a cell is the end result of a series of genetic changes that remove safeguards restricting cell growth and induce new features that enable the cell to metastasize, including surface receptors for binding to basement membranes, enzymes to poke holes in anatomic barriers, cytokines to facilitate mobility, and angiogenic factors to develop a new vascular lifeline for nutrients and oxygen. These genetic changes usually involve increased or abnormal expression or activity of certain genes known as *proto-oncogenes* (often growth factors or their receptors, enzymes in growth pathways, or transcription factors), deletion or inactivation of tumor-suppressor genes, and defects in DNA repair enzymes. These genetic changes may occur by point mutation, gene amplification, gene rearrangement, or epigenetic changes such as altered gene methylation.

Once cells are malignant, their growth kinetics are similar to those of normal cells but lack regulation. For unclear reasons, tumor growth kinetics follow a Gompertzian curve: as the tumor mass increases, the fraction of dividing cells declines. Thus, by the time a cancer is large enough to be detected clinically, its growth fraction is often small. Unfortunately, tumor growth usually does not stop altogether before the tumor reaches a lethal tumor burden. Cancer cells proceed through the same cell-cycle stages as normal cycling cells: G_1 (period of preparation for DNA synthesis), S (DNA synthesis), G_2 (tetraploid phase preceding mitosis in which integrity of DNA replication is assessed), and M (mitosis). Some noncycling cells may remain in a G_o, or resting, phase for long periods. Certain chemotherapeutic agents are specific for cells in certain phases of the cell cycle, a fact that is important in designing effective chemotherapeutic regimens.

DEVELOPMENT OF DRUG RESISTANCE

Drug resistance can be divided into de novo resistance or acquired resistance. De novo resistance refers to the tendency of many of the most common solid tumors to be unresponsive to chemotherapeutic agents. In acquired resistance, tumors initially responsive to chemotherapy develop resistance during treatment, usually because resistant clones appear within tumor cell populations (Table 68-1).

Resistance can be specific to single drugs because of (1) defective transport of the drug, (2) decreased activating enzymes, (3) increased drug inactivation, (4) increases in target enzyme levels, or (5) alterations in target molecules. Multiple drug resistance occurs in cells overexpressing the P glycoprotein, a membrane glycoprotein responsible for enhanced efflux of drugs from cells, but there are other mechanisms as well.

CATEGORIES OF CHEMOTHERAPEUTIC AGENTS AND MAJOR TOXICITIES

A partial list of toxicities is shown in Table 68-2; some toxicities may apply only to certain members of a group of drugs.

COMPLICATIONS OF THERAPY

While the effects of cancer chemotherapeutic agents may be exerted primarily on the malignant cell population, virtually all currently employed regimens have profound effects on normal tissues as well. Every side effect of treatment must be balanced against potential benefits expected, and pts must always be fully apprised of the toxicities they may encounter. While the duration of certain adverse effects may be short-lived, others, such as sterility and the risk of secondary malignancy, have long-term implications; consideration of these effects is of importance in the use of regimens as adjuvant therapy. The combined toxicity of regimens involving radiotherapy and chemotherapy is greater than that seen with each modality alone. Teratogenesis is a special concern in treating women of childbearing years with radiation or chemotherapy. The most serious late toxicities are sterility (common; from alkylating agents), secondary acute leukemia (rare; from alkylating agents and topoisomerase inhibitors), secondary

Table 68-1

Curability of Cancers with Chemotherapy

Advanced cancers with possible cure
Acute lymphoid and acute myeloid
 leukemia (pediatric/
 adult)
Hodgkin's disease (pediatric/adult)
Lymphomas—certain types (pediatric/
 adult)
Germ cell neoplasms
 Embryonal carcinoma
 Teratocarcinoma
 Seminoma or dysgerminoma
 Choriocarcinoma
Gestational trophoblastic neoplasia
Pediatric neoplasms
 Wilm's tumor
 Embryonal rhabdomyocarcinoma
 Ewing's sarcoma
 Peripheral neuroepithelioma
 Neuroblastoma
Small cell lung carcinoma
Ovarian carcinoma
Advanced cancers possibly cured by
 chemotherapy and radiation
Squamous carcinoma (head and neck)
Squamous carcinoma (anus)
Breast carcinoma
Carcinoma of the uterine cervix
Non-small cell lung carcinoma (stage
 III)
Small-cell lung carcinoma
Cancers possibly cured with chemo-
 therapy as adjuvant to surgery
Breast carcinoma
Colorectal carcinoma[a]
Osteogenic sarcoma
Soft tissue sarcoma

Cancers possibly cured with
 "high-dose" chemotherapy
 with stem cell support
Relapsed leukemias, lymphoid
 and myeloid
Relapsed lymphomas, Hodgkin's
 and non-Hodgkin's
Chronic myeloid leukemia
Multiple myeloma
Cancers responsive with useful
 palliation, but not cure, by
 chemotherapy
Bladder carcinoma
Chronic myeloid leukemia
Hairy cell leukemia
Chronic lymphocytic leukemia
Lymphoma—certain types
Multiple myeloma
Gastric carcinoma
Cervix carcinoma
Endometrial carcinoma
Soft tissue sarcoma
Head and neck cancer
Adrenocortical carcinoma
Islet-cell neoplasms
Breast carcinoma
Colorectal carcinoma
Tumor poorly responsive in ad-
 vanced stages to
 chemotherapy
Pancreatic carcinoma
Biliary-tract neoplasms
Renal carcinoma
Thyroid carcinoma
Carcinoma of the vulva
Non-small cell lung carcinoma
Prostate carcinoma
Melanoma
Hepatocellular carcinoma

[a] Rectum also receives radiation therapy.

solid tumors (0.5–1%/year risk for at least 25 years after treatment; from radiation therapy), premature atherosclerosis (3-fold increased risk of fatal MI;
from radiation therapy that includes the heart), heart failure (rare; from anthra-
cyclines), and pulmonary fibrosis (rare; from bleomycin).

MANAGEMENT OF ACUTE TOXICITIES

   NAUSEA AND VOMITING   Mildly to moderately emetogenic agents—
prochlorperazine, 5–10 mg PO or 25 mg PR before chemotherapy; effects are
enhanced by also administering dexamethasone, 10–20 mg IV. Highly emetogenic agents (such as cisplatin, mechlorethamine, dacarbazine, streptozocin)—

Table 68-2

Toxicities of Cancer Treatments

Agent	Toxicities
Alkylating agents (add alkyl groups to N-7 or O-6 of guanine) Busulfan Chlorambucil Cyclophosphamide Ifosfamide Dacarbazine Mechlorethamine Nitrosoureas Melphalan	Nausea, vomiting, myelosuppression, sterility, alopecia, acute leukemia (rare), hemorrhagic cystitis, pulmonary fibrosis
Antimetabolites (inhibit DNA or RNA synthesis) 5-Fluorouracil Capecitabine Fludarabine Cladribine Cytarabine Methotrexate Pemetrexed Hydroxyurea Pentostatin Azathioprine Thioguanine	Nausea, vomiting, myelosuppression, oral ulceration, hepatic toxicity, alopecia, neurologic symptoms
Tubulin poisons (block tubule polymerization or depolymerization) Vincristine Vinblastine Vinorelban Paclitaxel Docetaxel Estramustine	Nausea, vomiting, myelosuppression, vesicant, ileus, hypersensitivity reaction, peripheral neuropathy, SIADH
Topoisomerase inhibitors (interfere with DNA unwinding/repair) Doxorubicin Daunorubicin Idarubicin Epirubicin Etoposide Irinotecan Topotecan Mitoxantrone	Nausea, vomiting, myelosuppression, vesicant, cardiac failure, acute leukemia (rare)
Platinum compounds (form DNA adducts, disrupt repair) Cisplatin Carboplatin Oxaliplatin	Nausea, vomiting, myelosuppression, renal toxicity, neurotoxicity

(continued)

Table 68-2 *(Continued)*

Toxicities of Cancer Treatments

Agent	Toxicities
Antibiotics (diverse mechanisms)	
Bleomycin	Nausea, vomiting, myelosuppression, cardiac toxicity, lung fibrosis, hypocalcemia, hypersensitivity reaction
Dactinomycin	
Mithramycin	
Mitomycin	
Hormone and Nuclear Receptor Targeting Agents	
Tamoxifen	Nausea, vomiting, hot flashes, gynecomastia, impotence
Raloxifene	
Anastrazole	
Letrozole	
Exemestane	
Tretinoin	
Bexarotene	
Flutamide	
Leuprolide	
Diethylstilbestrol	
Medroxyprogesterone	
Biologic Agents	
Interferon	Nausea, vomiting, fever, chills, vascular leak, respiratory distress, skin rashes, edema
Interleukin 2	
Rituximab	
Herceptin	
Cetuximab	
Bevacizumab	
Gemtuzumab ogomicin	
Benileukin diftitox	
Bortezomib	
Imatinib	
Gefitinib	
Radiation therapy	
External beam (teletherapy)	Nausea, vomiting, myelosuppression, tissue damage, late second cancers, heart disease, sterility
Internal implants (brachytherapy)	
Ibritumomab tiuxetan	
Tositumomab	
Samarium-153 EDTMP	
Strontium-89	

ondansetron, 8 mg PO q6h the day before chemotherapy and IV at time of chemotherapy, plus dexamethasone, 20 mg IV at time of chemotherapy. Aprepitant (125 mg PO day 1, 80 mg PO days 2,3), a substance P/neurokinin 1 receptor blocker, decreases the risk of acute and delayed vomiting from cisplatin.

NEUTROPENIA Colony-stimulating factors are often used where they have been shown to have little or no benefit. Specific indications for the use of G-CSF or GM-CSF are provided in Table 68-3.

ANEMIA Quality of life is improved by maintaining Hb levels >90 g/L (9 g/dL). This is routinely done with packed RBC transfusions. Erythropoietin,

Table 68-3

Indications for the Clinical Use of G-CSF or GM-CSF

Preventive Uses
With the first cycle of chemotherapy (so-called primary CSF administration)
  Not needed on a routine basis
  Use if the probability of febrile neutropenia is ≥40%
  Use if patient has preexisting neutropenia or active infection
With subsequent cycles if febrile neutropenia has previously occurred (so-called
  secondary CSF administration)
  Not needed after short-duration neutropenia without fever
  Use if patient had febrile neutropenia in previous cycle
  Use if prolonged neutropenia (even without fever) delays therapy
Therapeutic Uses
Afebrile neutropenic patients
  No evidence of benefit
Febrile neutropenic patients
  No evidence of benefit
  May feel compelled to use in the face of clinical deterioration from sepsis,
    pneumonia, or fungal infection, but benefit unclear
To augment dose-intensity of chemotherapy in patients with curable malignan-
  cies
  No evidence of benefit
In bone marrow or peripheral blood stem cell transplantation
  Use to mobilize stem cells from marrow
  Use to hasten myeloid recovery
In acute myeloid leukemia
  G-CSF of minor or no benefit
  GM-CSF of no benefit and may be harmful
In myelodysplastic syndromes
  Not routinely beneficial
  Use intermittently in subset with neutropenia and recurrent infection
What Dose and Schedule Should Be Used?
G-CSF: 5 μg/kg per day subcutaneously
GM-CSF: 250 μg/m^2 per day subcutaneously
When Should Therapy Begin and End?
When indicated, start 24–72 h after chemotherapy
Continue until absolute neutrophil count is 10,000/μL
Do not use concurrently with chemotherapy or radiation therapy

---

Note: G-CSF, granulocyte colony-stimulating factor; GM-CSF, granulocyte-macrophage colony-stimulating factor.
Source: From the American Society of Clinical Oncology.

150 U thrice weekly, may improve quality-of-life scores independently of Hb level. Depot forms of erythropoietin may permit less frequent administration. Hb levels may take up to 2 mos to increase. Concerns have been raised about the ability of erythropoietin to protect hypoxic cells from dying, and at least one study found that its use resulted in poorer tumor control.

For a more detailed discussion, see Sausville EA, Longo DL: Principles of Cancer Treatment, Chap. 70, p. 464, in HPIM-16.

69

MYELOID LEUKEMIAS, MYELODYSPLASIA, AND MYELOPROLIFERATIVE SYNDROMES

ACUTE MYELOID LEUKEMIA

Acute myeloid leukemia (AML) is a clonal malignancy of myeloid bone marrow precursors in which poorly differentiated cells accumulate in the bone marrow and circulation.

Signs and symptoms occur because of the absence of mature cells normally produced by the bone marrow, including granulocytes (susceptibility to infection) and platelets (susceptibility to bleeding). In addition, if large numbers of immature malignant myeloblasts circulate, they may invade organs and rarely produce dysfunction. Distinct morphologic subtypes exist (Table 69-1) that have largely overlapping clinical features. Of note is the propensity of pts with acute promyelocytic leukemia (APL) (FAB M3) to develop bleeding and DIC, especially during induction chemotherapy, because of the release of procoagulants from their cytoplasmic granules.

INCIDENCE AND ETIOLOGY In the United States about 7000 cases occur each year. AML accounts for about 80% of acute leukemias in adults. Etiology is unknown for the vast majority. Three environmental exposures increase the risk: chronic benzene exposure, radiation exposure, and prior treatment with alkylating agents (especially in addition to radiation therapy) and topoisomerase II inhibitors (e.g., doxorubicin and etoposide). Chronic myeloid leukemia (CML), myelodysplasia, and myeloproliferative syndromes may all evolve into AML. Certain genetic abnormalities are associated with particular morphologic variants: t(15;17) with APL, inv(16) with eosinophilic leukemia; others occur in a number of types. Chromosome 11q23 abnormalities are often seen in leukemias developing after exposure to topoisomerase II inhibitors. Chromosome 5 or 7 deletions are seen in leukemias following radiation plus chemotherapy. The particular genetic abnormality has a strong influence on treatment outcome. Expression of MDR1 (multidrug resistance efflux pump) is common in older pts and adversely affects prognosis.

CLINICAL AND LABORATORY FEATURES Initial symptoms of acute leukemia have usually been present for <3 months; a preleukemic syndrome may be present in some 25% of pts with AML. Signs of anemia, pallor, fatigue, weakness, palpitations, and dyspnea on exertion are most common. WBC may be low, normal, or markedly elevated; circulating blast cells may or may not be present; with WBC > 100×10^9 blasts per liter, leukostasis in lungs and brain may occur. Minor pyogenic infections of the skin are common. Thrombocytopenia leads to spontaneous bleeding, epistaxis, petechiae, conjunctival hemorrhage, gingival bleeding, bruising, especially with platelet count <20,000/μL. Anorexia and weight loss are common; fever may be present.

Bacterial and fungal infection are common; risk is heightened with total neutrophil count <5000/μL, breakdown of mucosal and cutaneous barriers aggravates susceptibility; infections may be clinically occult in presence of severe leukopenia, and prompt recognition requires a high degree of clinical suspicion.

Hepatosplenomegaly occurs in about one-third of pts; leukemic meningitis may present with headache, nausea, seizures, papilledema, cranial nerve palsies.

Metabolic abnormalities may include hyponatremia, hypokalemia, elevated serum lactate dehydrogenase (LDH), hyperuricemia, and (rarely) lactic acidosis. With very high blast cell count in the blood, spurious hyperkalemia and hy-

Table 69-1

Acute Myeloid Leukemia (AML) Classification Systems

French-American-British (FAB) Classification[a]
M0: Minimally differentiated leukemia
M1: Myeloblastic leukemia without maturation
M2: Myeloblastic leukemia with maturation
M3: Hypergranular promyelocytic leukemia
M4Eo: Variant: Increase in abnormal marrow eosinophils
M4: Myelomonocytic leukemia
M5: Monocytic leukemia
M6: Erythroleukemia (DiGuglielmo's disease)
M7: Megakaryoblastic leukemia

World Health Organization Classification[b]
I. AML with recurrent cytogenetic translocations
   AML with t(8;21)(q22;q22); *AML1(CBFα)/ETO*
   Acute promyelocytic leukemia [AML with t(15;17)(q22;q12) and variants; *PML/RARα*]
   AML with abnormal bone marrow eosinophils [inv(16)(p13q22) or t(16;16)(p13;q22) *CBFβ/MYH1*]
   AML with 11q23 (*MLL*) abnormalities
II. AML with multilineage dysplasia
   With prior myelodysplastic syndrome
   Without prior myelodysplastic syndrome
III. AML and myelodysplastic syndrome, therapy-related
   Alkylating agent-related
   Epipodophyllotoxin-related
   Other types
IV. AML not otherwise categorized
   AML minimally differentiated
   AML without maturation
   AML with maturation
   Acute myelomonocytic leukemia
   Acute monocytic leukemia
   Acute erythroid leukemia
   Acute megakaryocytic leukemia
   Acute basophilic leukemia
   Acute panmyelosis with myelofibrosis

---

[a] JM Bennett et al: Ann Intern Med 103:620, 1985.
[b] NL Harris et al: J Clin Oncol 17:3835, 1999.

poglycemia may occur (potassium released from and glucose consumed by tumor cells after the blood was drawn).

 TREATMENT

Leukemic cell mass at time of presentation may be $10^{11}–10^{12}$ cells; when total leukemic cell numbers fall below $\sim 10^9$, they are no longer detectable in blood or bone marrow and pt appears to be in complete remission (CR). Thus aggressive therapy must continue past the point when initial cell bulk is reduced if leukemia is to be eradicated. Typical phases of chemotherapy include remission induction and postremission therapy, with treatment lasting about 1 year.

Supportive care with transfusions of red cells and platelets (from CMV-seronegative donors, if pt is a candidate for bone marrow transplantation) is very important, as are aggressive prevention, diagnosis, and treatment of infections. Colony-stimulating factors offer little or no benefit; some recommend their use in older pts and those with active infections. Febrile neutropenia should be treated with broad-spectrum antibiotics (e.g., ceftazidime 1 g q8h); if febrile neutropenia persists beyond 7 days, amphotericin B should be added.

60–80% of pts will achieve initial remission when treated with cytarabine 100–200 (mg/m^2)/d by continuous infusion for 7 days, and daunorubicin [45 (mg/ m^2)/d] or idarubicin [12–13 (mg/m^2)/d] for 3 days. Addition of etoposide may improve CR duration. Half of treated pts enter CR with the first cycle of therapy, and another 25% require two cycles. 10–30% of pts achieve 5-year disease-free survival and probable cure. Patients achieving a CR who have low risk of relapse [cells contain t(8;21) or inv(16)] receive 3–4 cycles of cytarabine. Those at high risk of relapse may be considered for allogeneic bone marrow transplantation.

Response to treatment after relapse is short, and prognosis for pts who have relapsed is poor. In APL, addition of *trans*-retinoic acid (tretinoin) to chemotherapy induces differentiation of the leukemic cells and may improve outcome. Arsenic trioxide also induces differentiation in APL cells.

Bone marrow transplantation from identical twin or HLA-identical sibling is effective treatment for AML. Typical protocol uses high-dose chemotherapy ± total-body irradiation to ablate host marrow, followed by infusion of marrow from donor. Risks are substantial (unless marrow is from identical twin). Complications include graft-versus-host disease, interstitial pneumonitis, opportunistic infections (especially CMV). Comparison between transplantation and high-dose cytarabine as postremission therapy has not produced a clear advantage for either approach. Up to 30% of otherwise end-stage pts with refractory leukemia achieve probable cure from transplantation; results are better when transplant is performed during remission. Results are best for children and young adults.

CHRONIC MYELOID LEUKEMIA

CML is a clonal malignancy usually characterized by splenomegaly and production of increased numbers of granulocytes; course is initially indolent but eventuates in leukemic phase (blast crisis) that has a poorer prognosis than de novo AML; rate of progression to blast crisis is variable; overall survival averages 4 years from diagnosis.

INCIDENCE AND ETIOLOGY In the United States, about 4000 cases occur each year. Over 90% of cases have a reciprocal translocation between chromosomes 9 and 22, creating the Philadelphia (Ph) chromosome and a fusion gene product called BCR-ABL (BCR is from 9, ABL from 22). The chromosome abnormality appears in all bone marrow–derived cells except T cells. The protein made by the chimeric gene is 210 kDa in chronic phase and 190 kDa in acute blast transformation. In some pts, the chronic phase is clinically silent and pts present with acute leukemia with the Ph chromosome.

CLINICAL AND LABORATORY FEATURES Symptoms develop gradually; easy fatigability, malaise, anorexia, abdominal discomfort and early satiety from the large spleen, excessive sweating. Occasional pts are found incidentally based upon elevated leukocyte count. WBC count is usually >25,000/ μL with the increase accounted for by granulocytes and their precursors back to the myelocyte stage; bands and mature forms predominate. Basophils may account for 10–15% of the cells in the blood. Platelet count is normal or increased. Anemia is often present. Neutrophil alkaline phosphatase score is low.

Marrow is hypercellular with granulocytic hyperplasia. Marrow blast cell count is normal or slightly elevated. Serum levels of vitamin B_{12}, B_{12}-binding proteins, and LDH are elevated in proportion to the WBC. With high blood counts, spurious hyperkalemia and hypoglycemia may be seen.

NATURAL HISTORY Chronic phase lasts 2–4 years. Accelerated phase is marked by anemia disproportionate to the disease activity or treatment. Platelet counts fall. Additional cytogenetic abnormalities appear. Blast cell counts increase. Usually within 6–8 months, overt blast crisis develops in which maturation ceases and blasts predominate. The clinical picture is that of acute leukemia. Half of the cases become AML, one-third have morphologic features of acute lymphoid leukemia, 10% are erythroleukemia, and the rest are undifferentiated. Survival in blast crisis is often <4 months.

℞ TREATMENT

Criteria for response are provided in Table 69-2. Allogeneic bone marrow transplantation has the potential to cure the disease in chronic phase. However, the first treatment is imatinib, a molecule that inhibits the activity of chimeric gene product's tyrosine kinase activity. A daily oral dose of 400 mg produces complete hematologic remission of >90% and cytogenetic remission in 76%. If a matched donor is available, it is best to transplant patients in complete remission. Several mechanisms of resistance to imatinib have emerged, and it is unlikely that it leads to permanent remissions when used alone; however, follow-up is not sufficient to draw firm conclusions.

Patients who no longer respond to imatinib may respond to interferon-α (IFN-α) at 3 million units SC daily or thrice weekly. Allopurinol, 300 mg/d, prevents urate nephropathy. The only curative therapy for the disease is HLA-matched allogeneic bone marrow transplantation. The optimal timing of transplantation is unclear, but transplantation in chronic phase is more effective than transplantation in accelerated phase or blast crisis. Transplantation appears most effective in pts treated within a year of diagnosis who have not received long-term IFN. Long-term disease-free survival may be obtained in

Table 69-2

Response Criteria in CML

Hematologic	
Complete response[a]	White blood cell count <10,000/μl, normal morphology
	Normal hemoglobin and platelet counts
Incomplete response	White blood cell count ≥ 10,000/μl
Cytogenetic	Percentage of bone marrow metaphases with t(9;22)
Complete response	0
Partial response	≤35
Minor response	36–85[b]
No response	85–100
Molecular	Presence of *BCR/ABL* transcript by RT-PCR
Complete response	None
Incomplete response	Any

[a] Complete hematologic response requires the disappearance of splenomegaly.
[b] Up to 15% normal metaphases are occasionally seen at diagnosis (when 30 metaphases are analyzed).
Note: RT-PCR, reverse transcriptase polymerase chain reaction.

50–60% of transplanted pts. Infusion of donor lymphocytes can restore remission in relapsing pts. In pts without a matched donor, autologous transplantation may be helpful using peripheral blood stem cells. Treatment of pts in blast crisis with imatinib can obtain responses, but their durability has not been established.

MYELODYSPLASTIC SYNDROMES (MDS)

These are clonal abnormalities of marrow cells characterized by varying degrees of cytopenias affecting one or more cell lines. These entities have been divided into five clinical syndromes (Table 69-3). Other terms that have been used to describe one or more of the entities include *preleukemia* and *oligoblastic leukemia*.

INCIDENCE AND ETIOLOGY   About 3000 cases occur each year, mainly in persons >50 years old. Like AML, exposure to benzene, radiation, and chemotherapeutic agents may lead to MDS. Chromosome abnormalities occur in up to 80% of cases, including deletion of part or all of chromosomes 5, 7, and 9 (20 or 21 less commonly) and addition of part or all of chromosome 8.

CLINICAL AND LABORATORY FEATURES   Symptoms depend on the affected lineages. 85% of pts are anemic, 50% have neutropenia, and about one-third have thrombocytopenia. The pathologic features of MDS are a cellular marrow with varying degrees of cytologic atypia including delayed nuclear maturation, abnormal cytoplasmic maturation, accumulation of ringed sideroblasts (iron-laden mitochondria surrounding the nucleus), uni- or bilobed megakaryocytes, micromegakaryocytes, and increased myeloblasts. Table 69-3 lists features used to identify distinct entities. Prognosis is defined by marrow blast %, karyotype, and lineages affected (see Table 69-4).

 TREATMENT

Allogeneic bone marrow transplantation is the only curative therapy and may cure 60% of those so treated. However, the majority of pts with MDS are too

Table 69-3

French-American-British (FAB) Classification of Myelodysplastic Syndromes

	FAB Types				
	RA	RARS	RAEB	CMML	RAEB-t
% Cases	28	24	23	16	9
% Blasts					
Marrow	<5	<5	5–20	1–20	20–30
Blood	<1	<1	<5	<5	>5
% Ringed sideroblasts	<15	>15	<15	<15	<15
Monocytes	Rare	Rare	Rare	>1000/μL	Variable
Dyspoiesis	+	+	++	++	++
% Leukemic transformation	11	5	23	20	48
Median survival, months	37	49	9	22	6

Note: RA, refractory anemia; RARS, refractory anemia with ringed sideroblasts; RAEB, refractory anemia with excess blasts; CMML, chronic myelomonocytic leukemia; RAEB- t, refractory anemia with excess blasts in transformation.

Table 69-4

International Prognostic Scoring System for Myelodysplastic Syndromes

Prognostic Factors
  % Marrow blasts <5 = 0 pts; 5–10 = 0.5 pts; 11–20 = 1.5 pts;
                     21–30 = 2 pts
  Karyotype*   good = 0 pts; intermediate = 0.5 pts; poor = 1.5 pts
  Cytopenias   0/1 = 0 pts; 2/3 = 0.5 pts

Risk Group	Low	Intermediate-1	Intermediate-2	High
Total Points	0	0.5–1.0	1.5–2.0	≥2.5
Risk of AML	19%	30%	33%	45%
Median survival(years)	5.7	3.5	1.2	0.4

* Good karyotypes: normal, $-Y$, del(5q), del(20q)
  Poor karyotypes: ≥3 abnormalities, chr 7 abnormalities
  Intermediate karyotypes: others

old to receive transplantation. 5-Azacytidine can delay transformation to AML by 8–10 months. Pts with low erythropoietin levels may respond to erythropoietin, and a minority of pts with neutropenia respond to granulocyte colony-stimulating factor. Supportive care is the cornerstone of treatment.

MYELOPROLIFERATIVE SYNDROMES

The three major myeloproliferative syndromes are polycythemia vera, idiopathic myelofibrosis, and essential thrombocytosis. All are clonal disorders of hematopoietic stem cells.

Polycythemia Vera

The most common myeloproliferative syndrome, this is characterized by an increase in RBC mass, massive splenomegaly, and clinical manifestations related to increased blood viscosity, including neurologic symptoms (vertigo, tinnitus, headache, visual disturbances) and thromboses (myocardial infarction, stroke, peripheral vascular disease; uncommonly, mesenteric and hepatic). It must be distinguished from other causes of increased RBC mass (Chap. 57). This is most readily done by assaying serum erythropoietin levels. Polycythemia vera is associated with very low erythropoietin levels; in other causes of erythrocytosis, erythropoietin levels are high. Pts are effectively managed with phlebotomy. Some pts require splenectomy to control symptoms, and those with severe pruritus may benefit from psoralens and UV light. 20% develop myelofibrosis, $<5\%$ acute leukemia.

Idiopathic Myelofibrosis

This rare entity is characterized by marrow fibrosis, myeloid metaplasia with extramedullary hematopoiesis, and splenomegaly. Evaluation of a blood smear reveals tear-drop shaped RBC, nucleated RBC, and some early granulocytic forms, including promyelocytes. However, many entities may lead to marrow fibrosis and extramedullary hematopoiesis, and the diagnosis of primary idiopathic myelofibrosis is made only when the many other potential causes are ruled out. The following diseases are in the differential diagnosis: CML, polycythemia vera, Hodgkin's disease, cancer metastatic to the marrow (especially from breast and prostate), infection (particularly granulomatous infections), and hairy cell leukemia. Supportive therapy is generally used; no specific therapy is known.

Essential Thrombocytosis

This is usually noted incidentally upon routine platelet count done in an asymptomatic person. Like myelofibrosis, many conditions can produce elevated platelet counts; thus, the diagnosis is one of exclusion. Platelet count must be >500,000/μL, and known causes of thrombocytosis must be ruled out including CML, iron deficiency, splenectomy, malignancy, infection, hemorrhage, polycythemia vera, myelodysplasia, and recovery from vitamin B$_{12}$ deficiency. Although usually asymptomatic, pts should be treated if they develop migraine headache, transient ischemic attack, or other bleeding or thrombotic disease manifestations. Interferon-a is effective therapy, as are anagrelide and hydroxyurea. Treatment should not be given just because the absolute platelet count is high in the absence of other symptoms.

For a more detailed discussion, see Young NS: Aplastic Anemia, Myelodysplasia, and Related Bone Marrow Failure Syndromes, Chap. 94, p. 617; Spivak JL: Polycythemia Vera and Other Myeloproliferative Diseases, Chap. 95, p. 626; and Wetzler M, Byrd JC, Bloomfield CD: Acute and Chronic Myeloid Leukemia, Chap. 96, p. 631, in HPIM-16.

70

LYMPHOID MALIGNANCIES

DEFINITION   Neoplasms of lymphocytes usually represent malignant counterparts of cells at discrete stages of normal lymphocyte differentiation. When bone marrow and peripheral blood involvement dominate the clinical picture, the disease is classified as a *lymphoid leukemia*. When lymph nodes and/or other extranodal sites of disease are the dominant site(s) of involvement, the tumor is called a *lymphoma*. The distinction between lymphoma and leukemia is sometimes blurred; for example, small lymphocytic lymphoma and chronic lymphoid leukemia are tumors of the same cell type and are distinguished arbitrarily on the basis of the absolute number of peripheral blood lymphocytes ($>5 \times 10^9$/L defines leukemia).

CLASSIFICATION   Historically, lymphoid tumors have had separate pathologic classifications based on the clinical syndrome—lymphomas according to the Rappaport, Kiel, or Working Formulation systems; acute leukemias according to the French-American-British (FAB) system; Hodgkin's disease according to the Rye classification. Myelomas have generally not been subclassified by pathologic features of the neoplastic cells. The World Health Organization (WHO) has proposed a unifying classification system that brings together all lymphoid neoplasms into a single framework. Although the new system bases the definitions of disease entities on histology, genetic abnormalities, immunophenotype, and clinical features, its organization is based upon cell of origin (B cell vs. T cell) and maturation stage (precursor vs. mature) of the tumor, features that are of limited value to the clinician. Table 70-1 lists the

Table 70-1

Clinical Schema of Lymphoid Neoplasms

Chronic lymphoid leukemias/lymphomas
  Chronic lymphocytic leukemia/small lymphocytic lymphoma (99% B cell, 1% T cell)
  Prolymphocytic leukemia (90% B cell, 10% T cell)
  Large granular lymphocyte leukemia [80% natural killer (NK) cell, 20% T cell]
  Hairy cell leukemia (99-100% B cell)
Indolent lymphoma
  Follicular center cell lymphoma, grades I and II (100% B cell)
  Lymphoplasmacytic lymphoma/Waldenström's macroglobulinemia (100% B cell)
  Marginal zone lymphoma (100% B cell)
    Extranodal [mucosa-associated lymphatic tissue (MALT) lymphoma]
    Nodal (monocytoid B cell lymphoma)
    Splenic marginal zone lymphoma
  Cutaneous T cell lymphoma (mycosis fungoides) (100% T cell)
Aggressive lymphoma
  Diffuse large cell lymphoma (85% B cell, 15% T cell), includes immuno-blastic
  Follicular center cell lymphoma, grade III (100% B cell)
  Mantle cell lymphoma (100% B cell)
  Primary mediastinal (thymic) large B cell lymphoma (100% B cell)
  Burkitt-like lymphoma (100% B cell)
  Peripheral T cell lymphoma (100% T cell)
  Angioimmunoblastic lymphoma (100% T cell)
  Angiocentric lymphoma (80% T cell, 20% NK cell)
  Intestinal T cell lymphoma (100% T cell)
  Anaplastic large cell lymphoma (70% T cell, 30% null cell)
Acute lymphoid leukemias/lymphomas
  Precursor lymphoblastic leukemia/lymphoma (80% T cell, 20% B cell)
  Burkitt's leukemia/lymphoma (100% B cell)
  Adult T cell leukemia/lymphoma (100% T cell)
Plasma cell disorders (100% B cell)
  Monoclonal gammopathy of uncertain significance
  Solitary plasmacytoma
  Extramedullary plasmacytoma
  Multiple myeloma
  Plasma cell leukemia
Hodgkin's disease (cell of origin mainly B cell)
  Lymphocyte predominant
  Nodular sclerosis
  Mixed cellularity
  Lymphocyte depleted

---

disease entities according to a more clinically useful schema based upon the clinical manifestations and natural history of the diseases.

INCIDENCE   Lymphoid tumors are increasing in incidence. Nearly 90,000 cases were diagnosed in 2004 in the United States.

ETIOLOGY   The cause(s) for the vast majority of lymphoid neoplasms is unknown. The malignant cells are monoclonal and often contain numerous genetic abnormalities. Some genetic alterations are characteristic of particular histologic entities: t(8;14) in Burkitt's lymphoma, t(14;18) in follicular lymphoma, t(11;14) in mantle cell lymphoma, t(2;5) in anaplastic large cell lymphoma, translocations or mutations involving *bcl*-6 on 3q27 in diffuse large cell lymphoma, and others. In most cases, translocations involve insertion of a distant chromosome segment into the antigen receptor genes (either immunoglobulin or T cell receptor) during the rearrangement of the gene segments that form the receptors.

Three viruses, EBV, human herpesvirus-8 (HHV-8) (both herpes family viruses), and human T-lymphotropic virus type I (HTLV-I, a retrovirus), may cause some lymphoid tumors. EBV has been strongly associated with African Burkitt's lymphoma and the lymphomas that complicate immunodeficiencies (disease-related or iatrogenic). EBV has an uncertain relationship to mixed cellularity Hodgkin's disease and angiocentric lymphoma. HHV-8 causes a rare entity, body cavity lymphoma, mainly in patients with AIDS. HTLV-I is associated with adult T cell leukemia/lymphoma. Both the virus and the disease are endemic to southwestern Japan and the Caribbean.

Gastric *Helicobacter pylori* infection is associated with gastric mucosa-associated lymphoid tissue (MALT) lymphoma and perhaps gastric large cell lymphoma. Eradication of the infection produces durable remissions in about half of pts with gastric MALT lymphoma. MALT lymphomas of other sites are associated with either infection (ocular adnexae, *Chlamydia psitacci*; small intestine, *Campylobacter jejuni*; skin, *Borrelia*) or autoimmunity (salivary gland, Sjögren's syndrome; thyroid gland, Hashimoto's thyroiditis).

Inherited or acquired immunodeficiencies and autoimmune disorders predispose individuals to lymphoma. Lymphoma occurs with increased incidence in farmers and meat workers; Hodgkin's disease is increased in wood workers.

DIAGNOSIS AND STAGING Excisional biopsy is the standard diagnostic procedure; adequate tissue must be obtained. Tissue undergoes three kinds of studies: (1) light microscopy to discern the pattern of growth and the morphologic features of the malignant cells, (2) flow cytometry for assessment of immunophenotype, and (3) genetic studies (cytogenetics, DNA extraction). Needle aspirates of nodal or extranodal masses are not adequate diagnostic procedures. Leukemia diagnosis and lymphoma staging include generous bilateral iliac crest bone marrow biopsies. Differential diagnosis of adenopathy is reviewed in Chap. 58.

Staging varies with the diagnosis. In acute leukemia, peripheral blood blast counts are most significant in assessing prognosis. In chronic leukemia, peripheral blood RBC and platelet counts are most significant in assessing prognosis. Non-Hodgkin's lymphomas have five clinical prognostic factors; indolent and aggressive lymphomas share three of these, advanced stage, high LDH levels, and age >60. In follicular lymphoma, the last two factors are Hb < 120 g/L (<12 g/dL) and more than four nodal sites of involvement. In aggressive lymphoma, more than one extranodal site and performance status predict outcome. In myeloma, serum levels of paraprotein, creatinine, and β_2-microglobulin levels predict survival.

CHRONIC LYMPHOID LEUKEMIAS/LYMPHOMAS

Most of these entities have a natural history measured in years (prolymphocytic leukemia is very rare and can be very aggressive). Chronic lymphocytic leukemia is the most common entity in this group (~7300 cases/year) and the most common leukemia in the western world.

CHRONIC LYMPHOCYTIC LEUKEMIA (CLL) Usually presents as asymptomatic lymphocytosis in pts >60 years. The malignant cell is a CD5+

B cell that looks like a normal small lymphocyte. Trisomy 12 is the most common genetic abnormality. Prognosis is related to stage; stage is determined mainly by the degree to which the tumor cells crowd out normal hematopoietic elements from the marrow (Table 70-2). Cells may infiltrate nodes and spleen as well as marrow. Nodal involvement may be related to the expression of an adhesion molecule that allows the cells to remain in the node rather than recirculate. Pts often have hypogammaglobulinemia. Up to 20% have autoimmune antibodies that may produce autoimmune hemolytic anemia, thrombocytopenia, or red cell aplasia. Death is from infection, marrow failure, or intercurrent illnesses. In 5%, the disease evolves to aggressive lymphoma (Richter's syndrome) that is refractory to treatment.

Subsets of CLL may exist based on whether the immunoglobulin expressed by the tumor cell contains mutations (more indolent course, good prognosis) or retains the germline sequence (more aggressive course, poor response to therapy). Methods to distinguish the two subsets clinically are not well defined; CD38+ tumors may have poorer prognosis. The expression of ZAP-70, an intracellular tyrosine kinase normally present in T cells and aberrantly expressed in about 45% of CLL cases, may be a better way to define prognostic subsets. ZAP-70+ cases usually need treatment within about 3–4 years from diagnosis; ZAP-70-negative cases usually don't require treatment for 8–11 years.

℞ TREATMENT

Supportive care is generally given until anemia or thrombocytopenia develop. At that time, tests are indicated to assess the cause of the anemia or thrombocytopenia. Decreased red blood cell and/or platelet counts related to peripheral destruction may be treated with splenectomy or glucocorticoids without cytotoxic therapy in many cases. If marrow replacement is the mechanism, cytotoxic therapy is indicated. Fludarabine, 25 $(mg/m^2)/d$ IV $\times$ 5 days every 4 weeks, induces responses in about 75% of pts, complete responses in half. Glucocorticoids increase the risk of infection without adding a substantial antitumor benefit. Monthly IV immunoglobulin (IVIg) significantly reduces risk of serious infection but is expensive and usually reserved for patients who have had a serious infection. Alkylating agents are also active against the tumor. Therapeutic intent is palliative in most pts. Young pts may be

Table 70-2

Staging of B Cell CLL and Relation to Survival

Stage	Clinical Features	Median Survival, Years
RAI		
0	Lymphocytosis	12
I	Lymphocytosis + adenopathy	9
II	Lymphocytosis + splenomegaly	7
III	Anemia	1–2
IV	Thrombocytopenia	1–2
BINET		
A	No anemia/thrombocytopenia, <3 involved sites	>10
B	No anemia/thrombocytopenia, >3 involved sites	5
C	Anemia and/or thrombocytopenia	2

candidates for high-dose therapy and autologous or allogeneic hematopoietic cell transplantation; long-term disease-free survival has been noted. Mini-transplant, in which the preparative regimen is immunosuppressive but not myeloablative, may be less toxic and as active or more active in disease treatment than high-dose therapy. Monoclonal antibodies alemtuzumab (anti-CD52) and rituximab (anti-CD20) are also active.

See Chap. 97 in HPIM-16 for discussion of the rarer entities.

INDOLENT LYMPHOMAS

These entities have a natural history measured in years. Median survival is about 10 years. Follicular center lymphoma is the most common indolent lymphoma, accounting for about one-third of all lymphoid malignancies.

FOLLICULAR CENTER LYMPHOMA   Usually presents with painless peripheral lymphadenopathy, often involving several nodal regions. "B symptoms" (fever, sweats, weight loss) occur in 10%, less common than with Hodgkin's disease. In about 25%, nodes wax and wane before the pt seeks medical attention. Median age is 55 years. Disease is widespread at diagnosis in 85%. Liver and bone marrow are commonly involved extranodal sites.

The tumor has a follicular or nodular growth pattern reflecting the follicular center origin of the malignant cell. The t(14;18) is present in 85% of cases, resulting in the overexpression of bcl-2, a protein involved in prevention of programmed cell death. The normal follicular center B cell is undergoing active mutation of the immunoglobulin variable regions in an effort to generate antibody of higher affinity for the selecting antigen. Follicular center lymphoma cells also have a high rate of mutation that leads to the accumulation of genetic damage. Over time, follicular center lymphomas acquire sufficient genetic damage (e.g., mutated p53) to accelerate their growth and evolve into diffuse large cell lymphomas that are refractory to treatment. The majority of pts dying from follicular lymphoma have undergone histologic transformation. This transformation occurs at a rate of about 7% per year and is an attribute of the disease, not the treatment.

℞ TREATMENT

Only 15% of pts have localized disease, but the majority of these pts are curable with radiation therapy. Although many forms of treatment induce tumor regression in advanced-stage pts, it is not clear that treatment of any kind alters the natural history of disease. No therapy, single-agent alkylators, nucleoside analogues (fludarabine, cladribine), combination chemotherapy, radiation therapy, and biologic agents [interferon (IFN)α, monoclonal antibodies such as rituxan, anti-CD20] are all considered appropriate. Over 90% of pts are responsive to treatment; complete responses are seen in about half of pts treated aggressively. Younger pts are being treated experimentally with high-dose therapy and autologous hematopoietic stem cells or mini-transplant. It is not yet clear whether this is curative. There is some evidence that combination chemotherapy with or without IFN maintenance may prolong survival and delay or prevent histologic progression, especially in pts with poor prognostic features. Remissions appear to last longer (i.e., >2 years) with chemotherapy plus rituximab; however, it is not clear that survival is extended as a consequence of any therapy.

See Chap. 97 in HPIM-16 for discussion of the other indolent lymphomas.

AGGRESSIVE LYMPHOMAS

A large number of pathologic entities share an aggressive natural history; survival untreated is 6–8 months, and nearly all untreated pts are dead within 1 year. Pts may present with asymptomatic adenopathy or symptoms referable to involvement of practically any nodal or extranodal site: mediastinal involvement may produce superior vena cava syndrome or pericardial tamponade; retroperitoneal nodes may obstruct ureters; abdominal masses may produce pain, ascites, or GI obstruction or perforation; CNS involvement may produce confusion, cranial nerve signs, headache, seizures, and/or spinal cord compression; bone involvement may produce pain or pathologic fracture. About 45% of pts have B symptoms.

Diffuse large B cell lymphoma is the most common histologic diagnosis among the aggressive lymphomas, accounting for ~30% of all lymphomas. Aggressive lymphomas together account for ~55% of all lymphoid tumors. About 85% of aggressive lymphomas are of mature B cell origin; 15% are derived from peripheral (postthymic) T cells.

──────────────── *Approach to the Patient* ────────────────

Early diagnostic biopsy is critical. Pt workup is directed by symptoms and known patterns of disease. Pts with Waldeyer's ring involvement should undergo careful evaluation of the GI tract. Pts with bone or bone marrow involvement should have a lumbar puncture to evaluate meningeal CNS involvement.

Rx TREATMENT

Localized aggressive lymphomas are usually treated with four cycles of CHOP (cyclophosphamide, doxorubicin, vincristine, prednisone) combination chemotherapy +/− involved-field radiation therapy. About 85% of these pts are cured. The specific therapy used for pts with more advanced disease is controversial. Treatment outcome with CHOP is influenced by tumor bulk (usually measured by LDH levels, stage, and number of extranodal sites) and physiologic reserve (usually measured by age and Karnofsky status). The influence of these factors on outcome is shown in Table 70-3. In most series, CHOP cures about one-third of pts. Some investigators have demonstrated cure rates about twice those achieved by CHOP using more aggressive combination chemotherapy regimens that do not require hematopoietic stem cell support. However, randomized trials have not shown significant outcome dif-

Table 70-3

The International Index and Prognosis in Diffuse Aggressive Non-Hodgkin's Lymphoma

Risk Group (Patients of All Ages)	Risk Factors[a]	Distribution of Cases, %	Complete Response Rate, %	5-Year Survival Rate, %
Low	0, 1	35	87	73
Low-intermediate	2	27	67	51
High-intermediate	3	22	55	43
High	4, 5	16	44	26

[a] Age (≤60 vs. >60); serum LDH (normal vs. >1 × normal); performance status (0 or 1 vs. 2–4); stage (I or II vs. III or IV); and extranodal involvement (≥1 site vs. >1 site)
Source: Adapted from MA Shipp: Blood 83:1165, 1994.

ferences. Furthermore, the use of a sequential high-dose chemotherapy regimen in pts with high-intermediate- and high-risk disease has yielded long-term survival in about 75% of pts in some institutions. Other studies fail to confirm a role for high-dose therapy. The use of rituximab plus CHOP chemotherapy improves response rates significantly and is the most commonly used therapy currently. At least 50% of patients are cured with this approach. Whether high-dose therapy and hematopoietic stem cell support can further improve results with CHOP + rituximab is under study.

About 30–45% of pts not cured with initial standard combination chemotherapy may be salvaged with high-dose therapy and autologous hematopoietic stem cell transplantation.

Specialized approaches are required for lymphomas involving certain sites (e.g., CNS, stomach) or under certain complicating clinical circumstances (e.g., concurrent illness, AIDS). Lymphomas occurring in iatrogenically immunosuppressed pts may regress when immunosuppressive medication is withheld. Lymphomas occurring postallogeneic marrow transplant may regress with infusions of donor leukocytes.

Pts with rapidly growing bulky aggressive lymphoma may experience tumor lysis syndrome when treated (Chap. 27); prophylactic measures (hydration, urine alkalinization, allopurinol, rasburicase) may be lifesaving.

ACUTE LYMPHOID LEUKEMIAS/LYMPHOMAS

ACUTE LYMPHOBLASTIC LEUKEMIA AND LYMPHOBLASTIC LYMPHOMA These are more common in children than adults (~3600 total cases/year). The majority of cases have tumor cells that appear to be of thymic origin, and pts may have mediastinal masses. Pts usually present with recent onset of signs of marrow failure (pallor, fatigue, bleeding, fever, infection). Hepatosplenomegaly and adenopathy are common. Males may have testicular enlargement reflecting leukemic involvement. Meningeal involvement may be present at diagnosis or develop later. Elevated LDH, hyponatremia, and hypokalemia may be present, in addition to anemia, thrombocytopenia, and high peripheral blood blast counts. The leukemic cells are more often FAB L2 in type in adults than in children, where L1 predominates. Leukemia diagnosis requires at least 30% lymphoblasts in the marrow. Prognosis is adversely affected by high presenting white count, age >35 years, and the presence of t(9; 22), t(1;19), and t(4;11) translocations. HOX11 expression identifies a more favorable subset of T-ALL.

R̲x̲ **TREATMENT**

Successful treatment requires intensive induction phase, CNS prophylaxis, and maintenance chemotherapy that extends for about 2 years. Vincristine, L-asparaginase, cytarabine, daunorubicin, and prednisone are particularly effective agents. Intrathecal or high-dose systemic methotrexate is effective CNS prophylaxis. Long-term survival of 60–65% of pts may be achieved. The role and timing of bone marrow transplantation in primary therapy is debated, but up to 30% of relapsed pts may be cured with salvage transplantation.

BURKITT'S LYMPHOMA/LEUKEMIA This is also more common in children. It is associated with translocations involving the c-*myc* gene on chromosome 8 rearranging with immunoglobulin heavy or light chain genes. Pts often have disseminated disease with large abdominal masses, hepatomegaly, and adenopathy. If a leukemic picture predominates, it is classified as FAB L3.

TREATMENT

Resection of large abdominal masses improves treatment outcome. Aggressive leukemia regimens that include vincristine, cyclophosphamide, 6-mercaptopurine, doxorubicin, and prednisone are active. CODOX-M and the BFM regimen are the most effective regimens. Cure may be achieved in 50–60%. The need for maintenance therapy is unclear. Prophylaxis against tumor lysis syndrome is important (Chap. 27).

ADULT T CELL LEUKEMIA/LYMPHOMA (ATL)   This is very rare, and only a small fraction (~2%) of persons infected with HTLV-I go on to develop the disease. Some HTLV-I-infected pts develop spastic paraplegia from spinal cord involvement without developing cancer. The characteristic clinical syndrome of ATL includes high white count without severe anemia or thrombocytopenia, skin infiltration, hepatomegaly, pulmonary infiltrates, meningeal involvement, and opportunistic infections. The tumor cells are CD4+ T cells with cloven hoof– or flower-shaped nuclei. Hypercalcemia occurs in nearly all pts and is related to cytokines produced by the tumor cells.

 TREATMENT

Aggressive therapy is associated with serious toxicity related to the underlying immunodeficiency. Glucocorticoids relieve hypercalcemia. The tumor is responsive to therapy, but responses are generally short-lived. Zidovudine and IFN may be palliative in some pts.

PLASMA CELL DISORDERS

The hallmark of plasma cell disorders is the production of immunoglobulin molecules or fragments from abnormal plasma cells. The intact immunoglobulin molecule, or the heavy chain or light chain produced by the abnormal plasma cell clone, is detectable in the serum and/or urine and is called the M (for monoclonal) component. The amount of the M component in any given pt reflects the tumor burden in that pt. In some, the presence of a clonal light chain in the urine (Bence Jones protein) is the only tumor product that is detectable. M components may be seen in pts with other lymphoid tumors, nonlymphoid cancers, and noncancerous conditions such as cirrhosis, sarcoidosis, parasitic infestations, and autoimmune diseases.

MULTIPLE MYELOMA   A malignant proliferation of plasma cells in the bone marrow (notably not in lymph nodes). About 14,000 new cases are diagnosed each year. Disease manifestations result from tumor expansion, local and remote actions of tumor products, and the host response to the tumor. About 70% of pts have bone pain, usually involving the back and ribs, precipitated by movement. Bone lesions are multiple, lytic, and rarely accompanied by an osteoblastic response. Thus, bone scans are less useful than radiographs. The production of osteoclast-activating cytokines by tumor cells leads to substantial calcium mobilization, hypercalcemia, and symptoms related to it. Decreased synthesis and increased catabolism of normal immunoglobulins leads to hypogammaglobulinemia, and a poorly defined tumor product inhibits granulocyte migration. These changes create a susceptibility to bacterial infections, especially the pneumococcus, *Klebsiella pneumoniae*, and *Staphylococcus aureus* affecting the lung and *Escherichia coli* and other gram-negative pathogens affecting the urinary tract. Infections affect at least 75% of pts at some time in their course. Renal failure may affect 25% of pts; its pathogenesis is multifactorial—hypercalcemia, infection, toxic effects of light chains, urate nephropathy, dehydration. Neurologic symptoms may result from hyperviscosity, cryoglobulins, and rarely amyloid deposition in nerves. Anemia occurs in 80% related to myelophthisis and inhibition of erythropoiesis by tumor products. Clotting abnormalities may produce bleeding.

Diagnosis Marrow plasmacytosis >10%, lytic bone lesions, and a serum and/or urine M component are the classic triad. Monoclonal gammopathy of uncertain significance (MGUS) is much more common than myeloma, affecting about 6% of people over age 70; in general, MGUS is associated with a level of M component <20 g/L, low serum β_2-microglobulin, <10% marrow plasma cells, and no bone lesions. Lifetime risk of progression of MGUS to myeloma is about 25%.

Staging Disease stage influences survival (Table 70-4).

℞ TREATMENT

About 10% of pts have very slowly progressive disease and do not require treatment until the paraprotein levels rise above 50 g/L or progressive bone disease occurs. Pts with solitary plasmacytoma and extramedullary plasmacytoma are usually cured with localized radiation therapy. Supportive care includes early treatment of infections; control of hypercalcemia with glucocorticoids, hydration, and natriuresis; chronic administration of bisphosphonates to antagonize skeletal destruction; and prophylaxis against urate nephropathy and dehydration. Therapy aimed at the tumor is usually palliative. Initial therapy is usually one of several approaches: thalidomide, 400 mg/d PO, plus dexamethasone, 40 mg/d on days 1–4 each month, with or without chemotherapy such as liposomal doxorubicin; melphalan, 8 mg/m² orally for 4–7 days every 4–6 weeks, plus prednisone. About 60% of pts have significant symptomatic improvement plus a 75% decline in the M component. Experimental approaches using sequential high-dose pulses of melphalan plus two successive autologous stem cell transplants have produced complete responses in about 50% of pts <65 years. Long-term follow-up is required to see whether survival is enhanced. Palliatively treated pts generally follow a chronic course for 2–5 years, followed by an acceleration characterized by organ infiltration with myeloma cells and marrow failure. New approaches to salvage treatment include bortezomib, 1.3 mg/m² on days 1, 4, 8, and 11 every 3 weeks, often used with dexamethasone, vincristine, and/or liposomal doxorubicin.

HODGKIN'S DISEASE About 8000 new cases are diagnosed each year. Hodgkin's disease (HD) is a tumor of Reed-Sternberg cells, aneuploid cells that usually express CD30 and CD15 but may also express other B or T cell markers. Most tumors are derived from B cells in that immunoglobulin genes are rearranged, but some tumors are of T cell phenotype. Most of the cells in an enlarged node are normal lymphoid, plasma cells, monocytes, and eosinophils. The etiology is unknown, but the incidence in both identical twins is 99-fold increased over the expected concordance, suggesting a genetic susceptibility. Distribution of histologic subtypes is 75% nodular sclerosis, 20% mixed cellularity, with lymphocyte predominant and lymphocyte depleted representing about 5%.

Clinical Manifestations Usually presents with asymptomatic lymph node enlargement or with adenopathy associated with fever, night sweats, weight loss, and sometimes pruritus. Mediastinal adenopathy (common in nodular sclerosing

Table 70-4

Myeloma Staging System

Stage	Criteria	Estimated Tumor Burden, $\times 10^{12}$ cells/m^2

I	All the following:
	1. Hemoglobin > 100 g/L (>10 g/dL)
	2. Serum calcium < 3 mmol/L
	3. Normal bone x-ray or solitary lesion
	4. Low M-component production
	   a. IgG level < 50 g/L (<5 g/dL)
	   b. IgA level < 30 g/L (<3 g/dL)
	   c. Urine light chain <4 g/24 h)
		<0.6 (low)

II	Fitting neither I nor III	0.6–1.20 (intermediate)

III	One or more of the following:
	1. Hemoglobin < 85 g/L (<8.5 g/dL)
	2. Serum calcium > 3 mmol/L (<12 mg/dL)
	3. Advanced lytic bone lesions
	4. High M-component production
	   a. IgG level > 70 g/L (>7 g/dL)
	   b. IgA level > 50 g/L (>5 g/dL)
	   c. Urine light chains > 12 g/24 h
		<1.20 (high)

SUBCLASSIFICATION BASED ON SERUM CREATININE LEVELS

Level	Stage	Median Survival Months
A < 177 μmol/L ($\leq$2 mg/dL)	IA	61
B > 177 μmol/L (>2 mg/dL)	IIA, B	55
	IIIA	30
	IIIB	15

STAGING BASED ON SERUM β_2-MICROGLOBULIN LEVELS

<0.004 g/L ($\leq$4 μg/mL)	I	43
>0.004 g/L (>4 μg/mL)	II	12

HD) may produce cough. Spread of disease tends to be to contiguous lymph node groups. SVC obstruction or spinal cord compression may be presenting manifestation. Involvement of bone marrow and liver is rare.

Differential Diagnosis

• Infection—mononucleosis, viral syndromes, toxoplasma, histoplasma, primary tuberculosis
• Other malignancies—especially head and neck cancers
• Sarcoidosis—mediastinal and hilar adenopathy

Immunologic and Hematologic Abnormalities

• Defects in cell-mediated immunity (remains even after successful treatment of lymphoma); cutaneous anergy; diminished antibody production to capsular antigens of *Haemophilus* and pneumococcus
• Anemia; elevated ESR; leukemoid reaction; eosinophilia; lymphocytopenia; fibrosis and granulomas in marrow

Staging The Ann Arbor staging classification is shown in Table 70-5. Disease is staged by performing physical exam, CXR, thoracoabdominal CT, bone

Table 70-5

Ann Arbor Staging System	
Stage I	Involvement in single lymph node region or single extralymphatic site
Stage II	Involvement of two or more lymph node regions on the same side of diaphragm
	Localized contiguous involvement of only one extralymphatic site and lymph node region (stage IIE)
Stage III	Involvement of lymph node regions on both sides of diaphragm; may include spleen
Stage IV	Disseminated involvement of one or more extralymphatic organs with or without lymph node involvement

marrow biopsy; ultrasound examinations, lymphangiogram. Staging laparotomy should be used, especially to evaluate the spleen, if pt has early-stage disease on clinical grounds and radiation therapy is being contemplated. Pathologic staging is unnecessary if the pt is treated with chemotherapy.

 TREATMENT

About 85% of pts are curable. Therapy should be performed by experienced clinicians in centers with appropriate facilities. Pts with stages I and II disease documented by negative laparotomy are treated with subtotal nodal radiation therapy. Increasingly, patients are not taken to laparotomy for staging and are being treated either with chemotherapy alone or combined modality therapy for early-stage disease. Those with stage III or IV disease receive six cycles of combination chemotherapy, usually either ABVD or MOPP-ABV hybrid therapy or MOPP/ABVD alternating therapy. Pts with any stage disease accompanied by a large mediastinal mass ($>1/3$ the greatest chest diameter) should receive combined modality therapy with MOPP/ABVD or MOPP-ABV hybrid followed by mantle field radiation therapy (radiation plus ABVD is too toxic to the lung). About two-thirds of pts not cured by their initial radiation therapy treatment are rescued by salvage combination chemotherapy. About one-half of pts (or more) not cured by their initial chemotherapy regimen may be rescued by high-dose therapy and autologous stem cell transplant.

With long-term follow-up, it has become clear that more pts are dying of late fatal toxicities related to radiation therapy (myocardial infarction, second cancers) than from HD. It may be possible to avoid radiation exposure by using combination chemotherapy in early-stage disease as well as in advanced-stage disease.

For a more detailed discussion, see Armitage JO, Longo DL: Malignancies of Lymphoid Cells, Chap. 97, p. 641; Longo DL, Anderson KC: Plasma Cell Disorders, Chap. 98, p. 656, in HPIM-16.

71

SKIN CANCER

MALIGNANT MELANOMA

Most dangerous cutaneous malignancy; high metastatic potential; poor prognosis with metastatic spread.

INCIDENCE Melanoma was diagnosed in 55,100 people in the United States in 2004 and caused 7910 deaths.

PREDISPOSING FACTORS Fair complexion, sun exposure, family history of melanoma, dysplastic nevus syndrome (autosomal dominant disorder with multiple nevi of distinctive appearance and cutaneous melanoma, may be associated with 9p deletion), and presence of a giant congenital nevus. Blacks have a low incidence.

PREVENTION Sun avoidance lowers risk. Sunscreens are not proven effective.

TYPES

1. *Superficial spreading melanoma*: Most common; begins with initial radial growth phase before invasion.
2. *Lentigo maligna melanoma*: Very long radial growth phase before invasion, lentigo maligna (Hutchinson's melanotic freckle) is precursor lesion, most common in elderly and in sun-exposed areas (esp. face).
3. *Acral lentiginous*: Most common form in darkly pigmented pts; occurs on palms and soles, mucosal surfaces, in nail beds and mucocutaneous junctions; similar to lentigo maligna melanoma but with more aggressive biologic behavior.
4. *Nodular*: Generally poor prognosis because of invasive growth from onset.

CLINICAL APPEARANCE Generally pigmented (rarely amelanotic); color of lesions varies, but red, white, and/or blue are common, in addition to brown and/or black. Suspicion should be raised by a pigmented skin lesion that is >6 mm in diameter, asymmetric, has an irregular surface or border, or has variation in color.

PROGNOSIS Best with thin lesions without evidence of metastatic spread; with increasing thickness or evidence of spread, prognosis worsens. Stage I and II (primary tumor without spread) have 85% 5-year survival. Stage III (palpable regional nodes with tumor) has a 50% 5-year survival when only one node is involved and 15–20% when four or more are involved. Stage IV (disseminated disease) has <5% 5-year survival.

℞ **TREATMENT**

Early recognition and local excision for localized disease is best; 1- to 2-cm margins are as effective as 4- to 5-cm margins and do not usually require skin grafting. Elective lymph node dissection offers no advantage in overall survival compared with deferral of surgery until clinical recurrence. Pts with stage II disease may have improved disease-free survival with adjuvant interferon (IFN) α 3 million units three times weekly for 12–18 months; no overall survival advantage has been shown. In one study, pts with stage III disease had improved survival with adjuvant IFN, 20 million units IV daily × 5 for 4 weeks, then 10 million units SC three times weekly for 11 months.

This result was not confirmed in a second study. Metastatic disease may be treated with chemotherapy or immunotherapy. Dacarbazine (250 mg/m^2 IV daily × 5 q3w) plus tamoxifen (20 mg/m^2 PO daily) may induce partial responses in one-third of patients. IFN and interleukin 2 (IL-2) at maximum tolerated doses induce partial responses in 15% of pts. Rare long remissions occur with IL-2. Temozolamide is an oral agent related to dacarbazine that has some activity. It can enter the CNS and is being evaluated with radiation therapy for CNS metastases. No therapy for metastatic disease is curative.

BASAL CELL CARCINOMA (BCC)

Most common form of skin cancer; most frequently on sun-exposed skin, esp. face.

PREDISPOSING FACTORS Fair complexion, chronic UV exposure, exposure to inorganic arsenic (i.e., Fowler's solution or insecticides such as Paris green), or exposure to ionizing radiation.

PREVENTION Avoidance of sun exposure and use of sunscreens lower risk.

TYPES Five general types: noduloulcerative (most common), superficial (mimics eczema), pigmented (may be mistaken for melanoma), morpheaform (plaquelike lesion with telangiectasia—with keratotic is most aggressive), keratotic (basosquamous carcinoma).

CLINICAL APPEARANCE Classically a pearly, translucent, smooth papule with rolled edges and surface telangiectasia.

 TREATMENT

Local removal with electrodesiccation and curettage, excision, cryosurgery, or radiation therapy; metastases are rare but may spread locally. Exceedingly unusual for BCC to cause death.

SQUAMOUS CELL CARCINOMA (SCC)

Less common than basal cell but more likely to metastasize.

PREDISPOSING FACTORS Fair complexion, chronic UV exposure, previous burn or other scar (i.e., scar carcinoma), exposure to inorganic arsenic or ionizing radiation. Actinic keratosis is a premalignant lesion.

TYPES Most commonly occurs as an ulcerated nodule or a superficial erosion on the skin. Variants include:

1. *Bowen's disease*: Erythematous patch or plaque, often with scale; non-invasive; involvement limited to epidermis and epidermal appendages (i.e., SCC in situ).

2. *Scar carcinoma*: Suggested by sudden change in previously stable scar, esp. if ulceration or nodules appear.

3. *Verrucous carcinoma*: Most commonly on plantar aspect of foot; low-grade malignancy but may be mistaken for a common wart.

CLINICAL APPEARANCE Hyperkeratotic papule or nodule or erosion; nodule may be ulcerated.

 TREATMENT

Local excision and Moh's micrographic surgery are most common; radiation therapy in selected cases. Metastatic disease may be treated with radiation therapy or with combination biologic therapy; 13-*cis*-retinoic acid 1 mg/d PO plus IFN 3 million units/d SC.

   PROGNOSIS   Favorable if secondary to UV exposure; less favorable if in sun-protected areas or associated with ionizing radiation.

SKIN CANCER PREVENTION

Most skin cancer is related to sun exposure. Encourage pts to avoid the sun and use sunscreen.

For a more detailed discussion, see Chiller KG et al: Melanoma and Other Skin Cancers, Chap. 73, p. 497, in HPIM-16.

72

HEAD AND NECK CANCER

Epithelial cancers may arise from the mucosal surfaces of the head and neck including the sinuses, oral cavity, nasopharynx, oropharynx, hypopharynx, and larynx. These tumors are usually squamous cell cancers. Thyroid cancer is discussed in Chap. 173.

Incidence and Epidemiology

About 40,000 cases are diagnosed each year. Oral cavity, oropharynx, and larynx are the most frequent sites of primary lesions in the United States; nasopharyngeal primaries are more common in the Far East and Mediterranean countries. Alcohol and tobacco (including smokeless) abuse are risk factors.

Pathology

Nasopharyngeal cancer in the Far East has a distinct histology, nonkeratinizing undifferentiated carcinoma with infiltrating lymphocytes called *lymphoepithelioma*, and a distinct etiology, Epstein-Barr virus. Squamous cell head and neck cancer may develop from premalignant lesions (erythroplakia, leukoplakia), and the histologic grade affects prognosis. Pts who have survived head and neck cancer commonly develop a second cancer of the head and neck, lung, or esophagus, presumably reflecting the exposure of the upper aerodigestive mucosa to similar carcinogenic stimuli.

Genetic Alterations

Chromosomal deletions and mutations have been found in chromosomes 3p, 9p, 17p, 11q, and 13q; mutations in p53 have been reported. Cyclin D1 may be overexpressed.

Clinical Presentation

Most occur in persons > 50 years. Symptoms vary with the primary site. Nasopharynx lesions do not usually cause symptoms until late in the course and then cause unilateral serous otitis media or nasal obstruction or epistaxis. Oral cavity cancers present as nonhealing ulcers, sometimes painful. Oropharyngeal lesions also present late with sore throat or otalgia. Hoarseness may be an early sign of laryngeal cancer. Rare pts present with painless, rock-hard cervical or supraclavicular lymph node enlargement. Staging is based upon size of primary tumor and involvement of lymph nodes. Distant metastases occur in <10% of pts.

 TREATMENT

Three categories of disease are common: localized, locally or regionally advanced, and recurrent or metastatic. *Local disease* is treated with curative intent by surgery or radiation therapy. Radiation therapy is preferred for localized larynx cancer to preserve organ function; surgery is used more commonly for oral cavity lesions. *Locally advanced disease* is the most common presentation. Surgery followed by radiation therapy is standard; however, the disease is responsive to chemotherapy, and the use of three cycles of cisplatin (100 mg/m^2 IV day 1) plus 5-fluorouracil (5-FU) [1000 (mg/m^2)/d by 96- to 120-h continuous infusion] before or during radiation therapy is as effective as (or more effective than) surgery plus radiation therapy. Cetuximab plus radiation therapy may be more effective than radiation therapy alone. Head and neck cancer pts are frequently malnourished and often have intercurrent illness. Concomitant chemotherapy and radiation therapy shows a survival advantage, but mucositis is worse. Pts with *recurrent* or *metastatic disease* are treated palliatively with cisplatin plus 5-FU or paclitaxel (200–250 mg/m^2 with G-CSF support) or with single-agent chemotherapy (a taxane, methotrexate, cisplatin, or carboplatin). Treatment outcome varies somewhat with primary site; in general, pts with localized disease have about 75% 5-year survival, those with locally advanced disease have about 35% 5-year survival, and those with metastatic disease have about 15% 5-year survival.

Prevention

Pts with head and neck cancer who are rendered disease free may benefit from chemopreventive therapy with *cis*-retinoic acid [3 months of 1.5 (mg/kg)/d followed by 9 months of 0.5 (mg/kg)/d PO]. Trial results are mixed. However, the most important intervention is to get the pts to stop smoking. Long-term survival is significantly better in those who stop smoking.

For a more detailed discussion, see Vokes EE: Head and Neck Cancer, Chap. 74, p. 503, in HPIM-16.

73

LUNG CANCER

Incidence

Lung cancer was diagnosed in about 93,000 men and 80,600 women in the United States in 2004, and 86% of pts die within 5 years. Lung cancer, the leading cause of cancer death, accounts for 32% of all cancer deaths in men and 25% in women. Peak incidence occurs between ages 55 and 65 years. Incidence is decreasing in men and increasing in women.

Histologic Classification

Four major types account for 88% of primary lung cancers: epidermoid (squamous), 29%; adenocarcinoma (including bronchioloalveolar), 35%; large cell, 9%; and small cell (or oat cell), 18%. Histology (small cell versus non-small cell types) is a major determinant of treatment approach. Small cell is usually widely disseminated at presentation, while non-small cell may be localized. Epidermoid and small cell typically present as central masses, while adenocarcinomas and large cell usually present as peripheral nodules or masses. Epidermoid and large cell cavitate in 20–30% of pts.

Etiology

The major cause of lung cancer is tobacco use, particularly cigarette smoking. Lung cancer cells may have ≥10 acquired genetic lesions, most commonly point mutations in *ras* oncogenes; amplification, rearrangement, or transcriptional activation of *myc* family oncogenes; overexpression of *bcl*-2, *Her*-2/*neu*, and telomerase; and deletions involving chromosomes 1p, 1q, 3p12-13, 3p14 (FHIT gene region), 3p21, 3p24-25, 3q, 5q, 9p (p16 and p15 cyclin-dependent kinase inhibitors), 11p13, 11p15, 13q14 (*rb* gene), 16q, and 17p13 (p53 gene). Loss of 3p and 9p are the earliest events, detectable even in hyperplastic bronchial epithelium; *p53* abnormalities and *ras* point mutations are usually found only in invasive cancers.

Clinical Manifestations

Only 5–15% are detected while asymptomatic. Central endobronchial tumors cause cough, hemoptysis, wheeze, stridor, dyspnea, pneumonitis. Peripheral lesions cause pain, cough, dyspnea, symptoms of lung abscess resulting from cavitation. Metastatic spread of primary lung cancer may cause tracheal obstruction, dysphagia, hoarseness, Horner's syndrome. Other problems of regional spread include superior vena cava syndrome, pleural effusion, respiratory failure. Extrathoracic metastatic disease affects 50% of pts with epidermoid cancer, 80% with adenocarcinoma and large cell, and >95% with small cell. Clinical problems result from brain metastases, pathologic fractures, liver invasion, and spinal cord compression. Paraneoplastic syndromes may be a presenting finding of lung cancer or first sign of recurrence (Chap. 80). Systemic symptoms occur in 30% and include weight loss, anorexia, fever. Endocrine syndromes occur in 12% and include hypercalcemia (epidermoid), syndrome of inappropriate antidiuretic hormone secretion (small cell), gynecomastia (large cell). Skeletal connective tissue syndromes include clubbing in 30% (most often non-small cell) and hypertrophic pulmonary osteoarthropathy in 1–10% (most often adenocarcinomas), with clubbing, pain, and swelling.

Staging See Table 73-1.

Two parts to staging are (1) determination of location (anatomic staging) and (2) assessment of pt's ability to withstand antitumor treatment (physiologic staging). Non-small cell tumors are staged by the TNM/International Staging System (ISS). The T (tumor), N (regional node involvement), and M (presence or absence of distant metastasis) factors are taken together to define different stage groups. Small cell tumors are staged by two-stage system: limited stage dis-

Table 73-1

Tumor, Node, Metastasis International Staging System for Lung Cancer

		5-Year Survival Rate, %	
Stage	TNM Descriptors	Clinical Stage	Surgical-Pathologic Stage
IA	T1 N0 M0	61	67
IB	T2 N0 M0	38	57
IIA	T1 N1 M0	34	55
IIB	T2 N1 M0	24	39
IIB	T3 N0 M0	22	38
IIIA	T3 N1 M0	9	25
	T1–2–3 N2 M0	13	23
IIIB	T4 N0–1–2 M0	7	<5
	T1–2–3–4 N3 M0	3	<3
IV	Any T any N M1	1	<1

TUMOR (T) STATUS DESCRIPTOR

T0	No evidence of a primary tumor
TX	Primary tumor cannot be assessed, or tumor proven by the presence of malignant cells in sputum or bronchial washings but not visualized by imaging or bronchoscopy
TIS	Carcinoma in situ
T1	Tumor <3 cm in greatest dimension, surrounded by lung or visceral pleura, without bronchoscopic evidence of invasion more proximal than lobar bronchus (i.e., not in main bronchus)
T2	Tumor with any of following: >3 cm in greatest dimension; involves main bronchus, ≥2 cm distal to the carcina; invades visceral pleura; associated with atelectasis or obstructive pneumonitis extending to hilum but does not involve entire lung
T3	Tumor of any size that directly invades any of the following: chest wall (including superior sulcus tumors), diaphragm, mediastinal pleura, parietal pericardium; or tumor in main bronchus <2 cm distal to carina but without involvement of carina; or associated atelectasis or obstructive pneumonitis of entire lung
T4	Tumor of any size that invades any of the following: mediastinum, heart, great vessels, trachea, esophagus, vertebral body, carina; or tumor with a malignant pleural or pericardial effusion[a], or with satellite tumor nodule(s) within the ipsilateral primary-tumor lobe of the lung.

(continued)

---

ease—confined to one hemithorax and regional lymph nodes; extensive disease—involvement beyond this. General staging procedures include careful ENT examination, CXR, chest and abdominal CT scanning, and PET scan. CT scans may suggest mediastinal lymph node involvement and pleural extension in non-small cell lung cancer, but definitive evaluation of mediastinal spread requires histologic examination. Routine radionuclide scans are not obtained in asymptomatic pts. If a mass lesion is on CXR and no obvious contraindications to curative surgical approach are noted, the mediastinum should be investigated. Major contraindications to curative surgery include extrathoracic metastases, superior vena cava syndrome, vocal cord and phrenic nerve paralysis, malignant pleural effusions, metastases to contralateral lung, and histologic diagnosis of small cell cancer.

Table 73-1 *(Continued)*

Tumor, Node, Metastasis International Staging System for Lung Cancer

LYMPH NODE (N) INVOLVEMENT DESCRIPTOR

NX	Regional lymph nodes cannot be assessed
N0	No regional lymph node metastasis
N1	Metastasis to ipsilateral peribronchial and/or ipsilateral hilar lymph nodes, and intrapulmonary nodes involved by direct extension of the primary tumor
N2	Metastasis to ipsilateral mediastinal and/or subcarinal lymph nodes(s)
N3	Metastasis to contralateral mediastinal, contralateral hilar, ipsilateral or contralateral scalene, or supraclavicular lymph node(s)

DISTANT METASTASIS (M) DESCRIPTOR

MX	Presence of distant metastasis cannot be assessed
M0	No distant metastasis
M1	Distant metastasis present[b]

[a] Most pleural effusions associated with lung cancer are due to tumor. However, in a few patients with multiple negative cytopathologic exams of a non-bloody, non-exudative pleural or pericardial effusion that clinical judgment dictates is not related to the tumor, the effusion should be excluded as a staging element and the patient's disease staged as T1, T2, or T3.

[b] Separate metastatic pulmonary tumor nodule(s) in the ipsilateral nonprimary tumor lobe(s) of the lung are classified as M1.

Source: Adapted from CF Mountain: Chest 111:1710, 1997, with permission.

TREATMENT

See Table 73-2.

1. Surgery in pts with localized disease and non-small cell cancer; however, majority initially thought to have curative resection ultimately succumb to metastatic disease. The role of adjuvant chemotherapy in patients with total resection is controversial. Cisplatin (four cycles at 100 mg/m^2) plus a second active agent (vinblastine, vinorelban, vindesine) may modestly extend survival.

Table 73-2

Summary of Treatment Approach to Patients with Lung Cancer

NON-SMALL CELL LUNG CANCER

Stages IA, IB, IIA, IIB, and some IIIA:
    Surgical resection for stages IA, IB, IIA, and IIB
    Surgical resection with complete-mediastinal lymph node dissection and consideration of neoadjuvant CRx for stage IIIA disease with "minimal N2 involvement" (discovered at thoracotomy or mediastinoscopy)
    Postoperative RT for patients found to have N2 disease if no neoadjuvant CRx given
    Discussion of risks/benefits of adjuvant CRx with individual patients
    Curative potential RT for "nonoperable" patients
Stage IIIA with selected types of stage T3 tumors:
    Tumors with chest wall invasion (T3): en bloc resection of tumor with involved chest wall and consideration of postoperative RT

(continued)

Table 73-2 *(Continued)*

Summary of Treatment Approach to Patients with Lung Cancer

Superior sulcus (Pancoast's) (T3) tumors: preoperative RT (30–45 Gy) followed by en bloc resection of involved lung and chest wall with consideration of postoperative RT or intraoperative brachytherapy

Proximal airway involvement (<2 cm from carina) without mediastinal nodes: sleeve resection if possible preserving distal normal lung or pneumonectomy

Stages IIIA "advanced, bulky, clinically evident N2 disease" (discovered preoperatively) and IIIB disease that can be included in a tolerable RT port:

Curative potential RT + CRx if performance status and general medical condition are reasonable; otherwise, RT alone

Consider neoadjuvant CRx and surgical resection for IIIA disease with advanced N2 involvement

Stage IIIB disease with carinal invasion (T4) but without N2 involvement:

Consider pneumonectomy with tracheal sleeve resection with direct reanastomosis to contralateral mainstem bronchus

Stage IV and more advanced IIIB disease:

RT to symptomatic local sites

CRx for ambulatory patients

Chest tube drainage of large malignant pleural effusions

Consider resection of primary tumor and metastasis for isolated brain or adrenal metastases

SMALL CELL LUNG CANCER

Limited stage (good performance status): combination CRx + chest RT

Extensive stage (good performance status): combination CRx

Complete tumor responders (all stages): consider prophylactic cranial RT

Poor-performance-status patients (all stages):

Modified-dose combination CRx

Palliative RT

BRONCHOALVEOLAR CARCINOMA (EGF RECEPTOR MUTATIONS)

Gefitinib, inhibitor of EGF receptor kinase activity

ALL PATIENTS

RT for brain metastases, spinal cord compression, weight-bearing lytic bony lesions, symptomatic local lesions (nerve paralyses, obstructed airway, hemoptysis, intrathoracic large venous obstruction, in non-small cell lung cancer and in small cell cancer not responding to CRx)

Appropriate diagnosis and treatment of other medical problems and supportive care during CRx

Encouragement to stop smoking

Entrance into clinical trial, if eligible

Abbreviations: CRx, chemotherapy; RT, radiotherapy.

2. Solitary pulmonary nodule: factors suggesting resection include cigarette smoking, age ≥35, relatively large (>2 cm) lesion, lack of calcification, chest symptoms, and growth of lesion compared to old CXR. See Fig. 73-1.

3. For unresectable stage II non-small cell lung cancer, combined thoracic radiation therapy and cisplatin-based chemotherapy reduces mortality by about 25% at 1 year.

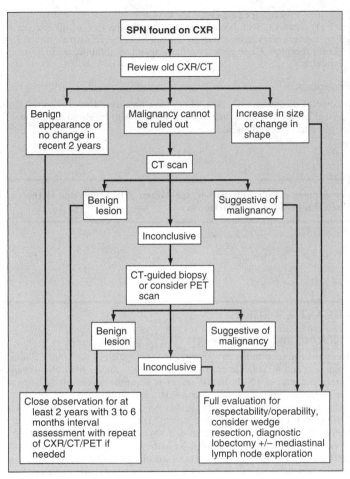

FIGURE 73-1 Algorithm for evaluation of a solitary pulmonary nodule (SPN). (CXR, chest x-ray; CT, computed tomography scan; PET, positron emission tomography.)

4. For unresectable non-small cell cancer, metastatic disease, or refusal of surgery: consider for radiation therapy; addition of cisplatin-based chemotherapy may reduce death risk by 13% at 2 years and improve quality of life.

5. Small cell cancer: combination chemotherapy is standard mode of therapy; response after 6–12 weeks predicts median- and long-term survival.

6. Addition of radiation therapy to chemotherapy in limited stage small cell lung cancer can increase 5-year survival from about 11% to 20%.

7. Prophylactic cranial irradiation improves survival of limited stage small cell lung cancer by another 5%.

8. Laser obliteration of tumor through bronchoscopy in presence of bronchial obstruction.

9. Radiation therapy for brain metastases, spinal cord compression, symptomatic masses, bone lesions.

10. Encourage cessation of smoking.

11. Patients with bronchioalveolar carcinoma (3% of all patients with lung cancer) often have activating mutations in the epidermal growth factor (EGF) receptor. These patients often respond to gefitinib, an EGF receptor inhibitor.

Prognosis

At time of diagnosis, only 20% of pts have localized disease. Overall 5-year survival is 30% for males and 50% for females with localized disease and 5% for pts with advanced disease.

For a more detailed discussion, see Minna JD: Neoplasms of the Lung, Chap. 75, p. 506, in HPIM-16.

74

BREAST CANCER

Incidence and Epidemiology

The most common tumor in women, 216,000 women in the United States are diagnosed and 40,000 die each year with breast cancer. Men also get breast cancer at a rate of 150:1. Breast cancer is hormone-dependent. Women with late menarche, early menopause, and first full-term pregnancy by age 18 have a significantly reduced risk. The average American woman has about a 1 in 9 lifetime risk of developing breast cancer. Dietary fat is a controversial risk factor. Oral contraceptives have little, if any, effect on risk and lower the risk of endometrial and ovarian cancer. Voluntary interruption of pregnancy does not increase risk. Estrogen replacement therapy may slightly increase the risk, but the beneficial effects of estrogen on quality of life, bone mineral density, and decreased risk of colorectal cancer appear to be somewhat outnumbered by increases in cardiovascular and thrombotic disease. Women who received therapeutic radiation before age 30 are at increased risk. Breast cancer risk is increased when a sister and mother also had the disease.

Genetics

Perhaps 8–10% of breast cancer is familial. *BRCA-1* mutations account for about 5%. *BRCA-1* maps to chromosome 17q21 and appears to be involved in transcription-coupled DNA repair. Ashkenazi Jewish women have a 1% chance of having a common mutation (deletion of adenine and guanine at position 185). The *BRCA-1* syndrome includes an increased risk of ovarian cancer in women and prostate cancer in men. *BRCA-2* on chromosome 11 may account for 2–3% of breast cancer. Mutations are associated with an increased risk of breast cancer in men and women. Germline mutations in p53 (Li-Fraumeni syndrome) are very rare, but breast cancer, sarcomas, and other malignancies occur in such families. Germline mutations in *hCHK2* may account for some familial breast cancer. Sporadic breast cancers show many genetic alterations including overexpression of *HER-2/neu* in 25% of cases, p53 mutations in 40%, and loss of heterozygosity at other loci.

Diagnosis

Breast cancer is usually diagnosed by biopsy of a nodule detected by mammogram or by palpation. Women should be strongly encouraged to examine their breasts monthly. In premenopausal women, questionable or nonsuspicious (small) masses should be reexamined in 2–4 weeks (Fig. 74-1). A mass in a premenopausal woman that persists throughout her cycle and any mass in a postmenopausal woman should be aspirated. If the mass is a cyst filled with non-bloody fluid that goes away with aspiration, the pt is returned to routine screening. If the cyst aspiration leaves a residual mass or reveals bloody fluid, the pt should have a mammogram and excisional biopsy. If the mass is solid, the pt should undergo a mammogram and excisional biopsy. Screening mammograms performed every other year beginning at age 50 have been shown to save lives. The controversy regarding screening mammograms beginning at age 40 relates to the following facts: (1) the disease is much less common in the 40- to 49-year age group; screening is generally less successful for less common problems; (2) workup of mammographic abnormalities in the 40- to 49-year age group less commonly diagnoses cancer; and (3) about 35% of women who are screened annually during their forties have an abnormality at some point that requires a diagnostic procedure (usually a biopsy); yet very few evaluations

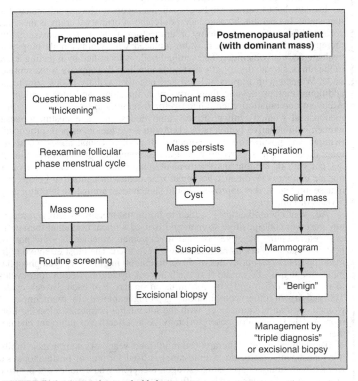

FIGURE 74-1   Approach to a palpable breast mass.

reveal cancer. However, many believe in the value of screening mammography beginning at age 40. After 13–15 years of follow-up, women who start screening at age 40 have a small survival benefit. Women with familial breast cancer more often have false-negative mammograms. MRI is a better screening tool in these women.

Staging

Therapy and prognosis are dictated by stage of disease (Table 74-1). Unless the breast mass is large or fixed to the chest wall, staging of the ipsilateral axilla is performed at the time of lumpectomy (see below). Within pts of a given stage, individual characteristics of the tumor may influence prognosis: expression of estrogen receptor improves prognosis, while overexpression of *HER-2/neu*, mutations in p53, high growth fraction, and aneuploidy worsen the prognosis. Breast cancer can spread almost anywhere but commonly goes to bone, lungs, liver, soft tissue, and brain.

 TREATMENT

Five-year survival rate by stage is shown in Table 74-2. Treatment varies with stage of disease.

Ductal carcinoma in situ is noninvasive tumor present in the breast ducts. Treatment of choice is wide excision with breast radiation therapy. In one study, adjuvant tamoxifen further reduced the risk of recurrence.

Invasive breast cancer can be classified as operable, locally advanced, and metastatic. In operable breast cancer, outcome of primary therapy is the same with modified radical mastectomy or lumpectomy followed by breast radiation therapy. Axillary dissection may be replaced with sentinel node biopsy to evaluate node involvement. The sentinel node is identified by injecting a dye in the tumor site at surgery; the first node in which dye appears is the sentinel node. Women with tumors <1 cm and negative axillary nodes require no additional therapy beyond their primary lumpectomy and breast radiation. Adjuvant combination chemotherapy for 6 months appears to benefit premenopausal women with positive lymph nodes, pre- and postmenopausal women with negative lymph nodes but with large tumors or poor prognostic features, and postmenopausal women with positive lymph nodes whose tumors do not express estrogen receptors. Estrogen receptor–positive tumors >1 cm with or without involvement of lymph nodes are treated with aromatase inhibitors. Women who began treatment with tamoxifen before aromatase inhibitors were approved should switch to an aromatase inhibitor after 5 years of tamoxifen.

Adjuvant chemotherapy is added to hormonal therapy in estrogen receptor–positive, node-positive women and is used without hormonal therapy in estrogen receptor–negative node-positive women, whether they are pre- or postmenopausal. Various regimens have been used. The most effective regimen appears to be four cycles of doxorubicin, 60 mg/m^2, plus cyclophosphamide, 600 mg/m^2, IV on day 1 of each 3-week cycle followed by four cycles of paclitaxel, 175 mg/m^2, by 3-h infusion on day 1 of each 3-week cycle. The activity of other combinations is being explored. In premenopausal women, ovarian ablation [e.g., with the luteinizing hormone–releasing hormone (LHRH) inhibitor goserelin] may be as effective as adjuvant chemotherapy.

Tamoxifen adjuvant therapy (20 mg/d for 5 years) or an aromatase inhibitor (anastrazole, letrozole, exemestane) is used for pre- or postmenopausal women with tumors expressing estrogen receptors whose nodes are positive or whose nodes are negative but with large tumors or poor prognostic features.

Table 74-1

Staging of Breast Cancer

PRIMARY TUMOR (T)

T0	No evidence of primary tumor
Tis	Carcinoma in situ
T1	Tumor ≤2 cm
T1a	≤0.5 cm in greatest dimension
T1b	>0.5 cm but ≤1 cm in greatest dimension
T1c	>1 cm but ≤2 cm in greatest dimension
T2	Tumor >2 cm but ≤5 cm
T3	Tumor >5 cm
T4	Extension to chest wall, inflammation
T4a	Extension to chest wall
T4b	Edema (including pean d'orange) or ulceration of the skin of the breast or satellite skin nodules confined to the same breast
T4c	Both (T4a and T4b)
T4d	Inflammatory carcinoma

REGIONAL LYMPH NODES (N)

N0	No tumor in regional lymph nodes
N1	Metastasis to movable ipsilateral nodes
N2	Metastasis to matted or fixed ipsilateral nodes
N3	Metastasis to ipsilateral internal mammary nodes

DISTANT METASTASIS (M)

M0	No distant metastasis
M1	Distant metastasis (includes spread to ipsilateral supraclavicular nodes)

STAGE GROUPING

Stage 0	Tis	N0	M0
Stage I	T1	N0	M0
Stage IIA	T0	N1	M0
	T1	N1	M0
	T2	N0	M0
Stage IIB	T2	N1	M0
	T3	N0	M0
Stage IIIA	T0	N2	M0
	T1	N2	M0
	T2	N2	M0
	T3	N1, N2	M0
Stage IIIB	T4	Any N	M0
	Any T	N3	M0
Stage IV	Any T	Any N	M1

Source: With the permission of the American Joint Committee on Cancer (AJCC), 1992, Chicago, IL. Original source for this material is the AJCC Manual for Staging of Cancer, 4th ed, 1992, published by Lippincott-Raven Publisher, PA.

Breast cancer will recur in about half of pts with localized disease. High-dose adjuvant therapy with marrow support does not appear to benefit even women with high-risk of recurrence.

Pts with locally advanced breast cancer benefit from neoadjuvant combination chemotherapy (e.g., CAF: cyclophosphamide 500 mg/m², doxorubicin

Table 74-2

5-Year Survival Rate for Breast Cancer by Stage

Stage	5-Year Survival (Percent of Patients)
0	99
I	92
IIA	82
IIB	65
IIIA	47
IIIB	44
IV	14

Source: Modified from data of the National Cancer Institute—Surveillance, Epidemiology, and End Results (SEER).

50 mg/m^2, and 5-fluorouracil 500 mg/m^2 all given IV on days 1 and 8 of a monthly cycle for 6 cycles) followed by surgery plus breast radiation therapy.

Treatment for metastatic disease depends upon estrogen receptor status and treatment philosophy. No therapy is known to cure pts with metastatic disease. Randomized trials do not show that the use of high-dose therapy with hematopoietic stem cell support improves survival. Median survival is about 16 months with conventional treatment: tamoxifen or aromatase inhibitors for estrogen receptor–positive tumors and combination chemotherapy for receptor-negative tumors. Pts whose tumors express *HER-2/neu* have somewhat higher response rates by adding trastuzumab (anti-*HER-2/neu*) to chemotherapy. Some advocate sequential use of active single agents in the setting of metastatic disease. Active agents in anthracycline- and taxane-resistant disease include capecitabine, vinorelbine, gemcitabine, irinotecan, and platinum agents. Pts progressing on adjuvant tamoxifen may benefit from an aromatase inhibitor such as letrozole or anastrazole. Bisphosphonates reduce skeletal complications and may promote antitumor effects of other therapy. Radiation therapy is useful for palliation of symptoms.

For a more detailed discussion, see Lippman ME: Breast Cancer, Chap. 76, p. 516, in HPIM-16.

75

TUMORS OF THE GASTROINTESTINAL TRACT

ESOPHAGEAL CARCINOMA

In 2004 in the United States, 14,250 cases and 13,300 deaths; less frequent in women than men. Highest incidence in focal regions of China, Iran, Afghanistan, Siberia, Mongolia. In United States, blacks more frequently affected than whites; usually presents sixth decade or later; 5-year survival <5% because most pts present with advanced disease.

PATHOLOGY 60% squamous cell carcinoma, most commonly in upper two-thirds; <40% adenocarcinoma, usually in distal third, arising in region of columnar metaplasia (Barrett's esophagus), glandular tissue, or as direct extension of proximal gastric adenocarcinoma; lymphoma and melanoma rare.

RISK FACTORS Major risk factors for squamous cell carcinoma: ethanol abuse, smoking (combination is synergistic); other risks: lye ingestion and esophageal stricture, radiation exposure, head and neck cancer, achalasia, smoked opiates, Plummer-Vinson syndrome, tylosis, chronic ingestion of extremely hot tea, deficiency of vitamin A, zinc, molybdenum. Barrett's esophagus is a risk for adenocarcinoma.

CLINICAL FEATURES Progressive dysphagia (first with solids, then liquids), rapid weight loss common, chest pain (from mediastinal spread), odynophagia, pulmonary aspiration (obstruction, tracheoesophageal fistula), hoarseness (laryngeal nerve palsy), hypercalcemia (parathyroid hormone–related peptide hypersecretion by squamous carcinomas); bleeding infrequent, occasionally severe; examination often unremarkable.

DIAGNOSIS Double-contrast barium swallow useful as initial test in dysphagia; flexible esophagogastroscopy most sensitive and specific test; pathologic confirmation by combining endoscopic biopsy and cytologic examination of mucosal brushings (neither alone sufficiently sensitive); CT and endoscopic ultrasonography valuable to assess local and nodal spread.

℞ TREATMENT

Surgical resection feasible in only 40% of pts; associated with high complication rate (fistula, abscess, aspiration). *Squamous cell carcinoma*: Surgical resection after chemotherapy [5-fluorouracil (5-FU), cisplatin] plus radiation therapy prolongs survival and may provide improved cure rate. *Adenocarcinoma*: Curative resection rarely possible; <20% of pts with resectable tumors survive 5 years. Palliative measures include laser ablation, mechanical dilatation, radiotherapy, and a luminal prosthesis to bypass the tumor. Gastrostomy or jejunostomy are frequently required for nutritional support.

GASTRIC CARCINOMA
Highest incidence in Japan, China, Chile, Ireland; incidence decreasing worldwide, eightfold in the United States over past 60 years; in 2004, 22,710 new cases and 11,780 deaths. Male:female = 2:1; peak incidence sixth and seventh decades; overall 5-year survival <15%.

RISK FACTORS Increased incidence in lower socioeconomic groups; environmental component is suggested by studies of migrants and their offspring. Several dietary factors correlated with increased incidence: nitrates, smoked foods, heavily salted foods; genetic component suggested by increased incidence in first-degree relatives of affected pts; other risk factors: atrophic gastritis, *Helicobacter pylori* infection, Billroth II gastrectomy, gastrojejunostomy, adenomatous gastric polyps, pernicious anemia, hyperplastic gastric polyps (latter two associated with atrophic gastritis), Ménétrier's disease, slight increased risk with blood group A.

PATHOLOGY Adenocarcinoma in 85%; usually focal (polypoid, ulcerative), two-thirds arising in antrum or lesser curvature, frequently ulcerative ("intestinal type"); less commonly diffuse infiltrative (linitis plastica) or superficial spreading (diffuse lesions more prevalent in younger pts; exhibit less geographic variation; have extremely poor prognosis); spreads primarily to local nodes, liver, peritoneum; systemic spread uncommon; lymphoma accounts for 15% (most frequent extranodal site in immunocompetent pts), either low-grade tumor of mucosa-associated lymphoid tissue (MALT) or aggressive diffuse large cell lymphoma; leiomyosarcoma or gastrointestinal stromal cell tumor (GIST) is rare.

CLINICAL FEATURES Most commonly presents with progressive upper abdominal discomfort, frequently with weight loss, anorexia, nausea; acute or chronic GI bleeding (mucosal ulceration) common; dysphagia (location in cardia); vomiting (pyloric and widespread disease); early satiety; examination often unrevealing early in course; later, abdominal tenderness, pallor, and cachexia most common signs; palpable mass uncommon; metastatic spread may be manifest by hepatomegaly, ascites, left supraclavicular or scalene adenopathy, periumbilical, ovarian, or prerectal mass (Blummer's shelf), low-grade fever, skin abnormalities (nodules, dermatomyositis, acanthosis nigricans, or multiple seborrheic keratoses). Laboratory findings: iron-deficiency anemia in two-thirds of pts; fecal occult blood in 80%; rarely associated with pancytopenia and microangiopathic hemolytic anemia (from marrow infiltration), leukemoid reaction, migratory thrombophlebitis, or acanthosis nigricans.

DIAGNOSIS Double-contrast barium swallow useful; gastroscopy most sensitive and specific test; pathologic confirmation by biopsy and cytologic examination of mucosal brushings; superficial biopsies less sensitive for lymphomas (frequently submucosal); important to differentiate benign from malignant gastric ulcers with multiple biopsies and follow-up examinations to demonstrate ulcer healing.

 TREATMENT

Adenocarcinoma: Gastrectomy offers only chance of cure; the rare tumors limited to mucosa are resectable for cure in 80%; deeper invasion, nodal metastases decrease 5-year survival to 20% of pts with resectable tumors in absence of obvious metastatic spread (Table 75-1); CT and endoscopic ultrasonography may aid in determining tumor resectability. Subtotal gastrectomy has similar efficacy to total gastrectomy for distal stomach lesions, but with less morbidity; no clear benefit for resection of spleen and a portion of the pancreas, or for radical lymph node removal. Adjuvant chemotherapy (5-FU/leucovorin) plus radiation therapy following primary surgery leads to a 7-month increase in median survival. Neoadjuvant chemotherapy with epirubicin, cisplatin and 5-FU may downstage tumors and increase the efficacy of surgery. Palliative therapy for pain, obstruction, and bleeding includes surgery, endoscopic dilatation, radiation therapy, chemotherapy.

Lymphoma: Low-grade MALT lymphoma is caused by *H. pylori* infection, and eradication of the infection causes complete remissions in 50% of pts; rest are responsive to combination chemotherapy including cyclophosphamide, doxorubicin, vincristine, prednisone (CHOP) plus rituximab. Diffuse large cell lymphoma may be treated with either CHOP plus rituximab or subtotal gastrectomy followed by chemotherapy; 50–60% 5-year survival.

Leiomyosarcoma: Surgical resection curative in most pts. Tumors expressing the *c-kit* tyrosine kinase (CD117)—GIST—respond to imatinib mesylate in a substantial fraction of cases.

BENIGN GASTRIC TUMORS

Much less common than malignant gastric tumors; hyperplastic polyps most common, with adenomas, hamartomas, and leiomyomas rare; 30% of adenomas and occasional hyperplastic polyps are associated with gastric malignancy; pol-

Table 75-1

Staging System for Gastric Carcinoma

| | | | Data from American College of Surgeons | |
Stage	TNM	Features	Number of Cases, %	5-Year Survival, %
0	TisN0M0	Node negative; limited to mucosa	1	90
IA	T1N0M0	Node negative; invasion of lamina propria or submucosa	7	59
IB	T2N0M0	Node negative; invasion of muscularis propria	10	44
II	T1N2M0 T2N1M0	Node positive; invasion beyond mucosa but within wall		
		or	17	29
	T3N0M0	Node negative; extension through wall		
IIIA	T2N2M0 T3N1-2M0	Node positive; invasion of muscularis propria or through wall	21	15
IIIB	T4N0-1M0	Node negative; adherence to surrounding tissue	14	9
IV	T4N2M0	Node positive; adherence to surrounding tissue		
		or	30	3
	T1-4N0-2M1	Distant metastases		

yposis syndromes include Peutz-Jeghers and familial polyposis (hamartomas and adenomas), Gardner's (adenomas), and Cronkhite-Canada (cystic polyps). See "Colonic Polyps," below.

CLINICAL FEATURES   Usually asymptomatic; occasionally present with bleeding or vague epigastric discomfort.

 TREATMENT

Endoscopic or surgical excision.

SMALL-BOWEL TUMORS

CLINICAL FEATURES   Uncommon tumors (~5% of all GI neoplasms); usually present with bleeding, abdominal pain, weight loss, fever, or intestinal obstruction (intermittent or fixed); increased incidence of lymphomas in pts with gluten-sensitive enteropathy, Crohn's disease involving small bowel, AIDS, prior organ transplantation, autoimmune disorders.

PATHOLOGY   Usually benign; most common are adenomas (usually duodenal), leiomyomas (intramural), and lipomas (usually ileal); 50% of malignant tumors are adenocarcinoma, usually in duodenum (at or near ampulla of Vater) or proximal jejunum, commonly coexisting with benign adenomas; primary intestinal lymphomas (non-Hodgkin's) account for 25% and occur as focal mass (western type), which is usually a T cell lymphoma associated with prior celiac disease, or diffuse infiltration (Mediterranean type), which is usually immunoproliferative small-intestinal disease (IPSID; α-heavy chain disease), a B cell

MALT lymphoma associated with *Campylobacter jejuni* infection, which can present as intestinal malabsorption; carcinoid tumors (usually asymptomatic) occasionally produce bleeding or intussusception (see below).

DIAGNOSIS   Endoscopy and biopsy most useful for tumors of duodenum and proximal jejunum; otherwise barium x-ray examination best diagnostic test; direct small-bowel instillation of contrast (enteroclysis) occasionally reveals tumors not seen with routine small-bowel radiography; angiography (to detect plexus of tumor vessels) or laparotomy often required for diagnosis; CT useful to evaluate extent of tumor (esp. lymphomas).

 TREATMENT

Surgical excision; adjuvant chemotherapy appears helpful for focal lymphoma; IPSID appears to be curable with combination chemotherapy used in aggressive lymphoma plus oral antibiotics (e.g., tetracycline); no proven role for chemotherapy or radiation therapy for other small-bowel tumors.

COLONIC POLYPS
Tubular Adenomas

Present in ~30% of adults; pedunculated or sessile; usually asymptomatic; ~5% cause occult blood in stool; may cause obstruction; overall risk of malignant degeneration correlates with size (<2% if <1.5 cm diam; >10% if >2.5 cm diam) and is higher in sessile polyps; 65% found in rectosigmoid colon; diagnosis by barium enema, sigmoidoscopy, or colonoscopy. *Treatment*: Full colonoscopy to detect synchronous lesions (present in 30%); endoscopic resection (surgery if polyp large or inaccessible by colonoscopy); follow-up surveillance by colonoscopy every 2–3 years.

Villous Adenomas

Generally larger than tubular adenomas at diagnosis; often sessile; high risk of malignancy (up to 30% when >2 cm); more prevalent in left colon; occasionally associated with potassium-rich secretory diarrhea. *Treatment*: As for tubular adenomas.

Hyperplastic Polyps

Asymptomatic; usually incidental finding at colonoscopy; rarely >5 mm; no malignant potential. No treatment required.

Hereditary Polyposis Syndromes

See Table 75-2.

1. *Familial polyposis coli* (FPC): Diffuse pancolonic adenomatous polyposis (up to several thousand polyps); autosomal dominant inheritance associated with deletion in adenomatous polyposis coli (*APC*) gene on chromosome 5; colon carcinoma from malignant degeneration of polyp in 100% by age 40. *Treatment*: Prophylactic total colectomy or subtotal colectomy with ileoproctostomy before age 30; subtotal resection avoids ileostomy but necessitates frequent proctoscopic surveillance; periodic colonoscopic or annual radiologic screening of siblings and offspring of pts with FPC until age 35; sulindac and other NSAIDs cause regression of polyps and inhibit their development.

2. *Gardner's syndrome*: Variant of FPC with associated soft tissue tumors (epidermoid cysts, osteomas, lipomas, fibromas, desmoids); higher incidence of

Table 75-2

Hereditable (Autosomal Dominant) Gastrointestinal Polyposis Syndromes

Syndrome	Distribution of Polyps	Histologic Type	Malignant Potential	Associated Lesions
Familial adenomatous polyposis	Large intestine	Adenoma	Common	None
Gardner's syndrome	Large and small intestine	Adenoma	Common	Osteomas, fibromas, lipomas, epidermoid cysts, ampullary cancers, congenital hypertrophy of retinal pigment epithelium
Turcot's syndrome	Large intestine	Adenoma	Common	Brain tumors
Nonpolyposis syndrome (Lynch syndrome)	Large intestine (often proximal)	Adenoma	Common	Endometrial and ovarian tumors
Peutz-Jeghers syndrome	Small and large intestines, stomach	Hamartoma	Rare	Mucocutaneous pigmentation; tumors of the ovary, breast, pancreas, endometrium
Juvenile polyposis	Large and small intestines, stomach	Hamartoma, rarely progressing to adenoma	Rare	Various congenital abnormalities

gastroduodenal polyps, ampullary adenocarcinoma. *Treatment*: As for FPC; surveillance for small-bowel disease with fecal occult blood testing after colectomy.

3. *Turcot's syndrome*: Rare variant of FPC with associated malignant brain tumors. *Treatment*: As for FPC.

4. *Nonpolyposis syndrome*: Familial syndrome with up to 50% risk of colon carcinoma; peak incidence in fifth decade; associated with multiple primary cancers (esp. endometrial); autosomal dominant; due to defective DNA mismatch repair.

5. *Juvenile polyposis*: Multiple benign colonic and small-bowel hamartomas; intestinal bleeding common. Other symptoms: abdominal pain, diarrhea; occasional intussusception. Rarely recur after excision; low risk of colon cancer from malignant degeneration of interspersed adenomatous polyps. Prophylactic colectomy controversial.

6. *Peutz-Jeghers syndrome*: Numerous hamartomatous polyps of entire GI tract, though denser in small bowel than colon; GI bleeding common; somewhat increased risk for the development of cancer at GI and non-GI sites. Prophylactic surgery not recommended.

COLORECTAL CANCER

Second most common internal cancer in humans; accounts for 10% of cancer-related deaths in United States, incidence increases dramatically above age 50, nearly equal in men and women. In 2004, 146,940 new cases, 56,730 deaths.

ETIOLOGY AND RISK FACTORS　Most colon cancers arise from adenomatous polyps. Genetic steps from polyp to dysplasia to carcinoma in situ to invasive cancer have been defined, including: point mutation in K-*ras* proto-oncogene, hypomethylation of DNA leading to enhanced gene expression, allelic loss at the *APC* gene (a tumor suppressor), allelic loss at the *DCC* (deleted in colon cancer) gene on chromosome 18, and loss and mutation of p53 on chromosome 17. Hereditary nonpolyposis colon cancer arises from mutations in the DNA mismatch repair genes, *hMSH2* gene on chromosome 2 and *hMLH1* gene on chromosome 3. Mutations lead to colon and other cancers. Diagnosis requires three or more relatives with colon cancer, one of whom is a first-degree relative; one or more cases diagnosed before age 50; and involvement of at least two generations. Environmental factors also play a role; increased prevalence in developed countries, urban areas, advantaged socioeconomic groups; increased risk in pts with hypercholesterolemia, coronary artery disease; correlation of risk with low-fiber, high animal fat diets, although direct effect of diet remains unproven; decreased risk with long-term dietary calcium supplementation and, possibly, daily aspirin ingestion. Risk increased in first-degree relatives of pts; families with increased prevalence of cancer; and pts with history of breast or gynecologic cancer, familial polyposis syndromes, >10-year history of ulcerative colitis or Crohn's colitis, >15-year history of ureterosigmoidostomy. Tumors in pts with strong family history of malignancy are frequently located in right colon and commonly present before age 50; high prevalence in pts with *Streptococcus bovis* bacteremia.

PATHOLOGY　Nearly always adenocarcinoma; 75% located distal to the splenic flexure (except in association with polyposis or hereditary cancer syndromes); may be polypoid, sessile, fungating, or constricting; subtype and degree of differentiation do not correlate with course. Degree of invasiveness at surgery (Dukes' classification) is single best predictor of prognosis (Table 75-3). Rectosigmoid tumors may spread to lungs early because of systemic paravertebral venous drainage of this area. Other predictors of poor prognosis: preoperative serum carcinoembryonic antigen (CEA) >5 ng/mL (>5 μg/L), poorly differentiated histology, bowel perforation, venous invasion, adherence

Table 75-3

Staging of and Prognosis for Colorectal Cancer

Stage				Approximate 5-Year
Dukes	TNM	Numerical	Pathologic Description	Survival, %
A	T1N0M0	I	Cancer limited to mucosa and submucosa	>90
B$_1$	T2N0M0	I	Cancer extends into muscularis	85
B$_2$	T3N0M0	II	Cancer extends into or through serosa	70–80
C	TxN1M0	III	Cancer involves regional lymph nodes	35–65
D	TxNxM1	IV	Distant metastases (liver, lung, etc.)	5

to adjacent organs, aneuploidy, specific deletions in chromosomes 5, 17, 18, and mutation of *ras* proto-oncogene. 15% have defects in DNA repair.

CLINICAL FEATURES Left-sided colon cancers present most commonly with rectal bleeding, altered bowel habits (narrowing, constipation, intermittent diarrhea, tenesmus), and abdominal or back pain; cecal and ascending colon cancers more frequently present with symptoms of anemia, occult blood in stool, or weight loss; other complications: perforation, fistula, volvulus, inguinal hernia; laboratory findings: anemia in 50% of right-sided lesions.

DIAGNOSIS Early diagnosis aided by screening asymptomatic persons with fecal occult blood testing (see below); >50% of all colon cancers are within reach of a 60-cm flexible sigmoidoscope; air-contrast barium enema will diagnose ~85% of colon cancers not within reach of sigmoidoscope; colonoscopy most sensitive and specific, permits tumor biopsy and removal of synchronous polyps (thus preventing neoplastic conversion), but is more expensive. Radiographic or virtual colonoscopy has not been shown to be a better diagnostic method than colonoscopy.

℞ TREATMENT

Local disease: Surgical resection of colonic segment containing tumor; preoperative evaluation to assess prognosis and surgical approach includes full colonoscopy, chest films, biochemical liver tests, plasma CEA level, and possible abdominal CT. Resection of isolated hepatic metastases possible in selected cases. Adjuvant radiation therapy to pelvis (with or without concomitant 5-FU chemotherapy) decreases local recurrence rate of rectal carcinoma (no apparent effect on survival); radiation therapy without benefit on colon tumors; preoperative radiation therapy may improve resectability and local control in pts with rectal cancer. Total mesorectal excision is more effective than conventional anteroposterior resection in rectal cancer. Adjuvant chemotherapy (5-FU/leucovorin plus oxaliplatin, or FOLFOX) decreases recurrence rate and improves survival of stage C (III) and stage B (II) tumors; periodic determination of serum CEA level useful to follow therapy and assess recurrence. *Follow-up after curative resection*: Yearly liver tests, CBC, follow-up radiologic or colonoscopic evaluation at 1 year—if normal, repeat every 3 years, with routine screening interim (see below); if polyps detected, repeat 1 year after resection. *Advanced tumor* (locally unresectable or metastatic): Systemic chemotherapy (5-FU/ leucovorin plus oxaliplatin plus bevacizumab), irinotecan usually used in second treatment; intraarterial chemotherapy [floxuridine (FUDR)] and/or radiation therapy may palliate symptoms from hepatic metastases.

PREVENTION Early detection of colon carcinoma may be facilitated by routine screening of stool for occult blood (Hemoccult II, Colo-Test, etc.); however, sensitivity only ~50% for carcinoma; specificity for tumor or polyp ~25–40%. False positives: ingestion of red meat, iron, aspirin; upper GI bleeding. False negatives: vitamin C ingestion, intermittent bleeding. Annual digital rectal exam and fecal occult blood testing recommended for pts over age 40, screening by flexible sigmoidoscopy every 3 years after age 50, earlier in pts at increased risk (see above); careful evaluation of all pts with positive fecal occult blood tests (flexible sigmoidoscopy and air-contrast barium enema or colonoscopy alone) reveals polyps in 20–40% and carcinoma in ~5%; screening of asymptomatic persons allows earlier detection of colon cancer (i.e., earlier Dukes' stage) and achieves greater resectability rate; decreased overall mortality from colon carcinoma seen only after 13 years of follow-up. More intensive evaluation of first-degree relatives of pts with colon carcinoma frequently includes screening air-contrast barium enema or colonoscopy after age 40. NSAIDs and cyclooxygenase-2 inhibitors appear to prevent polyp development and induce regression in high-risk groups but have not been recommended for average-risk pts at this time.

Anal Cancer

Accounts for 1–2% of large-bowel cancer, 4010 cases and 580 deaths in 2004; associated with chronic irritation, e.g., from condyloma accuminata, perianal fissures/fistulae, chronic hemorrhoids, leukoplakia, trauma from anal intercourse. Women are more commonly affected than men. Homosexual men are at increased risk. Presents with bleeding, pain, and perianal mass. Radiation therapy plus chemotherapy (5-FU and mitomycin) leads to complete response in 80% when the primary lesion is <3 cm. Abdominoperineal resection with permanent colostomy is reserved for those with large lesions or whose disease recurs after chemoradiotherapy.

BENIGN LIVER TUMORS

Hepatocellular adenomas occur most commonly in women in the third or fourth decades who take birth control pills. Most are found incidentally but may cause pain; intratumoral hemorrhage may cause circulatory collapse. 10% may become malignant. Women with these adenomas should stop taking birth control pills. Large tumors near the liver surface may be resected. Focal nodular hyperplasia is also more common in women but seems not to be caused by birth control pills. Lesions are vascular on angiography and have septae and are usually asymptomatic.

HEPATOCELLULAR CARCINOMA

About 18,920 cases in the United States in 2004, but worldwide this may be the most common tumor. Male:female = 4:1; tumor usually develops in cirrhotic liver in persons in fifth or sixth decade. High incidence in Asia and Africa is related to etiologic relationship between this cancer and hepatitis B and C infections. Aflatoxin exposure contributes to etiology and leaves a molecular signature, a mutation in codon 249 of the gene for p53. Surgical resection or liver transplantation is therapeutic option but rarely successful. Screening populations at risk has given conflicting results. Hepatitis B vaccine prevents the disease. Interferon α may prevent liver cancer in persons with chronic active hepatitis C disease and possibly in those with hepatitis B. Ribivarin $+/-$ interferon (IFN) α is most effective treatment of chronic hepatitis C.

PANCREATIC CANCER

In 2004 in the United States, about 31,860 new cases and 31,270 deaths. The incidence is decreasing somewhat, but nearly all diagnosed cases are fatal. The tumors are ductal adenocarcinomas and are not usually detected until the disease has spread. About 70% of tumors are in the pancreatic head, 20% in the body, and 10% in the tail. Mutations in K-*ras* have been found in 85% of tumors, and the p16 cyclin-dependent kinase inhibitor on chromosome 9 may also be implicated. Long-standing diabetes, chronic pancreatitis, and smoking increase the risk; coffee-drinking, alcoholism, and cholelithiasis do not. Pts present with pain and weight loss, the pain often relieved by bending forward. Jaundice commonly complicates tumors of the head, due to biliary obstruction. Curative surgical resections are feasible in about 10%. Adjuvant chemotherapy may benefit some patients after resection. Gemcitabine may palliate symptoms in pts with advanced disease.

ENDOCRINE TUMORS OF THE GI TRACT AND PANCREAS
Carcinoid Tumor

Carcinoid tumor accounts for 75% of GI endocrine tumors; incidence is about 15 cases per million population. 90% originate in Kulchitsky cells of the GI tract, most commonly the appendix, ileum, and rectum. Carcinoid tumors of the small bowel and bronchus have a more malignant course than tumors of other sites. About 5% of pts with carcinoid tumors develop symptoms of the carcinoid syndrome, the classic triad being cutaneous flushing, diarrhea, and valvular heart disease. For tumors of GI tract origin, symptoms imply metastases to liver.

Diagnosis can be made by detecting the site of tumor or documenting production of >15 mg/d of the serotonin metabolite 5-hydroxyindoleacetic acid (5-HIAA) in the urine. Octreotide scintigraphy identifies sites of primary and metastatic tumor in about 2/3 of cases.

℞ TREATMENT

Surgical resection where feasible. Symptoms may be controlled with histamine blockers and octreotide, 150–1500 mg/d in three doses. Hepatic artery embolization and chemotherapy (5-FU plus streptozotocin or doxorubicin) have been used for metastatic disease. IFN-α at 3–10 million units subcutaneously three times a week may relieve symptoms. Prognosis ranges from 95% 5-year survival for localized disease to 20% 5-year survival for those with liver metastases. Median survival of pts with carcinoid syndrome is 2.5 years from the first episode of flushing.

Pancreatic Islet-Cell Tumors

Gastrinoma, insulinoma, VIPoma, glucagonoma, and somatostatinoma account for the vast majority of pancreatic islet-cell tumors; their characteristics are shown in Table 75-4. The tumors are named for the dominant hormone they produce. They are generally slow-growing and produce symptoms related to hormone production. *Gastrinomas* and *peptic ulcer disease* comprise the Zollinger-Ellison syndrome. Gastrinomas are rare (4 cases per 10 million population), and in 25–50%, the tumor is a component of a MEN I syndrome (Chap. 179).

Insulinoma may present with Whipple's triad: fasting hypoglycemia, symptoms of hypoglycemia, and relief after intravenous glucose. Normal or elevated serum insulin levels in the presence of fasting hypoglycemia are diagnostic. Insulinomas may also be associated with MEN I.

Verner and Morrison described a syndrome of watery diarrhea, hypokalemia, achlorhydria, and renal failure associated with pancreatic islet tumors that produce vasoactive intestinal polypeptide (VIP). *VIPomas* are rare (1 case per 10 million) but often grow to a large size before producing symptoms.

Glucagonoma is associated with diabetes mellitus and necrolytic migratory erythema, a characteristic red, raised, scaly rash usually located on the face, abdomen, perineum, and distal extremities. Glucagon levels >1000 ng/L not suppressed by glucose are diagnostic.

The classic triad of *somatostatinoma* is diabetes mellitus, steatorrhea, and cholelithiasis.

Provocative tests may facilitate diagnosis of functional endocrine tumors: tolbutamide enhances somatostatin secretion by somatostatinomas; pentagastrin enhances calcitonin secretion from medullary thyroid (C cell) tumors; secretin enhances gastrin secretion from gastinomas. If imaging techniques fail to detect tumor masses, angiography or selective venous sampling for hormone deter-

Table 75-4

Gastrointestinal Endocrine Tumor Syndromes

Syndrome	Cell Type	Clinical Features	Percentage Malignant	Major Products
Carcinoid syndrome	Enterochromaffin, enterochromaffin-like	Flushing, diarrhea, wheezing, hypotension	~100	Serotonin, histamine, miscellaneous peptides
Zollinger-Ellison, gastrinoma	Non-β islet cell, duodenal G cell	Peptic ulcers, diarrhea	~70	Gastrin
Insulinoma	Islet β cell	Hypoglycemia	~10	Insulin
VIPoma (Verner-Morrison, WDHA)	Islet D_1 cell	Diarrhea, hypokalemia, hypochlorhydria	~60	Vasoactive intestinal peptide
Glucagonoma	Islet A cell	Mild diabetes mellitus, erythema necrolytica migrans, glossitis	>75	Glucagon
Somatostatinoma	Islet D cell	Diabetes mellitus, diarrhea, steatorrhea, gallstones	~70	Somatostatin

mination may reveal the site of tumor. Metastases to nodes and liver should be sought by CT or MRI.

 TREATMENT

Tumor is surgically removed, if possible. Octreotide inhibits hormone secretion in the majority of cases. IFN-α may reduce symptoms. Streptozotocin plus doxorubicin combination chemotherapy may produce responses in 60–90% of cases. Embolization of hepatic metastases may be palliative.

For a more detailed discussion, see Mayer RJ: Gastrointestinal Tract Cancer, Chap. 77, p. 523; Dienstag JL, Isselbacher KJ: Tumors of the Liver and Biliary Tract, Chap. 78, p. 533; Mayer RJ: Pancreatic Cancer, Chap. 79, p. 537; and Jensen RT: Endocrine Tumors of the Gastrointestinal Tract and Pancreas, Chap. 329, p. 2220, in HPIM-16.

76

GENITOURINARY TRACT CANCER

BLADDER CANCER

INCIDENCE AND EPIDEMIOLOGY Annual incidence in the United States is about 60,240 cases with 12,700 deaths. Median age is 65 years. Smoking accounts for 50% of the risk. Exposure to polycyclic aromatic hydrocarbons increases the risk, especially in slow acetylators. Risk is increased in chimney sweeps, dry cleaners, and those involved in aluminum manufacturing. Chronic cyclophosphamide exposure increases risk ninefold. *Schistosoma haematobium* infection also increases risk, especially of squamous histology.

ETIOLOGY Lesions involving chromosome 9q are an early event. Deletions in 17p (p53), 18q (the DCC locus), 13q (RB), 3p, and 5q are characteristic of invasive lesions. Overexpression of epidermal growth factor receptors and *HER-2/neu* receptors is common.

PATHOLOGY Over 90% of tumors are derived from transitional epithelium; 3% are squamous, 2% are adenocarcinomas, and <1% are neuroendocrine small cell tumors. Field effects are seen that place all sites lined by transitional epithelium at risk including the renal pelvis, ureter, bladder, and proximal two-thirds of the urethra. 90% of tumors are in the bladder, 8% in the renal pelvis, and 2% in the ureter or urethra. Histologic grade influences survival. Lesion recurrence is influenced by size, number, and growth pattern of the primary tumor.

CLINICAL PRESENTATION Hematuria is the initial sign in 80–90%; however, cystitis is a more common cause of hematuria (22% of all hematuria) than is bladder cancer (15%). Pts are initially staged and treated by endoscopy. Superficial tumors are removed at endoscopy; muscle invasion requires more extensive surgery.

℞ TREATMENT

Management is based on extent of disease: superficial, invasive, or metastatic. Frequency of presentation is 75% superficial, 20% invasive, and 5% metastatic. Superficial lesions are resected at endoscopy. Although complete resection is possible in 80%, 30–80% of cases recur; grade and stage progression occur in 30%. Intravesical instillation of bacille Calmette-Guérin (BCG) reduces the risk of recurrence by 40–45%. Recurrence is monitored every 3 months.

The standard management of muscle-invasive disease is radical cystectomy. 5-year survival is 70% for those without invasion of perivesicular fat or lymph nodes, 50% for those with invasion of fat but not lymph nodes, 35% for those with one node involved, and 10% for those with six or more involved nodes. Pts who cannot withstand radical surgery may have 30–35% 5-year survival with 5000- to 7000-cGy external beam radiation therapy. Bladder sparing may be possible in up to 45% of pts with two cycles of chemotherapy with CMV (methotrexate, 30 mg/m^2 days 1 and 8, vinblastine, 4 mg/m^2 days 1 and 8, cisplatin, 100 mg/m^2 day 2, q21d) followed by 4000-cGy radiation therapy given concurrently with cisplatin.

Metastatic disease is treated with combination chemotherapy. Useful regimens include CMV (see above), M-VAC (methotrexate, 30 mg/m^2 days 1, 15, 22; vinblastine, 3 mg/m^2 days 2, 15, 22; doxorubicin, 30 mg/m^2 day 2; cisplatin, 70 mg/m^2 day 2; q28d) or cisplatin (70 mg/m^2 day 2) plus gemcitabine (1000 mg/m^2 days 1, 8, 15 of a 28-day cycle) or carboplatin plus paclitaxel. About 70% of pts respond to treatment, and 20% have a complete response; 10–15% have long-term disease-free survival.

RENAL CANCER

INCIDENCE AND EPIDEMIOLOGY   Annual incidence in the United States is about 36,700 cases with 12,480 deaths. Cigarette smoking accounts for 20–30% of cases. Risk is increased in acquired renal cystic disease. There are two familial forms: a rare autosomal dominant syndrome and von Hippel–Lindau disease. About 35% of pts with von Hippel–Lindau disease develop renal cancer. Incidence is also increased in those with tuberous sclerosis and polycystic kidney disease.

ETIOLOGY   Most cases are sporadic; however, the most frequent chromosomal abnormality (occurs in 60%) is deletion or rearrangement of 3p21-26. The von Hippel–Lindau gene has been mapped to that region and appears to have novel activities, regulation of speed of transcription, and participation in turnover of damaged proteins. It is unclear how lesions in the gene lead to cancer.

PATHOLOGY   Five variants are recognized: clear cell tumors (75%), chromophilic tumors (15%), chromophobic tumors (5%), oncocytic tumors (3%), and collecting duct tumors (2%). Clear cell tumors arise from cells of the proximal convoluted tubules. Chromophilic tumors tend to be bilateral and multifocal and often show trisomy 7 and/or trisomy 17. Chromophobic and eosinophilic tumors less frequently have chromosomal aberrations and follow a more indolent course.

CLINICAL PRESENTATION   The classic triad of hematuria, flank pain, and flank mass is seen in only 10–20% of pts; hematuria (40%), flank pain (40%), palpable mass (33%), weight loss (33%) are the most common individual symptoms. Paraneoplastic syndromes of erythrocytosis (3%), hypercalcemia (5%), and nonmetastatic hepatic dysfunction (Stauffers' syndrome) (15%) may also occur. Workup should include IV pyelography, renal ultrasonography, CT of abdomen and pelvis, CXR, urinalysis, and urine cytology. Stage I is disease restricted to the kidney, stage II is disease contained within Gerota's fascia, stage III is locally invasive disease involving nodes and/or inferior vena cava, stage IV is invasion of adjacent organs or metastatic sites. Prognosis is related to stage: 66% 5-year survival for I, 64% for II, 42% for III, and 11% for IV.

 TREATMENT

> Radical nephrectomy is standard for stages I, II, and most stage III pts. Surgery may also be indicated in the setting of metastatic disease for intractable local symptoms (bleeding, pain). About 10–15% of pts with advanced stage disease may benefit from interleukin 2 and/or interferon α. Some remissions are durable. Chemotherapy is of little or no benefit.

TESTICULAR CANCER

INCIDENCE AND EPIDEMIOLOGY   Annual incidence is about 8900 cases with 300 deaths. Peak age incidence is 20–40. Occurs 4–5 times more frequently in white than black men. Cryptorchid testes are at increased risk. Early orchiopexy may protect against testis cancer. Risk is also increased in testicular femininization syndromes, and Klinefelter's syndrome is associated with mediastinal germ cell tumor.

ETIOLOGY   The cause is unknown. Disease is associated with a characteristic cytogenetic defect, isochromosome 12p.

PATHOLOGY   Two main subtypes are noted: seminoma and nonseminoma. Each accounts for ~50% of cases. Seminoma has a more indolent natural history and is highly sensitive to radiation therapy. Four subtypes of nonseminoma are defined: embryonal carcinoma, teratoma, choriocarcinoma, and endodermal sinus (yolk sac) tumor.

CLINICAL PRESENTATION   Painless testicular mass is the classic initial sign. In the presence of pain, differential diagnosis includes epididymitis or orchitis; a brief trial of antibiotics may be undertaken. Staging evaluation includes measurement of serum tumor markers α fetoprotein (AFP) and β-human chorionic gonadotropin (hCG), CXR, and CT scan of abdomen and pelvis. Lymph nodes are staged at resection of the primary tumor through an inguinal approach. Stage I disease is limited to the testis, epididymis, or spermatic cord; stage II involves retroperitoneal nodes; and stage III is disease outside the retroperitoneum. Among seminoma pts, 70% are stage I, 20% are stage II, and 10% are stage III. Among nonseminoma germ cell tumor pts, 33% are found in each stage. hCG may be elevated in either seminoma or nonseminoma, but AFP is elevated only in nonseminoma. 95% of pts are cured if treated appropriately. Primary nonseminoma in the mediastinum is associated with acute leukemia or other hematologic disorders and has a poorer prognosis than testicular primaries (~33%).

 TREATMENT

> For stages I and II seminoma, inguinal orchiectomy followed by retroperitoneal radiation therapy to 2500–3000 cGy is effective. For stages I and II nonseminoma germ cell tumors, inguinal orchiectomy followed by retroperitoneal lymph node dissection is effective. For pts of either histology with bulky nodes or stage III disease, chemotherapy is given. Cisplatin (20 mg/m^2 days 1–5), etoposide (100 mg/m^2 days 1–5), and bleomycin (30 U days 2,

9, 16) given every 21 days for four cycles is the standard therapy. If tumor markers return to zero, residual masses are resected. Most are necrotic debris or teratomas. Salvage therapy rescues about 25% of those not cured with primary therapy.

For a more detailed discussion, see Scher HI, Motzer RJ: Bladder and Renal Cell Carcinomas, Chap. 80, p. 539; and Motzer RJ, Bosl GL: Testicular Cancer, Chap. 82, p. 550, in HPIM-16.

77

GYNECOLOGIC CANCER

OVARIAN CANCER

INCIDENCE AND EPIDEMIOLOGY Annually in the United States, about 25,000 new cases are found and nearly 16,000 women die of ovarian cancer. Incidence begins to rise in the fifth decade, peaking in the eighth decade. Risk is increased in nulliparous women and reduced by pregnancy (risk decreased about 10% per pregnancy) and oral contraceptives. About 5% of cases are familial.

GENETICS Mutations in *BRCA-1* predispose women to both breast and ovarian cancer. Cytogenetic analysis of epithelial ovarian cancers that are not familial often reveals complex karyotypic abnormalities including structural lesions on chromosomes 1 and 11 and loss of heterozygosity for loci on chromosomes 3q, 6q, 11q, 13q, and 17. C-*myc*, H-*ras*, K-*ras*, and *HER2/neu* are often mutated or overexpressed. Unlike colon cancer, a stepwise pathway to ovarian carcinoma is not apparent.

SCREENING No benefit has been seen from screening women of average risk. Hereditary ovarian cancer accounts for 10% of all cases. Women with *BRCA-1* or *-2* mutations should consider prophylactic bilateral salpingo-oophorectomy by age 40.

CLINICAL PRESENTATION Most pts present with abdominal pain, bloating, urinary symptoms, and weight gain indicative of disease spread beyond the true pelvis. Localized ovarian cancer is usually asymptomatic and detected on routine pelvic examination as a palpable nontender adnexal mass. Most ovarian masses detected incidentally in ovulating women are ovarian cysts that resolve over one to three menstrual cycles. Adnexal masses in postmenopausal women are more often pathologic and should be surgically removed. CA-125 serum levels are $\geq$35 U/mL in 80–85% of women with ovarian cancer, but other conditions may also cause elevations.

PATHOLOGY Half of ovarian tumors are benign, one-third are malignant, and the rest are tumors of low malignant potential. These borderline lesions have cytologic features of malignancy but do not invade. Malignant epithelial tumors may be of five different types: serous (50%), mucinous (25%), endometrioid (15%), clear cell (5%), and Brenner tumors (1%, derived from urothelial or transitional epithelium). The remaining 4% of ovarian tumors are stromal or germ cell tumors, which are managed like testicular cancer in men (Chap. 76). Histologic grade is an important prognostic factor for the epithelial varieties.

STAGING Extent of disease is ascertained by a surgical procedure that permits visual and manual inspection of all peritoneal surfaces and the diaphragm. Total abdominal hysterectomy, bilateral salpingo-oopherectomy, partial omentectomy, pelvic and paraaortic lymph node sampling, and peritoneal washings should be performed. The staging system and its influence on survival is shown in Table 77-1.

 TREATMENT

Pts with stage I disease, no residual tumor after surgery, and well- or moderately differentiated tumors need no further treatment after surgery and have a 5-year survival >95%. For stage II pts totally resected and stage I pts with poor histologic grade, adjuvant therapy with single-agent cisplatin or cisplatin plus paclitaxel produces 5-year survival of 80%. Advanced-stage pts should receive paclitaxel, 175 mg/m^2 by 3-h infusion, followed by carboplatin dosed to an area under the curve (AUC) of 7.5 every 3 or 4 weeks. Carboplatin dose is calculated by the Calvert formula: dose = target AUC × (glomerular filtration rate + 25). The complete response rate is about 55%, and median survival is 38 months.

ENDOMETRIAL CANCER

INCIDENCE AND EPIDEMIOLOGY The most common gynecologic cancer, 40,000 cases are diagnosed in the United States and 7000 pts die annually. It is primarily a disease of postmenopausal women. Obesity, altered menstrual cycles, infertility, late menopause, and postmenopausal bleeding are commonly encountered in women with endometrial cancer. Women taking tamoxifen to prevent breast cancer recurrence and those taking estrogen replacement therapy are at a modestly increased risk. Peak incidence is in the sixth and seventh decades.

CLINICAL PRESENTATION Abnormal vaginal discharge (90%), abnormal vaginal bleeding (80%), and leukorrhea (10%) are the most common symptoms.

PATHOLOGY Endometrial cancers are adenocarcinomas in 75–80% of cases. The remaining cases include mucinous carcinoma; papillary serous carcinoma; and secretory, ciliate, and clear cell varieties. Prognosis depends on stage, histologic grade, and degree of myometrial invasion.

STAGING Total abdominal hysterectomy and bilateral salpingo-oopherectomy comprise both the staging procedure and the treatment of choice. The staging scheme and its influence on prognosis are shown in Table 77-1.

 TREATMENT

In women with poor histologic grade, deep myometrial invasion, or extensive involvement of the lower uterine segment or cervix, intracavitary or external beam radiation therapy is given. If cervical invasion is deep, preoperative radiation therapy may improve the resectability of the tumor. Stage III disease is managed with surgery and radiation therapy. Stage IV disease is usually

Table 77-1

Staging and Survival in Gynecologic Malignancies

Stage	Ovarian	5-Year Survival, %	Endometrial	5-Year Survival, %	Cervical	5-Year Survival, %
0	—		—		Carcinoma in situ	100
I	Confined to ovary	90	Confined to corpus	89	Confined to uterus	85
II	Confined to pelvis	70	Involves corpus and cervix	80	Invades beyond uterus but not pelvic wall	60
III	Intraabdominal spread	15–20	Extends outside the uterus but not outside the true pelvis	30	Extends to pelvic wall and/or lower third of vagina, or hydronephrosis	33
IV	Spread outside abdomen	1–5	Extends outside the true pelvis or involves the bladder or rectum	9	Invades mucosa of bladder or rectum or extends beyond the true pelvis	7

treated palliatively. Progestational agents such as hydroxyprogesterone or megastrol and the antiestrogen tamoxifen may produce responses in 20% of pts. Doxorubicin, 60 mg/m² IV day 1, and cisplatin, 50 mg/m² IV day 1, every 3 weeks for 8 cycles produces a 45% response rate.

CERVICAL CANCER

INCIDENCE AND EPIDEMIOLOGY In the United States about 10,500 cases of invasive cervical cancer are diagnosed each year and 50,000 cases of carcinoma in situ are detected by Pap smear. Cervical cancer kills 3900 women a year, 85% of whom never had a Pap smear. It is a major cause of disease in underdeveloped countries and is more common in lower socioeconomic groups, in women with early sexual activity and/or multiple sexual partners, and in smokers. Human papilloma virus (HPV) types 16 and 18 are the major types associated with cervical cancer. The virus attacks the G_1 checkpoint of the cell cycle; its E7 protein binds and inactivates Rb protein, and E6 induces the degradation of p53.

SCREENING Women should begin screening when they begin sexual activity or at age 20. After two consecutive negative annual Pap smears, the test should be repeated every 3 years. Abnormal smears dictate the need for a cervical biopsy, usually under colposcopy, with the cervix painted with 3% acetic acid, which shows abnormal areas as white patches. If there is evidence of carcinoma in situ, a cone biopsy is performed, which is therapeutic.

CLINICAL PRESENTATION Pts present with abnormal bleeding or postcoital spotting or menometrorrhagia or intermenstrual bleeding. Vaginal discharge, low back pain, and urinary symptoms may also be present.

STAGING Staging is clinical and consists of a pelvic exam under anesthesia with cystoscopy and proctoscopy. CXR, IV pyelography, and abdominal CT are used to search for metastases. The staging system and its influence on prognosis are shown in Table 77-1.

℞ **TREATMENT**

Carcinoma in situ is cured with cone biopsy. Stage I disease may be treated with radical hysterectomy or radiation therapy. Stages II–IV disease are usually treated with radiation therapy, often with both brachytherapy and teletherapy, or combined modality therapy. Pelvic exenteration is used uncommonly to control the disease, especially in the setting of centrally recurrent or persistent disease. Women with locally advanced (stage IIB to IVA) disease usually receive concurrent chemotherapy and radiation therapy. The chemotherapy acts as a radiosensitizer. Hydroxyurea, 5-fluorouracil (5-FU), and cisplatin have all shown promising results given concurrently with radiation therapy. Cisplatin, 75 mg/m² IV over 4 h on day 1, and 5-FU, 4 g given by 96-h infusion on days 1–5 of radiation therapy, is a common regimen. Relapse rates are reduced 30–50% by such therapy. Advanced stage disease is treated palliatively with single agents (cisplatin, irinotecan, ifosfamide).

For a more detailed discussion, see Young RC: Gynecologic Malignancies, Chap. 83, p. 553, in HPIM-16.

78

PROSTATE HYPERPLASIA AND CARCINOMA

PROSTATE HYPERPLASIA

Enlargement of the prostate is nearly universal in aging men. Hyperplasia usually begins by age 45 years, occurs in the area of the prostate gland surrounding the urethra, and produces urinary outflow obstruction. Symptoms develop on average by age 65 in whites and 60 in blacks. Symptoms develop late because hypertrophy of the bladder detrusor compensates for ureteral compression. As obstruction progresses, urinary stream caliber and force diminish, hesitancy in stream initiation develops, and postvoid dribbling occurs. Dysuria and urgency are signs of bladder irritation (perhaps due to inflammation or tumor) and are usually not seen in prostate hyperplasia. As the postvoid residual increases, nocturia and overflow incontinence may develop. Common medications such as tranquilizing drugs and decongestants, infections, or alcohol may precipitate urinary retention. Because of the prevalence of hyperplasia, the relationship to neoplasia is unclear.

On digital rectal exam (DRE), a hyperplastic prostate is smooth, firm, and rubbery in consistency; the median groove may be lost. Prostate-specific antigen (PSA) levels may be elevated but are ≤10 ng/mL unless cancer is also present (see below). Cancer may also be present at lower levels of PSA.

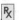 **TREATMENT**

Asymptomatic pts do not require treatment, and those with complications of urethral obstruction such as inability to urinate, renal failure, recurrent UTI, hematuria, or bladder stones clearly require surgical extirpation of the prostate, usually by transurethral resection (TURP). However, the approach to the remaining pts should be based on the degree of incapacity or discomfort from the disease and the likely side effects of any intervention. If the pt has only mild symptoms, watchful waiting is not harmful and permits an assessment of the rate of symptom progression. If therapy is desired by the pt, two medical approaches may be helpful: terazosin, an α_1-adrenergic blocker (1 mg at bedtime, titrated to symptoms up to 20 mg/d), relaxes the smooth muscle of the bladder neck and increases urine flow; finasteride (5 mg/d), an inhibitor of 5α-reductase, blocks the conversion of testosterone to dihydrotestosterone and causes an average decrease in prostate size of ~24%. TURP has the greatest success rate but also the greatest risk of complications. Transurethral microwave thermotherapy (TUMT) may be comparably effective to TURP. Direct comparison has not been made between medical and surgical management.

PROSTATE CARCINOMA

Prostate cancer was diagnosed in 230,110 men in 2004 in the U.S, comparable to the incidence of breast cancer. About 29,900 men died of prostate cancer in 2004. The early diagnosis of cancers in mildly symptomatic men found on screening to have elevated serum levels of PSA has complicated management. Like most other cancers, incidence is age-related. The disease is more common in blacks than whites. Symptoms are generally similar to and indistinguishable from those of prostate hyperplasia, but those with cancer more often have dysuria and back or hip pain. On histology, 95% are adenocarcinomas. Biologic behavior is affected by histologic grade (Gleason score).

In contrast to hyperplasia, prostate cancer generally originates in the periphery of the gland and may be detectable on DRE as one or more nodules on the posterior surface of the gland, hard in consistency and irregular in shape. An approach to diagnosis is shown in Fig. 78-1. Those with a negative DRE and PSA ≤ 4 ng/mL may be followed annually. Those with an abnormal DRE or a PSA > 10 ng/mL should undergo transrectal ultrasound-guided biopsy (TRUS). Those with normal DRE and PSA of 4.1–10 ng/mL may be handled differently in different centers. Some would perform transrectal ultrasound and biopsy any abnormality or follow if no abnormality is found. Some would repeat the PSA in a year and biopsy if the increase over that period was >0.75 ng/ mL. Other methods of using PSA to distinguish early cancer from hyperplasia include quantitating bound and free PSA and relating the PSA to the size of the prostate (PSA density). Perhaps 1/3 of persons with prostate cancer do not have PSA elevations.

Lymphatic spread is assessed surgically; it is present in only 10% of those with Gleason grade 5 or lower and in 70% of those with grade 9 or 10. PSA level also correlates with spread; only 10% of those with PSA < 10 ng/mL have lymphatic spread. Bone is the most common site of distant metastasis. Whitmore-Jewett staging includes A: tumor not palpable but detected at TURP; B: palpable tumor in one (B1) or both (B2) lobes; C: palpable tumor outside capsule; and D: metastatic disease.

℞ TREATMENT

For pts with stages A through C disease, surgery (radical retropubic prostatectomy) and radiation therapy (conformal 3-dimensional fields) are said to have similar outcomes; however, most pts are treated surgically. Both modalities are associated with impotence. Surgery is more likely to lead to incontinence. Radiation therapy is more likely to produce proctitis, perhaps with bleeding or stricture. Addition of hormonal therapy (goserelin) to radiation therapy of patients with localized disease appears to improve results. Patients usually must have a 5-year life expectancy to undergo radical prostatectomy. Stage A pts have survival identical to age-matched controls without cancer. Stage B and C pts have a 10-year survival of 82% and 42%, respectively.

Pts treated surgically for localized disease who develop rising PSA may undergo prostascint scanning (antibody to a prostate-specific membrane antigen). If no uptake is seen, the pt is observed. If uptake is seen in the prostate bed, local recurrence is implied and external beam radiation therapy is delivered to the site. (If the pt was initially treated with radiation therapy, this local recurrence may be treated with surgery.) However, in most cases, a rising PSA after local therapy indicates systemic disease. It is not clear when to intervene in such patients.

For pts with metastatic disease, androgen deprivation is the treatment of choice. Surgical castration is effective, but most pts prefer to take leuprolide, 7.5 mg depot form IM monthly (to inhibit pituitary gonadotrophin production), plus flutamide, 250 mg PO tid (an androgen receptor blocker). The value of added flutamide is debated. Alternative approaches include adrenalectomy, hypophysectomy, estrogen administration, and medical adrenalectomy with aminoglutethimide. The median survival of stage D pts is 33 months. Pts occasionally respond to withdrawal of hormonal therapy with tumor shrinkage. Rarely a second hormonal manipulation will work, but most pts who progress on hormonal therapy have androgen-independent tumors, often associated with genetic changes in the androgen receptor and new expression of *bcl*-2, which may contribute to chemotherapy resistance. Chemotherapy is used for palliation in prostate cancer. Mitoxantrone, estramustine, and taxanes appear to be active single agents, and combinations of drugs are being tested. Chemotherapy-treated pts are more likely to have pain relief than those re-

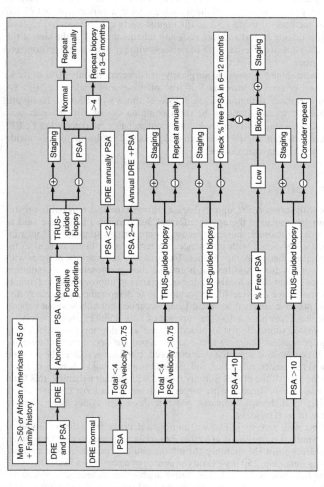

FIGURE 78-1 The use of the annual digital rectal examination (DRE) and measurement of prostate-specific antigen (PSA) as guides for deciding which men should have transrectal prostate biopsy under sonography (TRUS). There are at least three schools of thought about what to do if the DRE is negative and the PSA is equivocal (4.1 to 10 ng/mL).

ceiving supportive care alone. Bone pain from metastases may be palliated with strontium-89 or samarium-153. Bisphosphonates have not been adequately evaluated.

For a more detailed discussion, see Scher HI: Hyperplastic and Malignant Diseases of the Prostate, Chap. 81, p. 543, in HPIM-16.

79

CANCER OF UNKNOWN PRIMARY SITE

Cancer of unknown primary site (CUPS) is defined as follows: biopsy-proven malignancy; primary site unapparent after history, physical exam, CXR, abdominal and pelvic CT, CBC, chemistry survey, mammography (women), β-human chorionic gonadotropin (hCG) levels (men), α-fetoprotein (AFP) levels (men), and prostate-specific antigen (PSA) levels (men); and histologic evaluation not consistent with a primary tumor at the biopsy site. CUPS incidence is declining, probably because of better pathology diagnostic criteria; they account for about 3% of all cancers today, down from 10–15% 15 years ago. Most pts are over age 60. Cell lines derived from such tumors frequently have abnormalities in chromosome 1.

CLINICAL PRESENTATION Pts may present with fatigue, weight loss, pain, bleeding, abdominal swelling, subcutaneous masses, and lymphadenopathy. Once metastatic malignancy is confirmed, diagnostic efforts should be confined to evaluating the presence of potentially curable tumors, such as lymphoma, Hodgkin's disease, germ cell tumor, ovarian cancer, head and neck cancer, and primitive neuroectodermal tumor, or tumors for which therapy may be of significant palliative value such as breast cancer or prostate cancer. In general, efforts to evaluate the presence of these tumor types depends more on the pathologist than on expensive clinical diagnostic testing. Localizing symptoms, a history of carcinogen exposure, or a history of fulguration of skin lesion may direct some clinical testing; however, the careful light microscopic, ultrastructural, immunologic, karyotypic, and molecular biologic examination of adequate volumes of tumor tissue is the most important feature of the diagnostic workup in the absence of suspicious findings on history and physical exam (Table 79-1).

HISTOLOGY About 60% of CUPS tumors are adenocarcinomas, 10–20% are squamous cell carcinomas, and 20–30% are poorly differentiated neoplasms not further classified on light microscopy.

PROGNOSIS Pts with squamous cell carcinoma have a median survival of 9 months; those with adenocarcinoma or unclassifiable tumors have a median survival of 4–6 months. Pts in whom a primary site is identified usually have a better prognosis. Limited sites of involvement and neuroendocrine histology are favorable prognostic factors. Pts without a primary diagnosis should be treated palliatively with radiation therapy to symptomatic lesions. All-purpose

Table 79-1

Possible Pathologic Evaluation of Biopsy Specimens from Patients with Metastatic Cancer of Unknown Primary Site

Evaluation/Findings	Suggested Primary Site or Neoplasm
HISTOLOGY (HEMATOXYLIN AND EOSIN STAINING)	
Psammoma bodies, papillary configuration	Ovary, thyroid
Signet ring cells	Stomach
IMMUNOHISTOLOGY	
Leukocyte common antigen (LCA, CD45)	Lymphoid neoplasm
Leu-M1	Hodgkin's disease
Epithelial membrane antigen	Carcinoma
Cytokeratin	Carcinoma
CEA	Carcinoma
HMB45	Melanoma
Desmin	Sarcoma
Thyroglobulin	Thyroid carcinoma
Calcitonin	Medullary carcinoma of the thyroid
Myoglobin	Rhabdomyosarcoma
PSA/prostatic acid phosphatase	Prostate
AFP	Liver, stomach, germ cell
Placental alkaline phosphatase	Germ cell
B, T cell markers	Lymphoid neoplasm
S-100 protein	Neuroendocrine tumor, melanoma
Gross cystic fluid protein	Breast, sweat gland
Factor VIII	Kaposi's sarcoma, angiosarcoma
Thyroid transcription factor-1 (TTF-1)	Lung adenocarcinoma, thyroid
FLOW CYTOMETRY	
B, T cell markers	Lymphoid neoplasm
ULTRASTRUCTURE	
Actin-myosin filaments	Rhabdomyosarcoma
Secretory granules	Neuroendocrine tumors
Desmosomes	Carcinoma
Premelanosomes	Melanoma
CYTOGENETICS	
Isochromosome 12p; 12q($-$)	Germ cell
t(11;22)	Ewing's sarcoma, primitive neuro-ectodermal tumor
t(8;14)[a]	Lymphoid neoplasm
3p($-$)	Small cell lung carcinoma; renal cell carcinoma, mesothelioma
t(X;18)	Synovial sarcoma
t(12;16)	Myxoid liposarcoma
t(12;22)	Clear cell sarcoma (melanoma of soft parts)
t(2;13)	Alveolar rhabdomyosarcoma
1p($-$)	Neuroblastoma

(continued)

Table 79-1 *(Continued)*

Possible Pathologic Evaluation of Biopsy Specimens from Patients with Metastatic Cancer of Unknown Primary Site

Evaluation/Findings	Suggested Primary Site or Neoplasm
RECEPTOR ANALYSIS	
Estrogen/progesterone receptor	Breast
MOLECULAR BIOLOGIC STUDIES	
Immunoglobulin, *bcl*-2, T-cell receptor gene rearrangement	Lymphoid neoplasm

a Or any other rearrangement involving an antigen-receptor gene.
Note: CEA, carcinoembyronic antigen.

chemotherapy regimens rarely produce responses but always produce toxicity. Certain clinical features may permit individualized therapy.

Syndrome of Unrecognized Extragonadal Germ Cell Cancer

In pts <50 years with tumor involving midline structures, lung parenchyma, or lymph nodes and evidence of rapid tumor growth, germ cell tumor is a possible diagnosis. Serum tumor markers may or may not be elevated. Cisplatin, etoposide, and bleomycin (Chap. 76) chemotherapy may induce complete responses in ≥25%, and ~15% may be cured. A trial of such therapy should probably also be undertaken in pts whose tumors have abnormalities in chromosome 12.

Peritoneal Carcinomatosis in Women

Women who present with pelvic mass or pain and an adenocarcinoma diffusely throughout the peritoneal cavity, but without a clear site of origin, have primary peritoneal papillary serous carcinoma. The presence of psammoma bodies in the tumor or elevated CA-125 levels may favor ovarian origin. Such pts should undergo debulking surgery followed by paclitaxel plus cisplatin or carboplatin combination chemotherapy (Chap. 77). About 20% of pts will respond, and 10% will survive at least 2 years.

Carcinoma in an Axillary Lymph Node in Women

Such women should receive adjuvant breast cancer therapy appropriate for their menopausal status even in the absence of a breast mass on physical examination or mammography and undetermined or negative estrogen and progesterone receptors on the tumor (Chap. 74). Unless the ipsilateral breast is radiated, up to 50% of these pts will later develop a breast mass. Although this is a rare clinical situation, long-term survival similar to women with stage II breast cancer is possible.

Osteoblastic Bone Metastases in Men

The probability of prostate cancer is high; a trial of empirical hormonal therapy (leuprolide and flutamide) is warranted (Chap. 78).

Cervical Lymph Node Metastases

Even if panendoscopy fails to reveal a head and neck primary, treatment of such pts with cisplatin and 5-fluorouracil chemotherapy may produce a response; some responses are long-lived (Chap. 72).

For a more detailed discussion, see Stone RM: Metastatic Cancer of Unknown Primary Site, Chap. 85, p. 562, in HPIM-16.

80

PARANEOPLASTIC ENDOCRINE SYNDROMES

Both benign and malignant tumors of nonendocrine tissue can secrete a variety of hormones, principally peptide hormones, and many tumors produce more than one hormone (Table 80-1). At the clinical level, ectopic hormone production is important for two reasons.

First, endocrine syndromes that result may either be the presenting manifestations of the neoplasm or occur late in the course. The endocrine manifestations in some instances are of greater significance than the tumor itself, as in pts with benign or slowly growing malignancies that secrete corticotropin-releasing hormone and cause fulminant Cushing's syndrome. The frequency with

Table 80-1

Common Paraneoplastic Endocrine Syndromes

Syndrome	Proteins	Tumors Typically Associated with Syndrome
Hypercalcemia of malignancy	Parathyroid hormone–related peptide (PTHrP)	Non–small cell lung cancer
		Breast cancer
	Parathyroid hormone (PTH)	Renal cell carcinoma
		Head and neck cancer
		Bladder cancer
		Myeloma
Syndrome of inappropriate vasopressin secretion (SIADH)	Arginine vasopressin (AVP)	Small cell lung cancer
		Head and neck cancer
	Atrial natriuretic peptide	Non–small cell lung cancer
Cushing's syndrome	Adrenocorticotropic hormone (ACTH)	Small cell lung cancer
		Carcinoid tumors
	Corticotropin-releasing hormone (CRH)	
Acromegaly	Growth hormone–releasing hormone (GHRH)	Carcinoid
		Small cell lung cancer
		Pancreatic islet cell tumors
	Growth hormone (GH)	
Gynecomastia	Human chorionic gonadotropin (hCG)	Testicular cancer
		Lung cancer
		Carcinoid tumors of the lung and gastrointestinal tract
Non–islet cell tumor hypoglycemia	Insulin-like growth factor-2 (IGF-2)	Sarcomas

which ectopic hormone production is recognized varies with the criteria used for diagnosis. The most common syndromes of clinical import are those of ACTH hypersecretion, hypercalcemia, and hypoglycemia. Indeed, ectopic ACTH secretion is responsible for 15–20% of pts with Cushing's syndrome, and ~50% of pts with persistent hypercalcemia have a malignancy rather than hyperparathyroidism. Because of the rapidity of development of hormone secretion in some rapidly growing tumors, diagnosis may require a high index of suspicion, and hormone levels may be elevated out of proportion to the manifestations.

Second, ectopic hormones serve as valuable peripheral markers for neoplasia. Because of the broad spectrum of ectopic hormone secretion, screening measurements of plasma hormone levels for diagnostic purposes are not cost-effective. However, in pts with malignancies that are known to secrete hormones, serial measurements of circulating hormone levels can serve as markers for completeness of tumor excision and for effectiveness of radiation therapy or chemotherapy. Likewise, tumor recurrence may be heralded by reappearance of elevated plasma hormone levels before mass effects of the tumor are evident. However, some tumors at recurrence do not secrete hormones, so that hormone measurements cannot be relied on as the sole evidence of tumor activity.

 TREATMENT

Therapy of ectopic hormone-secreting tumors should be directed when possible toward removal of the tumor. When the tumor cannot be removed or is incurable, specific therapy can be directed toward inhibiting hormone secretion (octreotide for ectopic acromegaly or mitotane to inhibit adrenal steroidogenesis in the ectopic ACTH syndrome) or blocking the action of the hormone at the tissue level (demeclocycline for inappropriate vasopressin secretion).

Hypercalcemia

The most common paraneoplastic syndrome, hypercalcemia of malignancy accounts for 40% of all hypercalcemia. 80% of cancer pts with hypercalcemia have humoral hypercalcemia mediated by parathyroid hormone–related peptide; 20% have local osteolytic hypercalcemia mediated by cytokines such as interleukin 1 and tumor necrosis factor. Many tumor types may produce hypercalcemia (Table 80-1). Pts may have malaise, fatigue, confusion, anorexia, bone pain, polyuria, weakness, constipation, nausea, and vomiting. At high calcium levels, confusion, lethargy, coma, and death may ensue. Median survival of hypercalcemic cancer pts is 1–3 months. Treatment with saline hydration, furosemide diuresis, and pamidronate (60–90 mg IV) or zoledronate (4–8 mg IV) controls calcium levels within 2 days and suppresses calcium release for several weeks. Oral bisphosphonates can be used for chronic treatment.

Hyponatremia

Most commonly discovered in asymptomatic individuals as a result of serum electrolyte measurements, hyponatremia is usually due to tumor secretion of arginine vasopressin and is called *syndrome of inappropriate antidiuretic hormone* (SIADH). Atrial natriuretic hormone may also produce hyponatremia. SIADH occurs most commonly in small cell lung cancer (15%) and head and neck cancer (3%). A number of drugs may produce the syndrome. Symptoms of fatigue, poor attention span, nausea, weakness, anorexia, and headache may be controlled by restricting fluid intake to 500 mL/d or blocking the effects of the hormone with 600–1200 mg demeclocycline a day. With severe hyponatremia (<115 meq/L) or in the setting of mental status changes, normal saline infusion plus furosemide may be required; rate of correction should be <1 meq/L per hour to prevent complications.

Ectopic ACTH Syndrome

When pro-opiomelanocortin mRNA in the tumor is processed into ACTH, excessive secretion of glucocorticoids and mineralocorticoids may ensue. Pts develop Cushing's syndrome with hypokalemic alkalosis, weakness, hypertension, and hyperglycemia. About half the cases occur in small cell lung cancer. ACTH production adversely affects prognosis. Ketoconazole (400–1200 mg/d) or metyrapone (1–4 g/d) may be used to inhibit adrenal steroid synthesis.

For a more detailed discussion, see Jameson JL, Johnson BE: Paraneoplastic Syndromes: Endocrinologic/Hematologic, Chap. 86, p. 566, in HPIM-16.

81

NEUROLOGIC PARANEOPLASTIC SYNDROMES

Paraneoplastic neurologic disorders (PNDs) are remote effects of cancer, caused by mechanisms other than metastasis or by any of the complications of cancer such as coagulopathy, stroke, metabolic and nutritional conditions, infections, and side effects of cancer therapy. In 60% of pts the neurologic symptoms precede the cancer diagnosis. Overall, clinically disabling PNDs occur in 0.5–1% of all cancer pts, but they occur in 2–3% of pts with neuroblastoma or small cell lung cancer (SCLC), and in 30–50% of pts with thymoma or sclerotic myeloma. Recognition of a distinctive paraneoplastic syndrome (Table 81-1) should prompt a search for cancer, although these disorders also occur without cancer. Diagnosis is based upon the clinical pattern, exclusion of other cancer-related disorders, confirmatory serum or CSF antibodies (Table 81-2), or electrodiagnostic testing. Most PNDs are mediated by immune responses directed against common antigenic determinants expressed by tumor and neural cells.

PNDs of the Central Nervous System and Dorsal Root Ganglia

MRI and CSF studies are important to rule out neurologic complications due to the direct spread of cancer. CSF findings typically consist of mild to moderate pleocytosis (<200 mononuclear cells, predominantly lymphocytes), an increase in the protein concentration, intrathecal synthesis of IgG, and a variable presence of oligoclonal bands. A biopsy of affected tissue may be useful to rule out other disorders (e.g., metastasis, infection); neuropathologic findings are not specific for PNDs.

Limbic encephalitis is characterized by confusion, depression, agitation, anxiety, severe short-term memory deficits, partial complex seizures, and demen-

Table 81-1

Paraneoplastic Syndromes of the Nervous System

Syndromes of the brain, brainstem, and cerebellum
  Focal encephalitis
    Cortical encephalitis
    Limbic encephalitis
    Brainstem encephalitis
    Cerebellar dysfunction
    Autonomic dysfunction
  Paraneoplastic cerebellar degeneration
  Opsoclonus-myoclonus
Syndromes of the spinal cord
  Subacute necrotizing myelopathy
  Motor neuron dysfunction
  Myelitis
  Stiff-person syndrome
Syndromes of dorsal root ganglia
  Sensory neuronopathy
Multiple levels of involvement
  Encephalomyelitis[a], sensory neuronopathy, autonomic dysfunction
Syndromes of peripheral nerve
  Chronic and subacute sensorimotor peripheral neuropathy
  Vasculitis of nerve and muscle
  Neuropathy associated with malignant monoclonal gammopathies
  Peripheral nerve hyperexcitability
  Autonomic neuropathy
Syndromes of the neuromuscular junction
  Lambert-Eaton myasthenic syndrome
  Myasthenia gravis
Syndromes of the muscle
  Polymyositis/dermatomyositis
  Acute necrotizing myopathy
Syndromes affecting the visual system
  Cancer-associated retinopathy (CAR)
  Melanoma-associated retinopathy (MAR)
  Uveitis (usually in association with encephalomyelitis)

[a] Includes cortical, limbic, or brainstem encephalitis, cerebellar dysfunction, myelitis.

tia; the MRI usually shows unilateral or bilateral medial temporal lobe abnormalities. *Paraneoplastic cerebellar degeneration* begins as dizziness, oscillopsia, blurry or double vision, nausea, and vomiting; a few days or weeks later, dysarthria, gait and limb ataxia, and variable dysphagia can appear. *Opsoclonus-myoclonus syndrome* consists of involuntary, chaotic eye movements that occur in all directions of gaze; it is frequently associated with myoclonus and ataxia. *Dorsal root ganglionopathy* (sensory neuronopathy) is characterized by sensory deficits that may be symmetric or asymmetric, painful dysesthesias, radicular pain, and decreased or absent reflexes; all modalities of sensation can be involved.

These disorders generally respond poorly to treatment. Stabilization of symptoms or partial neurologic improvement may occasionally occur, particularly if there is a satisfactory response of the tumor to treatment. The roles of plasma exchange, intravenous immunoglobulin (IVIg), and immunosuppression have not been established. Rare pts with limbic encephalitis have shown dra-

Table 81-2

Paraneoplastic Antineuronal Antibodies, Associated Syndromes and Cancers

Antibody	Syndrome	Associated Cancers
Anti-Hu (ANNA-1)	PEM (including cortical, limbic, brainstem encephalitis, cerebellar dysfunction, myelitis), PSN, autonomic dysfunction	SCLC, neuroendocrine tumors
Anti-Yo (PCA-1)	PCD	Ovary and other gynecologic cancers, breast
Anti-Ri (ANNA-2)	PCD, brainstem encephalitis, opsoclonus-myoclonus	Breast, gynecological, SCLC
Anti-Tr	PCD	Hodgkin's lymphoma
Anti-Zic	PCD, encephalomyelitis	SCLC and other neuroendocrine tumors
Anti-CV$_2$/CRMP5	PEM, PCD, chorea, peripheral neuropathy, uveitis	SCLC, thymoma, other
Anti-Ma proteins[a]	Limbic, hypothalamic, brainstem encephalitis (infrequently PCD)	Germ cell tumors of testis, lung cancer, other solid tumors
Anti-amphiphysin	Stiff-person syndrome, PEM	Breast, SCLC
Anti-VGCC[b]	LEMS, PCD	SCLC, lymphoma
Anti-AChR[b]	MG	Thymoma
Anti-VGKC[b]	Peripheral nerve hyperexcitability (neuromyotonia)	Thymoma, SCLC, others
Anti-recoverin	Cancer-associated retinopathy (CAR)	SCLC and other
Anti-bipolar cells of the retina	Melanoma-associated retinopathy (MAR)	Melanoma

[a] Patients with antibodies to Ma2 are usually men with testicular cancer. Patients with additional antibodies to other Ma proteins are men or women with a variety of solid tumors.
[b] These antibodies can occur with or without a cancer association.
Note: PEM: paraneoplastic encephalomyelitis; PCD, paraneoplastic cerebellar degeneration; PSN, paraneoplastic sensory neuronopathy; LEMS, Lambert-Eaton myasthenic syndrome; MG, myasthenia gravis; VGCC, voltage-gated calcium channel; AChR, acetylcholine receptor; VGKC, voltage-gated potassium channel; SCLC, small cell lung cancer.

matic improvement after treatment, but it is not known whether remission of the cancer, glucocorticoids, or IVIg was responsible.

PNDs of Nerve and Muscle

The diagnosis of a specific PND is usually established based upon clinical and electrophysiologic criteria, biopsy results, and by antibody testing. Serum and urine immunofixation studies should be considered in patients with peripheral neuropathy of unknown cause; detection of a monoclonal gammopathy suggests the need for additional studies to uncover a B cell or plasma cell malignancy.

These neuropathies are often masked by concurrent neurotoxicity from chemotherapy and other cancer therapies. Neuropathies that develop in the early stages of cancer often show a rapid progression, sometimes with a relapsing and remitting course, and evidence of inflammatory infiltrates and axonal loss or demyelination in biopsy studies. If demyelinating features predominate, IVIg or glucocorticoids may improve symptoms. Plasma exchange or immunosuppression has been used successfully to treat Lambert-Eaton syndrome; myasthenia gravis is discussed in Chap. 198, and polymyositis/dermatomyositis is discussed in Chap. 199.

For a more detailed discussion, see Dalmau J, Rosenfeld MR: Paraneoplastic Neurologic Syndromes, Chap. 87, p. 571, in HPIM-16.

82

DIAGNOSIS OF INFECTIOUS DISEASES

The laboratory diagnosis of infection requires the demonstration—either direct or indirect—of viral, bacterial, fungal, or parasitic agents in tissues, fluids, or excreta of the host. The traditional detection methods of microscopy and culture are increasingly being complemented by more rapid and sensitive techniques, including serologic and nucleic acid probe assays.

BACTERIA, FUNGI, AND VIRUSES
Microscopy

• Wet mounts: The examination of wet mounts does not require fixation of the specimen before microscopy. Wet mounts are useful for certain large and/or motile organisms; e.g., with dark-field illumination, *Treponema* can be detected in genital lesions or *Leptospira* in blood. Fungal elements may be identified in skin scrapings with 10% KOH wet mount preparations. Some wet mounts use staining to enhance detection—e.g., India ink to visualize encapsulated cryptococci in CSF.

• Stains: Without staining, bacteria are difficult to visualize. *Gram's stain* differentiates between organisms with thick peptidoglycan cell walls (gram-positive) and those with outer membranes that can be dissolved with alcohol or acetone (gram-negative). This stain is particularly useful for sputum samples that have ≥ 25 PMNs and <10 epithelial cells. In normally sterile fluids (e.g., CSF), the detection of bacteria suggests the infectious etiology and correlates with the presence of $>10^4$ bacteria/mL. Sensitivity is increased by centrifugation of the sample. *Acid-fast stains* are useful for organisms that retain carbol fuchsin dye after acid/organic solvation (e.g., *Mycobacterium* spp.). Modification of this procedure permits the detection of weakly acid-fast organisms such as *Nocardia*. *Immunofluorescent stains* (antibody coupled directly or indirectly to a fluorescing compound) can detect viral inclusions (e.g., CMV, HSV) within cultured cells or reveal difficult-to-grow bacteria such as *Legionella*. Many other stains, such as toluidine blue for *Pneumocystis* or methenamine silver for fungal hyphae, are available to assist in the detection of organisms.

Macroscopic Antigen Detection

Latex agglutination assays and enzyme immunoassays (EIAs) are rapid and inexpensive tests that identify bacteria, viruses, or extracellular bacterial toxins by means of their protein or polysaccharide antigens. The assays are performed either directly on clinical specimens or after growth of the organisms in the laboratory.

Culture

The success of efforts to culture a specific pathogen often depends on the use of appropriate collection and transport procedures in conjunction with a laboratory-processing algorithm suitable for the specimen. Instructions for collection are listed in Table 82-1. Bacterial isolation relies on the use of artificial media that support bacterial growth in vitro. Once bacteria are isolated, different methods are used to characterize specific isolates (e.g., phenotyping, gas-liquid chromatography, and nucleic acid probes). Viruses are grown on a monolayer of cultured cells sensitive to infection with the suspected agent. After proliferation

Table 82-1

Instructions for Collection and Transport of Specimens for Culture[*]

Type of Culture (Synonyms)	Specimen	Minimum Volume	Container	Other Considerations
BLOOD				
Blood, routine (blood culture for aerobes, anaerobes, and yeasts)	Whole blood	10 mL in each of 2 bottles for adults and children; 5 mL, if possible, in each of 2 bottles for infants; less for neonates	See below.[a]	See below.[b]
Blood for fungi/*Mycobacterium* spp.	Whole blood	10 mL in each of 2 bottles, as for routine blood cultures, or in Isolator tube requested from laboratory	Same as for routine blood culture	Specify "hold for extended incubation," since fungal agents may require 4 weeks or more to grow.
Blood, Isolator (lysis centrifugation)	Whole blood	10 mL	Isolator tubes	Use mainly for isolation of fungi, *Mycobacterium*, or other fastidious aerobes and for elimination of antibiotics from cultured blood in which organisms are concentrated by centrifugation.

RESPIRATORY TRACT

Nose	Swab from nares	1 swab	Sterile culturette or similar transport system containing holding medium
Throat	Swab of posterior pharynx, ulcerations, or areas of suspected purulence	1 swab	Sterile culturette or similar swab specimen collection system containing holding medium See below.[c]
Sputum	Fresh sputum (not saliva)	2 mL	Commercially available sputum collection system or similar sterile container with screw cap	*Cause for rejection:* Care must be taken to ensure that the specimen is sputum and not saliva. Examination of Gram's stain, with number of epithelial cells and PMNs noted, can be an important part of the evaluation process. Induced sputum specimens should not be rejected.
Bronchial aspirates	Transtracheal aspirate, bronchoscopy specimen, or bronchial aspirate	1 mL of aspirate or brush in transport medium	Sterile aspirate or bronchoscopy tube, bronchoscopy brush in a separate sterile container	Special precautions may be required, depending on diagnostic considerations (e.g., *Pneumocystis*).

STOOL

Stool for routine culture; stool for *Salmonella*, *Shigella*, and *Campylobacter*	Rectal swab or (preferably) fresh, randomly collected stool	1 g of stool or 2 rectal swabs	Plastic-coated cardboard cup or plastic cup with tight-fitting lid. Other leak-proof containers are also acceptable.	If *Vibrio* spp. are suspected, the laboratory must be notified, and appropriate collection/transport methods should be used.
Stool for *Yersinia*, *Escherichia coli* O157	Fresh, randomly collected stool	1 g	Plastic-coated cardboard cup or plastic cup with tight-fitting lid	*Limitations:* Procedure requires enrichment techniques.

(continued)

Table 82-1 (Continued)

Instructions for Collection and Transport of Specimens for Culture[*]

Type of Culture (Synonyms)	Specimen	Minimum Volume	Container	Other Considerations
Stool for *Aeromonas* and *Plesiomonas*	Fresh, randomly collected stool	1 g	Plastic-coated cardboard cup or plastic cup with tight-fitting lid	*Limitations*: Stool should not be cultured for these organisms unless also cultured for other enteric pathogens.
UROGENITAL TRACT				
Urine	Clean-voided urine specimen or urine collected by catheter	0.5 mL	Sterile, leak-proof container with screw cap or special urine transfer tube	See below.[a]
Urogenital secretions	Vaginal or urethral secretions, cervical swabs, uterine fluid, prostatic fluid, etc.	1 swab or 0.5 mL of fluid	Transwab containing Amies transport medium or similar system containing holding medium for *Neisseria gonorrhoeae*; modified Todd-Hewitt broth for group B *Streptococcus* surveillance cultures	Vaginal swab samples for "routine culture" should be discouraged whenever possible unless a particular pathogen is suspected. For detection of multiple organisms (e.g., group B *Streptococcus*, *Trichomonas*, *Chlamydia*, or *Candida* spp.), 1 swab per test should be obtained.
BODY FLUIDS, ASPIRATES, AND TISSUES				
Cerebrospinal fluid (lumbar puncture)	Spinal fluid	1 mL for routine cultures; ≥5 mL for *Mycobacterium*	Sterile tube with tight-fitting cap	Do not refrigerate; transfer to laboratory as soon as possible.

Body fluids	Aseptically aspirated body fluids	Sterile tube with tight-fitting cap. Specimen may be left in syringe used for collection if the syringe is capped before transport.
	1 mL for routine cultures	For some body fluids (e.g., peritoneal lavage samples), increased volumes are helpful for isolation of small numbers of bacteria.
Biopsy and aspirated materials	Tissue removed at surgery, bone, anticoagulated bone marrow, biopsy samples, or other specimens from normally sterile areas	Sterile culturette-type swab or similar transport system containing holding medium. Sterile bottle or jar should be used for tissue specimens.
	1 mL of fluid or a 1-g piece of tissue	Accurate identification of specimen and source is critical. Enough tissue should be collected for both microbiologic and histopathologic evaluations.
Wounds	Purulent material or abscess contents obtained from wound or abscess without contamination by normal microflora	Culturette swab or similar transport system or sterile tube with tight-fitting screw cap. For simultaneous anaerobic cultures, send specimen in anaerobic transport device or closed syringe.
	2 swabs or 0.5 mL of aspirated pus	Collection: Abscess contents or other fluids should be collected in a syringe (see above) when possible to provide an adequate sample volume and an anaerobic environment.

SPECIAL RECOMMENDATIONS

Fungi	Specimen types listed above may be used. When urine or sputum is cultured for fungi, a first morning specimen is usually preferred.	Sterile, leak-proof container with tight-fitting cap
	1 mL or as specified above for individual listing of specimens. Large volumes may be useful for urinary fungi.	Collection: Specimen should be transported to microbiology laboratory within 1 h of collection. Contamination with normal flora from skin, rectum, vaginal tract, or other body surfaces should be avoided.

(continued)

Table 82-1 (*Continued*)

Instructions for Collection and Transport of Specimens for Culture[*]

Type of Culture (Synonyms)	Specimen	Minimum Volume	Container	Other Considerations
Mycobacterium (acid-fast bacilli)	Sputum, tissue, urine, body fluids	10 mL of fluid or small piece of tissue. Swabs should not be used.	Sterile container with tight-fitting cap	Detection of *Mycobacterium* spp. is improved by use of concentration techniques. Smears and cultures of pleural, peritoneal, and pericardial fluids often have low yields. Multiple cultures from the same patient are encouraged. Culturing in liquid media shortens the time to detection.
Legionella	Pleural fluid, lung biopsy, bronchoalveolar lavage fluid, bronchial/transbronchial biopsy. Rapid transport to laboratory is critical.	1 mL of fluid; any size tissue sample, although a 0.5-g sample should be obtained when possible	—	—
Anaerobic organisms	Aspirated specimens from abscesses or body fluids	1 mL of aspirated fluid or 2 swabs	An appropriate anaerobic transport device is required.[*e*]	Specimens cultured for obligate anaerobes should be cultured for facultative bacteria as well.

Viruses[f]	Respiratory secretions, wash aspirates from respiratory tract, nasal swabs, blood samples (including buffy coats), vaginal and rectal swabs, swab specimens from suspicious skin lesions, stool samples (in some cases)	1 mL of fluid, 1 swab, or 1 g of stool in each appropriate transport medium	Fluid or stool samples in sterile containers or swab samples in viral culturette devices (kept on ice but not frozen). Plasma samples and buffy coats in sterile collection tubes should be kept at 4 to 8°C. If specimens are to be shipped or kept for a long time, freezing at −80°C is usually adequate.	Most samples for culture are transported in holding medium containing antibiotics to prevent bacterial overgrowth and viral inactivation. Many specimens should be kept cool but not frozen, provided they are transported promptly to the laboratory. Procedures and transport media vary with the agent to be cultured and the duration of transport.

* *Note:* It is absolutely essential that the microbiology laboratory be informed of the site of origin of the sample to be cultured and of the infections that are suspected. This information determines the selection of culture media and the length of culture time.

[a] For samples from adults and children, two bottles (smaller for pediatric samples) should be used; one with dextrose phosphate, tryptic soy, or another appropriate broth and the other with thioglycollate or another broth containing reducing agents appropriate for isolation of obligate anaerobes. For special situations (e.g., suspected fungal infection, culture-negative endocarditis, or mycobacteremia), different blood collection systems may be used (Isolator systems).

[b] *Collection:* An appropriate disinfecting technique should be used on both the bottle septum and the pt. Do not allow air bubbles to get into anaerobic broth bottles. *Special considerations:* There is no more important clinical microbiology test than the detection of blood-borne pathogens. The rapid identification of bacterial and fungal agents is a major determinant of pts' survival. Bacteria may be present in blood either continuously (as in endocarditis, overwhelming sepsis, and the early stages of salmonellosis and brucellosis) or intermittently (as in most other bacterial infections, in which bacteria are shed into the blood on a sporadic basis). Most blood culture systems employ two separate bottles containing broth medium: one that is vented for the growth of facultative and aerobic organisms and a second that is maintained under anaerobic conditions. In cases of suspected continuous bacteremia/fungemia, two or three samples should be drawn before the start of therapy, with additional sets obtained if fastidious organisms are thought to be involved. For intermittent bacteremia, two or three samples should be obtained at least 1 h apart during the first 24 h.

[c] Normal microflora includes α-hemolytic streptococci, saprophytic *Neisseria* spp., diphtheroids, and *Staphylococcus* spp. Aerobic culture of the throat ("routine") includes screening for and identification of β-hemolytic *Streptococcus* spp. and other potentially pathogenic organisms. Although considered components of the normal microflora, organisms such as *Staphylococcus aureus*, *Haemophilus influenzae*, and *Streptococcus pneumoniae* will be identified by most laboratories, if requested. When *Neisseria gonorrhoeae* or *Corynebacterium diphtheriae* is suspected, a special culture request is recommended.

[d] (1) Clean-voided specimens, midvoid specimens, and Foley or indwelling catheter specimens that yield ≥50,000 organisms/mL and from which no more than three species are isolated should have organisms identified. (2) Straight-catheterized, bladder-tap, and similar urine specimens should undergo a complete workup (identification and susceptibility testing) for all potentially pathogenic organisms, regardless of colony count. (3) Certain clinical problems (e.g., acute dysuria in women) may warrant identification and susceptibility testing of isolates present at concentrations of <50,000 organisms/mL.

[e] Aspirated specimens in capped syringes or other transport devices designed to limit oxygen exposure are suitable for the cultivation of obligate anaerobes. A variety of commercially available transport devices may be used. Contamination of specimens with normal microflora from the skin, rectum, vaginal vault, or another body site should be avoided. Collection containers for aerobic culture (such as dry swabs) and inappropriate specimens (such as refrigerated samples; expectorated sputum; stool; gastric aspirates; and vaginal, throat, nose, and rectal swabs) should be rejected as unsuitable.

[f] Laboratories generally use diverse methods to detect viral agents, and the specific requirements for each specimen should be checked before a sample is sent.

of viral particles, cells are examined for cytopathic effects or immunofluorescent studies are performed to detect viral antigens.

Serology

The measurement of serum antibody provides an indirect marker for past or current infection with a specific viral agent or other pathogen. Quantitative assays detect increases in antibody titers, most often using paired serum samples obtained 10–14 days apart (i.e., acute- and convalescent-phase samples). Serology can also be used to document protective levels of antibody, particularly in diseases for which vaccines are available (e.g., rubella, varicella-zoster virus infections). Detection systems include agglutination reactions, immunofluorescence, EIAs, hemagglutination inhibition, and complement fixation.

Nucleic Acid Probes

Techniques for the detection and quantitation of specific DNA and RNA base sequences in clinical specimens have become powerful tools for the diagnosis of infection.

• Probes are available for directly detecting various pathogens (e.g., *Legionella pneumophila*, *Chlamydia trachomatis*, *Neisseria gonorrhoeae*) in clinical specimens and for confirming the identity of cultured pathogens (e.g., *Mycobacterium* and *Salmonella* spp.). These probes are often directed against highly conserved 16S ribosomal RNA sequences that have higher copy numbers than any single DNA sequence would. The sensitivity and specificity of probe assays for direct detection are comparable to those of more traditional assays, including EIA and culture.
• Amplification strategies (e.g., PCR, ligase chain reaction) enhance the sensitivity of RNA or DNA assays, but false-positive findings can result from even low levels of contamination.

Susceptibility Testing

Susceptibility testing allows the clinician to choose the optimal antimicrobial agents and to identify potential infection-control problems (e.g., the level of methicillin-resistant *Staphylococcus aureus* in a hospital). Susceptibility testing for fungi has only recently been standardized; several systems have now been approved.

PARASITES

Table 82-2 summarizes the diagnosis of some common parasitic infections. The cornerstone for the diagnosis of parasitic diseases, as for that of many other infections, is the elicitation of a thorough history of the illness and of epidemiologic factors such as travel, recreational activities, and occupation.

Intestinal Parasites

Most helminths and protozoa exit the body in the fecal stream. Feces should be collected in a clean cardboard container, with the time of collection recorded. Contamination with urine or water should be avoided. Fecal samples should be collected before the ingestion of barium or other contrast agents and before treatment with antidiarrheal agents; these substances alter fecal consistency and interfere with microscopic detection of parasites. The collection of three samples on alternate days is recommended because of the cyclic shedding of most parasites in the feces. Macroscopic examination involves a search for adult worms or tapeworm segments. Microscopic examination is not complete until direct wet mounts have been evaluated and concentration techniques as well as per-

Table 82-2

Diagnosis of Some Common Parasitic Infections

Parasite	Geographic Distribution	Parasite Stage	Body Fluid or Tissue	Serologic Tests	Other Tests/Comments
				Diagnosis	
Blood flukes					
Schistosoma mansoni	Africa, Central and South America, West Indies	Ova, adults	Feces	EIA, WB	Rectal snips, liver biopsy
S. haematobium	Africa	Ova, adults	Urine	WB	Liver, urine, or bladder biopsy
S. japonicum	Far East	Ova, adults	Feces	WB	Liver biopsy
Intestinal roundworms					
Strongyloides stercoralis (strongyloidiasis)	Moist tropics and subtropics	Larvae	Feces, sputum, duodenal fluid	EIA	Dissemination in immunodeficiency
Intestinal protozoans					
Entamoeba histolytica (amebiasis)	Worldwide, especially tropics	Troph, cyst	Feces, liver	EIA, ID, antigen detection	Ultrasound, liver CT, PCR
Giardia lamblia (giardiasis)	Worldwide	Troph, cyst	Feces	Antigen detection	String test
Isospora belli	Worldwide	Oocyst	Feces	—	Acid-fast
Cryptosporidium	Worldwide	Oocyst	Feces	Antigen detection	Acid-fast, biopsy, PCR
Blood and tissue protozoans					
Plasmodium spp. (malaria)	Subtropics and tropics	Asexual	Blood	Limited use	PCR
Babesia microti (babesiosis)	U.S., especially New England	Asexual	Blood	IIF	PCR
Toxoplasma gondii (toxoplasmosis)	Worldwide	Cyst, troph	CNS, eye, muscles, other	EIA, IIF	PCR/reactivation in immunosuppression

Note: WB, western blot; CT, computed tomography; CNS, central nervous system; EIA, enzyme immunoassay; ID, immunodiffusion by commercial kit; troph, trophozoite; IIF, indirect immunofluorescence; PCR, polymerase chain reaction. Serologic tests listed are available from the Centers for Disease Control and Prevention, Atlanta, GA.
Source: Adapted from Davis CE: HPIM-16, p. 1197.

manent stains applied. Sampling of duodenal contents may be needed to detect *Giardia lamblia*, *Cryptosporidium*, and *Strongyloides* larvae. "Scotch tape" methods may be needed to detect pinworm ova or *Taenia saginata*.

Blood and Tissue Parasites

Invasion of tissue by parasites may direct the evaluation of other samples; e.g., examination of urine sediment is the appropriate way to detect *Schistosoma haematobium*. The laboratory procedures for detection of parasites in other body fluids are similar to those used in the examination of feces. Wet mounts, concentration techniques, and permanent stains should all be used. The parasites most commonly detected in Giemsa-stained blood smears are the plasmodia, microfilariae, and African trypanosomes; however, wet mounts may be more sensitive for microfilariae and African trypanosomes because these active parasites cause movement of erythrocytes in microscopic fields. The timing of blood collection is crucial; e.g., the nocturnal periodicity of *Wuchereria bancrofti* correlates with diagnostic yields only when blood is drawn near midnight.

Antibody and Antigen Detection

In addition to direct detection techniques, antibody assays for many of the important tissue parasites are available, as are antigen detection techniques that make use of ELISA, fluorescent antibody assay, or PCR. Although a promising diagnostic tool, PCR is commercially available for only a limited number of parasites.

For a more detailed discussion, see Onderdonk AB: Laboratory Diagnosis of Infectious Diseases, Chap. 105A, *Harrison's Online*; and Davis CE: Laboratory Diagnosis of Parasitic Infections, Chap. 192, p. 1197, in HPIM-16.

83

ANTIBACTERIAL THERAPY

The development of vaccines and drugs that prevent and cure bacterial infections was one of the twentieth century's major contributions to human longevity and quality of life. Antibacterial agents are among the most commonly prescribed drugs worldwide.

PRINCIPLES OF ANTIBACTERIAL CHEMOTHERAPY

- When possible, obtain specimens to identify the etiologic agent prior to treatment.
- Be aware of local susceptibility patterns to help direct empirical treatment.
- Once etiology and susceptibility are known, change the therapeutic regimen to one that has the narrowest effective spectrum and (if possible) is least costly.

- Choose a therapeutic agent on the basis of pharmacokinetic data, adverse reaction profile, site of infection, immune status of the host, and evidence of efficacy in scientific trials.
- Check for dose adjustments in pts with renal or hepatic insufficiency.
- Check for drug interactions and contraindications before prescribing antibiotics.

MECHANISMS OF DRUG ACTION
Antibacterial agents act on unique targets not found in mammalian cells.

- Inhibition of cell-wall synthesis: Drugs that inhibit cell-wall synthesis are almost always bactericidal. Bacterial autolysins (cell-wall recycling enzymes) contribute to cell lysis in the presence of these agents.
- Inhibition of protein synthesis: Typically inhibition takes place through interaction with bacterial ribosomes. Except for aminoglycosides, these drugs are bacteriostatic.
- Inhibition of bacterial metabolism: Drugs interfere with bacterial folic acid synthesis.
- Inhibition of nucleic acid synthesis or activity
- Alteration of cell-membrane permeability

MECHANISMS OF ANTIBACTERIAL RESISTANCE
Bacteria can either be intrinsically resistant to an agent (e.g., anaerobic bacteria are resistant to aminoglycosides) or acquire resistance through mutation of resident genes or acquisition of new genes. The major mechanisms of resistance used by bacteria are drug inactivation, alteration or overproduction of the antibacterial target, acquisition of a new drug-insensitive target, decreased permeability to the agent, and active efflux of the agent.

SPECIFIC CLASSES OF ANTIBACTERIAL AGENTS
β-Lactam Drugs
MECHANISM   Inhibit cell-wall synthesis

ADVERSE REACTIONS

1. Allergy: anaphylaxis, drug fever, serum sickness, maculopapular eruptions, nephritis, hemolytic anemia, leukopenia, Stevens-Johnson syndrome; low-level cross-allergy between penicillins and cephalosporins; no cross-allergy between monobactams and other β-lactams
2. Miscellaneous reactions
   a. GI side effects (e.g., diarrhea, colitis, hepatitis)
   b. Ceftriaxone: sludging in the gallbladder, occasionally cholecystitis
   c. Impaired platelet aggregation (e.g., antipseudomonal penicillins)
   d. Seizures: response to especially high doses in pts with renal impairment

SPECTRUM OF ACTIVITY   *Penicillins*

- Penicillin: streptococci, enterococci, *Neisseria*, fastidious oral bacteria, *Actinomyces*, *Listeria*, spirochetes, *Clostridium* spp. except *C. difficile*, *Pasteurella*
- Ampicillin: extension of penicillin spectrum to more gram-negative organisms (e.g., susceptible strains of *Escherichia coli*, *Proteus mirabilis*, *Salmonella*, *Shigella*, *Haemophilus influenzae*); better coverage of *Listeria* and *Enterococcus* than is provided by penicillin
- Penicillinase-resistant penicillins (e.g., oxacillin): staphylococci, streptococci
- Antipseudomonal penicillins (e.g., piperacillin): ampicillin spectrum plus anaerobes, *Pseudomonas aeruginosa*, nonenteric gram-negative bacilli (e.g.,

Enterobacter, Serratia). Addition of β-lactamase inhibitors extends gram-negative, anaerobic, and *Staphylococcus aureus* spectrum, but gram-negative bacteria that produce chromosomal β-lactamases remain resistant.

Cephalosporins   No coverage of *Listeria* or *Enterococcus* or of methicillin-resistant *S. aureus* (MRSA), *Acinetobacter*, or *Stenotrophomonas*

1. First-generation (e.g., cefazolin): *S. aureus*, streptococci, *E. coli*, *P. mirabilis*, *Klebsiella pneumoniae*
2. Second-generation
   a. Cefuroxime: extends cefazolin spectrum plus *H. influenzae*, *Neisseria*
   b. Cefotetan, cefoxitin: good activity against gram-negative bacteria and *Bacteroides fragilis*, poor activity against gram-positive bacteria and *H. influenzae*
3. Third-generation: expanded gram-negative activity, poor anaerobic activity
   a. Ceftazidime: poor gram-positive activity, good *P. aeruginosa* activity
   b. Ceftriaxone: excellent activity against streptococci, *H. influenzae*, and *Neisseria*; not active against *P. aeruginosa*
   c. Cefepime: more stable to chromosomal β-lactamases of *Enterobacter* and *Serratia*; better *S. aureus* coverage than other third-generation drugs

Carbapenems

Imipenem, meropenem: broad coverage against most pathogens except *Stenotrophomonas*, methicillin-resistant staphylococci, and *Enterococcus faecium*; nosocomial *P. aeruginosa* isolates ~20% resistant
Ertapenem: Poor activity against enterococci, *P. aeruginosa*, and *Acinetobacter*; otherwise, similar spectrum to other carbapenems

Monobactams   Aztreonam, the only available monobactam, is active against aerobic gram-negative organisms.

Vancomycin

MECHANISM   Inhibits cell-wall synthesis

SPECTRUM OF ACTIVITY   Gram-positive cocci

ADVERSE REACTIONS   Red man syndrome (pruritus, flushing, erythema of head and upper torso; can be reduced by slower infusion or lower dose); phlebitis; nephrotoxicity (mild, uncommon); ototoxicity, leukopenia, skin rashes, true allergy (all rare)

Aminoglycosides

MECHANISM   Inhibit protein synthesis

SPECTRUM OF ACTIVITY   Aerobic gram-negative bacteria, staphylococci, *Mycobacterium tuberculosis*; synergistic with penicillins against enterococci, staphylococci, and viridans streptococci

ADVERSE REACTIONS   These drugs have a narrow therapeutic index.

- Nephrotoxicity: Proximal tubule damage, usually reversible, may be reduced by once-daily administration.
- Ototoxicity: auditory or vestibular damage, sometimes irreversible
- Neuromuscular depression: rare respiratory depression

Macrolides/ Ketolides

MECHANISM   Inhibit protein synthesis

SPECTRUM OF ACTIVITY Gram-positive bacteria, *Legionella*, *Mycoplasma*, *Campylobacter*, *Bordetella pertussis*, *Chlamydia*. Newer macrolides: *H. influenzae*, mycobacteria

ADVERSE REACTIONS Serious reactions are rare. GI side effects such as substernal burning, nausea, and vomiting are common. Hepatotoxicity, ototoxicity, and prolonged QT_c interval are less common and are usually mild and reversible.

Lincosamides (Clindamycin)

MECHANISM Inhibit protein synthesis

SPECTRUM OF ACTIVITY Anaerobes, gram-positive organisms; gram-positive spectrum similar to that of macrolides, but more active against susceptible staphylococci; drug of choice for toxigenic invasive group A streptococcal infections

ADVERSE REACTIONS GI distress, diarrhea. *C. difficile* colitis, although caused by most antibacterial agents, occurs most often with clindamycin (Chap. 87).

Chloramphenicol

MECHANISM Inhibits protein synthesis

SPECTRUM OF ACTIVITY Broad gram-positive and gram-negative spectrum, but rising rates of resistance

ADVERSE REACTIONS Bone marrow suppression (dose-related reversible pancytopenia or idiosyncratic, irreversible aplastic anemia); "gray syndrome" in premature newborns (neonatal inability to metabolize drug leading to cyanosis, hypotension, and death). Chloramphenicol is rarely used because more effective, safer alternatives are available.

Tetracyclines

Doxycycline is the tetracycline of choice in most instances.

MECHANISM Inhibit protein synthesis

SPECTRUM OF ACTIVITY Broad bacteriostatic activity against gram-positive and gram-negative organisms, including *Brucella* and *Francisella tularensis*; also spirochetes, *Chlamydia*, actinomycetes, *Rickettsia*, and *Mycobacterium marinum*

ADVERSE REACTIONS

- GI effects: nausea, erosive esophagitis. Food intake may improve tolerance, but absorption is impaired if these drugs are taken with food.
- Hepatotoxicity: occurs at high doses or during pregnancy
- Mottling of permanent teeth in children <8 years of age; contraindication to drugs' use
- Miscellaneous: phototoxic skin reactions, vertigo (most common among women given minocycline as meningococcal prophylaxis)

Sulfonamides and Trimethoprim

MECHANISM Inhibit folic acid synthesis

SPECTRUM OF ACTIVITY

- Broad activity against gram-positive and gram-negative organisms, including *H. influenzae* and *Moraxella catarrhalis*

• The combination trimethoprim-sulfamethoxazole (TMP-SMX) can be bactericidal against facultative gram-negative bacteria and staphylococci.
• TMP-SMX is active against causes of nosocomial infections (e.g., *Aeromonas*, *Stenotrophomonas*, *Burkholderia cepacia*, and *Acinetobacter*) and against *Nocardia*, *Mycobacterium leprae*, *Toxoplasma*, and *Pneumocystis*.

ADVERSE REACTIONS

• Allergic reactions: rash, erythema multiforme, Stevens-Johnson syndrome
• Hematologic reactions: agranulocytosis, hemolytic anemia (especially with G6PD deficiency), megaloblastic anemia, thrombocytopenia
• Renal insufficiency: crystalluria of drug metabolite
• Jaundice and kernicterus in newborns

Fluoroquinolones

MECHANISM Inhibit DNA gyrase and topoisomerase IV

SPECTRUM OF ACTIVITY Facultative gram-negative rods; best oral agents for *P. aeruginosa* (ciprofloxacin); variable gram-positive activity (e.g., ciprofloxacin has poor activity, while levofloxacin has good pneumococcal activity); active against mycobacteria

ADVERSE REACTIONS

• Nausea or diarrhea, insomnia, dizziness, phototoxicity, tendon rupture
• Not recommended for pts <18 years of age because of concern about cartilage damage in developing joints (based on data in animals)
• Contraindicated in pregnancy
• Can increase QT_c interval
• Hepatic, renal dysfunction

Rifampin

MECHANISM Inhibits nucleic acid synthesis

SPECTRUM OF ACTIVITY *Legionella*; prophylaxis against meningococcal disease; mycobacteria; used as synergistic agent for treatment of gram-positive infections

ADVERSE REACTIONS

• Increases serum levels of hepatic aminotransferases
• Turns secretions such as urine and tears orange
• Intermittent administration can be associated with flulike symptoms, hemolysis, thrombocytopenia, shock, and renal failure.

Metronidazole

MECHANISM Nitro group is reduced to reactive intermediate that causes DNA damage in bacteria. The unique redox of anaerobic bacteria is required for activity.

SPECTRUM OF ACTIVITY Anaerobic bacteria, particularly gram-negative anaerobes

ADVERSE REACTIONS

• Nausea, metallic taste, stomatitis, glossitis, peripheral neuropathy, seizures, encephalopathy in pts with hepatic failure, disulfiram-like reactions
• Possible mutagenicity, carcinogenicity. Use in pregnancy should be avoided.

Linezolid

MECHANISM Inhibits protein synthesis

SPECTRUM OF ACTIVITY Gram-positive bacteria, including vancomycin-resistant staphylococci and enterococci (including *E. faecalis*)

ADVERSE REACTIONS Nausea, vomiting, diarrhea, headache, reversible myelosuppression

Streptogramins

MECHANISM Inhibit protein synthesis

SPECTRUM OF ACTIVITY Gram-positive bacteria, including vancomycin-resistant staphylococci and *E. faecium* (not active against *E. faecalis*)

ADVERSE REACTIONS Poorly tolerated; venous irritation, arthralgias, myalgias, rash, increased bilirubin levels, GI distress

Nitrofurantoin

MECHANISM Urinary tract antiseptic, inhibits nucleic acid synthesis

SPECTRUM OF ACTIVITY Gram-negative enteric bacteria in UTIs; also active against enterococci, including those resistant to vancomycin

Mupirocin

MECHANISM Topical agent, inhibits protein synthesis

SPECTRUM OF ACTIVITY Active against staphylococci, streptococci; eradicates nasal carriage of *S. aureus*, including MRSA

For a more detailed discussion, see Archer GL, Polk RE: Treatment and Prophylaxis of Bacterial Infections, Chap. 118, p. 789, in HPIM-16. For discussion of antifungal therapy, see Chap. 113 in this manual; for antimycobacterial therapy, see Chap. 102; for antiviral therapy, see Chaps. 107 through 112; and for antiparasitic therapy, see Chaps. 115 and 116.

84

IMMUNIZATION AND ADVICE TO TRAVELERS

IMMUNIZATION

Vaccination is one of the greatest public health achievements of the twentieth century and one of the few cost-saving interventions to prevent infectious diseases.

Definitions

- Active immunization: administration of antigens to induce immune defenses
- Passive immunization: provision of temporary protection by the administration of exogenously produced immune substances
- Immunizing agents

1. Vaccine: a preparation of attenuated live or killed microorganisms or antigenic portions of those agents used to induce immunity and prevent disease
2. Toxoid: a modified bacterial toxin that has been rendered nontoxic but retains the capacity to stimulate the formation of antitoxin
3. Immune globulin: an antibody-containing protein fraction derived from human plasma that is used for maintaining immunity in immunodeficient persons or for passive immunization when active immunization is not possible
4. Antitoxin: an antibody derived from the serum of animals after stimulation with specific antigens that is used to provide passive immunity to the toxin protein to which it is directed

Vaccines for Routine Use

For the recommended immunization schedule for childhood and adolescence, see Fig. 84-1; for adults, see Fig. 84-2; and for adults with certain medical conditions, see Fig. 84-3.

ADVICE FOR TRAVELERS

Travelers should be aware of various health risks that might be associated with given destinations. Information regarding country-specific risks can be obtained from the CDC publication *Health Information for International Travel*, which is available at www.cdc.gov/travel.

Immunizations for Travel

There are three categories of immunization for travel.

- *Routine* immunizations (see Figs. 84-1, -2, and -3) are needed regardless of travel. However, travelers should be certain that their routine immunizations are up-to-date because certain diseases (e.g., diphtheria, tetanus, polio, measles) are more likely to be acquired outside the United States than at home.
- *Required* immunizations are mandated by international regulations for entry into certain areas. *Recommended* immunizations are advisable because they protect against illnesses for whose acquisition the traveler is at increased risk. Table 84-1 lists vaccines required or recommended for travel to different destinations.

Prevention of Malaria and Other Insect-Borne Diseases

Chemoprophylaxis against malaria and other measures may be recommended for travel. In the United States, 90% of cases of *Plasmodium falciparum* infection occur in persons returning or immigrating from Africa and Oceania. The destination helps determine the particular medication chosen (e.g., whether chloroquine-resistant *P. falciparum* is present), as does the traveler's preference and medical history. In addition, personal protective measures against mosquito bites, especially between dusk and dawn (e.g., the use of DEET-containing insect repellents, permethrin-impregnated bed-nets, and screened sleeping areas), can prevent malaria and other insect-borne disease (e.g., dengue fever).

Prevention of Gastrointestinal Illness

Diarrhea is the leading cause of illness in travelers. The incidence is highest in parts of Africa, Central and South America, and Southeast Asia. Travelers should eat only well-cooked hot foods, peeled or cooked fruits and vegetables, and bottled or boiled liquids. Although self-limited, diarrheal illness alters travel plans and confines 20% of pts to bed. Travelers should carry medications for self-treatment. Mild to moderate diarrhea can be treated with loperamide and

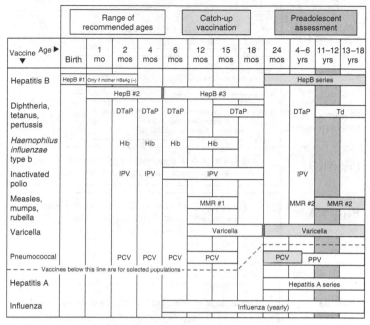

FIGURE 84-1 Recommended childhood and adolescent immunization schedule—United States, 2003. Any dose not given at the recommended age should be given at any subsequent time when indicated and feasible. Red bars indicate age groups that warrant special efforts to administer those vaccines not previously given. Infants born to mothers positive for hepatitis B surface antigen (HBsAg) should receive hepatitis B vaccine (HepB) and 0.5 mL of hepatitis B immune globulin (HBIG) at separate sites within 12 h of birth. The second dose of HepB is recommended at at age 1 to 2 months. The last dose in the series should not be administered before age 6 months. Infants born to mothers whose HBsAg status is unknown should receive the first dose of the HepB series within 12 h of birth. The mother's HBsAg status should be tested as soon as possible; if positive, the infant should receive HBIG as soon as possible. The number of *Haemophilus influenzae* type b (Hib) conjugate vaccine doses depends on the vaccine used. PRP-OMP (PedvaxHIB or ComVax) is administered just twice: at ages 2 and 4 months. Diphtheria/tetanus/acellular pertussis (DtaP)/Hib combination products should not be used for primary immunization but can be used as boosters following a primary series with any Hib vaccine. Influenza vaccine is now recommended annually for children age ≥6 months with certain risk factors (including but not limited to asthma, cardiac disease, sickle cell disease, HIV infection, and diabetes mellitus) and household members of persons in groups at high risk; it can be administered to all others wishing to obtain immunity. If feasible, influenza vaccination of healthy children age 6 to 23 months is encouraged because of a substantially increased risk for influenza-related hospitalizations in this group. Children ≥12 years old should receive influenza vaccine in a dosage appropriate for their age. Children ≤8 years old who are receiving influenza vaccine for the first time should receive two doses separated by at least 4 weeks. Hepatitis A vaccine is recommended for children and adolescents in selected states and regions and for certain high-risk groups; hepatitis A immunization can begin during any visit, and the two doses should be administered at least 6 months apart. The heptavalent pneumococcal conjugate vaccine (PCV) is recommended for all children age 2 to 23 months. It is also recommended for certain children age 24 to 59 months. Pneumococcal polysaccharide vaccine (PPV) is recommended in addition to the conjugate vaccine for certain high-risk groups. Further information can be obtained via the National Immunization Program website (www.cdc.gov/nip) or at the National Immunization Information Hotline (800-232-2522 for English and 800-232-0233 for Spanish). MMR, measles/mumps/rubella vaccine; IPV, inactivated poliovirus vaccine; Td, tetanus and diphtheria toxoids, adsorbed, for adult use. (*Adapted from recommendations approved by the Advisory Committee on Immunization Practices, the American Academy of Pediatrics, and the American College of Family Physicians.*)

Vaccine ▼ / Age ▶	19–49 Years	50–64 Years	65 Years and Older
Tetanus, diphtheria (Td)	1 dose booster every 10 years[1]		
Influenza	1 dose annually for persons with medical or occupational indications, or household contacts of persons with indications[2]	1 annual dose	
Pneumococcal (polysaccharide)	1 dose for persons with medical or other indications (1 dose revaccination for immunosuppressive conditions)[3,4]		1 dose for unvaccinated persons[3] / 1 dose revaccination[4]
Hepatitis B	3 doses (0, 1–2, 4–6 months) for persons with medical, behavioral, occupational, or other indications[5]		
Hepatitis A	2 doses (0, 6–12 months) for persons with medical, behavioral, occupational, or other indications[6]		
Measles, mumps, rubella (MMR)	1 dose if measles, mumps, or rubella vaccination history is unreliable; 2 doses for persons with occupational or other indications[7]		
Varicella	2 doses (0, 4–8 weeks) for persons who are susceptible[8]		
Meningococcal (polysaccharide)	1 dose for persons with medical or other indications[9]		

☐ For all persons in this group   ☐ Catch-up on childhood vaccinations   ☐ For persons with medical/ exposure indications

FIGURE 84-2 Recommended adult immunization schedule—United States, 2002–2003. (1) *Tetanus and diphtheria (Td)*: A primary series for adults is 3 doses, with the first 2 doses at least 4 weeks apart and the third dose 6 to 12 months after the second. One dose suffices if a primary series was completed >10 years before. In addition to a teenage/young adult booster, adults >50 years of age who have completed the full series plus booster should receive one more dose. (2) *Influenza vaccination*: Indications include chronic cardiovascular or pulmonary disease, asthma, diabetes, renal disease, hemoglobinopathy, immunosuppression (due to medications or HIV infection), pregnancy (second or third trimester during the influenza season), health care employment, residence in a nursing home or another long-term-care facility, and high likelihood of transmitting influenza to those at high risk. (3) *Pneumococcal polysaccharide vaccination*: Indications include chronic cardiovascular or pulmonary disease (except asthma), diabetes, chronic liver disease, chronic renal failure or nephrotic syndrome, asplenia, immunosuppression, certain cancer chemotherapy, and long-term systemic glucocorticoid therapy. Vaccination is also indicated in Alaskan natives, certain Native American populations, and residents of nursing homes and other long-term-care facilities. (4) *Revaccination with pneumococcal polysaccharide vaccine*: One-time revaccination after age 5 is indicated for persons with chronic renal failure or nephrotic syndrome, asplenia, immunosuppression, certain cancer chemotherapy, or long-term systemic glucocorticoid therapy. Persons >65 years old should undergo one-time revaccination if their prior vaccination was at least 5 years before and was given before age 65. (5) *Hepatitis B vaccination*: Vaccination is indicated for hemodialysis patients, patients receiving clotting factor concentrates, health care workers and public safety workers exposed to blood, students in the health professions, injection drug users, persons with multiple sex partners within 6 months, patients with recent sexually transmitted disease (STD), clients of STD clinics, men who have

(continued)

fluids. Moderate to severe diarrhea should be treated with a 3-day course or a single double dose of a fluoroquinolone. High rates of quinolone-resistant *Campylobacter* in Thailand make azithromycin a better choice for that country. Prophylaxis with bismuth subsalicylate is ~60% effective, and a single daily dose of a quinolone is very effective for travel of <1 month's duration; however, preventive treatment usually is not recommended.

Other Infections

Travelers are at high risk for (1) sexually transmitted diseases preventable by condom use; (2) schistosomiasis preventable by avoidance of swimming or bathing in freshwater lakes, streams, or rivers in endemic areas; and (3) hookworm and *Strongyloides* infections preventable by the avoidance of barefoot walking outside.

Travel during Pregnancy

The safest part of pregnancy in which to travel is between 18 and 24 weeks. Relative contraindications to international travel during pregnancy include a history of miscarriage, premature labor, incompetent cervix, or toxemia or the presence of other general medical problems (e.g., diabetes). Areas of excessive risk (e.g., where live virus vaccines are required for travel or where multidrug-resistant malaria is endemic) should be avoided throughout pregnancy.

The HIV-Infected Traveler

HIV-seropositive persons with CD4+ T cell counts that are normal or >500/ μL do not appear to be at increased risk during travel. However, persons with depressed CD4+ cell counts should seek counseling from a travel medicine practitioner before departure, particularly when traveling to the developing

---

sex with men, household contacts and sex partners of persons with chronic hepatitis B virus infection, clients and staff of institutions for the mentally disabled, inmates of correctional institutions, and international travelers to countries with high prevalence. (6) *Hepatitis A vaccination*: For the combined HepA/HepB vaccine, use 3 doses at 0, 1, and 6 months. Hepatitis A vaccination is indicated in persons with clotting factor disorders or chronic liver disease, men who have sex with men, users of injection and noninjection illegal drugs, persons working with hepatitis A virus–infected primates or working with the virus in a laboratory, and persons traveling to or working in countries with high prevalence. (7) *Measles/mumps/rubella vaccination (MMR): Measles component*: Adults born before 1957 are considered immune to measles. Adults born after 1957 should have at least 1 dose of MMR vaccine barring a medical contraindication or documentation of prior immunization. A second dose is recommended for adults who have recently been exposed to measles in an outbreak setting, who have previously received killed measles vaccine, who were vaccinated with an unknown measles vaccine between 1963 and 1967, who are students at a college or university, who work in health care facilities, or who plan to travel internationally. *Mumps component*: 1 dose of MMR vaccine is adequate. *Rubella component*: 1 dose of MMR vaccine should be given to women whose history is unreliable, with counseling to avoid becoming pregnant for 4 weeks. The rubella immune status of women of childbearing age should be ascertained and counseling provided regarding congenital rubella. (8) *Varicella vaccination*: Vaccination is recommended for all persons without a reliable clinical history of varicella or serologic evidence of immunity, health care workers, family contacts of immunosuppressed persons, those who live or work in high-risk settings (teachers of young children, daycare workers, residents and staff members working in institutional settings), adolescents and adults living in households with children, and women who are not pregnant but intend to become pregnant in the future. (9) *Meningococcal vaccine, quadrivalent*: Vaccination should be considered for adults with terminal complement component deficiencies, those with anatomical or functional asplenia, college freshmen (especially those living in dormitories), and travelers to the "meningitis belt" in sub-Saharan Africa or to Mecca for the Hajj. High-risk persons can be revaccinated in 5 years. (*Adapted from recommendations approved by the Advisory Committee on Immunization Practices and accepted by the American College of Obstetricians and Gynecologists and the American Academy of Family Physicians.*)

Medical conditions ▼ / Vaccine ▶	Tetanus-Diphtheria (Td)	Influenza	Pneumo-coccal (Poly-saccharide)	Hepatitis B	Hepatitis A	Measles, Mumps, Rubella (MMR)	Varicella
Pregnancy		A					
Diabetes, heart disease, chronic pulmonary disease, chronic liver disease, including chronic alcoholism		B	C		D		
Congenital immunodeficiency, leukemia, lymphoma, generalized malignancy, therapy with alkylating agents, antimetabolites, radiation or large amounts of glucocorticoids		E					F
Renal failure/end stage renal disease, recipients of hemodialysis or clotting factor concentrates		E	G				
Asplenia (including elective splenectomy) and terminal complement component deficiencies		E, H, I					
HIV infection		E, J				K	

☐ For all persons in this group   ☐ Catch-up on childhood vaccinations   ▨ For persons with medical/ exposure indications   ■ Contraindicated

FIGURE 84-3 Recommended immunizations for adults with medical conditions—United States, 2002–2003. **A.** Vaccine may be given if pregnancy is at second or third trimester during influenza season. **B.** Although chronic liver disease and alcoholism are not indicator conditions for influenza vaccination, give 1 dose annually if the patient is ≥50 years old, has other indications for influenza vaccine, or requests vaccination. **C.** Asthma is an indicator condition for influenza vaccination but not for pneumococcal vaccination. **D.** Vaccinate all persons with chronic liver disease. **E.** Revaccinate once after ≥5 years have elapsed since initial vaccination. **F.** Persons with impaired humoral (but not cellular) immunity may be vaccinated [*MMWR* 1999; 48 (RR-06), 1–5]. **G.** *Hemodialysis patients*: Use special formulation of vaccine (40 μg/mL) or two 1.0-mL, 20-μg doses given at one site. Vaccinate early in the course of renal disease. Assess antibody titers to hepatitis B surface antigen annually; administer additional doses if titers decline to <10 mIU/mL. **H.** Also administer meningococcal vaccine. **I.** In persons undergoing elective splenectomy, vaccinate at least 2 weeks before surgery. **J.** Vaccinate as close to diagnosis as possible, when CD4+ cell counts are highest. **K.** Withhold MMR or other measles-containing vaccines from HIV-infected persons with evidence of severe immunosuppression [*MMWR* 1996; 45, 603–606; *MMWR* 1992; 41 (RR-17), 1–19]. (*Approved by the Advisory Committee on Immunization Practices and accepted by the American College of Obstetricians and Gynecologists and the American Academy of Family Physicians.*)

Table 84-1

Vaccines Commonly Used for Travel

Vaccine	Primary Series	Booster Interval
Cholera, live oral (CVD 103 - HgR)	1 dose	6 months
Hepatitis A (Havrix), 1440 enzyme immu-noassay U/mL	2 doses, 6–12 months apart, IM	None required
Hepatitis A (VAQTA, AVAXIM, EPAXAL)	2 doses, 6–12 months apart, IM	None required
Hepatitis A/B com-bined (Twinrix)	3 doses at 0, 1, and 6–12 months *or* 0, 7, and 21 days plus booster of B at 1 year, IM	None required *except* 12 months (once only, for accelerated sched-ule)
Hepatitis B (Engerix B): accelerated sched-ule	3 doses at 0, 1, and 2 months *or* 0, 7, and 21 days plus booster at 1 year, IM	12 months, once only
Hepatitis B (Engerix B or Recombivax): stan-dard schedule	3 doses at 0, 1, and 6 months, IM	None required
Immune globulin (hep-atitis A prevention)	1 dose IM	Intervals of 3–5 months, depending on initial dose
Japanese encephalitis (JEV, Biken)	3 doses, 1 week apart, SC	12–18 months (first booster), then 4 years
Meningococcus, quad-rivalent	1 dose SC	>3 years (optimum booster schedule not yet determined)
Rabies (HDCV), rabies vaccine absorbed (RVA), or purified chick embryo cell vaccine (PCEC)	3 doses at 0, 7, and 21 or 28 days, IM	None required except with exposure
Typhoid Ty21a, oral live attenuated (Vivo-tif)	1 capsule every other day × 4 doses	5 years
Typhoid Vi capsular polysaccharide, inject-able (Typhim Vi)	1 dose IM	2 years
Yellow fever	1 dose SC	10 years

world. This consultation should include a discussion of the appropriate use of vaccines (e.g., live yellow fever vaccine is not recommended for HIV-infected persons), prophylactic medications, and particular risks for certain infections. Other important issues include the routine denial of entry to HIV-positive persons by several countries.

Problems after Return from Travel

• Diarrhea: After traveler's diarrhea, symptoms may persist because of the continued presence of pathogens (e.g., *Giardia lamblia* or *Cyclospora cayetanensis*) or, more often, because of postinfectious sequelae such as lactose intolerance or irritable bowel syndrome. A trial of metronidazole for giardiasis, a lactose-free diet, or a trial of high-dose hydrophilic mucilloid (plus lactulose for constipation) may relieve symptoms.

• Fever: Malaria should be the first diagnosis considered if a traveler returns from an endemic area with fever. Viral hepatitis, typhoid fever, bacterial enteritis, arbovirus infections, rickettsial infections, and amebic liver abscess are other possibilities.

• Skin conditions: Pyodermas, sunburn, insect bites, skin ulcers, and cutaneous larva migrans are the most common skin conditions in returning travelers.

For a more detailed discussion, see Keusch GT et al: Immunization Principles and Vaccine Use, Chap. 107, p. 713; and Keystone JS, Kozarsky PE: Health Advice for International Travel, Chap. 108, p. 725, in HPIM-16.

85

INFECTIVE ENDOCARDITIS

Acute endocarditis is a febrile illness that rapidly damages cardiac structures, seeds extracardiac sites hematogenously, and can progress to death within weeks. Subacute endocarditis follows an indolent course, rarely causes metastatic infection, and progresses gradually unless complicated by a major embolic event or a ruptured mycotic aneurysm.

Epidemiology

The incidence of endocarditis is increased among the elderly, IV drug users, and pts with prosthetic heart valves. The risk of endocarditis is 1.5–3% at 1 year after valve replacement and 3–6% at 5 years.

Etiology

The causative microorganisms vary, in part because of different portals of entry. In native valve endocarditis (NVE), viridans streptococci, staphylococci, and HACEK organisms (*Haemophilus* spp., *Actinobacillus actinomycetemcomitans*, *Cardiobacterium hominis*, *Eikenella corrodens*, *Kingella kingae*) enter the bloodstream from oral, skin, and upper respiratory tract portals, respectively. *Streptococcus bovis* originates from the gut and is associated with colon polyps or cancer. Enterococci originate from the genitourinary tract. Nosocomial endocarditis, frequently due to *Staphylococcus aureus*, arises most often from bacteremia related to intravascular devices. Prosthetic valve endocarditis (PVE) developing within 2 months of surgery is due to intraoperative contamination or a bacteremic postoperative complication and is typically caused by coagulase-negative staphylococci, *S. aureus*, facultative gram-negative bacilli, diphtheroids, or fungi. At 1 year after valve surgery, endocarditis is caused by the same organisms that cause community-acquired NVE. IV drug users are particularly prone to tricuspid valve endocarditis caused by *S. aureus* (often a methicillin-resistant strain); they are also at risk for left-sided endocarditis caused by *S. aureus, Pseudomonas aeruginosa,* or *Candida* spp. Fastidious organisms such as *Abiotrophia,* HACEK bacteria, *Bartonella* spp., *Coxiella burnetii, Brucella* spp., and *Tropheryma whipplei* can cause culture-negative endocarditis. β-Hemolytic streptococci, *S. aureus,* pneumococci, and enterococci typically cause acute endocarditis, while viridans streptococci and coagulase-negative staphylococci usually cause subacute disease.

Pathogenesis

If endothelial injury occurs, direct infection by pathogens such as *S. aureus* can result, or an uninfected platelet-fibrin thrombus may develop and become infected during transient bacteremia. The vegetation is the prototypic lesion at the site of infection: a mass of platelets, fibrin, and microcolonies of organisms, with scant inflammatory cells.

Clinical Features

The clinical syndrome is variable and spans a continuum between acute and subacute presentations. Nonspecific symptoms include fevers, chills, sweats, anorexia, myalgias, and back pain.

Cardiac Manifestations

• Heart murmurs, particularly new or worsened regurgitant murmurs, are ultimately heard in 85% of pts with acute NVE.
• CHF develops in 30–40% of pts and is usually due to valvular dysfunction.
• Extension of infection can result in perivalvular abscesses, which in turn may cause fistulae from the aortic root into cardiac chambers or may burrow through epicardium and cause pericarditis.
• Heart block may result when infection extends into the conduction system.
• Emboli to a coronary artery may result in myocardial infarcts.

Noncardiac Manifestations

• Hematogenous bacterial seeding (e.g., to the spleen, kidneys, and meninges) can cause abscesses in noncardiac tissues.
• Arterial emboli of vegetation fragments lead to infection or infarction of remote tissues such as the extremities, spleen, kidneys, bowel, or brain. Emboli most commonly arise from vegetations >10 mm in diameter and from those located on the mitral valve. With antibiotic treatment, the frequency of emboli decreases from 13 per 1000 pt-days during the first week of infection to 1.2 per 1000 pt-days during the third week.
• Neurologic complications are seen in up to 40% of pts and include embolic stroke, aseptic or purulent meningitis, intracranial hemorrhage due to ruptured mycotic aneurysms (focal dilations of arteries at points in the artery wall weakened by infection or where septic emboli have lodged) or hemorrhagic infarcts, seizures, encephalopathy, and microabscesses.
• Renal infarcts cause flank pain and hematuria without renal dysfunction.
• Immune complex deposition causes glomerulonephritis and renal dysfunction.
• Peripheral manifestations such as Osler's nodes, subungual hemorrhages, Janeway lesions, and Roth's spots are nonsuppurative complications seen in prolonged infection and are now rare because of early diagnosis and treatment.

Tricuspid Valve Endocarditis   This condition is associated with fever, faint or no heart murmur, and prominent pulmonary findings such as cough, pleuritic chest pain, and nodular pulmonary infiltrates.

Paravalvular Infection   This condition is common in PVE, resulting in partial valve dehiscence, regurgitant murmurs, CHF, or disruption of the conduction system.

Diagnosis

• The Duke criteria (Table 85-1) constitute a sensitive and specific diagnostic schema. *Definite* endocarditis is defined by 2 major, 1 major plus 3 minor, or 5 minor criteria. *Possible* endocarditis is defined by 1 major plus 1 minor criterion or by 3 minor criteria.

• If blood cultures are negative after 48–72 h, 2 or 3 additional cultures, including a lysis-centrifugation culture, should be performed, and the laboratory

Table 85-1

The Duke Criteria for the Clinical Diagnosis of Infective Endocarditis

MAJOR CRITERIA

1. Positive blood culture
   Typical microorganism for infective endocarditis from two separate blood cultures
      Viridans streptococci, *Streptococcus bovis*, HACEK group, *Staphylococcus aureus, or*
      Community-acquired enterococci in the absence of a primary focus, *or*
   Persistently positive blood culture, defined as recovery of a microorganism consistent with infective endocarditis from:
      Blood cultures drawn >12 h apart; *or*
      All of three or a majority of four or more separate blood cultures, with first and last drawn at least 1 h apart
      Single positive blood culture for *Coxiella burnetii* or phase I IgG antibody titer of >1:800
2. Evidence of endocardial involvement
   Positive echocardiogram
      Oscillating intracardiac mass on valve or supporting structures or in the path of regurgitant jets or in implanted material, in the absence of an alternative anatomic explanation, *or*
      Abscess, *or*
      New partial dehiscence of prosthetic valve, *or*
   New valvular regurgitation (increase or change in preexisting murmur not sufficient)

MINOR CRITERIA

1. Predisposition: predisposing heart condition or injection drug use
2. Fever ≥38.0°C (≥100.4°F)
3. Vascular phenomena: major arterial emboli, septic pulmonary infarcts, mycotic aneurysm, intracranial hemorrhage, conjunctival hemorrhages, Janeway lesions
4. Immunologic phenomena: glomerulonephritis, Osler's nodes, Roth's spots, rheumatoid factor
5. Microbiologic evidence: positive blood culture but not meeting major criterion as noted previously[a] or serologic evidence of active infection with organism consistent with infective endocarditis

---

[a] Excluding single positive cultures for coagulase-negative staphylococci and diphtheroids, which are common culture contaminants, and organisms that do not cause endocarditis frequently, such as gram-negative bacilli.

Note: HACEK, *Haemophilus* spp., *Actinobacillus actinomycetemcomitans, Cardiobacterium hominis, Eikenella corrodens, Kingella kingae.*

Source: Adapted from JS Li et al: Clin Infect Dis 30:633, 2000, with permission from the University of Chicago Press.

should be asked to seek fastidious microorganisms by prolonging incubation time and undertaking special subcultures.

- Serology is helpful in the diagnosis of *Bartonella*, *Legionella*, or *C. burnetii* endocarditis.
- Echocardiography should be performed to confirm the diagnosis, to verify the size of vegetations, to detect intracardiac complications, and to assess cardiac function. Transthoracic echocardiography (TTE) does not detect vegetations <2 mm in diameter and is not adequate to evaluate prosthetic valves or to detect intracardiac complications; however, TTE may be used in pts with a low pretest likelihood of endocarditis (<5%). In other pts, transesophageal echocardiography (TEE) is indicated. TEE detects vegetations in >90% of cases of definite endocarditis and is optimal for evaluation of prosthetic valves and detection of abscesses, valve perforation, or intracardiac fistulae.
- Other laboratory findings include anemia; leukocytosis; hematuria; elevations of ESR, rheumatoid factor level, and circulating immune complex titer; and a decrease in serum complement concentration.

℞ TREATMENT

Antimicrobial Therapy   Antimicrobial therapy must be bactericidal and prolonged. See Table 85-2 for organism-specific regimens. Most pts defervesce within 5–7 days. Blood cultures should be repeated until sterile and should be rechecked if there is recrudescent fever and at 4–6 weeks after therapy to document cure. If pts are febrile for 7 days despite antibiotic therapy, an evaluation for paravalvular or extracardiac abscesses should be performed.

- Pts with acute endocarditis require antibiotic treatment as soon as three sets of blood culture samples are obtained, but stable pts with subacute disease should have antibiotics withheld until a diagnosis is made. Pts treated with vancomycin or an aminoglycoside should have serum drug levels monitored.
- Enterococci require the synergistic activity of a cell wall–active agent and an aminoglycoside for killing. Enterococci must be tested for high-level resistance to streptomycin and gentamicin; if resistance is detected, the addition of an aminoglycoside will not produce a synergistic effect and the cell wall–active agent should be given alone for periods of 8–12 weeks. If treatment fails or the isolate is resistant to commonly used agents, surgical therapy is advised (see below and Table 85-3).
- Staphylococcal PVE is treated for 6–8 weeks with a multidrug regimen. Rifampin is important because it kills organisms adherent to foreign material. Two other agents in addition to rifampin help prevent the emergence of rifampin resistance in vivo. Susceptibility testing for gentamicin should be performed before rifampin is given; if the strain is resistant, another aminoglycoside or a fluoroquinolone should be substituted.
- Pts with negative blood cultures and without confounding prior antibiotic treatment should receive ceftriaxone plus gentamicin. If the pt has a prosthetic valve, those two drugs plus vancomycin should be given.

Surgical Treatment   Surgery should be considered early in the course of illness in pts with the indications listed in Table 85-3, although most of these indications are not absolute. However, pts who develop acute aortic regurgitation with preclosure of the mitral valve or a sinus of Valsalva abscess rupture into the right heart require emergent surgery. Likewise, surgery should not be delayed when severe valvular dysfunction with progressive CHF or uncontrolled or perivalvular infection is present. Cardiac surgery should be delayed for 2–3 weeks if possible when the pt has had a nonhemorrhagic

Table 85-2

Antibiotic Treatment for Infective Endocarditis Caused by Common Organisms[a]

Organism	Drug, Dose, Duration	Comments
Streptococci		
Penicillin-susceptible[b] streptococci, *S. bovis*	Penicillin G 2–3 million units IV q4h for 4 weeks	—
	Penicillin G 2–3 million units IV q4h *plus* gentamicin[c] 1 mg/kg IM or IV q8h, both for 2 weeks	Avoid penicillin plus gentamicin if risks of aminoglycoside toxicity are increased or case is complicated
	Ceftriaxone 2 g/d IV as single dose for 4 weeks	Can use ceftriaxone in patients with nonimmediate penicillin allergy
	Vancomycin[d] 15 mg/kg IV q12h for 4 weeks	Use vancomycin in patients with severe or immediate β-lactam allergy
Relatively penicillin-resistant[e] streptococci	Penicillin G 3 million units IV q4h for 4–6 weeks *plus* gentamicin[c] 1 mg/kg IV q8h for 2 weeks	Preferred for treatment of prosthetic valve endocarditis caused by penicillin-susceptible streptococci; continue penicillin for 6 weeks in this setting
Moderately penicillin-resistant[f] streptococci, pyridoxal-requiring streptococci (*Abiotrophia* spp.)	Penicillin G 3–4 million units IV q4h *plus* gentamicin[c] 1 mg/kg IV q8h, both for 4–6 weeks	—
Enterococci[g]	Penicillin G 3–4 million units IV q4h *plus* gentamicin[c] 1 mg/kg IV q8h, both for 4–6 weeks	Can use streptomycin 7.5 mg/kg q12h in lieu of gentamicin if there is not high-level resistance to streptomycin
	Ampicillin 2 g IV q4h *plus* gentamicin[c] 1 mg/kg IV q8h, both for 4–6 weeks	Do not use cephalosporins or carbapenems for treatment of enterococcal endocarditis
	Vancomycin[d] 15 mg/kg IV q12h *plus* gentamicin[c] 1 mg/kg IV q8h, both for 4–6 weeks	Use vancomycin plus gentamicin for penicillin-allergic patients or desensitize to penicillin
Staphylococci		
Methicillin-susceptible, infecting native valves (no foreign devices)	Nafcillin or oxacillin 2 g IV q4h for 4–6 weeks *plus* (optional) gentamicin[c] 1 mg/kg IM or IV q8h for 3–5 days	May use penicillin 3–4 million units q6h if isolate is penicillin-susceptible (does not produce β-lactamase)

376

Condition	Regimen	Comments
	Cefazolin 2 g IV q8h for 4–6 weeks *plus* (optional) gentamicin[c] 1 mg/kg IM or IV q8h for 3–5 days	Can use cefazolin regimen for patients with nonimmediate penicillin allergy
	Vancomycin[d] 15 mg/kg IV q12h for 4–6 weeks	Use vancomycin for patients with immediate (urticarial) or severe penicillin allergy
Methicillin-resistant, infecting native valves (no foreign devices)	Vancomycin[d] 15 mg/kg IV q12h for 4–6 weeks	No role for routine use of rifampin
Methicillin-susceptible, infecting prosthetic valves	Nafcillin or oxacillin 2 g IV q4h for 6–8 weeks *plus* gentamicin[c] 1 mg/kg IM or IV q8h for 2 weeks *plus* rifampin[h] 300 mg PO q8h for 6–8 weeks	Use gentamicin during initial 2 weeks; determine susceptibility to gentamicin before initiating rifampin (see text); if patient is highly allergic to penicillin, use regimen for methicillin-resistant staphylococci; if β-lactam allergy is of the minor, nonimmediate type, can substitute cefazolin for oxacillin/nafcillin
Methicillin-resistant, infecting prosthetic valves	Vancomycin[d] 15 mg/kg IV q12h for 6–8 weeks *plus* gentamicin[c] 1 mg/kg IM or IV q8h for 2 weeks *plus* rifampin[h] 300 mg PO q8h for 6–8 weeks	Use gentamicin during initial 2 weeks; determine gentamicin susceptibility before initiating rifampin.
HACEK organisms	Ceftriaxone 2 g/d IV as single dose for 4 weeks	May use another third-generation cephalosporin at comparable dosage
	Ampicillin 2 g IV q4h *plus* gentamicin[c] 1 mg/kg IM or IV q8h, both for 4 weeks	Determine ampicillin susceptibility; do not use ampicillin if β-lactamase is produced

[a] Doses are for adults with normal renal function. Doses of gentamicin, streptomycin, and vancomycin must be adjusted for reduced renal function. Ideal body weight is used to calculate doses per kilogram (men = 50 kg + 2.3 kg per 2.5 cm over 150 cm; women = 45.5 kg + 2.3 kg per 2.5 cm over 150 cm).

[b] MIC ≤ 0.1 μg/mL.

[c] Aminoglycosides should not be administered as single daily doses and should be introduced as part of the initial treatment. Target peak and trough serum concentrations of gentamicin 1 h after a 20- to 30-min infusion or IM injection are 3–5 μg/mL and ≤1 μg/mL, respectively; the target peak serum concentration of streptomycin (timing as with gentamicin) is 20–25 μg/mL.

[d] Desirable peak vancomycin level 1 h after completion of a 1-h infusion is 30–45 μg/mL.

[e] MIC > 0.1 μg/mL and <0.5 μg/mL.

[f] MIC ≥ 0.5 μg/mL and <8.0 μg/mL.

[g] Antimicrobial susceptibility must be evaluated.

[h] Rifampin increases warfarin and dicumarol requirements for anticoagulation.

Table 85-3

Indications for Cardiac Surgical Intervention in Patients with Endocarditis

Surgery required for optimal outcome
    Moderate to severe CHF due to valve dysfunction
    Partially dehisced unstable prosthetic valve
    Persistent bacteremia despite optimal antimicrobial therapy
    Lack of effective microbicidal therapy (e.g., fungal or *Brucella* endocarditis)
    S. aureus PVE with an intracardiac complication
    Relapse of PVE after optimal antimicrobial therapy
Surgery to be strongly considered for improved outcome[a]
    Perivalvular extension of infection
    Poorly responsive *S. aureus* endocarditis involving the aortic or mitral valve
    Large (>10-mm diameter) hypermobile vegetations with increased risk of embolism
    Persistent unexplained fever (≥10 days) in culture-negative NVE
    Poorly responsive or relapsed endocarditis due to highly antibiotic-resistant enterococci or gram-negative bacilli

[a] Surgery must be carefully considered; findings are often combined with other indications to prompt surgery.

Table 85-4

Procedures for which Endocarditis Prophylaxis Is Advised in Patients at High or Moderate Risk for Endocarditis[a]

Dental procedures
    Extractions
    Periodontal procedures, cleaning causing gingival bleeding
    Implant placement, reimplantation of avulsed teeth
    Endodontic instrumentation (root canal) or surgery beyond the apex
    Subgingival placement of antibiotic fibers or strips
    Placement of orthodontic bands but not brackets
    Intraligamentary injections (anesthetic)
Respiratory procedures
    Operations involving the mucosa
    Bronchoscopy with rigid bronchoscope
Gastrointestinal procedures[b]
    Esophageal: Sclerotherapy of varices, stricture dilation
    Biliary tract: Endoscopic retrograde cholangiography with biliary obstruction, biliary tract surgery
    Intestinal tract: Surgery involving the mucosa
Genitourinary procedures
    Urethral dilation, prostate or urethral surgery
    Cystoscopy

[a] Prophylaxis is optional for high-risk patients undergoing bronchoscopy or GI endoscopy with/without biopsy, vaginal delivery, vaginal hysterectomy, or TEE.
[b] Prophylaxis is recommended for high-risk patients and optional for moderate-risk group (see Table 85-5).
Source: Adapted from AS Dajani et al: JAMA 277:1794, 1997; with permission.

Table 85-5

Cardiac Lesions for which Endocarditis Prophylaxis Is Advised

High Risk	Moderate Risk
Prosthetic heart valves	Congenital cardiac malformations (other than high-/low-risk lesions), ventricular septal defect, bicuspid aortic valve
Prior bacterial endocarditis	
Complex cyanotic congenital heart disease; other complex congenital lesions after correction	Acquired aortic and mitral valve dysfunction
Patent ductus arteriosus	Hypertrophic cardiomyopathy (asymmetric septal hypertrophy)
Coarctation of the aorta	Mitral valve prolapse with valvular regurgitation and/or thickened leaflets
Surgically constructed systemic-pulmonary shunts	

Table 85-6

Antibiotic Regimens for Prophylaxis of Endocarditis in Adults at Moderate or High Risk[a]

I. Oral cavity, respiratory tract, or esophageal procedures[b]
   A. Standard regimen
      1. Amoxicillin 2.0 g PO 1 h before procedure
   B. Inability to take oral medication
      1. Ampicillin 2.0 g IV or IM within 30 min of procedure
   C. Penicillin allergy
      1. Clarithromycin 500 mg PO 1 h before procedure
      2. Cephalexin[c] or cefadroxil[c] 2.0 g PO 1 h before procedure
      3. Clindamycin 600 mg PO 1 h before procedure or IV 30 min before procedure
   D. Penicillin allergy, inability to take oral medication
      1. Cefazolin[c] 1.0 g IV or IM 30 min before procedure
II. Genitourinary and GI[d] procedures
   A. High-risk patients
      1. Ampicillin 2.0 g IV or IM *plus* gentamicin 1.5 mg/kg (not to exceed 120 mg) IV or IM within 30 min of procedure; repeat ampicillin 1.0 g IV or IM or amoxicillin 1.0 g PO 6 h later
   B. High-risk, penicillin-allergic patients
      1. Vancomycin 1.0 g IV over 1–2 h *plus* gentamicin 1.5 mg/kg (not to exceed 120 mg) IV or IM within 30 min before procedure; no second dose recommended
   C. Moderate-risk patients
      1. Amoxicillin 2.0 g PO 1 h before procedure or ampicillin 2.0 g IV or IM within 30 min before procedure
   D. Moderate-risk, penicillin-allergic patients
      1. Vancomycin 1.0 g IV infused over 1–2 h and completed within 30 min of procedure

[a] Dosing for children: for amoxicillin, ampicillin, cephalexin, or cefadroxil, use 50 mg/kg PO; cefazolin, 25 mg/kg IV; clindamycin, 20 mg/kg PO, 25 mg/kg IV; clarithromycin, 15 mg/kg PO; gentamicin, 1.5 mg/kg IV or IM; and vancomycin, 20 mg/kg IV.
[b] For patients at high risk (Table 85-5), administer a half-dose 6 h after the initial dose.
[c] Do not use cephalosporins in patients with immediate hypersensitivity (urticaria, angioedema, anaphylaxis) to penicillin.
[d] Excludes esophageal procedures.
Source: Adapted from AS Dajani et al: JAMA 277:1794, 1997; with permission.

embolic stroke and for 4 weeks when the pt has had a hemorrhagic embolic stroke. Ruptured mycotic aneurysms should be clipped and cerebral edema allowed to resolve prior to cardiac surgery.

Prevention

The American Heart Association has identified procedures that may cause bacteremia with organisms prone to cause endocarditis (Table 85-4), pts who should receive antibiotic prophylaxis based on their relative risk of developing endocarditis (Table 85-5), and regimens for prophylaxis (Table 85-6).

For a more detailed discussion, see Karchmer AW: Infective Endocarditis, Chap. 109, p. 731, in HPIM-16.

86

INTRAABDOMINAL INFECTIONS

Intraperitoneal infections result when normal anatomical barriers are disrupted. Organisms contained within the bowel or an intraabdominal organ enter the sterile peritoneal cavity, causing peritonitis and—if the infection goes untreated and the pt survives—abscesses.

PERITONITIS

Peritonitis is a life-threatening event that is often accompanied by bacteremia and sepsis. Peritonitis is either primary (without an apparent source) or secondary (bacterial contamination resulting from spillage from an intraabdominal viscus).

Primary (Spontaneous) Bacterial Peritonitis (PBP)

PBP is most common among pts with cirrhosis (usually due to alcoholism) and preexisting ascites, although it is also described in other settings (e.g., malignancy, hepatitis). PBP is due to hematogenous spread of organisms to ascitic fluid in pts in whom a diseased liver and altered portal circulation compromise the usual filtration function of the liver.

   Clinical Features   Pts experience an acute onset of symptoms, with fever, abdominal pain, and signs of peritoneal irritation. The diagnosis is established by sampling of peritoneal fluid, which contains >300 PMNs/μL. Enteric gram-negative bacilli such as *Escherichia coli* or gram-positive organisms such as streptococci, enterococci, and pneumococci are the most common etiologic agents; a single organism is typically isolated. The organism burden is low, but the culture yield is improved if 10 mL of peritoneal fluid is placed directly into blood culture bottles. Because bacteremia is common, blood cultures should also be performed.

Rx TREATMENT

Empirical therapy should be directed against likely etiologic organisms, such as gram-negative bacilli and gram-positive cocci. Ceftriaxone (2 g/d IV) or piperacillin/tazobactam (3.375 g qid IV) constitutes appropriate empirical treatment. The regimen should be narrowed after the etiology is identified. Treatment should continue for 5–14 days, depending on how quickly the pt's condition improves.

Prevention Up to 70% of pts have a recurrence of PBP within 1 year. Fluoroquinolones (e.g., ciprofloxacin, 750 mg weekly) or trimethoprim-sulfamethoxazole (TMP-SMX; one double-strength tablet daily) provides effective prophylaxis. However, the risk of serious staphylococcal or antibiotic-resistant infections increases over time.

Secondary Peritonitis

Secondary peritonitis almost always involves a mixed aerobic and anaerobic flora, especially when the contaminating source is colonic. This infection can result primarily from chemical irritation (e.g., a ruptured gastric ulcer) or from bacterial contamination (e.g., a ruptured appendix).

Clinical Features Initial symptoms may be localized or vague and depend on the primary organ involved. Once infection has spread to the peritoneal cavity, pain increases; pts lie motionless, often with knees drawn up to avoid stretching the nerve fibers of the peritoneal cavity. Coughing or sneezing causes severe, sharp pain. There is marked voluntary and involuntary guarding of anterior abdominal musculature, tenderness (often with rebound), and fever.

Diagnosis and Treatment There is marked leukocytosis with a left shift. Studies to find the source of peritonitis are central to treatment. Abdominal taps are done only to exclude hemoperitoneum in trauma cases. The selected antibiotics are aimed at aerobic gram-negative bacilli and anaerobes—e.g., penicillin/β-lactamase inhibitor combinations or, in critically ill pts in the ICU, imipenem (500 mg q6h IV) or drug combinations such as ampicillin plus metronidazole plus ciprofloxacin. Surgical intervention is often needed.

Peritonitis in Pts Undergoing Chronic Ambulatory Peritoneal Dialysis

Common etiologic agents include coagulase-negative staphylococci (~30% of cases), *Staphylococcus aureus*, gram-negative bacilli, and fungi such as *Candida* spp. Several hundred milliliters of removed dialysis fluid should be centrifuged and sent for culture, preferably in blood culture bottles to improve the diagnostic yield. Empirical therapy should be directed against staphylococcal species and gram-negative bacilli (e.g., cefazolin plus ceftazidime, with an initial loading dose of each administered IP). If methicillin resistance is prevalent, vancomycin (2 g) can be administered and should be allowed to remain in the peritoneal cavity for 6 h. Severely ill pts should be given the same regimen IV. Catheter removal should be considered if the pt's condition does not improve within 48 h.

INTRAPERITONEAL ABSCESSES

Abscesses develop in untreated peritonitis as an extension of the disease process and as an attempt by the host's defenses to contain the infection. Most abscesses arise from colonic sources. *Bacteroides fragilis* accounts for only 0.5% of the normal colonic flora, but it is the anaerobe most frequently isolated from intraabdominal abscesses and the most common anaerobic bloodstream isolate. Scanning procedures facilitate the diagnosis; abdominal CT has the highest yield. Ultrasonography is useful for the RUQ, the kidneys, and the pelvis. Indium-labeled WBCs and gallium localize in abscesses; however, because the bowel takes up gallium, the indium scan may be preferable. Occasionally, exploratory laparotomy is still needed to identify an abscess.

Intraperitoneal and Retroperitoneal Abscesses

These abscesses account for three-quarters of all intraabdominal abscesses. Pts are febrile and may have localizing abdominal pain and leukocytosis. Antimicrobial therapy is adjunctive to drainage and/or surgical correction of an underlying lesion or process. Antimicrobial agents with activity against gramnegative bacilli and anaerobic organisms are indicated (see "Secondary Peritonitis," above).

Visceral Abscesses

LIVER ABSCESS Liver abscesses account for up to half of visceral intraabdominal abscesses and are caused most commonly by biliary tract disease (due to aerobic gram-negative bacilli, enterococci) and less often by local spread from other contiguous sites of infection (mixed aerobic and anaerobic infection) or hematogenous seeding (infection with a single species, usually staphylococci or streptococci). Pts have fever, anorexia, weight loss, nausea, and vomiting, but only ~50% have signs localized to the RUQ, such as pain, tenderness, hepatomegaly, and jaundice. Serum levels of alkaline phosphatase are elevated in ~70% of pts, and leukocytosis is common. About one-third of pts are bacteremic. Amebic liver abscesses are not uncommon; amebic serology has yielded positive results in >95% of affected pts. Drainage remains the mainstay of treatment, but medical management with long courses of antibiotics can be successful. Percutaneous drainage tends to fail when there are multiple, sizable abscesses; viscous abscess contents that plug the pigtail catheter; associated disease (e.g., of the biliary tract); or lack of response in 4–7 days.

SPLENIC ABSCESS Splenic abscesses usually develop by hematogenous spread of infection (e.g., due to endocarditis). Abdominal pain or splenomegaly occurs in ~50% of cases, and pain localized to the LUQ in ~25%. Fever and leukocytosis are common. CXR may show infiltrates or left-sided pleural effusions. Splenic abscesses are most often caused by streptococci; *S. aureus* is the next most common cause. Gram-negative bacilli can cause splenic abscess in pts with urinary tract foci, and *Salmonella* can be responsible in pts with sickle cell disease. The diagnosis is often made only after the pt's death; the condition is frequently fatal if left untreated. Most pts undergo splenectomy and receive adjunctive antibiotics, although percutaneous drainage has been successful.

PERINEPHRIC AND RENAL ABSCESSES More than 75% of these abscesses are due to ascending infection and are preceded by pyelonephritis. Areas of abscess within the renal parenchyma may rupture into the perinephric space. The most important risk factor is the presence of renal calculi that produce local obstruction to urinary flow. Other risk factors include structural abnormalities of the urinary tract, a history of urologic surgery, trauma, or diabetes. *E. coli*, *Proteus* spp. (associated with struvite stones), and *Klebsiella* spp. are the most common etiologic agents. Clinical signs are nonspecific and include flank pain, abdominal pain, and fever. The diagnosis should be considered if pts with pyelonephritis have persistent fever after 4 or 5 days of treatment, a urine culture yields a polymicrobial flora in pts with known renal stone disease, or fever and pyuria occur in conjunction with a sterile urine culture. Treatment includes drainage and the administration of antibiotics active against the organisms recovered. Percutaneous drainage is usually successful.

PSOAS ABSCESS Psoas abscesses arise from hematogenous seeding or from contiguous spread from an intraabdominal or pelvic source or from nearby bony structures (e.g., vertebral bodies). *S. aureus* is most common when the source is hematogenous or bony; a mixed enteric flora is likely with an abdominal source. Pts have fever, lower abdominal or back pain, or pain referred to the hip or knee.

For a more detailed discussion, see Kasper DL, Zaleznik DF: Intraabdominal Infections and Abscesses, Chap. 112, p. 749, in HPIM-16.

87

INFECTIOUS DIARRHEAS

Infectious diarrheas are the second most common group of diseases worldwide and are a significant cause of morbidity and mortality in developing countries. Disease is mediated by toxins and/or direct invasion of the GI mucosa. Infections with pathogens that induce acute inflammation tend to involve the lower GI tract, cause small-volume purulent or bloody stools, and are accompanied by fever. Infections due to noninflammatory pathogens tend to involve the upper GI tract and cause more voluminous but nonbloody stools that do not contain PMNs.

Approach to the Patient

The history should include inquiries about fever (which may suggest invasive disease), abdominal pain, nausea, vomiting, frequency and character of stools, duration of diarrhea, food recently ingested (seafood; possible common food sources, such as a picnic), travel (location, duration, and nature of trip), sexual exposures, and general medical history (immunosuppression, treatment with antibiotics or gastric-acid inhibitors). On physical examination, particular attention to signs of dehydration and abdominal findings is warranted. Stool specimens should be examined grossly (e.g., grossly visible blood or mucus in stools suggests an inflammatory process) and microscopically. A fecal leukocyte test can be done but has an unclear predictive value; fecal lactoferrin, a marker for fecal leukocytes, is more sensitive. Whether stool cultures and other tests should be performed depends on the clinical circumstances.

NONINFLAMMATORY DIARRHEA
Traveler's Diarrhea

Of people traveling to Asia, Africa, or Central or South America, 20–50% experience the sudden onset of abdominal cramps, anorexia, and watery diarrhea. Disease usually begins within 3–5 days of arrival, is associated with ingestion of contaminated food or water, lasts 1–5 days, and is most often due to enterotoxigenic *Escherichia coli* (ETEC). Bismuth subsalicylate [2 tablets (525 mg) every 30–60 min, up to 8 doses] can be used prophylactically. Hydration usually constitutes adequate treatment, but, if desired, a 1- to 3-day course of a fluoroquinolone (or azithromycin in children or in travelers to Thailand) can decrease the duration of illness to 24–36 h. Antimotility agents (e.g., loperamide, 4 mg at onset, then 2 mg after each loose stool, to 16 mg in a 24-h period) can control diarrhea.

Bacterial Food Poisoning

Evidence of a common-source outbreak is often found.

1. *Staphylococcus aureus*: Enterotoxin is elaborated in food left at room temperature (e.g., at picnics). The incubation period is 1–6 h. Disease lasts <12 h and consists of diarrhea, nausea, vomiting, and abdominal cramping, usually without fever.
2. *Bacillus cereus*
    a. Emetic form: presents like *S. aureus* food poisoning, is associated with contaminated fried rice
    b. Diarrheal form: incubation period of 8–16 h; diarrhea, cramps, no vomiting
3. *Clostridium perfringens*: Heat-resistant spores in undercooked meat, poultry, or legumes; incubation period, 8–14 h; 24-h illness of diarrhea and abdominal cramps, without vomiting or fever

Cholera

Etiology   *Vibrio cholerae* serogroups O1 (classical and El Tor biotypes) and O139

Epidemiology   Occurs in Ganges delta on Indian subcontinent and in Southeast Asia, Africa, and occasionally coastal Texas and Louisiana; spread by fecal contamination of water and food sources. Infection requires ingestion of a large inoculum (10^5–10^8 organisms). Toxin production causes disease manifestations.

Clinical Manifestations

• Incubation period of 24–48 h followed by painless watery diarrhea and vomiting that can cause profound, rapidly progressive dehydration and death within hours
• "Rice-water" stool: gray, cloudy fluid with flecks of mucus

Diagnosis   Stool cultures on selective medium (e.g., TCBS agar)

Rx TREATMENT

Rapid replacement of fluid, electrolytes, and base, with high Na levels (90 mmol/L) to correct for Na losses in stool or Ringer's lactate for pts with >10% weight loss. Antibiotics can be used in conjunction: doxycycline, 300 mg once; ciprofloxacin in a single dose not to exceed 1 g/d; or erythromycin, 40 mg/kg qd in three divided doses for 3 days.

Vibrio parahaemolyticus and Non-O1 *V. cholerae*

These infections are linked to ingestion of seawater or contaminated, under-cooked seafood. After an incubation period of 4 h to 4 days, watery diarrhea, abdominal cramps, nausea, vomiting, and occasionally fever and chills develop. The disease lasts 3–7 days and requires only supportive measures. Pts with comorbid disease (e.g., liver disease), sometimes have extraintestinal infections that require antibiotics.

Norwalk Virus and Related Human Caliciviruses

These viruses are common causes of traveler's diarrhea and of viral gastroen-teritis in pts of all ages as well as of epidemics worldwide, with a higher prev-alence in cold-weather months. Shellfish concentrate the viruses through filtra-tion and pose a special risk. Very small inocula are required for infection. Thus, although the fecal-oral route is the primary mode of transmission, aerosoliza-tion, fomite contact, and person-to-person contact can also result in infection.

Clinical Manifestations   After a 24-h incubation period (range, 12–72 h), pts experience the sudden onset of nausea, vomiting, diarrhea, and/or abdominal cramps with constitutional symptoms. Stools are loose, watery, and without blood, mucus, or leukocytes. Disease lasts 12–60 h.

 TREATMENT

Only supportive measures are required.

Rotavirus

Most infections occur by 3–5 years of age, but adults can become infected if exposed. Reinfections are progressively less severe. Large quantities of virus are shed in the stool during the first week of infection, and transmission takes place both via the fecal-oral route and from person to person. Disease incidence peaks in the cooler fall and winter months. Rotavirus is common in both in-dustrialized and developing nations.

Clinical Manifestations   After an incubation period of 1–3 days, disease onset is abrupt. Vomiting often precedes diarrhea (loose, watery stools without blood or fecal leukocytes), and about one-third of pts are febrile. Symptoms resolve within 3–7 days, but life-threatening dehydration is more common than with most other types of gastroenteritis.

Diagnosis   Enzyme immunoassays (EIAs) or viral RNA detection tech-niques, such as PCR, can identify rotavirus in stool samples.

 TREATMENT

Only supportive treatment is needed. Antimotility agents should be avoided.

Prevention   A rotavirus vaccine was withdrawn shortly after approval by the U.S. Food and Drug Administration (FDA) because it was causally linked to intussusception.

Giardiasis

Giardia lamblia inhabits the small intestines of humans and other mammals. Cysts are ingested from the environment, excyst in the small intestine, and release flagellated trophozoites. Infection results from as few as 10 cysts. Transmission occurs via the fecal-oral route, by ingestion of contaminated food and water, or from person to person in settings with poor fecal hygiene (e.g., day-care centers, institutional settings) or via sexual contact. Standard chlorination techniques used to control bacteria do not destroy cysts. People at the extremes of age, those newly exposed, and pts with hypogammaglobulinemia are at increased risk—a pattern suggesting a role for humoral immunity in resistance.

Clinical Manifestations

• Incubation period of 5 days to 3 weeks. Disease ranges from asymptomatic carriage (most common) to fulminant diarrhea and malabsorption.
• Diarrhea, abdominal pain, bloating, belching, flatus, nausea, vomiting lasting >1 week. Fever is rare, as is blood or mucus in stool.
• Chronic disease is often dominated by symptoms of malabsorption.

Diagnosis Giardiasis can be diagnosed by parasite antigen detection in feces and/or examination of several samples of freshly collected stool specimens, with concentration methods used to identify cysts (oval, with four nuclei) or trophozoites (pear-shaped, flattened parasites with two nuclei and four pairs of flagella).

 TREATMENT

1. Metronidazole, 250 mg tid for 5 days
2. Quinacrine, 100 mg tid for 5 days (limited availability in United States)
3. Furazolidone (for children)
4. Treatment failure: Repeat therapy for up to 21 days at higher doses (e.g., metronidazole at 750 mg tid). Seek possible sources of reinfection

Cryptosporidiosis

Disease is acquired by ingestion of oocysts that subsequently excyst, enter intestinal cells, and generate oocysts that are excreted in feces. Person-to-person transmission of infectious oocysts can occur among close contacts and in day-care settings. Waterborne transmission is common. Oocysts are not killed by routine chlorination.

Clinical Manifestations

• Incubation period: ~1 week
• Asymptomatic infection or watery, nonbloody diarrhea, occasionally with abdominal pain, nausea, anorexia, fever, and/or weight loss lasting 1–2 weeks
• Immunocompromised hosts, especially HIV-infected pts: Disease can be chronic and can cause severe dehydration, weight loss, and wasting, with biliary tract involvement.

Diagnosis On multiple days, examine fecal samples for oocysts (4–5 μm in diameter, smaller than most parasites). Modified acid-fast staining, direct immunofluorescent techniques, and EIAs can enhance diagnosis.

 TREATMENT

No good treatments exist, but immunologic status has improved with the use of antiretroviral agents, along with antidiarrheal agents and supportive care to replace fluid and electrolytes. Paromomycin (500–750 mg qid) may be partially effective. Nitazoxanide has been approved for the treatment of children.

Isosporiasis

Isospora belli infection is acquired by oocyst ingestion and is most common in tropical and subtropical countries. Acute infection can begin suddenly with fever, abdominal pain, and watery, nonbloody diarrhea and can last for weeks to months. Eosinophilia may occur. Compromised (e.g., HIV-infected) pts may have chronic disease.

Diagnosis Detection of large oocysts in stool by modified acid-fast staining

 TREATMENT

Responds to trimethoprim-sulfamethoxazole (TMP-SMX;160/800 mg qid for 10 days, then tid for 3 weeks). Pyrimethamine (50–75 mg/d) or ciprofloxacin (500 mg bid) for 1 week are alternatives.

Cyclosporiasis

Cyclospora cayetanensis can be transmitted through water or food (e.g., basil, raspberries). Clinical symptoms include diarrhea, flulike symptoms, flatulence, and burping. Disease can be self-limited or can persist for >1 month.

Diagnosis Detection of oocysts in stool (studies must be specifically requested)

 TREATMENT

TMP-SMX (160/800 mg bid for 1 week). Ciprofloxacin (500 mg bid for 1 week) may be used instead.

Microsporidiosis

Enterocytozoon bieneusi and *E. intestinalis* are obligate intracellular spore-forming protozoa that cause chronic diarrhea, wasting, biliary tract disease, and (in the case of *E. intestinalis*) disseminated disease in immunocompromised hosts, especially HIV-infected pts.

Diagnosis Identification of intracellular spores in tissue samples

 TREATMENT

No known treatment.

INFLAMMATORY DIARRHEAS
Salmonellosis

Etiology and Pathogenesis Salmonellae cause infection when 10^3–10^6 organisms are ingested. Conditions that reduce gastric acidity or decrease intestinal integrity increase susceptibility to infection. Organisms penetrate the small-intestinal mucosa and traverse the intestinal layer through cells within Peyer's patches. *S. typhi* and *S. paratyphi* survive within macrophages, then disseminate throughout the body via lymphatics, and ultimately colonize reticuloendothelial tissues. Nontyphoidal salmonellae most commonly cause gastroenteritis, invading the large- and small-intestinal mucosa and resulting in massive PMN infiltration.

Epidemiology and Clinical Manifestations

1. *Typhoid (enteric) fever:* Humans are the only hosts for *S. typhi* and *S. paratyphi* (enteric fever, typhoid fever). Disease results from ingestion of contaminated food or water and is rare in developed nations. After an incubation period of 3–21 days, prolonged fever is the most prominent symptom. Additional nonspecific symptoms include chills, headache, anorexia, cough, weakness, sore throat, dizziness, and muscle pain. GI symptoms are variable and can include either diarrhea or constipation. Abdominal pain occurs in 20–40% of pts. Physical findings include rash ("rose spots"), hepatosplenomegaly, epistaxis, and relative bradycardia. Late complications include intestinal perforation and/or GI hemorrhage, presumably due to necrosis of infiltrated Peyer's patches. Long-term *Salmonella* carriage in urine or stool develops in 1–5% of pts, usually in association with disease in the bladder or biliary and GI tracts.

2. *Nontyphoidal salmonellosis:* The incidence of nontyphoidal salmonellosis has doubled in the United States over the past two decades, with 2 million cases and 500–2000 deaths each year. Most disease is caused by *S. typhimurium* or *S. enteritidis*. Disease is acquired from multiple animal reservoirs. The main mode of transmission is from contaminated food products, such as eggs (*S. enteritidis*), poultry, undercooked meat, unpasteurized dairy products, seafood, and fresh produce. Infection is also acquired during exposure to pets, especially reptiles.

a. *Gastroenteritis*: Nausea, vomiting, diarrhea, abdominal cramping, and fever occur 6–48 h after exposure. Diarrhea is usually loose, non-bloody, and moderate in volume, but stools are sometimes bloody. Diarrhea is usually self-limited, abating within 3–7 days, and fever resolves within 72 h in most cases. Stool cultures may remain positive for ≥4–5 weeks.

b. *Extraintestinal infections*
Up to 5% of pts are bacteremic, and 5–10% of bacteremic pts may develop localized infections, particularly in vascular sites (e.g., aortic aneurysms). *S. choleraesuis* and *S. dublin* are unusual serotypes that cause high rates of bacteremia and invasive infection.

Localized infections caused by nontyphoidal salmonellae are rare and include abscesses, meningitis, pneumonia, UTIs, and osteomyelitis (particularly in pts with sickle cell disease, hemoglobinopathies, or preexisting bone disease).

Reactive arthritis (Reiter's syndrome) can follow *Salmonella* gastroenteritis in persons with the HLA-B27 histocompatibility antigen.

Diagnosis   Positive cultures of blood, stool, or other specimens are required for diagnosis. If blood cultures are positive for nontyphoidal salmonellae, high-grade bacteremia should be ruled out by obtaining multiple blood cultures.

℞ TREATMENT

1. *Typhoid fever*: A fluoroquinolone (e.g., ciprofloxacin, 500 mg PO bid) or a third-generation cephalosporin (e.g., ceftriaxone, 1–2 g/d IV or IM) for 10–14 days is recommended. Ofloxacin may be more potent and need to be administered for only 2 or 3 days. For susceptible strains, a fluoroquinolone is more efficacious than a ß-lactam. Dexamethasone may be of benefit in severe cases.

2. *Nontyphoidal salmonellosis*: Antibiotic treatment is not recommended in most cases. However, infants, the elderly, and the immunocompromised may require antibiotic treatment, hydration, and hospitalization.

Fluoroquinolones or third-generation cephalosporins can be given in the same doses as for typhoid fever until defervescence (if the pt is immunocompetent) or for 1–2 weeks (if the pt is immunocompromised). Pts with HIV infection are at high risk for *Salmonella* bacteremia and should receive 4 weeks of oral quinolone therapy after 1–2 weeks of IV treatment. In cases of relapse, long-term suppression with a quinolone or TMP-SMX should be considered. Pts with endovascular infections or endocarditis should receive 6 weeks of treatment with a third-generation cephalosporin. Infected aneurysms or endovascular lesions may require surgical resection.

Campylobacteriosis

Etiology *Campylobacter* is the most common bacterial cause of gastroenteritis in the United States. Most cases are caused by *C. jejuni.*

Epidemiology Campylobacters are common commensals in the GI tract of many food animals and household pets. In the United States, ingestion of contaminated poultry accounts for 50–70% of cases. Transmission to humans occurs via contact with or ingestion of raw or undercooked food products or direct contact with infected animals.

Clinical Manifestations

1. Gastroenteritis: An incubation period of 2–4 days (range, 1–7 days) is followed by a prodrome of fever, headache, myalgia, and/or malaise. Within the next 12–24 h, diarrhea (with stools containing blood, mucus, and leukocytes), cramping abdominal pain, and fever develop. Most cases are self-limited, but illness persists for >1 week in 10–20% of pts and may be confused with inflammatory bowel disease.
2. Extraintestinal infections: Other species (e.g., *C. fetus*) can cause a similar illness or prolonged relapsing systemic disease without a primary focus in compromised pts. The course may be fulminant, with bacterial seeding of many organs, particularly vascular sites. Fetal death can result from infection in a pregnant pt.
3. Complications
   a. Severe, persistent, disseminated disease in pts with AIDS or hypogammaglobulinemia
   b. Local suppurative complications (e.g., cholecystitis)
   c. Reactive arthritis in persons with HLA-B27 phenotype
   d. Guillain-Barré syndrome (campylobacters are associated with 20–40% of cases)

Diagnosis Confirmation of diagnosis is based on cultures of stool, blood, or other specimens on special media and/or with selective techniques (e.g., growth at 42°C).

℞ TREATMENT

1. Fluid and electrolyte replacement
2. Avoid antimotility agents, which may prolong symptoms and are associated with toxic megacolon
3. Antibiotic treatment benefits fewer than half of pts but is indicated in cases with high fever, bloody and/or severe diarrhea, disease persistence for >1 week, or worsening symptoms.
   a. Erythromycin (250 mg qid for 5–7 days) or newer macrolides
   b. Ciprofloxacin (500 mg bid) or another fluoroquinolone for 5–7 days (although resistance is increasing)

Shigellosis and Enterohemorrhagic *E. coli* (EHEC) Infection

Etiology Shigellae are small, gram-negative, nonmotile bacilli that are very closely related to *E. coli*. There are no animal reservoirs other than higher primates. Shigellae survive the low pH of the gastric acid barrier, and as few as 10–100 organisms can cause infection. These bacteria are transmitted from person to person via the fecal-oral route and occasionally via intermediate vectors such as food, water, flies, and fomites. Shigellosis is associated with a high rate of secondary household transmission. The four most common *Shigella* serotypes are *S. dysenteriae* type 1, *S. flexneri*, *S. boydii*, and *S. sonnei* (the cause of most shigellosis cases in the United States). Shiga toxin and related toxins produced by some strains of *E. coli* (including O157:H7) are important factors in disease severity. The toxins target endothelial cells and play a significant role in the microangiopathic complications of *Shigella* and *E. coli* infections, such as hemolytic-uremic syndrome (HUS) and thrombotic thrombocytopenic purpura (TTP). *Shigella* causes extensive ulceration of the epithelial surface of the colonic mucosa.

Clinical Manifestations

1. Pts can remain asymptomatic, develop fever, develop fever and diarrhea, or experience a progression to bloody diarrhea and dysentery. Dysentery is characterized by the passage of 10–30 stools per day in small volumes containing blood, mucus, and pus, with associated severe abdominal cramping and tenesmus.
2. Without treatment, fever lasts for 3–4 days and diarrhea for 1–2 weeks.
3. Complications
   a. Severe cases may progress to toxic dilatation, colonic perforation, and death.
   b. HUS is more frequent with *E. coli* O157:H7 but also occurs with *S. dysenteriae* type 1. The syndrome is characterized by oliguria, a marked drop in hematocrit, renal failure, and a mortality rate of 5–10%.

Diagnosis

• The yield of stool cultures is increased if stools contain leukocytes or blood. Most bloody diarrhea in the United States is due to *E. coli* O157:H7 or *C. jejuni*.
• Commercial EIAs to detect Shiga toxins in stool identify most pts infected with *S. dysenteriae* type 1 (rare in the United States) and EHEC within 3 h.

℞ TREATMENT

1. Rehydration and supportive measures. Use of antimotility agents is contraindicated in the dysenteric phase of disease.
2. Antibiotics are given only in severe cases, in which they can decrease illness duration and shorten the carrier state. Fluoroquinolones are effective (e.g., ciprofloxacin, 500 mg bid for 3 days). In domestically acquired U.S. cases, TMP-SMX (160/800 mg bid for 3–5 days) can still be used, as can ampicillin (but not amoxicillin). Azithromycin (1 g in a single dose) is effective in adults. Antibiotics for EHEC treatment are controversial and may worsen prognosis.

Yersiniosis

Etiology *Y. enterocolitica* and *Y. pseudotuberculosis* are nonmotile gram-negative rods that cause enteritis or enterocolitis with self-limited diarrhea that lasts an average of 2 weeks (especially common with *Y. enterocolitica*) as well as mesenteric adenitis and terminal ileitis that can resemble acute appendicitis (especially common with *Y. pseudotuberculosis*). Septicemia and metastatic focal infections can occur in pts with chronic liver disease, malignancy, diabetes mellitus, and other underlying illnesses. Infection has been linked to reactive arthritis in HLA-B27-positive pts.

Diagnosis The organisms are present in stool for almost a month; stool culture studies must be specifically requested.

 TREATMENT

Antibiotics are not indicated for diarrhea caused by yersiniae; supportive measures suffice.

Amebiasis

Amebiasis is caused by *Entamoeba histolytica* and is the third most common cause of death from parasitic disease worldwide. The incidence is high in developing countries and among travelers, recent immigrants, homosexual men, and inmates of institutions in developed nations. Infection follows ingestion of cysts from fecally contaminated water, food, or hands. Motile trophozoites are released from cysts in the small intestine and then cause infection in the large bowel. Trophozoites may be shed in stool (in active dysentery) or encyst. Excreted cysts survive for weeks in a moist environment.

Clinical Manifestations

• *Asymptomatic infection*: 90% of cases
• *Colitis*: Develops in 10% of pts 2–6 weeks after ingestion of infectious cysts, with lower abdominal pain, mild diarrhea, malaise, weight loss, and diffuse lower abdominal or back pain. Dysentery may develop, with daily passage of 10–12 small stools consisting mostly of blood and mucus. Fewer than 40% of pts have fever. Toxic megacolon is a rare complication. Pts taking glucocorticoids are at greater risk for severe disease. Chronic amebiasis may be confused with inflammatory bowel disease. Amebomas—inflammatory mass lesions—may develop in chronic amebic intestinal disease.
• *Extraintestinal infection*: Liver abscess is the most common type of extraintestinal infection; trophozoites invade veins to reach the liver through the portal venous system. Most pts are febrile and have RUQ pain that can radiate to the shoulder, point tenderness over the liver, and right-sided pleural effusion. Fewer than one-third have active diarrhea. Abscesses can occur elsewhere (e.g., lung, brain).

Diagnosis Barium rapidly kills trophozoites. At least three fresh stool specimens should be examined for amebic cysts or trophozoites. Sigmoidoscopy with biopsy of ulcers (often flask-shaped) may aid in the diagnosis but poses a risk of perforation. Serologic assays (ELISA and agar gel diffusion) are positive in >90% of pts with colitis, amebomas, or liver abscess. Serology reverts to negative within 6–12 months after active disease resolves. Imaging of the liver may assist in the diagnosis of liver abscess.

 TREATMENT

Iodoquinol (650 mg tid for 20 days) and paromomycin (500 mg tid for 10 days) are luminal agents that eradicate cysts in pts with colitis or liver abscess and in asymptomatic carriers. Tissue amebicides include nitroimidazole compounds (e.g., metronidazole,750 mg PO or IV tid for 5–10 days) and should be given with a luminal agent for colitis or liver abscess. Other nitroimidazoles (e.g, tinidazole, ornidazole) are not available in the United States. A clinical response occurs within 72 h in >90% of pts with liver abscess. Aspiration of liver abscesses usually does not accelerate healing. Indications for aspiration include the need to rule out pyogenic abscess, a lack of response to treatment after 3–5 days, an imminent threat of liver-abscess rupture, or the need to prevent left-lobe abscess rupture into the pericardium.

Clostridium difficile–Associated Disease (CDAD)

CDAD is the diarrheal illness most commonly diagnosed in the hospital. The disease is acquired almost exclusively in association with antimicrobial use; virtually all antibiotics carry a risk of CDAD. After *C. difficile* colonizes the gut, its spores vegetate, multiply, and secrete toxin A (an enterotoxin) and toxin B (a cytotoxin), causing diarrhea and pseudomembranous colitis. Spores can persist on environmental hospital surfaces for months and on the hands of hospital personnel who do not practice adequate hand hygiene.

Clinical Manifestations Diarrhea is the usual manifestation, with up to 20 bowel movements per day. Stools usually are not grossly bloody and are soft to watery, with a characteristic odor. Fever, abdominal pain, and leukocytosis are common. Pts with unexplained leukocytosis, particularly in the presence of adynamic colon, should be evaluated for CDAD. CDAD may become fulminant, and toxic megacolon or ileus may develop. Surgical intervention is often required if perforation is suspected or disease does not respond to medical management. Surgical mortality may exceed 50% in this setting.

Diagnosis If clinically suspected, CDAD should be diagnosed by means of stool studies. Stool culture for toxin-producing *C. difficile* is most sensitive; if the isolate tests positive for toxin, this test is also specific. However, the test takes at least 48 h. The cell culture cytotoxin test is specific but less sensitive and also takes 48 h. EIA or latex tests for toxin A or toxins A and B are less sensitive and specific than culture or cell culture cytotoxin testing but yield results more rapidly.

 TREATMENT

Treatment with the inciting antimicrobial agent should be discontinued if possible. Clinical response rates to different treatments are largely equivalent, although bacitracin is inferior to other agents. Metronidazole (250–500 mg tid for 10 days) should be given because of efficacy and low cost. Oral therapy is preferable, given that IV therapy is less effective as diarrhea abates or in the presence of adynamic ileus. Oral administration of vancomycin is effective but expensive and may increase the incidence of vancomycin-resistant enterococci. Infection control and restrictive antibiotic policies may be needed to preclude further cases within a hospital. Relapse is documented in 15–25% of cases and should prompt a repeat course of metronidazole. Other approaches have been described, but for persistent disease, the combination of vancomycin (125 mg qid) with rifampin (300 mg bid) for 10 days is one preferred option.

For a more detailed discussion, see Butterton JR, Calderwood SB: **Acute Infectious Diarrheal Diseases and Bacterial Food Poisoning,** Chap. 113, p. 754; Gerding DN, Johnson S: *Clostridium difficile*–Associated Disease, Including **Pseudomembranous Colitis, Chap. 114, p. 760; Lesser CF, Miller SI: Salmonellosis, Chap. 137, p. 897; Keusch GT, Kopecko DJ: Shigellosis, Chap. 138, p. 902; Blaser MJ: Infections Due to** *Campylobacter* **and Related Species, Chap. 139, p. 907; Waldor MK, Keusch GT: Cholera and Other Vibrioses, Chap. 140, p. 909; Dennis DT, Campbell GL: Plague and Other** *Yersinia* **Infections, Chap. 143, p. 921; Parashar UD, Glass RI: Viral Gastroenteritis, Chap. 174, p. 1140; Reed SL: Amebiasis and Infections with Free-Living Amebas, Chap. 194, p. 1214; Weller PF: Protozoal Intestinal Infections and Trichomoniasis, Chap. 199, p. 1248, in HPIM-16.**

88

SEXUALLY TRANSMITTED DISEASES AND REPRODUCTIVE TRACT INFECTIONS

GENERAL CLINICAL APPROACH

• Assess risk factors and obtain basic demographic data.
• Assess specific symptoms and signs, and perform confirmatory diagnostic tests.
• Institute syndrome-based treatment to cover most likely causes.
• Prevention and control ("4 C's"): contact tracing, compliance with treatment, counseling on risk reduction, condom promotion and provision

SPECIFIC SYNDROMES
Urethritis in Men

Etiology and Epidemiology

• Most cases are caused by either *Neisseria gonorrhoeae* or *Chlamydia trachomatis*. The incidence of nongonococcal urethritis (NGU) is increasing. *Chlamydia* causes more than one-third of NGU cases among heterosexual men.
• Other causative organisms include *Ureaplasma urealyticum*, *Trichomonas vaginalis*, herpes simplex virus (HSV), and *Mycoplasma genitalium*.

Clinical Considerations

• Pts present with mucopurulent urethral discharge that can usually be expressed by milking the urethra.
• Exclude both local complications (e.g., epididymitis) and systemic complications (e.g., disseminated gonorrhea).
• Apply Gram's stain to a smear of urethral exudates containing ≥5 PMNs/ 1000× field to look for intracellular gram-negative diplococci (diagnostic of *N. gonorrhoeae*). Alternatively, examine a Gram's-stained preparation of centrifuged sediment of the day's first 20–30 mL of voided urine.
• Perform tests for *N. gonorrhoeae* and *C. trachomatis* (culture or nucleic acid amplification tests; see specific pathogens below).

℞ TREATMENT

Treat gonorrhea (unless excluded) with cefpodoxime (400 mg PO once) or ceftriaxone (125 mg IM once) or a fluoroquinolone such as ciprofloxacin (500

Table 88-1

Diagnostic Features and Management of Vaginal Infection

Feature	Normal Vaginal Examination	Vulvovaginal Candidiasis	Trichomonal Vaginitis	Bacterial Vaginosis
Etiology	Uninfected; lactobacilli predominant	*Candida albicans*	*Trichomonas vaginalis*	Associated with *Gardnerella vaginalis*, various anaerobic bacteria, and mycoplasmas
Typical symptoms	None	Vulvar itching and/or irritation	Profuse purulent discharge; vulvar itching	Malodorous, slightly increased discharge
Discharge				
Amount	Variable; usually scant	Scant	Often profuse	Moderate
Color[a]	Clear or white	White	White or yellow	White or gray
Consistency	Nonhomogeneous, floccular	Clumped; adherent plaques	Homogeneous	Homogeneous, low viscosity; uniformly coats vaginal walls
Inflammation of vulvar or vaginal epithelium	None	Erythema of vaginal epithelium, introitus; vulvar dermatitis common	Erythema of vaginal and vulvar epithelium; colpitis macularis	None
pH of vaginal fluid[b]	Usually ≤4.5	Usually ≤4.5	Usually ≥5.0	Usually >4.5
Amine ("fishy") odor with 10% KOH	None	None	May be present	Present
Microscopy[c]	Normal epithelial cells; lactobacilli predominant	Leukocytes, epithelial cells; mycelia or pseudomycelia in up to 80% of *C. albicans* culture-positive persons with typical symptoms	Leukocytes; motile trichomonads seen in 80 to 90% of symptomatic pts, less often in the absence of symptoms	Clue cells; few leukocytes; no lactobacilli or only a few outnumbered by profuse mixed flora, nearly always including *G. vaginalis* plus anaerobic species on Gram's stain

394

Usual treatment	None	Azole cream, tablet, or suppository—e.g., miconazole 100-mg vaginal suppository or clotrimazole 100-mg vaginal tablet, once daily for 7 days / Fluconazole, 150 mg orally (single dose)	Metronidazole, 2 g orally (single dose) / Metronidazole, 500 mg PO bid for 7 days	Metronidazole, 500 mg PO bid for 7 days / Clindamycin, 2% cream, one full applicator vaginally each night for 7 days / Metronidazole gel, 0.75%, one full applicator vaginally twice daily for 5 days / Metronidazole, 2 g PO (single dose)[d]
Usual management of sexual partner	None	None; topical treatment if candidal dermatitis of penis is detected	Examination for STD; treatment with metronidazole, 2 g PO (single dose)	Examination for STD; no treatment if normal

[a] Color of discharge is best determined by examination against the white background of a swab.

[b] pH determination is not useful if blood is present.

[c] To detect fungal elements, vaginal fluid is digested with 10% KOH prior to microscopic examination; to examine for other features, fluid is mixed (1:1) with physiologic saline. Gram's stain is also excellent for detecting yeasts and pseudomycelia and for distinguishing normal flora from the mixed flora seen in bacterial vaginosis, but it is less sensitive than the saline preparation for detection of *T. vaginalis*.

[d] Single-dose regimen is less effective than 7-day metronidazole regimen.

mg PO once), plus treat *Chlamydia* with azithromycin (1 g PO once) or doxycycline (100 mg bid for 7 days).

For recurrent symptoms: With reexposure, re-treat pt and partner. If no reexposure, exclude *T. vaginalis* (with culture or nucleic acid amplification of early-morning first-voided urine or urethral swab prior to voiding) and doxycycline-resistant *U. urealyticum*, and consider metronidazole or azithromycin treatment.

Epididymitis

Etiology

• In sexually active young men, *C. trachomatis* and *N. gonorrhoeae* are most common, and epididymitis is often associated with urethritis.
• In older men or after urinary tract instrumentation, consider urinary pathogens.
• In men who practice insertive rectal intercourse, consider Enterobacteriaceae.

Clinical Considerations

• Usually unilateral testicular pain of acute onset, intrascrotal swelling, tenderness, and fever
• Rule out testicular torsion, tumor, and trauma.
• If symptoms persist after treatment, consider testicular tumor.

 TREATMENT

• Ceftriaxone (250 mg IM once) followed by 10 days of doxycycline (100 mg PO bid)
• Alternative: ofloxacin (300 mg PO bid for 10 days) or levofloxacin (500 mg PO daily) for 10 days

Urethritis and the Urethral Syndrome in Women

Etiology   *C. trachomatis*, *N. gonorrhoeae*, occasionally HSV

Clinical Considerations

• Internal vs. external dysuria (the latter seen with vulvovaginitis)
• Usually no urinary urgency or frequency, distinct from bacterial cystitis
• Pyuria with culture demonstrating <100 uropathogens/mL of urine supports the urethral syndrome rather than cystitis.
• Evaluate *N. gonorrhoeae* or *C. trachomatis* with nucleic acid amplification test on the first 10 mL of voided urine or culture.

 TREATMENT

See "Urethritis in Men," above.

Vulvovaginal Infections   (See Table 88-1)

• Unsolicited reporting of abnormal vaginal discharge suggests vaginosis or trichomoniasis.
• Genital herpes, which can cause vulvar pruritus, burning, irritation, and lesions as well as external dysuria and vulvar dyspareunia, must be considered in the diagnosis.
• Vulvovaginal infections are associated with increased risk of HIV acquisition.

• Vaginal trichomoniasis and bacterial vaginosis early in pregnancy are associated with premature onset of labor.
• Vulvovaginal candidiasis develops with increased frequency among women with systemic illnesses (e.g., diabetes, HIV disease).
• New DNA probe test (the Affirm test) can detect *T. vaginalis*, *Candida albicans*, and increased concentrations of *Gardnerella vaginalis*.

Mucopurulent Cervicitis

• Inflammation of the columnar epithelium and subepithelium of the endocervix
• "Silent partner" of urethritis in men
• Major etiologies: *N. gonorrhoeae*, *C. trachomatis*, *M. genitalium*; many cases idiopathic
• Yellow mucopurulent discharge from cervical os, with ≥20 PMNs/1000× field on Gram's stain of cervical mucus
• HSV cervicitis produces ulcerative lesions on the exocervix.
• Intracellular gram-negative diplococci on Gram's stain of cervical mucus are specific but <50% sensitive for gonorrhea.

 TREATMENT

See "Urethritis in Men," above.

Pelvic Inflammatory Disease (PID)

Definition　Infection ascending from the cervix or vagina to the endometrium and/or fallopian tubes (or beyond) to cause peritonitis, perihepatitis, or pelvic abscess

Etiology　*N. gonorrhoeae*, *C. trachomatis*, *M. genitalium*, and other genital mycoplasmas, anaerobic and facultative organisms such *Prevotella* species, group B streptococci

Epidemiology

• More than 200,000 cases per year in the United States, with ~66,000 hospitalizations in 2002
• Risk factors: cervicitis, bacterial vaginosis, vaginal douching, menstruation, intrauterine contraceptive device (IUD) use. Oral contraceptive pills decrease risk.
• *N. gonorrhoeae* presentation usually more acute than that of *C. trachomatis*

Clinical Manifestations

1.　Endometritis: pain and vaginal bleeding; lower quadrant, adnexal, and cervical motion pain not severe if this is the only manifestation of PID
2.　Salpingitis: bilateral lower abdominal and pelvic pain, nausea, vomiting, progression to peritoneal signs
　　a.　Mucopurulent cervicitis with discharge; cervical motion, uterine, and adnexal tenderness or swelling on examination
　　b.　Fever (one-third of cases), elevated ESR (75%), elevated peripheral WBC count (60%)
3.　Perihepatitis and periappendicitis
　　a.　Fitz-Hugh–Curtis syndrome: perihepatitis associated with salpingitis, seen in 3–10% of PID cases, most often due to *Chlamydia* but also caused by *N. gonorrhoeae*; right or bilateral upper quadrant pain, occasional hepatic friction rub
　　b.　Periappendicitis in ~5% of pts with PID due to gonococci or chlamydiae

Diagnosis

• Predictors of PID: pelvic pain, tenderness, endocervical discharge with increased PMNs, onset with menses, history of abnormal menstrual bleeding preceding or coincident with pain in ~40% of women, presence of an IUD, sexual exposure to a man with urethritis
• Perform ultrasonography or MRI if tuboovarian or pelvic abscess is a concern.
• Evaluate for pregnancy with human β-chorionic gonadotropin test.
• Unilateral pain or pelvic mass is an indication for laparoscopy, as are atypical clinical findings or poor response to appropriate treatment.
• Gram's staining of endocervical swabs for PMNs; nucleic acid amplification tests for *N. gonorrhoeae* and *C. trachomatis*; aerobic and anaerobic cultures

℞ **TREATMENT**

1. Parenteral
   a. Cefotetan (2 g IV q12h) or cefoxitin (2 g IV q6h) plus doxycycline (100 mg IV or PO q12h) until 48 h after improvement; then doxycycline PO to complete 14-day course
   b. Alternative: clindamycin (900 mg IV q8h) plus gentamicin (2.0 mg/kg IV or IM load followed by 1.5 mg/kg q8h) until 48 h after improvement; then complete 14-day course with either oral doxycycline (100 mg bid) or oral clindamycin (450 mg qid). Once-daily aminoglycoside dosing may be used instead.
2. Outpatient regimens: (1) ofloxacin (400 mg PO bid for 14 days) or levofloxacin (500 mg PO once daily for 14 days) plus metronidazole (500 mg PO bid for 14 days); or (2) ceftriaxone (250 mg IM once) plus doxycycline (100 mg PO bid) and metronidazole (500 mg PO bid) for 14 days
3. Consider hospitalization if the diagnosis is uncertain, an abscess is suspected, the illness is severe, nausea and vomiting preclude outpatient treatment, or the pt is infected with HIV, is unlikely to follow an outpatient regimen, or has already had an unsuccessful course of outpatient treatment.
4. Evaluate in 72 h for treatment response.

Prognosis   Late sequelae include infertility (11% after one episode of PID, 23% after two, and 54% after three or more); ectopic pregnancy (7-fold increase in risk); chronic pelvic pain (8-fold increase in rate of hysterectomy); and recurrent salpingitis.

Prevention   Risk-based chlamydial screening of young women can reduce PID incidence.

Ulcerative Genital Lesions

• Most common etiologies in the United States are genital herpes, syphilitic ulcers, and chancroid.
• All pts with genital ulcerations should undergo HIV serologic testing.

Clinical Manifestations, Evaluation, and Treatment   (See "Individual Pathogens," below)   Immediate treatment (before all test results are available) is often appropriate to improve response, reduce transmission, and cover pts who might not return for follow-up visits.

Proctitis, Proctocolitis, Enterocolitis, Enteritis

Definitions

• *Proctitis*: inflammation limited to rectal mucosa from direct inoculation of typical sexually transmitted disease (STD) pathogens; associated with pain, mucopurulent discharge, tenesmus, and constipation

• Ingestion of typical intestinal pathogens through oral-anal exposure during sexual contact can result in the following syndromes, often associated with diarrhea: (1) *proctocolitis*: inflammation from rectum to colon, (2) *enterocolitis*: inflammation involving both large and small intestine, and (3) *enteritis*: inflammation of small intestine alone.

Etiology and Epidemiology

• *N. gonorrhoeae*, HSV, and *C. trachomatis* are the chief causes of proctitis; symptoms are minimal and usually not systemic.
• HSV proctitis and lymphogranuloma venereum (LGV) proctocolitis can cause severe pain, fever, and systemic manifestations. Sacral nerve root radiculopathies, with urinary retention or anal sphincter dysfunction, are associated with primary HSV proctitis.
• LGV and syphilis can be associated with granulomata and inflammation.
• *Giardia lamblia* is a common cause of enteritis in homosexual men.
• *Campylobacter* or *Shigella* spp. can cause sexually acquired proctocolitis.

 TREATMENT

1. Anoscopy to examine mucosa and obtain specimens for diagnosis
2. Ceftriaxone (125 mg IM once) followed by doxycycline (100 mg bid for 7 days) if gonorrhea or chlamydial infection is suspected; syphilis or herpes therapy as indicated

INDIVIDUAL PATHOGENS
Gonorrhea

Etiology Gram-negative, nonmotile, non-spore-forming organisms that grow in pairs and are shaped like coffee beans

Epidemiology

• 362,000 cases reported in the United States in 2002; actual case numbers higher
• U.S. incidence of 120 cases per 100,000 population—the highest among industrialized nations
• 75% of cases in 20- to 24-year age group; highest risk among sexually active 15- to 19-year-old women and among African Americans
• Efficient male-to-female transmission; 40–60% rate with a single unprotected encounter; 20% rate to women who practice fellatio with infected partners; chance of HIV acquisition increased if infected person also has gonorrhea
• Drug-resistant strains are widespread. Penicillin, ampicillin, and tetracycline are no longer reliable agents. Third-generation cephalosporins remain effective. Fluoroquinolones are useful, but resistance is increasing, particularly in Southeast Asia, parts of the western continental United States, and Hawaii.

Clinical Syndromes

1. *Urethritis* (see above): incubation period, 2–7 days. Uncommon complications include epididymitis, prostatitis, penile edema, abscess or fistulae, seminal vesiculitis, and balanitis in uncircumcised men.
2. *Cervicitis* (see above): incubation period, ~10 days. Co-infection with *N. gonorrhoeae* and *C. trachomatis* is seen in up to 40% of genital gonococcal infections.
3. *Anorectal gonorrhea*: spreads from cervical exudates in women; rarely the sole site of infection or the cause of symptomatic proctitis; rates in homosexual men decreasing in the AIDS era, despite recent resurgence. Strains in this population tend to be more resistant to antibiotics.

4. *Pharyngeal gonorrhea*: usually asymptomatic infection resulting from oral-genital sexual exposure; transmission from the pharynx rare; almost always coexists with genital infection. Rate may increase during pregnancy because of altered sexual practices. Most cases resolve spontaneously. If symptomatic, pharyngeal gonorrhea is harder to eradicate than genital disease. Follow-up cultures are needed.

5. *Ocular gonorrhea*: caused by autoinoculation; swollen eyelid, hyperemia, chemosis, profuse purulent discharge, occasional corneal ulceration and perforation. Rule out associated genital infection.

6. *Gonorrhea in pregnancy*: Salpingitis and PID in first trimester can cause fetal loss. Other STDs must be ruled out. Third-trimester disease can cause prolonged rupture of membranes, premature delivery, chorioamnionitis, funisitis, neonatal sepsis, and perinatal distress and death. Ophthalmia neonatorum, the most common form of gonorrhea in neonates, is preventable by prophylactic 1% silver nitrate drops, but treatment requires systemic antibiotics.

7. *Gonococcal arthritis and disseminated gonococcal infection* (DGI)
   a. DGI strains resist bactericidal action of human serum and often do not incite inflammation at genital sites.
   b. Up to 13% of pts with DGI have terminal complement deficiencies.
   c. Menstruation is a risk factor for DGI; two-thirds of DGI cases are in women.
   d. A bacteremic phase, often not clinically recognized, precedes arthritis.
   e. Arthritis presents with painful joints in conjunction with tenosynovitis, skin lesions, and polyarthralgias of knees, elbows, and distal joints. Skin lesions develop in 75% of pts and include papules and pustules, often with hemorrhage. Suppurative arthritis affects one or two joints, most often knees, wrists, ankles, and elbows.

Laboratory Diagnosis

- Intracellular gram-negative cocci in urethral discharge collected from a male pt with Dacron or rayon swabs
- Culture on Thayer-Martin or other media selective for gonococci. Process immediately or store in candle extinction jars prior to incubation. Use special transport systems or culture media with CO_2-generating systems.
- Single culture of endocervical discharge has a sensitivity of 80–90%.
- DNA probe that hybridizes gonococcal 16S ribosomal RNA has good sensitivity, particularly in high-risk men, but no ability to provide susceptibility information.

℞ TREATMENT See Table 88-2.

Infections with *Chlamydia trachomatis*

Etiology

- Obligate intracellular bacteria in their own order, Chlamydiales
- Serovars D through K are associated with STDs. Serovars L1, L2, and L3 produce LGV. LGV strains are unique: they are unusually invasive, produce disease in lymphatic tissue, and grow in cell culture systems and macrophages.

Epidemiology

- Most common STDs in the United States; ~4 million cases per year
- Clinical spectrum parallels that of *N. gonorrhoeae*.
- Asymptomatic or mild clinical disease more common, but morbidity greater with *Chlamydia* than with *N. gonorrhoeae*

Table 88-2

Recommended Treatment for Gonococcal Infections: 2002 Guidelines of the Centers for Disease Control and Prevention

Diagnosis	Treatment of Choice
Uncomplicated gonococcal infection of the cervix, urethra, pharynx, or rectum[a]	
First-line regimens	Ceftriaxone (125 mg IM, single dose) *or* Ciprofloxacin (500 mg PO, single dose)[b] *or* Ofloxacin (400 mg PO, single dose)[b] *or* Levofloxacin (250 mg PO, single dose)[b] *or* Cefixime (400 mg PO, single dose)[c] *plus* If chlamydial infection is not ruled out: Azithromycin (1 g PO, single dose) *or* Doxycycline (100 mg PO bid for 7 days)
Alternative regimens	Spectinomycin (2 g IM, single dose) *or* Ceftizoxime (500 mg IM, single dose) *or* Cefotaxime (500 mg IM, single dose) *or* Cefotetan (1 g IM, single dose) plus probenecid (1 g PO, single dose) *or* Cefoxitin (2 g IM, single dose) plus probenecid (1 g PO, single dose)
Epididymitis	See text and Chap. 115, HPIM-16
Pelvic inflammatory disease	See text and Chap. 115, HPIM-16
Gonococcal conjunctivitis in an adult	Ceftriaxone (1 g IM, single dose)[d]
Ophthalmia neonatorum[e]	Ceftriaxone (25–50 mg/kg IV, single dose, not to exceed 125 mg)
Disseminated gonococcal infection[f] Initial therapy[g]	
Patient tolerant of β-lactam drugs	Ceftriaxone (1 g IM or IV q24h; recommended) *or* Cefotaxime (1 g IV q8h) *or* Ceftizoxime (1 g IV q8h)
Patients allergic to β-lactam drugs	Ciprofloxacin (500 mg IV q12h)[b] *or* Ofloxacin (400 mg IV q12h)[b] *or* Levofloxacin (500 mg IV q24h)[b] *or* Spectinomycin (2 g IM q12h)
Continuation therapy	Ciprofloxacin (500 mg PO bid)[b] *or* Ofloxacin (400 mg PO bid)[b] *or* Levofloxacin (500 mg PO qd)[b] *or* Cefixime (400 mg PO bid)[c]
Meningitis or endocarditis	See Chap. 128, HPIM-16[h]

[a] True failure of treatment with a recommended regimen is rare and should prompt an evaluation for reinfection or consideration of an alternative diagnosis. In cases of quinolone failure, the isolate should be tested for drug resistance if possible.

[b] Quinolones should not be used for infections acquired in Asia or the Pacific, including Hawaii and California. The use of quinolones is also inadvisable for treating infections acquired in other areas where the prevalence of quinolone-resistant *N. gonorrhoeae* (QRNG) is >1%, or in areas that are reporting increasing numbers of QRNG strains.

[c] Cefixime, a first-line recommendation for treatment of uncomplicated gonococcal infection (or continuation therapy for DGI), is currently unavailable in the United States.

[d] Plus lavage of the infected eye with saline solution (once).

[e] Prophylactic regimens are discussed in Chap. 128, HPIM-16.

[f] Hospitalization is indicated if the diagnosis is uncertain, if the pt has frank arthritis with an effusion, or if the pt cannot be relied on to adhere to treatment.

[g] All initial regimens should be continued for 24 to 48 h after clinical improvement begins, at which time therapy may be switched to one of the continuation regimens to complete a full week of antimicrobial treatment.

[h] Hospitalization is indicated to exclude suspected meningitis or endocarditis.

• *C. trachomatis* has been identified in the fallopian tubes or endometrium of up to half of women with PID. Infertility due to fallopian tube scarring has been strongly linked to antecedent *C. trachomatis* infection.

Clinical Syndromes

1. Urethritis, epididymitis, cervicitis, salpingitis, PID, and proctitis (discussed above)
2. Associated with Reiter's syndrome (conjunctivitis, urethritis or cervicitis, arthritis, mucocutaneous lesions). *C. trachomatis* is recovered from the urethra of up to 70% of men with nondiarrheal Reiter's and associated urethritis. More than 80% of pts have the HLA-B27 phenotype.
3. LGV: Primary genital lesion is noted in about one-third of heterosexual men, occasionally in women. The lesion is small and painless and heals in a few days. Local lymphadenitis then spreads to regional nodes; inguinal syndrome is the most common presentation in heterosexual men. Painful inguinal adenopathy develops 2–6 weeks after exposure. In two-thirds of cases, nodes are unilateral, matted, fluctuant, and suppurative, with overlying inflamed skin and draining fistulae. LGV is associated with systemic symptoms. Painful adenopathy above and below inguinal ligament presents with the "sign of the groove."

Diagnosis

• Direct microscopic examination of tissue scrapings is unreliable.
• Isolation of the organism in cell culture has low sensitivity with high cost.
• Chlamydial antigens or nucleic acid can be detected by direct immunofluorescent antibody (DFA) slide tests, ELISA, DNA-RNA hybridization, and PCR. Tests surpass culture in sensitivity and allow use of urine specimens rather than urethral or cervical swabs. In LGV, aspirate fluctuant buboes through normal skin for testing.
• Detection of antibody in serum or in local secretions is of limited usefulness except in LGV.

[Rx] **TREATMENT**

• See "Specific Syndromes," above.
• LGV: Doxycycline (100 mg PO bid) or erythromycin base (500 mg PO qid) for at least 3 weeks

Infections Due to Mycoplasmas

Etiology and Epidemiology

• Smallest free-living organisms known, lack a cell wall, resist in vitro cultivation
• *Mycoplasma hominis* and *Ureaplasma urealyticum* are the most prevalent genital mycoplasmas.
• Higher colonization rates in disadvantaged populations

Clinical Syndromes and Diagnosis

• Cause nongonococcal urethritis (NGU) and bacterial vaginosis; associated with PID
• Can be associated with reactive arthritis and Reiter's syndrome, which are usually due to *C. trachomatis*
• Ubiquity of the organism in the lower genital tract makes isolation attempts unnecessary in most cases. Microbiologic diagnosis is beyond the capability of most laboratories. Nucleic acid amplification tests have been developed.

TREATMENT

Current recommendations for treatment of NGU and PID are appropriate for genital mycoplasmas.

Syphilis

Etiology and Epidemiology

- Caused by *Treponema pallidum* subspecies *pallidum*, a thin, delicate organism with 6–14 spirals and tapered ends (6–15 μm long, 0.2 μm wide)
- Cases acquired by sexual contact with infectious lesions (chancre, mucous patch, skin rash, condyloma latum); nonsexual acquisition through close personal contact, infection in utero, and blood transfusion
- 31,575 reported cases in the United States in 2000
- High-risk populations changing—previously homosexual or bisexual men; 1990 peak among African-American heterosexuals in urban areas, correlated with exchange of sex for crack cocaine
- One-half of sexual contacts of persons with infectious syphilis become infected. All recently exposed sexual contacts are treated.

Pathogenesis Untreated syphilis penetrates intact mucous membranes or microscopic abrasions, entering lymphatics and blood within hours. Systemic infection and metastatic foci result. The primary lesion appears at the site of inoculation within 4–6 weeks and heals spontaneously. Generalized parenchymal (CNS, liver, lymph node), constitutional, and mucocutaneous manifestations of secondary syphilis appear 6–8 weeks later despite high antibody titers, subsiding in 2–6 weeks. A latent period follows. Eventually one-third of pts develop tertiary disease (syphilitic gummas, cardiovascular disease, neurologic disease), and one-quarter of those pts die.

Clinical Manifestations

1. *Primary*: chancre at site of inoculation (penis, rectum or anal canal, mouth, cervix, labia) after an incubation period of 9–90 days. The typical primary chancre is a painless papule progressing to a nontender, indurated ulcer with firm, nontender, bilateral inguinal adenopathy that can persist long after the chancre heals. Serology can be negative; repeat in 1–2 weeks.
2. *Secondary*: diffuse mucocutaneous lesions of variable morphologies, generalized nontender lymphadenopathy. Primary chancre may still be present. Initial lesions are bilaterally symmetric, pale red or pink, nonpruritic macules that progress to papules and may become necrotic. Lesions are widely distributed over the trunk and extremities, including the palms and soles. In moist intertriginous areas, papules can enlarge and erode to produce broad, highly infectious lesions called *condylomata lata*. Superficial mucosal erosions are called *mucous patches*. Constitutional symptoms are often present. The CNS is seeded by organisms in ≥30% of cases, although no clinical meningitis is evident. Less common findings include hepatitis, nephropathy, arthritis, optic neuritis, and anterior uveitis.
3. *Latent*: positive syphilis serology without clinical manifestations. Early latent syphilis develops within the first year of infection. Late latent syphilis, which develops >1 year after infection, is unlikely to cause infectious relapse. However, women with latent syphilis can infect the fetus in utero.
4. *Late*
   a. *CNS disease*: a continuum throughout syphilis. Asymptomatic CSF abnormalities exist in up to 40% of pts with primary or secondary syphilis and in 25% of those with latent disease. Symptomatic neurosyphilis develops only in this subset. Meningeal findings, including headache, nausea, vomiting, change in mental status, and neck stiff-

ness, often with associated uveitis or iritis, present within 1 year of infection. Meningovascular involvement (5–10 years after infection) usually presents as a subacute encephalitic prodrome and is followed by a gradually progressive vascular syndrome. Parenchymatous involvement presents at 20 years for general paresis and 25–30 years for tabes dorsalis. A general mnemonic for paresis is *p*ersonality, *af*fect, *r*eflexes (hyperactive), *e*ye (Argyll Robertson pupils, which react to accommodation but not to light), *s*ensorium (illusions, delusions, hallucinations), *i*ntellect (decrease in recent memory and orientation, judgment, calculations, insight), and *s*peech. Tabes dorsalis is a demyelination of posterior columns, dorsal roots, and dorsal root ganglia, with ataxic, wide-based gait and footslap; paresthesia; bladder disturbances; impotence; areflexia; and loss of position, deep pain, and temperature sensations. Trophic joint degeneration (Charcot's joints), optic atrophy, and Argyll Robertson pupils are also present.

b. *Cardiovascular syphilis*: About 10% of pts with untreated late latent syphilis develop cardiovascular symptoms 10–40 years later. Endarteritis obliterans of the vasa vasorum providing the blood supply to large vessels results in aortitis, aortic regurgitation, saccular aneurysm, and coronary ostial stenosis.

c. *Late benign syphilis (gumma)*: Usually solitary lesions showing granulomatous inflammation with central necrosis are found most often in the skin and skeletal system, mouth, upper respiratory tract, liver, and stomach.

5. *Congenital*: Syphilis can be transmitted throughout pregnancy. Lesions begin to be manifest in the fetus at ~4 months of gestation. All pregnant women should be tested for syphilis early in pregnancy.

Diagnosis

- Dark-field microscopy of lesion exudates or direct fluorescent antibody *T. pallidum* (DFA-TP) test in fixed smears from suspect lesions
- Nontreponemal serologic tests that measure IgG and IgM directed against a cardiolipin-lecithin-cholesterol antigen complex [e.g., rapid plasmin reagin (RPR), VDRL]
- Treponemal serologic tests: agglutination assay (e.g., the Serodia TP-PA test) and the fluorescent treponemal antibody–absorbed (FTA-ABS) test. Results remain positive even after successful treatment.
- Three uses of serology: screening or diagnosis, quantitation of titers (e.g., with RPR) to monitor response to treatment, and confirmation of the diagnosis in a pt with a positive nontreponemal test
- LP is recommended for pts with syphilis and neurologic signs or symptoms, other late syphilis manifestations, or suspected treatment failure and for HIV-infected pts with untreated syphilis of unknown or >1 year's duration. CSF exam demonstrates pleocytosis and increased protein. A positive CSF VDRL test is specific but not sensitive; an unabsorbed FTA test is sensitive but not specific. A negative unabsorbed FTA test excludes neurosyphilis.
- Pts with syphilis should be evaluated for HIV disease.

⟦Rx⟧ **TREATMENT**   See Table 88-3.

- Jarisch-Herxheimer reaction: a dramatic reaction to treatment most commonly seen with initiation of therapy for primary (~50% of pts) or secondary (~90%) syphilis. The reaction is associated with fever, chills, myalgias, tachycardia, headache, tachypnea, and vasodilation. Symptoms subside within 12–24 h without treatment.

Table 88-3

Recommendations for the Treatment of Syphilis[a]

Stage of Syphilis	Patients without Penicillin Allergy	Patients with Confirmed Penicillin Allergy
Primary, secondary, or early latent	Penicillin G benzathine (single dose of 2.4 mU IM)	Tetracycline hydrochloride (500 mg PO qid) *or* doxycycline (100 mg PO bid) for 2 weeks

Late latent (or latent of uncertain duration), cardiovascular, or benign tertiary	Lumbar puncture
	    CSF normal: Penicillin G benzathine (2.4 mU IM weekly for 3 weeks)
	    CSF abnormal: Treat as neurosyphilis
		Lumbar puncture
		    CSF normal and pt not infected with HIV: Tetracycline hydrochloride (500 mg PO qid) *or* doxycycline (100 mg PO bid) for 4 weeks
		    CSF normal and pt infected with HIV: Densensitization and treatment with penicillin if compliance cannot be ensured
		    CSF abnormal: Treat as neurosyphilis

Neurosyphilis (asymptomatic or symptomatic)	Aqueous penicillin G (18–24 mU/d IV, given as 3–4 mU q4h or continuous infusion) for 10–14 days *or* Aqueous penicillin G procaine (2.4 mU/d IM) plus oral probenecid (500 mg qid), both for 10–14 days	Desensitization and treatment with penicillin
Syphilis in pregnancy	According to stage	Desensitization and treatment with penicillin

[a] See Chap. 153, HPIM-16, for full discussion of syphilis therapy in HIV-infected individuals.
NOTE: mU, million units.
Source: These recommendations are based on those issued by the Centers for Disease Control and Prevention in 2002.

- Response to treatment should be monitored with RPR or VDRL titers at 6 and 12 months (every 3 months in HIV-infected persons) in early syphilis and at 6, 12, and 24 months for late or latent syphilis. If the titer rises by 4-fold or fails to fall by 4-fold in primary or secondary syphilis or in pts with latent or late syphilis whose initial titers are ≥1:32, or if symptoms persist or recur, the pt should be re-treated and evaluated with LP to exclude neurosyphilis. In treated neurosyphilis, CSF cell counts should be monitored every

6 months for 2 years or until normal, and quantitative RPR or VDRL should be monitored every 6 months for 2 years.

Herpes Simplex Virus Infections

Etiology and Epidemiology

• HSV is a linear, double-strand DNA virus packaged in a regular icosahedral protein shell (capsid) composed of 162 capsomers.
• More than 90% of adults in the United States have antibodies to HSV-1 by age 50; ~20% of the U.S. population has antibodies to HSV-2.
• A large reservoir of unidentified carriers of HSV-2 and frequent asymptomatic reactivations of virus from the genital tract foster the continued spread of HSV disease.
• Genital lesions caused by HSV-1 have lower recurrence rates in the first year (~55%) than those caused by HSV-2 (~90%).

Clinical Manifestations First episodes of genital herpes can be associated with fever, headache, malaise, and myalgias. Lesions, which typically develop after an incubation period of 2–7 days, consist of bilateral vesicles or pustules or a cluster of painful ulcers on the external genitalia. More than 80% of women with primary genital herpes have cervical or urethral involvement. Local symptoms include pain, dysuria, vaginal and urethral discharge, and tender inguinal lymphadenopathy.

Diagnosis

• Staining of scrapings with Wright's or Giemsa's (Tzanck preparation) to detect giant cells or intranuclear inclusions is well described, but most clinicians are not skilled in these techniques, which furthermore do not differentiate between HSV and varicella-zoster virus.
• Isolation of HSV in tissue culture or demonstration of HSV antigens or DNA in scrapings from lesions is the most accurate diagnostic method. PCR is increasingly being used for detection of HSV DNA and is more sensitive than culture at mucosal sites.

℞ TREATMENT

• *First episodes*: acyclovir (400 mg tid), valacyclovir (1 g bid), or famciclovir (250 mg bid) for 10–14 days
• *Recurrent episodes*: acyclovir (800 mg bid for 2 days), valacyclovir (500 mg bid for 3–5 days), or famciclovir (125 mg bid for 5 days)
• *Suppression*: acyclovir (400 mg bid or 800 mg qd), valacyclovir (500 mg qd for pts with <9 episodes per year; otherwise, 1g qd or 500 mg bid), or famciclovir (250 mg bid)

Chancroid (*Haemophilus ducreyi* Infection)

Epidemiology Significant problem in developing countries, increasing incidence in the United States, associated with HIV infection because of genital ulcerations

Clinical Manifestations After an incubation period of 4–7 days, a papule with surrounding erythema appears and evolves into a pustule that ruptures and forms a sharply circumscribed, nonindurated ulcer. Lesions bleed easily. Half of pts develop tender inguinal adenopathy. Nodes become fluctuant and can rupture. Multiple ulcers can coalesce to form giant ulcers.

Diagnosis PCR or culture for *H. ducreyi*

TREATMENT

Azithromycin (1 g PO once), ciprofloxacin (500 mg PO bid for 3 days), ceftriaxone (250 mg IM once), or erythromycin base (500 mg tid for 1 week)

Donovanosis (*Calymmatobacterium granulomatis* Infection)

Etiology and Epidemiology Also known as *granuloma inguinale* and *granuloma venereum*, donovanosis is caused by *C. granulomatis*, an intracellular, gram-negative, pleomorphic, encapsulated bacterium that is closely related to *Klebsiella* species. The infection is endemic in the Caribbean, southern Africa, and southeastern India and among Aborigines in Australia. Fewer than 20 cases are reported annually in the United States.

Clinical Manifestations An incubation period of 1–4 weeks is followed by SC nodules that erode through the skin to produce granulomatous, sharply demarcated, painless ulcers that bleed easily. Lesions slowly enlarge, causing genital swelling (especially of the labia), with occasional progression to pseudoelephantiasis. Extragenital lesions occur in 6% of pts.

Diagnosis Typical intracellular Donovan bodies are seen within large mononuclear cells in smears from lesions or biopsy specimens. PCR and serology are available.

 TREATMENT

Azithromycin (1 g weekly until healing of lesions, usually 3–5 weeks). Doxycycline (100 mg bid) is an alternative.

Human Papillomavirus (HPV) Infections

Etiology Papillomaviruses are nonenveloped, double-strand DNA viruses with icosahedral capsids composed of 72 capsomers. HPV-6 and HPV-11 are associated with anogenital warts (condylomata acuminata). HPV types 16, 18, 31, 33, and 45 have been most strongly associated with cervical cancers. Most infections, including those with oncogenic types, are self-limited.

Clinical Manifestations
- Incubation period of 3–4 months (range, 1 month to 2 years)
- Common warts and plantar warts
- Anogenital warts on the skin and mucosal surfaces of genitalia and perianal areas

Diagnosis
- Direct visualization (may be aided by application of 3–5% acetic acid solution to lesions)
- Papanicolaou smears from cervical or anal scrapings show cytologic evidence of HPV infection.
- PCR or hybrid-capture assays of lesions

 TREATMENT

Many lesions resolve spontaneously. Current treatment is not completely effective, and some agents have significant side effects.

1. *Provider-administered therapy* includes: cryotherapy, podophyllin resin (10–25%), trichloroacetic acid or bichloroacetic acid (80–90%), surgical excision, intralesionally administered interferon, laser surgery.

2. *Patient-administered therapy* includes: podofilox (0.5% solution or gel) or imiquimod (topically applied interferon inducer; 5% cream).

For a more detailed discussion, see Holmes KK: Sexually Transmitted Diseases: Overview and Clinical Approach, Chap. 115, p. 762; Ram S, Rice PA: Gonococcal Infections, Chap. 128, p. 855; Murphy TF: *Haemophilus* **Infections, Chap. 130, p. 864; Hart G: Donovanosis, Chap. 145, p. 932; Lukehart SA: Syphilis, Chap. 153, p. 977; McCormack WM: Infections Due to Mycoplasmas, Chap. 159, p. 1008; Stamm WE: Chlamydial Infections, Chap. 160, p. 1011; Corey L: Herpes Simplex Viruses, Chap. 163, p. 1035; and Reichman RC: Human Papillomavirus Infections, Chap. 169, p. 1056, in HPIM-16.**

89

INFECTIONS OF THE SKIN, SOFT TISSUES, JOINTS, AND BONES

SKIN AND SOFT TISSUE INFECTIONS

Protection of the avascular epithelium of the skin against infection depends on the mechanical barrier afforded by the stratum corneum. If this barrier is disrupted, infections of deeper tissue can result. Infection can also spread via hair follicles and lymphatics. The rich capillary plexus below the dermal papillae is the site of infective vasculitic findings (e.g., petechiae, purpura) and metastatic infection (e.g., meningococcal infection). This plexus gives organisms access to the circulation, facilitating local spread and bacteremia.

Skin and soft tissue infections are diagnosed principally by a careful history (e.g., temporal progression, travel history, animal exposure, bites, trauma, underlying medical conditions) and physical examination (appearance of lesions and distribution). Types of skin and soft tissue manifestations include the following.

1. *Vesicles*: due to proliferation of organisms, usually viruses, within the epidermis (e.g., varicella; herpes simplex; infections with coxsackievirus, poxviruses, *Rickettsia akari*)

2. *Bullae*: caused by toxin-producing organisms. Different entities affect different skin levels (e.g., staphylococcal scalded-skin syndrome and toxic epidermal necrolysis cause cleavage of the stratum corneum and the stratum germinativum, respectively). Bullae are also seen in necrotizing fasciitis, gas gangrene, and *Vibrio vulnificus* infection in pts with cirrhosis who have ingested contaminated raw seafood or been exposed to Gulf of Mexico or Atlantic seaboard waters.

3. *Crusted lesions*: Impetigo caused by either *Streptococcus pyogenes* (impetigo contagiosa) or *Staphylococcus aureus* (bullous impetigo) usually starts with a bullous phase before crusting. It is important to recognize impetigo contagiosa because of its relation to poststreptococcal glomerulonephritis. Crusted lesions are also seen in some systemic fungal infections, dermatophytic infections, and cutaneous mycobacterial infection.

4.   *Folliculitis*: Localized infection of hair follicles is usually due to *S. aureus*. "Hot-tub folliculitis" is a diffuse condition caused by *Pseudomonas aeruginosa*. Freshwater avian schistosomes cause swimmer's itch.

5.   *Papular and nodular lesions*: can be caused by *Bartonella* (cat-scratch disease), *Treponema pallidum*, papillomavirus, mycobacteria, and helminths

6.   *Ulcers, with or without eschars*: can be caused by cutaneous anthrax, ulceroglandular tularemia, plague, mycobacterial infection, and (in the case of genital lesions) chancroid or syphilis

7.   *Erysipelas*: Lymphangitis of the dermis, with abrupt onset of fiery red swelling of the face or extremities, well-defined indurated margins, intense pain, and rapid progression. *S. pyogenes* is the exclusive cause (see Chap. 95).

Cellulitis

DEFINITION   Cellulitis, an acute inflammatory condition of the skin, is characterized by localized pain, erythema, swelling, and heat.

ETIOLOGY

• May be caused by indigenous skin flora (e.g., *S. aureus*, *S. pyogenes*). *S. aureus* cellulitis spreads from a central localized infection site. *S. pyogenes* can cause a rapidly spreading, diffuse process, often with fever and lymphangitis; recurrent episodes occur in association with chronic venous stasis and lymphedema. Group B streptococcal cellulitis is associated with older age, diabetes, and peripheral vascular disease.

• May also be caused by exogenous bacteria. A thorough history and epidemiologic data may help identify the cause.

1.   *Pasteurella multocida*: cat and dog bites
2.   *Capnocytophaga canimorsus*, *Streptococcus intermedius*: dog bites
3.   Anaerobes (e.g., *Fusobacterium*, *Bacteroides*, streptococci, *Eikenella corrodens*): dog and human bites
4.   *Aeromonas hydrophila*: lacerations sustained in fresh water
5.   *P. aeruginosa*: penetrating injury (stepping on a nail), "hot-tub" folliculitis, or ecthyma gangrenosum in neutropenic pts
6.   *Erysipelothrix rhusiopathiae*: contact with domestic swine and fish

DIAGNOSIS   If there is a wound or portal of entry, Gram's staining and culture may identify the etiology. If both a wound and a portal of entry are lacking, aspiration or biopsy of the leading edge of the cellulitis tissue yields a diagnosis in only about one-fifth of cases.

 TREATMENT

See Table 89-1. A typical course is 2 weeks. IV therapy is usually given until inflammation and systemic signs and symptoms have improved.

Necrotizing Fasciitis

DEFINITION   Necrotizing fasciitis is caused by either *S. pyogenes* or mixed aerobic and anaerobic bacteria, usually of GI or genitourinary origin. Infection, either apparent or inapparent, results from a breach in integrity of skin or mucous membrane barriers.

Clinical Features

• Onset of severe pain and fever, with minimal physical findings; rapid progression to swelling; brawny edema; dark red induration; bullae; friable, necrotic skin

Table 89-1

Treatment of Common Infections of the Skin

Diagnosis/Condition	Primary Treatment
Animal bite (prophylaxis or early infection)[a]	Amoxicillin/clavulanate, 875/125 mg PO bid
Animal bite[a] (established infection)	Ampicillin/sulbactam, 1.5–3.0 g IV q6h
Bacillary angiomatosis	Erythromycin, 500 mg PO qid
Herpes simplex (primary genital)	Acyclovir, 400 mg PO tid for 10 days
Herpes zoster (immunocompetent host >50 years of age)	Acyclovir, 800 mg PO 5 times daily for 7–10 days
Cellulitis (staphylococcal or streptococcal[b,c])	Nafcillin or oxacillin, 2 g IV q4–6h
Necrotizing fasciitis (group A streptococcal[b])	Clindamycin, 600–900 mg IV q6–8h *plus* Penicillin G, 4 million units IV q4h
Necrotizing fasciitis (mixed aerobes and anaerobes)	Ampicillin, 2 g IV q4h *plus* Clindamycin, 600–900 mg IV q6–8h *plus* Ciprofloxacin, 400 mg IV q6–8h
Gas gangrene	Clindamycin, 600–900 mg IV q6–8h *plus* Penicillin G, 4 million units IV q4–6h

[a] *Pasteurella multocida*, a species commonly associated with both dog and cat bites, is resistant to cephalexin, dicloxacillin, clindamycin, and erythromycin. *Eikenella corrodens*, a bacterium commonly associated with human bites, is resistant to clindamycin, penicillinase-resistant penicillins, and metronidazole but is sensitive to trimethoprim-sulfamethoxazole and fluoroquinolones.

[b] The frequency of erythromycin resistance in group A *Streptococcus* is currently ~5% in the United States but has reached 70 to 100% in some other countries. Most, but not all, erythromycin-resistant group A streptococci are susceptible to clindamycin. Approximately 90 to 95% of *Staphylococcus aureus* strains are sensitive to clindamycin.

[c] Severe hospital-acquired *S. aureus* infections or community-acquired *S. aureus* infections that are not responding to the β-lactam antibiotics recommended in this table may be caused by methicillin-resistant strains, requiring a switch to vancomycin or linezolid.

Alternative Treatment	See Also HPIM-16 Chap(s).
Doxycycline, 100 mg PO bid	. . .
Clindamycin, 600–900 mg IV q8h *plus* Ciprofloxacin, 400 mg IV q12h *or* Cefoxitin, 2 g IV q6h	. . .
Doxycycline, 100 mg PO bid	144
Famciclovir, 250 mg PO tid for 5–10 days *or* Valacyclovir, 1000 mg PO bid for 10 days	163
Famciclovir, 500 mg PO tid for 7–10 days *or* Valacyclovir, 1000 mg PO tid for 7 days	164
Cefazolin, 1–2 g q8h *or* Ampicillin/sulbactam, 1.5–3.0 g IV q6h *or* Erythromycin, 0.5–1.0 g IV q6h *or* Clindamycin, 600–900 mg IV q8h	120, 121
Clindamycin, 600–900 mg IV q6–8h *plus* Cephalosporin (first- or second-generation)	121
Vancomycin, 1 g IV q6h *plus* Metronidazole, 500 mg IV q6h *plus* Ciprofloxacin, 400 mg IV q6–8h	148
Clindamycin, 600–900 mg IV q6–8h *plus* Cefoxitin, 2 g IV q6h	126

- Thrombosis of blood vessels in dermal papillae leads to ischemia of peripheral nerves and anesthesia of the affected area.
- Infection spreads to deep fascia and along fascial planes through venous channels and lymphatics.
- Pts are toxic and develop shock and multiorgan failure.

DIAGNOSIS Diagnosis is based on clinical presentation. Other findings may include: (1) renal failure, often preceding shock and hypotension; (2) gas in tissue (in mixed infections but rarely with *S. pyogenes*); and (3) markedly elevated serum creatine phosphokinase levels.

TREATMENT

> • Emergent surgical exploration to deep fascia and muscle, with removal of necrotic tissue.
> • For antibiotic choices, see Table 89-1.

Myositis/Myonecrosis

DEFINITIONS

• *Myositis*: can be caused by viruses (influenza virus, dengue virus, coxsackievirus), parasites (*Trichinella*, cysticerci, *Toxoplasma*), or bacteria (clostridia, streptococci). This condition usually manifests with myalgias, but pain can be severe in coxsackievirus, *Trichinella*, and bacterial infections.
• *Pyomyositis*: localized muscle infection, usually due to *S. aureus*
• *Myonecrosis*: caused by clostridial species (*C. perfringens, C. septicum, C. histolyticum*) or by mixed aerobic and anaerobic bacteria. Myonecrosis is usually related to trauma; however, spontaneous gangrene—usually due to *C. septicum*—can occur in pts with neutropenia, GI malignancy, or diverticulosis. Myonecrosis can also occur with necrotizing fasciitis in ~50% of cases.

DIAGNOSIS AND TREATMENT

• Emergent surgical intervention to remove necrotic tissue, provide visualization of deep structures, obtain materials for culture and sensitivity testing, and reduce compartment pressure
• For antibiotic choices, see Table 89-1.

INFECTIOUS ARTHRITIS

Joints become infected by hematogenous seeding (the most common route), spread from a contiguous site of infection, or direct inoculation (e.g., during trauma or surgery).

ETIOLOGY AND CLINICAL FEATURES

• Children <5 years: *S. aureus, S. pyogenes, Kingella kingae*
• Young adults: *Neisseria gonorrhoeae, S. aureus*
• Adults: *S. aureus, N. gonorrhoeae*, gram-negative bacilli, pneumococci, streptococci (groups A, B, C, F, and G)

Nongonococcal Bacterial Arthritis Risk is increased in pts with rheumatoid arthritis, diabetes mellitus, glucocorticoid therapy, hemodialysis, malignancy, and IV drug use. An extraarticular focus is found in ~25% of pts.

In 90% of pts, one joint is involved—most often the knee, which is followed in frequency by the hip, shoulder, wrist, and elbow. IV drug users often have spinal, sacroiliac, or sternoclavicular joint involvement. Pts have moderate to severe pain, effusion, decreased range of motion, and fever. Gram-positive cocci (most commonly *S. aureus*, followed by streptococci of groups A and G) cause 75% of cases.

Gonococcal Arthritis Women are more likely than men to develop disseminated gonococcal disease, particularly during menses and during pregnancy (see Chap. 88). True gonococcal arthritis usually affects a single joint: hip, knee, ankle, or wrist.

Prosthetic Joint Infection

• Complicates 1–4% of joint replacements
• Usually acquired intra- or perioperatively
• Acute presentations are seen in infections caused by *S. aureus*, pyogenic streptococci, and enteric bacilli.

- Indolent presentations are seen in infections caused by coagulase-negative staphylococci and diphtheroids.

Miscellaneous Etiologies Other causes of septic arthritis include Lyme disease, tuberculosis and other mycobacterial infections, fungal infections (coccidioidomycosis, histoplasmosis), and viral infections (rubella, mumps, hepatitis B, parvovirus).

Reiter's Arthritis Reiter's arthritis follows ~1% of cases of nongonococcal urethritis and 2% of enteric infections due to *Yersinia enterocolitica, Shigella flexneri, Campylobacter jejuni,* and *Salmonella* species in genetically susceptible pts.

DIAGNOSIS Infection of the joint is evidenced by clinical signs and symptoms. Examination of synovial fluid from the affected joint is essential. *Normal* synovial fluid contains <180 cells (mostly mononuclear)/μL. *Acute bacterial infection* of joints results in synovial fluid cell counts averaging 100,000/μL (range, 25,000 to 250,000/μL), with >90% PMNs. Synovial fluid in *gonococcal arthritis* contains >50,000 cells/μL, but results of Gram's staining are usually negative, and cultures of synovial fluid are positive in <40% of cases. Other mucosal sites should be cultured to diagnose gonorrhea. Pts with septic arthritis due to *mycobacteria* or *fungi* can have 10,000 to 30,000 cells/μL in synovial fluid, with 50–70% PMNs. Synovial fluid cell counts in *noninfectious inflammatory arthritides* are typically 30,000 to 50,000/μL.

Gram's staining of synovial fluid should be performed, and injection of fluid into blood culture bottles can increase the yield of synovial fluid cultures. Fluid should be examined for crystals to rule out gout or pseudogout, and an attempt should be made to identify the extraarticular source of hematogenous seeding.

Blood for cultures should be taken before initiation of antibiotic therapy. Blood cultures are positive in up to 50% of cases due to *S. aureus* and are less common with other organisms.

Plain radiographs show soft tissue swelling, joint space widening, and displacement of tissue planes by distended capsule. Narrowing of the joint space and bony erosions suggest advanced disease.

℞ TREATMENT

Drainage of pus and necrotic debris is needed to cure infection and to prevent destruction of cartilage, postinfectious degenerative arthritis, and joint deformity or instability.

Empirical antibiotics can include oxacillin (2 g q4h) if gram-positive cocci are seen in synovial fluid; vancomycin (1 g q12h) if methicillin-resistant *S. aureus* is a concern; or ceftriaxone (1 g q24h) if no organism is evident (to cover community-acquired organisms). In IV drug users, treatment for gram-negative organisms such as *P. aeruginosa* should be considered. After definitive diagnosis, treatment should be adjusted. Treatment for *S. aureus* should be given for 4 weeks, that for enteric gram-negative bacilli for 3–4 weeks, and that for pneumococci or streptococci for 2 weeks. Treatment of gonococcal arthritis should commence with ceftriaxone (1 g/d) until improvement and can be completed with an oral fluoroquinolone (e.g., ciprofloxacin, 500 mg bid). If fluoroquinolone resistance is not prevalent, a fluoroquinolone can be given for the entire course.

Prosthetic joint infections should be treated with surgery and high-dose IV antibiotics for 4–6 weeks. The prosthesis often has to be removed; to avoid joint removal, antibiotic suppression of infection may be tried. A 3- to 6-month course of ciprofloxacin and rifampin has been successful in *S. aureus* prosthetic joint infections of relatively short duration.

OSTEOMYELITIS
DEFINITIONS

1. *Osteomyelitis*: infection of bone caused by pyogenic bacteria and myco-bacteria that gain access to bone by the hematogenous route (20% of cases, primarily in children), via direct spread from a contiguous focus of infec-tion, or by a penetrating wound
2. *Sequestra*: ischemic necrosis of bone resulting in the separation of large devascularized bone fragments; caused when pus spreads into vascular channels
3. *Involucrum*: elevated periosteum deposits of new bone around a sequestrum

CLINICAL FEATURES *Acute Hematogenous Osteomyelitis* This condition usually involves a single bone (long bones in children), presenting as an acute febrile illness with localized pain and tenderness. Restriction of move-ment or difficulty bearing weight is often evident. Infection may extend to joint spaces. In adults, vertebral bodies are most often involved. Organisms seed the end plate and extend into the disk space and thence to adjacent vertebral bodies. A prior history of degenerative disease or trauma is common. Diabetic pts, pts undergoing hemodialysis, and IV drug users are at increased risk. Bacteremic infections or UTIs are common sources in older men. The lumbar and cervical spine is often involved in pyogenic infections and the thoracic spine in tuber-culosis. Pts can present either acutely, with ongoing bacteremia, or indolently, with vague dull pain that increases over weeks and low-grade or no fever.

Spinal epidural abscess may complicate vertebral osteomyelitis, presenting as spinal pain and progressing to radicular pain and/or weakness; it is best diagnosed by MRI and must be treated urgently to prevent neurologic compli-cations.

Usually, a single organism causes acute hematogenous osteomyelitis; *S. au-reus* accounts for ~50% of cases. Other common pathogens include gram-negative bacilli. Less common causes include *Mycobacterium tuberculosis*, *Brucella*, and fungi.

Osteomyelitis from a Contiguous Focus of Infection

• Accounts for ~80% of all cases
• Includes osteomyelitis in the setting of bites, puncture wounds, open frac-tures, peripheral vascular disease (particularly in diabetic adults), and foreign bodies
• Although *S. aureus* is one of the pathogens in more than half of cases, infections are often polymicrobial and involve gram-negative and anaerobic bacteria as well.

Chronic Osteomyelitis

• More likely to develop after infection from a contiguous source of infection than is acute hematogenous osteomyelitis
• The presence of a foreign body also increases risk.
• The clinical course is prolonged and is characterized by quiescent periods with acute exacerbations, lack of fever, and development of sinus tracts that can occasionally drain pus or bits of necrotic bone.

DIAGNOSIS ESR and C-reactive protein levels are usually increased in acute infection and can be used to monitor the response to treatment.

Imaging studies are important in the diagnosis of osteomyelitis, but there is a lack of consensus about their optimal use (see Table 89-2). Conditions due to noninfectious etiologies can be distinguished from osteomyelitis by imaging studies because the former do not usually cross the disk space.

Table 89-2

Diagnostic Imaging Studies for Osteomyelitis

Type of Study	Comments
Plain radiographs	Insensitive, especially in early osteomyelitis. May show periosteal elevation after 10 days, lytic changes after 2–6 weeks. Useful to look for anatomical abnormalities (e.g., fractures, bony variants, or deformities), foreign bodies, and soft tissue gas.
Three-phase bone scan (^{99m}Tc-MDP)	Characteristic finding in osteomyelitis: increased uptake in all three phases of scan. Highly sensitive ($\sim$95%) in acute infection; somewhat less sensitive if blood flow to bone is poor. Specificity moderate if plain films are normal, but poor in presence of neuropathic arthropathy, fractures, tumor, infarction.
Other radionuclide scans	Examples: ^{67}Ga-citrate, ^{111}In-labeled WBCs. ^{111}In-WBCs more specific than gallium but not always available. Often used in conjunction with bone scan because its greater specificity for inflammation than ^{99m}Tc-MDP helps to distinguish infectious from noninfectious processes. Lack of consensus over role in routine evaluation.
Ultrasound	May detect subperiosteal fluid collection or soft tissue abscess adjacent to bone, but largely supplanted by CT and MRI.
CT	Limited role in acute osteomyelitis. In chronic osteomyelitis, excellent for detection of sequestra, cortical destruction, soft tissue abscesses, and sinus tracts. Use may be limited by metallic foreign body.
MRI	As sensitive as ^{99m}Tc-MDP bone scan for acute osteomyelitis ($\sim$95%); detects changes in water content of marrow before disruption of cortical bone. High specificity ($\sim$87%), with better anatomical detail than nuclear studies. Procedure of choice for vertebral osteomyelitis because of high sensitivity for epidural abscess. Use may be limited by metallic foreign body.

Abbreviations: CT, computed tomography; MDP, monodiphosphonate; MRI, magnetic resonance imaging; WBCs, white blood cells.

If at all possible, appropriate samples for microbiologic studies should be obtained before antibiotic treatment. Blood should be cultured in acute hematogenous osteomyelitis. The results of cultures from sinus tracts do not correlate well with organisms infecting the bone; thus bone samples for cultures must be obtained either percutaneously or intraoperatively.

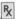 **TREATMENT**

Antibiotics used for therapy (see Table 89-3) should be bactericidal and given at high doses, usually commencing with IV administration.

1. *Acute hematogenous osteomyelitis in children*: 4–6 weeks of treatment. After 5–10 days, high-dose oral treatment can be used.

Table 89-3

Selection of Antibiotics for Treatment of Acute Osteomyelitis

Organism	Suggested Regimen[a]	
	Primary	Alternative[b]
Staphylococcus aureus		
Penicillin-resistant, methicillin-sensitive (MSSA)	Nafcillin or oxacillin, 2 g IV q4h	Cefazolin, 1 g IV q8h; ceftriaxone, 1 g IV q24h; clinda-mycin, 900 mg IV q8h[c]
Penicillin-sensitive	Penicillin, 3–4 million U IV q4h	Cefazolin, ceftriaxone, clindamycin (as above)
Methicillin-resistant (MRSA)	Vancomycin, 15 mg/kg (up to 1 g) IV q12h	Clindamycin (as above); linezolid, 600 mg IV or PO q12h[d]; daptomycin, 4–6 mg/kg per day IV[d]
Streptococci (including *S. milleri*, β-hemolytic streptococci)	Penicillin (as above)	Cefazolin, ceftriaxone, clindamycin (as above)
Gram-negative aerobic bacilli		
Escherichia coli, other "sensitive" species	Ampicillin, 2 g IV q4h; cefazolin, 1 g IV q8h	Ceftriaxone, 1 g IV q24h; parenteral or oral fluoroquino-lone (e.g., ciprofloxacin, 400 mg IV or 750 mg PO q12h[e]
Pseudomonas aeruginosa	Extended-spectrum β-lactam agent (e.g., piperacillin, 3–4 g IV q4–6h, or ceftazidime, 2 g IV q12h) *plus* tobramy-cin, 5–7 mg/kg q24h[f]	May substitute parenteral or oral fluoroquinolone for β-lactam agent
Enterobacter spp., other "resistant" species	Extended-spectrum β-lactam agent IV or fluoroquinolone IV or PO[e] (as above)	
Mixed infections possibly involving anaerobic bac-teria	Ampicillin/sulbactam, 1.5–3 g IV q6h; piperacillin/tazo-bactam, 3.375 g IV q6h	Cefotetan, 1–2 g IV q12h; combination of fluoroquino-lone plus clindamycin (as above)

[a] Duration of treatment is discussed in the text.
[b] Cephalosporins may be used for the treatment of patients allergic to penicillin whose reaction did not consist of anaphylaxis or urticaria (immediate-type hypersensitivity).
[c] Because of the possibility of inducible resistance, clindamycin must be used with caution for the treatment of strains resistant to erythromycin. Consult clinical microbiology laboratory.
[d] Experience is limited; there are anecdotal reports of efficacy.
[e] Oral fluoroquinolones must not be coadministered with divalent cations (calcium, magnesium, iron, aluminum), which block the drugs' absorption.
[f] Tobramycin levels and renal function must be monitored closely to minimize the risks of nephro- and ototoxicity.

2. *Vertebral osteomyelitis*: 4–6 weeks of treatment. Consider a longer course if the ESR does not decline by at least two-thirds. The majority of epidural abscesses require surgical intervention.

3. *Contiguous-focus osteomyelitis*: surgical debridement and 4–6 weeks of treatment unless only the outer cortex of bone is involved. In the latter situation, a 2-week course of antibiotic treatment after thorough debridement has had excellent success.

4. *Chronic osteomyelitis*: It should be decided whether aggressive treatment is warranted or intermittent antibiotic therapy to suppress exacerbations is adequate. Otherwise, surgery and 4–6 weeks of antibiotic therapy can be tried. The value of further suppressive antibiotic treatment remains unproven.

For a more detailed discussion, see Stevens DL: Infections of the Skin, Muscle, and Soft Tissues, Chap. 110, p. 740; Parsonnet J, Maguire JH: Osteomyelitis, Chap. 111, p. 745; and Madoff LC et al: Infectious Arthritis, Chap. 314, p. 2050, in HPIM-16.

90

INFECTIONS IN THE IMMUNOCOMPROMISED HOST

The immunocompromised pt is at increased risk for infection with both common and opportunistic pathogens. Acquired disease, loss of physical barriers, or inborn immune defects lower a person's immunity. Cancer pts and transplant recipients are at particular risk.

INFECTIONS IN CANCER PTS

Table 90-1 lists the normal barriers to infection whose disruption may permit infections in cancer pts.

SYSTEM-SPECIFIC SYNDROMES

- Skin infections

  1. Cellulitis caused by streptococci or staphylococci or by unusual (in this setting) organisms such as *Escherichia coli*, *Pseudomonas*, or fungi
  2. Macules or papules due to bacteria (e.g., *Pseudomonas aeruginosa* causing ecthyma gangrenosum) or fungi (*Candida*)
  3. Sweet's syndrome or febrile neutrophilic dermatosis: most often seen in neutropenic leukemic pts; red or bluish-red papules or nodules that form sharply bordered plaques
  4. Erythema multiforme with mucous membrane involvement due to herpes simplex virus (HSV)
  5. Drug-associated Stevens-Johnson syndrome

- Catheter-related infections: If a red streak develops over the SC part of a "tunneled" catheter, the device must be removed to prevent extensive cellulitis and tissue necrosis. Exit-site infections caused by coagulase-negative staphylococci can be treated with vancomycin without catheter removal. Infections

Table 90-1

Normal Barriers to Infections

Type of Defense	Specific Lesion	Cells Involved	Organism	Cancer Association	Disease
Physical barrier	Breaks in skin	Skin epithelial cells	Staphylococci, streptococci	Head and neck, squamous cell carcinoma	Cellulitis, extensive skin infection
Emptying of fluid collections	Occlusion of orifices: ureters, bile duct, colon	Luminal epithelial cells	Gram-negative bacilli	Renal, ovarian, biliary tree, metastatic diseases of many cancers	Rapid, overwhelming bacteremia, urinary tract infection
Lymphatic disease	Node dissection	Lymph nodes	Staphylococci, streptococci	Breast cancer surgery	Cellulitis
Splenic clearance of microorganisms	Splenectomy	Splenic reticuloendothelial cells	*Streptococcus pneumoniae, Haemophilus influenzae, Neisseria meningitidis, Babesia, Capnocytophaga canimorsus*	Hodgkin's disease, leukemia, idiopathic thrombocytopenic purpura	Rapid, overwhelming sepsis
Phagocytosis	Lack of granulocytes	Granulocytes (neutrophils)	Staphylococci, streptococci, enteric organisms, fungi	Hairy cell, acute myelocytic, and acute lymphocytic leukemias	Bacteremia
Humoral immunity	Lack of antibody	B cells	*S. pneumoniae, H. influenzae, N. meningitidis*	Chronic lymphocytic leukemia, multiple myeloma	Infections with encapsulated organisms, sinusitis, pneumonia
Cellular immunity	Lack of T cells	T cells and macrophages	*Mycobacterium tuberculosis, Listeria,* herpesviruses, fungi, other intracellular parasites	Hodgkin's disease, leukemia, T cell lymphoma	Infections with intracellular bacteria, fungi, parasites

caused by other organisms, including *Staphylococcus aureus*, *P. aeruginosa*, *Candida* species, *Stenotrophomonas*, or *Bacillus*, usually require catheter removal.

- Upper GI infections: mouth ulcerations (viridans streptococci, anaerobic bacteria, and HSV); thrush (*Candida albicans*); and esophagitis (*C. albicans* and HSV)

- Lower GI infections
    1. Hepatic candidiasis results from seeding of the liver during neutropenia in pts with hematologic malignancy but presents when neutropenia resolves. Pts have fever, abdominal pain, nausea, and increased alkaline phosphatase levels. CT may reveal bull's-eye lesions. MRI is also helpful in the diagnosis. Amphotericin B is usually prescribed initially, but fluconazole may be useful for outpatient treatment.
    2. Typhlitis/neutropenic colitis is more common among children than among adults and among pts with acute myelocytic leukemia or acute lymphocytic leukemia (ALL) than among pts with other forms of cancer. Pts have fever, RLQ tenderness, and diarrhea that is often bloody. The diagnosis is confirmed by the documentation of a thickened cecal wall via CT, MRI, or ultrasound. Treatment should be directed against gram-negative bacteria and bowel flora.

- CNS infections
    1. Meningitis: Consider *Cryptococcus* or *Listeria*. Splenectomized pts and those with hypogammaglobulinemia are also at risk for infection with encapsulated bacteria such as *Streptococcus pneumoniae*, *Haemophilus influenzae*, and *Neisseria meningitidis*.
    2. Encephalitis can develop in pts receiving high-dose cytotoxic treatment or chemotherapy that affects T cell function. Consider varicella-zoster virus (VZV), JC virus (progressive multifocal leukoencephalopathy), cytomegalovirus (CMV), *Listeria*, HSV, and human herpesvirus 6 (HHV-6).
    3. Brain masses: Consider *Nocardia*, *Cryptococcus*, *Aspergillus*, and *Toxoplasma gondii*. Epstein-Barr virus–associated lymphoproliferative disease (EBV-LPD) may present as a mass lesion.

- Pulmonary infections
    1. Localized: bacterial pneumonia, *Legionella*, mycobacteria
    2. Nodular: suggests fungal etiology. *Aspergillus* causes invasive disease in neutropenic pts, presenting as a thrombotic event due to blood vessel invasion, pleuritic chest pain, and fever. Hemoptysis is an ominous sign. *Mucor* or *Nocardia* can also cause nodular lesions.
    3. Diffuse: Consider viruses (CMV), *Chlamydia*, *Pneumocystis*, mycobacteria, and *T. gondii*. Viruses that cause URI in normal hosts (e.g., influenza, respiratory syncytial) may cause fatal pneumonitis.

- Renal and ureteral infections: usually associated with obstructing tumor masses. *Candida* has a predilection for the kidneys, reaching this site via either hematogenous seeding or retrograde spread from the bladder. Adenovirus can cause hemorrhagic cystitis.

APPROACH TO DIAGNOSIS AND TREATMENT OF FEBRILE NEUTROPENIC PTS Figure 90-1 is an algorithm for the diagnosis and treatment of febrile neutropenic pts. The initial regimen can be refined on the basis of culture data. Adding antibiotics is not appropriate unless there is a clinical or microbiologic reason to do so. Other than the use of a β-lactam antibiotic together with an aminoglycoside, "double coverage" has not been shown to be of benefit and may add toxicities and side effects. Although am-

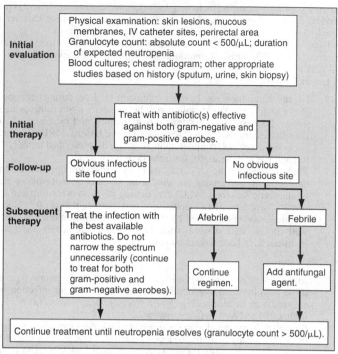

FIGURE 90-1 Algorithm for the diagnosis and treatment of febrile neutopenic pts. Several general guidelines are useful in the initial treatment of these pts: (1) It is necessary to use antibiotics active against both gram-negative and gram-positive bacteria in the initial regimen. (2) An aminoglycoside or an antibiotic without good activity against gram-positive organisms (e.g., ciprofloxacin or aztreonam) alone is not adequate in this setting. (3) The agents used should reflect both the epidemiology and the antibiotic resistance pattern of the hospital. For example, in hospitals where there is gentamicin resistance, amikacin-containing regimens should be considered; in hospitals with frequent *P. aeruginosa* infections, a regimen with the highest level of activity against this pathogen (such as tobramycin plus a semisynthetic penicillin) would be reasonable for initial therapy. (4) A single third-generation cephalosporin constitutes an appropriate initial regimen in many hospitals (if the pattern of resistance justifies its use). (5) Most standard regimens are designed for pts who have not previously received prophylactic antibiotics. The development of fever in a pt receiving antibiotics affects the choice of subsequent therapy (which should target resistant organisms and organisms known to cause infections in pts being treated with the antibiotics already administered). (6) Randomized trials have indicated that it is safe to use oral antibiotic regimens to treat "low-risk" pts with fever and neutropenia. Outpatients who are expected to remain neutropenic for <10 days and who have no concurrent medical problems (such as hypotension, pulmonary compromise, or abdominal pain) can be classified as low-risk and treated with a broad-spectrum oral regimen. On the basis of large studies, it can be concluded that this therapy is safe and effective, at least when delivered in the inpatient setting. Outpatient treatment has been assessed in small studies, but data from large randomized trials demonstrating the safety of outpatient treatment of fever and neutropenia are not yet available.

photericin B remains the standard agent for the treatment for fungal disease, newer azoles such as voriconazole may supplant it. Each azole has a different spectrum, and no drug can be assumed to be efficacious against all fungi. Antiviral agents may be appropriate, particularly those directed against the herpes group viruses HSV and CMV. Prophylactic antibiotics (e.g., fluoroquinolones) or antifungal agents (e.g., fluconazole) may prevent infections but may also increase the number of infections caused by resistant organisms. Prophylaxis should be reserved for pts at greatest risk—i.e., those who will be neutropenic for prolonged periods. *Pneumocystis* prophylaxis is mandatory for pts with ALL and for those receiving glucocorticoid-containing regimens.

INFECTIONS IN TRANSPLANT RECIPIENTS

Evaluation of infections in transplant recipients must involve consideration of both donor and recipient and of the immunosuppressive drugs required to reduce rejection of the transplanted organ.

BONE MARROW TRANSPLANTATION (BMT)   Infections occur in a predictable time frame after BMT (Table 90-2).

• *Bacterial infections*: Neutropenia-related infectious complications are most common during the first month. Some centers give prophylactic antibiotics (e.g., levofloxacin) to decrease the risk of gram-negative bacteremia.

• *Fungal infections*: Infections with resistant fungi are more common when pts are given prophylactic fluconazole. The risk for infection with *Candida* or *Aspergillus* increases, as does the risk for reactivation of endemic fungi, in pts requiring prolonged treatment with glucocorticoids or other immunosuppressive agents. Maintenance prophylaxis with trimethoprim-sulfamethoxazole (TMP-SMX; 160/800 mg/d starting 1 month after engraftment and continuing for at least 1 year) is recommended to prevent *Pneumocystis* pneumonia.

• *Parasitic infections*: The regimen just described for *Pneumocystis* pneumonia is also protective against disease caused by *Toxoplasma* as well as against some bacterial infections, including *Nocardia* and *Listeria* infections and late infections with *S. pneumoniae* or *H. influenzae*.

• *Viral infections*: Prophylactic acyclovir or valacyclovir for HSV-seropositive pts reduces rates of mucositis and prevents pneumonia and other HSV manifestations. Zoster is usually managed readily with acyclovir. HHV-6 can

Table 90-2

Infections After Bone Marrow Transplantation

Infection Site	Period after Transplantation		
	Early (<1 Month)	Middle (1–4 Months)	Late (>6 Months)
Disseminated	Bacteria (aerobic gram-negative, gram-positive)	Bacteria (*Nocardia*, agents of actinomycosis) Fungi (*Candida*, *Aspergillus*)	Encapsulated bacteria (*Streptococcus pneumoniae*, *Haemophilus influenzae*, *Neisseria meningitidis*)
Skin and mucous membranes	Herpes simplex virus	Human herpesvirus type 6	Varicella-zoster virus
Lungs	Herpes simplex virus	Viruses (cytomegalovirus, human herpesvirus type 6) Parasites (*Toxoplasma gondii*) Fungi (*Pneumocystis*)	
Kidneys			Viruses (BK)
Brain			Parasites (*T. gondii*) Viruses (JC)

prolong neutropenia. CMV causes interstitial pneumonia, bone marrow suppression, colitis, and graft failure. The risk is highest with a CMV-seropositive donor and a CMV-seronegative recipient. Severe disease is more common among allogeneic transplant recipients and is often associated with graft-versus-host disease. Many centers give prophylactic IV ganciclovir or oral valganciclovir from engraftment to day 120 after allogeneic BMT. In addition, preemptive therapy is given when CMV is detected in blood by an antigen or DNA test. EBV-LPD as well as infections caused by respiratory syncytial virus, parainfluenza virus, influenza virus, and adenovirus can occur. BK virus, a polyomavirus, has been found in the urine of pts after BMT.

SOLID ORGAN TRANSPLANTATION   After solid organ transplantation, pts do not go through a stage of neutropenia like that seen after BMT; thus the infections in these two groups of pts differ. However, solid organ transplant recipients are immunosuppressed for longer periods with agents that chronically impair T cell immunity.

1. Infection risk depends on the interval since transplantation.
   a. Early infections (<1 month): Infections are related to surgery and wounds.
   b. Middle-period infections (1–6 months): Infections are the same as those seen in pts with chronically impaired T cell immunity. CMV causes severe systemic disease or infection of transplanted organs, which increases organ rejection, prompting increased immunosuppression that, in turn, increases CMV replication. Diagnosis, treatment, and prophylaxis for CMV infection are the keys to interrupting this cycle.
   c. Late infections (>6 months): *Listeria*, *Nocardia*, various fungi, and other intracellular organisms associated with defects in cell-mediated immunity may pose problems. When EBV-LPD occurs (often within the transplanted organ), immunosuppression should be decreased or discontinued, if possible.
2. Kidney transplantation: TMP-SMX prophylaxis for the first 4 months decreases infection rates. Valacyclovir or valganciclovir may be considered for prophylactic treatment of high-risk pts to prevent primary or reactivation CMV infection and other herpesvirus disease.
3. Heart transplantation
   a. Early period: sternal wound infection and mediastinitis due to common skin organisms, gram-negative bacteria, fungi, and *Mycoplasma hominis*
   b. Middle period: The risk of *T. gondii* infection is high. TMP-SMX prophylaxis, which also protects the pt against *Pneumocystis*, *Nocardia*, and other organisms, is warranted. CMV disease due to reactivation or primary infection is associated with poor outcomes.
   c. Late period: EBV-LPD, *Pneumocystis* infection
4. Lung transplantation
   a. Early period: pneumonia, mediastinitis
   b. Middle period: CMV disease is most severe in lung or heart-lung transplant recipients; it is very common if either the donor or the recipient is seropositive. Prophylaxis is indicated.
   c. Late period: EBV-LPD, *Pneumocystis* infection. Prophylaxis is given for 1 year.
5. Liver transplantation
   a. Early period: peritonitis, intraabdominal abscesses. Fungal infections are frequent and correlate with preoperative glucocorticoid use or long-term antimicrobial use.
   b. Middle period: cholangitis, viral hepatitis due to reactivation of hepatitis B and C infections. High dose IV hepatitis B immune globulin is given; other agents are being studied for hepatitis B and C. CMV

Table 90-3

Vaccination of Cancer Patients Receiving Chemotherapy

Vaccine	Use in Indicated Patients			Bone Marrow Transplantation
	Intensive Chemotherapy	Hodgkin's Disease		
Diphtheria-tetanus (diphtheria, pertussis, tetanus; DPT) for children <7 years old	Primary series and boosters as necessary	No special recommendation		12, 14, and 24 months after transplantation
Poliomyelitis[a]	Complete primary series and boosters	No special recommendation		12, 14, and 24 months after transplantation
Haemophilus influenzae type b conjugate	Primary series and booster for children	Immunization before treatment and booster 3 months afterward		12, 14, and 24 months after transplantation
Hepatitis A	Not routinely recommended	Not routinely recommended		Not routinely recommended
Hepatitis B	Complete series	No special recommendation		12, 14, and 24 months after transplantation
23-Valent pneumococcal	Every 5 years	Immunization before treatment and booster 3 months afterward		12 and 24 months after transplantation
4-Valent meningococcal	Should be administered to splenectomized pts and pts living in endemic areas, including college students in dormitories	Should be administered to splenectomized pts and pts living in endemic areas, including college students in dormitories		Should be administered to splenectomized pts and pts living in endemic areas, including college students in dormitories
Influenza	Seasonal immunization	Seasonal immunization		Seasonal immunization
Measles/mumps/rubella	Contraindicated	Contraindicated		After 24 months in pts without graft-versus-host disease
Varicella-zoster virus	Contraindicated[b]	Contraindicated		Contraindicated

[a] Live-virus vaccine is contraindicated; inactivated vaccine should be used.

[b] Contact the manufacturer for more information on use in children with acute lymphocytic leukemia.

infection occurs in seronegative recipients of organs from seropositive donors; disease is not usually as severe as in other types of transplantation.

IMMUNIZATIONS IN IMMUNOSUPPRESSED PATIENTS

Recommendations for vaccination of cancer pts and bone marrow transplant recipients are listed in Table 90-3. In solid organ transplant recipients, the usual vaccines and boosters should be given before immunosuppression. Pneumococcal vaccination should be repeated every 5 years; this vaccine can be given with meningococcal vaccine. Solid organ transplant recipients receiving immunosuppressive agents should not receive live vaccines.

For a more detailed discussion, see Finberg R: Infections in Patients with Cancer, Chap. 72, p. 489; Madoff LC, Kasper DL: Introduction to Infectious Diseases: Host-Pathogen Interactions, Chap. 104, p. 695; and Finberg R, Fingeroth J: Infections in Transplant Recipients, Chap. 117, p. 781, in HPIM-16.

91

HIV INFECTION AND AIDS

Definition

AIDS was originally defined empirically by the Centers for Disease Control and Prevention (CDC) as "the presence of a reliably diagnosed disease that is at least moderately indicative of an underlying defect in cell-mediated immunity." Following the recognition of the causative virus, HIV (formerly called HTLV-III/LAV), and the development of sensitive and specific tests for HIV infection, the definition of AIDS has undergone substantial revision. The current surveillance definition categorizes HIV-infected persons on the basis of clinical conditions associated with HIV infection and CD4+T lymphocyte counts (Tables 173-1 and 173-2, p. 1076, in HPIM-16). From a practical standpoint, the clinician should view HIV infection as a spectrum of disorders ranging from primary infection, with or without the acute HIV syndrome, to the asymptomatic infected state to advanced disease.

Etiology

AIDS is caused by infection with the human retroviruses HIV-1 or -2. HIV-1 is the most common cause worldwide; HIV-2 has about 40% sequence homology with HIV-1, is more closely related to simian immunodeficiency viruses, and has been identified predominantly in western Africa. HIV-2 infection has now, however, been reported in Europe, South America, Canada, and the United States. These viruses are passed through sexual contact; through contact with blood, blood products, or other bodily fluids (as in drug abusers who share contaminated intravenous needles); intrapartum or perinatally from mother to infant; or via breast milk. There is no evidence that the virus can be passed through casual or family contact or by insects such as mosquitoes. There is a definite, though small, occupational risk of infection for health care workers and laboratory personnel who work with HIV-infected specimens. The risk of transmission of HIV from an infected health care worker to his or her pts through invasive procedures is extremely low.

Epidemiology

As of January 1, 2003, an estimated 886,575 cumulative cases of AIDS had been diagnosed in the United States; ~57% of those have died. However, the death rate from AIDS has decreased substantially in the past 10 years primarily due to the increased use of potent antiretroviral drugs. It has been estimated that there are between 850,000 and 950,000 HIV-infected people living in the United States. Major risk groups continue to be men who have had sex with men and men and women injection drug users (IDUs). However, the number of cases that are transmitted heterosexually, particularly among women, is increasing rapidly (see Table 173-5, p. 1085; Figs. 173-10 through 173-13, pp. 1085, 1086, in HPIM-16). As the majority of IDU-associated cases are among inner-city minority populations, the burden of HIV infection and AIDS falls increasingly and disproportionately on minorities, especially in the cities of the northeast and southeast United States. Cases of AIDS are still being found among individuals who have received contaminated blood products in the past, although the risk of acquiring new infection through this route is extremely small in the United States. HIV infection/AIDS is a global pandemic, especially in developing countries. The current estimate of the number of cases of HIV infection worldwide is ~ 40 million, two-thirds of whom are in sub-Saharan Africa; 50% of cases are in women (Fig. 173-9, p. 1083, and Table 173-3, p. 1084, in HPIM-16).

Pathophysiology and Immunopathogenesis

The hallmark of HIV disease is a profound immunodeficiency resulting from a progressive quantitative and qualitative deficiency of the subset of T lymphocytes referred to as helper or inducer T cells. This subset of T cells is defined phenotypically by the expression on the cell surface of the CD4 molecule, which serves as the primary cellular receptor for HIV. A co-receptor must be present with CD4 for efficient entry of HIV-1 into target cells. The two major co-receptors for HIV-1 are CCR5 and CXCR4. Both of these receptors belong to the seven-transmembrane-domain G protein–coupled family of receptors. Although the CD4+ T lymphocyte and CD4+ monocyte lineage are the principal cellular targets of HIV, virtually any cell that expresses CD4 along with one of the co-receptors can potentially be infected by HIV.

PRIMARY INFECTION   Following initial transmission, the virus infects CD4+ cells, probably T lymphocytes, monocytes, or bone marrow–derived dendritic cells. Both during this initial stage and later in infection, the lymphoid system is a major site for the establishment and propagation of HIV infection. Initially, lymph node architecture is preserved, but ultimately it is completely disrupted and the efficiency of the node in trapping virions declines, leading to equilibration of the viral burden between peripheral blood cells and lymph node cells.

Most pts undergo a viremic stage during primary infection; in some pts this is associated with the "acute retroviral syndrome," a mononucleosis-like illness (see below). This phase is important in disseminating virus to lymphoid and other organs throughout the body, and it is ultimately contained partially by the development of an HIV-specific immune response and the trapping of virions in lymphoid tissue.

ESTABLISHMENT OF CHRONIC AND PERSISTENT INFECTION Despite the robust immune response that is mounted following primary infection, the virus, with very few exceptions, is not cleared from the body. Instead, a chronic infection develops that persists for a median time of 10 years before the patient becomes clinically ill. During this period of clinical latency, the number of CD4+ T cells gradually declines but few, if any, clinical findings are evident; however, active viral replication can almost always be detected by measurable plasma viremia and the demonstration of virus replication in lymphoid tissue. The level of steady-state viremia (referred to as the *viral set point*) at approximately 1 year postinfection has important prognostic implications for the progression of HIV disease; individuals with a low viral set point at 6 months to 1 year after infection progress to AIDS more slowly than those whose set point is very high at this time (see Fig. 173-17, p. 1088, in HPIM-16).

ADVANCED HIV DISEASE In untreated pts or in pts in whom therapy has not controlled viral replication (see below), after some period of time (often years), CD4+ T cell counts will fall below a critical level (~$200/\mu L$) and pts become highly susceptible to opportunistic disease. However, control of plasma viremia by effective antiretroviral therapy, even in individuals with extremely low CD4+ T cell counts, has increased survival in these pts despite the fact that their CD4+ T cell counts may not increase significantly as a result of therapy.

Immune Abnormalities in HIV Disease

A broad range of immune abnormalities has been documented in HIV-infected pts. These include both quantitative and qualitative defects in lymphocyte, monocyte/macrophage, and natural killer (NK) cell function, as well as the development of autoimmune phenomena.

Immune Response to HIV Infection

Both humoral and cellular immune responses to HIV develop soon after primary infection (see summary in Table 173-8, p. 1098, and Fig. 173-21, p. 1099, in HPIM-16). Humoral responses include antibodies with HIV binding and neutralizing activity, as well as antibodies participating in antibody-dependent cellular cytotoxicity (ADCC). Cellular immune responses include the generation of HIV-specific CD4+ and CD8+ T lymphocytes, as well as NK cells and mononuclear cells mediating ADCC. CD8+ T lymphocytes may also suppress HIV replication in a noncytolytic, non-MHC restricted manner. This effect is mediated by soluble factors such as the CC-chemokines RANTES, MIP-1α, and MIP-1β.

Diagnosis of HIV Infection

Laboratory diagnosis of HIV infection depends on the demonstration of anti-HIV antibodies and/or the detection of HIV or one of its components.

The standard screening test for HIV infection is the detection of anti-HIV antibodies using an enzyme immunoassay (EIA). This test is highly sensitive (>99.5%) and is quite specific. Most commercial EIA kits are able to detect antibodies to both HIV-1 and -2. Western blot is the most commonly used confirmatory test and detects antibodies to HIV antigens of specific molecular weights. Antibodies to HIV begin to appear within 2 weeks of infection, and the period of time between initial infection and the development of detectable antibodies is rarely >3 months. The HIV p24 antigen can be measured using a capture assay, an EIA-type assay. Plasma p24 antigen levels rise during the first few weeks following infection, prior to the appearance of anti-HIV antibodies. A guideline for the use of these serologic tests in the diagnosis of HIV infection is depicted in Fig. 91-1.

HIV can be cultured directly from tissue, peripheral blood cells, or plasma, but this is most commonly done in a research setting. HIV genetic material can be detected using reverse transcriptase PCR (RT-PCR), branched DNA (bDNA), or nucleic acid sequence-based assay (NASBA). These tests are useful in pts with a positive or indeterminate EIA and an indeterminate Western blot or in pts in whom serologic testing may be unreliable (such as those with hypogammaglobulinemia).

Laboratory Monitoring of Patients with HIV Infection

Measurement of the CD4+ T cell count and level of plasma HIV RNA are important parts of the routine evaluation and monitoring of HIV-infected individuals. The CD4+ T cell count is a generally accepted indicator of the immunologic competence of the pt with HIV infection, and there is a close relationship between the CD4+ T cell count and the clinical manifestations of AIDS (Fig. 173-26, p. 1103, in HPIM-16). Pts with CD4+ T cell counts < 200/μL are at high risk of infection with *Pneumocystis carinii*, while pts with CD4+ T cell counts < 50/μL are at high risk for developing CMV disease and infection with *Mycobacterium avium intracellulare*. Pts should have the CD4+ T cell count measured at the time of diagnosis and every 3–6 months thereafter (measurements may be done more frequently in pts with declining counts). According to most practice guidelines, a CD4+ T cell count < 350/μL is an indication to initiate antiretroviral therapy. While the CD4+ T cell count provides information on the current immunologic status of the pt, the HIV RNA level predicts what will happen to the CD4+ T cell count in the near future and hence predicts

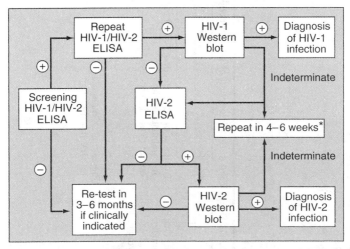

FIGURE 91-1 Algorithm for the use of serologic tests in the diagnosis of HIV-1 or HIV-2 infection. * Stable indeterminate Western blot 4 to 6 weeks later makes HIV infection unlikely. However, it should be repeated twice at 3-month intervals to rule out HIV infection. Alternatively, one may test for HIV-1 p24 antigen on HIV RNA.

Table 91-1

Antiretroviral Drugs Used in the Treatment of HIV Infection[a]

Drug	Indication	Dose in Combination	Supporting Data	Toxicity
REVERSE TRANSCRIPTASE INHIBITORS				
Zidovudine (AZT, azidothymidine, Retrovir, 3'-azido-3'-deoxythymidine)	Treatment of HIV infection in combination with other antiretroviral agents	200 mg q8h or 300 mg bid	19 vs 1 death in original placebo-controlled trial in 281 pts with AIDS or ARC. Decreased progression to AIDS in pts with CD4+ T cell counts <500/μL, n = 2051	Anemia, granulocytopenia, myopathy, lactic acidosis, hepatomegaly with steatosis, headache, nausea
	Prevention of maternal-fetal HIV transmission		In pregnant women with CD4+ T cell count ≥200/μL, AZT PO beginning at weeks 14–34 of gestation plus IV drug during labor and delivery plus PO AZT to infant for 6 wk decreased transmission of HIV by 67.5% (from 25.5% to 8.3%), n = 363	

428

| Didanosine (Videx, Videx EC, ddI, dideoxyinosine, 2',3'-dideoxyinosine) | For treatment of HIV infection in combination with other antiretroviral agents | Buffered: Requires 2 tablets to achieve adequate buffering of stomach acid; should be administered on an empty stomach ≥60 kg: 200 mg bid <60 kg: 125 mg bid Enteric coated: ≥60 kg: 400 mg qd < 60 kg: 250 mg qd | Clinically superior to AZT as monotherapy in 913 pts with prior AZT therapy. Clinically superior to AZT and comparable to AZT + ddI and AZT + ddC in 1067 AZT-naive pts with CD4+ T cell counts of 200–500/μL | Pancreatitis, peripheral neuropathy, abnormalities on liver function tests, lactic acidosis, hepatomegaly with steatosis |
| Zalcitabine (ddC, HIVID, 2'3'-dideoxycytidine) | In combination with other antiretroviral agents for the treatment of HIV infection | 0.75 mg tid | Clinically inferior to AZT monotherapy as initial treatment. Clinically as good as ddI in advanced pts intolerant to AZT. In combination with AZT, was clinically superior to AZT alone in pts with AIDS or CD4+ T cell count <350/μL | Peripheral neuropathy, pancreatitis, lactic acidosis, hepatomegaly with steatosis, oral ulcers |

(continued)

Table 91-1 (Continued)

Antiretroviral Drugs Used in the Treatment of HIV Infection[a]

Drug	Indication	Dose in Combination	Supporting Data	Toxicity
Stavudine (d4T, Zerit, 2′,3′-didehydro-3′-dideoxy-thymidine)	Treatment of HIV-infected pts in combination with other antiretroviral agents	≥60 kg: 40 mg bid <60 kg: 30 mg bid	Superior to AZT with respect to changes in CD4+ T cell counts in 359 pts who had received ≥24 wk of AZT. Following 12 wk of randomization, the CD4+ T cell count had decreased in AZT-treated controls by a mean of 22/μL, while in stavudine-treated pts, it had increased by a mean of 22/μL	Peripheral neuropathy, pancreatitis, lactic acidosis, hepatomegaly with steatosis, ascending neuromuscular weakness, lipodystrophy
Lamivudine (Epivir, 2′,3′-dideoxy-3′-thiacytidine, 3TC)	In combination with other antiretroviral agents for the treatment of HIV infection	150 mg bid 300 mg qd	Superior to AZT alone with respect to changes in CD4 counts in 495 pts who were zidovudine-naïve and 477 pts who were zidovudine-experienced. Overall CD4+ T cell counts for the zidovudine group were at baseline by 24 wk, while in the group treated with zidovudine plus lamivudine, they were 10–50 cells/μL above baseline. 54% decrease in progression to AIDS/death compared to AZT alone	

430

Entricitabine (FTC, Emtriva)	In combination with other antiretroviral agents for the treatment of HIV infection	200 mg qd	Comparable to d4T in combination with ddI and efavirenz in 571 treatment-naive pts. Similar to 3TC in combination with 2DV or d4T + NNRT1 or PI in 440 pts doing well for at least 12 weeks on a 3TC regimen.
Abacavir (Ziagen)	For treatment of HIV infection in combination with other antiretroviral agents	300 mg bid	Abacavir + AZT + 3TC equivalent to indinavir + AZT + 3TC with regard to viral load suppression ($\sim$60% in each group with <400 HIV RNA copies/mL plasma) and CD4 cell increase ($\sim$100/μL in each group) at 24 weeks	Hypersensitivity reaction (can be fatal); fever, rash, nausea, vomiting, malaise or fatigue, and loss of appetite
Tenofovir (Viread)	For use in combination with other antiretroviral agents when treatment is indicated	300 mg qd	Reduction of $\sim$0.6 log in HIV-1 RNA levels when added to background regimen in treatment-experienced pts	Potential for renal toxicity

(continued)

431

Table 91-1 (*Continued*)

Antiretroviral Drugs Used in the Treatment of HIV Infection[a]

Drug	Indication	Dose in Combination	Supporting Data	Toxicity
Delavirdine (Rescriptor)	For use in combination with appropriate antiretrovirals when treatment is warranted	400 mg tid	Delavirdine + AZT superior to AZT alone with regard to viral load suppression at 52 weeks	Skin rash, abnormalities in liver function tests
Nevirapine (Viramune)	In combination with other antiretroviral agents for treatment of progressive HIV infection	200 mg/d $\times$ 14 days then 200 mg bid	Increases in CD4+ T cell count, decrease in HIV RNA when used in combination with nucleosides	Skin rash, hepatotoxicity
Efavirenz (Sustiva)	For treatment of HIV infection in combination with other antiretroviral agents	600 mg qhs	Efavirenz + AZT + 3TC comparable to indinavir + AZT + 3TC with regard to viral load suppression (a higher percentage of the efavirenz group achieved viral load <50 copies/mL; however, the discontinuation rate in the indinavir group was unexpectedly high, accounting for most treatment "failures") and CD4 cell increase ($\sim$140/μL in each group) at 24 weeks	Rash, dysphoria, elevated liver function tests, drowsiness, abnormal dreams, depression

PROTEASE INHIBITORS

Saquinavir mesylate (Invirase—hard gel capsule)	In combination with other antiretroviral agents when therapy is warranted	600 mg q8h	Increases in CD4+ T cell counts, reduction in HIV RNA most pronounced in combination therapy with ddC. 50% reduction in first AIDS-defining event or death in combination with ddC compared to either agent alone	Diarrhea, nausea, headaches, hyperglycemia, fat redistribution, lipid abnormalities
(Fortovase—soft gel capsule)	For use in combination with other antiretroviral agents when treatment is warranted	1200 mg tid	Reduction in the mortality rate and AIDS-defining events for pts who received hard-gel formulation in combination with ddC	Diarrhea, nausea, abdominal pain, headaches, hyperglycemia, fat redistribution, lipid abnormalities
Ritonavir (Norvir)	In combination with other antiretroviral agents for treatment of HIV infection when treatment is warranted	600 mg bid	Reduction in the cumulative incidence of clinical progression or death from 34 to 17% in pts with CD4+ T cell count <100/μL treated for a median of 6 months	Nausea, abdominal pain, hyperglycemia, fat redistribution, lipid abnormalities, may alter levels of many other drugs, including saquinavir

(continued)

Table 91-1 *(Continued)*

Antiretroviral Drugs Used in the Treatment of HIV Infection[a]

Drug	Indication	Dose in Combination	Supporting Data	Toxicity
Indinavir sulfate (Crixivan)	For treatment of HIV infection in combination with other antiretroviral agents when antiretroviral treatment is warranted	800 mg q8h	Increase in CD4+ T cell count by 100/μL and 2-log decrease in HIV RNA levels when given in combination with zidovudine and lamivudine. Decrease of 50% in risk of progression to AIDS or death when given with zidovudine and lamivudine compared with zidovudine and lamivudine alone	Nephrolithiasis, indirect hyperbilirubinemia, hyperglycemia, fat redistribution, lipid abnormalities
Nelfinavir mesylate (Viracept)	For treatment of HIV infection in combination with other antiretroviral agents when antiretroviral therapy is warranted	750 mg tid or 1250 mg bid	2.0-log decline in HIV RNA when given in combination with stavudine	Diarrhea, loose stools, hyperglycemia, fat redistribution, lipid abnormalities

434

| Amprenavir (Agenerase) | In combination with other antiretroviral agents for treatment of HIV infection | 1200 mg bid or 600 mg bid + Ritonavir 100 mg bid or 1200 mg qd + Ritonavir 200 mg qd | In treatment-naïve pts, amprenavir + AZT + 3TC superior to AZT + 3TC with regard to viral load suppression (53% vs 11% with <400 HIV RNA copies/mL plasma at 24 weeks). CD4+ T cell responses similar between treatment groups. In treatment-experienced pts, amprenavir + NRTIs similar to indinavir + NRTIs with regard to viral load suppression (43% vs 53% with <400 HIV RNA copies/mL plasma at 24 weeks). CD4+ T cell responses superior in the indinavir + NRTIs group | Nausea, vomiting, diarrhea, rash, oral paresthesias, elevated liver function tests, hyperglycemia, fat redistribution, lipid abnormalities |
| Fosamprenavir (Lexiva) | | 1400 mg bid or 700 mg bid + Ritonavir 100 mg bid | | |

435

(continued)

Table 91-1 (Continued)

Antiretroviral Drugs Used in the Treatment of HIV Infection[a]

Drug	Indication	Dose in Combination	Supporting Data	Toxicity
Lopinavir/ritonavir (Kaletra)	For treatment of HIV infection in combination with other antiretroviral agents	400 mg/100 mg bid	In treatment of naïve pts, lopinavir/ritonavir + d4T + 3TC superior to nelfinavir + d4T + 3TC with regard to viral load suppression (79% vs 64% with <400 HIV RNA copies/mL at 40 weeks). CD4+ T cell increases similar in both groups.	Diarrhea, hyperglycemia, fat redistribution, lipid abnormalities
Atazanavir (Reyataz)	For treatment of HIV infection in combination with other antiretroviral agents	400 mg qd or 300 mg qd + Ritonavir 100 mg qd when given with efavirenz	Comparable to efavirenz when given in combination with AZT + 3TC in a study of 810 treatment-naive pts. Comparable to nelfinavir when given in combination with d4T + 3TC in a study of 467 treatment-naive pts.	Hyperbilirubinemia, PR prolongation, nausea, vomiting, hyperglycemia, fat maldistribution
FUSION INHIBITOR				
Enfuvirtide (Fuzeon)	In combination with other agents in treatment-experienced pts with evidence of HIV-1 replication despite ongoing antiretroviral therapy	90 mg SC bid	In treatment of experienced pts, superior to placebo when added to new optimized background (37% vs 16% with <400 HIV RNA copies/mL at 24 weeks; + 71 vs + 35 CD4+ T cells at 24 weeks)	Local injection reactions, hypersensitivity reactions, increased rate of bacterial pneumonia

[a] All drugs in this table are licensed.

Note: ARC, AIDS-related complex; NRTIs, nonnucleoside reverse transcriptase inhibitors.

the clinical prognosis. Measurements of plasma HIV RNA levels should be made at the time of HIV diagnosis and every 3–4 months thereafter in the untreated pt. Measurement of plasma HIV RNA is also useful in making therapeutic decisions about antiretroviral therapy (see below). Following the initiation of therapy or any change in therapy, HIV RNA levels should be monitored approximately every 4 weeks until the effectiveness of the therapeutic regimen is determined by the development of a new steady-state level of HIV RNA. During therapy, levels of HIV RNA should be monitored every 3–4 months to evaluate the continuing effectiveness of therapy.

The sensitivity of an individual's HIV virus(es) to different antiretroviral agents can be tested by either genotypic or phenotypic assays. These tests are good at identifying those antiretroviral agents a given pt has received in the past. In the hands of experts the use of resistance testing enhances the short-term ability to achieve ~0.5-log declines in viral load compared to changing drugs merely on the basis of drug history. The clinical value of HIV resistance testing in selecting an initial treatment regimen is still under investigation.

Clinical Manifestations of HIV Infection

A complete discussion is beyond the scope of this chapter. The major clinical features of the various stages of HIV infection are summarized below (see also Chap. 173, HPIM-16).

ACUTE HIV (RETROVIRAL) SYNDROME Approximately 50 to 70% of infected individuals experience an acute syndrome following primary infection. The acute syndrome follows infection by 3 to 6 weeks. It is characterized by fevers, pharyngitis, arthralgias, myalgias, lymphadenopathy, maculopapular rash, mucocutaneous ulceration, nausea, vomiting, diarrhea, and aseptic meningitis; lasts 1 to 2 weeks and resolves spontaneously as immune response to HIV develops. Most pts will then enter a phase of clinical latency, although an occasional pt will experience progressive immunologic and clinical deterioration.

ASYMPTOMATIC INFECTION The length of time between infection and development of disease varies greatly, but the median is estimated to be 10 years. HIV disease with active viral replication usually progresses during this asymptomatic period, and CD4+ T cell counts fall. The rate of disease progression is directly correlated with plasma HIV RNA levels. Pts with high levels of HIV RNA progress to symptomatic disease faster than do those with low levels of HIV RNA.

SYMPTOMATIC DISEASE Symptoms of HIV disease can develop at any time during the course of HIV infection. In general, the spectrum of illness changes as the CD4+ T cell count declines. The more severe and life-threatening complications of HIV infection occur in patients with a CD4+ T cell count < 200/μl. Approximately 60% of the deaths among AIDS pts are a direct result of infection other than HIV, with bacterial infections heading the list. Overall, the clinical spectrum of HIV disease is constantly changing as pts live longer and new and better approaches to treatment and prophylaxis of opportunistic infections are developed. The key element to treating symptomatic complications of HIV disease, whether primary or secondary, is achieving good control of HIV replication through the use of combination antiretroviral therapy and instituting primary and secondary prophylaxis as indicated. Major clinical syndromes seen in the symptomatic stage of HIV infection are summarized below.

• *Persistent generalized lymphadenopathy*: Palpable adenopathy at two or more extrainguinal sites that persists for >3 months without explanation other than HIV infection. Many pts will go on to disease progression.
• *Constitutional symptoms*: Fever persisting for >1 month, involuntary weight loss of >10% of baseline, diarrhea for >1 month in absence of explainable cause.
• *Neurologic disease*: Most common is HIV encephalopathy (AIDS dementia complex); other neurologic complications include opportunistic infections, primary CNS lymphoma, CNS Kaposi's sarcoma, aseptic meningitis, myelopathy, peripheral neuropathy and myopathy.
• *Secondary infectious diseases*: *P. carinii* pneumonia is most common opportunistic infection, occurring in ~80% of individuals during the course of their illness. Other common pathogens include CMV (chorioretinitis, colitis, pneumonitis, adrenalitis), *Candida albicans* (oral thrush, esophagitis), *M. avium intracellulare* (localized or disseminated infection), *M. tuberculosis, Cryptococcus neoformans* (meningitis, disseminated disease), *Toxoplasma gondii* (encephalitis, intracerebral mass lesion), herpes simplex virus (severe mucocutaneous lesions, esophagitis), diarrhea due to *Cryptosporidium* spp. or *Isospora belli*, bacterial pathogens (especially in pediatric cases).
• *Secondary neoplasms*: Kaposi's sarcoma (cutaneous and visceral, more fulminant course than in non-HIV-infected pts), lymphoid neoplasms (especially B cell lymphomas of brain, marrow, GI tract).
• *Other diseases*: A variety of organ-specific syndromes can be seen in HIV-infected pts, either as primary manifestations of the HIV infection or as complications of treatment.

 TREATMENT   (See Chap. 173, HPIM-16)

General principles of pt management include counseling, psychosocial support, and screening for infections and require comprehensive knowledge of the disease processes associated with HIV infection.

Antiretroviral Therapy (See Table 91-1)

The cornerstone of medical management of HIV infection is combination antiretroviral therapy, or HAART. Suppression of HIV replication is an important component in prolonging life as well as in improving the quality of life of pts with HIV infection. However, several important questions related to the treatment of HIV disease lack definitive answers. Among them are questions of when antiretroviral therapy should be started, what is the best HAART regimen, when should a given regimen be changed, and what drugs in a regimen should be changed when a change is made. The drugs that are currently licensed for the treatment of HIV infection are listed in Table 91-1. These drugs fall into three main categories: those that inhibit the viral reverse transcriptase enzyme, those that inhibit the viral protease enzyme, and those that inhibit viral entry. There are numerous drug-drug interactions that must be taken into consideration when using these medications (see Table 173-21, pp. 1130–1132, in HPIM-16). One of the main problems that has been encountered with the widespread use of HAART regimens has been a syndrome of hyperlipidemia and fat distribution often referred to as *lipodystrophy syndrome* (Chap. 173, HPIM-16).

Nucleoside Analogues   These should only be used in combination with other antiretroviral agents. The only exception is the use of zidovudine as monotherapy for preventing mother-to-child transmission of HIV when the mother does not require antiretroviral therapy based on the stage of her disease (see Chap. 173, HPIM-16). The most common usage is together with another nucleoside analogue, a nonnucleoside reverse transcriptase inhibitor, or a protease inhibitor (see below).

Nonnucleoside Reverse Transcriptase Inhibitors These agents interfere with the function of HIV-1 reverse transcriptase by binding to regions outside the active site and causing conformational changes in the enzyme that render it inactive. These agents are very potent; however, when they are used as monotherapy, they induce rapid emergence of drug-resistant mutants. Three members of this class, *nevirapine, delavirdine*, and *efavirenz*, are currently available for clinical use. These drugs are licensed for use in combination with other antiretrovirals.

Protease Inhibitors These drugs are potent and selective inhibitors of the HIV-1 protease enzyme and are active in the nanomolar range. Unfortunately, as in the case of the nonnucleoside reverse transcriptase inhibitors, this potency is accompanied by the rapid emergence of resistant isolates when these drugs are used as monotherapy. Thus, the protease inhibitors should be used only in combination with other antiretroviral drugs.

HIV Entry Inhibitors The newest class of antiretroviral drugs are the entry inhibitors. These agents act by interfering with the binding of HIV to its receptor or co-receptor or by interfering with the process of fusion. A variety of small molecules that bind to HIV-1 co-receptors are currently in clinical trials. The first drug in this class to be licensed is the fusion inhibitor *enfuvirtide*.

Choice of Antiretroviral Treatment Strategy

The large number of available antiretroviral agents coupled with a relative paucity of clinical end-point studies make the subject of antiretroviral therapy one of the more controversial in the management of HIV-infected pts.

The principles of therapy for HIV infection have been articulated by a panel sponsored by the U.S. Department of Health and Human Services (Table 91-2). Treatment decisions must take into account the fact that one is dealing with a chronic infection and that complete eradication of HIV infection is probably not possible with currently available HAART regimens. Thus, immediate treatment of HIV infection upon diagnosis may not be prudent, and therapeutic decisions must take into account the balance between risks and benefits. At present a reasonable course of action is to initiate antiretroviral therapy in anyone with the acute HIV syndrome; pts with symptomatic disease; pts with asymptomatic infection and CD4+ counts < $350/\mu L$ or with >50,000 copies/mL of HIV RNA. In addition, one may wish to administer a 4-week course of therapy to uninfected individuals immediately following a high-risk exposure to HIV (see below).

When the decision to initiate therapy is made, the physician must decide which drugs to use in the initial regimen. The two options for initial therapy most commonly in use today are: two nucleoside analogues (one of which is usually lamivudine) combined with a protease inhibitor; or two nucleoside analogues and a nonnucleoside reverse transcriptase inhibitor. There are no clear data at present on which to base distinctions between these two approaches. Following the initiation of therapy, one should expect a 1-log (tenfold) reduction in plasma HIV RNA within 1–2 months and eventually a decline in plasma HIV RNA to <50 copies/mL. There should also be a rise in CD4+ T cell count of $100-150/\mu L$. Many physicians feel that failure to achieve this end point is an indication for a change in therapy. Other reasons for changing therapy are listed in Table 91-3. When changing therapy because of treatment failure, it is important to attempt to provide a regimen with at least two new drugs. In the pt in whom a change is made for reasons of drug toxicity, a simple replacement of one drug is reasonable.

Treatment of Secondary Infections and Neoplasms

Specific for each infection and neoplasm (see Chap. 173, in HPIM-16).

Table 91-2

Principles of Therapy of HIV Infection

1. Ongoing HIV replication leads to immune system damage and progression to AIDS.
2. Plasma HIV RNA levels indicate the magnitude of HIV replication and the rate of CD4+ T cell destruction. CD4+ T cell counts indicate the current level of competence of the immune system.
3. Rates of disease progression differ among individuals, and treatment decisions should be individualized based upon plasma HIV RNA levels and CD4+ T cell counts.
4. Maximal suppression of viral replication is a goal of therapy; the greater the suppression the less likely the appearance of drug-resistant quasispecies.
5. The most effective therapeutic strategies involve the simultaneous initiation of combinations of effective anti-HIV drugs with which the patient has not been previously treated and that are not cross-resistant with antiretroviral agents that the patient has already received.
6. The antiretroviral drugs used in combination regimens should be used according to optimum schedules and dosages.
7. The number of available drugs is limited. Any decisions on antiretroviral therapy have a long-term impact on future options for the patient.
8. Women should receive optimal antiretroviral therapy regardless of pregnancy status.
9. The same principles apply to children and adults. The treatment of HIV-infected children involves unique pharmacologic, virologic, and immunologic considerations.
10. Compliance is an important part of ensuring maximal effect from a given regimen. The simpler the regimen, the easier it is for the patient to be compliant.

Source: Modified from *Principles of Therapy of HIV Infection*, USPHS and the Henry J. Kaiser Family Foundation.

> **Prophylaxis against Secondary Infections** (Table 173-11, pp. 1106, 1107, in HPIM-16)   Primary prophylaxis is clearly indicated for *P. carinii* pneumonia (especially when CD4+ T cell counts fall to <200 cells/μL), *M. avium* complex infections, and *M. tuberculosis* infections in pts with a positive PPD or anergy if at high risk of TB. Vaccination with the influenza and pneumococcal polysaccharide vaccines is generally recommended for all pts with CD4+ T cell counts >200/μl (see Table 173-11, pp. 1106, 1107, in HPIM-16). Secondary prophylaxis, when available, is indicated for virtually every infection experienced by HIV-infected pts.

HIV and the Health Care Worker

There is a small but definite risk to health care workers of acquiring HIV infection via needle stick exposures, large mucosal surface exposures, or exposure of open wounds to HIV-infected secretions or blood products. The risk of HIV transmission after a skin puncture by an object contaminated with blood from a person with documented HIV infection is ~0.3%, compared to 20–30% risk for hepatitis B infection from a similar incident. The role of antiretroviral agents in postexposure prophylaxis is still controversial. However, a U.S. Public Health Service working group has recommended that chemoprophylaxis be given as soon as possible after occupational exposure. While the precise regimen remains a subject of debate, the U.S. Public Health Service guidelines recommend (1) a combination of two nucleoside analogue reverse transcriptase inhibitors given

Table 91-3

Indications for Changing Antiretroviral Therapy in Patients with HIV Infection[a]

Less than a 1-log drop in plasma HIV RNA by 4 weeks following the initiation of therapy

A reproducible significant increase (defined as 3-fold or greater) from the nadir of plasma HIV RNA level not attributable to intercurrent infection, vaccination, or test methodology

Persistently declining CD4+ T cell numbers

Clinical deterioration

Side effects

---

[a] Generally speaking, a change should involve the initiation of at least 2 drugs felt to be effective in the given patient. The exception to this is when change is being made to manage toxicity, in which case a single substitution is reasonable.

Source: *Guidelines for the Use of Antiretroviral Agents in HIV-Infected Adults and Adolescents.* USPHS.

---

for 4 weeks for routine exposures, or (2) a combination of two nucleoside analogue reverse transcriptase inhibitors plus a third drug given for 4 weeks for high-risk or otherwise complicated exposures. Most clinicians administer the latter regimen in all cases in which a decision to treat is made. Regardless of which regimen is used, treatment should be initiated as soon as possible after exposure.

Prevention of exposure is the best strategy and includes following universal precautions and proper handling of needles and other potentially contaminated objects.

Transmission of TB is another potential risk for all health care workers, including those dealing with HIV-infected pts. All workers should know their PPD status, which should be checked yearly.

Vaccines

Development of a safe and effective HIV vaccine is the object of active investigation at present. Extensive animal work is ongoing, and clinical trials of candidate vaccines have begun in humans.

Prevention

Education, counseling, and behavior modification remain the cornerstones of HIV prevention efforts. While abstinence is an absolute way to prevent sexual transmission, other strategies include "safe sex" practices such as use of condoms together with the spermatocide nonoxynol-9. Avoidance of shared needle use by IDUs is critical. If possible, breast feeding should be avoided by HIV-positive women, as the virus can be transmitted to infants via this route.

For a more detailed discussion, see Fauci AS, Lane HC: Human Immunodeficiency Virus (HIV) Disease: AIDS and Related Disorders, Chap. 173, p. 1076, in HPIM-16.

92

HOSPITAL-ACQUIRED INFECTIONS

Hospital-acquired (nosocomial) infections are defined as those not present or incubating at the time of admission to the hospital. Nosocomial infections are estimated to affect >2 million pts, cost \$4.5 billion, and contribute to 88,000 deaths in U.S. hospitals each year. In recent years, nosocomial infections have become even more problematic because of increased numbers of immunocompromised pts, increasing antibiotic resistance in pathogenic bacteria, increased rates of fungal and viral superinfections, and increased numbers of invasive procedures and invasive devices.

Prevention of Hospital-Acquired Infections

Hospital infection-control programs use several mechanisms to prevent nosocomial infections.

- Surveillance: review of microbiology laboratory results, surveys of nursing wards, and use of other mechanisms to keep track of infections acquired after hospital admission. Infections that are associated with the greatest morbidity (e.g., nosocomial pneumonia), incur the highest costs (e.g., cardiac surgical wounds), are the most difficult to treat (e.g., antibiotic-resistant infections), cause recurrent epidemic problems (e.g., *Clostridium difficile*–related diarrhea), and/or are preventable (e.g., vascular-access infections) are the primary focus of hospital infection-control programs.
- Prevention and control measures: Hand hygiene is the single most important measure to prevent cross-infection. Other measures include identification and eradication of reservoirs of infection and minimizing use of invasive procedures and catheters.
- Isolation techniques to limit the spread of infection

  1. Standard precautions are used for all pts when there is a potential for contact with blood, body fluids, nonintact skin, and mucous membranes. Hand hygiene and use of gloves are central components of standard precautions; in certain cases masks, eye protection, and gowns are used as well.
  2. Transmission-based guidelines: Airborne precautions, droplet precautions, and contact precautions are used to prevent transmission of disease from infected pts. More than one precaution can be combined for diseases such as varicella that have more than one mode of transmission. Because antibiotic-resistant bacteria can be present on intact skin of infected pts, any contact with sick pts who may be harboring those bacteria should involve hand hygiene and use of gloves. Gowns are frequently used as well, although their importance in preventing cross-infection is less clear.

Nosocomial and Device-Related Infections

Urinary Tract Infections   Up to 40–45% of nosocomial infections are UTIs. Most nosocomial UTIs are associated with prior instrumentation or indwelling bladder catheterization. There is a 3–10% risk of infection for each day a catheter remains in place. Pts become infected with bacteria ascending from the periurethral area or via intraluminal contamination of the catheter. The pt should be assessed for symptoms of upper tract disease, such as flank pain, fever, and leukocytosis. Lower tract symptoms, such as dysuria, are unreliable as markers of infection in catheterized pts. If infection is suspected, the catheter should be replaced and a freshly voided urine specimen obtained for culture; repeat cultures should confirm the persistence of infection at the time therapy is initiated. Urinary sediment should be examined for evidence of infection (e.g., pyuria). Catheters should be placed (by aseptic techniques) only when they are essential, should be manipulated as infrequently as possible, and should be removed as soon as possible. In men, condom catheters—unless carefully maintained—are as strongly associated with infection as indwelling catheters.

Pneumonia Accounting for 15–20% of nosocomial infections, pneumonia increases the duration of hospital stay and costs. Pts aspirate endogenous or hospital-acquired flora. Risk factors include events that increase colonization with potential pathogens, such as prior antibiotic use, contaminated ventilator equipment, or increased gastric pH; events that increase risk of aspiration, such as intubation, decreased levels of consciousness, or nasogastric or endotracheal tubes; and conditions that compromise host defense mechanisms in the lung, such as chronic obstructive pulmonary disease. Diagnosis should depend on clinical criteria such as fever, leukocytosis, purulent secretions, and new or changing pulmonary infiltrates on CXR. An etiology should be sought by studies of lower respiratory tract samples protected from upper-tract contamination; quantitative cultures have diagnostic sensitivities in the range of 80%. Febrile pts with nasogastric tubes should also have sinusitis or otitis media ruled out. Organisms, particularly in ICU pts, include *Streptococcus pneumoniae* and *Haemophilus influenzae* early during hospitalization and *Staphylococcus aureus*, *Pseudomonas aeruginosa*, *Klebsiella*, *Enterobacter*, *Acinetobacter*, and other gram-negative bacilli later in the hospital stay. Prevention efforts should focus on minimal use of aspiration-prone supine positioning and meticulous aseptic care of respirator equipment.

Surgical Wound Infections Making up 20–30% of nosocomial infections, surgical wound infections increase the length of hospital stay as well as costs. These infections have an average incubation period of 5–7 days and often become evident after pts have left the hospital; thus it is difficult to assess the true incidence. Common risk factors include deficits in the surgeon's technical skill, the pt's underlying conditions (e.g., diabetes mellitus or obesity), and inappropriate timing of antibiotic prophylaxis. Other factors include the presence of drains, prolonged preoperative hospital stays, shaving of the operative site the day before surgery, long duration of surgery, and infection at remote sites. An area of erythema with a diameter of >2 cm around the wound margin, local pain and induration, fluctuance, pus, or dehiscence of the wound suggests infection. *S. aureus*, coagulase-negative staphylococci, and enteric and anaerobic bacteria are the most common pathogens. In rapidly progressing postoperative infections, group A streptococcal or clostridial infections should be considered. Treatment includes administration of appropriate antibiotics and drainage or excision of infected or necrotic material.

Intravascular Device Infections Infections of intravascular devices cause up to 50% of nosocomial bacteremias; central vascular catheters account for 80–90% of these infections. As many as 250,000 bloodstream infections associated with central vascular catheters occur each year in the United States, with attributable mortality rates of 12–25% and a cost of $25,000 per episode. Pts often present with fever, erythema, purulent drainage, induration, and tenderness at the exit site. Bacteremia without another source suggests a vascular access infection. Coagulase-negative staphylococci, *S. aureus*, enterococci, nosocomial gram-negative bacilli, and *Candida* are the pathogens most frequently associated with these bacteremias. The diagnosis is confirmed by isolation of the same bacteria from peripheral blood cultures and from semiquantitative or quantitative cultures of samples from the vascular catheter tip. In addition to the initiation of appropriate antibiotic treatment, other considerations should include the risk for endocarditis (relatively high in pts with *S. aureus* bacteremia), whether to use the "antibiotic lock" technique (instillation of concentrated antibiotic solution into the catheter lumen along with systemic antibiotics), and whether to remove the catheter (given that its removal is usually necessary to cure infection). If the catheter is changed over a guide wire and cultures of the removed catheter tip are positive, the catheter should be moved to a new site. Meticulous aseptic technique during catheter placement and avoidance of femoral sites minimize the risk of vascular access infection. If a device is expected to remain in place for >5 days, an antibiotic-impregnated catheter may be useful.

Miscellaneous Infections Other common nosocomial infections include antibiotic-associated *C. difficile* diarrhea, decubitus ulcers, and sinusitis.

Epidemic and Emerging Problems

- *Chickenpox*: If varicella-zoster virus (VZV) exposure occurs, postexposure prophylaxis with varicella-zoster immune globulin (VZIg) is considered for immunocompromised or pregnant contacts (with preemptive administration of acyclovir an alternative for some susceptible persons), and susceptible employees are furloughed for 8–21 days (or for 28 days if VZIg has been given). Vaccine should be routinely offered to VZV-susceptible employees.
- *Tuberculosis*: Prompt recognition and isolation of cases, use of negative-pressure private rooms with 100% exhaust and 6–12 air changes per hour, use of approved face masks, and follow-up skin testing of exposed personnel are required.
- *Group A streptococcal infection*: A single nosocomial case should prompt an investigation for health care workers who are carriers. Employees identified as carriers should be removed from pt-care settings until carriage is eliminated.
- *Aspergillosis*: linked to hospital renovations and disturbance of dusty surfaces
- *Legionellosis*: linked to contamination of potable water supplies
- *Antibiotic-resistant bacterial infection*: Strict infection-control practices and aggressive antibiotic-control policies are cornerstones of resistance-control efforts.
- *Bioterrorism preparedness*: Education, effective systems of internal and external communication, and risk assessment capabilities are key features.

For a more detailed discussion, see Weinstein RA: Hospital-Acquired Infections, Chap. 116, p. 775, in HPIM-16.

93

PNEUMOCOCCAL INFECTIONS

Etiology

Streptococcus pneumoniae (the pneumococcus) is a gram-positive coccus that grows in chains and causes ∝-hemolysis on blood agar. Nearly every clinical isolate has a polysaccharide capsule. More than 90 distinct capsules have been identified.

Epidemiology

S. pneumoniae colonizes the nasopharynx of 5–10% of healthy adults and 20–40% of healthy children on any single occasion. Once colonization takes place, pneumococci usually persist in adults for 4–6 weeks but can persist for up to 6 months. The organisms are spread by direct or droplet transmission as a result of close contact, and their spread is enhanced by crowding or poor ventilation. Outbreaks among adults have occurred in military barracks, prisons, homeless shelters, and nursing homes. Rates of bacteremic infection are highest among children <2 years of age and drop to low levels until age 55, when incidence again begins to increase. Pneumococcal pneumonia occurs annually in an estimated 20 young adults per 100,000 and in 280 persons >70 years of age per 100,000. Native Americans, Native Alaskans, and African Americans are unusually susceptible to invasive disease.

Pathogenesis

Once the nasopharynx has been colonized, infection can result if pneumococci are carried into contiguous areas (e.g., the sinuses) or are inhaled or aspirated into the bronchioles or alveoli. Spread to meninges, joints, and other sites through the bloodstream usually arises from a respiratory tract focus of infection. Pneumococci cause an inflammatory response, but—in the absence of anticapsular antibodies, which provide the best specific protection against pneumococcal infection—the polysaccharide capsule renders the organisms resistant to phagocytosis and killing. Many conditions predispose to pneumococcal infection. Risk factors for disease include increased exposure to pneumococci (e.g., in day-care centers, military barracks, prisons, or homeless shelters); antecedent respiratory insult with inflammation (e.g., influenza or upper respiratory viral infection, air pollution, allergies, cigarette smoking, or chronic obstructive pulmonary disease); anatomical disruption (e.g., dural tear); defects in antibody production (e.g., in pts with hypo- or agammaglobulinemia, multiple myeloma, chronic lymphocytic leukemia, or lymphoma); defects in splenic function (e.g., asplenia, sickle cell disease); and other, multifactorial conditions (e.g., infancy or aging, chronic disease and hospitalizations, alcoholism, malnutrition, HIV infection, glucocorticoid treatment, cirrhosis, renal insufficiency, diabetes, anemia, coronary artery disease, fatigue, and stress). The absence of a spleen predisposes to fulminant pneumococcal disease.

Specific Infections

OTITIS MEDIA AND SINUSITIS *S. pneumoniae* is the most common bacterial isolate from middle-ear fluid in acute otitis media and from paranasal sinus fluid during acute sinusitis. See Chap. 60 for more detail.

PNEUMONIA Pts usually present with fever, cough, and sputum production. Nausea and vomiting or diarrhea may be prominent. The "classic" presentation—an acute onset of a shaking chill, fever, and cough productive of blood-tinged sputum—is actually uncommon. On examination, pts usually appear ill and anxious, with fever, tachypnea, and tachycardia. Dullness to percussion, increased vocal fremitus, and bronchial or tubular breath sounds or crackles can be heard on pulmonary examination. Pleural effusions are common and may cause dullness to percussion, decreased breath sounds, and lack of fremitus. Hypoxemia may cause confusion, but meningitis should be considered as well. Empyema complicates ~2% of cases. On CXR, air-space consolidation is the predominant finding; disease is multilobar in about half of pts. Air bronchograms are evident in fewer than half of cases but are more common in bacteremic disease. Leukocytosis (>12,000 WBCs/μL) is usually present; WBC counts of <6000/μL may be associated with a poor prognosis. Pneumococcal pneumonia is strongly suggested by a sputum Gram's stain with >25 PMNs and <10 squamous epithelial cells along with slightly elongated gram-positive cocci in pairs and chains. Sputum culture may be more sensitive than sputum Gram's stain for identifying *S. pneumoniae*. Blood cultures are positive in ~25% of cases.

MENINGITIS *S. pneumoniae* is the most common cause of meningitis in adults. Infection results from direct extension (e.g., from the sinuses or middle ear) or from seeding during bacteremia. *S. pneumoniae* is also the most common cause of recurrent meningitis due to head trauma, CSF leak, and/or dural tear. Clinical and laboratory features resemble those of meningitis due to other bacteria. Pts have fever, headache, and neck stiffness, and disease progresses over 24–48 h to confusion and obtundation. On examination, the pt is acutely ill with a rigid neck. CSF findings consist of pleocytosis with ≥85% PMNs, elevated protein levels [1.0–5.0 g/L (100–500 mg/dL)], and decreased glucose content [1.7 mmol/L (<30 mg/dL)]. Organisms can be seen on a gram-stained specimen of CSF if antibiotics have not yet been given.

OTHER SYNDROMES *S. pneumoniae* can seed ordinarily sterile body sites via hematogenous spread, usually during pneumonia or occasionally from an inapparent focus. Pneumococcal endocarditis (an acute infection that results in rapid destruction of heart valves), pericarditis, septic arthritis, osteomyelitis, peritonitis, salpingitis, epidural and brain abscesses, and cellulitis have been described. Unusual manifestations of pneumococcal infection should prompt consideration of testing for HIV infection.

 TREATMENT

Penicillin has been the cornerstone of treatment, but resistance has been slowly increasing over the past two decades. Resistance to other antibiotics is often present as well. In the United States, ~20% of pneumococcal isolates are intermediately susceptible to penicillin (MIC, 0.1–1.0 μg/mL), and 15% are resistant (MIC, ≥2.0 μg/mL). These definitions are based on levels achievable in the CSF to treat meningitis. Pneumonia caused by a penicillin-resistant strain often still responds to 24 mU of penicillin daily. Most penicillin-intermediate strains are susceptible to ceftriaxone, cefotaxime, cefepime, and cefpodoxime, but penicillin-resistant pneumococci are often resistant to those cephalosporins as well. One-quarter of pneumococcal isolates in the United States are resistant to macrolides, with particularly high rates among strains that are also resistant to penicillin; however, >90% of isolates retain sensitivity to clindamycin. The newer quinolones have excellent activity against pneumococci, but resistance is emerging because of the widespread use of these agents.

Pneumonia

• Outpatient treatment: Amoxicillin (1 g q8h) should be effective except against strains highly resistant to penicillin. In those cases, a newer fluoroquinolone (e.g., gatifloxacin, 400 mg/d) can be used. Clindamycin will be effective in 90% of cases; doxycycline, azithromycin, or clarithromycin is likely to be efficacious in 75% of cases.

• Inpatient treatment: For strains susceptible or intermediately resistant to penicillin, β-lactam antibiotics are recommended—e.g., penicillin (3–4 mU q4h), ampicillin (1–2 g q6h), or ceftriaxone (1 g q12–24h). Fluoroquinolones (e.g., gatifloxacin, 400 mg/d) offer a good alternative, and clindamycin adequately treats >90% of cases. Pneumonia due to highly antibiotic-resistant pneumococci should be treated with either vancomycin (500 mg q6h) or a quinolone together with a third-generation cephalosporin. Treatment should initially be given by the IV route in most cases, and therapy should continue until at least 5 days after the pt becomes afebrile.

Meningitis

Initial treatment should include ceftriaxone (1–2 g q12h) plus vancomycin (500 mg q6h or 1 g q12h). Both drugs are used because the cephalosporin is likely to be effective in most cases and penetrates well into the CSF, while vancomycin covers all isolates (including those resistant to penicillin and cephalosporins) but displays unpredictable CSF penetration. If the isolate is susceptible to ceftriaxone, vancomycin should be discontinued; if it is resistant to ceftriaxone, both agents should be continued. Treatment for 10 days is recommended. Glucocorticoids should be given before or in conjunction with the first dose of antibiotics.

Endocarditis

Treatment with ceftriaxone and vancomycin, pending susceptibility testing, is indicated. Aminoglycosides can be used for synergy, but rifampin or fluoroquinolones are antagonistic with β-lactam antibiotics.

Prevention

Pneumococcal polysaccharide vaccine contains capsular polysaccharide from the 23 most prevalent serotypes of *S. pneumoniae*. It is at least 85% efficacious for ≥5 years in persons <55 years of age, but the level and duration of protection decrease with advancing age. Pts at high risk for pneumococcal disease (e.g., debilitated pts, pts with chronic lung disease, and pts with depressed IgG response) may not respond well to the vaccine. However, because of the safety and low cost of the vaccine, its administration is still recommended. Candidates for the vaccine include pts >2 years of age who are at risk for a serious complication of pneumococcal infection (e.g., asplenic pts; pts >65 years of age; pts with CSF leak, diabetes, alcoholism, cirrhosis, chronic renal insufficiency, chronic pulmonary disease, or advanced cardiovascular disease); pts who have an immunocompromising condition associated with increased risk of pneumococcal disease, such as multiple myeloma or HIV infection; pts who are at genetically increased risk, such as Native Americans and Native Alaskans; and pts who live in environments where outbreaks are likely, such as nursing homes. Recommendations for revaccination are less clear; most experts recommend at least one revaccination 5 years after initial vaccination. Children <2 years of age should receive the conjugate pneumococcal vaccine, which reduces invasive pneumococcal illness in this age group and (through a "herd effect") in the population as a whole.

For a more detailed discussion, see Musher DM: Pneumococcal Infections, Chap. 119, p. 806, in HPIM-16.

94

STAPHYLOCOCCAL INFECTIONS

Etiology

Staphylococci are gram-positive cocci that form grapelike clusters on Gram's stain and are catalase-positive (unlike streptococci), nonmotile, aerobic, and facultatively anaerobic. *Staphylococcus aureus* is the most virulent of the 33 staphylococcal species, causing disease through both toxin-mediated and non-toxin-mediated mechanisms. *S. aureus* is distinguished from other staphylococci (with few exceptions) by its production of coagulase, a surface enzyme that converts fibrinogen to fibrin.

S. aureus Infections

EPIDEMIOLOGY *S. aureus* is a component of the normal human flora, most frequently colonizing the anterior nares but also colonizing the skin (particularly if damaged), vagina, axilla, perineum, and oropharynx. Of healthy persons, 25–50% may be persistently or transiently colonized with *S. aureus*, and the rate is especially high among insulin-dependent diabetics, HIV-infected persons, injection drug users, hemodialysis pts, and pts with skin damage. Sites of colonization are reservoirs for future infection. *S. aureus* is an important cause of nosocomial as well as community-acquired infections. Methicillin-resistant *S. aureus* (MRSA) is common in hospitals, and its prevalence is increasing in community settings. Community MRSA isolates remain susceptible to non-β-lactam agents, whereas nosocomial strains are usually resistant to multiple agents.

PATHOGENESIS *Invasive* **S. aureus** *Disease* *S. aureus* is a pyogenic pathogen known for its capacity to induce abscess formation. For invasive *S. aureus* infection to occur, some or all of the following steps are necessary.

- Inoculation and local colonization of tissue surfaces: The anterior nares are the principal site of staphylococcal colonization in humans. Staphylococci may also be introduced directly into tissue—e.g., as a result of minor abrasions or via IV access catheters. The bacteria adhere to different tissue surfaces, such as those with exposed fibronectin, fibrinogen, or collagen. *S. aureus* can form a biofilm similar to that formed by coagulase-negative staphylococci.
- Invasion: The bacteria replicate at the site of infection, elaborate enzymes that facilitate survival and local spread across tissue surfaces, or elaborate toxins.
- Evasion of the host response and metastatic spread: *S. aureus* possesses an antiphagocytic polysaccharide microcapsule that facilitates evasion of host defenses and plays a role in abscess formation. *S. aureus* also has the capacity to survive intracellularly. Recurrences are relatively frequent because the organisms can survive in a quiescent state in various tissues and then cause recrudescent infections when conditions are suitable.

Host Response to **S. aureus** *Infection* PMNs constitute the primary host response to *S. aureus* infection.

Groups at Increased Risk of **S. aureus** *Infection*

• Hosts at increased risk for *S. aureus* infection include those with the following.

1. Frequent or chronic disruptions in epithelial integrity (e.g., pts with eczema)
2. Impaired leukocyte function or phagocytes defective in oxidative killing (e.g., neutropenic pts, pts with chronic granulomatous disease)
3. Indwelling foreign bodies

• At-risk populations often have multiple factors that increase susceptibility to *S. aureus* infections—e.g., diabetics have increased rates of colonization; use injectable insulin, which can introduce the organism into tissue; and may have impaired leukocyte function.

Toxin-Mediated Disease *S. aureus* produces three types of toxins: cytotoxins, pyrogenic toxins, and exfoliative toxins. Antitoxin antibodies are protective against toxin-mediated staphylococcal illness. Enterotoxins and toxic shock syndrome toxin 1 (TSST-1) act as "superantigens" or T cell mitogens and cause the release of large amounts of inflammatory mediators (such as interferon), producing multisystem disease that includes fever, rash, and hypotension.

DIAGNOSIS *S. aureus* infections are readily diagnosed by Gram's stain and microscopic examination of infected tissue. The organisms appear as large gram-positive cocci in pairs or clusters. Routine cultures are usually positive. PCR assays are being developed for rapid testing.

CLINICAL SYNDROMES *Skin and Soft Tissue Infection* Predisposing factors include skin disease, skin damage, injections, and poor personal hygiene. These infections are characterized by pus-containing blisters.

• *Folliculitis* involves hair follicles.
• *Furuncles* (boils) extend from follicles to cause true abscesses and more extensive, painful lesions.
• *Carbuncles* are often located in the lower neck, are even more severe and painful, and are due to coalesced lesions extending to deeper SC tissue.
• *Mastitis* occurs in nursing mothers.
• *S. aureus* also causes impetigo, cellulitis, hidradenitis suppurativa, and surgical wound infections (see Chap. 89).

Musculoskeletal Infections

• *S. aureus* is the most common cause of *osteomyelitis*, both from hematogenous dissemination and from contiguous spread from a soft tissue site (e.g., diabetic or vascular ulcers). Hematogenous osteomyelitis in children involves long bones and presents with fever, bone pain, and reluctance to bear weight. Leukocytosis, increased ESR, and positive blood cultures are typical. Hematogenous osteomyelitis in adults is often vertebral and occurs in pts with endocarditis, pts undergoing hemodialysis, injection drug users, or diabetics. Intense back pain and fever can occur. *Epidural abscess* is a serious complication that can present as trouble voiding or walking or as radicular pain in addition to symptoms of osteomyelitis; neurologic compromise can develop in the absence of timely treatment. Osteomyelitis from contiguous soft tissue infections is suggested by exposure of bone, a draining fistulous tract, failure to heal, or continued drainage.

- *S. aureus* is also the most common cause of *septic arthritis* among children. *S. aureus* septic arthritis in adults is associated with trauma or surgery or is due to hematogenous dissemination.
- *Pyomyositis*, an infection of skeletal muscles that is seen in tropical climates and in seriously compromised pts (including HIV-infected pts), causes fever, swelling, and pain overlying involved muscle and is usually due to *S. aureus* as well.

Respiratory Tract Infections

- Newborns and infants: serious infections characterized by fever, dyspnea, respiratory failure. Pneumatoceles may be seen on CXR. Pneumothorax and empyema may occur.
- Nosocomial pneumonia: occurs primarily in intubated pts in ICUs. Clinical presentations resemble those of other nosocomial pneumonias. Pts have an increased volume of purulent sputum, fever, and new pulmonary infiltrates and can develop respiratory distress.
- Community-acquired pneumonia: usually postviral (e.g., after influenza). Pts may present with fever, bloody sputum production, and midlung-field pneumatoceles or multiple patchy pulmonary infiltrates.

Bacteremia and Sepsis   The incidence of metastatic seeding during bacteremia has been estimated to be as high as 31%. Bones, joints, kidneys, and lungs are most commonly infected. Diabetes, HIV infection, and renal insufficiency are often seen in association with *S. aureus* bacteremia and increase the risk of complications.

Infective Endocarditis   (See also Chap. 85) *S. aureus* accounts for 25–35% of cases of bacterial endocarditis. The incidence is increasing as a result of injection drug use, hemodialysis, intravascular prosthetic devices, and immunosuppression. Mortality rates range from 20 to 40% despite the availability of effective antibiotics. There are four clinical settings in which *S. aureus* endocarditis is encountered.

- Right-sided endocarditis in association with injection drug use: Pts have high fever, a toxic appearance, and pleuritic chest pain and produce purulent sputum that is sometimes bloody. CXR can reveal septic emboli: small, peripheral, circular lesions that may cavitate.
- Left-sided native-valve endocarditis: Compared with pts with right-sided disease, those with left-sided native-valve endocarditis tend to be older, to have a worse prognosis, and to have a higher incidence of complications, including peripheral emboli, cardiac decompensation, and metastatic seeding.
- Prosthetic-valve endocarditis: This infection, which is particularly fulminant if it occurs in the early postoperative period, is associated with a high mortality rate. Valve replacement is usually an urgent priority. Pts are prone to develop valvular insufficiency and myocardial abscesses.
- Nosocomial endocarditis: makes up 15–30% of *S. aureus* endocarditis cases and is related to the increased use of intravascular devices. Pts are often critically ill before the infection, with many comorbid conditions, and the disease can be difficult to recognize.

Urinary Tract Infections   UTIs are infrequently caused by *S. aureus*. Unlike UTIs caused by other urinary pathogens, those caused by *S. aureus* are most often due to hematogenous dissemination.

Prosthetic Device–Related Infections   In contrast with coagulase-negative staphylococci, *S. aureus* causes more acute disease with localized and systemic manifestations that tend to be rapidly progressive. Successful treatment usually involves removal of the prosthetic device.

Toxin-Mediated Diseases

• Toxic shock syndrome (TSS): Pts with staphylococcal TSS may not have a clinically evident staphylococcal infection. TSS results from elaboration of an enterotoxin (many nonmenstrual TSS cases) or TSST-1 (some nonmenstrual cases and >90% of menstrual cases). Menstrual cases occur 2–3 days after menses begin. Diagnosis is based on a constellation of clinical findings. Case definition includes a fever $\geq$ 38.9°C ($\geq$102°F); hypotension; a diffuse macular rash that involves the palms and soles, with subsequent desquamation 1–2 weeks after disease onset; multisystem involvement—e.g., hepatic (bilirubin or aminotransferase levels $\geq$ 2 times normal), hematologic (platelet count $\leq$ 100,000/μL), renal (BUN or creatinine $\geq$ 2 times normal), mucous membranes (vaginal, oropharyngeal, or conjunctival hyperemia), GI (vomiting or diarrhea at the onset of illness), muscular (myalgias or serum creatine phosphokinase $\geq$ 2 times normal), CNS (disorientation or altered consciousness without focal findings); and no evidence of other illnesses.

• Food poisoning: results from inoculation of toxin-producing *S. aureus* into food by colonized food handlers. Toxin is then elaborated in growth-promoting foods, such as custard, potato salad, or processed meat. The heat-stable toxin is not destroyed even if heating kills the bacteria. Disease onset is rapid and explosive, occurring within 1–6 h of ingestion of contaminated food. The chief signs and symptoms are nausea and vomiting, but diarrhea, hypotension, and dehydration may occur. Fever is absent. Symptoms resolve within 8–10 h.

• Staphylococcal scalded-skin syndrome (SSSS): most often affects newborns and infants. Disease ranges from localized blisters to exfoliation of most of the skin surface. Skin is fragile, with tender, thick-walled, fluid-filled bullae. Nikolsky's sign is diagnosed when gentle pressure of bullae causes rupture of lesions and leaves denuded underlying skin.

PREVENTION   Hand washing and careful attention to appropriate isolation procedures prevent the spread of *S. aureus* infection. Mupirocin treatment to eliminate nasal carriage of *S. aureus* has reduced rates of infection among hemodialysis and peritoneal dialysis pts. Reduction in rates of wound infection among pts undergoing surgery is less evident and appears to be limited to pts proven to be nasally colonized with *S. aureus*.

Infections Caused by Coagulase-Negative Staphylococci (CoNS)

CoNS are less virulent than *S. aureus* but are important and common causes of prosthetic-device infections. Of CoNS species, *S. epidermidis* causes most disease. This organism is a normal component of the skin, oropharyngeal, and vaginal flora. *S. saprophyticus* is a cause of UTIs. Two other species of CoNS, *S. lugdunensis* and *S. schleiferi*, are more virulent and cause serious infections such as native-valve endocarditis and osteomyelitis.

PATHOGENESIS   CoNS are uniquely adapted to cause prosthetic-device infections because they can elaborate extracellular polysaccharide (slime) that forms a protective biofilm on the device surface, protecting bacteria from host defenses as well as from antibiotic treatment while allowing bacterial survival.

CLINICAL SYNDROMES   CoNS cause diverse prosthetic device–related infections. Signs of localized infection are usually subtle, disease progression is slow, and systemic findings are limited. Fever and mild leukocytosis may be documented. Infections not associated with prosthetic devices are infrequent, but up to 5% of native-valve endocarditis cases have been due to CoNS in some series.

Table 94-1

Antimicrobial Therapy for Serious _S. aureus_ Infections[a]

Sensitivity/Resistance of Isolate	Drug of Choice	Alternative(s)	Comments
Sensitive to penicillin	Penicillin G (4 mU q4h)	Nafcillin (2 g q4h) or oxacillin (2 g q4h), cefazolin (2 g q8h), vancomycin (1 g q12h[b])	Fewer than 5% of isolates are sensitive to penicillin.
Sensitive to methicillin	Nafcillin or oxacillin (2 g q4h)	Cefazolin (2 g q8h[b]), vancomycin (1 g q12h[b])	Patients with penicillin allergy can be treated with a cephalosporin if the allergy does not involve an anaphylactic or accelerated reaction; vancomycin is the alternative. Desensitization to β-lactams may be indicated in selected cases of serious infection where maximal bactericidal activity is needed (e.g., prosthetic-valve endocarditis[c]). Type A β-lactamase may rapidly hydrolyze cefazolin and reduce its efficacy in endocarditis.
Resistant to methicillin	Vancomycin (1 g q12h[b])	TMP-SMX (TMP, 5 mg/kg q12h[b]), minocycline (100 mg PO q12h[b]), ciprofloxacin (400 mg q12h[b]), levofloxacin (500 mg q24h[b]), quinupristin/dalfopristin (7.5 mg/kg q8h), linezolid (600 mg q12h _except:_ 400 mg q12h for uncomplicated skin infections); daptomycin (4 mg/kg q24h[b]) for complicated skin infections; investigational drugs: oritavancin, tigecycline	Sensitivity testing is necessary before an alternative drug is used. Adjunctive drugs (those that should be used only in combination with other antimicrobial agents) include gentamicin (1 mg/kg q8h[b]), rifampin (300 mg PO q8h), and fusidic acid (500 mg q8h; not readily available in the United States). Quinupristin/dalfopristin is bactericidal against methicillin-resistant isolates unless the strain is resistant to erythromycin or clindamycin. The newer quinolones may retain in vitro activity against ciprofloxacin-resistant isolates; resistance may develop during therapy. The efficacy of adjunctive therapy is not well established in many settings. Both linezolid and quinupristin/dalfopristin have had in vitro activity against most VISA and VRSA strains. See footnote for treatment of prosthetic-valve endocarditis.[c]

452

| Resistant to methicillin with intermediate or complete resistance to vancomycin[a] | Uncertain | Same as for methicillin-resistant strains; check antibiotic susceptibilities |
| Not yet known (i.e., empirical therapy) | Vancomycin (1 g q12h) | — | Empirical therapy is given when the susceptibility of the isolate is not known. Vancomycin with or without an aminoglycoside is recommended for suspected community- or hospital-acquired S. aureus infections because of the increased frequency of methicillin-resistant strains in the community. |

[a] Recommended dosages are for adults with normal renal and hepatic function. The route of administration is intravenous unless otherwise indicated.

[b] The dosage must be adjusted in patients with reduced creatinine clearance.

[c] For the treatment of prosthetic-valve endocarditis, the addition of gentamicin (1 mg/kg q8h) and rifampin (300 mg PO q8h) is recommended, with adjustment of the gentamicin dosage if the creatinine clearance rate is reduced.

[d] Vancomycin-resistant S. aureus isolates from clinical infections have recently been reported.

Note: TMP-SMX, trimethoprim-sulfamethoxazole; VISA, vancomycin-intermediate S. aureus; VRSA, vancomycin-resistant S. aureus.

Source: Modified with permission of the *New England Journal of Medicine* (Lowy, 1998). Copyright 1998 Massachusetts Medical Society. All rights reserved.

453

DIAGNOSIS CoNS are readily detected by standard methods, but distinguishing infection from colonization is often problematic. CoNS are frequent contaminants of cultures of blood and other sites, with true infection in a fraction of cases.

℞ TREATMENT

In the treatment of staphylococcal infections, suppurative collections should be surgically drained. In most cases of prosthetic-device infections, the device should be removed, although some CoNS infections can be managed medically. Antibiotic therapy for *S. aureus* infection is generally prolonged, particularly if blood cultures remain positive 48–96 h after initiation of therapy, infection is acquired in the community, a removable focus of infection is not removed, or cutaneous or embolic manifestations of infection occur. The selection of antimicrobial agents is increasingly difficult because of the prevalence of multidrug-resistant strains. Antimicrobial therapy for serious *S. aureus* infections is summarized in Table 94-1. Fewer than 5% of isolates are sensitive to penicillin, but when strains are susceptible, penicillin is still the drug of choice. Penicillinase-resistant penicillins, such as nafcillin or first-generation cephalosporins, are highly effective against penicillin-resistant strains. The incidence of MRSA is high in hospital settings, and strains intermediately or fully resistant to vancomycin have now been described. In general, vancomycin is less bactericidal than the β-lactams and should be used only when absolutely indicated. Among newer antistaphylococcal agents, quinupristin/dalfopristin displays bactericidal activity against all strains, including those intermediately sensitive to vancomycin, but is bacteriostatic against isolates resistant to erythromycin or clindamycin; linezolid is bacteriostatic and has not yet been established as efficacious in deep-seated infections such as osteomyelitis; and daptomycin is bactericidal and approved by the FDA for complicated skin infections. Other alternatives to β-lactam agents or vancomycin include the quinolones, trimethoprim-sulfamethoxazole, and minocycline, but these agents generally have weaker antistaphylococcal activity. Resistance to fluoroquinolones is increasing. Synergy has been demonstrated for certain antimicrobial combinations: β-lactams and aminoglycosides; vancomycin and gentamicin; vancomycin, gentamicin, and rifampin (against CoNS); and vancomycin and rifampin.

Special considerations are applicable in selected settings.

- Uncomplicated skin and soft tissue infections: Oral agents are usually adequate.
- Native-valve endocarditis: A β-lactam for 4–6 weeks plus gentamicin (1 mg/kg q8h) for 3–5 days. (Addition of gentamicin does not alter clinical outcome but reduces the duration of bacteremia.) If infection is due to MRSA, vancomycin (1 g q12h) is recommended. Treatment should continue for 4–6 weeks.
- Prosthetic-valve endocarditis: Surgery is often needed in addition to antibiotics. A β-lactam (or vancomycin if MRSA is involved) with gentamicin and rifampin is indicated.
- Hematogenous osteomyelitis or septic arthritis: A 4-week treatment course is adequate for children, but adults require longer courses. Joint infections require repeated aspiration or arthroscopy to prevent damage from inflammatory cells.
- Chronic osteomyelitis: Surgical debridement is needed in most cases.
- Prosthetic-joint infections: The combination of ciprofloxacin plus rifampin has been used successfully, particularly when the prosthesis cannot be removed.

• TSS: Supportive therapy and removal of tampons or other packing material or debridement of an infected site are most important. The role of antibiotics is less clear, but a clindamycin/semisynthetic penicillin combination is recommended. Clindamycin is used because it is a protein synthesis inhibitor and has been shown to decrease toxin synthesis in vitro. IV immunoglobulin may be helpful. The role of glucocorticoids is uncertain.

For a more detailed discussion, see Lowy FD: Staphylococcal Infections, Chap. 120, p. 814, in HPIM-16.

95

STREPTOCOCCAL/ENTEROCOCCAL INFECTIONS, DIPHTHERIA, AND OTHER CORYNEBACTERIAL INFECTIONS

STREPTOCOCCAL/ENTEROCOCCAL INFECTIONS

Many varieties of streptococci are part of the normal human flora, colonizing the respiratory, GI, and genitourinary tracts. Streptococci are gram-positive cocci that form chains when grown in liquid media. Most are facultative anaerobes and are relatively fastidious, requiring enriched media to grow. When streptococci are cultured on blood agar, three types of hemolytic patterns occur.

• β-Hemolysis: complete hemolysis around a colony. In humans, the most common streptococcal pathogens are β-hemolytic streptococci of Lancefield groups A, B, C, and G. Lancefield grouping depends on cell-wall carbohydrate antigens.
• α-Hemolysis: partial hemolysis imparting a greenish appearance to agar. This pattern is seen with *S. pneumoniae* and viridans streptococci.
• γ-Hemolysis: no hemolysis. This pattern is typical of enterococci, *S. bovis*, and anaerobic streptococci.

Group A *Streptococcus* (GAS)

ETIOLOGY AND PATHOGENESIS GAS causes suppurative infections and is associated with postinfectious syndromes such as acute rheumatic fever (ARF) and poststreptococcal glomerulonephritis (PSGN). The major surface protein, M protein, and the hyaluronic acid polysaccharide capsule protect against phagocytic ingestion and killing. GAS produces a large number of extracellular products that may contribute to local and systemic toxicity; these include streptolysins S and O, streptokinase, DNases, and pyrogenic toxins that cause the rash of scarlet fever and contribute to the pathogenesis of toxic shock syndrome (TSS) and necrotizing fasciitis.

CLINICAL FEATURES *Pharyngitis* GAS pharyngitis is among the most common bacterial infections in children; GAS accounts for 20–40% of all cases of exudative pharyngitis in children >3 years of age. Respiratory droplets spread infection. After an incubation period of 1–4 days, pts develop sore throat, fever, chills, malaise, and GI manifestations. Examination reveals an erythematous pharyngeal mucosa, swelling, purulent exudates over the posterior pharynx and tonsillar pillars, and tender anterior cervical adenopathy. Viral pharyngitis is the more likely diagnosis when patients have coryza, hoarseness, conjunctivitis, or mucosal ulcers. Rapid diagnosis by latex agglutination or enzyme immunoassay is variably sensitive but highly specific. Throat culture is the "gold standard" for diagnosis. Serologic tests (e.g., antistreptolysin O) confirm past infection in pts with suspected ARF but are not useful for the acute diagnosis of pharyngitis. Symptoms resolve spontaneously in most pts after 3–5 days.

 TREATMENT

The primary goal of treatment is to prevent suppurative complications (e.g., lymphadenitis, abscess, sinusitis, bacteremia, pneumonia) and ARF; therapy does not seem to prevent PSGN. Benzathine penicillin G (1.2 mU IM once) or penicillin V (250 mg PO tid or 500 mg bid for 10 days) is the recommended regimen. Macrolides such as erythromycin may be used, but resistance to these agents is increasing. Asymptomatic GAS carriage is usually not treated; however, when the pt is the source of infection in others, penicillin V (500 mg qid for 10 days) with rifampin (600 mg bid for the final 4 days) is used.

Scarlet Fever Scarlet fever is the designation for GAS pharyngitis associated with a characteristic rash (perhaps a hypersensitivity reaction from prior exposure to pyrogenic exotoxin A, B, or C). The rash typically appears in the first 2 days of illness over the upper trunk and spreads to the extremities but not to the palms and soles. The skin has a sandpaper feel. Other findings include strawberry tongue (enlarged papillae on a coated tongue) and Pastia's lines (accentuation of rash in skin folds). Rash improves in 6–9 days with desquamation on palms and soles. Scarlet fever is much less common than in the past.

Skin and Soft Tissue Infections See Chap. 89 for further discussion of clinical manifestations and treatment.

1. *Impetigo*: A superficial skin infection, impetigo is also occasionally caused by *Staphylococcus aureus*. The disease is most often seen in young children in warmer months or climates and under poor hygienic conditions. The facial areas around the nose and mouth and the legs are the sites most commonly involved. Red papular lesions evolve into pustules that crust. Pts are usually afebrile. Treatment should cover GAS and *S. aureus*; thus dicloxacillin or cephalexin (250 mg qid for 10 days) is used. Topical mupirocin ointment is also effective. GAS impetigo is associated with PSGN.

2. *Cellulitis*: GAS cellulitis develops at anatomic sites where normal lymphatic drainage has been disrupted (e.g., areas of prior cellulitis, the ipsilateral arm after mastectomy and axillary node dissection). Organisms may enter at sites distant from the area of cellulitis where there is a breach of skin integrity. GAS may cause rapidly developing postoperative wound infection. *Erysipelas*, a form of cellulitis that usually involves the malar facial area or the lower extremities, is caused almost exclusively by GAS. Pts experience an acute onset of bright red swelling that is sharply demarcated from normal skin as well as pain and fever. The illness develops over hours, and blebs or bullae may form after 2 or 3 days. Empirical treatment for cellulitis is directed against GAS and *S. aureus*. However, erysipelas or cellulitis known to be due to GAS is treated with penicillin (1–2 mU IV q4h). Mild to moderate disease may be treated with procaine penicillin (1.2 mU IM bid).

3. *Necrotizing fasciitis*: GAS causes ~60% of cases of necrotizing fasciitis. Immediate surgical debridement is key, as is the administration of penicillin G (2–4 mU IV q4h) plus clindamycin (600–900 mg q8h).

Pneumonia and Empyema GAS occasionally causes pneumonia. The onset can be gradual or abrupt. Pts have pleuritic chest pain, fever, chills, and dyspnea; ~50% have accompanying pleural effusions that are almost always infected and should be drained quickly to avoid loculation. Cough may not be a prominent symptom.

Bacteremia In most cases of bacteremia, a focus is readily identifiable. Bacteremia occurs occasionally with cellulitis and frequently with necrotizing fasciitis. If a focus is not evident, a diagnosis of endocarditis, occult abscess, or osteomyelitis should be considered.

Puerperal Sepsis Common in the preantibiotic era, puerperal sepsis is now rare. Outbreaks are associated with asymptomatic carriage of GAS by delivery room personnel.

Toxic Shock Syndrome Table 95-1 presents a proposed case definition for streptococcal TSS. Pyrogenic exotoxin A and other exotoxins associated with this syndrome act as superantigens to trigger release of inflammatory cy-

Table 95-1

Proposed Case Definition for the Streptococcal Toxic Shock Syndrome[a]

I. Isolation of group A streptococci (*Streptococcus pyogenes*)
  A. From a normally sterile site (e.g., blood, cerebrospinal fluid, pleural or peritoneal fluid, tissue biopsy, surgical wound)
     From a nonsterile site (e.g., throat, sputum, vagina, superficial skin lesion)
II. Clinical signs of severity
  A. Hypotension: Systolic blood pressure of ≤90 mmHg in adults or in the 5th percentile for age in children *and*
     Two or more of the following signs:
     1. Renal impairment: Serum creatinine level of ≥177 μmol/L (≥2 mg/dL) for adults or at least twice the upper limit of normal for age; in patients with preexisting renal disease, elevation over baseline by a factor of at least 2
     2. Coagulopathy: Platelet count of ≤100 × 10^9/L (100,000/μL) *or* DIC, defined by prolonged clotting times, low fibrinogen level, and the presence of fibrin degradation products
     3. Liver involvement: Alanine aminotransferase (SGOT), aspartate aminotransferase (SGPT), or total bilirubin level at least twice the upper limit of normal for age; in patients with preexisting liver disease, elevation over baseline by a factor of at least 2
     4. ARDS, defined by acute onset of diffuse pulmonary infiltrates and hypoxemia in the absence of cardiac failure; *or* evidence of diffuse capillary leak manifested by acute onset of generalized edema; *or* pleural or peritoneal effusions with hypoalbuminemia
     5. Generalized erythematous macular rash that may desquamate
     6. Soft tissue necrosis, including necrotizing fasciitis or myositis; *or* gangrene

[a] An illness fulfilling criteria IA, IIA, and IIB is defined as a *definite* case. An illness fulfilling criteria IB, IIA, and IIB is defined as a *probable* case if no other etiology for the illness is identified.
Source: Working Group on Severe Streptococcal Infections, 1993.

tokines from T lymphocytes. Unlike TSS due to *S. aureus*, streptococcal TSS includes bacteremia in most pts, does not usually cause the development of a rash, and commonly includes a soft tissue infection (cellulitis, necrotizing fasciitis, or myositis). The mortality rate for streptococcal TSS is ~30%, with most deaths due to shock and respiratory failure. Penicillin G (2–4 mU IV q4h) and clindamycin (600–900 mg q8h) are given. A single dose of IV immunoglobulin (2 g/kg) is given as adjunctive therapy in severe cases.

Streptococci of Groups C and G

Streptococci of groups C and G cause infections similar to those caused by GAS. Group C streptococci commonly cause infections in domesticated animals (e.g., horses and cattle), and contact with the infected animals or consumption of unpasteurized milk accounts for some infections. Group G organisms cause bacteremia and septic arthritis more commonly than do group C streptococci. Bacteremia occurs more frequently in elderly or chronically ill pts. Treatment is the same as for GAS infection. Septic arthritis should be treated with penicillin (1–4 mU IV q4h). Although it has not been shown to be superior, gentamicin (1 mg/kg q8h) is recommended by some experts for endocarditis or septic arthritis due to group C or G streptococci because of a poor clinical response to penicillin alone. Joint infections can require repeated aspiration or open drainage for cure.

Group B *Streptococcus* (GBS)

GBS is a major cause of meningitis and sepsis in neonates and a frequent cause of peripartum fever in women.

NEONATAL INFECTION *Early-onset infection* occurs within the first week of life (median age, 20 h). The infection is acquired within the maternal genital tract during birth. Neonates have respiratory distress, lethargy, hypotension, bacteremia, pneumonia (one-third to one-half of cases), and meningitis (one-third of cases).

Late-onset infection develops between 1 week and 3 months of age (mean age, 3–4 weeks). Meningitis is the most common manifestation. Infants are lethargic, febrile, and irritable; feed poorly; and may have seizures.

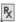 TREATMENT

Penicillin or ampicillin is the agent of choice and is administered with gentamicin while cultures are pending. Pts with bacteremia or soft tissue infection should receive penicillin at a dosage of 200,000 units/kg per day in divided doses; those with meningitis should receive 400,000 units/kg per day in divided doses for 14 days. Many physicians continue to give gentamicin until the pt improves clinically.

Prevention About half of the infants delivered vaginally to mothers colonized with GBS (5–40% of women) become colonized, but only 1–2% develop infection. The risk of neonatal GBS is high if delivery is preterm or if the mother has an early rupture of membranes (>24 h before delivery), prolonged labor, fever, or chorioamnionitis. Identification of high-risk mothers and prophylactic administration of ampicillin or penicillin during delivery reduce the risk of neonatal infection. Screening for anogenital colonization with GBS at 35–37 weeks of pregnancy is currently recommended. Women who have previously given birth to an infant with GBS disease, who have a history of GBS bacteriuria during pregnancy, or who have an unknown culture status but risk factors noted above should receive intrapartum prophylaxis (usually 5 mU of penicillin G followed by 2.5 mU q4h until delivery). Cefazolin can be used as well. If the mother is at risk for anaphylaxis and the GBS isolate is known to be susceptible, clindamycin or erythromycin can be used; otherwise, vancomycin is indicated.

ADULT INFECTION Most GBS infections in adults are related to pregnancy and parturition. Other GBS infections are seen in the elderly, especially those with underlying conditions such as diabetes mellitus or cancer. Cellulitis and soft tissue infection, UTI, pneumonia, endocarditis, and septic arthritis are most common. Penicillin (12 mU/d for localized infections and 18–24 mU/d for endocarditis or meningitis, in divided doses) is recommended. Vancomycin is an acceptable alternative for penicillin-allergic pts.

Enterococci and Nonenterococcal Group D Streptococci

ENTEROCOCCI *Epidemiology* *E. faecalis* and *E. faecium* are significant pathogens that tend to produce infection in elderly or debilitated pts and in those whose mucosal or epithelial barriers are disrupted or whose normal flora is perturbed by antibiotic treatment.

Clinical Features Enterococci cause UTIs, especially in pts who have received antibiotics or have undergone instrumentation; bacteremia related to intravascular catheters; bacterial endocarditis of both native and prosthetic valves (10–20% of cases, usually with a subacute presentation but sometimes with an acute presentation and rapidly progressive valve destruction); biliary tract infections; and mixed infections, including those arising from bowel flora (e.g., abdominal surgical wounds and diabetic foot ulcers).

℞ TREATMENT

Therapy is complicated by the fact that penicillin alone does not reliably kill enterococci except in UTIs as well as by increasing drug resistance.

- Endocarditis and meningitis: penicillin (3–4 mU q4h) or ampicillin (2 g q4h) *plus* gentamicin (1 mg/kg q8h) for 4–6 weeks. Vancomycin may be substituted in penicillin-allergic pts.
- Gentamicin resistance (MIC > 2000 μg/mL) is increasingly common. If gentamicin-resistant strains are susceptible to streptomycin, the latter agent should be substituted.
- Penicillin or ampicillin resistance: If resistance is due to β-lactamase production, then β-lactam/β-lactamase inhibitor combinations or imipenem may be used along with gentamicin. Otherwise, vancomycin is recommended along with gentamicin.
- Vancomycin and penicillin resistance: Quinupristin/dalfopristin is effective against *E. faecium* with this resistance pattern. Linezolid, an oxazolidinone antibiotic, is effective against nearly all enterococci with such resistance.

OTHER GROUP D STREPTOCOCCI *S. bovis* has been associated with GI malignancies and other bowel lesions, which are found in ≥60% of pts presenting with *S. bovis* endocarditis. Penicillin alone constitutes adequate therapy.

Viridans Streptococci

Many viridans streptococcal species are part of the normal oral flora, residing in close association with the teeth and gingiva. Minor trauma such as flossing or brushing teeth can cause transient bacteremia. Viridans streptococci have a predilection to cause endocarditis. Moreover, they are often part of a mixed flora in sinus infections and brain and liver abscesses. Bacteremia is common in neutropenic pts, who can develop a sepsis syndrome with high fever and shock. Risk factors in those pts include trimethoprim-sulfamethoxazole or fluoroquinolone prophylaxis, mucositis, or antacids or histamine-antagonist therapy. *S. milleri* (also known as *S. intermedius* or *S. anginosus*) differs from other viridans streptococci in both hemolytic pattern and clinical syndromes; this organism commonly causes suppurative infections, especially abscesses of brain and viscera, as well as respiratory tract infections such as pneumonia, empyema, and lung abscess. Neutropenic pts should receive vancomycin pending susceptibility testing; other pts may be treated with penicillin.

Nutritionally Variant Streptococci

The organisms formerly known as nutritionally variant streptococci are now classified as the separate genus *Abiotrophia*. These fastidious organisms require media that are enriched (e.g., with vitamin B_6) for growth. They are associated with more frequent treatment failure and relapse in cases of endocarditis than are viridans streptococci. Addition of gentamicin (1 mg/kg q8h) to the penicillin regimen is recommended when *Abiotrophia* is present.

DIPHTHERIA

DEFINITION Diphtheria, a localized infection of mucous membranes or skin, is caused by *Corynebacterium diphtheriae* and is associated with a characteristic pseudomembrane at the site of infection. Some strains produce diphtheria toxin, which can cause myocarditis, polyneuropathy, and other toxicities.

ETIOLOGY *C. diphtheriae* is a club-shaped, aerobic, nonmotile, grampositive rod that is often arranged in clusters (Chinese letters) or parallel arrays (palisades) in culture.

EPIDEMIOLOGY *C. diphtheriae* is transmitted via close personal contact. Fewer than 5 cases due to routine immunization are diagnosed per year in the United States. Disease in the United States occurs in elderly and alcoholic individuals—often those of low socioeconomic status—as well as in Native Americans.

CLINICAL FEATURES *Respiratory Diphtheria* Upper respiratory tract illness due to *C. diphtheriae* typically has a 2- to 5-day incubation period that is followed by the gradual onset of sore throat, low-grade fever, and an adherent membrane of the tonsils, pharynx, and/or nose. Unlike that of GAS pharyngitis, the pseudomembrane often extends beyond the margin of the tonsils onto the tonsillar pillars, palate, and uvula, and extension is associated with severe toxicity. Dislodging the membrane usually causes bleeding. Fewer than half of pts have dysphagia, headache, and voice alteration. Fewer than 10% have neck edema and trouble breathing—findings associated with increased mortality risk.

Complications

• Respiratory tract obstruction due to swelling and sloughing of pseudomembrane
• Myocarditis (dysrhythmias, conduction disturbances, and cardiomyopathy) is seen in almost one-quarter of hospitalized pts; those who die usually do so within 4 or 5 days.

• Polyneuropathy occurs 3–5 weeks after diphtheria and follows an indolent course, usually beginning with gingival, lingual, or facial numbness; dysphonia; dysphagia; and paresthesias of the extremities. Cranial nerve dysfunction, muscle weakness, and sensory disturbances may occur. Hypotension due to autonomic dysfunction may occur 7–9 weeks after onset of polyneuropathy. Most survivors recover completely.

• Pneumonia develops in more than half of pts who succumb to diphtheria.

PROGNOSIS The death rate is highest in the first week of disease among pts with bull-neck diphtheria (extensive pseudomembrane formation, foul breath, massive swelling of tonsils and uvula, thick speech, cervical lymphadenopathy, striking edematous swelling of the submandibular region and anterior neck, and severe toxicity); pts with myocarditis who develop ventricular tachycardia, atrial fibrillation, or complete heart block; pts with laryngeal or tracheobronchial involvement; infants; pts >60 years of age; and alcoholics.

DIAGNOSIS A definitive diagnosis is based on compatible clinical findings and isolation of *C. diphtheriae* from local lesions or its identification by histopathology. Samples from the nose, throat, and membrane (from beneath the membrane if possible) should be submitted for culture. In addition to nonselective media, appropriate selective media must be used.

 TREATMENT

Diphtheria antitoxin is the most important component of treatment and should be given as soon as possible. Because antitoxin is produced in horses, preparations must be made to treat potential allergic reactions, and pts with immediate hypersensitivity should be desensitized before receiving a full dose. To obtain antitoxin, contact the National Immunization Program at the CDC (404-639-8255 during the day; 404-639-2888 at any time). Treatment for 14 days with erythromycin (IM or PO; maximal dose, 2 g/d) or procaine penicillin G (600,000 U/d IM for pts weighing >10 kg) is used to prevent transmission to contacts. Rifampin and clindamycin are other options. Cultures should document eradication of the organism. Supportive care and isolation should be instituted.

PREVENTION DTaP (diphtheria and tetanus toxoids and acellular pertussis vaccine adsorbed) is recommended for primary immunization of children up to age 7 years. Td (tetanus and diphtheria toxoids) is recommended for routine booster use in adults at 10-year intervals or for tetanus-prone wounds. Close contacts of pts with respiratory diphtheria should have throat and nasal specimens cultured for *C. diphtheriae*, should receive a 7- to 10-day course of benzathine penicillin or oral erythromycin, and should receive antitoxin if they become ill.

OTHER CORYNEBACTERIAL INFECTIONS

Corynebacterium species are common components of the normal human flora. Corynebacterial infections have increased in frequency over the past several decades. If isolated, these organisms cannot immediately be dismissed as contaminants. Corynebacteria should be identified to the species level if they are isolated from a normally sterile site, if they predominate in an appropriately collected specimen, or if they are the only organisms in urine. *C. jeikeium* colonizes pts with cancer or severe immunodeficiency and can cause severe sepsis, endocarditis, device-related infections, pneumonia, and soft tissue infections. *C. urealyticum* is a cause of nosocomial UTI. *Arcanobacterium haemolyticum* can cause pharyngitis and chronic skin ulcers.

 TREATMENT

C. jeikeium and C. urealyticum are resistant to most antibiotics. Vancomycin is usually the empirical drug of choice pending susceptibility testing. Removal of the device is recommended if the infection is device-related. A. haemolyticum infection is treated with erythromycin because penicillin failures have occurred.

For a more detailed discussion, see Wessels MR : Streptococcal and Enterococcal Infections, Chap. 121, p. 823; and Holmes RK: Diphtheria and Other Corynebacterial Infections, Chap. 122, p. 832, in HPIM-16.

96

MENINGOCOCCAL AND LISTERIAL INFECTIONS

MENINGOCOCCAL INFECTIONS

ETIOLOGY AND EPIDEMIOLOGY   *Neisseria meningitidis* (the meningococcus) causes two life-threatening diseases: meningitis and fulminant meningococcemia. Meningococci are gram-negative aerobic diplococci with a polysaccharide capsule. Five serogroups—A, B, C, Y, and W-135—account for >90% of the 300,000 to 500,000 cases of meningococcal disease that occur worldwide each year. Serogroup A causes recurrent epidemics in sub-Saharan Africa. In the United States, serogroup B causes most sporadic disease and serogroup C causes most outbreaks. Disease rates are highest among infants and children; a second peak in teenagers is due to residence in barracks, dormitories, or other crowded situations. Meningococci are transmitted via respiratory secretions. Colonization of the nasopharynx or pharynx can persist asymptomatically for months. In nonepidemic situations, 10% of the population is colonized. Household contact with a meningococcal disease pt or a meningococcal carrier, household or institutional crowding, exposure to tobacco smoke, and a recent viral URI are risk factors for meningococcal colonization and invasive disease.

PATHOGENESIS   Meningococci colonize the upper respiratory tract, are internalized by nonciliated mucosal cells, enter the submucosa, and reach the bloodstream. If bacterial multiplication is slow, the bacteria may seed local sites such as the meninges. If multiplication is rapid, meningococcemia develops. Morbidity and mortality from meningococcemia have been directly correlated with the amount of circulating endotoxin, which can be 10- to 1000-fold higher than levels seen in bacteremias caused by other gram-negative organisms. Marked deficiencies in antithrombin and proteins C and S can occur during meningococcal disease, and there is a strong negative correlation between protein C activity and mortality risk. Antibodies to serogroup-specific capsular polysaccharide constitute the major host defense. Protective antibodies are induced by colonization with nonpathogenic bacteria possessing cross-reactive antigens. Deficiency of late-complement components C5–C9 can result in recurrent infections.

CLINICAL FEATURES

• Respiratory tract disease: Clinically apparent respiratory disease is most common among adults. Serogroup Y pneumonia is particularly likely in military populations.
• Meningococcemia without meningitis occurs in ∼10–30% of pts with meningococcal disease. Clinical manifestations include:

1. Fever, chills, nausea, vomiting, myalgias, prostration
2. Rash (erythematous macules, primarily on the trunk and extremities, that become petechial and—in severe cases—purpuric and may coalesce into hemorrhagic bullae that necrose and ulcerate)
3. Fulminant disease is associated with hemorrhagic skin lesions and DIC and is perhaps the most rapidly fatal form of septic shock in humans. Waterhouse-Friderichsen syndrome consists of DIC-induced microthrombosis, hemorrhage, tissue injury, and adrenal insufficiency.
4. Long-term morbidity includes loss of skin, limbs, or digits from ischemic necrosis and infarction.
5. Chronic meningococcemia is a rare syndrome of episodic fever, rash, and arthralgias lasting for weeks to months. If treated with steroids, this condition may become fulminant or evolve into meningitis.

• Meningitis pts usually present after >24 h of illness with headache, nausea and vomiting, neck stiffness, lethargy, and confusion. Petechial or purpuric skin lesions help distinguish this form of bacterial meningitis from other types. CSF examination reveals an increased protein concentration, a low glucose level, and neutrophilic leukocytosis. Sequelae include mental retardation, deafness, and hemiparesis.
• Arthritis occurs in ∼10% of pts with meningococcal disease.

DIAGNOSIS Definitive diagnosis relies on isolation of the organism from normally sterile body fluids. Gram's staining of CSF yields positive results in ∼85% of pts with meningococcal meningitis; if positive results are obtained in the absence of CSF leukocytosis, the prognosis is poor. PCR tests on buffy coat or CSF are more sensitive than Gram's staining or latex agglutination tests for meningococcal polysaccharides and are unaffected by prior antibiotic therapy.

 TREATMENT

See Table 96-1.
Glucocorticoid therapy (10 mg IV 15 min before the first antibiotic dose and then q6h for 4 days) is controversial, but many experts recommend it. Pts with fulminant meningococcemia need aggressive supportive therapy that can include vigorous fluid resuscitation, elective ventilation, pressor agents, fresh-frozen plasma (in pts with abnormal clotting parameters), and supplemental glucocorticoid treatment (hydrocortisone, 1 mg/kg q6h) for impaired adrenal reserve. Activated protein C (24 μg/kg per hour in a continuous infusion for 96 h) is recommended for pts with severe sepsis of any cause and an APACHE II score of >25; pts with meningococcemia may be one group most likely to benefit from this treatment. If the platelet count is <50,000/μL or if there is active bleeding, activated protein C should not be given.

Table 96-1

Antibiotic Treatment, Chemoprophylaxis, and Vaccinations for Invasive Meningococcal Disease

ANTIBIOTIC TREATMENT[a]

1. Ceftriaxone 2 g IV q12h (100 mg/kg per day) or cefotaxime 2 g IV q4h
2. For penicillin-sensitive *N. meningitidis*: Penicillin G 18–24 million units per day in divided doses q4h (250,000 units/kg per day)
3. Chloramphenicol 75–100 mg/kg per day in divided doses q6h
4. Meropenem 1.0 g (children, 40 mg) IV q8h
5. In an outbreak setting in developing countries: Long-acting chloramphenicol in oil suspension (Tifomycin), single dose
    Adults: 3.0 g (6 mL)
    Children 1–15 years old: 100 mg/kg
    Children <1 year old: 50 mg/kg

CHEMOPROPHYLAXIS[b]

Rifampin (oral)
    Adults: 600 mg bid for 2 days
    Children ≥1 month old: 10 mg/kg bid for 2 days
    Children <1 month old: 5 mg/kg bid for 2 days
Ciprofloxacin (oral)
    Adults: 500 mg, 1 dose
Ofloxacin (oral)
    Adults: 400 mg, 1 dose
Ceftriaxone (IM)
    Adults: 250 mg, 1 dose
    Children <15 years old: 125 mg, 1 dose
Azithromycin (oral)
    500 mg, 1 dose

VACCINATION[c]

A, C, Y, W-135 vaccine (Memomune, Aventis Pasteur) or A, C vaccine
    Single 0.5-mL subcutaneous injection
New C; A, C; and A, C, Y, W-135 meningococcal conjugate vaccines[d]

[a] Patients with meningococcal meningitis should receive antimicrobial therapy for at least 5 days.
[b] Use is recommended for close contacts of cases.
[c] At present, use is generally limited to the control of epidemics and to individuals with increased risk of meningococcal disease. Vaccine efficacy wanes after 3–5 years, and vaccine is not effective in recipients <2 years of age.
[d] These vaccines appear to provide immunity in young children, a prolonged immune response, and herd immunity (decreased transmission and colonization).

PROGNOSIS   Shock, purpuric or ecchymotic rash, low or normal blood leukocyte count, age ≥60 years, coma, absence of meningitis, thrombocytopenia, and low ESR are all associated with increased mortality risk. Receipt of antibiotics prior to hospital admission has been associated with a better outcome in some studies.

PREVENTION

• Vaccine: Immunizes against serogroups A, C, W-135, and Y but not serogroup B. Protection lasts <5 years. Vaccination is recommended for persons with late-complement-component deficiency, sickle cell anemia, or splenectomy as well as to military recruits, travelers to areas with epidemic disease, and college freshmen who will live in dormitories.

• Antimicrobial chemoprophylaxis: See Table 96-1 for prophylaxis options. Household and other close contacts (e.g., day-care center contacts, persons exposed to a pt's oral secretions) have a >400-fold higher risk of meningococcal disease than the population as a whole.

• Respiratory isolation: Hospitalized pts require respiratory isolation during the first 24 h of treatment.

LISTERIAL INFECTIONS

ETIOLOGY AND EPIDEMIOLOGY Unlike other food-borne pathogens, *Listeria monocytogenes* causes primarily invasive syndromes. The organism is a gram-positive bacillus with characteristic tumbling motility when cultured at 20° to 25°C. This intracellular organism is particularly likely to cause disease in pts with deficient cell-mediated immunity—e.g., in the setting of pregnancy or immunosuppression. The organism is both a veterinary and a human pathogen. It causes invasive disease in ~3–5 people per 1 million population each year in the United States. Perinatal disease complicates 9 births per 100,000. Most human disease is caused by ingestion of contaminated food. Many foods, such as hot dogs, soft cheeses, contaminated coleslaw, and food from delicatessen counters, have been implicated in sporadic and epidemic disease. The incubation period ranges from 2 to 6 weeks.

CLINICAL FEATURES

• Pregnancy-associated listeriosis: Most cases are diagnosed in the third trimester and are mild. Pts have fever, myalgias, malaise, and occasionally abdominal pain, nausea, and diarrhea. Chorioamnionitis, premature labor, intrauterine fetal death, or disease of the newborn can result from transplacental spread.

• Neonatal listeriosis: Early-onset disease usually presents within 2 days of birth, with sepsis, respiratory distress, skin lesions, and granulomatosis infantisepticum (disseminated abscesses of liver, spleen, adrenal glands, lungs, and other sites). Late-onset disease is more likely to present as meningitis.

• Listeriosis in nonpregnant adults: Pts usually are receiving chronic glucocorticoid therapy and/or have solid or hematologic malignancies, diabetes, renal disease, liver disease, or AIDS. Elderly immunocompetent adults can develop invasive listeriosis.

1. Sepsis: Bacteremic infection without a focus is the most common presentation.

2. CNS infection (usually acute meningitis): Pts present with fever, headache, and an altered level of consciousness. CSF examination reveals pleocytosis, increased protein concentrations, and normal glucose levels. Other CNS disease includes cerebritis, spinal cord or intracranial abscesses, and meningoencephalitis. Pts can have fever, ataxia, seizures, personality changes, and coma.

3. Endocarditis: damaged or prosthetic valves; frequent systemic embolization

4. Focal infections: Endophthalmitis, osteomyelitis, and abscesses can occur.

5. GI illness: *Listeria* occasionally causes acute gastroenteritis.

DIAGNOSIS Listeriosis is diagnosed when the organism is cultured from a usually sterile site, such as blood or CSF. Listeriae grow readily on routine media, but biochemical tests are needed to distinguish the organism from diphtheroids.

℞ TREATMENT

Cephalosporins are not effective against *Listeria* and should not be used alone as empirical treatment for meningitis or other invasive disease if the involvement of *Listeria* is being considered.

• Nonpregnant adults: ampicillin (2 g q4h) or penicillin (15–20 mU/d). Alternative: trimethoprim-sulfamethoxazole (15/75 mg/kg IV daily in 3 divided doses). Immunocompetent pts with meningitis should receive 2–3 weeks of therapy after defervescence. Compromised hosts should be treated for 4–6 weeks for meningitis or invasive disease. Gentamicin may be used for synergy.

• Pregnant adults: ampicillin (4–6 g/d in divided doses for 2 weeks). If the pt has a severe penicillin allergy, erythromycin may be used in the last month of pregnancy.

• Neonates: Ampicillin for 2 weeks with gentamicin for synergy.

PROGNOSIS Treatment of maternal bacteremia can prevent neonatal infection. Treatment of the newborn can limit sequelae, but disseminated disease is often fatal. Compromised hosts have a worse prognosis than healthy hosts.

For a more detailed discussion, see Stephens DS et al: Meningococcal Infections, Chap. 127, p. 849; and Schuchat A, Broome CV: Infections Caused by *Listeria monocytogenes*, Chap. 123, p. 837, in HPIM-16.

97

INFECTIONS CAUSED BY *HAEMOPHILUS*, *BORDETELLA*, *MORAXELLA*, AND HACEK GROUP ORGANISMS

HAEMOPHILUS INFLUENZAE

ETIOLOGY AND EPIDEMIOLOGY   *H. influenzae* is a small, gram-negative, pleomorphic coccobacillus. Strains with a polysaccharide capsule are serotyped *a* through *f*. *H. influenzae* type b (Hib) is most important clinically, causing systemic invasive disease in infants and children <6 years of age. Use of Hib conjugate vaccine has dramatically decreased rates of Hib colonization and invasive disease. Nontypable strains (NTHi), which are unencapsulated, cause disease by locally invading mucosal surfaces. Nontypable strains colonize the upper respiratory tract of up to 75% of healthy adults. *H. influenzae* is spread by airborne droplets or through direct contact with secretions or fomites.

CLINICAL FEATURES

• Hib: seen primarily in unvaccinated or underimmunized children

  1. Meningitis is associated with high morbidity; 6% of pts have sensorineural hearing loss; one-fourth have some significant sequelae; mortality is ~5%.

2. Epiglottitis, which occurs in older children and occasionally in adults, involves cellulitis of the epiglottis and supraglottic tissues that begins with a sore throat and progresses rapidly to dysphagia, drooling, and airway obstruction.
3. Miscellaneous: cellulitis, pneumonia, osteomyelitis

- NTHi

1. Community-acquired pneumonia in adults—especially those with chronic obstructive pulmonary disease (COPD) or AIDS—and exacerbations of COPD
2. Miscellaneous: childhood otitis media, puerperal sepsis, neonatal bacteremia, sinusitis, and—less commonly—invasive infections (e.g., empyema, adult epiglottitis, pericarditis, cellulitis, septic arthritis, osteomyelitis, endocarditis)

DIAGNOSIS   Gram's staining and culture of clinical samples

Ｒx **TREATMENT**

- Hib meningitis in adults: ceftriaxone (2 g q12h for 1–2 weeks)
- Hib meningitis in children: ceftriaxone (75–100 mg/kg per day, split into two doses given q12h) plus dexamethasone (0.6 mg/kg per day in four divided doses for 2 days at initiation of antibiotic treatment to prevent hearing loss)
- Epiglottitis: ceftriaxone (50 mg/kg daily for 1–2 weeks)
- NTHi: About one-fourth of clinical isolates produce β-lactamase. Many agents are useful: trimethoprim-sulfamethoxazole (TMP-SMX), amoxicillin/clavulanate, extended-spectrum cephalosporins, newer macrolides (azithromycin or clarithromycin), and fluoroquinolones (in nonpregnant adults).

PREVENTION   Hib vaccine is recommended for all children; the immunization series should be started at ~2 months of age. Secondary attack rates are high among household contacts of pts with Hib disease. In households where at least one member is incompletely vaccinated and <4 years of age, all household contacts should receive rifampin (20 mg/kg daily, up to 600 mg for 4 days). The index case should also receive rifampin to eradicate nasopharyngeal carriage of the organism. Children in the household should be immunized.

PERTUSSIS

ETIOLOGY   *Bordetella pertussis* causes pertussis, an acute respiratory tract infection. *B. pertussis* is a fastidious gram-negative aerobic bacillus that attaches to ciliated epithelial cells of the nasopharynx, multiplies locally, and produces a wide array of toxins and biologically active products.

EPIDEMIOLOGY   Pertussis is highly communicable. In households, attack rates are 80% among unimmunized contacts and 20% among immunized contacts. The incidence has been increasing slowly since 1976, particularly among adolescents and adults. Persistent cough of >2 weeks' duration in an adult may be due to *B. pertussis* in 12–30% of cases. Severe morbidity and mortality, however, are restricted to infants <6 months of age.

CLINICAL FEATURES   After an incubation period of 7–10 days, a prolonged coughing illness begins. Symptoms are usually more severe in infants and young children.

- The *catarrhal* phase is similar to the common cold and lasts 1–2 weeks.
- The *paroxysmal* phase follows and lasts 2–4 weeks. It is characterized by cough that at times occurs in spasmodic fits of 5–10 coughs each. Episodes are

worse at night. Vomiting or a "whoop" may follow a coughing fit. Apnea and cyanosis can occur during spasms. Pts become increasingly fatigued.
- In the *convalescent* phase, symptoms resolve over 1–3 months.

DIAGNOSIS

- Cultures of nasopharyngeal secretions remain positive in untreated cases for a mean of 3 weeks after illness onset. Secretions must be inoculated immediately onto selective media.
- PCR of nasopharyngeal specimens, especially in antibiotic-treated pts
- Although serology can be useful in pts with symptoms lasting >4 weeks, diagnostic criteria are not agreed upon, and antibody tests are not widely available.

 TREATMENT

- Macrolides: erythromycin (1–2 g/d for 1–2 weeks); clarithromycin (250 mg bid for 1 week); azithromycin (500-mg load on day 1, then 250 mg/d for 4 days)
- TMP-SMX in macrolide-intolerant pts
- Respiratory isolation for hospitalized pts until antibiotics have been given for 5 days

PREVENTION

- Chemoprophylaxis: Macrolide treatment for household contacts of pts, especially children <1 year of age
- Immunization: In the United States, acellular vaccines are safe for older children and adults.

MORAXELLA CATARRHALIS

ETIOLOGY *M. catarrhalis* is a gram-negative coccus that resembles *Neisseria*. It can retain crystal violet on Gram's staining and be confused with *Staphylococcus aureus*. Part of the normal flora of the upper airways, *M. catarrhalis* colonizes up to 50% of healthy children and up to 7% of healthy adults. Infection rates peak in late winter/early spring.

CLINICAL FEATURES

- Otitis media and sinusitis: *M. catarrhalis* is the third most common cause of otitis media in children and is a prominent isolate from cases of acute and chronic sinusitis.
- Purulent tracheobronchitis and pneumonia: Most pts are >50 years of age and have COPD (often with lung cancer as well).
- Symptoms are mild to moderate; invasive disease (e.g., empyema) is rare.

DIAGNOSIS Gram's staining of sputum is helpful, along with sputum cultures.

 TREATMENT

Because 85% of isolates produce β-lactamase, penicillin or ampicillin is often inadequate. Moraxellae are susceptible to second- and third-generation cephalosporins, penicillin/β-lactamase inhibitor combinations, tetracycline, newer macrolides, TMP-SMX, and quinolones. A 5-day course is adequate for respiratory infections.

Table 97-1

Treatment of Endocarditis Caused by HACEK Group Organisms[a]

Organism	Initial Therapy	Alternative Agents	Comments
Haemophilus species	Ceftriaxone (2 g/d)	Fluoroquinolones,[b] ampicillin/sulbactam	Ampicillin ± aminoglycoside can be used if organism does not produce β-lactamase.
Actinobacillus actinomycetemcomitans	Ceftriaxone (2 g/d)	Semisynthetic penicillins (e.g., mezlocillin), TMP-SMX, fluoroquinolones,[b] azithromycin	Limited data exist on efficacy of regimens other than semisynthetic penicillins or third-generation cephalosporins.
Cardiobacterium hominis	Penicillin (16–18 mU/d in 6 divided doses) ± gentamicin (5–6 mg/kg per day in 3 divided doses)	Ceftriaxone, ampicillin/sulbactam	Value of aminoglycoside has not been proven. Organism is usually pan-sensitive, but high-level resistance to penicillin has been reported.
Eikenella corrodens	Ampicillin (2 g q4h)	Ceftriaxone, fluoroquinolones[b]	Organism is resistant to clindamycin and metronidazole.
Kingella kingae	Ceftriaxone (2 g/d) or ampicillin/sulbactam (3 g of ampicillin q6h)	Fluoroquinolones,[b] vancomycin, clindamycin, macrolides, TMP-SMX	Prevalence of β-lactamase-producing strains is increasing. Efficacy for invasive infections is best demonstrated for first-line treatments.

[a] Susceptibility testing should be performed to guide therapy.
[b] Fluoroquinolones are not recommended for treatment of children <17 years of age.
NOTE: TMP-SMX, trimethoprim-sulfamethoxazole.

THE HACEK GROUP

ETIOLOGY The HACEK group consists of fastidious, slow-growing, gram-negative bacteria whose growth requires carbon dioxide. Normal residents of the oral cavity, HACEK bacteria can cause both local oral infections and severe systemic disease, particularly endocarditis. Several *Haemophilus* species, *Actinobacillus actinomycetemcomitans*, *Cardiobacterium hominis*, *Eikenella corrodens*, and *Kingella kingae* make up this group.

CLINICAL FEATURES

- HACEK endocarditis: Up to 3% of cases of infective endocarditis are caused by HACEK organisms; most of these cases are due to *Haemophilus* species, *A. actinomycetemcomitans*, or *C. hominis*. Pts often have underlying valvular disease. Embolization is common, even in subacute presentations. Major emboli are found in 28–71% of pts, and vegetations—often very large—in 85%. Cultures can take 30 days to become positive, although most cultures that ultimately yield HACEK bacteria become positive in the first week, especially with newer detection systems such as BACTEC.
- *Haemophilus* species: *H. aphrophilus*, *H. parainfluenzae*, and *H. paraphrophilus* cause more than half of all cases of HACEK endocarditis. Pts usually present within the first 2 months of illness and are usually anemic at presentation; about half develop CHF.
- *A. actinomycetemcomitans*: This organism is isolated from soft tissue infections in association with *Actinomyces israelii*. It is associated with severe destructive periodontal disease, which also is frequently evident in pts with endocarditis.
- *C. hominis*: Unlike other HACEK bacteria, *C. hominis* most often affects the aortic valve. Long-standing infection usually precedes diagnosis.
- *E. corrodens*: Usually a component of mixed infections, *E. corrodens* is common in human bite wounds, head and neck soft-tissue infections, endocarditis, and infections in IV drug users.
- *K. kingae*: *K. kingae* is the third most common cause of septic arthritis in children <2 years old and a common cause of osteomyelitis in the same age group. *K. kingae* bacteremia is seen in association with stomatitis (e.g., due to herpes simplex virus infection). Unlike other *K. kingae* infections, endocarditis due to this organism occurs in older children and adults.

℞ TREATMENT

See Table 97-1 for antibiotic regimens used to treat HACEK endocarditis. Native-valve endocarditis should be treated for 4 weeks and prosthetic-valve endocarditis for 6 weeks. Unlike prosthetic-valve endocarditis caused by other gram-negative organisms, that due to HACEK bacteria can often be cured with antibiotics alone (i.e., without surgery).

For a more detailed discussion, see Musher DM: *Moraxella catarrhalis* and Other *Moraxella* Species, Chap. 129, p. 862; Murphy TF: *Haemophilus* Infections, Chap. 130, p. 864; Kasper DL, Barlam TF: Infections Due to HACEK Group and Miscellaneous Gram-Negative Bacteria, Chap. 131, p. 867; and Halperin SA: Pertussis and Other *Bordetella* Infections, Chap. 133, p. 874, in HPIM-16.

98

DISEASES CAUSED BY GRAM-NEGATIVE ENTERIC BACTERIA, *PSEUDOMONAS*, AND *LEGIONELLA*

INFECTIONS CAUSED BY GRAM-NEGATIVE ENTERIC BACTERIA

Intestinal Infections Caused by *Escherichia coli*

At least six "pathotypes" of *E. coli* exclusively cause intestinal infections. (For further discussion, see Chap. 87.)

1. Shiga toxin–producing *E. coli* (STEC)/enterohemorrhagic *E. coli* (EHEC) is most common in developed countries. *E. coli* O157:H7 belongs to this pathotype. EHEC is associated with ingestion of contaminated food and water or person-to-person transmission. Ground beef is a common food source.
2. Pathotypes most common in developing countries
   a. Enterotoxigenic *E. coli* (ETEC): the most common agent of traveler's diarrhea
   b. Enteropathogenic *E. coli* (EPEC): an important cause of diarrhea among infants
   c. Enteroinvasive *E. coli* (EIEC): causes inflammatory colitis similar to that caused by *Shigella*
   d. Enteroaggregative and diffusely adherent *E. coli* (EAEC/DAEC): causes prolonged watery diarrhea

Diagnosis   Specific diagnosis is usually not necessary except when EHEC is involved. Bloody diarrhea can be screened for *E. coli* strains that do not ferment sorbitol, and strains can then be typed for *E. coli* O157:H7, but testing for Shiga toxins or toxin genes is more sensitive, specific, and rapid.

 TREATMENT

Supportive care, replacement of water and electrolytes, and avoidance of antibiotics in EHEC infection (since antibiotic use may increase the risk of hemolytic-uremic syndrome) are indicated.

Extraintestinal Pathogens

GENERAL CONSIDERATIONS   Enterobacteriaceae and *Acinetobacter* are normal components of the human colonic flora and can colonize mucosal and skin surfaces of pts in long-term-care and hospital settings. Virtually every organ or body cavity can be infected with these gram-negative bacilli. *E. coli*, *Klebsiella*, and *Proteus* account for most infections. The bacteria grow readily on standard media. Isolation of gram-negative bacilli from any sterile site almost always implies infection. Isolation from nonsterile sites requires clinical correlation.

EXTRAINTESTINAL PATHOGENIC *E. COLI* (ExPEC)   Most *E. coli* isolates from symptomatic infections outside the GI tract are distinct from commensal strains and from pathogenic strains that cause intestinal infections.

Clinical Features

- UTI: *E. coli* is the most prevalent pathogen in all genitourinary syndromes and causes 85–95% of acute uncomplicated UTIs.

- Abdominal and pelvic infection: the second most common site of ExPEC infection. Syndromes include peritonitis, intraabdominal abscesses, and cholangitis.
- Pneumonia: Gram-negative bacilli only transiently colonize the oropharynx in healthy people. In pts with underlying illnesses and antibiotic exposure, colonization and pneumonia rates increase. ExPEC is a common cause of pneumonia in long-term-care residents and hospitalized pts. *E. coli* can cause multifocal nodular infiltrates with tissue necrosis. Mortality rates are high.
- Meningitis: occurs mostly in neonates; caused by strains with the K1 capsular serotype
- Cellulitis/musculoskeletal infection: usually occurs as part of a polymicrobial picture. Cellulitis and burn-site or surgical-site infections can be due to *E. coli* when close to the perineum. Osteomyelitis, particularly vertebral, is more common than is generally appreciated; *E. coli* accounts for up to 10% of cases in some series.
- Bacteremia: can arise from primary infection at any site but originates most commonly from the urinary tract and next most commonly from the bowel and biliary tract. Endovascular infections are rare but have been described.

 TREATMENT

Resistance to ampicillin, piperacillin and β-lactam/β-lactamase inhibitor agents, first-generation cephalosporins, and trimethoprim-sulfamethoxazole (TMP-SMX) is increasing. Extended-spectrum β-lactamases (ESBLs) are increasingly common in *E. coli*. Currently, cephalosporins (particularly second-, third-, and fourth-generation agents), fluoroquinolones, monobactams, carbapenems, and aminoglycosides retain good activity.

KLEBSIELLA   Etiology   *K. pneumoniae* colonizes the colon in 5–35% of healthy individuals and causes most *Klebsiella* infections. *K. oxytoca* causes infections in long-term-care and hospital settings. *K. rhinoscleromatis* and *K. ozaenae* infect pts in tropical climates.

Clinical Features

- Pneumonia: occurs primarily in pts with underlying disease (e.g., alcoholism, diabetes, COPD). Long-term-care facility residents and hospitalized pts have higher rates of oropharyngeal colonization and more frequent *K. pneumoniae* pulmonary infections. The presentation is similar to that of pneumococcal pneumonia, with purulent sputum production and pulmonary infiltrates on CXR. Infection can progress to pulmonary necrosis, pleural effusion, and empyema.
- UTI: *K. pneumoniae* causes 1–2% of cases of uncomplicated cystitis and 5–17% of complicated UTIs.
- Abdominal infections: spectrum similar to that of *E. coli* but less frequent occurrence
- Cellulitis and soft tissue infections: most often involve devitalized tissues in compromised hosts. *K. pneumoniae* causes a significant minority of surgical-site infections.
- Miscellaneous: Bacteremia can arise from a primary infection at any site.
- Other infections: include endophthalmitis, nosocomial sinusitis, osteomyelitis

 TREATMENT

Klebsiellae are resistant to ampicillin and ticarcillin. Their resistance to third-generation cephalosporins is increasing, as is the frequency of ESBL-containing isolates. In general, fluoroquinolones, cephamycins (cefoxitin), fourth-generation cephalosporins, and amikacin retain broad activity against *Klebsiella*, with carbapenems being the most active agents.

PROTEUS Etiology *P. mirabilis* is part of the colonic flora in up to half of healthy people and causes 90% of *Proteus* infections. *P. vulgaris* and *P. penneri* are isolated primarily from pts in hospitals and long-term-care facilities.

Clinical Features *Proteus* causes 1–2% of uncomplicated UTIs, 5% of hospital-acquired UTIs, and 10–15% of complicated UTIs, especially those associated with urinary catheters. Pts with long-term catheterization have *Proteus* infection prevalence rates of 20–45%. *Proteus* produces high levels of urease, alkalinizes urine, and causes formation of struvite calculi. Infections in other sites occur but are uncommon.

Diagnosis *Proteus* exhibits swarming motility on agar plates. *P. mirabilis* is indole-negative, whereas most other *Proteus* strains are indole-positive.

 TREATMENT

P. mirabilis is susceptible to most agents. Resistance to ampicillin and first-generation cephalosporins is increasing. *P. vulgaris* and *P. penneri* are more resistant. Imipenem, fourth-generation cephalosporins, aminoglycosides, TMP-SMX, and quinolones have excellent activity. Infected struvite stones often require surgical removal.

MORGANELLA* AND *PROVIDENCIA Infections due to *M. morganii*, *P. stuartii*, and *P. rettgeri* resemble *Proteus* infections in epidemiology, pathogenicity, and clinical manifestations but occur almost exclusively in persons in long-term-care facilities and, to a lesser degree, in hospitalized pts. These species are particularly associated with long-term urinary catheterization (>30 days). Treatment with imipenem, fourth-generation cephalosporins, and amikacin is most reliable.

OTHER GRAM-NEGATIVE ENTERIC PATHOGENS *Enterobacter* (e.g., *E. cloacae, E. aerogenes*), *Acinetobacter* (e.g., *A. baumannii*), *Serratia* (e.g., *S. marcescens*), and *Citrobacter* (e.g., *C. freundii, C. koseri*) usually cause nosocomial infections. These organisms are associated with moist environmental foci. Risk factors include immunosuppression, comorbid disease, prior antibiotic use, and ICU stays.

Clinical Features

• Pneumonia, particularly ventilator-associated
• UTI, especially catheter-related
• Intravascular device–related infection, surgical-site infection, and abdominal infection
• *Enterobacter* species are associated with biliary disease.

 TREATMENT

Significant antibiotic resistance makes therapy challenging. Imipenem, fourth-generation cephalosporins, aminoglycosides (amikacin > gentamicin), TMP-SMX, and quinolones often have excellent activity. *Enterobacter* is commonly resistant to third-generation cephalosporins and monobactams. *Acinetobacter* may be susceptible to β-lactam/β-lactamase inhibitor agents, but these agents do not have enhanced activity against *Enterobacter* or *Citrobacter*.

AEROMONAS *A. hydrophila* is the most common *Aeromonas* species causing infection. *Aeromonas* organisms proliferate in potable and fresh water and are a putative cause of gastroenteritis. *Aeromonas* causes bacteremia and sepsis in infants and compromised hosts, especially those with cancer, hepatobiliary disease, trauma, or burns. The organisms can produce skin lesions similar to the ecthyma gangrenosum lesions seen with *P. aeruginosa*. Infection with *Aeromonas* can occur in trauma victims whose wounds are contaminated with water or soil. Because leeches are colonized with *Aeromonas*, their medical use necessitates the administration of antibiotics active against *Aeromonas*.

 TREATMENT

Aeromonas is usually susceptible to fluoroquinolones (e.g., ciprofloxacin at a dose of 500 mg PO q12h or 400 mg IV q12h), TMP-SMX (10 mg of TMP/kg per day in 3 or 4 divided doses), third-generation cephalosporins, and aminoglycosides.

INFECTIONS DUE TO *PSEUDOMONAS* AND RELATED SPECIES
Pseudomonas aeruginosa

Microbiology *P. aeruginosa* is an aerobic gram-negative rod; more than half of isolates produce the blue-green pigment pyocyanin. *P. aeruginosa* differs from enteric gram-negative bacilli in that it oxidizes indophenol and does not ferment lactose.

Epidemiology *P. aeruginosa* has a predilection for moist environments. The many factors that predispose to *P. aeruginosa* infection include disruption of cutaneous or mucosal barriers (e.g., due to burns or trauma), immunosuppression (e.g., due to neutropenia, AIDS, or diabetes), and disruption of the normal bacterial flora (e.g., due to broad-spectrum antibiotic therapy).

Clinical Features

- Respiratory tract infections
  1. Primary or nonbacteremic pneumonia: common cause of ventilator-associated pneumonia, especially in pts with AIDS, COPD, or CHF. *P. aeruginosa* pneumonia is an acute, often severe or even life-threatening infection with fever, cough, dyspnea, and severe systemic toxicity. CXR shows bilateral bronchopneumonia, and pleural effusions are common. AIDS pts frequently have cavitary lesions.
  2. Bacteremic pneumonia: A *P. aeruginosa* respiratory infection, usually associated with neutropenia, progresses to bloodstream invasion, metastatic spread, and gram-negative sepsis. Alveolar hemorrhage, necrosis, and diffuse necrotizing bronchopneumonia with cavity formation can occur. Death within 3 or 4 days is typical.
  3. Chronic respiratory infections with mucoid strains occur in pts with cystic fibrosis, bronchiectasis, or AIDS. Recurrent infection results in progressive pulmonary disease and ultimately in fibrosis and pulmonary insufficiency.

- Bacteremia
  1. *P. aeruginosa* is an important cause of life-threatening bacteremia in compromised pts, particularly those with hematologic malignancy com-

plicated by neutropenia. Clinical features resemble those of other types of bacteremia and sepsis.
2. Pathognomonic skin lesions, called *ecthyma gangrenosum*, develop in a small minority of pts with *P. aeruginosa* bacteremia, beginning as hemorrhagic vesicles and undergoing central necrosis with a rim of erythema and subsequent ulceration.

- Endocarditis: occurs mostly in IV drug users and pts with prosthetic valves
- CNS infections: Meningitis or brain abscess follows extension from an infected parameningeal structure (e.g., ear, mastoid, sinus) or direct inoculation (e.g., surgical), usually in compromised hosts. Mortality rates are high.
- Ear infections

  1. External otitis ("swimmer's ear")
  2. Malignant external otitis: occurs mostly in elderly diabetic pts. Otorrhea and severe otalgia are common presenting symptoms. The infection progresses, slowly invading underlying soft tissue and bone. Facial-nerve paralysis occurs early; other palsies appear later. Constitutional symptoms are usually absent.

- Eye infections: bacterial keratitis or corneal ulcer and endophthalmitis resulting from injury, contact lens use, or contaminated lens solutions and in burn pts. These infections are rapidly progressing entities that demand immediate therapeutic intervention.
- Bone and joint infections

  1. Sternoclavicular pyarthrosis: a complication of injection drug use
  2. Symphysis pubis infections: associated with pelvic surgery and injection drug use
  3. Osteochondritis of the foot: follows plantar puncture wounds
  4. Vertebral osteomyelitis: associated with complicated respiratory infection, genitourinary instrumentation, or injection drug use

- UTIs: complicated or nosocomial
- Skin and soft tissue infections

  1. Primary infections in the setting of skin breakdown and burns. Pts are systemically ill and have signs of sepsis and multiorgan system failure.
  2. Hot-tub folliculitis: diffuse pruritic, maculopapular, and vesiculopustular rashes upon exposure to contaminated hot tubs

℞ TREATMENT

See Table 98-1 for antibiotic options and schedules. Severe or life-threatening infections are generally treated with two antibiotics sensitive to the infecting strain, although evidence that this course is more efficacious than monotherapy has been lacking since the advent of more active β-lactam agents. The duration of therapy depends on the location and severity of infection. Chronic infections with extensive tissue damage or prosthetic material may need weeks to months of treatment, whereas more acute infections may be treated aggressively for shorter periods.

Other *Pseudomonas* Species and Related Bacteria

BURKHOLDERIA CEPACIA AND STENOTROPHOMONAS MALTOPHILIA *B. cepacia* is primarily an opportunistic pathogen implicated in sporadic endemic infections and nosocomial outbreaks. The latter are most often associated with a liquid reservoir or a moist environmental surface. Clinical syndromes include pneumonia, UTI, meningitis, peritonitis, surgical and burn wound infections, bacteremia, and endocarditis related to injection drug

Table 98-1

Antimicrobial Agents Active Against *Pseudomonas aeruginosa* and Available in the United States

Agent	Dose,[a] Route	Comments
ANTIPSEUDOMONAL PENICILLINS		
Piperacillin	3–4 g q4–6h IV	Drugs in class are listed in order of decreasing in vitro activity. Piperacillin/tazobactam or ticarcillin/clavulanate has little more activity against *P. aeruginosa* than piperacillin or ticarcillin alone. Monotherapy should not be used for serious infections.
Piperacillin/ tazobactam	3.375 g q4h IV	
Mezlocillin	3 g q4h IV	
Ticarcillin	3 g q3–6h IV	
Ticarcillin/ clavulanate	3.1 g q4–6h IV	
ANTIPSEUDOMONAL CEPHALOSPORINS		
Ceftazidime[b]	2 g q8–12h IV	Use more frequent indicated doses for CNS infections or infections in neutropenic or severely immunocompromised patients. The antipseudomonal activity of cefepime is equivalent to that of ceftazidime, with less potential for β-lactamase induction in gram-negative enteric bacteria.
Cefoperazone[b]	2 g q6h IV	
Cefepime	2 g q8–12h IV	
CARBAPENEMS[b,c]		
Imipenem/ cilastatin	0.5 g q6h IV	Class is active against strains producing β-lactamases. Imipenem may cause seizures in patients with renal failure (avoid by reducing dose) or CNS infections or lesions. Meropenem is slightly more active in vitro against *P. aeruginosa* than imipenem.
Meropenem	1 g q8h IV	
MONOBACTAMS		
Aztreonam	2 g q6–8h IV	Drug can usually be administered to patients with β-lactam hypersensitivity.
AMINOGLYCOSIDES[b]		
Tobramycin	MD: 2 mg/kg load, then 1.7 mg/kg q8h IV; ODD: 5–7 mg/kg q24h IV	Tobramycin has greater in vitro activity against *P. aeruginosa* than gentamicin, but the drugs' clinical efficacies are probably equivalent. Some *P. aeruginosa* isolates that are resistant to tobramycin or gentamicin may be susceptible to amikacin. Except in urinary tract infection, this class should not be used for monotherapy. ODD may reduce adverse effects. Serum levels must be monitored.
Gentamicin	MD: Same as tobramycin; ODD: Same as tobramycin	
Amikacin	MD: 7.5 mg/kg load, then 7.5 mg/kg q12h IV; ODD: 15 mg/kg q24h IV	

(continued)

Table 98-1 *(Continued)*

Antimicrobial Agents Active Against *Pseudomonas aeruginosa* and Available in the United States

Agent	Dose,[a] Route	Comments
FLUOROQUINOLONES[b,d]		
Ciprofloxacin	0.4 g q12h IV or 0.5–0.75 g bid PO	Ciprofloxacin is the most active of the available quinolones against *P. aeruginosa*. Serum levels attained with oral therapy approximate those after IV therapy; thus oral formulations are useful for long-duration therapy in selected patients.
Levofloxacin	0.75 g q24h IV or PO	
OTHER AGENTS		
Polymyxin B	0.75–1.25 mg/kg q12h IV	These drugs are reserved for use in multidrug-resistant infections. Nephrotoxicity and neurotoxicity occur. Colistin inhalational therapy consists of 75 mg in 3 mL of normal saline via nebulizer, given twice daily.
Colistin	1.5 mg/kg q8h IV	

[a] Indicated dosages are for the treatment of infections due to *P. aeruginosa* in adults. Doses should be adjusted in renal insufficiency. Higher doses may be required in patients with cystic fibrosis, and lower doses may be adequate for the treatment of uncomplicated UTIs.

[b] Some strains of *P. aeruginosa* may rapidly develop resistance to these agents during therapy.

[c] Ertapenem, an additional drug in this class, has less in vitro activity and should not be used for the treatment of *Pseudomonas* infections.

[d] Trovafloxacin, an additional fluoroquinolone with antipseudomonal activity, has limited usefulness because of its hepatotoxicity. Gatifloxacin and moxifloxacin have in vitro activity against *P. aeruginosa* (albeit less than ciprofloxacin and levofloxacin), but there are no clinical studies to support their use in *Pseudomonas* or nosocomial infections.

Abbreviations: MD, multidose; ODD, once-daily dosing; CNS, central nervous system.

use. *B. cepacia* also causes chronic infections (e.g., in pts with cystic fibrosis). *S. maltophilia* is an important nosocomial pathogen, especially at cancer centers and in ICUs. Risk factors include prolonged hospitalization, malignancy and neutropenia, instrumentation, and prior therapy with broad-spectrum antibiotics. *S. maltophilia* causes pneumonia and a host of other infections. Bacteremic *S. maltophilia* pneumonia is a devastating disease seen in debilitated ICU pts.

 TREATMENT

Intrinsic resistance to many antibiotics limits treatment. TMP-SMX (15–20 mg of TMP/kg per day) is the preferred agent.

MISCELLANEOUS ORGANISMS   Melioidosis is endemic to Southeast Asia and is caused by *Burkholderia pseudomallei*. Glanders is associated with close contact with horses or other equines and is caused by *Burkholderia mallei*. These diseases present as acute or chronic pulmonary or extrapulmonary suppurative illnesses or as acute septicemia.

LEGIONELLA INFECTIONS

Microbiology Legionellaceae are intracellular aerobic gram-negative bacilli that grow on buffered charcoal yeast extract (BCYE) agar. *L. pneumophila* causes 80–90% of cases of human *Legionella* disease; serogroups 1, 4, and 6 are most common. A total of 17 other species, including *L. micdadei*, have been linked to human infections.

Epidemiology *Legionella* is found in fresh water and human-constructed water sources. Outbreaks have been traced to cooling towers and potable-water distribution systems. The organisms are transmitted to individuals primarily via aspiration but can also be transmitted by aerosolization and direct instillation into the lung during respiratory tract manipulations. *Legionella* is the fourth most common cause of community-acquired pneumonia, accounting for 3–15% of cases. It causes 10–50% of cases of nosocomial pneumonia if the hospital's water system is colonized with the organism. Pts who have chronic lung disease, smoke, and/or are elderly or immunosuppressed are at particular risk for disease. Cell-mediated immunity is the primary mechanism of host defense.

Clinical Features

• Pontiac fever: a flulike illness with a 24- to 48-h incubation period. Pneumonia does not develop, but malaise, fatigue, myalgias, and fever are frequent. The disease is self-limited, and recovery takes place in a few days.
• Legionnaires' disease: more severe than other atypical pneumonias and more likely to result in ICU admission

   1. After an incubation period of 2–10 days, nonspecific symptoms (e.g., malaise, fatigue, headache, fever) develop and are followed by a cough that is usually mild and nonproductive.
   2. Chest pain (pleuritic or nonpleuritic) can be prominent, and dyspnea is common. Sputum is usually scant and may be blood-streaked.
   3. GI manifestations (pain, nausea, vomiting, diarrhea) may be pronounced.
   4. Diarrhea, confusion, high fevers, hyponatremia, increased values in LFTs, hematuria, hypophosphatemia, and elevated CPK levels are documented more frequently than in other pneumonias.
   5. The heart is the most common extrapulmonary site of disease (myocarditis, pericarditis, and occasionally prosthetic valve endocarditis).
   6. CXR reveals pulmonary infiltrates, multilobar involvement in many instances, and pleural effusion in up to 63% of cases. In compromised hosts, nodular infiltrates, abscesses, and cavities can be seen.

Diagnosis

• Sputum or bronchoalveolar samples are subjected to direct fluorescent antibody (DFA) staining and culture. DFA testing is rapid and specific but less sensitive than culture.
• Cultures on BCYE media require 3–5 days to become positive.
• Diagnosis by antibody testing can take 12 weeks.
• Urinary antigen assay is rapid, inexpensive, easy to perform, second only to culture in terms of sensitivity, and highly specific. It is useful only for *L. pneumophila* serogroup 1, which causes 80% of disease cases. Urinary antigen is detectable 3 days after disease onset, with positive results persisting for weeks.

℞ TREATMENT

   • Fluoroquinolones (e.g., levofloxacin at 750 mg IV or 500 mg PO daily or moxifloxacin at 400 mg PO daily) or newer macrolides (e.g., azithromycin at

500 mg/d or clarithromycin at 500 mg bid, IV or PO) are most effective. Rifampin (300–600 mg bid) combined with either class of drug in severe cases is recommended.
• Tetracyclines (doxycycline at 100 mg bid, IV or PO) or TMP-SMX (160/ 800 mg IV q8h or PO bid) are alternatives.
• Immunocompetent hosts can receive 10–14 days of therapy, but immunocompromised hosts should receive 3 weeks of treatment. A 5- to 10-day course of azithromycin is adequate because of this drug's long half-life.

Prognosis Mortality approaches 80% among compromised hosts who do not receive timely therapy. Among immunocompetent hosts, mortality can approach 31% without treatment but ranges from 0 to 11% if pts receive appropriate therapy. Fatigue, weakness, and neurologic symptoms can persist for >1 year in survivors.

For a more detailed discussion, see Kasper DL, Barlam TF: Infections due to HACEK Group and Miscellaneous Gram-Negative Bacteria, Chap. 131, p. 867; Chang FY, Yu VL: *Legionella* Infection, Chap. 132, p. 870; Russo TA: Diseases Caused by Gram-Negative Enteric Bacilli, Chap. 134, p. 878; and Ohl CA, Pollack M: Infections due to *Pseudomonas* Species and Related Organisms, Chap. 136, p. 889, in HPIM-16.

99

INFECTIONS CAUSED BY OTHER GRAM-NEGATIVE BACILLI

BRUCELLOSIS

ETIOLOGY Brucellae are facultative intracellular parasites in a genus that includes four major species: *B. melitensis* (acquired by humans most commonly from goats, sheep, and camels), *B. suis* (from swine), *B. abortus* (from cattle or buffalo), and *B. canis* (from dogs). Brucellosis is transmitted via exposure to infected animals or their products in either occupational settings (e.g., butchering, slaughterhouse work) or domestic settings (e.g., consumption of contaminated foods, especially dairy products and raw meat).

CLINICAL FEATURES An incubation period of 1 week to several months is followed by the development of undulating fever; night sweats; increasing apathy, fatigue, and anorexia; and nonspecific symptoms such as headache, myalgias, low back pain, constipation, sore throat, and dry cough. Brucellosis can present as a febrile illness similar to but less severe than typhoid fever. However, the most common findings are musculoskeletal pain and involvement of the peripheral and axial skeleton—i.e., vertebral osteomyelitis (fever and low back or hip pain in an older man) or septic arthritis (fever and acute monarthritis, typically of the hip or knee). *Brucella* infection can cause lymphadenopathy, hepatosplenomegaly, and focal abscess.

DIAGNOSIS Laboratory personnel must be alerted to the potential diagnosis to ensure that they take precautions to prevent occupational exposure. The organism is successfully cultured in 50–70% of cases, but culture identification usually takes up to 6 weeks. Cultures using the BACTEC systems can be deemed negative at 3 weeks. IgM assays by standard agglutination test are positive early in infection. Single titers of ≥1:160 and 1:320–1:640 are diagnostic in nonendemic and endemic areas, respectively. Brucellosis must be distinguished from tuberculosis; if this distinction is not possible, the regimen should be tailored to avoid inadvertent monotherapy for tuberculosis (see below). Brucellosis tends to cause less bone and joint destruction than tuberculosis (Table 99-1).

R̄x **TREATMENT**

• Streptomycin at a dosage of 750 mg to 1 g daily (or gentamicin at 5–6 mg/kg daily) for 14–21 days plus doxycycline at a dosage of 100 mg bid for 6 weeks. Complex or focal disease requires at least 3 months of treatment.
• Alternative: rifampin (600–900 mg/d) plus doxycycline (100 mg bid) for 6 weeks. Trimethoprim-sulfamethoxazole (TMP-SMX) can be given instead to children.
• Neurologic involvement: Include ceftriaxone in the regimen; treat for 6–12 months.
• Relapse occurs in ~30% of cases, usually because of poor compliance. Pts should be monitored for at least 2 years.

TULAREMIA

EPIDEMIOLOGY Human infections caused by *Francisella tularensis* occur via interaction with biting or blood-sucking insects (especially ticks and tabanid flies), wild or domestic animals (e.g., wild rabbits, squirrels), or the environment. The organism can persist for months in mud, water, and decaying animal carcasses. More than half of U.S. cases occur in Arkansas, Oklahoma, and Missouri. The organism gains entry into the skin or mucous membranes through bites or inapparent abrasions (75–85% of U.S. cases) or is acquired via

Table 99-1

Radiology of the Spine: Differentiation of Brucellosis from Tuberculosis

	Brucellosis	Tuberculosis
Site	Lumbar and others	Dorsolumbar
Vertebrae	Multiple or contiguous	Contiguous
Diskitis	Late	Early
Body	Intact until late	Morphology lost early
Canal compression	Rare	Common
Epiphysitis	Anterosuperior	General: upper, lower disk region, central, subperiosteal
Osteophyte	Anterolateral	Unusual
Deformity	Wedging uncommon	Anterior wedge, gibbus
Recovery	Sclerosis, whole body	Variable
Paravertebral abscess	Small, well-localized	Common and discrete loss, transverse process
Psoas abscess	Rare	More likely

inhalation or ingestion. *F. tularensis* is a potential agent of bioterrorism (see Chap. 31).

CLINICAL FEATURES After a 2- to 10-day incubation period, there is an acute onset of fever, chills, headache, and myalgias. One of several syndromes then develops.

1. *Ulceroglandular/glandular tularemia* (75–85% of cases)
   a. The hallmark is an indurated, erythematous, nonhealing ulcer lasting 1–3 weeks (ulceroglandular form) that begins as a pruritic papule, ulcerates, has sharply demarcated edges and a yellow exudate, and develops a black base. A primary skin lesion may not be apparent in 5–10% of cases (glandular form).
   b. Lymphadenopathy is related to the location of the tick bite; inguinal/femoral nodes are most often affected in adults because of the frequency of bites on the legs. Lymph nodes can become fluctuant and drain spontaneously.
2. *Oculoglandular tularemia*: Infection of the conjunctiva, usually by contact with contaminated fingers, results in purulent conjunctivitis with regional adenopathy and debilitating pain. Painful preauricular lymphadenopathy is unique to tularemia.
3. *Oropharyngeal and GI tularemia*: Acquired via ingestion, infection can present with pharyngitis and cervical adenopathy, intestinal ulcerations, mesenteric adenopathy, diarrhea, nausea, vomiting, and abdominal pain.
4. *Pulmonary tularemia*: Infection is acquired via inhalation or hematogenous spread. Pts present with a nonproductive cough, dyspnea, pleuritic chest pain, bilateral patchy or lobar infiltrates, cavities, and occasional pleural effusions and empyema on CXR.
5. *Typhoidal tularemia*: consists of fever and signs of sepsis without focal findings

DIAGNOSIS

- Polychromatic staining of clinical specimens (Gram staining of little help)
- Serology via standard tube agglutination test. A single titer of ≥1:160 or a fourfold increase in titer after 2–3 weeks is considered positive. Microagglutination tests and ELISAs are more sensitive. Antigen testing (e.g., of urine) looks promising.
- Culture is difficult and poses a significant risk to laboratory personnel.

℞ **TREATMENT**

- Streptomycin (7.5–10 mg/kg q12h) is the drug of choice for adults. Gentamicin is an acceptable alternative, but tobramycin is not. Defervescence occurs within 1–2 days, but healing of skin lesions and lymph nodes may take 1–2 weeks. Late lymph-node suppuration can occur, with sterile necrotic tissue.
- Rapidly responding mild to moderate disease can be treated for 5–7 days; otherwise, treatment is given for 7–10 days.
- Alternatives include tetracyclines or chloramphenicol (relapse rates of up to 20%).
- Fluoroquinolones have shown promise and are candidates for primary or alternative treatment, pending clinical trials.

PLAGUE

EPIDEMIOLOGY *Yersinia pestis* causes plague, one of the most virulent and lethal of all bacterial diseases. Most often seen in Asia, Africa, and the Americas, plague occurs in the United States, primarily in New Mexico, Arizona, Colorado, and California. Wild rodents and rats are the usual hosts; ground squirrels, prairie dogs, and chipmunks are the main epizootic hosts in the United States. Fleabites or direct contact with infected tissues or airborne droplets can cause human infections. *Y. pestis* is a potential agent of bioterrorism (see Chap. 31).

CLINICAL FEATURES   There are three major presentations.

1. *Bubonic plague*: the most common form, caused by the bite of an infected flea
   a. After an incubation period of 2–6 days, the pt develops chills, fever, myalgias and arthralgias, headache, weakness, and signs of toxemia.
   b. Within 24 h, adenopathy proximal to the inoculation site occurs. An enlarging node or bubo becomes painful and tender. Edema and erythema—but not cellulitis or lymphangitis—develop in the surrounding tissue.
   c. The primary inoculation site may have a papule, pustule, ulcer, or eschar.
   d. Disease progresses to lethargy, convulsions, shock, organ failure, and death.
2. *Septicemic plague*
   a. Overwhelming infection (no bubo) with disease progression to multiorgan failure, DIC, hypotension, and death
   b. GI symptoms (diarrhea, nausea and vomiting, abdominal pain) are common.
3. *Pneumonic plague*: the most rapidly progressive form of disease, often fatal
   a. After an incubation period of 3–5 days, there is a sudden onset of chills, fever, headache, myalgias, weakness, and dizziness.
   b. Pulmonary signs include tachypnea, dyspnea, cough, sputum production, chest pain, hemoptysis, and circulatory collapse. Auscultatory findings are minimal. Sputum is watery, frothy, and blood-tinged or frankly bloody.
   c. Bronchopneumonia progresses rapidly to involve multiple lobes and both lungs, with liquefaction necrosis and cavitation of consolidated areas.
   d. The pt is toxic and at risk for sudden death.
   e. Secondary pneumonic plague is a diffuse interstitial process and may be less infectious because sputum is tenacious and scant.

DIAGNOSIS   A diagnosis of plague should be considered when acute regional lymphadenitis, sepsis, or acute severe pneumonia occurs in an otherwise-healthy person who has recently traveled or resided in the rural western United States or abroad.

Smear and culture of specimens of blood, lymph node aspirates, pulmonary aspirates, and other sites should be prepared as appropriate. Smears should be examined immediately with Wayson or Giemsa stain (*Y. pestis* has a bipolar appearance resembling closed safety pins) and with Gram's stain and should be submitted for direct fluorescent antibody testing, ELISA, or PCR. Acute-phase—and, if possible, convalescent-phase—serum samples should undergo serologic testing. Either a single titer of >128 or seroconversion (as documented by a fourfold or greater rise in titer) is considered diagnostic. Confirm with the F1 antigen hemagglutination-inhibition test, which is positive in most cases by 1–2 weeks.

℞ **TREATMENT**

- More than half of bubonic plague pts and virtually all pts with septicemic or pneumonic plague die if not treated.

• As for tularemia, streptomycin or gentamicin is the drug of choice.
• Doxycycline and chloramphenicol are alternative agents.
• National bioterrorism-response protocols recommend administration of gentamicin, ciprofloxacin, and doxycycline in the event of a *Y. pestis* attack.
• Persons who are exposed to pts with pneumonic plague or who have traveled to an area where a plague outbreak is in progress should receive short-term prophylaxis with doxycycline (adult dose, 100–200 mg q12–24h), ciprofloxacin (1 g q12h), or TMP-SMX (320 mg of TMP q12h).
• Pts hospitalized with pneumonic plague should be placed on respiratory droplet precautions until treatment has been given for at least 48 h.

BARTONELLA INFECTIONS

Bartonella species can adhere to and invade mammalian cells, including endothelial cells and erythrocytes, causing severe anemia. Clinical syndromes, risk factors, and therapy are summarized in Table 99-2.

Oroya Fever and Verruga Peruana

These infections, caused by *B. bacilliformis*, are transmitted by a sandfly vector (*Phlebotomus*) found in river valleys of the Andes Mountains. Pts present with fever; profound anemia follows. Without treatment, mortality is high. During convalescence, nodular dermal eruptions, or *verrugas*, may develop. The diagnosis is based on positive blood cultures and formation of new blood vessels at sites of bacterial replication.

Cat-Scratch Disease

This infection, caused by *B. henselae*, is associated with exposure to young cats with flea infestation. About 60% of cases affect children.

CLINICAL FEATURES   Appearance of a localized lesion (papule, pustule) is followed 1–2 weeks later by tender lymphadenopathy. Nodes may suppurate; malaise and anorexia—and, less often, fever—occur. Encephalitis, seizures and coma, and other signs of dissemination are more common in children. Untreated pts can have adenopathy that persists for weeks to months.

DIAGNOSIS

• Warthin-Starry silver staining of biopsy samples
• Serologic testing positive in 70–90% of pts
• Cultures rarely positive
• PCR under development

Trench Fever

In this infection due to *B. quintana*, there is a sudden onset of headache, aseptic meningitis, persistent or relapsing fever, and malaise and other nonspecific symptoms. Bacteremia can persist for weeks. The diagnosis is made by blood culture; bacteria grow slowly over 1–4 weeks.

Bacillary Angiomatosis

CLINICAL FEATURES   This disease, caused by *B. henselae* and *B. quintana*, is manifest by skin lesions (epithelioid angiomatosis) that are sites of angiogenesis and are seen as vascular nodules, papules, or tumors ranging in size from tiny to large, pedunculated, exophytic masses. Lesions are typically red or purple and can resemble Kaposi's sarcoma. They may be found anywhere on the skin, may involve mucous membranes, may ulcerate, and may invade underlying bone. Dissemination may occur in compromised hosts (e.g., HIV-

Table 99-2

Bartonella Infections: Clinical Syndromes, Risk Factors, and Therapy

Bartonella Species	Clinical Syndrome	Risk Factors	Therapy[a]
Bartonella henselae	Cat-scratch disease	Cat scratch or bite	Azithromycin for 5 days (500 mg on day 1, 250 mg on days 2–5); or variable duration of rifampin (300 mg daily or bid), doxycycline (100 mg/d), or ciprofloxacin (500 mg/d)
	Bacillary angiomatosis/peliosis	Cat scratch or bite	Erythromycin (500 mg qid) or doxycycline (100 mg/d) for 3–6 weeks
	Endocarditis	Cat exposure	If patient is Bartonella culture-positive or seropositive: Give azithromycin (250 mg/d) or doxycycline (100 mg/d) for 4–6 months (surgery may be required) If Bartonella is suspected but unconfirmed: Treat for culture-negative endocarditis with ceftriaxone (2 g/d IV) plus gentamicin for 6–8 weeks[b]
Bartonella quintana	Trench fever	Homelessness; alcoholism; body lice	Doxycycline (100 mg bid) or azithromycin (500 mg/d) for 4–6 weeks
	Bacillary angiomatosis	Homelessness ± body lice; HIV infection	Same as for bacillary angiomatosis due to B. henselae
	Endocarditis	Same as for other B. quintana infections	Same as for endocarditis due to B. henselae
Bartonella bacilliformis	Oroya fever	Lack of immunity; sandfly bite	Chloramphenicol for 10 days (in South America); ampicillin (1 g q6h IV or PO) or cephalexin (500 mg qid PO) for 10–14 days
	Verruga peruana	Previous exposure to B. bacilliformis	Rifampin (300 mg bid) or ciprofloxacin (500 mg/d) for 7–10 days

[a] Azithromycin therapy for cat-scratch disease is based on clinical-trial data; all other recommendations are based on case reports or case series.

[b] If culture results confirm Bartonella infection, ceftriaxone may be discontinued and therapy with azithromycin or doxycycline given for a prolonged period.

infected pts), primarily affecting the liver and spleen, bone marrow, lymph nodes, and CNS. Skin lesions are usually absent in disseminated infection.

DIAGNOSIS

- Histopathologic findings and a positive Warthin-Starry silver stain
- CT or MRI may show nodular vascular lesions of organs.
- Blood cultures using lysis-centrifugation techniques or PCR

Culture-Negative Endocarditis

Bartonella species cause a proportion of cases of culture-negative endocarditis. The diagnosis is based on positive blood cultures and/or serologic tests. In some tests, *Bartonella* antibodies may cross-react with *Chlamydia pneumoniae*. *B. quintana* antibodies may cross-react with *Coxiella burnetii* (the cause of Q fever).

For a more detailed discussion, see Corbel MJ, Beeching NJ: Brucellosis, Chap. 141, p. 914; Jacobs RF: Tularemia, Chap. 142, p. 917; Dennis DT, Campbell GL: Plague and Other *Yersinia* Infections, Chap. 143, p. 921; and Tompkins LS: *Bartonella* Infections, Including Cat-Scratch Disease, Chap. 144, p. 929, in HPIM-16.

ANAEROBIC INFECTIONS

TETANUS

ETIOLOGY, EPIDEMIOLOGY, AND PATHOGENESIS   Tetanus is a neurologic disorder characterized by increased muscle tone and spasms caused by tetanospasmin, a toxin produced by *Clostridium tetani*. *C. tetani* is a drumstick-shaped, spore-forming, anaerobic gram-positive rod that is ubiquitous in soil. Disease in the United States occurs in inadequately immunized persons—primarily nonwhites and the elderly—following an acute injury (e.g., a puncture wound) that becomes contaminated with *C. tetani* spores. Spores germinate in wounds with low oxidation-reduction potential (e.g., those with devitalized tissue or foreign bodies) and produce toxin. The toxin then binds to peripheral motor neurons and spreads by retrograde intraneuronal transport. Rigidity results from an increased resting firing rate of the α-motor neurons due to blockage of release of inhibitory neurotransmitters (glycine and γ-aminobutyric acid) in presynaptic terminals.

CLINICAL FEATURES

- *Generalized tetanus*: A median of 7 days after injury (range, 3–14 days), pts develop trismus—increased tone of the masseter muscles (lockjaw)—as well as sustained facial muscle contraction (risus sardonicus), dysphagia, neck stiffness or pain, back muscle contraction (opisthotonus), and rigidity of the abdominal wall and proximal limb muscles. Mentation is clear. Pts are often afebrile. Paroxysmal generalized spasms, either entirely spontaneous or provoked by even the slightest stimulation, may result in cyanosis and ventilatory compromise. Autonomic dysfunction can cause labile hypertension, tachycardia, arrhythmias, and sudden cardiac arrest.

• *Local tetanus*: Only muscles near the wound are affected.

• *Neonatal tetanus*: Usually fatal if not treated, neonatal tetanus occurs in children of unimmunized mothers, often after contamination of the umbilical cord stump.

DIAGNOSIS   The diagnosis is made primarily on clinical grounds. Muscle enzyme levels can be elevated.

 TREATMENT

• Monitor and give supportive care in a quiet ICU room.

• Give metronidazole (500 mg q6h) to eliminate vegetative cells and a source of further toxin. Penicillin, clindamycin, and erythromycin are alternatives.

• Give one dose of human tetanus immune globulin (TIG), 3000 to 6000 units IM, to neutralize unbound toxin; divide the dose because of the large volume.

• Control muscle spasms using benzodiazepines such as diazepam. Therapeutic paralysis with neuromuscular blocking agents may be necessary. However, prolonged paralysis may follow discontinuation of those agents.

• Immunize recovering pts. Natural disease does not induce immunity.

PREVENTION

• Primary vaccination: Adults should receive two doses 4–8 weeks apart and a third dose 6–12 months later. Pts >7 years of age should receive booster vaccines every 10 years with adsorbed tetanus and diphtheria toxoid (Td).

• Wound management: Administer Td if immune status is unknown, immunization was incomplete, or >10 years have elapsed since the last booster. In contaminated or severe wounds, administer Td if >5 years have elapsed since the last vaccination. Consider TIG (250 units IM) for all but clean or minor wounds if the pt's immune status is unknown or immunization was incomplete. TIG and Td must be given at separate sites.

PROGNOSIS   Mortality is <10% with optimal management. Recovery is usually complete but extends over 4–6 weeks. Prolonged ventilator support may be needed. Increased muscle tone and minor spasms may last for months.

BOTULISM

ETIOLOGY, EPIDEMIOLOGY, AND PATHOGENESIS   Botulism is a paralytic disease caused by neurotoxins elaborated by *Clostridium botulinum*, an anaerobic spore-forming bacterium. The neurotoxin enters the vascular system, travels to peripheral cholinergic nerve terminals, and inhibits release of the neurotransmitter acetylcholine. *C. botulinum* is found in soil and marine environments worldwide. In the United States, *C. botulinum* type A is found west of the Rocky Mountains, type B is more common in the East, and type E is found in the Pacific Northwest, the Great Lakes region, and Alaska. Most U.S. food-borne cases are associated with home-canned food, especially vegetables, fruits, and condiments. Type E is associated with fish products. Disease occurs when (1) spores contaminate food; (2) the food is subsequently preserved in a manner that kills other bacteria but not the spores and provides anaerobic conditions at a pH and temperature permissive for germination and toxin production; and (3) the food is ingested before being heated to a temperature adequate for toxin destruction. Toxin is heat-labile (inactivated when heated for 10 min at 100°C), and spores are heat-resistant (inactivated at 116°–121°C or with steam sterilizers or pressure cookers).

CLINICAL FEATURES

- *Food-borne botulism* occurs 18–36 h after ingestion of food contaminated with toxin and ranges in severity from mild to fatal (within 24 h). The characteristic presentation is symmetric descending paralysis with early cranial nerve involvement (diplopia, dysarthria, dysphonia, ptosis, and/or dysphagia) that can progress to paralysis, respiratory failure, and death. Sensory findings are absent. Nausea, abdominal pain, and vomiting may occur. Fever is uncommon. Pts are usually alert and oriented but may be drowsy or agitated.
- *Wound botulism* occurs when spores contaminate a wound and germinate. This form occurs in wounds of black-tar heroin users. Wound botulism has a longer incubation period (~10 days) than food-borne botulism and causes no GI symptoms. Otherwise, the two diseases are similar.
- In *intestinal botulism*, spores germinate in the intestine and produce toxin, which is absorbed and causes illness. This form has been associated with contaminated honey. Infants <6 months of age are at risk.
- *Bioterrorism-related botulism* is the potential result of the intentional dispersal (as an aerosol or as a contaminant in ingested material) of the most potent bacterial toxin known.

DIAGNOSIS The clinical symptoms should suggest the diagnosis. The definitive test is the demonstration of the toxin in serum with a mouse bioassay, but this test may yield a negative result, particularly in wound and infant intestinal botulism. Demonstration of the organism or the toxin in clinical samples strongly suggests the diagnosis.

Rx TREATMENT

- Supportive care with intubation and mechanical ventilation as needed
- Routine administration of bivalent equine antitoxin to types A and B; use of an investigational monovalent antitoxin if exposure to type E toxin (i.e., through seafood ingestion) is suspected
- Infants should receive human botulism immune globulin.
- Wound botulism: exploration, debridement, penicillin treatment (to eradicate the organism from the site), and administration of equine antitoxin
- For antitoxin and management advice, contact state health departments or the CDC at 404-639-2206 (emergency number: 404-639-2888).

PROGNOSIS Mortality has been reduced to ~7.5%. Type A disease tends to be the most severe. Respiratory support may be required for months. Residual weakness and autonomic dysfunction may persist for as long as a year.

OTHER CLOSTRIDIAL INFECTIONS

ETIOLOGY AND PATHOGENESIS Clostridia are gram-positive, spore-forming obligate anaerobes. In humans, they reside in the GI and female genital tracts. *Clostridium perfringens* is the most common clostridial species isolated from tissue infections and bacteremias; next in frequency are *C. novyi* and *C. septicum*. Tissue necrosis and low oxidation-reduction potential are factors that allow rapid growth and toxin production and are essential for the development of severe disease. *C. perfringens* produces multiple virulence factors and toxins, including ∝ toxin, which causes hemolysis, destroys platelets and PMNs, causes widespread capillary damage, and is probably important in the initiation of muscle infections that can progress to gas gangrene.

CLINICAL FEATURES

I. Intestinal disorders: Food poisoning and antibiotic-associated colitis (see Chap. 87)

II. Bacteremia: fever, bacteremia from a focus in the GI or biliary tract or uterus. Fever resolves within 1–2 days without treatment.

III. Suppurative deep-tissue infections: severe local inflammation without systemic signs (e.g., intraabdominal infection, empyema, pelvic abscess). Clostridia are isolated from two-thirds of pts with intraabdominal infections resulting from intestinal perforation. *C. perfringens* is isolated from 20% of diseased gallbladders at surgery and from at least 50% of pts with emphysematous cholecystitis. Clostridia can be identified in association with other anaerobic and aerobic bacteria or as the sole isolate. The isolation of *C. septicum* often takes place in the setting of leukemia or other solid tumors, especially of the GI tract (and in particular the colon).

IV. Clostridial sepsis: an uncommon but usually fatal clostridial infection, primarily of the uterus, colon, or biliary tract. The majority of cases follow septic abortion within 1–3 days. Pts are hyperalert and have fever, chills, malaise, headache, severe myalgias, abdominal pain, nausea, vomiting, oliguria, hypotension, hemolysis with jaundice, and hemoglobinuria. Pts with sepsis due to *C. septicum* have hemolysis only 20–30% of the time. Death occurs within 12 h.

V. Skin and soft tissue infections

A. Localized infection without systemic signs (also called *anaerobic cellulitis*) is caused by clostridia alone or with other organisms. An indolent infection that may spread to contiguous areas, it causes little pain or edema and does not involve the muscles. Gas production may be more noticeable than in more severe infections because of the lack of edema. If not treated appropriately, infection may progress to severe systemic toxic illness.

B. The onset of spreading cellulitis and fasciitis with systemic toxicity is abrupt, with rapid spread through fascial planes. On examination, SC crepitus with little localized pain is evident. The infection can be rapidly fatal (within 48 h) despite aggressive treatment. It is associated with malignancy, especially of the sigmoid or cecum. The tumor probably invades fascia, and colonic contents invade the abdominal wall. This infection differs from necrotizing fasciitis by its rapid mortality, rapid tissue invasion, and massive hemolysis.

C. Gas gangrene (clostridial myonecrosis) is characterized by rapid and extensive necrosis of muscle accompanied by gas formation and systemic toxicity. It is typically associated with traumatic wounds that are deep, necrotic, and without communication to the surface. *C. perfringens* causes 80% of cases.

1. Incubation period: <3 days and often <24 h

2. Sudden onset of pain that is localized to the infected area and increases steadily. Infection progresses with swelling; edema; cool, tense, white skin; and profuse serous discharge with a sweetish, mousy odor. Gram's stain reveals few white cells and many gram-positive rods. Pts have a heightened sense of awareness.

DIAGNOSIS Isolation of clostridia from clinical sites does not alone indicate severe disease. Clinical findings and presentation must be taken into account.

Rx TREATMENT

- Surgical intervention and debridement are the mainstays of treatment.
- Antibiotics: Penicillin (3–4 million units q4h) in conjunction with clindamycin (600 mg q6h) is indicated for severe clostridial disease. Clostridial wound contamination alone does not require antibiotics, and localized skin and soft tissue infections without systemic signs can be treated by debridement alone. Because suppurative infections are often mixed, they require broader-spectrum treatment. Use of hyperbaric oxygen for gas gangrene is controversial.

MIXED ANAEROBIC INFECTIONS

DEFINITIONS

- *Anaerobic bacteria:* require reduced oxygen tension for growth; do not grow on the surface of solid media in 10% CO_2 in air
- *Microaerophilic bacteria:* grow in an atmosphere of 10% CO_2 in air or under anaerobic or aerobic conditions but grow best if only a small amount of atmospheric oxygen is present
- *Facultative bacteria:* grow in the presence or absence of air

ETIOLOGY AND PATHOGENESIS Nonsporulating anaerobic bacteria are components of the normal flora of mucosal surfaces of the mouth, lower GI tract, skin, and female genital tract. Infection results when a disruption in the balance between host and colonizing organisms causes reduced tissue redox potentials—e.g., from tissue ischemia, trauma, surgery, perforated viscus, shock, or aspiration. Infections often involve multiple species of anaerobes combined with microaerophilic and facultative bacteria. Most anaerobes associated with human infections are relatively aerotolerant and can survive for as long as 72 h in the presence of oxygen. Anaerobic bacteria produce exoproteins that enhance virulence; e.g., *Bacteroides fragilis* has a polysaccharide capsule that promotes abscess formation. Major anaerobic gram-positive cocci include *Peptostreptococcus* spp. Major anaerobic gram-positive rods include spore-forming clostridia and non-spore-forming *Propionibacterium acnes*. (The latter organism is an uncommon cause of human infections.) Major anaerobic gram-negative bacilli include the *B. fragilis* group (normal bowel flora), *Fusobacterium* spp. (oral cavity and GI tract), *Prevotella* spp. (oral cavity and female genital tract), and *Porphyromonas* spp. (oral flora).

CLINICAL FEATURES *Anaerobic Infections of the Mouth, Head, and Neck*

- Gingivitis and periodontal disease: Supragingival plaque acquires pathogenic bacteria, with consequent inflammation, caries, and infection. Periodontal disease can progress to involve bone, sinuses, and adjacent soft tissue.
- Necrotizing ulcerative gingivitis (trench mouth, Vincent's angina): When gingivitis becomes necrotizing, the pt has a sudden onset of bleeding tender gums, foul breath, and ulceration with gray exudates. Infection can cause widespread destruction of bone and soft tissue (acute necrotizing ulcerative mucositis; cancrum oris, noma) after a debilitating illness, in malnourished children, or in leukemic pts. Lesions heal but leave disfiguring defects.
- Acute necrotizing infections of the pharynx: associated with ulcerative gingivitis. Pts have sore throat, foul breath, fever, a choking sensation, and tonsillar pillars that are swollen, red, ulcerated, and covered with a gray membrane. Lymphadenopathy and leukocytosis are common. Infections can result in aspiration and lung abscesses or in soft tissue infection. *Ludwig's angina* is an infection arising from the third molar and associated with submandibular soft

tissue infection, swelling, pain, trismus, and displacement of the tongue. Swelling can cause respiratory obstruction.
• Sinusitis and otitis: Anaerobes are important, especially in chronic infections.
• Lemierre syndrome: acute oropharyngeal *F. necrophorum* infection causing septic thrombophlebitis of the internal jugular vein and metastatic infections
• Other complications of anaerobic mouth, head, and neck infections: osteomyelitis, brain abscess, subdural empyema, mediastinitis or pleuropulmonary infection, hematogenous dissemination

CNS Infections Up to 85% of brain abscesses yield anaerobic bacteria, usually gram-positive cocci such as peptostreptococci.

Pleuropulmonary Infections

• Aspiration pneumonia: Mendelson's syndrome is characterized by aspiration of the stomach contents, with consequent destruction of the alveolar lining and rapid transudation of fluid into the alveolar space. This condition initially represents a chemical injury and not an infection, and antibiotics should be withheld until evidence of bacterial superinfection is found.
• Bacterial aspiration pneumonia: due to depressed gag reflex, impaired swallowing, or altered mental status. Illness develops over days with low-grade fevers, malaise, and sputum production. Sputum reveals a mixed flora, and cultures are usually unreliable because of contamination by oral flora components.
• Necrotizing pneumonitis: numerous small abscesses throughout the lung. The clinical course can be either indolent or fulminant.
• Anaerobic lung abscess: usually a subacute infection, often from a dental source. Pts have constitutional symptoms and foul-smelling sputum.
• Empyema: usually follows long-standing anaerobic pulmonary infection. Pts have symptoms resembling other anaerobic pulmonary infections but may report pleuritic chest pain and marked chest-wall tenderness.

Intraabdominal Infections See Chap. 86.

Pelvic Infections Most infections of the female genital tract and pelvis are mixed infections that include anaerobes and coliforms. Pure anaerobic infections occur more often in pelvic infections than at other intraabdominal sites. Pts may have foul-smelling drainage or pus from the uterus, generalized uterine or local pelvic tenderness, and fever. Suppurative thrombophlebitis of the pelvic veins may complicate the picture and lead to septic pulmonary emboli.

Skin and Soft Tissue Infections

• Trauma, ischemia, or surgery may create a suitable environment for skin or soft tissue infections caused by anaerobic bacteria, usually as part of a mixed etiology. There is a higher frequency of fever, foul-smelling drainage, gas in the tissues, and visible foot ulcer in cases involving anaerobic bacteria.
• Meleney's gangrene (synergistic gangrene) is characterized by exquisite pain, redness, swelling, and induration with erythema around a central zone of necrosis, usually at the site of a surgical wound or an ulcer on an extremity.
• Necrotizing fasciitis is a rapidly destructive disease that is usually due to group A *Streptococcus* but can be a mixed anaerobic-aerobic infection. *Fournier's gangrene* involves the scrotum, perineum, and anterior abdominal wall.

Bone and Joint Infections Anaerobic bone and joint infections usually occur adjacent to soft tissue infections.

Bacteremia *B. fragilis* is the most common cause of significant anaerobic bacteremia. The clinical course can resemble septic shock, and pts can become extremely ill.

Table 100-1

Doses and Schedules for Treatment of Serious Infections Due to Commonly Encountered Anaerobic Gram-Negative Rods

First-Line Therapy	Dose	Schedule[a]
Metronidazole[b]	500 mg	q6h
Ticarcillin/clavulanic acid	3.1 g	q4h
Piperacillin/tazobactam	3.375 g	q6h
Imipenem	0.5 g	q6h
Meropenem	1.0 g	q8h

[a] See disease-specific chapters in HPIM-16 for recommendations on duration of therapy.
[b] Should generally be used in conjunction with drugs active against aerobic or facultative organisms.
Note: All drugs are given by the intravenous route.

DIAGNOSIS   When infections develop in close proximity to mucosal surfaces normally harboring anaerobic flora, the involvement of anaerobes should be considered. The three critical steps in successfully culturing anaerobic bacteria from clinical samples are (1) proper specimen collection, with avoidance of contamination by normal flora; (2) rapid transport to the microbiology laboratory in anaerobic transport media; and (3) proper specimen handling.

 TREATMENT

Appropriate treatment requires antibiotic administration (Table 100-1), surgical resection or debridement of devitalized tissues, and drainage.

1. Infections above the diaphragm: Metronidazole treatment gives unpredictable results in infections caused by peptostreptococci, and penicillin resistance is increasing because of ß-lactamase production. Either clindamycin or a penicillin/metronidazole combination is an option.
2. Infections below the diaphragm must be treated with agents active against *Bacteroides* spp., such as metronidazole, ß-lactam/ß-lactamase inhibitor combinations, or carbapenems. Aerobic gram-negative flora should also be treated, with coverage for enterococci when indicated.

For a more detailed discussion, see Abrutyn E: Tetanus, Chap. 124, p. 840; Abrutyn E: Botulism, Chap. 125, p. 842; Kasper DL, Madoff LC: Gas Gangrene and Other Clostridial Infections, Chap. 126, p. 845; and Kasper DL: Infections Due to Mixed Anaerobic Organisms, Chap. 148, p. 940, in HPIM-16.

101

NOCARDIOSIS AND ACTINOMYCOSIS

NOCARDIOSIS

Nocardiae are saprophytic aerobic actinomycetes common in soil. Several species are associated with human disease. *N. asteroides* is the species most commonly associated with invasive disease. *N. brasiliensis* is most often associated with localized skin lesions.

EPIDEMIOLOGY In the United States, ~1000 cases of nocardial infection occur annually, of which 85% are pulmonary or systemic.

PATHOLOGY AND PATHOGENESIS Invasive disease is acquired after inhalation of bacterial mycelia. Nocardiosis causes abscesses with neutrophilic infiltration and necrosis. Organisms survive within phagocytes. Cell-mediated immunity (CMI) is important for control of disease; persons with deficient CMI (e.g., transplant recipients and pts who have lymphoma, are receiving glucocorticoid treatment, or are infected with HIV) are at higher than usual risk of nocardiosis.

CLINICAL FEATURES

- Pulmonary disease: Pneumonia is usually subacute, presenting over days to weeks. Extrapulmonary disease is documented in >50% of cases, and some pulmonary involvement is evident in 80% of pts with extrapulmonary disease. A prominent cough productive of small amounts of thick purulent sputum, fever, anorexia, weight loss, and malaise can develop. Dyspnea, hemoptysis, and pleuritic chest pain are less common. CXR typically shows single or multiple nodular infiltrates of varying sizes that tend to cavitate. Empyema is noted in one-third of cases. Infection may spread to adjacent tissues, such as pericardium or mediastinum.
- Extrapulmonary disease: The most common sites are brain, skin, kidneys, bone, and muscle, and the typical presentation is a subacute abscess. Some abscesses form fistulae and discharge small amounts of pus, but not those in the lungs or brain. Brain abscesses are usually supratentorial, are often multiloculated, can be single or multiple, and tend to burrow into ventricles or extend into the subarachnoid space.
- Disease after transcutaneous inoculation
  1. Cellulitis: Subacute cellulitis may present 1–3 weeks after a break in the skin (often contaminated with soil). The firm, tender, erythematous, warm, and nonfluctuant lesions may involve underlying structures.
  2. Lymphocutaneous syndrome: A pyodermatous lesion develops at the inoculation site, with central ulceration and purulent discharge. This lesion is often drained by SC nodules along lymphatics. This form resembles sporotrichosis.
  3. Actinomycetoma: A nodular swelling forms at the site of local trauma, typically on the feet or hands. Fistulae form and discharge serous or purulent drainage that can contain granules consisting of masses of mycelia. Lesions, which spread slowly along fascial planes to involve adjacent skin and SC tissue and bone, can cause extensive deformity.
- Keratitis: usually follows eye trauma

DIAGNOSIS

- Sputum or pus should be examined for branching, beaded, gram-positive filaments. Nocardiae usually give positive results with modified acid-fast stains.

Sputum smears are often negative, and bronchoscopy may be needed to obtain adequate specimens.
- Cultures take 2–4 weeks to grow the organism. The laboratory should be alerted if nocardiosis is being considered. Sputum cultures positive for nocardiae should be assumed to reflect disease in immunocompromised hosts but may represent colonization in immunocompetent pts. If indicated, samples of CSF and urine should be cultured.

℞ **TREATMENT**   Table 101-1 lists the drugs, dosages, and durations used for treatment of nocardiosis.

- Sulfonamides are the drugs of choice. For serious disease, serum sulfonamide levels should be monitored and maintained at 100–150 μg/mL. Once disease is controlled, the sulfonamide dose may be decreased to 1 g qid, or the trimethoprim-sulfamethoxazole dose may be decreased by 50%.
- Susceptibility testing can identify other treatment options.
- Therapy for nocardiosis should continue while pts remain immunosuppressed.
- Surgical management of abscesses is similar to that in other bacterial diseases. For example, abscesses that are large or not responsive to antibiotics should be aspirated.

Table 101-1

Treatment for Nocardiosis

Disease	Duration	Drugs (Daily Dose)[a]
Pulmonary or systemic		Systemic therapy
Intact host defenses	6–12 mo	Oral
Deficient host defenses	12 mo[b]	1. Sulfonamides (6–8 g) or
CNS disease	12 mo[c]	combination of trimethoprim (10–20 mg/kg)
Cellulitis, lymphocutaneous syndrome	2 mo	and sulfamethoxazole (50–100 mg/kg)
Osteomyelitis, arthritis, laryngitis, sinusitis	4 mo	2. Minocycline (200–400 mg)
Actinomycetoma	6–12 mo after clinical cure	Parenteral
		1. Amikacin (10–15 mg/kg)
		2. Cefotaxime (6 g), ceftizoxime (6 g), ceftriaxone (2 g), or imipenem (2 g)
Keratitis	Topical: Until apparent cure	1. Sulfonamide drops
		2. Amikacin drops
	Systemic: Until 2–4 mo after apparent cure	Drugs for systemic therapy as listed above

[a] For each category, choices are numbered in order of preference.
[b] In some patients with AIDS or chronic granulomatous disease, therapy for pulmonary or systemic disease must be continued indefinitely.
[c] If all apparent CNS disease has been excised, the duration of therapy may be reduced to 6 months.

• Pts should be followed for at least 6 months after therapy is complete. Mortality rates are high among pts with nocardiosis of the brain.

ACTINOMYCOSIS

Actinomycosis is an indolent, slowly progressive infection caused by anaerobic or microaerophilic bacteria primarily of the genus *Actinomyces* (e.g., *A. israelii*). This diagnosis should be considered when a chronic progressive process with masslike features crosses tissue boundaries, a sinus tract develops, and/or the pt has evidence of a refractory or relapsing infection despite short courses of antibiotics. Most infections are polymicrobial, but the role of other species in the pathogenesis of the disease is unclear.

EPIDEMIOLOGY   Actinomycosis is associated with poor dental hygiene, use of intrauterine contraceptive devices (IUCDs), and immunosuppression. Its incidence is decreasing, probably as result of better dental hygiene and earlier initiation of antibiotic treatment.

PATHOGENESIS   The agents of actinomycosis are members of the normal oral flora and are commonly cultured from the GI and female genital tracts. Disease occurs only after disruption of the mucosal barrier. Local infection spreads contiguously in a slow, progressive manner, ignoring tissue planes. In vivo growth produces clumps called *grains* or *sulfur granules*. Central necrosis of lesions with neutrophils and sulfur granules is virtually diagnostic of the disease. The fibrotic walls of the mass are often described as "wooden."

CLINICAL FEATURES

• Oral-cervicofacial disease: Infection starts as a soft tissue swelling, abscess, or mass, often at the angle of the jaw with contiguous extension to the brain, cervical spine, or thorax. Pain, fever, and leukocytosis are variable.

• Thoracic disease: The pulmonary parenchyma and/or pleural space is usually involved. Chest pain, fever, and weight loss occur. CXR shows a mass lesion or pneumonia. Cavitary disease or hilar adenopathy may occur, and >50% of pts have pleural thickening, effusion, or empyema. Lesions cross fissures or pleura and may involve the mediastinum, contiguous bone, or the chest wall.

• Abdominal disease: The diagnosis is challenging and may not be made until months after the initial event (e.g., diverticulitis, bowel surgery). The disease usually presents as an abscess, mass, or lesion fixed to underlying tissue and is often mistaken for cancer. Sinus tracts to the abdominal wall, perianal region, or other organs may develop and mimic inflammatory bowel disease. Involvement of the urogenital tract can present as pyelonephritis or perinephric abscess.

• Pelvic disease: Pelvic actinomycosis is often associated with IUCDs. The presentation is indolent and may follow removal of the device. Pts have fever, weight loss, abdominal pain, and abnormal vaginal bleeding. Endometritis progresses to pelvic masses or tuboovarian abscess. When there are no symptoms and actinomycosis-causing organisms are isolated, it is not clear whether an IUCD should be removed, but the pt should be carefully observed over time.

• Miscellaneous sites: Actinomycosis can involve musculoskeletal, soft tissue, CNS, and other sites. Hematogenous dissemination is rare and usually involves lungs and liver.

DIAGNOSIS   Aspirations, biopsies, or surgical excision may be required to obtain material for diagnosis. Microscopic identification of sulfur granules in pus or tissues makes the diagnosis. Sulfur granules can occasionally be grossly identified from draining sinus tracts or pus. Cultures require 5–7 days but may take 2–4 weeks to become positive and are often rendered useless by prior antibiotic treatment.

TREATMENT

Like nocardiosis, actinomycosis requires prolonged treatment. For serious infection, IV therapy for 2–6 weeks (usually with penicillin) followed by oral therapy for 6–12 months (e.g., with penicillin or ampicillin) is suggested. If treatment is extended beyond the point of resolution of measurable disease (as quantified by CT or MRI), relapse is minimized.

For a more detailed discussion, see Filice GA: Nocardiosis, Chap. 146, p. 934; and Russo TA: Actinomycosis, Chap. 147, p. 937, in HPIM-16.

102

TUBERCULOSIS AND OTHER MYCOBACTERIAL INFECTIONS

TUBERCULOSIS

Tuberculosis (TB) is caused by organisms of the *Mycobacterium tuberculosis* complex. The complex includes *M. tuberculosis* (MTB), the most frequent and important agent of human mycobacterial disease, and *M. bovis*, previously an important cause of disease acquired via ingestion of unpasteurized milk. MTB is a thin aerobic bacterium that is neutral on Gram's staining but that, once stained, is acid-fast—i.e., it cannot be decolorized by acid alcohol because of the cell wall's high content of mycolic acids and other lipids.

EPIDEMIOLOGY

- It is estimated that >8.5 million new cases of TB occurred worldwide in 2001, mostly in developing countries. In 2000, 1.8 million deaths due to TB are estimated to have occurred. The HIV epidemic has had a major impact on TB, increasing the number of cases by several fold in the developing world. Increased rates of TB in the United States during the late 1980s were related to immigration, HIV disease, social problems (e.g., homelessness), and the emergence of multidrug-resistant (MDR) MTB. Rates have since decreased as a result of strong TB control programs. In the United States, TB tends to be a disease of elderly persons, HIV-infected young adults, immigrants, and the poor.
- MDR TB is defined as that caused by strains resistant to isoniazid and rifampin, but it is often associated with resistance to other drugs as well. MDR TB cases are generally few in North America and Europe but are more common among immigrants from certain developing areas (e.g., the former Soviet Union, Southeast Asia).
- Disease from a pt with infectious pulmonary TB is most commonly spread by droplet nuclei that are aerosolized by coughing, sneezing, or speaking. Droplets may be suspended in air for several hours. Transmission is determined by the intimacy and duration of contact with a pt with TB, the degree of infectiousness of that pt, and the shared environment. Pts with cavitary disease are usually most infectious, with as many as 10^5 acid-fast bacilli (AFB) per milliliter of sputum.

- Risk factors for development of active disease after MTB infection include recent acquisition (within the preceding year), comorbidity (e.g., HIV disease, diabetes, silicosis, immunosuppression, gastrectomy), malnutrition, and presence of fibrotic lesions.

PATHOGENESIS   AFB that reach alveoli are ingested by activated macrophages. If the bacilli are not contained, they multiply, lyse the macrophages, and spread to nonactivated monocytes. Macrophages may transport bacilli to regional lymph nodes, from which dissemination throughout the body may occur. About 2–4 weeks after infection, delayed-type hypersensitivity (DTH) destroys nonactivated macrophages that contain multiplying bacilli, and a macrophage-activating response activates cells capable of killing AFB. DTH is the basis for the PPD skin test. A granuloma forms at the site of the primary lesion and at sites of dissemination. The lesions can then either heal by fibrosis or undergo further evolution. Despite "healing," viable bacilli can remain dormant within macrophages or in the necrotic material for years. Cell-mediated immunity confers partial protection against TB. Cytokines secreted by alveolar macrophages contribute to disease manifestations, granuloma formation, and mycobacterial killing.

CLINICAL FEATURES   *Pulmonary TB*   TB is limited to the lungs in >80% of cases in HIV-negative pts.

1. *Primary* disease: The initial infection is frequently located in the middle and lower lobes. The primary lesion usually heals spontaneously, and a calcified nodule (Ghon lesion) remains. Hilar and paratracheal lymphadenopathy are common. In immunosuppressed pts and children, primary disease may progress rapidly to clinical disease, with cavitation, pleural effusions, and hematogenous dissemination.
2. *Postprimary* (adult-type, reactivation, or secondary) disease: Usually localized to the apical and posterior segments of the upper lobes and the superior segments of the lower lobes.
   a. Early symptoms of fever, night sweats, weight loss, anorexia, malaise, and weakness are nonspecific and insidious.
   b. Cough and purulent sputum production, often with blood streaking, occur. Occasionally, massive hemoptysis follows erosion of a vessel located in the wall of a cavity.
   c. Disease can be limited, or extensive cavitation may develop. Extensive disease may cause dyspnea and respiratory distress.

Extrapulmonary TB   Any site in the body can be involved. Up to two-thirds of HIV-infected pts with TB have extrapulmonary disease.

1. *Lymphadenitis* occurs in >25% of extrapulmonary TB cases, especially among HIV-infected pts. Painless swelling of cervical and supraclavicular nodes (*scrofula*) is typical. Early on, nodes are discrete but can be inflamed with a fistulous tract. Fine-needle aspiration or surgical biopsy of the node is required for diagnosis. AFB smears are positive in ~50% of cases and cultures in 70–80%.
2. *Pleural involvement* is common in primary TB, resulting from penetration of bacilli into the pleural space.
   a. DTH in response to these bacilli can result in effusion. Fluid is straw-colored and exudative, with protein levels >50% of those in serum, normal to low glucose levels, a usual pH of <7.2, and pleocytosis (500–2500 cells per microliter). Mononuclear cells are most common, although neutrophils may be present early in disease, and mesothelial cells are rare or absent. Pleural biopsy is often required for diagnosis, with up to 70% of biopsy cultures positive.

b. Empyema is less common and is usually a result of the rupture of a cavity with many bacilli into the pleural space.

3. In *genitourinary* disease, local symptoms predominate (e.g., frequency and dysuria). Calcifications and ureteral strictures can be seen. In >90% of cases, urinalysis shows pyuria and hematuria with negative bacterial cultures; in 90% of cases, culture of three morning urine specimens is diagnostic. Genital TB is more common among women than among men. Fallopian tube and uterine disease can cause infertility.

4. *Skeletal* disease: The spine, hips, and knees are the most common sites. Spinal TB (Pott's disease) often involves three or more adjacent vertebral bodies; in adults, lower thoracic/upper lumbar vertebrae are usually affected. Disease spreads to adjacent vertebral bodies, destroying the intervertebral disk and causing collapse of vertebral bodies in advanced disease (kyphosis, gibbus). Paravertebral cold abscesses may form.

5. *Meningitis* occurs most often in young children and HIV-seropositive pts. Disease typically evolves over 1–2 weeks.
   a. Cranial nerve involvement (particularly of the ocular nerve) and hydrocephalus are common.
   b. The CSF has a high lymphocyte count, an elevated protein level, and a low glucose concentration. Cultures are positive in 80% of cases.
   c. Neurologic sequelae can be reduced with adjunctive glucocorticoids administered along with treatment for TB.

6. *Gastrointestinal* disease affects the terminal ileum and cecum, causing abdominal pain and diarrhea, and can present with a clinical picture similar to that of Crohn's disease. A palpable mass and bowel obstruction may occur. Peritonitis presents with fever, abdominal pain, and ascites that is exudative with a high protein content and lymphocytic leukocytosis. Peritoneal biopsy is usually required for diagnosis.

7. *Pericarditis* is characterized by an acute or subacute onset of fever, dull retrosternal pain, and sometimes a friction rub. Effusion is common. Chronic constrictive pericarditis is a potentially fatal complication, even in treated pts. Adjunctive glucocorticoids may help manage acute disease but do not seem to reduce constriction.

8. *Miliary* disease arises from hematogenous spread of MTB throughout the body. Lesions are small (1- to 2-mm) granulomas, and symptoms are nonspecific. Hepatomegaly, splenomegaly, lymphadenopathy, and choroidal tubercles of the eye may occur.

HIV-Associated TB The manifestations of TB vary with the stage of HIV infection. When cell-mediated immunity is only partly compromised, pulmonary TB presents as typical upper-lobe cavitary disease. In late HIV infection, a primary TB-like pattern may be evident, with diffuse interstitial or miliary infiltrates, little or no cavitation, and intrathoracic lymphadenopathy. An immune reconstitution syndrome may occur when antiretroviral therapy is initiated. Symptoms and signs of TB are exacerbated as a consequence of improving immune function.

DIAGNOSIS

• Maintain a high index of suspicion, perform appropriate radiographic studies, and obtain appropriate clinical specimens.
• Examine diagnostic specimens for AFB with auramine-rhodamine stain and fluorescence microscopy.
• Isolate and identify MTB on culture. New liquid media and nucleic acid probes for species identification have decreased the time for diagnostic confirmation to 2–3 weeks.

- Nucleic acid amplification is useful to confirm MTB as the species in AFB-positive sputa. It may be useful in other settings but is hampered by a sensitivity lower than that of culture (although higher than that of AFB smear microscopy).
- The results of drug susceptibility testing are most rapid if liquid medium is used.
- PPD skin testing is of limited value in active disease because of low sensitivity and specificity.

℞ TREATMENT

Drugs

First-Line Agents

- *Rifampin*: the most important and potent antituberculous agent. The standard dosage in adults is 600 mg/d. The drug distributes well throughout body tissues, including inflamed meninges. It turns body fluids (e.g., urine, saliva, tears) red-orange and is excreted through bile and the enterohepatic circulation. Rifampin is usually well tolerated but may cause GI upset. In pts with underlying chronic liver disease (e.g., alcoholics, the elderly), the drug can cause hepatitis. Rash, anemia, and thrombocytopenia are less common side effects. Of note, rifampin is a potent inducer of hepatic microsomal enzymes and decreases the half-life of many other drugs. Although relevant clinical data are less abundant than for rifampin, rifabutin—a closely related agent—may be as effective, eliciting fewer drug interactions.
- *Isoniazid (INH)*: the best agent available after rifampin. The usual adult dosage is 300 mg/d or 900 mg 2 or 3 times per week. INH is distributed well throughout the body and infected tissues, including CSF and caseous granulomas. The most important toxicities are hepatotoxicity and peripheral neuropathy. INH-associated hepatitis is idiosyncratic and increases with age, alcohol use, pregnancy or the postpartum period, and concomitant use of rifampin. Because peripheral neuropathy can result from interference with pyridoxine metabolism, pyridoxine (25–50 mg/d) should be given.
- *Pyrazinamide*: The usual dosage is 25 mg/kg daily. The drug distributes well throughout the body, including the CSF. At current doses, hepatotoxicity is no greater than with INH or rifampin. Hyperuricemia and—in rare cases—gout can occur.
- *Ethambutol*: The least potent first-line agent, ethambutol is usually given at a dosage of 15 mg/kg daily. It is distributed throughout the body but reaches only low levels in CSF. At higher doses, retrobulbar optic neuritis can occur, causing central scotoma and impairing both visual acuity and the ability to see green.

Other Effective Agents

- *Fluoroquinolones*: Levofloxacin, ciprofloxacin, moxifloxacin, and gatifloxacin have good, broad antimycobacterial activity.
- *Streptomycin*: The usual adult dose is 0.5–1.0 g IM daily or 5 times per week. Streptomycin is similar to other aminoglycosides but is less nephrotoxic. Ototoxicity affects both hearing and vestibular function.
- Second-line agents are uncommonly used but may be needed in disease caused by MDR strains of MTB.

Regimens

See Table 102-1.

- Bacteriologic evaluation is the preferred method of monitoring response to treatment. Virtually all pts should have negative sputum cultures by the

Table 102-1

Recommended Antituberculosis Treatment Regimens

Indication	Initial Phase		Continuation Phase	
	Duration, Months	Drugs	Duration, Months	Drugs
New smear- or culture-positive cases	2	HRZE[a,b]	4	HR[a,c,d]
New culture-negative cases	2	HRZE[a]	2	HR[a]
Pregnancy	2	HRE[e]	7	HR
Failure and relapse[f]	—	—	—	—
Resistance (or intolerance) to H	Throughout (6)	RZE[g]		
Resistance to H + R	Throughout (18–24)	ZEQ + S (or another injectable agent[h])		
Resistance to all first-line drugs	Throughout (24)	1 injectable agent[h] + 3 of these 4: ethionamide, cycloserine, Q, PAS		
Standardized re-treatment (susceptibility testing unavailable)	3	HRZES[i]	5	HRE
Drug intolerance to R	Throughout (12)[j]	HZE		
Drug intolerance to Z	2	HRE	7	HR

[a] All drugs can be given daily or intermittently (three times weekly throughout or twice weekly after 2 to 8 weeks of daily therapy during the initial phase).

[b] Streptomycin can be used in place of ethambutol but is no longer considered to be a first-line drug by ATS/IDSA/CDC.

[c] The continuation phase should be extended to 7 months for patients with cavitary pulmonary tuberculosis who remain sputum culture–positive after the initial phase of treatment.

[d] HIV-negative patients with noncavitary pulmonary tuberculosis who have negative sputum AFB smears after the initial phase of treatment can be given once-weekly rifapentine/isoniazid in the continuation phase.

[e] The 6-month regimen with pyrazinamide can probably be used safely during pregnancy and is recommended by the WHO and the International Union Against Tuberculosis and Lung Disease. If pyrazinamide is not included in the initial treatment regimen, the minimum duration of therapy is 9 months.

[f] Regimen is tailored according to the results of drug susceptibility tests.

[g] A fluoroquinolone (Q) may strengthen the regimen for patients with extensive disease.

[h] Amikacin, kanamycin, or capreomycin. All these agents should be discontinued after 2 to 6 months, depending upon tolerance and response.

[i] Streptomycin should be discontinued after 2 months. This regimen is less effective for patients in whom treatment has failed, who have an increased probability of rifampin-resistant disease. In such cases, the re-treatment regimen might include second-line drugs chosen in light of the likely pattern of drug resistance.

[j] Streptomycin for the initial 2 months or a fluoroquinolone might strengthen the regimen for patients with extensive disease.

Note: H, isoniazid; R, rifampin; Z, pyrazinamide; E, ethambutol; S, streptomycin; Q, a quinolone antibiotic; PAS, para-aminosalicylic acid.

end of 2–3 months of treatment. If the culture remains positive, treatment failure and drug resistance should be suspected.

• Drug resistance may be either primary (i.e., infection caused by a strain resistant prior to therapy) or acquired (i.e., resistance arising during treatment because of an inadequate regimen or the pt's noncompliance).

• Nonadherence to the regimen is the most important impediment to cure. Use of directly observed treatment and fixed-drug-combination products should be considered.
• Close monitoring for drug toxicity should take place during treatment and should include baseline LFTs and monthly questioning about possible hepatitis symptoms. High-risk pts should have LFTs monitored during treatment if baseline results are abnormal.

PREVENTION

• Vaccination: An attenuated strain of *M. bovis*, bacille Calmette-Guérin (BCG), protects infants and young children from serious forms of TB. Its efficacy is unclear in other situations.
• Treatment of latent infection: Candidates for chemoprophylaxis are usually identified by PPD skin testing. Positive skin tests are determined by reaction size and risk group (Table 102-2), and, if the test is positive, drug treatment is considered (Table 102-3). INH should not be given to persons with active liver disease.

LEPROSY

ETIOLOGY AND EPIDEMIOLOGY Leprosy, a nonfatal chronic infectious disease caused by *M. leprae*, is a disease of the developing world; its global prevalence is difficult to assess and is variously estimated at 0.6–8 million. Africa has the highest prevalence, and Asia has the most cases, with especially high numbers in India, China, Myanmar, and Nepal. Leprosy is associated with poverty and rural residence. The route of transmission is uncertain but may be via nasal droplets, contact with infected soil, or insect vectors.

CLINICAL, HISTOLOGIC, AND IMMUNOLOGIC SPECTRUM The spectrum of clinical and histologic manifestations of leprosy is attributable to variability in the immune response to *M. leprae*. The spectrum from tuberculoid leprosy (TL) to lepromatous leprosy (LL) is associated with an evolution from localized to more generalized disease manifestations and an increasing bacterial load. Prognosis, complications, and intensity of antimicrobial therapy

Table 102-2

Tuberculin Reaction Size, Treatment of Latent Tuberculosis Infection

Risk Group	Tuberculin Reaction Size, mm
HIV-infected persons or persons receiving immunosuppressive therapy	≥5
Close contacts of tuberculosis patients	≥5[a]
Persons with fibrotic lesions on chest radiography	≥5
Recently infected persons (≤2 years)	≥10
Persons with high-risk medical conditions[b]	≥10
Low-risk persons[c]	≥15

[a] Tuberculin-negative contacts, especially children, should receive prophylaxis for 2 to 3 months after contact ends and should then be retested with PPD. Those whose results remain negative should discontinue prophylaxis. HIV-infected contacts should receive a full course of treatment regardless of PPD results.

[b] Includes diabetes mellitus, some hematologic and reticuloendothelial diseases, injection drug use (with HIV seronegativity), end-stage renal disease, and clinical situations associated with rapid weight loss.

[c] Decision to treat should be based on individual risk/benefit considerations.

Table 102-3

Revised Drug Regimens for Treatment of Latent Tuberculosis Infection (LTBI) in Adults

Drug	Interval and Duration	Comments[a]	Rating[b] (Evidence[c]) HIV-Negative	HIV-Infected
Isoniazid	Daily for 9 months[d,e]	In HIV-infected persons, isoniazid may be administered concurrently with nucleoside reverse transcriptase inhibitors, protease inhibitors, or nonnucleoside reverse transcriptase inhibitors (NNRTIs).	A (II)	A (II)
	Twice weekly for 9 months[d,e]	Directly observed therapy (DOT) must be used with twice-weekly dosing.	B (II)	B (II)
	Daily for 6 months[e]	Regimen is not indicated for HIV-infected persons, those with fibrotic lesions on chest radiographs, or children.	B (I)	C (I)
	Twice weekly for 6 months[e]	DOT must be used with twice-weekly dosing.	B (II)	C (I)
Rifampin[f]	Daily for 4 months	Regimen is used for contacts of pts with isoniazid-resistant, rifampin-susceptible TB. In HIV-infected pts, most protease inhibitors and delavirdine should not be administered concurrently with rifampin. Rifabutin, with appropriate dose adjustments, can be used with protease inhibitors (saquinavir should be augmented with ritonavir) and NNRTIs (except delavirdine). Consult web-based updates for the latest specific recommendations.	B (II)	B (III)

(continued)

Table 102-3 *(Continued)*

Revised Drug Regimens for Treatment of Latent Tuberculosis Infection (LTBI) in Adults

Drug	Interval and Duration	Comments[a]	Rating[b] (Evidence[c]) HIV-Negative	HIV-Infected
Rifampin plus pyrazinamide (RZ)	Daily for 2 months	Regimen generally should not be offered for treatment of LTBI in either HIV-infected or HIV-negative pts.	D (II)	D (II)
	Twice weekly for 2–3 months		D (III)	D (III)

[a] Interactions with HIV-related drugs are updated frequently and are available at http://www.aidsinfo.nih.gov/guidelines.

[b] Strength of the recommendation: A. Both strong evidence of efficacy and substantial clinical benefit support recommendation for use. Should always be offered. B. Moderate evidence for efficacy or strong evidence for efficacy, but only limited clinical benefit, supports recommendation for use. Should generally be offered. C. Evidence for efficacy is insufficient to support a recommendation for or against use, or evidence for efficacy might not outweigh adverse consequences (e.g., drug toxicity, drug interactions) or cost of the treatment or alternative approaches. Optional. D. Moderate evidence for lack of efficacy or for adverse outcome supports a recommendation against use. Should generally not be offered. E. Good evidence for lack of efficacy or for adverse outcome supports a recommendation against use. Should never be offered.

[c] Quality of evidence supporting the recommendation: I. Evidence from at least one properly randomized controlled trial. II. Evidence from at least one well-designed clinical trial without randomization, from cohort or case-controlled analytic studies (preferably from more than one center), from multiple time-series studies, or from dramatic results in uncontrolled experiments. III. Evidence from opinions of respected authorities based on clinical experience, descriptive studies, or reports of expert committees.

[d] Recommended regimen for persons aged <18 years.

[e] Recommended regimen for pregnant women.

[f] The substitution of rifapentine for rifampin is not recommended because rifapentine's safety and effectiveness have not been established for pts with LTBI.

Source: Adapted from CDC: MMWR 49(RR-6), 2000.

depend on where a pt presents on the clinical spectrum. The incubation period ranges from 2 to 40 years but is usually 5–7 years.

Tuberculoid Leprosy

• Disease is confined to the skin and peripheral nerves. AFB are few or absent.
• One or several hypopigmented macules or plaques with sharp margins that are hypesthetic and have lost sweat glands and hair follicles are present.
• There is asymmetric enlargement of one or several peripheral nerves—most often the ulnar, posterior auricular, peroneal, and posterior tibial nerves—associated with hypesthesia and myopathy.

Lepromatous Leprosy

• Symmetrically distributed skin nodules, raised plaques, and diffuse dermal infiltration that can cause leonine facies, loss of eyebrows and lashes, pendulous earlobes, and dry scaling
• Numerous bacilli in skin, nerves, and all organs except lungs and CNS
• Nerve enlargement and damage are usually symmetric; symmetric nerve-trunk enlargement and acral distal peripheral neuropathy are seen.

Complications

• Reactional states: inflammatory conditions at the site of lesions. Erythema nodosum leproticum (ENL) occurs in pts near the LL end of the disease spectrum as they tend toward TL after treatment.
• Extremities: Neuropathy results in insensitivity and affects fine touch, pain, and heat receptors. Ulcerations, trauma, secondary infections, and (at times) a profound osteolytic process can take place.
• Nose: chronic nasal congestion and epistaxis, destruction of cartilage with saddle-nose deformity or anosmia
• Eye: trauma, secondary infection, corneal ulcerations, opacities, uveitis, cataracts, glaucoma, sometimes blindness
• Testes: orchitis, aspermia, impotence, infertility

DIAGNOSIS   Biopsy the advancing edge of a skin lesion in TT. In LL, biopsy even of normal-appearing skin often yields positive results.

 TREATMENT

Drugs

• Rifampin (600 mg daily or monthly) is the only bactericidal *M. leprae* agent.
• Dapsone (50–100 mg/d). Hemolysis and methemoglobinemia are common adverse effects. G6PD deficiency must be ruled out before therapy to avoid hemolytic anemia. GI intolerance, headache, pruritus, peripheral neuropathies, and rash can occur.
• Clofazimine (50–100 mg/d, 100 mg 3 times per week, or 300 mg monthly). A phenazine iminoquinone dye, clofazimine is weakly active against *M. leprae*. Adverse effects include skin discoloration and GI intolerance.

Regimens

• Paucibacillary disease in adults (<6 skin lesions)

  1. Dapsone (100 mg/d) and rifampin (600 mg monthly) for 6 months or dapsone (100 mg/d) for 5 years
  2. With a single lesion: a single dose of rifampin (600 mg), ofloxacin (400 mg), and minocycline (100 mg)

• Multibacillary disease in adults (≥6 skin lesions)

  1. Dapsone (100 mg/d) plus clofazimine (50 mg/d) unsupervised as well as rifampin (600 mg monthly) plus clofazimine (300 mg monthly) supervised for 1 year, per the World Health Organization
  2. Relapse can occur years later; prolonged follow-up is needed.
  3. Some experts prefer rifampin (600 mg/d for 3 years) and dapsone (100 mg/d) for life.

• Reactional states

  1. Mild reactions: glucocorticoids (40–60 mg/d for at least 3 months)
  2. If ENL is present and persists despite two courses of steroids, thalidomide (100–300 mg nightly) should be given.

INFECTIONS WITH NONTUBERCULOUS MYCOBACTERIA (NTM)

Mycobacteria other than MTB and *M. leprae* are distributed widely throughout the environment in water, biofilms, and soil as well as in numerous animal species. Isolation of NTM from a clinical specimen requires an assessment of the organism's significance. For example, *M. kansasii* is usually pathogenic, but *M. gordonae* is seldom so.

MICROBIOLOGY *M. abscessus*, *M. fortuitum*, and *M. chelonae* grow rapidly (within 7 days). Other NTM species, such as *M. avium* and *M. intracellulare* (the *M. avium* complex, or MAC), *M. kansasii*, *M. ulcerans*, and *M. marinum*, more typically grow within 2–3 weeks, although newer broth culture systems can isolate these organisms more quickly.

CLINICAL FEATURES *MAC* Infections with MAC are probably acquired via the oral route.

1. Pulmonary disease: Compared with MTB, MAC organisms more commonly cause lung disease in pts born in the United States.
    a. Pts present with chronic cough, dyspnea, and fatigue but no fever. Nodules, pneumonitis, bronchiectasis, or cavity formation may result. Disease is found in apparently healthy nonsmokers who might have a subtle defect in cell-mediated immunity. Disease is also seen in pts with underlying lung disease, such as COPD, cystic fibrosis, or prior TB.
    b. CT of the chest should be performed to document the extent of disease and establish a treatment baseline.
    c. Most pts with cavitary disease or progression should be treated. If disease is indolent, the adverse effects of treatment can be more debilitating than the disease itself and treatment can be deferred. Agents include ethambutol (15 mg/kg daily), rifabutin (150–300 mg/d), and a macrolide—either clarithromycin (500 mg bid) or azithromycin (600 mg 3 times per week). Streptomycin (500–1000 mg 2 or 3 times per week) can be included in the first 2 months for severe disease, and a fluoroquinolone can be considered if one of the first-line agents (usually rifabutin) cannot be tolerated. A macrolide-containing regimen should be given for at least 12 months after sputum cultures become negative.
2. Disseminated disease occurs primarily in pts with advanced HIV disease who are not receiving highly active antiretroviral treatment (HAART). It can also occur in other immunocompromised pts—e.g., transplant recipients and leukemia pts, particularly those with hairy cell leukemia.
    a. Pts present with fever, weakness, wasting, and adenopathy. Laboratory studies reveal anemia, hypoalbuminemia, increased alkaline phosphatase levels, and blood cultures positive for MAC.
    b. Pts in whom HAART is initiated may experience immune reconstitution syndrome 1–12 weeks later and develop localized or generalized culture-positive lymphadenitis.
    c. Blood cultures performed with the liquid BACTEC system yield positive results within 7–14 days. AFB staining of bone marrow and/or liver can provide more rapid results. Liver biopsies provide a diagnosis in >50% of pts with abnormal LFTs.
    d. Treatment should consist of a macrolide—clarithromycin (500 mg bid) or azithromycin (500 mg/d)—plus ethambutol (15 mg/kg daily) and HAART. Rifabutin may be included as well. Therapy can be stopped after 12 months if CD4+ T cell counts have been >100/μL for at least 6 months.
    e. Chemoprophylaxis with azithromycin (1200 mg weekly) or clarithromycin (500 mg bid) is indicated to prevent MAC disease in pts with CD4+ T cell counts of <50/μL or when another AIDS-defining illness occurs.

M. kansasii *M. kansasii* is the second most common cause of lung disease due to NTM in the United States. The average age of onset is 60 years, and most pts have COPD, lung cancer, silicosis, or prior TB. Clinical features resemble those of pulmonary TB. A sputum culture positive for *M. kansasii* is usually clinically significant, especially in HIV-positive pts. Treatment with rifampin (600 mg/d), isoniazid (300 mg/d), and ethambutol (25 mg/kg daily for 2 months, then 15 mg/kg daily) should be administered for at least 18–24 months. Disseminated disease can occur in pts with advanced AIDS and resembles disseminated MAC infection but has more prominent pulmonary findings. Treatment is the same as for pulmonary disease, but if pts are receiving HAART, rifabutin (150 mg) or clarithromycin (500 mg) bid can be substituted for rifampin to avoid drug interactions.

M. abscessus, M. chelonae, and M. fortuitum Disseminated cutaneous disease is the most common clinical manifestation of infection with the rapidly growing NTM species. Lesions are cellulitic or nodular, erythematous, indurated, and tender. They may ulcerate and exude purulent drainage and may spread proximally along lymphatics. These organisms may infect surgical or traumatic wounds, contaminated injection sites, body piercing sites, or prosthetic materials. Pulmonary infections, usually due to *M. abscessus*, are the next most common manifestation and occur in pts with an underlying lung disease such as cystic fibrosis. Susceptibility testing should be performed, although all three species are usually susceptible to clarithromycin (500 mg bid) and amikacin (5–7.5 mg/kg q12h). Cefoxitin (3 g q6h) is effective for most *M. abscessus* and *M. fortuitum* infections. Treatment for 6–12 months for bacteremic or disseminated cutaneous disease or pulmonary disease is recommended. Localized cutaneous lesions may respond to a single agent, such as clarithromycin, administered for 2 weeks.

M. marinum *M. marinum* is widely distributed in water and causes chronic cutaneous infections when open wounds are exposed to a colonized water source, usually via fish tanks, shellfish, or marine settings. *M. marinum* grows best at 30°C, a temperature lower than that at which other mycobacteria thrive. After a median incubation period of 21 days, a granulomatous or ulcerating skin lesion develops, with subsequent proximal spread along lymphatics; extension to deeper structures may occur in pts receiving immunosuppressive therapy, resulting in tenosynovitis or osteomyelitis. Administration of clarithromycin and ethambutol for 1–2 months after lesion resolution (usually a 4-month course) is recommended.

M. ulcerans Buruli ulcer caused by *M. ulcerans* is a painless nodule that progresses to a deep ulcer with sloughing of skin and SC tissue. Osteomyelitis may occur, and deforming scarring and contractures may result from extensive necrosis. This infection is seen primarily in the tropics. Antimycobacterial treatment has not yet been shown to be helpful.

For a more detailed discussion, see Wallace RJ Jr, Griffith DE: Antimycobacterial Agents, Chap. 149, p. 946; Raviglione MC, O'Brien RJ: Tuberculosis, Chap. 150, p. 953; Gelber RH: Leprosy (Hansen's Disease), Chap. 151, p. 966; and von Reyn CF: Nontuberculous Mycobacteria, Chap. 152, p. 972, in HPIM-16.

103

LYME DISEASE AND OTHER NONSYPHILITIC SPIROCHETAL INFECTIONS

LYME BORRELIOSIS

ETIOLOGY AND EPIDEMIOLOGY   Lyme disease, caused by the spirochete *Borrelia burgdorferi*, is the most common vector-borne illness in the United States. *B. burgdorferi sensu stricto* causes disease in North America; *B. garinii* and *B. afzelii* are more common in Europe. *Ixodes* ticks transmit the disease: *I. scapularis*, which also transmits babesiosis and anaplasmosis, is found in the northeastern and midwestern United States; *I. pacificus* is found in the western United States. The white-footed mouse is the preferred host for larval and nymphal ticks. Adult ticks prefer the white-tailed deer as host. The tick must feed for 24 h to transmit the disease.

CLINICAL FEATURES   *Early Infection, Stage 1: Localized Infection*
After an incubation period of 3–32 days, erythema migrans (EM) develops at the site of the tick bite in 80% of pts. The classic presentation is a red macule that expands slowly to form an annular lesion with a bright red outer border and central clearing; central erythema, induration, necrosis, or vesicular changes or many red rings within an outer ring are also possible.

Early Infection, Stage 2: Disseminated Infection

• Hematogenous spread occurs within days to weeks after infection. Secondary annular lesions, similar in appearance to EM, may develop.
• Pts develop headache, mild neck stiffness, fever, chills, migratory musculoskeletal pain, arthralgias, malaise, and fatigue. These symptoms subside within a few weeks, even in untreated pts.
• Meningeal irritation: CSF is initially normal; however, weeks to months later, ~15% of pts progress to frank neurologic abnormalities (meningitis; encephalitis; cranial neuritis, including bilateral facial palsy; motor or sensory radiculoneuropathy; mononeuritis multiplex; ataxia; and myelitis).
• Cardiac involvement occurs in ~8% of pts. Atrioventricular (AV) block of fluctuating degree is most common, but acute myopericarditis is possible.

Late Infection, Stage 3: Persistent Infection

• Lyme arthritis develops in ~60% of untreated pts in the United States. It usually consists of intermittent attacks of oligoarticular arthritis in large joints (especially the knees) lasting weeks to months. Joint fluid cell counts range from 500 to 110,000/μL. Recurrent attacks decrease yearly, but a few pts have chronic arthritis with bony and cartilage erosion. Arthritis can persist despite eradication of spirochetes.
• Chronic neurologic involvement is less common. Encephalopathy affecting memory, mood, or sleep can be accompanied by axonal polyneuropathy manifested as either distal paresthesia or spinal radicular pain. In Europe, severe encephalomyelitis is seen with *B. garinii* infection.
• Acrodermatitis chronica atrophicans, a late skin manifestation, is seen in Europe and Asia and is associated with *B. afzelii* infection.

DIAGNOSIS

• Culture of the organism in Barbour-Stoenner-Kelly medium is largely a research tool. Cultures are positive only early in illness, with the organism isolated primarily from EM skin lesions.

- PCR is most useful for joint fluid, somewhat useful for CSF, and of little use for plasma or urine testing.
- Serology can be problematic because tests do not clearly distinguish between active and inactive infection. Serologic testing should be undertaken when the pt has at least an intermediate pretest likelihood of having Lyme disease.
- Two-step testing: ELISA screening with Western blot testing in cases with positive or equivocal results. IgM and IgG testing should be done in the first 4 weeks of illness; after 1 month, IgG testing alone is adequate.

℞ TREATMENT

Except for neurologic and cardiac disease, most treatment can be oral.

1. Doxycycline (100 mg bid) is the agent of choice for men and nonpregnant women.
2. Amoxicillin (500 mg tid), cefuroxime (500 mg bid), erythromycin (250 mg qid), and newer macrolides are alternative agents, in that order.
3. More than 90% of pts have good outcomes with a 14-day course of treatment for localized infection or a 21-day course for disseminated infection.
4. Neuroborreliosis: IV treatment with ceftriaxone (2 g/d for 14–28 days) should be given. Cefotaxime or penicillin is an alternative.
5. Pts with high-degree AV block should receive a 28-day course that commences with IV ceftriaxone (or alternative IV drugs) until the block has resolved; oral agents can then be used to complete treatment.
6. Lyme arthritis: 30–60 days of PO antibiotic or 14–28 days of IV ceftriaxone

PROPHYLAXIS If an attached, engorged *I. scapularis* nymph is found or if follow-up will be difficult, a single 200-mg dose of doxycycline, given within 72 h of the tick bite, effectively prevents the disease. This measure is not routinely recommended.

PROGNOSIS Early treatment results in an excellent prognosis. Although convalescence is longer the later antibiotics are given, the overall prognosis remains excellent, with minimal or no residual deficits. Reinfection can occur. No vaccine is commercially available.

ENDEMIC TREPONEMATOSES

ETIOLOGY AND EPIDEMIOLOGY The endemic treponematoses—yaws, endemic syphilis, and pinta—are nonvenereal chronic childhood diseases caused by organisms closely related to the agent of syphilis, *Treponema pallidum*. A World Health Organization eradication program was very effective, and only pockets of resurgence, primarily in Africa, remain. Early skin lesions are infectious; disease is transmitted by direct contact.

CLINICAL FEATURES Disease is manifest by primary skin lesions that become disseminated with time. After a latency phase, destructive gummas in skin, bone, and joints occur as late manifestations. Pinta causes dyschromic macules but not destructive lesions.

DIAGNOSIS Diagnosis is based on clinical presentation and dark-field microscopy of scrapings from lesions. Serologic tests used for syphilis are also used for diagnosis of endemic treponematoses.

TREATMENT

Benzathine penicillin (600,000 units for children <10 years of age, 1.2 million units for pts >10 years of age) is the treatment of choice. Doxycycline is probably an effective alternative.

LEPTOSPIROSIS

ETIOLOGY AND EPIDEMIOLOGY   Leptospires are spirochetal organisms that cause an important zoonosis with a broad spectrum of clinical manifestations. Rodents, particularly rats, are the most important disease reservoir, but at least 160 mammalian species can harbor the organisms. Transmission can occur during contact with urine, blood, or tissue from infected animals or during exposure to contaminated environments. Organisms are found in urine and can survive in water for many months. The disease is particularly common in developing tropical nations. Approximately 40–120 cases are reported each year in the United States, but these numbers are likely to represent significant underestimates. Risk factors in the United States include recreational water activities, occupational activities that result in exposure to animals or animal waste (e.g., sewage work), and residence in urban settings with expanding rat populations.

PATHOGENESIS   Entry of the organisms via skin abrasions or intact mucous membranes is followed by leptospiremia and widespread dissemination. Organisms can be isolated from blood and CSF for the first 4–10 days of illness. Leptospires damage blood vessel walls and cause vasculitis, leakage, and extravasation, including hemorrhages. Vasculitis is responsible for most manifestations.

CLINICAL FEATURES
- Incubation period, 1–2 weeks (range, 2–20 days)
- Anicteric leptospirosis, a biphasic illness, is the milder form and is found in 90% of symptomatic cases.
  1. Flulike illness: fever, severe headache, nausea, vomiting. Myalgias, especially of the calves, back, and abdomen, are a dominant feature.
  2. Conjunctival suffusion and fever are the most common physical findings; rash develops occasionally. Symptoms subside within 1 week and recur after 1–3 days in conjunction with antibody development.
  3. Symptoms are generally milder in phase 2, but 15% of pts can develop clinically evident aseptic meningitis. A higher percentage of pts have asymptomatic CSF pleocytosis. Iritis, chorioretinitis, and uveitis can occur. Symptoms usually subside in days but can persist for weeks to months.
- Icteric leptospirosis (Weil's syndrome) is severe, with a mortality rate of 5–15%.
  1. After 4–9 days of mild illness, more severe symptoms develop; however, this is not a truly biphasic disease.
  2. Pts have jaundice, hepatosplenomegaly, and abdominal tenderness.
  3. Renal failure with acute tubular necrosis may develop.
  4. Cough, dyspnea, chest pain, and hemoptysis can occur.
  5. Hemorrhagic manifestations commonly include epistaxis, petechiae, purpura, and ecchymoses.
  6. Rhabdomyolysis, hemolysis, myocarditis, pericarditis, CHF, shock, ARDS, pancreatitis, and multiorgan failure have all been described.
- Laboratory findings
  1. Renal dysfunction, abnormal urinary sediment, proteinuria
  2. Elevated ESR, marked leukocytosis, thrombocytopenia

3. Elevated bilirubin and alkaline phosphatase levels, mild aminotransferase increases
4. Prolonged prothrombin time, elevated creatine phosphokinase level
5. Patchy alveolar pattern due to hemorrhage on CXR

DIAGNOSIS

• Serology: Microscopic agglutination test (MAT) done at CDC; ELISA available at reference laboratories
• Organism cultured from blood or CSF in the first 10 days of illness or from urine after the first week. Cultures most often become positive within 2–4 weeks (range, 1 week to 4 months).
• Differential: dengue, malaria, viral hepatitis, hantavirus disease, rickettsial disease

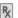 **TREATMENT**

Treatment should be started as early as possible but should be given even if delayed. IV penicillin G (1.5 million units qid), ampicillin (1 g qid), and erythromycin (500 mg qid) are all effective. Milder cases can be treated with oral doxycycline (100 mg bid) or amoxicillin (500 mg qid).

RELAPSING FEVER

ETIOLOGY *Borrelia recurrentis* causes louse-borne relapsing fever (LBRF), a disease transmitted from person to person by the body louse. Tick-borne relapsing fever (TBRF), a zoonosis usually transmitted from rodents to humans via the bite of various *Ornithodoros* ticks, is caused by multiple *Borrelia* species. DNA rearrangement within *vmp* genes on linear plasmids in borreliae results in variation in expression of surface antigens, allowing organisms to evade host immune responses.

EPIDEMIOLOGY Rates of LBRF have decreased markedly with improvements in the standard of living. TBRF is still present worldwide and often goes unrecognized or underreported. About 35 cases per year are reported in the United States, mostly in forested mountainous areas of far western states and among persons sleeping in rustic mountain cabins and vacation homes. Ticks feed painlessly and quickly (20–45 min).

CLINICAL FEATURES Symptoms are similar in the two types of relapsing fever.

1. Mean incubation period, 7 days; range, 2–18 days
2. Sudden onset of high fever, headache, shaking chills, sweats, dizziness, nausea, vomiting, myalgias, arthralgias (sometimes severe); no arthritis
3. Tachycardia, tachypnea, dehydration, scleral icterus, and petechiae can occur. Conjunctivae are often injected, and photophobia is common.
4. Epistaxis, blood-tinged sputum, and GI or CNS hemorrhage can occur.
5. Symptoms increase for 2–7 days, then end in a crisis with two phases.
   a. *Chill phase*: rigors, rising temperature, hypermetabolism
   b. *Flush phase*: falling temperature, diaphoresis, decreased effective circulating blood volume
6. Spirochetemia and symptoms recur after days to weeks. LBRF is associated with 1 or 2 relapses, TBRF with up to 10. Each episode is less severe and is followed by a longer afebrile interval than the last.

DIAGNOSIS Spirochetes can be demonstrated in blood, bone marrow aspirates, or CSF by dark-field microscopy or in thick or thin smears of peripheral blood or buffy-coat preparations using Wright, Giemsa, or acridine orange stain. Organisms are most numerous before the crisis and during high fevers.

 TREATMENT

One dose of doxycycline (100 mg), erythromycin (500 mg), or chloramphenicol (500 mg) is effective for LBRF. A 7-day course is recommended for TBRF. A Jarisch-Herxheimer-like reaction within 1–4 h of the first dose occurs in >50% of TBRF cases but is more severe in LBRF cases or when high numbers of spirochetes are circulating at treatment outset. The reaction can last up to 8 h, and pts should be closely monitored.

PROGNOSIS Untreated LBRF has a high case-fatality rate, but the mortality rate is <5% with therapy. TBRF is generally a milder disease.

For a more detailed discussion, see Lukehart SA: Endemic Treponematoses, Chap. 154, p. 985; Speelman P: Leptospirosis, Chap. 155, p. 988; Dennis DT, Hayes EB: Relapsing Fever, Chap. 156, p. 991; and Steere AC: Lyme Borreliosis, Chap. 157, p. 995, in HPIM-16. For a discussion of syphilis, see Chap. 88 in this manual.

104

RICKETTSIAL DISEASES

Rickettsiae are obligate intracellular organisms appearing as gram-negative coccobacilli and short bacilli. These organisms have mammalian reservoirs and are transmitted by insects or ticks. Except in the case of louse-borne typhus, humans are incidental hosts.

TICK- AND MITE-BORNE SPOTTED FEVERS
Rocky Mountain Spotted Fever (RMSF)

Epidemiology Caused by *R. rickettsii*, RMSF is the most severe rickettsial disease. In the United States, the prevalence is highest in the south-central and southeastern states. Most cases occur between May and September. The American dog tick, *Dermacentor variabilis*, transmits RMSF in the eastern two-thirds of the nation and in California; *D. andersoni*, the Rocky Mountain wood tick, transmits the disease in the western region. In 2001, the incidence of RMSF was 0.20 persons infected per 100,000 population.

Pathogenesis Rickettsiae are inoculated by the tick after ≥6 h of feeding, spread lymphohematogenously, become intracellularly located, and then spread from cell to cell, creating numerous foci of contiguous infected endothelial cells. *R. rickettsii* is more invasive than other *Rickettsia* spp. and spreads to vascular smooth-muscle cells, causing increased vascular permeability.

Clinical Features The incubation period averages 7 days (range, 2–14 days). Symptoms in the first 3 days of illness are nonspecific and include fever, headache, malaise, myalgias, nausea, vomiting, and anorexia. By day 3, macules typically appear on the wrists and ankles, subsequently spreading to the rest of the extremities and the trunk. Lesions initially blanch, but, because of vascular damage, central hemorrhage later develops and the lesions become petechial. Such petechiae eventually develop in 41–59% of pts, appearing on or after day 6 of illness in ~74% of cases that include a rash. The palms and soles become involved after day 5 in 43% of pts but do not become involved at all in 18–64%. The microcirculation, both systemic and pulmonary, is damaged in RMSF, causing edema, decreased plasma volume, hypoalbuminemia, reduced serum oncotic pressure, prerenal azotemia, hypotension, noncardiogenic pulmonary edema, and cardiac involvement with dysrhythmias. Pulmonary disease is an important factor in fatal cases and develops in 17% of cases overall, of which 12% are considered to represent severe respiratory disease. CNS involvement is the other important determinant of outcome. Encephalitis can progress to stupor or delirium, ataxia, coma, seizures, cranial nerve palsy, hearing loss, severe vertigo, nystagmus, dysarthria, aphasia, and other CNS signs. Meningoencephalitis can develop, with CSF notable for pleocytosis, mononuclear cell predominance, and increased protein and normal glucose levels. Renal and hepatic injury can occur, and bleeding is a potentially life-threatening effect of severe vascular damage. Other laboratory findings may include a normal WBC count with increased immature myeloid cells, increased plasma levels of acute-phase reactants such as C-reactive protein, hyponatremia, and myositis with elevated levels of creatine kinase.

Prognosis Without treatment, the pt usually dies in 8–15 days; a rare fulminant presentation can result in death within 5 days. Mortality ~5% despite the availability of effective antibiotics, mostly because of delayed diagnosis.

Diagnosis Within the first 3 days, diagnosis is difficult, since only 3% of pts have the classic triad of fever, rash, and known history of tick exposure. When the rash appears, the diagnosis should be considered. Immunohistologic examination with immunofluorescence or immunoenzyme staining of a cutaneous biopsy sample from a rash lesion is the only diagnostic test of use during acute illness. Serology, most commonly the indirect immunofluorescence assay (IFA), is usually positive 7–10 days after the onset of disease, and a diagnostic titer ≥ 1:64 is usually documented.

 TREATMENT

Doxycycline (100 mg bid PO or IV) is the treatment of choice for both children and adults but not for pregnant women and pts allergic to the drug, who should receive chloramphenicol (50–75 mg/kg daily, in 4 divided oral doses, for 7 days). In the latter pts, the CBC should be monitored during treatment. Treatment is given until the pt is afebrile and has been improving for 2 or 3 days.

Rickettsialpox

Epidemiology Rickettsialpox is caused by *R. akari* and is maintained by mice and their mites. Currently a rare disease that is recognized principally in New York City, rickettsialpox has also been reported in North Carolina, Virginia, Maryland, Arizona, Utah, and Ohio.

Clinical Features A papule forms at the site of the mite bite and develops a central vesicle that becomes a painless black-crusted eschar surrounded by an erythematous halo. Lymph nodes draining the region of the eschar appear. After an incubation period of 10–17 days, malaise, chills, fever, headache, and myalgia mark disease onset. A macular rash appears on day 2–6 of illness and evolves sequentially into papules, vesicles, and crusts that heal without scarring. Some pts have nausea, vomiting, abdominal pain, cough, conjunctivitis, or photophobia. Disease resolves within 6–10 days and is not fatal.

 TREATMENT

Treatment options are doxycycline (100 mg bid for 1–5 days), ciprofloxacin (750 mg bid for 1–5 days), or chloramphenicol (500 mg qid for 7–10 days).

FLEA- AND LOUSE-BORNE TYPHUS GROUP RICKETTSIOSES
Endemic Murine Typhus (Flea-Borne)

Epidemiology   Caused by *R. typhi*, endemic murine typhus has a rat reservoir and is transmitted by fleas. Humans become infected when rickettsia-laden flea feces are scratched into pruritic bite lesions; less often, the flea bite itself transmits the organisms. Fewer than 100 cases of endemic typhus are reported each year in the United States, with most cases occurring in southern Texas and southern California. Flea bites are not often recalled by pts, but exposure to animals such as cats, opossums, raccoons, skunks, and rats is reported by ~40%.

Clinical Features   The incubation period averages 11 days (range, 8–16 days). Prodromal symptoms 1–3 days before the abrupt onset of chills and fever include headache, myalgia, arthralgia, nausea, and malaise. Nausea and vomiting are common early in illness. The duration of untreated disease averages 12 days (range, 9–18 days). Rash is apparent at presentation (usually ~4 days after symptom onset) in 13% of pts; 2 days later, half of the remaining pts develop a maculopapular rash that involves the trunk more than the extremities, is seldom petechial, and rarely involves the face, palms, or soles. Pulmonary disease is common, causing a hacking, nonproductive cough. Almost one-fourth of pts who undergo CXR have pulmonary densities due to interstitial pneumonia, pulmonary edema, and pleural effusions. Abdominal pain, confusion, stupor, seizures, ataxia, coma, and jaundice occur less commonly. Laboratory abnormalities include anemia, leukocytosis, thrombocytopenia, hyponatremia, hypoalbuminemia, increased hepatic aminotransferase levels, and prerenal azotemia. Disease can be severe enough for admission to an ICU, and complications include respiratory failure requiring intubation and mechanical ventilation, hematemesis, cerebral hemorrhage, and hemolysis. The disease is more severe in older pts, those with underlying disease, and those treated with a sulfonamide drug.

Diagnosis   The diagnosis can be based on an immunofluorescence assay that detects a fourfold serum antibody increase to a titer ≥ 1:64 or a single titer ≥ 1:128, immunohistology, skin biopsy, or PCR amplification of *R. typhi* from blood.

 TREATMENT

Doxycycline (100 mg bid for 7–15 days) or chloramphenicol (500 mg qid for 7–15 days) is effective.

Epidemic Typhus (Louse-Borne)

Epidemiology   Epidemic typhus is caused by *R. prowazekii* and is transmitted by the human body louse. The louse lives on clothes and is found in poor hygienic conditions, particularly in colder climates and classically at times of war or natural disaster. In the United States, the disease is seen sporadically and is transmitted by flying-squirrel fleas. Lice feed on pts with epidemic typhus and then defecate the organism into the bite at their next meal. The pt autoinoculates the organism while scratching. Because lice abandon corpses and pts with high fevers, they effectively spread disease. *Brill-Zinsser disease* is a recrudescent and mild form of the disease whose occurrence years after acute illness suggests that *R. prowazekii* remains dormant in the host, reactivating when immunity wanes.

Clinical Features   After an incubation period of ~1 week (range, 7–14 days), there is an abrupt onset of high fevers, prostration, severe headache, cough, and severe myalgias. Rash appears on the upper trunk around the fifth day of illness and spreads to involve all body-surface areas except the face, palms, and soles. Photophobia with conjunctival injection and eye pain is also common. Confusion and coma, skin necrosis, and gangrene of the digits are noted in severe cases. Untreated, the disease is fatal in 7–40% of cases. Pts develop renal failure, multiorgan involvement, and prominent neurologic manifestations.

Diagnosis   The diagnosis can be based on an immunofluorescence assay that detects an antibody titer of ≥1:128 in the appropriate clinical setting.

 TREATMENT

Doxycycline (a 200-mg dose once or daily until the pt has been afebrile for 24 h) is the treatment of choice.

Scrub Typhus

A member of the family Rickettsiaceae that is classified in a separate genus, *Orientia tsutsugamushi*, the agent of scrub typhus, is transmitted by larval mites or chiggers in environments of heavy scrub vegetation. Disease occurs during the wet season. It is endemic in Asia, northern Australia, and the Pacific islands. Clinical manifestations range from mild to fatal disease. Pts have an eschar at the site of chigger feeding, regional lymphadenopathy, and maculopapular rash. Severe cases include encephalitis and interstitial pneumonia. Scrub typhus can be diagnosed by serologic or PCR tests. A 7- to 15-day course of doxycycline (100 mg bid) or chloramphenicol (500 mg qid) is effective.

EHRLICHIOSES AND ANAPLASMOSIS

Ehrlichiae are small intracellular bacteria with a gram-negative–type cell wall that grow in cytoplasmic vacuoles to form clusters called *morulae*. Two distinct *Ehrlichia* species and one *Anaplasma* species cause human infections (Table 104-1).

Human Monocytotropic Ehrlichiosis (HME)

Most cases of HME occur in southeastern, south-central, and mid-Atlantic states. Most pts are male, with a median pt age of 44 years. After a median incubation period of 8 days, pts develop fever, headache, myalgia, and malaise. Nausea, vomiting, diarrhea, cough, rash, and confusion may be noted. Disease can be severe: up to 62% of pts are hospitalized. Complications include a toxic shock–like syndrome, respiratory distress, meningoencephalitis, fulminant infection, and hemorrhage. Leukopenia, thrombocytopenia, and elevated serum aminotransferase levels are common. The diagnosis is usually based on clinical

Table 104-1

Comparison of Three Human Ehrlichioses: Human Monocytotropic Ehrlichiosis (HME), Human Anaplasmosis, and Ehrlichiosis Ewingii

Variable	HME	Human Anaplasmosis	Ehrlichiosis Ewingii
Etiologic agent	*E. chaffeensis*	*A. phagocytophila*	*E. ewingii*
Tick vector(s)	*Amblyomma americanum, Dermacentor variabilis* (dog tick)	*Ixodes scapularis* (deer tick), *I. ricinus, I. pacificus*	*A. americanum*
Seasonality	April through September	Year-round (peak: May, June, and July)	April through September
Major target cell	Monocyte	Granulocyte	Neutrophil
Morulae seen	Rarely	Frequently	Rarely
Antigen used in IFA test	*E. chaffeensis*	*A. phagocytophila*	*E. chaffeensis* as surrogate
Diagnostic titer	Fourfold rise or a single titer of ≥1:128; cutoff for negative titer, 1:64	Fourfold rise; cutoff for negative titer, 1:80	No established criteria
Treatment of choice	Doxycycline	Doxycycline	Doxycycline
Mortality	2–3%	<1%	None reported

Note: IFA, indirect immunofluorescence assay.

presentation, but PCR testing before initiation of antibiotic therapy or retrospective IFA to detect increased antibody titers can be performed. Bone marrow examination reveals hypercellular marrow, and noncaseating granulomas may be evident. Morulae are rarely seen in peripheral blood. Treatment with tetracycline (250–500 mg q6h) or doxycycline (100 mg bid) is effective and should be continued for 3–5 days after defervescence.

Ehrlichiosis Ewingii

Ehrlichiosis ewingii resembles HME but is less severe. Most cases are diagnosed in immunocompromised pts. Treatment is the same as for HME.

Human Anaplasmosis

Most cases of human anaplasmosis occur in northeastern and upper midwestern states. After an incubation period of 4–8 days, pts develop fever, myalgia, headache, and malaise—i.e., an influenza-like illness. A minority of pts develop nausea, vomiting, diarrhea, cough, or confusion. Respiratory insufficiency, a toxic shock–like syndrome, and opportunistic infections are troubling complications. Although the mortality rate is low, nearly 7% of pts require intensive care. On laboratory examination, pts are found to have leukopenia, thrombocytopenia, and elevated serum aminotransferase levels. Bone marrow is normo- or hypercellular without granulomas. Anaplasmosis should be considered in pts with atypical severe presentations of Lyme disease. Co-infection with either *Borrelia burgdorferi* (the agent of Lyme disease) or *Babesia microti* should be considered in all cases because these three agents share the *Ixodes scapularis* vector and have the same geographic distribution. Peripheral blood films may reveal morulae in neutrophils in 20–75% of infections. PCR testing before antibiotic therapy or retrospective IFA for antibody rises can confirm the diagnosis. Treatment with doxycycline (100 mg bid) is effective, and most pts defervesce within 24–48 h. Pregnant women may be treated with rifampin.

Prevention

These diseases are prevented by avoidance of ticks in endemic areas, use of protective clothing and tick repellents, careful tick searches after exposures, and prompt removal of attached ticks.

Q FEVER

Etiology *Coxiella burnetii*, a small gram-negative organism, causes Q fever. The organism can exist as a highly infectious or phase I form within humans and animals or as an avirulent phase II form. It can form spores that allow its survival in harsh environments for prolonged periods.

Epidemiology Q fever is a zoonosis that occurs worldwide. The primary sources of human infection are infected cattle, sheep, and goats, but cats, rabbits, pigeons, and dogs can transmit disease as well. *C. burnetii* localizes to the uterus and mammary glands of infected female mammals. It is reactivated in pregnancy and is found at high concentrations in the placenta. At parturition, the organism is dispersed as an aerosol, and infection usually follows inhalation. Abattoir workers, veterinarians, and others persons who have contact with infected animals are at risk. Exposure to newborn animals or infected products of conception poses the highest risk. *C. burnetii* is shed in the milk for weeks to months after parturition; transmission from infected mother to infant is rare. Ingestion of contaminated milk is believed to be an important route of transmission in some areas, although the evidence is contradictory.

Clinical Features

- Acute Q fever: The incubation period ranges from 3 to 30 days. Clinical presentations include flulike syndromes, prolonged fever, pneumonia, hepatitis, pericarditis, myocarditis, meningoencephalitis, and infection during pregnancy. Symptoms are often nonspecific (e.g., fever, fatigue, headache, chills, sweats, nausea, vomiting, diarrhea, cough, and occasionally rash). Multiple rounded opacities on CXR are common and are highly suggestive of Q fever pneumonia. The WBC count is usually normal, but thrombocytopenia occurs. During recovery, reactive thrombocytosis can develop and cause deep vein thrombosis.
- Chronic Q fever: This uncommon entity almost always implies endocarditis, occurring in pts with prior valvulvar heart disease, immunosuppression, or chronic renal failure. Fever is absent or low grade; nonspecific symptoms may be present for a year before diagnosis. Vegetations are seen in only 12% of cases and manifest as nodules on the valve. Hepatomegaly and/or splenomegaly in combination with a positive rheumatoid factor, high ESR, high C-reactive protein level, and/or increased γ-globulin concentration, suggests the diagnosis. Although *C. burnetii* can be isolated by a shell-vial technique, most laboratories are not permitted to attempt isolation because of its highly contagious nature. PCR testing of tissue or biopsy specimens can be used, but serology is the most common diagnostic tool; IFA is the method of choice, but complement fixation and ELISA are also used. In chronic Q fever, titers of antibody to phase I antigen are much higher than those to phase II; the reverse is true in acute infection. Acute infection can be diagnosed by a fourfold rise in antibody titer. Chronic infection is associated with an IgG titer $\geq$ 1:800.

℞ TREATMENT

Acute Q fever is treated with doxycycline (100 mg bid for 14 days). Quinolones are also efficacious. If Q fever is diagnosed during pregnancy, trimethoprim-sulfamethoxazole should be administered up to term. Treatment for chronic Q fever should include at least two agents active against *C. burnetii*. The combination of rifampin (300 mg once daily) plus doxycycline (100 mg bid) or ciprofloxacin (750 mg bid) has been used with success, but the required duration of treatment is undetermined. Treatment should be given for at least 3 years and discontinued only if phase I IgA and IgG antibody titers are ≤1:50 and ≤1:200, respectively. The administration of doxycycline (100 mg bid) with hydroxychloroquine (600 mg once daily) for 18 months is under investigation. In vitro, hydroxychloroquine renders doxycycline bactericidal against *C. burnetii*. Hydroxychloroquine is given at a dose that maintains plasma concentrations at 0.8–1.2 μg/mL.

For a more detailed discussion, see Walker DH et al: Rickettsial Diseases, Chap. 158, p. 999, in HPIM-16.

105

MYCOPLASMA INFECTIONS

Mycoplasmas are the smallest free-living organisms. Lacking a cell wall and bounded only by a plasma membrane, they colonize mucosal surfaces of the respiratory and urogenital tracts.

M. pneumoniae

Epidemiology   *M. pneumoniae* causes upper and lower respiratory tract disease, with the highest attack rates among persons 5–20 years old. Infection is acquired by inhalation of aerosols. Children <5 years old usually have only upper respiratory tract disease; children >5 years old and adults usually have bronchitis and pneumonia. Infection can be severe in pts with sickle cell disease as a result of functional asplenia.

Clinical Features   The incubation period is longer than those for other respiratory infections, typically lasting for 2–3 weeks. Pts often have antecedent upper respiratory tract symptoms and then develop fever, sore throat, and prominent headache and cough. Myalgias, arthralgias, and GI symptoms may occur. Sputum production is lacking or minimal. If present, sputum is usually white but may be blood-tinged. Pharyngeal injection is common. Bullous myringitis (blisters on the tympanic membrane) is an uncommon but unique manifestation. Physical findings are minimal, and pleural effusion is documented in <20% of pts. Extrapulmonary manifestations suggest *M. pneumoniae* infection because, although unusual in the latter illness, they are even rarer in other respiratory illnesses. These manifestations include erythema multiforme, digital necrosis (due to high titers of cold agglutinins) in pts with sickle cell disease, myocarditis, pericarditis, encephalitis, cerebellar ataxia, Guillain-Barré syndrome, transverse myelitis, peripheral neuropathy, hemolytic anemia, coagulopathies, and arthritis (in pts with hypogammaglobulinemia).

Diagnosis CXR may show reticulonodular or interstitial infiltrates, primarily in the lower lobes. Most infections are not definitively diagnosed. Gram's staining gives negative results because mycoplasmas lack a cell wall; culture is possible but very difficult; and serologic tests are not positive early enough to help guide clinical decisions (although they may be helpful retrospectively when acute- and convalescent-phase sera are available). Cold agglutinins are nonspecific but develop within the first 7–10 days in >50% of pts with *M. pneumoniae* pneumonia. A titer ≥ 1:32 suggests the diagnosis. Antigen detection tests have been developed but are not yet widely available.

 TREATMENT

URIs due to *M. pneumoniae* do not require antibiotic treatment. Pneumonia is usually self-limited, but effective antibiotics shorten the duration of illness and reduce coughing and therefore may also reduce transmission. If the diagnosis is known, doxycycline (100 mg bid), macrolides (e.g., clarithromycin, 500 mg bid, or azithromycin, 500 mg/d), or fluoroquinolones (e.g., levofloxacin, 500 mg/d) are effective and should be administered for 14–21 days. For empirical treatment of community-acquired pneumonia, a fluoroquinolone alone or a macrolide plus ceftriaxone (1 g/d) is recommended for better coverage of *Streptococcus pneumoniae* and *Haemophilus influenzae*.

Genital Mycoplasmas
See Chap. 88.

For a more detailed discussion, see McCormack WM: Infections Due to Mycoplasmas, Chap. 159, p. 1008, in HPIM-16.

106

CHLAMYDIAL INFECTIONS

The genus *Chlamydia* contains three species that infect humans: *C. trachomatis, C. psittaci,* and *C. pneumoniae* (formerly the TWAR agent). Chlamydiae are obligate intracellular bacteria, possess both DNA and RNA, and have a cell wall and ribosomes similar to those of gram-negative bacteria. They have a complex reproductive cycle and exist in two forms. The *elementary body* is adapted for extracellular survival and is the infective form. It attaches to target cells—usually columnar or transitional epithelial cells—and enters the cell inside a phagosome. Within 8 h, elementary bodies reorganize into *reticulate bodies*, which are adapted for intracellular survival and multiplication. After replication, the reticulate bodies condense into elementary bodies that are released to infect other cells or people. *C. trachomatis*, *C. psittaci*, and *C. pneumoniae* share genus-specific group antigens; the micro-IF test can differentiate among the three species.

C. TRACHOMATIS INFECTIONS

Genital Infections, Including Lymphogranuloma Venereum

See Chap. 88.

Trachoma and Adult Inclusion Conjunctivitis (AIC)

Definitions and Etiology   Trachoma is a chronic conjunctivitis caused by *C. trachomatis* serovars A, B, Ba, and C. AIC is an acute eye infection in adults exposed to infected genital secretions and in their newborns; this infection is caused by sexually transmitted *C. trachomatis* strains, usually serovars D through K.

Epidemiology   Trachoma causes ~20 million cases of blindness worldwide, primarily in northern and sub-Saharan Africa, the Middle East, and parts of Asia. Transmission occurs from eye to eye via hands, flies, towels, and other fomites, particularly among young children in rural communities with limited water supplies.

Clinical Features   Both diseases present initially as conjunctivitis, with small lymphoid follicles in the conjunctiva. Trachoma usually starts insidiously before 2 years of age. Reinfection and persistent infection are common. With progression, there is inflammatory leukocytic infiltration and superficial vascularization (pannus formation) of the cornea. Scarring eventually distorts the eyelids, turning lashes inward and abrading the eyeball. Eventually, the corneal epithelium ulcerates, with subsequent scarring and blindness. Destruction of goblet cells, lacrimal ducts, and glands causes dry-eye syndrome, with resultant corneal opacity and secondary bacterial corneal ulcers. AIC is an acute unilateral follicular conjunctivitis with preauricular lymphadenopathy. Corneal inflammation is evidenced by discrete opacities, punctate epithelial erosions, and superficial corneal vascularization.

Diagnosis   Clinical diagnosis is based on the presence of two of the following signs: lymphoid follicles on the upper tarsal conjunctiva, typical conjunctival scarring, vascular pannus, or limbal follicles. Intracytoplasmic chlamydial inclusions are found in 10–60% of Giemsa-stained conjunctival smears. Chlamydial PCR or ligase chain reaction is more sensitive and often gives positive results when smears or cultures are negative.

 TREATMENT

Public health programs consist of mass application of tetracycline or erythromycin ointment into the eyes of all children in affected communities for 21–60 days or on an intermittent schedule in conjunction with surgical correction of inturned eyelids. AIC responds to a 3-week course of oral tetracycline or erythromycin and treatment of sexual partners to prevent reinfection. Untreated, it persists for 6 weeks to 2 years.

C. PSITTACI INFECTIONS

Epidemiology and Pathogenesis   Psittacosis is primarily an infection of birds and mammals. Most avian species can harbor *C. psittaci*, but psittacine birds (e.g., parrots, parakeets) are most often infected. Psittacosis is an occupational disease in pet-shop owners, poultry workers, and other individuals with regular avian contact. Present in nasal secretions, excreta, tissues, and feathers of infected birds, *C. psittaci* is transmitted to humans mainly by the respiratory route, gains access to the upper respiratory tract, spreads hematogenously, and localizes in the pulmonary alveoli and reticuloendothelial cells of the spleen and liver. The pathognomonic histologic finding is the presence of macrophages with typical cytoplasmic inclusion bodies in alveoli filled with fluid, erythrocytes, and lymphocytes.

Clinical Features After an incubation period of 7–14 days or longer, disease onset may be gradual or may be abrupt with shaking chills and fever to 40.6°C (105°F). Headache is prominent, and many pts have a dry, hacking, nonproductive cough. Small amounts of mucoid or bloody sputum may be produced as disease progresses. An increased respiratory rate and dyspnea with cyanosis can develop with extensive pulmonary involvement. Pts also report myalgias, spasm and stiffness of back and neck muscles, lethargy, depression, agitation, insomnia, and disorientation. Occasionally pts are comatose at presentation. GI symptoms can occur. Physical findings are less prominent than symptoms and x-ray findings would suggest. Splenomegaly is evident in 10–70% of pts.

Diagnosis The diagnosis, which should be considered in a pt with pneumonia and splenomegaly, is confirmed by serologic studies. A rise in the titer of CF antibody between acute- and convalescent-phase serum samples suggests the diagnosis.

 TREATMENT

Tetracycline (2–4 g/d in four divided doses) is consistently effective, resulting in defervescence and symptom alleviation within 24–48 h. Treatment is continued for 7–14 days to avoid relapse. Erythromycin is an alternative agent.

C. PNEUMONIAE INFECTIONS

Epidemiology Infections are most common among young adults but can occur throughout life, and reinfection is common. Seroprevalence exceeds 40% in the many adult populations tested throughout the world. Epidemics occur in close residential quarters such as military barracks. There is an epidemiologic association between serologic evidence of *C. pneumoniae* infection and atherosclerotic disease. *C. pneumoniae* has been identified in atherosclerotic plaques by electron microscopy, DNA hybridization, immunocytochemistry, and culture. It is hypothesized that the organism's presence accelerates atherosclerosis, especially in the setting of high cholesterol levels.

Clinical Features Manifestations of *C. pneumoniae* infection include pharyngitis, sinusitis, bronchitis, and pneumonitis. Primary infection is more severe than reinfection. Pneumonia due to *C. pneumoniae* resembles that due to *Mycoplasma pneumoniae*: pts have antecedent upper respiratory tract symptoms, fever, dry cough, minimal findings on auscultation, small segmental infiltrates on CXR, and no leukocytosis. Elderly pts can have severe disease.

Diagnosis Diagnosis is difficult. Serology does not reliably distinguish *C. pneumoniae* from *C. trachomatis* or *C. psittaci*.

 TREATMENT

Erythromycin or tetracycline (2 g/d for 10–14 days) is recommended. Other macrolides (e.g., azithromycin) or quinolones (e.g., levofloxacin) are alternative agents.

For a more detailed discussion, see Stamm WE: Chlamydial Infections, Chap. 160, p. 1011, in HPIM-16.

107

HERPESVIRUS INFECTIONS

HERPES SIMPLEX VIRUSES

ETIOLOGY AND PATHOGENESIS The herpes simplex viruses HSV-1 and HSV-2 are linear, double-stranded DNA viruses. There is ~50% sequence homology between HSV-1 and HSV-2. Unique type-specific regions exist and are the basis for serologic assays to distinguish between the two viral subtypes. Exposure to HSV at mucosal surfaces or abraded skin sites permits viral entry and replication in cells of the epidermis and dermis. HSV enters sensory or autonomic neuronal cells and is transported to nerve cell bodies in ganglia, where it can cause latency. The virus is maintained in a repressed state compatible with the survival and normal activities of the cell. Reactivation occurs when normal viral gene expression resumes, with reappearance of the virus on mucosal surfaces. Both antibody-mediated and cell-mediated immunity (including type-specific immunity) are clinically important.

EPIDEMIOLOGY HSV-1 is acquired more frequently and at an earlier age than HSV-2. More than 90% of adults have antibodies to HSV-1 by the fifth decade of life. Antibodies to HSV-2 are usually not detected until adolescence and correlate with sexual activity. In the United States, ~20% of the population has antibody to HSV-2. Infection with HSV-2 is an independent risk factor for the acquisition and transmission of infection with HIV-1. HIV-1 can be shed from genital herpes lesions. During the first years after primary infection with HSV-1 or HSV-2, viral shedding from mucosal sites of immunocompetent and immunocompromised adults can occur on 30–50% and up to 70% of days, respectively. Pts with long-term infection can shed virus on as many as 20–30% of days. HSV is transmitted most efficiently by contact with active lesions but can also be spread by asymptomatic persons excreting the virus. The large reservoir of unidentified carriers and the frequent asymptomatic reactivation of HSV-2 have fostered the continued spread of HSV throughout the world.

CLINICAL SPECTRUM The incubation period for primary infection is 1–26 days (median, 6–8 days). Reactivation depends on anatomical site and virus type as well as the pt's age and immune status. Overall, genital HSV-2 is twice as likely to reactivate as genital HSV-1 and recurs 8–10 times more often. In contrast, oral-labial HSV-1 recurs more frequently than oral-labial HSV-2.

Oral-Facial Infections

• Primary infection: Gingivostomatitis and pharyngitis, seen in children and young adults, are common manifestations of primary HSV-1 infection. Pts have up to 2 weeks of fever, malaise, myalgia, inability to eat, and cervical adenopathy with lesions on the palate, gingiva, tongue, lip, face, posterior pharynx, and/or tonsillar pillars. Exudative pharyngitis may occur.
• Reactivation: Viral excretion in the saliva, intraoral mucosal ulcerations, or ulcers on the vermillion border of the lip or external facial skin can occur with

reactivation of latent virus in the trigeminal ganglia. Pts undergoing trigeminal nerve root decompression or dental extraction can develop oral-labial herpes a median of 3 days after the procedure.

• Infection in compromised hosts: Compromised hosts (e.g., AIDS pts, pts undergoing induction chemotherapy or in the early phases of transplantation) can have a severe infection that extends into the mucosa and skin, causing friability, necrosis, bleeding, pain, and inability to eat or drink.

• Eczema herpeticum: This severe oral-facial HSV infection, with extensive skin lesions and occasional visceral dissemination, may develop in pts with atopic eczema.

• Erythema multiforme: HSV infection is the precipitating event in ~75% of cases.

• Bell's palsy: A flaccid paralysis of the mandibular portion of the facial nerve, Bell's palsy has been linked to HSV and varicella-zoster virus (VZV). Antiviral therapy and a short course of glucocorticoids may be helpful.

Genital Infections

• Primary infection: Primary HSV genital infection is characterized by fever, headache, malaise, myalgias, widely spaced bilateral lesions (vesicles, pustules, or painful erythematous ulcers) of the external genitalia, pain, itching, dysuria, vaginal and urethral discharge, and tender inguinal adenopathy. Pts with prior HSV-1 infection have milder cases. About 15% of cases are associated with other clinical syndromes, such as aseptic meningitis, cervicitis, and urethritis.

• Reactivation: Reactivation infections are often subclinical or can cause genital lesions or urethritis with dysuria. Even without a history of rectal intercourse, perianal lesions can occur as a result of latency established in the sacral dermatome from prior genital tract infection. Proctitis can cause anorectal pain, discharge, tenesmus, and constipation. Ulcerative lesions can be seen in the distal 10 cm of the rectal mucosa.

Whitlow In HSV infection of the finger, pts experience an abrupt onset of edema, erythema, pain, and vesicular or pustular lesions of the fingertips that are often confused with the lesions of pyogenic bacterial infection. Fever and lymphadenitis are common.

Herpes Gladiatorum HSV infection caused by trauma to the skin during wrestling can occur anywhere on the body but commonly affects the thorax, ears, face, and hands.

Eye Infections HSV is the most frequent cause of corneal blindness in the United States.

• Keratitis: acute onset of pain, blurred vision, chemosis, conjunctivitis, and dendritic lesions of the cornea. Topical glucocorticoids may exacerbate disease. Recurrences are common.

• Chorioretinitis: usually seen with disseminated HSV infection

• Acute necrotizing retinitis: a rare, serious manifestation of HSV or VZV infection

Central and Peripheral Nervous System Infections

• Encephalitis: In the United States, HSV causes 10–20% of all cases of sporadic viral encephalitis, and 95% of these cases are due to HSV-1. The estimated incidence is 2.3 cases per 1 million persons per year. Encephalitis can occur during primary infection or in pts already seropositive for HSV-1. Pts present with an acute onset of fever and focal neurologic symptoms and signs, especially in the temporal lobe. Neurologic sequelae are common, especially in pts >50 years of age. Antiviral treatment should be started empirically until the diagnosis is confirmed or an alternative diagnosis is made. IV treatment is recommended until CSF levels of viral DNA are reduced or undetectable.

- Aseptic meningitis: HSV DNA is found in CSF from 3–15% of pts with aseptic meningitis, usually in association with primary genital HSV infection. This acute, self-limited disease without sequelae is manifested by headache, fever, and photophobia. Pts have symptoms for 2–7 days. Lymphocytic pleocytosis in the CSF is documented. HSV is the most common cause of recurrent lymphocytic meningitis (Mollaret's meningitis).
- Autonomic dysfunction caused by either HSV or VZV most commonly affects the sacral region. Numbness, tingling of the buttocks or perineal areas, urinary retention, constipation, and impotence can occur. Symptoms take days to weeks to resolve. Hypesthesia and/or weakness of the lower extremities may develop and persist for months. Rarely, transverse myelitis or Guillain-Barré syndrome follows HSV infection.

Visceral Infections

- Multiorgan involvement caused by viremia can be evident.
- Esophagitis: HSV esophagitis is marked by odynophagia, dysphagia, substernal pain, and weight loss. Ulcers are most common in the distal esophagus. Cytologic examination and culture of secretions obtained by endoscopy are indicated to distinguish this entity from esophagitis of other etiologies (e.g., *Candida* esophagitis).
- Pneumonitis: Focal necrotizing pneumonitis occurs in rare instances and is due to extension of herpetic tracheobronchitis into the lung parenchyma in severely immunocompromised pts. Hematogenous dissemination from other sites can cause bilateral interstitial pneumonitis. Mortality rates exceed 80% in compromised pts.

Neonatal Infections
The frequency of neonatal visceral and/or CNS infection is highest among pts <6 weeks of age. The mortality rate is 65% without therapy but drops to 25% with IV acyclovir treatment. Fewer than 10% of neonates with CNS disease develop normally. Infection is usually acquired perinatally from contact with infected genital secretions during delivery. More than two-thirds of cases are due to HSV-2. The risk is 10 times higher for infants born to a mother who has recently acquired HSV.

DIAGNOSIS

- Tzanck preparation: This method entails Wright's, Giemsa's, or Papanicolaou's staining of scrapings from the base of lesions to detect giant cells or intranuclear inclusions, which are typical of both HSV and VZV infection. Few clinicians are skilled in the technique.
- Culture: Positive results are seen within 48–96 h after inoculation. Spin-amplified culture with HSV antigen staining can yield a diagnosis in <24 h.
- PCR detection of HSV DNA: This method is more sensitive than culture for detection of HSV in CSF and at mucosal sites. Its sensitivity is higher in vesicular rather than ulcerative lesions, in primary rather than recurrent disease, and in compromised rather than immunocompetent hosts. PCR examination of CSF for viral DNA is the most sensitive noninvasive method for early diagnosis of HSV encephalitis. Examination of tissue obtained by brain biopsy for HSV antigen, DNA, or replication is also highly sensitive and has a low complication rate.
- Serologic assays can identify carriers of HSV-1 or HSV-2.

℞ TREATMENT

Table 107-1 details antiviral chemotherapy for HSV infection. Acyclovir and other drugs of its class serve as substrates for the HSV enzyme thymidine kinase. These drugs are phosphorylated to the monophosphate form in herpesvirus-infected cells. Cellular enzymes then convert the monophosphate form into the triphosphate form, which incorporates into the viral DNA chain and inhibits viral DNA polymerase. Acyclovir-resistant strains of HSV have been identified. Almost all resistance—more often to HSV-2 than to HSV-1—has been seen in strains from immunocompromised pts. These strains are infrequent, but clinical suspicion of resistance should rise if HSV persists despite adequate acyclovir dosages and blood levels.

• Acyclovir: This agent is available for IV, oral, and topical administration. IV acyclovir is associated with transient renal insufficiency due to crystallization of the compound in the renal parenchyma. The drug should be given slowly over 1 h to a well-hydrated pt. CSF levels are 30–50% of plasma levels, so doses are doubled for treatment of CNS infection over those used to treat mucocutaneous disease. Even higher doses are used for neonatal infections.
• Valacyclovir: The L-valyl ester of acyclovir, this agent is converted to acyclovir by intestinal and hepatic hydrolysis after oral administration, with greater bioavailability, higher blood levels, and less frequent dosing than acyclovir. Thrombotic thrombocytopenic purpura has been reported in compromised pts who have received high doses (8 g/d).
• Famciclovir: This drug offers excellent bioavailability and a twice-daily dosing schedule.

PREVENTION   The use of barrier forms of contraception, especially condoms, decreases the likelihood of HSV transmission, particularly during asymptomatic viral excretion.

VARICELLA-ZOSTER VIRUS

VZV causes two distinct entities: primary infection (varicella or chickenpox) and reactivation infection (herpes zoster or shingles). Primary infection is transmitted by the respiratory route. The virus replicates and causes viremia, which is reflected by the diffuse and scattered skin lesions in varicella; it then establishes latency in the dorsal root ganglia.

CHICKENPOX

• VZV causes disease only in humans. Chickenpox is highly contagious, with an attack rate of 90% among susceptible persons. Household attack rates among susceptible siblings are 70–90%. Before vaccine became available, children 5–9 years old accounted for half of all cases, but the epidemiology of chickenpox is now changing.
• The incubation period ranges from 10 to 21 days, but most pts evince disease within 14–17 days. Pts are infectious for 48 h before onset of rash and remain infectious until all vesicles have crusted.
• Pts present with fever, rash, and malaise. In immunocompetent hosts, the disease is benign and lasts 3–5 days. Skin lesions include maculopapules, vesicles, and scabs in various stages of evolution. Most lesions are small and have an erythematous base of 5–10 mm. Successive crops appear over 2–4 days. Lesions can occur on the mucosa of the pharynx or vagina. Severity varies from person to person, but older pts tend to have more severe disease.
• Compromised hosts (e.g., leukemic pts) have numerous lesions (often with a hemorrhagic base) that take longer to heal. These pts are more likely than immunocompetent pts to have visceral complications that, if not treated, are fatal in 15% of cases.

Table 107-1

Antiviral Chemotherapy for HSV Infection

I. Mucocutaneous HSV infections

A. Infections in immunosuppressed patients:

1. Acute symptomatic first or recurrent episodes: IV acyclovir (5 mg/kg q8h) or oral acyclovir (400 mg qid), famciclovir (500 mg tid), or valacyclovir (500 mg tid). Treatment duration may vary from 7 to 14 days.

2. Suppression of reactivation disease: IV acyclovir (5 mg/kg q8h) or oral valacyclovir (500 mg bid) or acyclovir (400–800 mg 3–5 times per day) prevents recurrences during the 30-day period immediately after transplantation. Longer-term HSV suppression is often used for persons with continued immunosuppression. In bone marrow and renal transplant recipients, oral valacyclovir (2 g/d) is also effective in preventing cytomegalovirus infection. Oral valacyclovir at a dose of 4 g/d has been associated with thrombotic thrombocytopenic purpura after extended use in HIV-positive persons. In HIV-infected persons, oral famciclovir (500 mg bid) is effective in reducing clinical and subclinical reactivations of HSV-1 and HSV-2.

B. Genital herpes:

1. First episodes: Oral acyclovir (200 mg 5 times per day or 400 mg tid), valacyclovir (1 g bid), or famciclovir (250 mg bid) for 10–14 days is effective. IV acyclovir (5 mg/kg q8h for 5 days) is given for severe disease or neurologic complications such as aseptic meningitis.

2. Symptomatic recurrent genital herpes: Oral acyclovir (200 mg 5 times per day for 5 days, 800 mg tid for 2 days), valacyclovir (500 mg bid for 3 or 5 days), or famciclovir (125 mg bid for 5 days) is effective in shortening lesion duration.

3. Suppression of recurrent genital herpes: Oral acyclovir (200-mg capsules tid or qid, 400 mg bid, or 800 mg qd), famciclovir (250 mg bid), or valacyclovir (500 mg or 1 g qd or 500 mg bid) prevents symptomatic reactivation. Persons with frequent reactivation but <9 episodes per year can take valacyclovir (500 mg PO daily); those with >9 episodes per year should take 1 g PO daily or 500 mg PO bid.

C. Oral-labial HSV infections:

1. First episode: Oral acyclovir (200 mg) is given 4 or 5 times per day. Oral famciclovir (250 mg bid) or valacyclovir (1 g bid) has been used clinically.

2. Recurrent episodes: Oral valacyclovir (1 g bid for 1 day or 500 mg bid for 3 days) is effective in reducing pain and speeding healing. Self-initiated therapy with 6-times-daily topical penciclovir cream is effective in speeding the healing of oral-labial HSV. Topical acyclovir cream has also been shown to speed healing.

3. Suppression of reactivation of oral-labial HSV: Oral acyclovir (400 mg bid), if started before exposure and continued for the duration of exposure (usually 5–10 days), will prevent reactivation of recurrent oral-labial HSV infection associated with severe sun exposure.

D. Herpetic whitlow: Oral acyclovir (200 mg) is given 5 times daily for 7–10 days.

E. HSV proctitis: Oral acyclovir (400 mg 5 times per day) is useful in shortening the course of infection. In immunosuppressed patients or in patients with severe infection, IV acyclovir (5 mg/kg q8h) may be useful.

524

F. Herpetic eye infections: In acute keratitis, topical trifluorothymidine, vidarabine, idoxuridine, acyclovir, penciclovir, and interferon are all beneficial. Debridement may be required; topical steroids may worsen disease.

II. CNS HSV infections
A. HSV encephalitis: IV acyclovir (10 mg/kg q8h; 30 mg/kg per day) for at least 10 days.
B. HSV aseptic meningitis: No studies of systemic antiviral chemotherapy exist. If therapy is to be given, IV acyclovir (15–30 mg/kg per day) should be used.
C. Autonomic radiculopathy: No studies are available. Most authorities recommend a trial of IV acyclovir.

III. Neonatal HSV infections
Oral acyclovir (60 mg/kg per day, divided into 3 doses) is given. The recommended duration of treatment is 21 days. Monitoring for relapse should be undertaken, and some authorities recommend continued suppression with oral acyclovir suspension for 3 to 4 months.

IV. Visceral HSV infections
A. HSV esophagitis: IV acyclovir (15 mg/kg per day). In some patients with milder forms of immunosuppression, oral therapy with valacyclovir or famciclovir is effective.
B. HSV pneumonitis: No controlled studies exist. IV acyclovir (15 mg/kg per day) should be considered.

V. Disseminated HSV infections
No controlled studies exist. Intravenous acyclovir nevertheless should be tried. No definite evidence indicates that therapy will decrease the risk of death.

VI. Erythema multiforme–associated HSV
Anecdotal observations suggest that oral acyclovir (400 mg bid or tid) or valacyclovir (500 mg bid) will suppress erythema multiforme.

VII. Surgical prophylaxis
Several surgical procedures (e.g., laser skin resurfacing, trigeminal nerve root decompression, and lumbar disk surgery) have been associated with HSV reactivation. Intravenous or oral acyclovir (800 mg bid) or oral valacyclovir (500 mg bid) or famciclovir (250 mg bid) is effective in reducing reactivation. Therapy should be initiated 48 h before surgery and continued for 3–7 days.

VIII. Infections due to acyclovir-resistant HSV
IV foscarnet (40 mg/kg q8h) should be given until lesions heal. The optimal duration of therapy and the usefulness of its continuation to suppress lesions are unclear. Some patients may benefit from cutaneous application of trifluorothymidine or 5% cidofovir gel.

525

Complications

- Bacterial superinfection is usually caused by *Streptococcus pyogenes* or *Staphylococcus aureus*. Necrotizing fasciitis has been associated with varicella.
- The CNS is the most common extracutaneous site of VZV disease in children. Acute cerebellar ataxia and meningeal irritation usually appear ~21 days after the onset of rash and run a benign course. CSF contains lymphocytes and has elevated protein levels. Aseptic meningitis, encephalitis, transverse myelitis, Guillain-Barré syndrome, or Reye's syndrome (which mandates the avoidance of aspirin administration to children) can occur. There is no specific therapy other than supportive care.
- The most common serious complication of chickenpox, pneumonia develops more frequently among adults (occurring in up to 20% of cases) than among children. The onset comes 3–5 days into illness, with tachypnea, cough, dyspnea, and fever. Cyanosis, pleuritic chest pain, and hemoptysis are common. CXR shows nodular infiltrates and interstitial pneumonitis.
- Perinatal varicella has a high mortality rate when maternal disease occurs within 5 days before delivery or within 48 h afterward. Congenital varicella causing birth defects is rare.

HERPES ZOSTER (SHINGLES)   Herpes zoster represents a reactivation of VZV from dorsal root ganglia.

- The incidence is highest among pts ≥60 years of age.
- There is usually a unilateral vesicular eruption within a dermatome, often associated with severe pain. Dermatomes T3 to L3 are most frequently involved. Dermatomal pain may precede lesions by 48–72 h. The usual duration of disease is 7–10 days, but it may take as long as 2–4 weeks for the skin to return to normal.

Complications

- Zoster ophthalmicus: Zoster of the ophthalmic division of the trigeminal nerve is a debilitating condition that can cause blindness if not treated.
- Ramsay Hunt syndrome is characterized by pain and vesicles in the external auditory canal, loss of taste in the anterior two-thirds of the tongue, and ipsilateral facial palsy.
- Postherpetic neuralgia (PHN) is a debilitating complication of shingles. Pain persists for months after resolution of cutaneous disease. At least 50% of pts over age 50 report this complication to some degree.
- Abnormal CSF in the absence of symptoms is not uncommon. Symptomatic meningoencephalitis can also occur.
- Compromised pts—particularly those with Hodgkin's disease and non-Hodgkin's lymphoma—are at greatest risk for severe zoster and progressive disease. Cutaneous dissemination occurs in up to 40% of these pts; among those with dissemination, the risk of visceral and other complications increases by 5–10%. Bone marrow transplant recipients are also at high risk of VZV infection, and 45% of these pts have cutaneous or visceral dissemination (pneumonitis, meningoencephalitis, hepatitis). Mortality rates are 10%. PHN, scarring, and bacterial superinfection are common in VZV infection developing within 9 months of transplantation. Concomitant graft-versus-host disease increases the chance of dissemination and/or death.

DIAGNOSIS

- Isolation of VZV in tissue-culture cell lines, detection of VZV DNA by PCR, or direct immunofluorescent staining of cells from the lesion base
- Seroconversion or a fourfold or greater rise in antibody titer between convalescent- and acute-phase serum specimens. The fluorescent antibody to membrane antigen (FAMA) test, immune adherence hemagglutination test, and en-

zyme-linked immunosorbent assay (ELISA) are the most frequently used techniques.

$\boxed{\text{R}_{\text{x}}}$ TREATMENT

- Chickenpox
  1. Adolescents and adults: acyclovir, 800 mg five times daily for 5–7 days for chickenpox of ≤24 h duration
  2. Children: acyclovir, 20 mg/kg q6h (may be beneficial if initiated early in disease)
  3. Good hygiene, meticulous skin care, and antipruritic drugs are important to relieve symptoms and prevent bacterial superinfection of skin lesions.

- Zoster: Lesions heal more quickly with antiviral treatment: acyclovir, 800 mg five times daily for 7–10 days; famciclovir, 500 mg tid for 7 days (one study also showed twofold faster resolution of PHN with this agent); or valacyclovir, 1 g tid for 5–7 days.
- Compromised hosts: IV acyclovir (10–12.5 mg/kg q8h for 7 days) should be given for chickenpox and herpes zoster to reduce complications, although this regimen does not speed the healing or relieve the pain of skin lesions.
- Pneumonia: This complication may require ventilatory support in addition to antiviral treatment.
- Zoster ophthalmicus: In addition to antiviral treatment, a consult with an ophthalmologist is required.
- PHN: Gabapentin, amitriptyline, lidocaine patches, and fluphenazine may relieve pain and can be given along with routine analgesic agents. Prednisone (administered at a dosage of 60 mg/d for the first week of zoster, tapered over 21 days, and given with antiviral therapy) can accelerate quality-of-life improvements, including a return to usual activity; this treatment is indicated only for healthy elderly persons with moderate or severe pain at presentation.

PREVENTION

- Vaccine: One dose of a live attenuated vaccine is recommended for all children at 1–12 years of age. VZV-seronegative adults should receive two doses of vaccine.
- VZIg: See Table 107-2.
- Antiviral treatment: Prophylaxis can be given to high-risk pts who are ineligible for vaccine or beyond the 96-h window after direct contact. Therapy is instituted 7 days after intense exposure; although it decreases disease severity, it may not prevent illness.

HUMAN HERPESVIRUS (HHV) TYPES 6, 7, AND 8

- HHV-6 causes exanthem subitum (roseola infantum), a common childhood febrile illness with rash, and is a major cause of febrile seizures without rash in infancy. Older pts can have an infectious mononucleosis syndrome or encephalitis. Compromised hosts can have disseminated disease and pneumonitis. More than 80% of adults are seropositive for HHV-6. This virus has been implicated in graft dysfunction in transplant recipients and may contribute to the pathogenesis of multiple sclerosis.
- HHV-7 is found in the saliva of healthy adults and has no proven association with human disease.
- HHV-8 is associated with Kaposi's sarcoma, body cavity–based lymphoma in AIDS pts, and multicentric Castleman's disease. The virus appears to be sexually spread and may also be transmitted in saliva, by

Table 107-2

Recommendations for VZIg Administration

Exposure criteria
1. Exposure to person with chickenpox or zoster
   a. Household: residence in the same household
   b. Playmate: face-to-face indoor play
   c. Hospital
      Varicella: same 2- to 4-bed room or adjacent beds in large ward, face-to-face contact with infectious staff member or patient, visit by a person deemed contagious
      Zoster: intimate contact (e.g., touching or hugging) with a person deemed contagious
   d. Newborn infant: onset of varicella in the mother ≤5 days before delivery or ≤48 h after delivery; VZIg is not indicated if the mother has zoster
2. Patient should receive VZIg as soon as possible but not >96 h after exposure

Candidates (provided they have significant exposure) include:
1. Immunocompromised susceptible children without history of varicella or varicella immunization
2. Susceptible pregnant women
3. Newborn infants whose mother had onset of chickenpox within 5 days before or within 48 h after delivery
4. Hospitalized premature infant (≥28 weeks of gestation) whose mother lacks a reliable history of chickenpox or serologic evidence of protection against varicella
5. Hospitalized premature infant (<28 weeks of gestation or ≤1000-g birth weight), regardless of maternal history of varicella or varicella-zoster virus serologic status

Source: Adapted from American Academy of Pediatrics, *Red Book, Report of the Committee on Infectious Diseases*, G Peter (ed), Elk Grove Village, IL, American Academy of Pediatrics, 2003, pp 678–679; with permission.

organ transplantation, and through IV drug use. Neoplastic disorders develop only after immunocompromise.

For a more detailed discussion, see Baden LR, Dolin R: Antiviral Chemotherapy, Excluding Antiretroviral Drugs, Chap. 162, p. 1027; Corey L: Herpes Simplex Viruses, Chap. 163, p. 1035; Whitley RJ: Varicella-Zoster Virus Infections, Chap. 164, p. 1042; and Hirsch MS: Cytomegalovirus and Human Herpesvirus Types 6, 7, and 8, Chap. 166, p. 1049, in HPIM-16.

108

CYTOMEGALOVIRUS AND EPSTEIN-BARR VIRUS INFECTIONS

CYTOMEGALOVIRUS (CMV)

ETIOLOGY   CMV is a herpesvirus that is so named because it renders cells 2–4 times the size of surrounding cells. These cytomegalic cells contain an eccentrically placed intranuclear inclusion surrounded by a clear halo, with an "owl's-eye" appearance.

EPIDEMIOLOGY   CMV disease is found worldwide. In the United States, ~1% of newborns are infected. The virus may be spread in breast milk, saliva, feces, and urine. Transmission requires repeated or prolonged contact. In adolescents and adults, sexual transmission is common, and CMV has been identified in semen and cervical secretions. Latent CMV infection persists throughout life unless reactivation is triggered by depressed cell-mediated immunity (e.g., in transplant recipients or HIV-infected pts).

PATHOGENESIS   Primary CMV infection is associated with a vigorous T lymphocyte response; atypical lymphocytes are predominantly activated CD8+ T cells. Latent infection occurs in multiple cell types and various organs. Chronic antigen stimulation in the presence of immunosuppression, as in the transplant setting, or certain immunosuppressant agents, such as antithymocyte globulin, promote CMV reactivation. CMV disease increases the risk of infection with opportunistic pathogens by depressing T lymphocyte responsiveness.

CLINICAL FEATURES   *Congenital CMV Infection*   Cytomegalic inclusion disease occurs in ~5% of infected fetuses in the setting of primary maternal CMV infection in pregnancy. Pts have petechiae, hepatosplenomegaly, and jaundice. Other findings include microcephaly with or without cerebral calcifications, intrauterine growth retardation, prematurity, and chorioretinitis. Laboratory findings include abnormal LFTs, thrombocytopenia, hemolysis, and increased CSF protein levels. The prognosis is poor for infants with severe disease; the mortality rate is 20–30%, and survivors have intellectual or hearing difficulties.

Perinatal CMV Infection   Perinatal infection with CMV is acquired by breast-feeding or contact with infected maternal secretions. Most pts are asymptomatic, but interstitial pneumonitis and other opportunistic infections can occur, particularly in premature infants.

CMV Mononucleosis   This heterophile antibody–negative illness is the most common CMV syndrome in normal hosts. The incubation period ranges from 20 to 60 days. Symptoms last 2–6 weeks and include fevers, profound fatigue and malaise, myalgias, headache, and splenomegaly; pharyngitis and cervical lymphadenopathy are rare. Laboratory findings include a relative lymphocytosis with >10% atypical lymphocytes. Increased serum levels of aminotransferases and alkaline phosphatase and immunologic abnormalities (e.g., the presence of cryoglobulins or cold agglutinins) can be evident. Recovery is complete, but postviral asthenia can persist for months. CMV excretion in urine, genital secretions, and/or saliva can continue for months or years.

CMV Infection in the Immunocompromised Host   Pts develop fever, malaise, anorexia, fatigue, night sweats, arthralgias, or myalgias. Tachypnea, hypoxia, and unproductive cough precede respiratory involvement. CMV involvement in the GI tract may be localized or extensive, with ulcers in any part of the GI tract that can bleed or perforate. Hepatitis is frequent. CNS disease sometimes develops, most often affecting HIV-infected pts and taking one of two forms: encephalitis with dementia or ventriculoencephalitis with cranial nerve deficits, disorientation, and lethargy. Subacute progressive polyradiculopathy has also been described. CMV retinitis can result in blindness. Lesions begin as small white areas of granular retinal necrosis, with later development of hemorrhages, vessel sheathing, and retinal edema. Fatal infection is associated with persistent viremia and multiorgan involvement. Extensive adrenal necrosis is often seen at autopsy.

1. *Transplant recipients*: CMV is the most common and important viral pathogen complicating organ transplantation. This virus is a risk factor for graft loss and death. The risk of infection is greatest 1–4 months after transplantation, but retinitis can occur later. Primary CMV infection is more likely to cause severe disease with high viral loads. Seropositive recipients can develop reinfection with a new, donor-derived strain of CMV. Reactivation infection is common but less important clinically. The transplanted organ is at particular risk; e.g., CMV pneumonitis tends to follow lung transplantation. Around 15–20% of bone marrow transplant recipients develop CMV pneumonia 5–13 weeks after transplantation; this disease has a case-fatality rate of 84–88%.

2. *HIV-infected pts*: CMV is an important pathogen when CD4+ cell counts fall below $50–100/\mu L$, producing retinitis, colitis, and disseminated disease.

DIAGNOSIS

• Viral culture using fibroblast monolayers: A shell vial assay entailing centrifugation and an immunocytochemical detection method using monoclonal antibodies to immediate-early CMV antigen give more rapid results from tissue culture.

• Detection of CMV antigens (pp65) in peripheral-blood leukocytes or of CMV DNA in blood, CSF, or tissues (e.g., with PCR assays): Positive results may be obtained days sooner than with culture methods, allowing earlier interventions.

• Serology: Antibodies may not be detectable for up to 4 weeks in primary infection and may remain elevated for years. IgM may be useful in diagnosing acute infection.

℞ TREATMENT

When possible, seronegative donors should be used for seronegative transplant recipients. Antiviral options include the following.

• Ganciclovir (or valganciclovir, the oral prodrug of ganciclovir) produces response rates of 70–90% among HIV-infected pts with CMV retinitis or colitis. Induction therapy with ganciclovir (5 mg/kg bid IV) or valganciclovir (900 mg qd PO) is given for 14–21 days. In bone marrow transplant recipients, CMV pneumonia should be treated with both ganciclovir and CMV immune globulin; clinical response rates are 50–70% with combination therapy. Neutropenia is an adverse reaction to ganciclovir treatment that may require administration of colony-stimulating factors. Maintenance therapy (ganciclovir, 5 mg/kg qd IV, or valganciclovir, 900 mg qd PO) is needed for prolonged periods except in AIDS pts receiving antiretroviral treatment who have a sustained (>6-month) increase in CD4+ cell counts to levels of $>100–150/\mu L$. Prophylactic or suppressive ganciclovir can be given to high-risk transplant recipients (those who are seropositive before transplantation or culture positive afterward).

- Foscarnet is active against CMV infection but is reserved for cases of ganciclovir failure or intolerance because of its toxicities, which include renal dysfunction, hypomagnesemia, hypokalemia, hypocalcemia, and paresthesia. This drug must be given via an infusion pump, and its administration must be closely monitored. An induction regimen of 60 mg/kg q8h or 90 mg/kg q12h for 2 weeks is followed by maintenance regimens of 90–120 mg/kg daily.
- Ganciclovir can be administered via a slow-release pellet sutured into the eye, but this intervention does not provide treatment for the contralateral eye or systemic disease.
- Cidofovir has a long intracellular half-life. Induction regimens of 5 mg/kg per week for 2 weeks are followed by maintenance regimens of 3–5 mg/kg every 2 weeks. Cidofovir causes severe nephrotoxicity by proximal tubular cell injury. The use of saline hydration and probenecid reduces this adverse effect.

EPSTEIN-BARR VIRUS (EBV)

EPIDEMIOLOGY   EBV is a herpesvirus that infects >90% of persons by adulthood. Infectious mononucleosis (IM) is a disease of young adults and is more common in areas with higher standards of hygiene; infection occurs at a younger age in poorer areas. EBV is spread by contact with oral secretions (e.g., by transfer of saliva during kissing) and is shed in oropharyngeal secretions by >90% of asymptomatic seropositive individuals.

PATHOGENESIS   EBV infects the epithelium of the oropharynx and salivary glands as well as B cells in tonsillar crypts. The virus spreads through the bloodstream. Reactive T cells proliferate, and there is polyclonal activation of B cells. During IM, there is clonal expansion of CD8+ T cells. Memory B cells are the reservoir for EBV. Cellular immunity is more important than humoral immunity in controlling infection. If T cell immunity is compromised, EBV-infected B cells may proliferate—a step toward neoplastic transformation.

CLINICAL FEATURES

I. Infants and young children: asymptomatic or mild pharyngitis
II. Adolescents and adults: IM, with an incubation period of ~4–6 weeks
   A. A prodrome of fatigue, malaise, and myalgia may last for 1–2 weeks before fever onset.
   B. Illness lasts for 2–4 weeks and is characterized by fever, sore throat, and lymphadenopathy, especially of the posterior cervical nodes. Other symptoms include headache, abdominal pain, nausea, or vomiting. Signs include pharyngitis or exudative tonsillitis that can resemble streptococcal infection, splenomegaly (usually in the second or third week), hepatomegaly, rash, periorbital edema, palatal enanthem, and jaundice. Ampicillin treatment can cause a rash that does not represent a true penicillin allergy. Erythema nodosum or erythema multiforme can occur.
   C. Malaise and difficulty with concentration can persist for months.
   D. Laboratory findings: Lymphocytosis occurs in the second or third week, with >10% atypical lymphocytes (enlarged cells with abundant cytoplasm and vacuoles). Most atypical lymphocytes are CD8+ T cells. Neutropenia, thrombocytopenia, and abnormal LFTs are common.
   E. Complications
      1. CNS: In the first 2 weeks of IM, meningitis or encephalitis can present as headache, meningismus, cerebellar ataxia, acute hemiplegia, or psychosis. The CSF contains lymphocytes. Most cases resolve without sequelae.

2. Autoimmune hemolytic anemia (Coombs'-test positive, with cold agglutinins directed against the i RBC antigen) can last for 1–2 months. Severe disease (red cell aplasia, severe granulocytopenia or pancytopenia, or hemophagocytic syndrome) can occur.

3. Splenic rupture is more common among males than among females and may manifest as abdominal pain, referred shoulder pain, or hemodynamic compromise.

4. Upper airway obstruction due to hypertrophy of lymphoid tissue may occur.

5. Hepatitis, myocarditis, pericarditis, pneumonia, interstitial nephritis, and vasculitis are rare complications.

III. EBV-associated lymphoproliferative disease occurs in immunodeficient pts (e.g., pts infected with HIV, transplant recipients, pts receiving immunosuppressive therapy). Proliferating EBV-infected B cells infiltrate lymph nodes and multiple organs; there is B cell hyperplasia or lymphoma. Pts have fever and lymphadenopathy or GI symptoms.

IV. Oral hairy leukoplakia consists of white corrugated lesions on the tongue in HIV-infected pts.

V. EBV-associated malignancies include Burkitt's lymphoma, anaplastic nasopharyngeal carcinoma, Hodgkin's disease (especially the mixed-cellularity type), and CNS lymphoma (especially HIV-related).

DIAGNOSIS Serologic features of EBV infection are summarized in Table 108-1.

• Heterophile test: Human serum is absorbed with guinea pig kidney, and the heterophile titer is defined as the highest serum dilution that agglutinates sheep, horse, or cow erythrocytes. A titer ≥ 40-fold is diagnostic of acute EBV infection. Heterophile titers are positive in 40% of pts during the first week and in 80–90% of pts by the third week. The test remains positive for 3 months—or as long as a year—after the onset of acute infection. The monospot test for heterophile antibodies is ~75% sensitive and ~90% specific compared with EBV-specific serologies.

• EBV-specific antibody testing: Specific antibody testing can be useful in heterophile-negative pts (a group that includes many young children) and pts

Table 108-1

Serologic Features of EBV-Associated Diseases

Condition	Result in Indicated Test[a]					
		Anti-VCA		Anti-EA		
	Heterophile	IgM	IgG	EA-D	EA-R	Anti-EBNA
Acute infectious mononucleosis	+	+	+ +	+	−	−
Convalescence	±	−	+	−	±	+
Past infection	−	−	+	−	−	+
Reactivation with immunodeficiency	−	−	+ +	+	+	±
Burkitt's lymphoma	−	−	+ + +	±	+ +	+
Nasopharyngeal carcinoma	−	−	+ + +	+ +	±	+

[a] VCA, viral capsid antigen; EA, early antigen; EA-D antibody, antibody to early antigen in diffuse pattern in nucleus and cytoplasm of infected cells; EA-R antibody, antibody to early antigen restricted to the cytoplasm; and EBNA, Epstein-Barr nuclear antigen.
Source: Adapted from M. Okano et al: Clin Microbiol Rev 1:300, 1988.

with atypical disease. Antibodies to viral capsid antigen occur in >90% of cases. IgM titers are elevated only during the first 2–3 months of disease and are most useful in diagnosing acute infection. Documented seroconversion to EBNA is also useful. EBNA antibodies are not detected until 3–6 weeks after symptom onset and then persist for life. Other antibodies may be elevated but are less useful diagnostically.

• Other studies: Detection of EBV DNA by PCR is useful in demonstrating the association with various malignancies (e.g., positive EBV DNA of the CSF in HIV-associated CNS lymphoma). PCR is used to monitor EBV DNA levels in the blood of pts with lymphoproliferative disease.

 TREATMENT

IM is treated with supportive measures. Excessive physical activity should be avoided in the first month of illness to reduce the possibility of splenic rupture. Splenectomy is required if rupture occurs. Administration of glucocorticoids may be indicated for some complications of IM—e.g., these agents may be given to prevent airway obstruction or for autoimmune hemolytic anemia. Antiviral therapy (e.g., with acyclovir) is generally not effective. Treatment of posttransplantation EBV lymphoproliferative syndrome is generally directed toward reduction of immunsuppression, although other treatments— e.g., with interferon α or antibody to CD20 (rituximab)—and donor lymphocyte infusions have been used with varying success.

For a more detailed discussion, see Baden LR, Dolin R: Antiviral Chemotherapy, Excluding Antiretroviral Drugs, Chap. 162, p. 1027; Cohen JI: Epstein-Barr Virus Infections, Including Infectious Mononucleosis, Chap. 165, p. 1046; and Hirsch MS: Cytomegalovirus and Human Herpesvirus Types 6, 7, and 8, Chap. 166, p. 1049, in HPIM-16.

109

INFLUENZA AND OTHER VIRAL RESPIRATORY DISEASES

INFLUENZA

Etiology Influenza viruses are RNA viruses and members of the Orthomyxoviridae family. Influenza A, B, and C viruses constitute separate genera distinguished by antigenic characteristics of the nucleoprotein (NP) and matrix (M) proteins. Influenza A viruses are further subtyped by surface hemagglutinin (H) and neuraminidase (N) antigens. Strains are designated according to site of origin, isolate number, and subtype. Influenza A and B viruses are the major human pathogens and are morphologically similar. Virus attaches to cell receptors via the hemagglutinin. Neuraminidase degrades the receptor and plays a role in the release of virus from infected cells after replication has occurred. Antibodies to the H antigen are the major determinants of immunity, while antibodies to the N antigen limit viral spread and contribute to reduction of the infection.

Epidemiology Influenza outbreaks occur each year but vary in extent and severity. Until 25 years ago, there were influenza A epidemics or pandemics every 10–15 years due in part to the propensity of the H and N antigens to undergo periodic antigenic variation. Major changes are called *antigenic shifts* and are associated with pandemics. Minor variations are called *antigenic drifts*. The segmented genome of influenza virus allows for reassortment. It is believed that pandemic strains may result from reassortment between human and animal strains of influenza virus. Infection due to avian strains has been documented (e.g., recent infections due to influenza virus A/H5N1), but disease spread has been limited. Epidemics begin abruptly, peak over 2–3 weeks, last 2–3 months, and then subside rapidly. They take place almost exclusively during the winter months in temperate climates but occur year-round in the tropics. The morbidity and mortality associated with influenza outbreaks continue to be substantial, particularly among persons with comorbid disease. Chronic cardiac and pulmonary disease and old age are prominent risk factors for severe illness. Influenza B viruses have a more restricted host range and do not undergo antigenic shifts, although they do exhibit antigenic drift. Outbreaks are less extensive and less severe than those of influenza A, occurring most commonly in schools and military camps. Influenza C causes subclinical infection.

Pathogenesis Influenza is acquired from respiratory secretions of acutely ill individuals through aerosols generated by coughs and sneezes and possibly by hand-to-hand contact or other personal or fomite contact. Virus then infects the respiratory epithelium. Ciliated columnar epithelial cells are initially involved; the virus replicates within 4–6 h and spreads quickly to infect other respiratory cells. Cells undergo degenerative changes, become necrotic, and desquamate. Extrapulmonary sites of infection are rare, but cytokine induction causes systemic symptoms. The host response involves production of humoral antibody (detectable by the second week of infection), local IgA antibody, cell-mediated immunity, and interferon. Host defenses are responsible for cessation of viral shedding 2–5 days after disease onset.

Clinical Features

- Systemic symptoms: abrupt onset of headache, fever, chills, myalgia, malaise
- Respiratory tract symptoms: cough and sore throat that can become more prominent as systemic symptoms subside
- Physical findings are minimal in uncomplicated disease.
- Pts with uncomplicated influenza improve over 2–5 days and have largely recovered at 1 week, although cough can persist for 1–2 weeks. Postinfluenzal asthenia may persist for weeks.

Complications Complications are more common among pts >64 years old, pregnant women, and pts with chronic disorders (e.g., cardiac or pulmonary disease, diabetes, renal diseases, hemoglobinopathies, or immunosuppression).

- Pneumonia: the most significant complication of influenza. Pts can have tachypnea, cyanosis, diffuse rales, and signs of consolidation.
  1. Primary viral: least common but most severe. Acute influenza progresses relentlessly, with persistent fever, dyspnea, cyanosis, and hemoptysis; CXR may show diffuse infiltrates. ARDS can result. Cultures of respiratory secretions yield high viral titers. Primary pneumonia is especially common among pts with cardiac disease, particularly mitral stenosis.

2. Secondary bacterial: usually due to *Streptococcus pneumoniae, Staphylococcus aureus,* or *Haemophilus influenzae.* Pts improve over 2–3 days of illness and then have a recurrence of fever and clinical signs of bacterial pneumonia (e.g., cough, sputum production, and consolidation on CXR).

3. Pts can have features of both primary and secondary pneumonia.

- Extrapulmonary complications

1. Reye's syndrome: associated with influenza B more often than with influenza A; also associated with varicella-zoster virus infection and with aspirin use. Aspirin should not be given to children with acute viral respiratory infections.

2. Miscellaneous: Myositis, rhabdomyolysis, and myoglobinuria are rare despite the prevalence of severe myalgia. Myocarditis and pericarditis, encephalitis, transverse myelitis, and Guillain-Barré syndrome have been reported.

Laboratory Findings During acute influenza, tissue culture of virus from throat swabs, nasopharyngeal washes, or sputum usually gives a positive result within 48–72 h. Rapid tests for viral nucleoprotein or neuraminidase are highly sensitive, with a specificity of 60–90%. Serology requires the availability of acute- and convalescent-phase sera and is useful only retrospectively.

℞ TREATMENT

- Symptom-based therapy (e.g., acetaminophen, rest, hydration)

- Antiviral agents

1. Amantadine and rimantadine (200 mg/d for 3–7 days) are used to treat influenza A; if their administration is begun within 48 h, the duration of systemic and respiratory symptoms is reduced by ~50%. Amantadine causes mild CNS side effects (e.g., jitteriness, anxiety, insomnia, difficulty concentrating) in ~5–10% of pts. Rimantadine has fewer CNS side effects and is equally efficacious.

2. The neuraminidase inhibitors zanamivir (10 mg inhaled bid for 5 days) and oseltamivir (75 mg bid PO with food for 5 days) are used to treat influenza A and B. The drugs decrease the duration of signs and symptoms by 1–1.5 days if therapy is begun within 2 days of illness onset. Zanamivir may exacerbate bronchospasm in asthmatic pts, while oseltamivir has been associated with nausea and vomiting (reactions whose incidence is reduced if the drug is given with food).

3. Antiviral resistance is common with amantadine and rimantadine but infrequent with neuraminidase inhibitors.

4. Antiviral treatment has been tested in healthy adults with uncomplicated influenza but not in pts with severe disease.

Prophylaxis

- Vaccination: Influenza vaccine is derived from the influenza A and B viruses that have circulated during the previous influenza season. If the currently circulating virus is similar to the vaccine strain, 50–80% protection is expected. Influenza vaccination is recommended for any individual >6 months of age who is at increased risk for complications (Table 109-1). The commercially available vaccines are inactivated and may be given to immunocompromised pts. A live attenuated influenza vaccine given by intranasal spray has recently been approved and can be used for healthy children and adults up to 49 years of age.

Table 109-1

Recommendations for Influenza Vaccination[a]

Persons at increased risk for complications
  Persons ≥65 years of age
  Residents of nursing homes and other chronic-care facilities that house persons of any age who have chronic medical conditions
  Adults and children (≥6 months) who have chronic disorders of the pulmonary or cardiovascular systems, including asthma
  Adults and children (≥6 months) who have required regular medical follow-up or hospitalization during the preceding year because of chronic metabolic diseases (including diabetes mellitus), renal dysfunction, hemoglobinopathies, or immunosuppression (including immunosuppression caused by medications or by HIV)
  Children and adolescents (6 months to 18 years old) who are receiving long-term aspirin therapy and therefore may be at risk for developing Reye's syndrome after influenza infection
  Women who will be in the second or third trimester of pregnancy during the influenza season
Persons 50 to 64 years of age
  Included because of increased prevalence of high-risk conditions
Persons who can transmit influenza to those at high risk
  Physicians, nurses, and other personnel in both hospital and outpatient-care settings, including medical emergency response workers (e.g., paramedics and emergency medical technicians)
  Employees of nursing homes and chronic-care facilities who have contact with patients or residents
  Employees of assisted-living and other residences for persons in groups at high risk
  Persons who provide home care to individuals in groups at high risk
  Household members (including children) of persons in groups at high risk

---

[a] Vaccination of healthy children 6 to 23 months of age is encouraged.
Source: Centers for Disease Control and Prevention: MMWR S1(RR-3):1, 2002.

- Chemoprophylaxis: Efficacy rates in preventing illness are 70–100% for amantadine or rimantadine (100–200 mg/d) and are 84–89% for oseltamivir (75 mg/d PO) or zanamivir (10 mg/d inhaled). Prophylaxis is useful for high-risk individuals who have not received vaccine and are exposed to influenza; it can be administered simultaneously with the inactivated vaccine.

OTHER COMMON VIRAL RESPIRATORY INFECTIONS (See also Chap. 60)

Rhinoviruses

Rhinoviruses are RNA viruses of the Picornaviridae family.

- Major cause of the "common cold" (15–40% of adult cases)
- Spread by direct contact with infected secretions, usually respiratory droplets
- Short incubation period (1–2 days). Pts develop rhinorrhea, sneezing, nasal congestion, and sore throat. Fever and systemic symptoms are unusual.
- Severe disease is rare but is described in bone marrow transplant recipients.
- Diagnosis is not usually attempted. PCR and tissue culture methods are available.

Coronaviruses

GENERAL INFORMATION   Coronaviruses are RNA viruses that account for 10–35% of common colds and cause typical presentations. A novel group of coronaviruses was recently identified as the cause of severe acute respiratory syndrome (SARS).

THE SARS OUTBREAK *Epidemiology* SARS began in China in 2002. Although 8422 cases were ultimately identified by the World Health Organization in 28 countries of Asia, Europe, and North America, ~90% of all cases occurred in China and Hong Kong. Case-fatality rates were ~11% overall. Transmission appeared to take place by both large and small aerosols and perhaps also by the fecal-oral route.

Pathogenesis SARS virus probably enters and infects cells of the respiratory tract but also causes viremia and is found in the urine and in the stool. Viral titers in the respiratory tract peak ~10 days after the onset of illness. Pulmonary pathology consists of hyaline membrane formation, pneumocyte desquamation in alveolar spaces, and an interstitial infiltrate with lymphocytes and mononuclear cells.

Clinical Features The incubation period lasts 2–7 days. A systemic illness with fever, malaise, headache, and myalgias is followed in 1–2 days by nonproductive cough, dyspnea, diarrhea, and abnormal CXR. Respiratory function deteriorates in the second week of illness and can progress to ARDS and multiorgan dysfunction. A worse prognosis is associated with an age >50 years and with comorbidities such as cardiovascular disease, diabetes, and hepatitis. Pregnant women have particularly severe disease.

Diagnosis Lymphopenia affecting mostly CD4+ T cells, thrombocytopenia, and increased serum levels of aminotransferases, creatine kinase, and LDH are described. Diagnosis is based on clinical, epidemiologic, and laboratory features. Virus can be isolated from respiratory tract secretions. A rapid diagnosis can be made by reverse-transcriptase PCR of respiratory tract samples and plasma early in illness and of urine and stool later in the course. Serum antibodies are detectable by ELISA or immunofluorescence and develop within 28 days of illness onset.

 TREATMENT

Ribavirin and glucocorticoids were used during the outbreak, but their benefit is uncertain. Aggressive supportive care is most important.

Prevention A worldwide public health response resulted from the outbreak. Case definitions were established, travel advisories issued, and quarantines imposed in certain locales. Transmission to health care workers was frequent; strict infection control measures were found to be essential.

Respiratory Syncytial Virus (RSV)

Respiratory syncytial virus is so named because its replication in vitro leads to fusion of neighboring cells into large multinucleated syncytia. RSV is an RNA virus and a member of the Paramyxoviridae family. It is a major respiratory pathogen among young children and the foremost cause of lower respiratory disease among infants. Rates of illness peak at 2–3 months of age, when attack rates among susceptible individuals approach 100%. RSV accounts for 20–25%

of hospital admissions of infants and young children for pneumonia and for up to 75% of cases of bronchiolitis in this age group. It is transmitted efficiently via contact with contaminated fingers or fomites and by spread of coarse aerosols. The incubation period is 4–6 days. Viral shedding can last for >2 weeks in children and compromised hosts. RSV is an important nosocomial pathogen.

Clinical Features

- Infants and young children: Around 20–25% of infections result in lower tract disease, including pneumonia, bronchiolitis, and tracheobronchitis. Mild disease begins with rhinorrhea, low-grade fever, cough, and wheezing, and recovery comes within 1–2 weeks. Severe disease is marked by tachypnea and dyspnea; hypoxia, cyanosis, and apnea can ensue. Examination reveals wheezing, rhonchi, and rales. CXR may reveal hyperexpansion, peribronchial thickening, and variable infiltrates. Mortality rates can be high, especially among infants with prematurity, bronchopulmonary dysplasia, CHD, nephrotic syndrome, or immunosuppression.
- Milder disease results from reinfection among older children and adults.
- The common cold is the most common presentation in adults, but RSV can cause severe pneumonia in immunocompromised or elderly pts.

Diagnosis

Diagnosis   Immunofluorescence, ELISA, and other techniques can identify RSV isolates in tissue culture. Rapid viral diagnosis is available by immunofluorescence or ELISA of nasopharyngeal washes, aspirates, or swabs. Serologic testing is also available.

 TREATMENT

For upper tract disease, treatment is symptom-based. For severe lower tract disease, aerosolized ribavirin is beneficial to infants, but its efficacy in older children and adults (including immunocompromised pts) has not been established. Health care workers exposed to the drug have experienced minor toxicity, including eye and respiratory tract irritation. Ribavirin is mutagenic, teratogenic, and embryotoxic; its use is contraindicated in pregnancy, and its aerosolized administration is a risk to pregnant health care workers. IVIg, immunoglobulin with high titers of antibody to RSV (RSVIg), and monoclonal IgG antibody to RSV (palivizumab) are available but have not been shown to be beneficial.

Prevention   Monthly RSVIg or palivizumab is approved for prophylaxis in children <2 years of age who have bronchopulmonary dysplasia or who were born prematurely.

Metapneumovirus

Metapneumovirus is an RNA virus of the Paramyxoviridae family. This newly described respiratory pathogen causes disease in a wide variety of age groups, with clinical manifestations similar to those caused by RSV.

Parainfluenza Virus

This RNA virus of the Paramyxoviridae family ranks second only to RSV as a cause of lower respiratory tract disease among young children and is the most common cause of croup (laryngotracheobronchitis). Infections are milder among older children and adults, but severe, prolonged, and fatal infection is reported among pts with severe immunosuppression, including transplant recipients. Tissue culture, rapid testing, or PCR of respiratory tract secretions or nasopharyngeal washings can detect the virus. Glucocorticoids are beneficial in severe cases. Ribavirin has been used on occasion, and anecdotal reports indicate some efficacy.

Adenoviruses

Adenoviruses are DNA viruses that cause ~10% of acute respiratory infections among children but <2% of respiratory illnesses among civilian adults. Some serotypes are associated with outbreaks among military recruits. Transmission can take place via inhalation of aerosolized virus, through inoculation of the conjunctival sacs, and probably via the fecal-oral route.

• In children, adenovirus causes acute upper (most common) and lower respiratory tract infections. The virus causes outbreaks of pharyngoconjunctival fever, which often occur at summer camps; this illness is characterized by bilateral conjunctivitis, granular conjunctivae, rhinitis, sore throat, and cervical adenopathy.
• In adults, adenovirus causes sore throat, fever, cough, coryza, and regional adenopathy.
• Other manifestations include diarrheal illness, hemorrhagic cystitis, and epidemic keratoconjunctivitis.
• Immunocompromised pts, especially transplant recipients, can develop disseminated disease, pneumonia, hepatitis, nephritis, colitis, encephalitis, and hemorrhagic cystitis. Adenovirus may involve the transplanted organ.
• Definitive diagnosis can be made by isolation in tissue culture; by rapid testing (with immunofluorescence or ELISA) of nasopharyngeal aspirates, conjunctival or respiratory secretions, urine, or stool; or by PCR testing.
• Treatment is supportive. Ribavirin and cidofovir exhibit in vitro activity against adenovirus.

For a more detailed discussion, see Baden LR, Dolin R: Antiviral Chemotherapy, Excluding Antiretroviral Drugs, Chap. 162, p. 1027; Dolin R: Common Viral Respiratory Infections and Severe Acute Respiratory Syndrome (SARS), Chap. 170, p. 1059; and Dolin R: Influenza, Chap. 171, p. 1066, in HPIM-16.

110

RUBEOLA, RUBELLA, MUMPS, AND PARVOVIRUS INFECTIONS

MEASLES (RUBEOLA)

DEFINITION AND ETIOLOGY Measles is a highly contagious, acute, exanthematous respiratory disease with a characteristic clinical picture and a pathognomonic enanthem (Koplik's spots). Measles is caused by an RNA virus of the genus *Morbillivirus* and the family Paramyxoviridae.

EPIDEMIOLOGY Humans are the only natural host for measles. Routine administration of the measles vaccine has markedly decreased the number of cases in the United States. Most of the 116 U.S. cases reported in 2001 were attributable to international importation of the virus. The disease is spread by respiratory secretions through exposure to aerosols and through direct contact with larger droplets. Pts are contagious from 1–2 days before symptom onset until 4 days after the rash appears; infectivity peaks during the prodromal phase.

CLINICAL FEATURES

I. Symptoms and rash occur a mean of 10 and 14 days, respectively, after infection.

II. Prodrome: 2–4 days of malaise, cough, coryza, conjunctivitis, nasal discharge, and fever. Fever starts to resolve by day 4 or 5 after rash onset.

III. Koplik's spots: 1- to 2-mm blue-white spots on a bright red background; typically occur on the buccal mucosa, alongside the second molars, 1–2 days before rash

IV. An erythematous, nonpruritic, maculopapular rash begins at the hairline and behind the ears, spreads down the trunk and limbs to include the palms and soles, can become confluent, and begins to fade by day 4. Rash is often more severe in adults.

V. Lymphadenopathy, diarrhea and vomiting, and splenomegaly are common.

VI. Pts with defects in cell-mediated immunity are at risk for severe, protracted, and fatal disease and may have no rash.

VII. Complications

    A. Respiratory tract: otitis media in children, croup in infants. Adults and compromised children can develop primary viral giant cell pneumonia.

    B. CNS disease

        1. Acute encephalitis: headache, drowsiness, coma, seizures; 10% mortality; retardation, epilepsy, and other sequelae in survivors

        2. Risk of progressive fatal encephalitis 1–6 months after illness in immunocompromised pts

        3. Subacute sclerosing panencephalitis: protracted, chronic, rare form of encephalitis with progressive dementia over several months; more common among children who contract measles at <2 years of age; rare in the United States because of widespread vaccination

    C. GI tract: hepatitis, colitis, adenitis, appendicitis

    D. Myocarditis, glomerulonephritis, thrombocytopenic purpura

VIII. Atypical measles occurs in pts who contract measles after receiving inactivated vaccine (in use before 1967). The rash appears peripherally, moves centrally, and can be urticarial, maculopapular, hemorrhagic, and/or vesicular. Pts have high fevers, edema of the extremities, interstitial pulmonary infiltrates, hepatitis, and occasionally pleural effusions. Full recovery is typical, but convalescence may be prolonged.

DIAGNOSIS Lymphopenia and neutropenia are common. Immunofluorescent staining of respiratory secretions for measles antigen or examination of secretions for multinucleated giant cells can help establish the diagnosis. Virus can be isolated from respiratory secretions or urine. PCR is available as well. IgM antibody appears 1–2 days before rash.

℞ TREATMENT

- Supportive care; antibiotics for bacterial superinfections (e.g., otitis or pneumonia)
- Vitamin A for young children hospitalized with measles and for pediatric measles pts with immunodeficiency, vitamin A deficiency, impaired intestinal

absorption, malnutrition, or immigration from areas with high measles mortality
- Ribavirin may be considered for use in immunocompromised pts.

PREVENTION   Live attenuated vaccine containing measles, mumps, and rubella (MMR) antigens is given routinely at 12–15 months; a second dose is given to school-age children at 4–12 years of age. Older individuals without documented illness or vaccination should be immunized. Asymptomatic HIV-infected children should receive MMR vaccine, but pts with severe immunosuppression, others with impaired cell-mediated immunity, pregnant women, and persons with anaphylaxis to egg protein or neomycin should not receive the vaccine.

Postexposure prophylaxis with immunoglobulin should be considered in susceptible children or adults exposed to measles; 0.25 mL/kg is given to healthy pts and 0.5 mL/kg to compromised hosts, with a maximal dose of 15 mL.

RUBELLA (GERMAN MEASLES)

ETIOLOGY AND EPIDEMIOLOGY   Rubella is a contagious infectious disease caused by an RNA togavirus of the genus *Rubivirus*. Virus is shed in respiratory secretions during the prodromal phase, and shedding continues for a week after symptom onset. Transmission occurs via droplets or direct contact with nasopharyngeal secretions. Infants with congenital disease can shed virus from the respiratory tract and urine for 2 years. Rubella vaccine, introduced in 1969, has eliminated most disease. Only 23 cases of postnatally acquired rubella and 3 confirmed cases of congenital rubella syndrome were reported to the CDC in 2001. Young immigrants from Latin America and the Caribbean, where childhood vaccination against the disease is not routine, are at increased risk.

CLINICAL FEATURES

- Incubation period: average, 18 days; range, 12–23 days
- Usually mild or subclinical illness; may be more severe in adults
- A prodrome of malaise, fever, and anorexia is followed by posterior auricular, cervical, and suboccipital lymphadenopathy; fever; mild coryza; and conjunctivitis.
- Rash follows, beginning on the face, spreading down the body, and lasting 3–5 days.
- Women are more prone to arthritis of the fingers, wrists, and/or knees; this condition can take weeks to resolve.
- Congenital rubella is the most serious manifestation of rubella infection and can include cataracts, heart disease, deafness, and other deficits. Maternal infection results in fetal infection in ~50% of cases in the first trimester and in about one-third of cases in the second trimester. Fetal disease is more severe the earlier infection occurs.

DIAGNOSIS

- ELISA testing for IgG and IgM antibodies
- Congenital rubella can be diagnosed by isolation of the virus, detection of IgM antibodies, or persistence of antibodies beyond 1 year of age.
- Biopsy tissue samples or blood or CSF samples can be analyzed for rubella antigen with monoclonal antibodies or for rubella RNA via in situ hybridization or PCR.

PREVENTION   See MMR recommendations under "Measles (Rubeola)," above. Pregnancy should be avoided for at least 3 months after vaccination. However, the occurrence of vaccine-related congenital rubella has not been proven in women inadvertently vaccinated during pregnancy.

MUMPS

DEFINITION AND ETIOLOGY   Mumps is an acute systemic communicable viral infection whose most distinctive feature is swelling of one or both parotid glands. It is caused by the mumps virus, an RNA paramyxovirus with only one antigenic type.

EPIDEMIOLOGY   The introduction of mumps vaccine in 1967 resulted in a marked decline in new mumps cases in the United States. In 2001, 266 cases were reported. Pts may shed virus before clinical disease onset or during subclinical infection (which occurs in one-third of pts). The virus is transmitted by droplet nuclei, saliva, and fomites. Transmission occurs 1–2 days before parotitis onset and can continue up to 5 days afterward. Viral replication in the upper respiratory tract leads to viremia, which is followed by infection of glandular tissues and/or the CNS.

CLINICAL FEATURES

- The incubation period is generally 14–18 days (range, 7–23 days).
- A prodrome of fever, malaise, myalgia, and anorexia is followed 1–7 days later by tender parotitis that is bilateral in two-thirds of pts. Pts have trouble eating, swallowing, or talking. Swelling slowly resolves within a week. Submaxillary and sublingual glands are involved less often.
- After parotitis, orchitis is the most common manifestation among postpubertal males, occurring in about one-fifth of cases. The testes are painful, tender, and enlarged, and atrophy can develop in half of affected men. Orchitis is bilateral in <15% of cases, and sterility is rare. Oophoritis can occur but does not lead to sterility.
- Aseptic meningitis: CSF pleocytosis can occur in half of mumps cases, but clinical meningitis is evident in only 5–25%. CSF glucose levels may be very low, and PMNs may predominate in the first 24 h, leading to a consideration of bacterial meningitis. Disease is self-limited; cranial nerve palsies occasionally lead to permanent sequelae, particularly deafness.
- Pancreatitis, myocarditis, and other unusual manifestations can occur. High serum amylase levels due to parotitis make pancreatitis difficult to diagnose. First-trimester maternal infection can cause spontaneous abortions but not congenital malformations.

DIAGNOSIS   Mumps virus is easily isolated and rapidly identified when grown in shell vials and stained with fluorescein-labeled monoclonal antibodies. Virus can be recovered from saliva, throat, urine (in which it is shed for up to 2 weeks), and CSF. PCR is also available. ELISA is useful for serologic diagnosis.

PREVENTION   See MMR recommendations under "Measles (Rubeola)," above.

PARVOVIRUS INFECTION

ETIOLOGY   Parvovirus B19, a DNA virus, is a human pathogen with a propensity to infect and lyse erythroid precursor cells in bone marrow.

PATHOGENESIS   Viremia occurs ~6 days after infection with B19 and lasts ~1 week; its clearance is associated with the development of antibodies. Around day 17 to 18 after infection, a second phase of illness, with rash and/or arthritis, occurs in the healthy host in the presence of rising antibody titers, consistent with an immune-complex disorder.

EPIDEMIOLOGY   Antibody prevalence rises between 5 and 18 years of age and continues to increase with age. Disease is most common in winter and spring.

CLINICAL FEATURES

• Erythema infectiosum (fifth disease), which mostly affects children, is a mild viral illness with a facial "slapped-cheek" rash and low-grade fever. A lacy, reticular erythematous rash develops primarily on the arms and legs; it usually resolves in a week but can recur.

• Arthropathy: Adults most often have acute arthralgias and arthritis, occasionally with rash. The arthritis is typically symmetric, peripheral (wrists, hands, knees), and nondestructive. Most cases resolve in 3 weeks, but some persist for months.

• Transient aplastic crisis: Pts with chronic hemolytic conditions (e.g., sickle cell disease) can develop aplastic crisis with B19 infection that can be life-threatening. Pts display weakness, lethargy, and pallor in association with severe anemia. Pts are viremic and can transmit B19 to others.

• Chronic anemia in immunodeficient pts: These pts are unable to eliminate B19 infection and have persistent infection of erythroid precursor cells and chronic transfusion-dependent anemia. HIV-infected pts, transplant recipients, and pts with other immunodeficiencies are at risk.

• Fetal and congenital infection: There is usually no adverse effect of maternal B19 infection; <10% of infections in the first 20 weeks of pregnancy lead to fetal death (usually due to nonimmune hydrops fetalis, in which the fetus succumbs to severe anemia and CHF). Some reports have described late-second-trimester and third-trimester nonhydropic fetal deaths due to B19.

DIAGNOSIS   Diagnosis relies on measurement of B19-specific IgM and IgG antibodies. The virus or its DNA or antigens can be detected in serum or infected tissues of some pts, particularly those with transient aplastic crisis and high virus titers. Bone marrow examination demonstrates characteristic giant pronormoblasts and hypoplasia.

℞ TREATMENT

Aplastic crisis should be treated with transfusions as needed. Commercial IV immunoglobulin should be given to immunodeficient anemic pts to control and possibly cure B19 infection.

PROPHYLAXIS   Pts with chronic hemolysis or immunodeficiency and some pregnant women may be candidates for immunoglobulin prophylaxis. Hospitalized pts with chronic B19 infection or transient aplastic crisis pose a risk of nosocomial transmission and should be placed on contact and respiratory isolation precautions.

For a more detailed discussion, see Blacklow NR: Parvovirus, Chap. 168, p. 1054; Gershon A: Measles (Rubeola), Chap. 176, p. 1148; Rubella (German Measles), Chap. 177, p. 1152; and Mumps, Chap. 178, p. 1154, in HPIM-16.

ENTEROVIRAL INFECTIONS

Etiology

Enteroviruses are so named because of their ability to multiply in the GI tract, but they do not typically cause gastroenteritis. This group of viruses includes 3 serotypes of poliovirus, 23 serotypes of coxsackievirus A, 6 serotypes of coxsackievirus B, 28 serotypes of echovirus, and enteroviruses 68–71. In the United States, echovirus causes most enteroviral infections.

Pathogenesis and Immunity

Of the enteroviruses, poliovirus is best characterized. After ingestion, poliovirus infects GI tract mucosal epithelial cells, spreads to regional lymph nodes, causes viremia, and replicates in the reticuloendothelial system; in some cases, a second round of viremia occurs. Virus gains CNS access either via the bloodstream or via direct spread from neural pathways. Virus is present in blood for 3–5 days. It is shed from the oropharynx for up to 3 weeks and from the GI tract for up to 12 weeks after infection. Immunocompromised pts can shed virus for >1 year. Infection is controlled by humoral and secretory immunity in the GI tract.

Epidemiology

Enteroviruses cause disease worldwide, especially in areas with crowded conditions and poor hygiene. Infants and young children are most often infected and are the most frequent shedders. Transmission takes place mainly by the fecal-oral route, but airborne transmission and placental transmission have been described. Pts are most infectious shortly before or after the onset of symptoms. The incubation period is 3–6 days.

Clinical Features

Poliovirus

- Most infections are asymptomatic. Mild illness resolves in 3 days and is manifest by fever, malaise, sore throat, myalgias, and headache.
- Aseptic meningitis (nonparalytic) occurs in ~1% of pts. CSF reveals normal glucose and protein concentrations and lymphocytic pleocytosis (with PMNs sometimes predominating early).
- Paralytic disease is least common. Risk factors include older age, pregnancy, and trauma or strenuous exercise at the onset of CNS symptoms. Aseptic meningitis is followed ≥1 day later by severe back, neck, and muscle pain as well as a gradual development of motor weakness. This weakness is usually asymmetric and proximal and is most common in the legs; the arms and the abdominal, thoracic, and bulbar muscles are other commonly involved sites. Paralysis occurs only during the febrile phase. Physical examination reveals weakness, fasciculations, decreased muscle tone, and reduced or absent reflexes in affected areas; hyperreflexia may precede the loss of reflexes. Bulbar paralysis is associated with dysphagia, difficulty handling secretions, or dysphonia. Respiratory insufficiency due to aspiration or neurologic involvement may develop. Severe medullary infection may lead to circulatory collapse. Most pts recover some function, but around two-thirds have residual neurologic sequelae.
- Live poliovirus vaccine–associated disease: The risk is estimated to be 1 case per 2.5 million doses and is ~2000 times higher among immunodeficient persons.

• Postpolio syndrome: new weakness 20–40 years after poliomyelitis. Onset is insidious, progression is slow, and plateau periods can last 1–10 years. This syndrome is not thought to be secondary to persistent or reactivated infection.

Coxsackievirus, Echovirus, and Other Enteroviruses   In the United States, 5–10 million cases of symptomatic enteroviral disease other than poliomyelitis occur each year.

• Nonspecific febrile illness (summer grippe) occurs during the summer and early fall. Pts have an acute onset of fever, malaise, and headache; upper respiratory symptoms; nausea; and vomiting. Disease resolves within a week.
• Generalized disease of the newborn occurs from the first week of life to 3 months of age. The illness resembles bacterial sepsis and has a high associated mortality rate. Myocarditis, hypotension, hepatitis, DIC, meningitis, and pneumonia are complications.
• Aseptic meningitis and encephalitis: Enteroviruses cause 90% of aseptic meningitis cases among children and young adults. Pts have an acute onset of fever, chills, headache, photophobia, nausea, and vomiting, with meningismus on examination. Diarrhea, rashes, myalgias, pleurodynia, myocarditis, and herpangina may occur. CSF examination reveals pleocytosis, with PMNs sometimes predominating early but a shift to lymphocyte predominance within 24 h. Total cell counts do not usually exceed 1000/μL. CSF glucose and protein levels are typically normal. Symptoms resolve within a week, but CSF abnormalities persist longer. Encephalitis is much less common, and the disease is usually mild, with an excellent prognosis in healthy hosts. However, pts with γ globulin defects can develop chronic meningitis or encephalitis. Pts receiving γ globulin replacement may develop neurologic disease due to echovirus.
• Pleurodynia (Bornholm disease): Pts have an acute onset of fever associated with spasms of pleuritic chest pain (more common among adults) or upper abdominal pain (more common among children). Fever subsides when pain resolves. A pleural rub may be present. Coxsackievirus B is the most common cause. Disease lasts for several days. NSAID administration and the application of heat to the affected muscles may help.
• Myocarditis and pericarditis: Enteroviruses (e.g., coxsackievirus B) cause up to one-third of cases of acute myocarditis. Disease is more common among males and occurs most often in newborns (most severe disease), adolescents, and young adults. Pts have upper respiratory symptoms, followed by fever, chest pain, dyspnea, arrhythmias, and occasionally CHF. A pericardial friction rub, ST segment and T-wave abnormalities on ECG, and elevated serum levels of myocardial enzymes can be present. Up to 10% of pts develop chronic dilated cardiomyopathy. Constrictive pericarditis may occur.
• Exanthems: Enteroviral infection is a leading cause of exanthems among children in the summer and fall. Echoviruses 9 and 16 are common causes.
• Hand-foot-and-mouth disease: Pts present with fever, anorexia, and malaise, followed by sore throat and vesicles on the buccal mucosa, tongue, and dorsum or palms of the hands and occasionally on the palate, uvula, tonsillar pillars, or feet. Lesions can become bullous and ulcerate. The disease is highly infectious, with attack rates of almost 100% among young children. Symptoms resolve within a week. Coxsackievirus A16 and enterovirus 71 are the most common etiologic agents. A Taiwan epidemic of enterovirus 71 infection was associated with CNS disease, myocarditis, and pulmonary hemorrhage. Deaths occurred primarily among children ≤5 years old.
• Herpangina: associated with coxsackievirus A infection. Pts have fever, sore throat, and dysphagia and develop grayish-white papulovesicular lesions that ulcerate and are concentrated in the posterior portion of the mouth. Lesions can persist for weeks. In contrast to herpes simplex stomatitis, enteroviral herpangina is not associated with gingivitis.

- Acute hemorrhagic conjunctivitis: associated with enterovirus 70 and coxsackievirus A24. Pts have an acute onset of severe eye pain, blurred vision, photophobia, watery eye discharge, fever, and headache. Edema, chemosis, and subconjunctival hemorrhage are evident. Symptoms resolve within 10 days.

Diagnosis

Enterovirus can be isolated from throat or rectal swabs or stool and from normally sterile body fluids. Stool and throat cultures may reflect colonization, but throat cultures are more likely to be associated with disease because virus is shed for shorter periods from the throat. Positive results for normally sterile body fluids, such as CSF and serum, reflect disease. Serotyping is not clinically useful. PCR detects >92% of the serotypes that infect humans. PCR of the CSF is sensitive and specific and is more rapid than culture. PCR of the serum is also useful. Tests are more likely to be positive early in disease.

 TREATMENT

Most enteroviral illness resolves spontaneously, but immunoglobulin may be helpful in pts with γ globulin defects and chronic infection and in neonates with severe disease. Pleconaril reduced symptoms in a placebo-controlled trial of enteroviral meningitis and is available on a compassionate-use basis for severe enteroviral illness. Glucocorticoids are contraindicated.

Prevention

Hand hygiene, use of gowns and gloves, and enteric precautions (for 7 days after disease onset) prevent nosocomial transmission of enteroviruses during epidemics. The availability of poliovirus vaccines and the implementation of polio eradication programs have eliminated disease due to wild-type poliovirus except in 11 countries (all in Asia and Africa). Outbreaks and sporadic disease due to vaccine-derived poliovirus occur. Both oral poliovirus vaccine (OPV) and inactivated poliovirus vaccine (IPV) induce IgG and IgA antibodies that persist for at least 5 years. OPV causes less viral shedding, reduces the risk of community transmission of wild-type virus, costs less, and is easier to administer than IPV. Most developing countries, particularly those with persistent wild-type poliomyelitis, use OPV. Developed countries without wild-type disease but with cases of vaccine-associated polio have adopted all-IPV childhood vaccination programs. Doses are given at 2, 4, and 6–18 months and at 4–6 years of age. Unvaccinated adults in the United States do not need routine poliovirus vaccination but should receive three doses of IPV (the second dose 1–2 months after the first and the final dose 6–12 months later) if they are traveling to polio-endemic areas or might be exposed to wild-type poliovirus in their communities or workplaces. Adults at increased risk of exposure who have received their primary vaccination series should receive a single dose of IPV.

For a more detailed discussion, see Cohen JI: Enteroviruses and Reoviruses, Chap. 175, p. 1143, in HPIM-16.

112

INSECT- AND ANIMAL-BORNE VIRAL INFECTIONS

RABIES

Rabies viruses are bullet-shaped, enveloped, single-stranded RNA viruses in the family Rhabdoviridae of the genus *Lyssavirus*. Isolates vary in antigenic and biologic properties depending on animal species and locale.

EPIDEMIOLOGY   Rabies causes >30,000 deaths each year, mostly in Southeast Asia, the Philippines, Africa, India, and tropical South America.

- Urban rabies: propagated primarily by unimmunized domestic dogs
- Sylvatic rabies: propagated by skunks, foxes, raccoons, coyotes, wolves, bats
- In the United States, rabies in domestic dogs has been largely eliminated by vaccination, and cats are now a more frequent cause of the disease. Because of the decreased risk, dog bites are appropriately managed with a 10-day observation of the animal. The major rabies hosts in the United States are bats (which have caused 90% of the 30 human cases described in this country since 1980), raccoons, skunks, foxes, and coyotes.

PATHOGENESIS   Rabies virus is inoculated through the skin, usually via a bite that delivers virus-laden saliva. Virus replicates within striated muscle cells at the inoculation site and spreads to peripheral nerves and then to the CNS. The virus continues to replicate within gray matter and passes along autonomic nerves to other tissues and from there into saliva, whence it may be transmitted to another host. Within the CNS, rabies virus causes nerve cell destruction and microglial infiltration. *Negri bodies*—characteristic eosinophilic cytoplasmic inclusions within neurons—are made up of a finely fibrillar matrix and rabies virus particles. The incubation period varies from 7 days to >1 year (mean, 1–2 months). Bites on the face are associated with the highest rates of infection and mortality, bites on the legs with the lowest rates.

CLINICAL FEATURES   Clinical rabies can be divided into four stages.

- *Prodromal period* (1–4 days): Pts have fever, headache, malaise, myalgias, anorexia, nausea, vomiting, sore throat, and nonproductive cough. Paresthesia and/or fasciculations at or near the site of viral inoculation are found in 50–80% of cases and are suggestive of rabies.
- *Encephalitic phase*: Pts develop periods of excessive motor activity, excitation, and agitation. Confusion, combativeness, muscle spasms, seizures, focal paralysis, and fever are interspersed with shortening periods of lucidity. Hyperesthesia is common. Hydrophobia or aerophobia is seen in approximately two-thirds of pts and helps in making the diagnosis. Hyperthermia, autonomic dysfunction, upper motor neuron paralysis, and vocal cord paralysis can occur.
- *Brainstem dysfunction*: This stage is characterized by cranial nerve involvement (e.g., diplopia, facial palsies, optic neuritis, and difficulty with deglutition); deglutition problems combined with excessive salivation produce characteristic foaming at the mouth. Hydrophobia—painful violent involuntary contractions of the diaphragm and of accessory respiratory, pharyngeal, and laryngeal muscles initiated by swallowing liquids—can occur, as can priapism. Prominent early brainstem dysfunction distinguishes rabies from other viral encephalitides.
- *Coma and death*: The median survival period after symptom onset is 4 days; the maximum is 20 days. Even with aggressive supportive measures, recovery is rare.

DIAGNOSIS

- CSF examination can show a mild pleocytosis and a slightly increased protein level.
- Rabies virus–specific antibodies in serum and CSF develop late in the clinical course and, if the pt dies during the acute phase, may remain undetectable.
- Reverse-transcription PCR (RT-PCR) can reveal viral shedding in fresh saliva, which directly precedes the onset of clinical signs and continues throughout the course.
- Because the virus spreads centrifugally from the CNS, a skin biopsy sample from the nape of the neck may be positive in DFA testing and RT-PCR.
- Differential diagnosis: Other viral encephalitides [e.g., those due to herpes simplex virus (HSV) type 1, varicella-zoster virus, and enteroviruses as well as arboviruses] should be considered.

 TREATMENT

Treatment is palliative and supportive. Death is virtually inevitable.

PREVENTION

- The wound should be thoroughly scrubbed with soap and flushed with water.
- Postexposure prophylaxis (PEP) with a modern cell-culture vaccine (Table 112-1) should be administered as appropriate.
- Preexposure prophylaxis is occasionally given to persons at high risk. After receiving a series of 1-mL doses of a modern cell-culture vaccine IM on days 0, 7, 21, and 28, high- and moderate-risk pts should have their rabies virus–neutralizing antibody titers monitored every 6 months and every 2 years, respectively.

INFECTIONS CAUSED BY ARTHROPOD- AND RODENT-BORNE VIRUSES

More than 500 distinct RNA viruses are maintained in arthropods or chronically infected rodents. Arthropod-borne viruses infect their vector after a blood meal from a viremic vertebrate; the viruses penetrate the gut and spread throughout the vector; when in the salivary glands, they can be transmitted to another vertebrate during a blood meal. The rodent-borne viruses cause chronic infections transmitted between rodents. Humans become infected by inhalation of aerosols containing the viruses and through close contact with rodents and their excreta. These infections are most common in the tropics but also occur in temperate and frigid climates.

CLINICAL FEATURES   Infection usually causes one of four major clinical syndromes: fever and myalgia, encephalitis, arthritis and rash, and hemorrhagic fever (HF).

Fever and Myalgia   This is the most common syndrome associated with these viruses. Typically, pts have an acute onset of fever, severe myalgia, and headache. Complete recovery is usual. Important examples include the following.

- *Lymphocytic choriomeningitis* (LCM): This infection is transmitted from the common house mouse and pet hamsters via aerosols of excreta and secreta. Unlike other viral infections that cause fever and myalgia, LCM has a gradual onset. Other manifestations include transient alopecia, arthritis, cough, maculopapular rash, and orchitis. About one-fourth of infected pts have a biphasic illness. After a 3- to 6-day febrile phase, there is a remission followed by recurrent fever, headache, nausea, vomiting, and meningeal signs lasting

Table 112-1

Rabies Postexposure Prophylaxis Guide—United States

Animal Type	Evaluation and Disposition of Animal	Postexposure Prophylaxis Recommendations
Dogs, cats, and ferrets	Healthy and available for 10 days observation	No treatment is necessary unless animal develops clinical signs of rabies.[a]
	Rabid or suspected rabid	Begin PEP.
	Unknown (e.g., escaped)	Consult public health officials.
Skunks, raccoons, foxes, and most other carnivores; bats	Regarded as rabid unless animal proven negative by laboratory tests[b]	Consider immediate vaccination.
Livestock, small rodents, lagomorphs (rabbits and hares), large rodents (woodchucks and beavers), and other mammals	Consider individually	Consult public health officials. Bites of squirrels, hamsters, guinea pigs, gerbils, chipmunks, rats, mice, other small rodents, rabbits, and hares almost never require postexposure prophylaxis.

[a] During the 10-day observation period, begin postexposure prophylaxis at the first sign of rabies in a dog, cat, or ferret that has bitten someone. If the animal exhibits clinical signs of rabies, it should be euthanized immediately and tested.

[b] The animal should be euthanized and tested as soon as possible. Holding for observation is not recommended. Discontinue vaccine if immunofluorescence test results of the animal are negative.

Source: Human rabies prevention—United States, 1999. Recommendations of the Advisory Committee on Immunization Practices (ACIP). MMWR Recomm Rep 48(RR-1):1-21, 1999; erratum in MMWR 48(1):16, 1999; MMWR 49(32):737, 2000.

~1 week. Pregnant women can have mild infection yet pass on the virus to the fetus, who can develop hydrocephalus and chorioretinitis. The diagnosis should be considered in adult pts who have aseptic meningitis in the autumn months and who have had a febrile prodrome. CSF examination reveals mononuclear cell counts that can exceed 1000/μL and low glucose levels. Marked leukopenia and thrombocytopenia are common. Recovery of LCM virus from blood or CSF is most likely in the initial phase of illness. Diagnosis can be made by IgM-capture ELISA of serum or CSF or by RT-PCR of CSF (if this test is available).

• *Dengue fever*: The vector of all four distinct dengue viruses (serotypes 1–4) is *Aedes aegypti*, which is also a vector for yellow fever. A second infection with a different dengue serotype can lead to dengue hemorrhagic fever (DHF; see "Hemorrhagic Fever," below). Year-round transmission occurs between latitudes 25°N and 25°S. After an incubation period of 2–7 days, pts have sudden onset of fever, headache, retroorbital pain, back pain, severe myalgia (breakbone fever), adenopathy, palatal vesicles, and scleral injection. Illness usually lasts 1 week, and a maculopapular rash often appears near the time of defervescence. Epistaxis, petechiae, and GI bleeding may occur. Leukopenia, thrombocytopenia, and increased serum aminotransferase levels may be documented. IgM ELISA, antigen-detection ELISA, or RT-PCR during the acute phase permits the diagnosis. Virus is easily isolated from blood during the acute phase.

Encephalitis   Depending on the causative virus, there is much variability in the ratio of clinical to subclinical disease, mortality, and residua (Table 112-2). The pt usually presents with a prodrome of nonspecific symptoms followed quickly by headache, meningeal signs, photophobia, and vomiting. Complications include deepening lethargy and ultimately coma, tremors, cranial nerve palsies, and focal neurologic signs and seizures. Acute encephalitis usually lasts from a few days to 2–3 weeks, but recovery may be slow. Treatable causes of encephalitis (e.g., HSV) should be ruled out quickly. Many viruses cause arboviral encephalitis. Some important examples follow.

- *Japanese encephalitis*: This infection is present throughout Asia and is occasionally found in the western Pacific islands. An effective vaccine (given on days 0, 7, and 30) is available and is indicated for summer travelers to rural Asia, where the risk can be as high as 2.1 cases per 10,000 per week. Expatriates have an especially high risk of severe and often fatal disease. There is a 0.1–1% chance of a vaccine reaction (which may be severe but is rarely fatal) beginning 1–9 days after vaccination. Spinal and motor neuron disease can be seen in addition to the encephalitis.
- *West Nile encephalitis*: Usually a mild or asymptomatic disease, West Nile virus infection can cause aseptic meningitis or encephalitis and is also associated with spinal and motor neuron disease. First diagnosed in New York City, the disease has been most severe among the elderly and is associated with muscle weakness and even flaccid paralysis. It has now spread throughout the United States.
- *Eastern equine encephalitis*: This disease is found primarily within endemic swampy foci along the eastern coast of the United States, with inland foci as distant as Michigan. It is most common in the summer and early fall. Horses are the primary targets for the virus. Contact with unimmunized horses is a risk factor for human disease. One of the most severe arboviral conditions, eastern equine encephalitis has a rapid onset, rapid progression, high mortality, and frequent residua. Necrotic lesions and PMN infiltrates are found in the brain at autopsy. PMN-predominant pleocytosis of the CSF within the first 3 days of disease is common, as is leukocytosis with a left shift in peripheral blood.

Arthritis and Rash   Arboviruses are common causes of true arthritis accompanied by a febrile illness and maculopapular rash. Examples include *Sindbis virus*, which is found in northern Europe and the independent states of the former Soviet Union; *chikungunya virus*, which is of African origin; and *Ross River virus*, a cause of epidemic polyarthritis in Australia since the start of the twentieth century.

Hemorrhagic Fever   The viral HF syndrome is a constellation of findings based on vascular instability and decreased vascular integrity. Pts develop local hemorrhage, hypotension, and—in severe cases—shock. All HF syndromes begin with the abrupt onset of fever and myalgia and can progress to severe prostration, headache, dizziness, photophobia, abdominal and/or chest pain, anorexia, and GI disturbances. On initial physical examination, there is conjunctival suffusion, muscle or abdominal tenderness to palpation, hypotension, petechiae, and periorbital edema. Laboratory examination usually reveals elevated serum aminotransferase levels, proteinuria, and hemoconcentration. Shock, multifocal bleeding, and CNS involvement (encephalopathy, coma, convulsions) are poor prognostic signs. Early recognition is important; appropriate supportive measures and, in some cases, virus-specific therapy can be instituted.

I. *Lassa fever*: Endemic and epidemic in West Africa, Lassa fever virus is spread to humans by aerosols from chronically infected rodents. Transmission by close person-to-person contact can occur. A gradual onset gives way to more severe constitutional symptoms and prostration. Bleeding is evident in 15–30% of cases. CNS dysfunction is marked by confusion, tremors of the upper extremity and tongue, and cerebellar signs; effusions, including pericarditis in men, are common. Pregnant women have higher mortality rates, and the fetal death rate is 92% in the last trimester. Pts who are pregnant should consider termination of the pregnancy. Pts with high-level viremia or a serum aspartate aminotransferase level of >150 IU/mL are at an elevated risk of death, and the administration of ribavirin, which appears to reduce mortality, should be considered. Ribavirin is given by slow IV infusion; an initial dose of 32 mg/kg is followed by 16 mg/kg q6h for 4 days and then by 8 mg/kg q8h for 6 days.

II. *South American HF syndromes* (Argentine, Bolivian, Venezuelan, Brazilian): These syndromes resemble Lassa fever; however, thrombocytopenia and bleeding are common, whereas CNS dysfunction is not. Passive antibody treatment for Argentine HF is effective, and an effective vaccine exists. Ribavirin is likely to be effective in all South American HF syndromes.

III. *Rift Valley fever*: Antibody or ribavirin therapy is likely to be effective.

IV. *Crimean-Congo HF*: This disease is similar to other HF syndromes but causes extensive liver damage and jaundice. Ribavirin should be given in severe cases.

V. *HF with renal syndrome*
   A. This entity is most often caused in Europe by Puumala virus (rodent reservoir, the bank vole) and in Asia by Hantaan virus (rodent reservoir, the striped field mouse). More than 100,000 cases of severe disease occur annually in endemic areas of Asia. Severe classic Hantaan disease has four stages.
      1. Febrile period: abrupt onset of fever, headache, myalgia, thirst
      2. Hypotensive phase: falling blood pressure; relative bradycardia; laboratory findings including leukocytosis with a left shift, atypical lymphocytosis, proteinuria, vascular leakage causing hemoconcentration, and renal tubular necrosis
      3. Oliguric phase: continuing hemorrhage; oliguria persisting for 3–10 days before renal function returns
      4. Polyuric stage: As renal function returns, there is a danger of dehydration and electrolyte abnormalities.
   B. Diagnosis can be made by IgM-capture ELISA, which should yield a positive result within 48 h of admission. RT-PCR of a blood clot gives a positive result early in the clinical course.
   C. Treatment: Expectant management of shock and renal failure is crucial. Ribavirin may reduce mortality and morbidity in severe cases if treatment is begun within the first 4 days of illness.

VI. *Hantavirus pulmonary syndrome* (HPS): The disease is linked to rodent exposure and particularly affects rural residents in dwellings permeable to rodent entry. Sin Nombre virus infects the deer mouse and is the most important virus causing HPS in the United States.
   A. Clinical findings include the following:
      1. Prodrome (3–4 days; range, 1–11 days): fever, myalgia, dizziness, vertigo, malaise, nausea, vomiting, abdominal pain
      2. Cardiopulmonary phase: tachycardia, hypotension, tachypnea, early signs of pulmonary edema
      3. Final phase: rapid decompensation with hypoxemia, respiratory failure, low cardiac output, myocardial depression, increased pulmonary vascular permeability, shock

Table 112-2

Prominent Features of Arboviral Encephalitis

Virus	Natural Cycle	Incubation Period, Days	Annual No. of Cases
La Crosse	*Aedes triseriatus*— chipmunk (transovarial component in mosquito also important)	~3–7	70 (U.S.)
St. Louis	*Culex tarsalis, C. pipiens, C. quinquefasciatus*— birds	4–21	85, with hundreds to thousands in epidemic years (U.S.)
Japanese	*Culex tritaeniorhyncus*— birds	5–15	>25,000
West Nile	*Culex* mosquitoes—birds	3–6	?
Central European	*Ixodes ricinus*—rodents, insectivores	7–14	Thousands
Russian spring-summer	*I. persulcatus*—rodents, insectivores	7–14	Hundreds
Powassan	*I. cookei*—wild mammals	~10	~1 (U.S.)
Eastern equine	*Culiseta melanura*—birds	~5–10	5 (U.S.)
Western equine	*Culex tarsalis*—birds	~5–10	~20 (U.S.)
Venezuelan equine (epidemic)	Unknown (multiple mosquito species and horses in epidemics)	1–5	?

   B. Laboratory findings include thrombocytopenia (an important early clue), atypical lymphocytes, and a left shift, often with leukocytosis; hemoconcentration; hypoalbuminemia; and proteinuria. IgM testing of acute-phase serum can yield positive results, even during the prodromal stage. RT-PCR of blood clots or tissue usually gives a positive result in the first 7–9 days of illness.
   C. Treatment: Intensive respiratory management and other supportive measures are crucial in the first few hours after presentation. Shock should be managed with pressor agents and modest amounts of fluid.

Case-to-Infection Ratio	Age of Cases	Case-Fatality Rate, %	Residua
<1:1000	<15 years	<0.5	Recurrent seizures in ~10%; severe deficits in rare cases; decreased school performance and behavioral change suspected in small proportion
<1:200	Milder cases in the young; more severe cases in adults >40 years old, particularly the elderly	7	Common in the elderly
1:200–300	All ages; children in highly endemic areas	20–50	Common (approximately half of cases); may be severe
Very low	Mainly the elderly	5–10	Uncommon
1:12	All ages; milder in children	1–5	20%
—	All ages; milder in children	20	Approximately half of cases; often severe; limb-girdle paralysis
—	All ages; some predilection for children	~10	Common (approximately half of cases)
1:40 adult 1:17 child	All ages; predilection for children	50–75	Common
1:1000 adult 1:50 child 1:1 infant	All ages; predilection for children <2 years old (increased mortality in elderly)	3–7	Common only among infants <1 year old
1:250 adult 1:25 child (approximate)	All ages; predilection for children	~10	—

    D. Prognosis: Most pts who survive for 48 h recover without residua. Mortality rates are ~30–40% despite optimal management.

VII. *Yellow fever*: Yellow fever is a former cause of major epidemics. Hundreds of cases in South America and thousands of cases in Africa still occur. Yellow fever causes a typical HF syndrome with prominent hepatic necrosis. Pts are viremic for 3–4 days and can have jaundice, hemorrhage, black vomit, anuria, and terminal delirium. Vaccination of visitors to endemic areas and control of the mosquito vector *A. aegypti* prevent disease.

VIII. *Dengue hemorrhagic fever (DHF)/dengue shock syndrome (DSS)*: Previous infection with a heterologous dengue virus serotype may elicit nonprotective antibodies and enhanced disease if pts are reinfected. The risk decreases considerably after age 12; DHF/DSS is more common among females than among males, more severe among Caucasians than among blacks, and less common among malnourished than among well-nourished persons. DHF is marked by bleeding tendencies. DSS is more serious because of vascular permeability leading to shock. In mild cases, lethargy, thrombocytopenia, and hemoconcentration occur 2–5 days after typical dengue fever, usually at the time of defervescence. In severe cases, frank shock occurs with cyanosis, hepatomegaly, ascites and pleural effusions, and GI bleeding. Shock lasts for 1–2 days and usually responds to supportive measures. With good care, the overall mortality rate is as low as 1%. Control of *A. aegypti*, the mosquito vector, is the key to control of the disease.

EBOLA AND MARBURG VIRUS INFECTIONS

ETIOLOGY   Marburg and Ebola viruses are two distinct single-stranded RNA viruses of the family Filoviridae. Almost all Filoviridae are African viruses that cause severe disease with high mortality rates. Both Marburg virus and Ebola virus are biosafety level 4 pathogens because of the high mortality rate from infection and the aerosol infectivity of the agents.

EPIDEMIOLOGY   The first human cases of Marburg virus infection occurred in laboratory workers exposed to infected African green monkeys from Uganda. Ebola virus has been associated with epidemics of severe hemorrhagic fever. The first two epidemics were due to different subtypes: Zaire, with 90% mortality, and Sudan, with 50% mortality. Interhuman spread was noted. However, epidemiologic studies in humans have failed to yield evidence for an important role of airborne particles in human Ebola virus disease unlike that seen for monkeys. The reservoir is unknown but is believed to be nonprimate.

PATHOGENESIS   Both viruses replicate well in virtually all cell types, and viral replication is associated with cellular necrosis. Acute infection is associated with high levels of circulating virus and viral antigen until antibody development, evidence of which is usually lacking in fatal cases. Virions are abundant in fibroblasts, interstitium, and SC tissues and may escape through breaks in the skin or through sweat glands—a potential scenario that may be correlated with the risk of transmission through close pt contact or by touching of deceased pts. High levels of circulating proinflammatory cytokines contribute to disease severity.

CLINICAL FEATURES   After a 7- to 10-day incubation period, pts experience an abrupt onset of fever, headache, severe myalgia, nausea, vomiting, diarrhea, prostration, and depressed mentation. A maculopapular rash may appear at day 5–7 and be followed by desquamation. Bleeding can occur from any mucosal site and into the skin. After 10–12 days, the fever breaks and the pt recovers, but recrudescence and secondary bacterial infection may occur.

LABORATORY FINDINGS   Leukopenia is common early on and is followed by neutrophilia. Thrombocytopenia, DIC, and increases in serum aminotransferase and amylase levels can develop. Proteinuria and renal failure are proportional to shock.

DIAGNOSIS   High concentrations of virus in blood can be documented by antigen detection ELISA, virus isolation, or RT-PCR. Antibodies can be detected in recovering pts.

TREATMENT

Supportive measures may not be as useful as had been hoped, but studies in rhesus monkeys suggest that an inhibitor of factor VIIa/tissue factor may improve survival rates.

For a more detailed discussion, see Hanlon CA, Corey L: Rabies Virus and Other Rhabdoviruses, Chap. 179, p. 1155; Peters CJ: Infections Caused by Arthropod- and Rodent-Borne Viruses, Chap. 180, p. 1161; and Peters CJ: Marburg and Ebola Viruses, Chap. 181, p. 1174, in HPIM-16.

FUNGAL INFECTIONS

GENERAL CONSIDERATIONS

Yeasts (e.g., *Candida*, *Cryptococcus*) appear microscopically as round, budding forms; *molds* (e.g., *Aspergillus*, *Rhizopus*) appear microscopically as hyphae; and *dimorphic fungi* (e.g., *Histoplasma*) are spherical in tissue but appear as molds in culture. Fungi that are pathogenic for humans are saprophytic in nature and infect hosts preferentially by one route—e.g., inhalation or inoculation into the skin or cornea. Person-to-person transmission of fungal infections (except for ringworm) is rare.

ANTIFUNGAL TREATMENTS
Topical Agents

1. Imidazoles and triazoles (e.g., clotrimazole, ketoconazole, miconazole): inhibit ergosterol synthesis in the fungal cell wall
2. Polyene macrolides (e.g., nystatin, amphotericin B suspensions): bind to sterol in the fungal cytoplasmic membrane, increasing membrane permeability
3. Other topical agents (e.g., terbinafine, ciclopirox olamine)

Systemic Agents

GRISEOFULVIN Treats some dermatophytes; interacts with warfarin, phenobarbital

TERBINAFINE A dose of 250 mg/d is as effective as itraconazole and superior to griseofulvin against onychomycosis and ringworm. Terbinafine treatment decreases cyclosporine levels. Cimetidine increases and rifampin decreases terbinafine levels.

IMIDAZOLES AND TRIAZOLES Ketoconazole is the most widely used imidazole. The triazoles are fluconazole, itraconazole, voriconazole, and investigational agents posaconazole and ravuconazole. Triazoles have less impact on human hormonal synthesis and are less hepatotoxic than imidazoles.

Drug interactions are most common with ketoconazole and itraconazole. All azoles have the potential for embryotoxicity and teratogenicity.

Itraconazole Useful for blastomycosis, histoplasmosis, cutaneous candidiasis, coccidioidomycosis, sporotrichosis, pseudallescheriasis, onychomycosis, ringworm, tinea versicolor, and indolent aspergillosis

- Metabolized by liver; hydroxyl metabolite responsible for half of antifungal activity in serum
- The multiple drug interactions and contraindicated agents should be checked before prescribing.
- Capsules are less expensive and cause less GI distress than the oral solution, but their absorption is problematic.
- Cyclodextrin, used in oral solution and IV formulation, is renally excreted but is not absorbed from the GI tract.
- Food increases absorption of capsules by threefold but reduces absorption of oral suspension.
- Minimal CSF penetration
- Blood levels can be used to document absorption of oral drug.

Fluconazole Useful in candidal and cryptococcal infections; less effective than itraconazole in blastomycosis, histoplasmosis, sporotrichosis; not active against aspergillosis or mucormycosis

- Can be given daily because of 31-h half-life
- Unlike itraconazole, is absorbed independent of food or gastric acid; has less effect on hepatic metabolism of other agents
- Of the dose given, 80% is excreted unchanged in urine. Reduce doses in pts with significant decreases in creatinine clearance rate (CCR).
- Penetrates CSF and other body fluids well

Voriconazole Active against fungi that fluconazole and itraconazole treat

- Multiple drug interactions similar to those of itraconazole. These and contraindicated agents should be checked before prescribing.
- Well absorbed, metabolized completely by liver; dose adjustments in pts with hepatic dysfunction
- Because of renal excretion of cyclodextrin in the IV formulation, oral treatment is indicated in pts with a CCR <50 mL/min.
- Good CSF penetration

ECHINOCANDINS

- Caspofungin, the only echinocandin on the market, is for IV administration only. It inhibits synthesis of $(1,3)\beta$-D-glucan in the cell wall and is useful against all *Candida* species except *C. parapsilosis* (variable activity).
- Minor drug interactions: Cyclosporine increases caspofungin levels.
- Poor CSF penetration

AMPHOTERICIN B

- Most active against histoplasmosis, blastomycosis, paracoccidioidomycosis, candidiasis, cryptococcosis; medium activity against aspergillosis, coccidioidomycosis, extraarticular sporotrichosis, aspergillosis, mucormycosis
- Administration is associated with febrile reactions. Premedication with aspirin, acetaminophen, or hydrocortisone decreases chills and fever. The drug should be infused in 5% dextrose over 2–4 h.
- Azotemia is usual; prehydrate pt with saline solutions.
- Side effects: anemia, hypokalemia, renal tubular acidosis
- Lipid formulations reduce nephrotoxicity but not infusion-related reactions. There is no evidence that these formulations are more effective against any mycosis than conventional amphotericin B.

CANDIDIASIS

ETIOLOGY *Candida* species (except *C. glabrata*) are seen in tissue as yeast forms with pseudohyphae (elongated branching structures with constrictions at the septae). *C. albicans* and the closely related *C. dubliniensis* are most common; they cause mucosal disease and half of cases of invasive disease and form germ tubes in serum that can be used for rapid diagnostic testing. *C. tropicalis*, *C. parapsilosis*, *C. glabrata*, *C. krusei*, and other species cause the remaining cases of invasive disease, usually associated with intravascular catheters.

PATHOGENESIS

- Common commensals of mouth, vagina, stool. Broad-spectrum antibiotic treatment increases colonization.
- Invasive infections are often preceded by increased colonization. Colonizing organisms pass to deep tissues when mucosal or skin integrity is violated.
- Neonates of low birth weight, neutropenic pts, pts taking high-dose glucocorticoids, and pts with other impairments of host defenses are especially susceptible to hematogenous seeding, which commonly affects the retina, kidney, spleen, and liver.

CLINICAL FEATURES

1. *Oral thrush*: discrete or confluent adherent white plaques on oral/pharyngeal mucosa; seen in neonatal period, diabetes, and HIV infection and after antibiotic treatments
2. *Vulvovaginal thrush*: pruritus, discharge, dyspareunia; associated with HIV disease and third trimester of pregnancy as well as antibiotic treatments
3. *Cutaneous candidiasis*: red macerated intertriginous areas, paronychia, balanitis, pruritus ani
4. *Esophageal candidiasis*: substernal pain or sense of blockage on swallowing
5. *Urinary tract candidiasis*: Candidal colonization secondary to indwelling catheters is common; if the urinary tract is obstructed, *Candida* causes cystitis and upper tract disease.
6. *Candidemia*: often originating from intravascular catheter
   a. Nonneutropenic pts: Candidemia can clear with catheter removal. Retina may become seeded, causing enlarging lesions that can result in retinal detachment, vitreous abscess, or extension to the anterior chamber. Pts note blurred vision, pain, or scotoma. Risk of retinal disease is the main reason for systemic therapy in these pts.
   b. Neutropenic pts: *Hepatosplenic candidiasis* usually occurs in pts with acute leukemia who are recovering from profound neutropenia, arising from intestinal seeding of the portal and venous circulation. Fever, alkaline phosphatase elevation, and multiple small abscesses on imaging are consistent with the diagnosis. *Skin lesions* consist of erythematous papules that may develop a necrotic center.
7. *Other*: pneumonia, endocarditis, indolent arthritis after glucocorticoid injections, peritonitis in association with peritoneal dialysis catheter

DIAGNOSIS

- Demonstration of pseudohyphae on wet smear with culture confirmation
- *Candida* yeast cells and pseudohyphae are the only fungi that stain grampositive.
- *Candida* grows well in culture on simple media. Exclude colonization (as opposed to true infection).
- Positive cultures from multiple sites are associated with invasive candidiasis in at-risk pts.

℞ TREATMENT

- *Cutaneous*: topical azoles or nystatin
- *Vulvovaginal*: vaginal azole suppositories or fluconazole (150 mg PO once)
- *Oropharyngeal*: clotrimazole troches (5 times daily) or fluconazole (100 mg/d)
- *Esophageal*: fluconazole (100–200 mg/d). Itraconazole or amphotericin B can be used if fluconazole treatment fails.
- *Deeply invasive candidiasis*

  1. Nonneutropenic pts: catheter removal and fluconazole (400 mg/d for 2 weeks after pt becomes afebrile). Alternatives: amphotericin B (0.5 mg/kg daily) or caspofungin (70 mg once, then 50 mg/d IV)
  2. Neutropenic pts: amphotericin B (0.5–0.7 mg/kg daily). Treatment should continue until the pt has been afebrile and nonneutropenic for 2 weeks. Relapse during the next bout of neutropenia is common.
  3. Foreign materials (e.g., catheters) should be removed and infected tissue debrided when possible.

- *C. krusei* and *C. inconspicua* are resistant to fluconazole in vitro; *C. glabrata* exhibits intermediate sensitivity.

PREVENTION

- Allogeneic bone marrow transplant recipients have a decreased incidence of invasive candidal infections if prophylaxis with fluconazole (400 mg/d) is given daily either for 70 days or until engraftment.
- Prophylaxis in acute leukemic and other neutropenic pts is controversial. Prophylaxis may be useful in high-risk postoperative pts.
- HIV-infected pts generally should not receive chronic prophylaxis against recurrent mucocutaneous disease because of the potential for emergence of fluconazole resistance.

ASPERGILLOSIS

ETIOLOGY *Aspergillus* is a mold with septate branching hyphae ~2–4 μm in diameter. *A. fumigatus* is the most common cause of aspergillosis.

PATHOGENESIS

- All disease-causing *Aspergillus* species are ubiquitous in the environment.
- Inhalation is common; disease is rare.
- More than 90% of pts with aspergillosis have 2 of 3 risk factors: (1) neutropenia ($<500/\mu$L), (2) treatment with supraphysiologic doses of glucocorticoids, (3) history of treatment with other immunosuppressive agents.
- Invasive disease is characterized by hyphal invasion of blood vessels, thrombosis, necrosis, and hemorrhagic infarction.

CLINICAL FEATURES

1. *Allergic bronchopulmonary aspergillosis* (ABPA)
   a. Seen in glucocorticoid-dependent asthmatics and cystic fibrosis pts
   b. Intermittent wheezing, infiltrates due to bronchial plugging, eosinophilia, sputum
2. *Aspergilloma*: hyphal ball in preexisting pulmonary cyst or cavity, usually upper lobe, without tissue invasion
3. *Endobronchial saprophytic pulmonary aspergillosis*: chronic cough with hemoptysis due to endobronchial *Aspergillus* colonization in pts with chronic pulmonary disease

4. *Invasive aspergillosis*
   a. Rapidly progressive pulmonary infiltrate extending across tissue planes and spreading hematogenously to lung, brain, and other organs; nodules with central core of infarcted tissue surrounded by edema or hemorrhage (*halo sign*); cavitation of core when bone marrow function returns (*crescent sign*)
   b. Nasal lesions with rapid extension into paranasal sinuses, orbit, or face
5. *Aspergillus sinusitis in immunocompetent pts*: three presentations
   a. Fungal ball without invasion in a diseased, chronically infected sinus
   b. Chronic granulomatous inflammation invasive to orbit and brain
   c. Allergic fungal sinusitis
6. *Aspergillosis and HIV*: usually pulmonary disease with fever, cough, dyspnea

DIAGNOSIS

- Repeated isolation of *Aspergillus* from sputum or bronchoalveolar lavage fluid suggests colonization or infection. In compromised pts with pneumonia (see risk factors above), even a single positive specimen should be considered indicative of invasive disease.
- Biopsy of involved sites demonstrating organism on histology and culture
- IgE antibody to *Aspergillus* antigens seen in ABPA
- Galactomannan antigen in serum has low sensitivity early in disease; false-positive tests occur.

R̲x̲ TREATMENT

- Endobronchial or endocavitary aspergillosis (aspergilloma) pts do not benefit from treatment with antifungal agents. Consider lobectomy in cases of severe hemoptysis.
- ABPA: Use a short course of glucocorticoids as needed. Prophylactic itraconazole may be of some benefit in select pts.
- Invasive aspergillosis: IV voriconazole (6 mg/kg bid for 2 doses, then 4 mg/kg bid) is more efficacious than amphotericin B treatment. After clinical improvement, oral voriconazole (200 mg bid) can be considered. Liposomal amphotericin (5 mg/kg per day) is equivalent to conventional amphotericin B in efficacy but is less toxic. Itraconazole (200 mg bid) may be used in less severely immunosuppressed pts with indolent or slowly progressive disease. Caspofungin (70 mg once, then 50 mg/d) can be considered only if other treatments fail.
- Fungus ball of sinus or allergic fungal sinusitis may be treated surgically. Systemic therapy is not helpful, but chronic suppression has been used postoperatively in allergic sinusitis.

CRYPTOCOCCOSIS

ETIOLOGY   *Cryptococcus neoformans* reproduces by budding to form round, yeastlike cells. In the host and on some culture media, a large polysaccharide capsule surrounds each cell.

EPIDEMIOLOGY   Found in pigeon droppings (serotypes A and D) and in litter around eucalyptus trees (*C. neoformans* var. *gattii*, serotype B); strongly associated with HIV infection, treatment with glucocorticoids or immunosuppressive drugs, and other cellular immunosuppression

PATHOGENESIS   Most cases are acquired via inhalation, with consequent pulmonary infection. Silent hematogenous spread to the brain can occur.

CLINICAL FEATURES

1. *Pulmonary manifestations*
   a. Lesions with granulomatous reactions
   b. Usually asymptomatic but chest pain in 40%, cough in 20%
   c. One or more dense, well-circumscribed infiltrates on CXR
   d. Cryptococcomas: usually in immunocompetent pts; associated with *C. neoformans* var. *gattii* infections
2. *Meningoencephalitis*: most common presentation. HIV pts often have a paucity of clinical findings (beyond headache and fever).
   a. Early: headache, nausea, dementia, irritability, confusion, blurred vision, staggering gait
   b. Papilledema in one-third of pts at diagnosis; cranial nerve palsies in one-fourth
   c. Deepening coma, brainstem compression with disease progression
3. *Skin lesions*
   a. Seen in 10% of pts
   b. Associated with disseminated cryptococcosis
   c. Papular lesions that enlarge, with central softening and ulceration
4. *Other findings*: osteolytic lesions, prostatitis, endophthalmitis, hepatitis, pericarditis, endocarditis, renal abscess

DIAGNOSIS

- India ink smear of centrifuged CSF sediment demonstrates encapsulated yeast in >50% of cases. Pts without HIV disease have low glucose and high protein levels in CSF, with lymphocyte-predominant pleocytosis.
- Obtain tissue samples for methenamine silver or periodic acid–Schiff staining and for cultures. Culture CSF, blood, urine, and sputum as indicated.
- Cryptococcal capsular antigen testing by latex agglutination of CSF, serum

℞ TREATMENT

1. HIV-infected pts: amphotericin B (0.7–1.0 mg/kg daily) for at least 2 weeks. When clinically stable, pts can switch to fluconazole (400 mg/d). Negativity of CSF cultures should be documented. After a total course of at least 10 weeks of therapy, fluconazole (200 mg/d) should be given indefinitely.
2. HIV-seronegative pts
   a. Meningitis: amphotericin B (0.6–0.7 mg/d) until cultures become negative (at least 10 weeks). Fluconazole (400 mg/d) to finish a course of 6–12 months is generally recommended. Culture conversion, normalization of CSF glucose levels, and a fall in CSF antigen titers are minimal end points that should be reached before the discontinuation of therapy.
   b. Pulmonary cryptococcosis: fluconazole for 6–12 months

MUCORMYCOSIS

ETIOLOGY Mucormycosis is caused primarily by *Rhizopus*, *Rhizomucor*, and *Cunninghamella*, fungi that have broad, rarely septate hyphae of uneven diameter in tissue.

EPIDEMIOLOGY *Rhizopus* and *Rhizomucor* species are ubiquitous in the environment. Pts at risk are those with diabetes, organ transplantation, or hematologic malignancy and those receiving long-term deferoxamine therapy (which chelates iron to a form the fungus can use).

PATHOLOGY Fungal hyphae cause vascular invasion and ischemic or hemorrhagic necrosis.

CLINICAL FEATURES

1. *Nose and paranasal sinus disease*
   a. Low-grade fever, dull sinus pain, nasal congestion, thin bloody discharge
   b. Progression to double vision, fever, obtundation, blindness
   c. Unilateral reduction of ocular motion, chemosis, proptosis, dusky or necrotic nasal turbinates on involved side
   d. Sharply delineated area of necrosis respecting the midline on the hard palate
2. *Pulmonary mucormycosis*
   a. Progressive severe pneumonia with high fever and toxicity
   b. Large infiltrates may have central necrosis and cavitation.
   c. Fatal hemoptysis may result from cavities near hilum.
   d. Hematogenous spread within lung, to brain and other organs
   e. Death within 2 weeks is usual.
3. *GI and cutaneous manifestations* have been described.

DIAGNOSIS Biopsy sites of infection for histology and culture (although cultures are often negative). In sinusitis, use imaging studies to assess the extent of disease before surgery.

 TREATMENT

- Control diabetes and reduce use of immunosuppressive agents, if possible.
- Perform extensive surgical debridement.
- Use the maximal tolerated dose of IV amphotericin B deoxycholate (1.0–1.5 mg/kg daily) or liposomal amphotericin B (5 mg/kg daily) until progression is halted (course, 10–12 weeks).
- Survival is rare among pts with pulmonary, GI, or disseminated disease. Craniofacial infections are cured half the time with appropriate therapy.

HISTOPLASMOSIS

ETIOLOGY *Histoplasma capsulatum* var. *capsulatum* is an unencapsulated dimorphic fungus with hyphae that bear large and small spores.

EPIDEMIOLOGY Histoplasmosis is endemic in the southeastern, mid-Atlantic, and central United States and in Latin America. The fungus is found in moist soil, particularly that enriched by droppings of certain birds and bats.

PATHOGENESIS AND PATHOLOGY Microconidia or small spores are inhaled, reach the alveoli, and are transformed to budding forms. A granulomatous reaction results that can mimic tuberculosis; it progresses or becomes disseminated in a small minority of pts.

CLINICAL FEATURES

1. *Acute pulmonary histoplasmosis*
   a. Asymptomatic or mild respiratory disease with cough, fever, hilar adenopathy, pneumonitis
   b. Occasionally associated with erythema nodosum or erythema multiforme, subacute pericarditis
2. *Mediastinal fibrosis associated with histoplasmosis* (rare): Hilar nodes caseate and fibrose, and mediastinal structures become encased by progressive fibrosis.
3. *Chronic pulmonary histoplasmosis*
   a. Most often affects men >40 years old with a smoking history or emphysema

     b. Increasing cough, weight loss, night sweats, fibronodular apical infiltrates, cavitation, emphysema, and bulla formation

     c. One-third of pts have spontaneous stabilization or improvement. Others die of cor pulmonale, bacterial pneumonia, or histoplasmosis in months to years.

4. *Disseminated histoplasmosis*

     a. Fever, emaciation, lymphadenopathy, hepatosplenomegaly, pancytopenia

     b. Other findings: skin lesions (particularly in HIV infection), indurated mucosal ulcers, ocular disease

DIAGNOSIS Isolation of *Histoplasma* from blood is difficult. For culture, use lysis-centrifugation technique with plates held at 30°C for at least 2 weeks. Culture lung or other sites in disseminated disease.

• Giemsa-stained smears of blood or bronchoalveolar lavage fluid or methenamine silver staining of infected tissue
• *Histoplasma* antigen assay of blood or urine is useful in diagnosis and in monitoring the response to treatment.

℞ **TREATMENT**

• Acute disease: no therapy necessary
• Mediastinal fibrosis: vascular stent placement, prognosis poor
• Disseminated or chronic pulmonary disease in immunosuppressed, severely ill pts or those with CNS disease: IV amphotericin B (0.5 mg/kg daily), with change to itraconazole (200 mg bid) after clinical improvement. HIV pts should receive lifelong treatment.
• Immunocompetent pts: itraconazole for 6–12 months or amphotericin B for 10 weeks

COCCIDIOIDOMYCOSIS

ETIOLOGY *Coccidioides immitis* is seen as a mold form on culture media and as a nonbudding spherical form (spherule) in tissue. Endospores, which form within mature spherules, go on to form mature spherules after rupture. Arthrospores are thick-walled, barrel-shaped spores in hyphae of the mold form.

EPIDEMIOLOGY Soil saprophyte in arid regions of the United States (California, Arizona, Texas), Mexico, Central and South America

PATHOGENESIS AND PATHOLOGY Infection, which results from inhalation of wind-borne arthrospores from soil, incites a chronic pyogranuloma in host tissue, often with caseating necrosis.

CLINICAL FEATURES

1. *Primary pulmonary infection*: develops 10–14 days after inhalation; symptomatic in 40% of cases

     a. Fever, cough, chest pain, malaise; also erythema nodosum, erythema multiforme, other hypersensitivity reactions

     b. CXR: infiltrate, hilar adenopathy, pleural effusion

     c. Mild peripheral-blood eosinophilia

     d. Improvement in days to 2 weeks

2. *Chronic fibrocavitary pulmonary disease*: chronic thin-walled cavity; asymptomatic in 50% of cases. Symptomatic pts have cough, hemoptysis, sputum production, and weight loss.

3. *Disseminated infection*

  a. More likely in pts with cell-mediated immunosuppression (e.g., Hodg-
     kin's disease, HIV infection), pregnant women, and certain racial and
     ethnic groups
  b. Fever, malaise, hilar or paratracheal lymphadenopathy, elevated ESR
  c. Bone, skin (maculopapular), SC, joint lesions
  d. Chronic meningitis: indolent onset; CSF smear and culture negative,
     but antibody detectable in CSF by CF

DIAGNOSIS

• Examine tissue by wet smear and culture. Alert laboratory of possible diagnosis to avoid exposure. Nucleic acid hybridization is a safe, accurate way to
identify the fungus.
• Serology: (1) latex agglutination and agar gel diffusion for screening sera;
(2) CF to confirm and quantify antibody and to test CSF; (3) positive tests most
common in disseminated disease, least common in solitary pulmonary cavities
or primary pulmonary infection

 TREATMENT

   • *Solitary cavity*: excision if there are problems with hemoptysis or recurrent
   infections
   • *Primary pneumonia*: observation or amphotericin B (0.5–0.7 mg/kg daily
   IV) followed by itraconazole (200 mg bid PO) or fluconazole (400 mg/d PO)
   • *Disseminated and/or rapidly progressive pneumonia*: amphotericin B ini-
   tially, then (after 2–3 months with improvement) itraconazole or fluconazole
   (see dosages above)
   • *Indolent disseminated infection*: can start therapy with oral medications
   • *Meningitis*: fluconazole (400–800 mg/d) +/− intrathecal amphotericin B

   PROGNOSIS   Prognosis for ultimate cure is guarded in most pts with
disseminated disease.

BLASTOMYCOSIS
Blastomyces dermatitidis is a dimorphic fungus that is found in the southeastern,
central, and mid-Atlantic states of the United States and in Ontario and Manitoba
in Canada. This fungus is an uncommon cause of disease. Its inhalation from
soil, decomposed vegetation, or rotting wood causes a primary pulmonary infection that spreads hematogenously, even if pneumonia resolves spontaneously. Indolent disseminated disease is associated with fever, cough, weight
loss, chest pain, skin lesions, and osteolytic lesions. Blastomycosis may present
with ARDS.

   DIAGNOSIS   Wet smears of clinical samples or culture of sputum, pus,
or urine. Nucleic acid hybridization testing is available.

 TREATMENT

Every pt should be treated because of the high risk of dissemination. Give
amphotericin B for rapidly progressive infections or severe illness; when condition stabilizes (10–12 weeks), switch to itraconazole (400 mg/d for 6–12
months). Treat CNS disease initially with amphotericin B; after 10–12 weeks
and a total dose of 2.5 g, switch to fluconazole (800 mg/d for 6–12 months).
More indolent infections can be treated with itraconazole (400 mg/d for 6–
12 months). Overall mortality is <15% for most cases; with ARDS presentation, mortality exceeds 50%.

PARACOCCIDIOIDOMYCOSIS

Paracoccidioidomycosis (South American blastomycosis) is caused by *Paracoccidioides brasiliensis*, a dimorphic fungus acquired by inhalation from environmental sources in South and Central America and Mexico. Pts have indurated ulcers of the mouth, oropharynx, larynx, and nose; draining, enlarged lymph nodes; skin and genital lesions; cough; weight loss; dyspnea; and patchy pneumonia on CXR.

DIAGNOSIS Histology and culture of infected tissue

 TREATMENT

For most cases, give itraconazole (200–400 mg/d) for at least 1 year. In severe cases, initiate amphotericin B therapy instead, and follow treatment response with serology.

PENICILLIOSIS MARNEFFEI

Penicillium marneffei, a leading cause of opportunistic infection in pts with advanced HIV disease in Southeast Asia, is acquired by spore inhalation. This dimorphic fungus resembles *Histoplasma* but does not bud. A red pigment forms under the organism as it grows in agar. At presentation in most cases, disease has already spread to bone marrow, liver, spleen, skin, or bone.

 TREATMENT

Amphotericin B until clinical improvement is seen; then itraconazole (400 mg/d for 8 weeks, then 200 mg/d as maintenance treatment)

FUSARIOSIS

Fusarium species cause cellulitis or necrotic lesions in immunocompetent pts at sites of trauma; they cause disseminated disease in immunocompromised pts, especially those who are severely neutropenic. The portal of entry is not apparent in most cases. Skin lesions develop in two-thirds of pts; these erythematous papules can have central necrosis. Blood cultures are positive in 59% of cases; in contrast, blood cultures are rarely positive in aspergillosis or mucormycosis.

 TREATMENT

Voriconazole or amphotericin B

MALASSEZIA INFECTION

Malassezia furfur, part of the normal skin flora, can cause tinea (pityriasis) versicolor. Catheter-acquired *Malassezia* sepsis is seen in pts (especially neonates) receiving IV lipids and is cured by catheter removal.

PSEUDALLESCHERIASIS

Pseudallescheria (*Petriellidium*) *boydii* causes clinical and histologic manifestations that are difficult to distinguish from those caused by *Aspergillus*. Both organisms exhibit intravascular hyphae in tissue.

DIAGNOSIS Tissue and culture confirmation

TREATMENT

The response to treatment is poor in compromised hosts. Amphotericin B has little activity. Voriconazole and itraconazole are the best choices. Surgical drainage or debridement may be helpful.

SPOROTRICHOSIS

Sporothrix schenckii is a dimorphic fungus that lives as a saprophyte on plants. Infection, which results from inoculation into SC tissue by minor trauma, is seen especially often in florists, gardeners, and nursery workers.

CLINICAL FEATURES

• *Lymphangitic disease*: most common presentation; painless red papule at site of inoculation, progressing to similar nodules along lymphatic channels proximally
• *Plaque sporotrichosis*: maculopapular granuloma confined to site of inoculation
• *Extracutaneous sites*: portal for infection thought to be lung

DIAGNOSIS Culture or skin biopsy

 TREATMENT

For cutaneous sporotrichosis, give itraconazole (100–200 mg/d) or potassium iodide solution. For extracutaneous disease, itraconazole (200 mg bid) can be given, but amphotericin B is more effective.

DERMATOPHYTOSIS

See "Common Skin Conditions," Chap. 62.

For a more detailed discussion, see Bennett JE: Diagnosis and Treatment of Fungal Infections, Chap. 182, p. 1176; Histoplasmosis, Chap. 183, p. 1179; Coccidioidomycosis, Chap. 184, p. 1180; Blastomycosis, Chap. 185, p. 1182; Cryptococcosis, Chap. 186, p. 1183; Candidiasis, Chap. 187, p. 1185; Aspergillosis, Chap. 188, p. 1188; Mucormycosis, Chap. 189, p. 1190; and Miscellaneous Mycoses and Algal Infections, Chap. 190, p. 1191, in HPIM-16.

PNEUMOCYSTIS INFECTION

Pneumocystis, an opportunistic fungal pulmonary pathogen, is an important cause of pneumonia in the immunocompromised host. In contrast to most fungi, *Pneumocystis* lacks ergosterol and is not susceptible to antifungal drugs that inhibit ergosterol synthesis. Developmental stages include the small trophic form; the cyst, which contains up to eight intracystic bodies; and the intermediate precyst stage.

Epidemiology

Pneumocystis is found worldwide. Most healthy children have been exposed to the organism by 3–4 years of age. Both airborne transmission and person-to-person transmission have been demonstrated.

Pathogenesis

Defects in cellular and humoral immunity predispose to *Pneumocystis* pneumonia. HIV-infected persons are at particular risk, and the risk rises dramatically when CD4+ T cell counts fall below $200/\mu L$. Other persons at risk include those receiving immunosuppressive therapy (particularly glucocorticoids) for cancer, organ transplantation, or other disorders; malnourished premature infants; and children with primary immunodeficiency disorders. The organisms are inhaled and attach tightly to type I cells in alveoli, although they remain extracellular. With immunosuppression, the organisms propagate and fill the alveoli, resulting in increased alveolar-capillary permeability and damage to alveolar type I cells. On histology, alveoli are seen to be filled with foamy, vacuolated exudates. Severe disease may cause interstitial edema, fibrosis, and hyaline membrane formation.

Clinical and Laboratory Features

Pts develop dyspnea, fever, and nonproductive cough. Pts without HIV infection often become symptomatic after their glucocorticoid dose has been tapered, and symptoms last 1–2 weeks. HIV-infected pts are usually ill for several weeks or longer with more subtle manifestations. On physical examination, pts are found to have tachypnea, tachycardia, and cyanosis, but findings on pulmonary examination are often unremarkable. Reduced arterial oxygen pressure, increased alveolar-arterial oxygen gradient, and respiratory alkalosis are evident. Gallium scans can be positive, with nonspecific uptake in the lungs. Serum LDH levels can be elevated, but this finding is nonspecific. CXR classically reveals bilateral diffuse infiltrates beginning in the perihilar regions. Other findings (e.g., nodular densities, cavitary lesions) have been described. Pneumothorax may occur. Rare cases of disseminated infection have been described, mainly in HIV pts taking aerosolized pentamidine. Lymph nodes, spleen, liver, and bone marrow are most often involved.

Diagnosis

Histopathologic staining makes the definitive diagnosis. Methenamine silver, toluidine blue, and cresyl echt violet selectively stain the wall of *Pneumocystis* cysts. Wright-Giemsa stains the nuclei of all developmental stages. Immunofluorescence with monoclonal antibodies increases diagnostic sensitivity, but DNA amplification by PCR is most sensitive. Proper specimens are key. HIV-infected pts have a higher organism burden, and their *Pneumocystis* infections can often be diagnosed by means of sputum induction. However, fiberoptic bronchoscopy with bronchoalveolar lavage (BAL) remains the mainstay of diagnosis. Transbronchial biopsy and open lung biopsy are used only when BAL is negative.

Course and Prognosis

Therapy is most effective if started early, before there is extensive alveolar damage. The mortality rate is 15–20% at 1 month and 50–55% at 1 year among

HIV-infected pts. The risk of early death remains high among people who need mechanical ventilation (60%) and among non-HIV pts (40%). The degree of hypoxemia predicts outcome.

℞ TREATMENT

Pts are classified as having disease that is mild (a $Pa_{O_2} > 70$ mmHg or a $PA_{O_2} - Pa_{O_2}$ gradient < 35 mmHg on room air) or moderate to severe (a $Pa_{O_2} \leq 70$ mmHg or a $PA_{O_2} - Pa_{O_2}$ gradient ≥ 35 mmHg). Trimethoprim-sulfamethoxazole (TMP-SMX) is the drug of choice for all pts. For doses and adverse effects of TMP-SMX and alternative regimens, see Table 114-1. For mild to moderate cases, alternatives include TMP plus dapsone or clindamycin plus primaquine. Atovaquone is less effective than TMP-SMX but is better tolerated. Parenteral pentamidine is given for moderate to severe infection but is highly toxic in both HIV-infected and HIV-uninfected pts. Other options include IV clindamycin plus primaquine or trimetrexate. Adjunctive administration of tapering doses of glucocorticoids to HIV-infected pts with moderate to severe disease reduces the risk of respiratory function deterio-

Table 114-1

Treatment of Pneumocystosis

Drug(s), Dose, Route	Adverse Effects
FIRST CHOICE[a]	
TMP-SMX (5 mg/kg TMP, 25 mg/kg SMX[b]) q6–8h PO or IV	Fever, rash, cytopenias, hepatitis, hyperkalemia, GI disturbances
OTHER AGENTS[a]	
TMP, 5 mg/kg q6–8h, plus dapsone, 100 mg qd PO	Hemolysis (G6PD deficiency), methemoglobinemia, fever, rash, GI disturbances
Atovaquone, 750 mg bid PO	Rash, fever, GI and hepatic disturbances
Clindamycin, 300–450 mg q6h PO or 600 mg q6–8h IV, plus primaquine, 15–30 mg qd PO	Hemolysis (G6PD deficiency), methemoglobinemia, rash, colitis, neutropenia
Pentamidine, 3–4 mg/kg qd IV	Hypotension, azotemia, cardiac arrhythmias, pancreatitis, dysglycemias, hypocalcemia, neutropenia, hepatitis
Trimetrexate, 45 mg/m² qd IV, plus leucovorin[c], 20 mg/kg q6h PO or IV	Cytopenias, peripheral neuropathy, hepatic disturbances
ADJUNCTIVE AGENT	
Prednisone, 40 mg bid × 5 d, 40 mg qd × 5 d, 20 mg qd × 11 d; PO or IV	Immunosuppression, peptic ulcer, hyperglycemia, mood changes, hypertension

[a] Therapy is administered for 14 days to non-HIV-infected patients and for 21 days to HIV-infected patients.

[b] Equivalent of 2 double-strength (DS) tablets. (One DS tablet contains 160 mg of TMP and 800 mg of SMX.)

[c] Leucovorin prevents bone marrow toxicity from trimetrexate.

Table 114-2

Prophylaxis of Pneumocystosis[a]

Drug, Dose, Route	Comments
FIRST CHOICE	
TMP-SMX, 1 DS tablet or 1 SS tablet qd PO[b]	TMP-SMX can be safely reintroduced in some patients who have experienced mild to moderate side effects.
OTHER AGENTS	
Dapsone, 50 mg bid or 100 mg qd PO	—
Dapsone, 50 mg qd PO, plus pyrimethamine, 50 mg weekly PO, plus leucovorin, 25 mg weekly PO	Leucovorin prevents bone marrow toxicity from pyrimethamine.
Dapsone, 200 mg weekly PO, plus pyrimethamine, 75 mg weekly PO, plus leucovorin, 25 mg weekly PO	Leucovorin prevents bone marrow toxicity from pyrimethamine.
Pentamidine, 300 mg monthly via Respirgard II nebulizer	Adverse reactions include cough, bronchospasm.
Atovaquone, 1500 mg qd PO	—
TMP-SMX, 1 DS tablet three times weekly PO	TMP-SMX can be safely reintroduced in some patients who have experienced mild to moderate side effects.

[a] For list of adverse effects, see Table 114-1.
[b] One DS tablet contains 160 mg of TMP and 800 mg of SMX.
Note: DS, double-strength; SS, single-strength.

ration shortly after initiation of treatment. The use of glucocorticoids in other pts remains to be evaluated.

Prevention

Primary prophylaxis is indicated for HIV-infected pts with CD4+ cell counts < 200/μL or a history of oropharyngeal candidiasis. Guidelines for other compromised hosts are less clear. Secondary prophylaxis is indicated for all pts who have recovered from pneumocystosis. In HIV infection, once CD4+ counts have risen to >200/μL and have remained above that cutoff for ≥3 months as a result of the institution of antiretroviral treatment, primary or secondary prophylaxis may be stopped. For prophylaxis regimens, see Table 114-2. TMP-SMX is the drug of choice for both primary and secondary prophylaxis and also protects against toxoplasmosis and some bacterial infections.

For a more detailed discussion, see Walzer PD: *Pneumocystis* **Infection, Chap. 191, p. 1194, in HPIM-16.**

115

PROTOZOAL INFECTIONS

MALARIA

EPIDEMIOLOGY   Malaria is the most important parasitic disease in humans, affecting >1 billion persons worldwide and causing between 1 and 3 million deaths each year.

ETIOLOGY   Four major species of *Plasmodium* cause nearly all human disease: *P. falciparum, P. vivax, P. ovale,* and *P. malariae. P. falciparum,* the cause of most cases of severe disease and most deaths, predominates in Africa, New Guinea, and Haiti. *P. vivax* is more common in Central America and the Indian subcontinent. *P. falciparum* and *P. vivax* are equally prevalent in South America, eastern Asia, and Oceania. *P. malariae* is less common but is found in most areas (especially throughout sub-Saharan Africa).

PATHOGENESIS

- Female anopheline mosquitoes inoculate *sporozoites* into humans during a blood meal. Sporozoites are carried to the liver, reproduce asexually, and produce *merozoites* that enter the bloodstream, invade RBCs, and become *trophozoites*. After progressively consuming and degrading intracellular proteins (principally hemoglobin), trophozoites become *schizonts*. When RBCs rupture, the cycle repeats with the invasion of new RBCs.
- In *P. vivax* or *P. ovale* infection, dormant forms called *hypnozoites* remain in liver cells and may cause disease 3 weeks to >1 year later.
- After a series of asexual cycles (*P. falciparum*) or immediately after release from the liver (*P. vivax, P. ovale, P. malariae*), some parasites develop into long-lived sexual forms called *gametocytes*. After ingestion by female anopheline mosquitoes during a blood meal, male and female gametocytes mature in the mosquito midgut to begin a new cycle of transmission.
- RBCs infected with *P. falciparum* may exhibit *cytoadherence* (attachment to venular and capillary endothelium), *rosetting* (adherence to uninfected RBCs), and *agglutination* (adherence to other infected RBCs). The result is sequestration of *P. falciparum* in vital organs, with consequent underestimation (through parasitemia determinations) of parasite numbers in the body. Sequestration is central to the pathogenesis of falciparum malaria but is not evident in the other three "benign" forms.
- In nonimmune individuals, infection triggers nonspecific host defense mechanisms such as splenic filtration. With repeated exposure to malaria, a specific immune response develops and limits the degree of parasitemia. Over time, pts are rendered immune to disease but remain susceptible to infection. Genetic disorders more common in endemic areas protect against death from malaria (e.g., sickle cell disease, thalassemia, and G6PD deficiency).

CLINICAL FEATURES

- Fever and nonspecific symptoms (headache, fatigue, muscle aches) occur at the onset of disease. Nausea, vomiting, and orthostasis are also common.
- Splenomegaly may develop along with mild anemia, hepatomegaly, and jaundice.
- Febrile paroxysms at regular intervals can occur with *P. vivax* or *P. ovale*.
- Severe falciparum malaria causes multiorgan dysfunction.

  1. Cerebral malaria: coma, obtundation, delirium, encephalopathy without focal neurologic signs. Seizures are common in children.

2. Blackwater fever: massive hemolysis with hemoglobinemia, renal failure
3. Poor prognostic signs: hypoglycemia, especially in children and pregnant women (may be exacerbated by quinine or quinidine treatment), lactic acidosis, noncardiogenic pulmonary edema, renal failure, severe anemia and coagulation abnormalities, severe jaundice and liver dysfunction

• Tropical splenomegaly: abnormal response to repeated infections. Pts have massive splenomegaly and, to a lesser degree, hepatomegaly. An abdominal mass is evident, and pts have a dragging sensation in the abdomen.
• Malaria in pregnancy: Pregnant women have unusually severe illness. Premature labor, stillbirths, delivery of low-birth-weight infants, and fetal distress are common.
• Malaria in children: Most persons who die of malaria are children. Convulsions, coma, hypoglycemia, acidosis, and severe anemia occur at high rates.
• Transfusion malaria: has a shorter incubation period than naturally acquired disease

DIAGNOSIS

• Demonstration of asexual forms of the parasite on peripheral blood smears is required for diagnosis. Giemsa is the preferred stain, but other stains (e.g., Wright's) can be used. Both thick and thin smears should be examined. Thick smears concentrate parasites by 20- to 40-fold compared with thin smears and increase diagnostic sensitivity. If the level of clinical suspicion is high and smears are initially negative, they should be repeated q12–24h for 2 days.
• Rapid antibody-based diagnostic stick or card tests are available for *P. falciparum*.
• The parasitemia level should be calculated from a thin smear and is expressed as the number of parasitized erythrocytes per 1000 RBCs or 200 WBCs.
• Other laboratory studies: anemia, elevated ESR, reduced platelet count (to $10^5/\mu L$)

 TREATMENT

See Table 115-1 for treatment options.

• *P. falciparum* should be treated with quinine or quinidine. Pts given quinidine should undergo cardiac monitoring; increased QT intervals (>0.6 s) and QRS widening by >25% are indications for slowing the infusion rate. Artemisinin derivatives are used instead as first-line agents in some areas but are not available in the United States.
• Pts with severe falciparum malaria should have intensive nursing care and monitoring. Ancillary drugs, including glucocorticoids or heparin, should not be given. Exchange transfusions can be considered for severely ill pts; indications for their use are not yet agreed upon, although most experts agree that pts with parasitemia levels of >15% should receive this treatment. Unconscious pts should have blood glucose levels measured q4–6h. Pts with glucose levels of <2.2 mmol/L (<40 mg/dL) should receive IV dextrose.
• Parasite counts and hematocrits should be measured q6–12h.
• Pts should be monitored for vomiting for 1 h after oral malaria treatment, and the dose should be repeated if vomiting occurs.
• Primaquine eradicates persistent liver stages and prevents relapse in *P. vivax* or *P. ovale* infection. G6PD deficiency must be ruled out before treatment.

PREVENTION *Personal Protection Measures* Measures that can protect against infection include avoidance of mosquito exposure at peak feeding

Table 115-1

Recommended Therapeutic Doses of Antimalarial Drugs

Drug	Uncomplicated Malaria (Oral)	Severe Malaria[a] (Parenteral)
Chloroquine[b]	10 mg of base/kg followed by 10 mg/kg at 24 h and 5 mg/kg at 48 h *or* by 5 mg/kg at 12, 24, and 36 h (total dose, 25 mg/kg); for *P. vivax* or *P. ovale*, primaquine (0.25 mg of base/kg per day for 14 days[d]) added for radical cure	10 mg of base/kg by constant-rate infusion over 8 h followed by 15 mg/kg over 24 h *or* by 3.5 mg of base/kg by IM or SC injection every 6 h (total dose, 25 mg/kg)[c]
Amodiaquine[b]	15 mg of base/kg followed by 10 mg/kg per day at 24 and 48 h (total dose, 35 mg/kg)	—
Sulfadoxine/pyrimethamine[b]	25/1.25 mg/kg, single oral dose (3 tablets for adults)	—
Mefloquine[b]	15 mg/kg followed 8–12 h later by second dose of 10 mg/kg	—
Quinine	10 mg of salt/kg q8h for 7 days combined with tetracycline[e] (4 mg/kg qid) or doxycycline (3 mg/kg once daily) or clindamycin (10 mg/kg bid) for 7 days	20 mg of salt/kg by IV infusion over 4 h[f] followed by 10 mg/kg infused over 2–8 h every 8 h
Quinidine gluconate	—	10 mg of base/kg by constant-rate infusion over 1–2 h followed by 0.02 mg/kg per min, with ECG monitoring[g]
Artesunate	In combination with 25 mg of mefloquine/kg, 12 mg/kg given in divided doses over 3–5 days (e.g., 4 mg/kg for 3 days or 4 mg/kg followed by 2 mg/kg per day for 4 days); if used alone or in combination with clindamycin or doxycycline, give for 7 days (usually 4 mg/kg initially followed by 2 mg/kg daily)	2.4 mg/kg IV or IM stat followed by 1.2 mg/kg at 12 and 24 h and then daily (or 2.4 mg/kg once daily)
Artemether	Same regimen as for artesunate	3.2 mg/kg IM stat followed by 1.6 mg/kg per day
Atovaquone-proguanil (Malarone)	For adults >40 kg, each dose comprises 4 tablets (each tablet containing atovaquone 250 mg and proguanil 100 mg) taken once daily for 3 days with food	—

(continued)

Table 115-1 *(Continued)*

Recommended Therapeutic Doses of Antimalarial Drugs

Drug	Uncomplicated Malaria (Oral)	Severe Malaria[a] (Parenteral)
Artemether-lumefantrine	For adults ≥35 kg, each dose comprises 4 tablets (each tablet containing artemether 20 mg and lumefantrine 120 mg) at 0, 8, 24, 36, 48, and 60 h, taken after food	—

[a] Oral treatment should be substituted for parenteral therapy as soon as the patient can take tablets by mouth.

[b] These drugs should be combined with either artesunate or artemether when used to treat falciparum malaria. Where there is full susceptibility to both drugs, chloroquine or amodiaquine can be combined with sulfadoxine/pyrimethamine.

[c] Chloroquine-resistant *P. falciparum* is now very widespread, so this regimen should not be used unless there is confirmed full susceptibility in the area.

[d] In Oceania and Southeast Asia, the dose should be 0.33 to 0.5 mg of base/kg. This regimen should not be used in patients with severe variants of G6PD deficiency.

[e] Neither tetracycline nor doxycycline should be given to pregnant women or to children <8 years old.

[f] Alternatively, infusion of 7 mg of salt/kg over 30 min can be followed by 10 mg of salt/kg over 4 h.

[g] Some authorities recommend a lower dose of intravenous quinidine: 6.2 mg of base/kg over 1–2 h followed by 0.0125 mg/kg per min.

Note: In severe malaria, quinine or quinidine should be used if there is any doubt about the infecting strain's sensitivity to chloroquine.

times (dusk and dawn) and use of insect repellents containing DEET, suitable clothing, and insecticide-impregnated bed nets.

Chemoprophylaxis   See Table 115-2.

• Pregnant women have limited chemoprophylaxis options.
• Prophylaxis should begin 1 week before departure to and continue for 4 weeks after departure from the endemic area. If atovaquone-proguanil or primaquine prophylaxis is used, it can be stopped 1 week after departure from the endemic area.
• Mefloquine is the usual agent of choice for much of the tropics but is associated with acute reversible neuropsychiatric reactions.
• The CDC offers 24-h travel and malaria information at 888-232-3228.

BABESIOSIS
ETIOLOGY

• United States: *Babesia microti*
• Europe: *B. divergens*

EPIDEMIOLOGY   In the United States, infections occur most frequently along the northeastern coast. Hard-bodied ticks (*Ixodes scapularis* or *I. ricinus*) transmit the parasite.

CLINICAL FEATURES

• The incubation period is usually 1–4 weeks. Immunocompromised hosts (e.g., HIV-infected, splenectomized, or elderly pts) have the most severe disease.

• There is a gradual onset of fevers, chills, muscle pains, fatigue, mild hepatosplenomegaly, and anemia. The parasitemia level may range from 1 to 50%.
• *B. divergens* causes severe—often fatal—disease in splenectomized pts. This illness is characterized by high fevers, hemolytic anemia, jaundice, and renal failure.

DIAGNOSIS   Giemsa-stained thick and thin smears identify intraerythrocytic parasites. *B. microti* parasites appear as small ring forms resembling *P. falciparum* but without pigment; no schizonts or gametocytes are formed. Tetrads—four daughter parasites attached by strands of cytoplasm—can be seen. *B. microti* infection can be diagnosed by an indirect immunofluorescence antibody test. The antibody titer rises 2–4 weeks after disease onset.

℞ TREATMENT

• Atovaquone (750 mg bid PO) plus azithromycin (600 mg/d PO) *or* quinine (650 mg tid PO) plus clindamycin (1200 mg bid IV or 600 mg tid PO) for 7–10 days
• Severe infections, particularly those caused by *B. divergens*, should be treated with a regimen including quinine, clindamycin, and atovaquone at the doses noted above.
• Exchange transfusions may be beneficial in pts with severe disease.

LEISHMANIASIS

ETIOLOGY   *Leishmania* spp. are obligate intracellular protozoa endemic in the tropics, subtropics, and southern Europe. Organisms of the *L. donovani* complex usually cause visceral leishmaniasis; *L. tropica*, *L. major*, and *L. aethiopica* cause Old World cutaneous leishmaniasis; and the *L. mexicana* complex causes New World or American cutaneous leishmaniasis. Rodents and canines are common reservoirs, while humans are incidental hosts. Leishmaniasis is typically a vector-borne zoonosis caused by the bite of female phlebotomine sandflies. The parasite's flagellated promastigote is introduced into the mammalian host and transforms into the nonflagellated amastigote within macrophages. Host defenses depend upon a T cell response, IFN-γ production, and macrophage activation.

CLINICAL FEATURES, DIAGNOSIS, AND TREATMENT

Visceral Leishmaniasis

• Around 90% of cases occur in Bangladesh, India, Nepal, Sudan, and Brazil.
• The incubation period can range from weeks to months or even years. Disease ranges from subclinical (most common) to an acute, subacute, or chronic course. Malnutrition increases the risk for development of clinical disease.
• Kala-azar: The classic picture is of cachectic, febrile pts with massive splenomegaly, hepatomegaly, lymphadenopathy, and life-threatening disease.
• Abnormal laboratory findings include pancytopenia (with anemia that can be due to bone marrow infiltration, hypersplenism, autoimmune hemolysis, and bleeding), hypergammaglobulinemia, and hypoalbuminemia.
• Co-infection with HIV often leads to severe, disseminated infections.
• *Diagnosis*: Identification of amastigotes on stained slides (e.g., with Giemsa) or by culture of tissue aspirates or biopsy samples of spleen, liver, bone marrow, or lymph node yields the diagnosis. Spleen aspiration poses a high risk of hemorrhage.
• *Treatment*: The pentavalent antimonial compounds (Sb^v) sodium stibogluconate and meglumine antimonate (20 mg/kg per day IV or IM for 28 days) are the first-line therapeutic agents outside of India, where amphotericin B (either

Table 115-2

Prophylaxis and Self-Treatment for Malaria

Drug	Usage	Adult Dosage	Child Dosage
Prophylaxis			
Mefloquine	Used in areas where chloroquine-resistant malaria has been reported	228 mg of base (250 mg of salt) orally, once/week[a]	<15 kg: 4.6 mg of base/kg (5 mg of salt/kg) 15–19 kg: 1/4 tablet/week 20–30 kg: 1/2 tablet/week 31–45 kg: 3/4 tablet/week >45 kg: 1 tablet/week
Doxycycline[b]	Used as alternative to mefloquine or atovaquone-proguanil	100 mg orally, once/day	>8 years of age: 2 mg/kg per day orally; maximum dose, 100 mg/d
Atovaquone-proguanil (Malarone)[c]	Used as alternative to mefloquine or doxycycline	250/100 mg orally, once/day	11–20 kg: 62.5 mg/25 mg 21–30 kg: 125 mg/50 mg 31–40 kg: 187.5 mg/75 mg >40 kg: 250 mg/100 mg
Chloroquine	Used in areas where chloroquine-resistant malaria has *not* been reported	300 mg of base (500 mg of salt) orally, once/week	5 mg of base/kg (8.3 mg of salt/kg) orally, once/week; maximum dose, 300 mg of base
Proguanil (not available in U.S.)	Used simultaneously *with* chloroquine as alternative to mefloquine or doxycycline	200 mg orally, once/day, in combination with weekly chloroquine	<2 years: 50 mg/d 2–6 years: 100 mg/d 7–10 years: 150 mg/d >10 years: 200 mg/d
Primaquine[c]	Used for travelers only after testing for G6PD deficiency; postexposure prevention for relapsing malaria or prophylaxis	Postexposure: 15 mg of base (26.3 mg of salt) orally, once/day for 14 days Prophylaxis: 30 mg of base daily	0.3 mg of base/kg (0.5 mg of salt/kg) orally, once/day for 14 days

574

Self-treatment		
Atovaquone-proguanil (Malarone)[d]	In areas with chloroquine-resistant malaria, should be carried during travel to very remote areas by persons taking mefloquine or doxycycline	4 tablets (1000 mg of atovaquone and 400 mg of proguanil orally, as a single daily dose for 3 consecutive days
	Used as alternative to atovaquone-proguanil for self-treatment	11–20 kg: 1 adult tablet 21–30 kg: 2 adult tablets 31–40 kg: 3 adult tablets >40 kg: 4 adult tablets
Sulfadoxine/ pyrimethamine[e]		3 tablets (75 mg of pyrimethamine and 1500 mg of sulfadoxine) orally, as a single dose
		5–10 kg: $\frac{1}{2}$ tablet 11–20 kg: 1 tablet 21–30 kg: $1\frac{1}{2}$ tablets 31–45 kg: 2 tablets >45 kg: 3 tablets

[a] Tablets manufactured outside the United States contain 250 mg of base.

[b] Not in pregnant women or children <8 years old.

[c] Primaquine and atovaquone-proguanil have both proved safe and effective for antimalarial chemoprophylaxis in areas with chloroquine-resistant falciparum malaria, but more data are needed, particularly in children. These drugs should not be used in pregnancy.

[d] Not for patients on atovaquone-proguanil prophylaxis.

[e] Regimen is used for treatment only (*not* prophylaxis) in areas with known susceptibility.

deoxycholate or a lipid formulation) is recommended (total dose, 15–20 mg/kg). The oral agent miltefosine (50 or 100 mg daily for 28 days) was highly effective in phase 3 trials in India but is not available in the United States. Sb^v treatment is associated with significant but reversible toxicity (myalgia, arthralgia, fatigue, elevated LFT values, chemical pancreatitis) whose incidence increases as treatment continues. Amphotericin B and pentamidine are alternatives that are more likely to cause serious or irreversible toxicity.

Cutaneous Leishmaniasis

- More than 90% of cases occur in Afghanistan, the Middle East, Brazil, and Peru.
- After an incubation period of weeks to months, a papule at the site of the sandfly bite develops and progresses first to a nodular and then to an ulcerative lesion with a central depression and a raised indurated border. Lesions persist as nodules or plaques and cause significant morbidity. *L. aethiopica* or *L. mexicana* causes chronic, disseminated, nonulcerative skin lesions. Leishmaniasis recidivans, caused by *L. tropica*, manifests as a solitary cheek lesion that expands slowly with central healing.
- Regional adenopathy, multiple primary and satellite lesions, pain, pruritus, and bacterial superinfection can occur.
- *Diagnosis*: made by microscopic identification of amastigotes in histologic sections, a Giemsa-stained thin smear of dermal scrapings, or touch preparations of biopsy specimens. Culture or PCR of skin lesion aspirates and biopsy specimens can be useful.
- *Treatment*: The decision to treat cutaneous leishmaniasis should be based on the species involved, the possibility of mucosal dissemination, the likelihood of self-healing, and the location, number, size, evolution, and chronicity of the lesions. Administration of Sb^v (20 mg/kg daily for 20 days) constitutes the most effective treatment. Oral agents have given disparate results, depending on the parasite species.

Mucosal Leishmaniasis This rare form of disease usually becomes evident years after healing of the original cutaneous lesion. Persistent nasal symptoms, such as epistaxis with erythema and edema of the mucosa, are followed by progressive ulcerative destruction.

PREVENTION It is helpful to avoid outdoor activities from dusk to dawn, when sandflies are most active, and to use screens, bed nets, protective clothing, and insect repellent. Dogs are important reservoirs, and collars with insecticide may be useful.

TRYPANOSOMIASIS
Chagas' Disease

ETIOLOGY AND PATHOLOGY *Trypanosoma cruzi* causes Chagas' disease (also known as American trypanosomiasis) and is transmitted among mammalian hosts by hematophagous reduviid bugs. One week after parasitic invasion, an indurated inflammatory lesion appears at the portal of entry, and organisms disseminate through the lymphatics and the bloodstream, often parasitizing muscles particularly heavily.

EPIDEMIOLOGY Chagas' disease is the most important parasitic disease in Latin America. *T. cruzi* is found mostly among the poor in rural Mexico and Central and South America. An estimated 16–18 million persons are infected, with 45,000 deaths annually.

CLINICAL FEATURES

- *Acute disease*: An indurated area of erythema and swelling (the *chagoma*) with local lymphadenopathy may appear. *Romaña's sign*—unilateral painless edema of the palpebrae and periocular tissues—occurs when the conjunctiva is the portal of entry.

1. Malaise, fever, anorexia, rash, lymphadenopathy, and hepatosplenomegaly develop.
2. After symptoms resolve spontaneously, pts enter an asymptomatic phase.

• *Chronic disease*: becomes apparent years to decades after initial infection

1. Heart: rhythm disturbances, dilated cardiomyopathy, thromboembolism. RBBB and other conduction abnormalities may occur.
2. Megaesophagus: dysphagia, odynophagia, chest pain, and aspiration. Weight loss, cachexia, or pulmonary infection can cause death.
3. Megacolon: abdominal pain, chronic constipation. Advanced megacolon can cause obstruction, volvulus, septicemia, and death.

DIAGNOSIS Microscopic examination of fresh anticoagulated blood or the buffy coat may reveal motile organisms. Giemsa-stained thin and thick blood smears can also be used. If attempts to visualize the organism fail, PCR or hemoculture can be performed. Chronic Chagas' disease is diagnosed by detection of specific antibodies. The assays vary in specificity and sensitivity; false-positive results pose a particular problem. A positive result in one assay should be confirmed by two other tests.

℞ TREATMENT

Acute Chagas' disease is treated with nifurtimox, which reduces symptom duration, parasitemia level, and mortality rate but cures only ~70% of pts. Treatment should be initiated as early as possible in acute disease. Adults should receive 8–10 mg/kg daily in four divided oral doses for 90–120 days. Higher doses are given to children and adolescents. Adverse drug effects include abdominal pain, anorexia, nausea, vomiting, weight loss, and neurologic reactions such as restlessness, disorientation, insomnia, paresthesia, and seizures. In Latin America, the drug of choice is benznidazole (5 mg/kg per day for 60 days). Benznidazole is associated with peripheral neuropathy, rash, and granulocytopenia. Chronic Chagas' disease is usually treated because cardiac pathology may be lessened with treatment.

Sleeping Sickness

ETIOLOGY AND EPIDEMIOLOGY Sleeping sickness (human African trypanosomiasis) is caused by parasites of the *T. brucei* complex and is transmitted via tsetse flies. *T. b. rhodesiense* causes the East African form, and *T. b. gambiense* the West African form. During stage I of infection, the parasites disseminate through the lymphatics and the bloodstream. CNS invasion occurs during stage II. West African infection occurs primarily in rural populations and rarely develops in tourists. East African disease has reservoirs in antelope and cattle; tourists can be infected when visiting areas where infected game and vectors are present.

CLINICAL FEATURES A painful chancre sometimes appears at the site of inoculation. Stage I is marked by bouts of high fever alternating with afebrile periods and by lymphadenopathy with discrete, rubbery, nontender nodes. *Winterbottom's sign*—the enlargement of nodes of the posterior cervical triangle—is a classic sign. Pruritus and maculopapular rashes are common. Malaise, headache, arthralgias, hepatosplenomegaly, and other nonspecific manifestations can develop. In stage II, pts develop progressive indifference and daytime somnolence, a state that sometimes alternates with restlessness and insomnia. Extra-pyramidal signs may include choreiform movements, tremors, and fasciculations; ataxia is common. Progressive neurologic impairment may end in coma and death. East African disease is a more acute illness that, without treatment, generally leads to death in weeks or months.

DIAGNOSIS Examination of fluid from the chancre, thin or thick blood smears, lymph node aspirates, bone marrow biopsy specimens, or CSF samples can reveal the parasite. CSF should be examined whenever the diagnosis is being considered. Increased opening pressure, increased protein level, and increased mononuclear cell counts are common. Parasites can be visualized in the sediment of centrifuged CSF.

℞ TREATMENT

Treatment is toxic and must be closely supervised.

I. Stage I disease
   A. East and West African: suramin (1 g on days 1, 3, 7, 14, and 21). There is a high incidence of serious adverse effects. Fever, photophobia, pruritus, arthralgias, skin eruptions, and renal damage can occur. Severe reactions can be fatal.
   B. Alternatives
      1. East African: Pentamidine (4 mg/kg for 10 days)
      2. West African: Eflornithine (400 mg/kg per day in 4 divided doses for 2 weeks)
II. Stage II disease
   A. East African: Melarsoprol (2–3.6 mg/kg daily in 3 divided doses for 3 days; 1 week later, 3.6 mg/kg per day in 3 divided doses for 3 days; repeat latter course 10–21 days later). Reactive encephalopathy occurs in up to 18% of pts.
   B. West African: Eflornithine (400 mg/kg per day in 4 divided doses for 2 weeks)

TOXOPLASMOSIS

ETIOLOGY AND EPIDEMIOLOGY Toxoplasmosis is caused by the intracellular parasite *Toxoplasma gondii*. In the United States and most European countries, seroconversion rates increase with age and exposure. Cats and their prey are the definitive hosts. Transmission occurs when humans ingest oocysts from contaminated soil or tissue cysts from undercooked meat. About one-third of women who become acutely infected with *T. gondii* during pregnancy transmit the parasite to the fetus. Congenital infection can occur if the mother is infected <6 months before conception and becomes increasingly likely throughout pregnancy, with a 65% likelihood if the mother is infected in the third trimester.

PATHOGENESIS Both humoral and cellular immunity are important, but infection commonly persists. Such lifelong infection usually remains subclinical. Compromised hosts do not control infection; progressive focal destruction and organ failure occur.

CLINICAL FEATURES

• Disease in immunocompetent hosts is usually asymptomatic and self-limited and does not require therapy; 80–90% of cases go unrecognized. Cervical lymphadenopathy is the most common finding; nodes are nontender and discrete. Generalized lymphadenopathy can occur. Fever, headache, malaise, and fatigue are documented in 20–40% of pts with lymphadenopathy.

• Immunocompromised pts, including those with AIDS and those receiving immunosuppressive treatment for lymphoproliferative disorders, are at greatest risk. Most clinical disease is due to reactivated latent infection.

1. CNS: principal site of involvement. Findings include encephalopathy, meningoencephalitis, and mass lesions. Pts may exhibit changes in mental status, fever, seizures, headaches, and aphasia. The brainstem, basal ganglia, pituitary gland, and corticomedullary junction are most often involved.
2. Pneumonia: Dyspnea, fever, and nonproductive cough can progress to respiratory failure. *Toxoplasma* pneumonia is often confused with *Pneumocystis* pneumonia.
3. Miscellaneous sites: GI tract, pancreas, eyes, heart, liver

• Congenital infection affects 400–4000 infants each year in the United States. Severe disease, manifesting as hydrocephalus, microcephaly, mental retardation, and chorioretinitis, is more common the earlier the infection is contracted.
• Ocular infection: *T. gondii* is estimated to cause ~35% of all cases of chorioretinitis in the United States and Europe. Most cases are associated with congenital infection. Blurred vision, scotoma, photophobia, and eye pain are manifestations of infection; macular involvement can occur with loss of central vision. On examination, yellow-white cotton-like patches with indistinct margins of hyperemia are seen. Older lesions appear as white plaques with distinct borders and black spots.

DIAGNOSIS

• Acute toxoplasmosis can be diagnosed by the demonstration of tachyzoites in tissue or by documentation of the simultaneous presence of serum IgM and IgG antibodies to *T. gondii*.
• In AIDS pts, the infection is diagnosed presumptively on the basis of clinical presentation and a positive test for IgG antibody to *T. gondii*. In these pts, CT or MRI of the brain shows lesions that are often multiple and contrast enhancing. A single lesion may prove to be a CNS lymphoma rather than toxoplasmosis.
• Congenital toxoplasmosis is diagnosed by PCR of the amniotic fluid (to detect the B1 gene of the parasite) and by the detection of IgG antibody or a positive IgM titer after the first week of life; IgG antibody determinations should be repeated every 2 months.
• Ocular toxoplasmosis is diagnosed by the detection of typical lesions on ophthalmologic examination and the demonstration of a positive IgG titer.

Rx TREATMENT

• Congenital infection: daily pyrimethamine (0.5–1 mg/kg) and sulfadiazine (100 mg/kg) for 1 year. If infection is diagnosed and treated early, up to 70% of children can have normal findings at follow-up evaluations.
• Ocular disease: pyrimethamine and sulfadiazine or clindamycin for 1 month
• Immunocompromised pts: pyrimethamine (200-mg PO loading dose followed by 50–75 mg/d) plus sulfadiazine (4–6 g/d PO, divided into 4 doses) plus leucovorin (10–15 mg/d). Pyrimethamine (75 mg/d) plus clindamycin (450 mg tid) is an alternative. Glucocorticoids are often used to treat intracerebral edema. After 4–6 weeks (or after radiographic improvement), the pt may be switched to chronic suppressive therapy (secondary prophylaxis) with pyrimethamine (25–50 mg/d) plus sulfadiazine (2–4 g/d), pyrimethamine (75 mg/d) plus clindamycin (450 mg tid), or pyrimethamine alone (50–75 mg/d).

PREVENTION   *Personal Protection Measures*   *Toxoplasma* infection can be prevented by avoiding undercooked meats and oocyst-contaminated materials (e.g., cats' litter boxes).

Chemoprophylaxis   The risk of disease is very high among AIDS pts who are seropositive for *T. gondii* and have a CD4+ T lymphocyte count of <100/μL. Trimethoprim-sulfamethoxazole (one double-strength tablet daily) should be given to these pts as prophylaxis against both *Pneumocystis* pneumonia and toxoplasmosis. Primary or secondary prophylaxis can be stopped if, after institution of antiretroviral treatment, the CD4+ T lymphocyte count increases to >200/μL and remains above that cutoff for 3 months.

For a more detailed discussion, see Davis CE: Laboratory Diagnosis of Parasitic Infections, Chap. 192, p. 1197; Moore TA: Agents Used to Treat Infections Due to Parasites and *Pneumocystis*, Chap. 193, p. 1202; White NJ, Breman JG: Malaria and Babesiosis: Diseases Caused by Red Blood Cell Parasites, Chap. 195, p. 1218; Herwaldt BL: Leishmaniasis, Chap. 196, p. 1233; Kirchhoff LV: Trypanosomiasis, Chap. 197, p. 1238; and Kasper LH: *Toxoplasma* Infection, Chap. 198, p. 1243, in HPIM-16.

116

HELMINTHIC INFECTIONS

NEMATODES

The nematodes, or roundworms, that are of medical significance can be broadly classified as either tissue or intestinal parasites.

Tissue Nematode Infections

TRICHINELLOSIS   *Etiology*   *T. spiralis* and six other *Trichinella* species cause human infection.

Life Cycle and Epidemiology   Infection results when humans ingest meat (usually pork) that contains cysts with *Trichinella* larvae. During the first week of infection, the larvae invade the small-bowel mucosa; during the second and third weeks, they mature into adult worms, which release new larvae that migrate to striated muscle via the circulation and encyst.

Clinical Features   Light infections (<10 larvae per gram of muscle) are asymptomatic. A burden of >50 larvae per gram can cause fatal disease.

- Week 1: diarrhea, abdominal pain, constipation, nausea, and/or vomiting
- Week 2: hypersensitivity reactions with fever and hypereosinophilia; periorbital and facial edema; hemorrhages in conjunctivae, retina, and nail beds; maculopapular rash; headache; cough; dyspnea; dysphagia. Deaths are usually due to myocarditis with arrhythmias or CHF and are less often caused by pneumonitis or encephalitis.

• Weeks 2–3: myositis, myalgias, muscle edema, weakness (especially in extraocular muscles, biceps, neck, lower back, and diaphragm). Symptoms peak at 3 weeks; convalescence is prolonged.

Diagnosis

• Eosinophilia in >90% of pts, peaking at a level of >50% at 2–4 weeks
• Elevated IgE and muscle enzyme levels; increase in specific antibody titers by week 3
• A definitive diagnosis is made by the detection of larvae on biopsy of at least 1 g of muscle tissue. Yields are highest near tendon insertions.

 TREATMENT

Drugs are ineffective against muscle larvae, but mebendazole and albendazole may be active against enteric-stage parasites. Glucocorticoids (1 mg/kg daily for 5 days) may reduce severe myositis and myocarditis.

Prevention Cooking pork until it is no longer pink or freezing it at −15°C for 3 weeks kills larvae and prevents infection.

VISCERAL AND OCULAR LARVA MIGRANS *Etiology* Most cases of larva migrans are caused by *Toxocara canis*.

Life Cycle and Epidemiology Infection results when humans—most often preschool children—ingest soil contaminated by puppy feces that contain infective *T. canis* eggs. Larvae penetrate the intestinal mucosa and disseminate hematogenously to a wide variety of organs (e.g., liver, lungs, CNS), provoking intense eosinophilic granulomatous responses.

Clinical Features Heavy infections may cause fever, malaise, anorexia, weight loss, cough, wheezing, rashes, and hepatosplenomegaly. Ocular disease usually develops in older children or young adults and may cause an eosinophilic mass that mimics retinoblastoma, endophthalmitis, uveitis, or chorioretinitis.

Diagnosis

• No eggs are found in the stool because larvae do not develop into adult worms.
• Blood eosinophilia up to 90%, leukocytosis, and hypergammaglobulinemia may be evident.
• Toxocaral antibodies detected by ELISA can confirm the diagnosis.

 TREATMENT

Glucocorticoids can reduce inflammatory complications. Only ocular infections require treatment: albendazole (800 mg bid for adults and 400 mg bid for children) for 5–20 days in conjunction with glucocorticoids.

CUTANEOUS LARVA MIGRANS This disease is caused by larvae of animal hookworms, usually the dog and cat hookworm *Ancylostoma braziliense*. Larvae in contaminated soil penetrate human skin; erythematous lesions form along the tracks of their migration and advance several centimeters each day. Pruritus is intense. Vesicles or bullae may form. Ivermectin (a single dose of 200 μg/kg) or albendazole (200 mg bid for 3 days) can relieve the symptoms of this self-limited infestation.

Intestinal Nematode Infections

Intestinal nematodes infect >1 billion persons worldwide in regions with poor sanitation, particularly in developing countries in the tropics or subtropics. These parasites contribute to malnutrition and diminished work capacity.

ASCARIASIS   *Etiology*   Ascariasis is caused by *Ascaris lumbricoides*, the largest intestinal nematode, which reaches lengths up to 40 cm. The parasite is transmitted via fecally contaminated soil.

Life Cycle   Swallowed eggs hatch in the intestine, invade the mucosa, migrate to the lungs, break into the alveoli, ascend the bronchial tree, are swallowed, reach the small intestine, mature, and produce up to 240,000 eggs per day that pass in the feces.

Clinical Features   Most infections have a low worm burden and are asymptomatic. During lung migration of the parasite, pts may develop a cough and substernal discomfort, occasionally with dyspnea or blood-tinged sputum, fever, and eosinophilia. Eosinophilic pneumonitis (Löffler's syndrome) may be evident. Heavy infections occasionally cause pain, small-bowel obstruction, perforation, volvulus, biliary obstruction and colic, or pancreatitis.

Laboratory Findings   *Ascaris* eggs (65 by 45 μm) can be found in fecal samples. Adult worms can pass in the stool or through the mouth or nose. During the transpulmonary migratory phase, larvae can be found in sputum or gastric aspirates.

 TREATMENT

A single dose of albendazole (400 mg) or mebendazole (500 mg) is effective. Pyrantel pamoate (a single dose of 11 mg/kg, up to 1 g) is safe in pregnancy.

HOOKWORM   *Etiology*   One-fourth of the world's population is infected with one of two hookworm species: *Ancylostoma duodenale* or *Necator americanus*.

Life Cycle   Infectious larvae penetrate the skin, reach the lungs via the bloodstream, invade the alveoli, ascend the airways, are swallowed, reach the small intestine, mature into adult worms, attach to the mucosa, and suck blood and interstitial fluid.

Clinical Features   Most infections are asymptomatic. Chronic infection causes iron deficiency and—in marginally nourished persons—progressive anemia and hypoproteinemia, weakness, shortness of breath, and skin depigmentation.

Laboratory Findings   Hookworm eggs (40 by 60 μm) can be found in the feces. Stool concentration may be needed for the diagnosis of light infections.

 TREATMENT

Albendazole (400 mg once), mebendazole (500 mg once), or pyrantel pamoate (11 mg/kg daily for 3 days) is effective. Nutritional support, iron replacement, and deworming are undertaken as needed.

STRONGYLOIDIASIS   *Etiology and Epidemiology*   Unlike other helminths, *Strongyloides stercoralis* can replicate in the human host, permitting ongoing cycles of autoinfection from endogenously produced larvae. Autoinfection is most common among immunocompromised hosts, including those receiving glucocorticoids. Hyperinfection and widespread larval dissemination can occur in these pts. However, severe disease due to *Strongyloides* is unusual in HIV-infected pts.

Life Cycle Infection results when filariform larvae in fecally contaminated soil penetrate the skin or mucous membranes. Larvae travel through the bloodstream to the lungs, break through alveolar spaces, ascend the bronchial tree, are swallowed, reach the small intestine, mature into adult worms, and penetrate the mucosa of the proximal small bowel; eggs hatch in intestinal mucosa. Rhabditiform larvae can pass with the feces into the soil or can develop into filariform larvae that penetrate the colonic wall or perianal skin and enter the circulation to establish ongoing autoinfection.

Clinical Features Uncomplicated disease is associated with mild cutaneous and/or abdominal manifestations such as urticaria, larva currens (a pathognomonic serpiginous, pruritic, erythematous eruption along the course of larval migration that may advance up to 10 cm/h), abdominal pain, nausea, diarrhea, bleeding, and weight loss. Colitis, enteritis, or malabsorption can develop. Disseminated disease involves extraintestinal tissues, including the CNS, peritoneum, liver, and kidney. Bacteremia can develop when enteric flora components enter the bloodstream through disrupted mucosal barriers. Gram-negative sepsis, pneumonia, or meningitis can complicate the disease.

Diagnosis Eosinophilia is common, with levels that fluctuate over time. Eggs are rarely found in feces because they hatch in the colon. A single stool examination detects rhabditiform larvae (200–250 μm long) in about one-third of uncomplicated infections. If stool examinations are negative, duodenojejunal contents can be sampled. Antibodies can be detected by ELISA. In disseminated infection, filariform larvae (550 μm long) can be found in stool or at sites of larval migration.

 TREATMENT

Ivermectin (200 μg/kg daily for 1 or 2 days) is more effective than albendazole (400 mg daily for 3 days, repeated at 2 weeks) and is better tolerated than thiabendazole (25 mg/kg bid for 2 days). Disseminated disease should be treated for 5–7 days.

ENTEROBIASIS ***Etiology*** Enterobiasis (pinworm) is caused by *Enterobius vermicularis*.

Life Cycle Adult worms dwell in the bowel lumen and migrate nocturnally out into the perianal region, releasing immature eggs that become infective within hours. Autoinfection results from perianal scratching and transport of infective eggs to the mouth. Person-to-person spread occurs. Pinworm is common among schoolchildren and their household contacts and among institutionalized populations.

Clinical Features Perianal pruritus is the cardinal symptom and is often worst at night.

Diagnosis Eggs in the perianal region are detected by application of cellulose acetate tape in the morning. Eggs measure 55 by 25 μm and are flattened on one side.

TREATMENT

One dose of mebendazole (100 mg), albendazole (400 mg), or pyrantel pamoate (11 mg/kg; maximum, 1 g) is given, with the same treatment repeated after 10–14 days. Household members should also be treated.

Filarial and Related Infections

Filarial worms are nematodes that dwell in the SC tissue and lymphatics. More than 170 million people are infected worldwide. Infection is established only with repeated and prolonged exposures to infective larvae. Disease tends to be more intense and acute in newly exposed individuals than in natives of endemic areas.

Life Cycle   Insects transmit infective larvae to humans. Adult worms reside in lymphatics or SC tissues; their offspring are microfilariae (200–250 μm long, 5–7 μm wide) that either circulate in the blood or migrate through the skin. *Subperiodic* forms are those that are present in peripheral blood at all times and peak in the afternoon. *Nocturnally periodic* forms are scarce in peripheral blood by day and increase by night. Adult worms live for years; microfilariae live for 3–36 months. A rickettsia-like endosymbiont of *Wolbachia* has been found in all stages of the four major filarial species that cause human disease and may prove to be a target for future antifilarial chemotherapy.

LYMPHATIC FILARIASIS ***Etiology***   *Wuchereria bancrofti*, *Brugia malayi*, or *B. timori* can reside in lymphatic channels or lymph nodes. *W. bancrofti* is most common and usually is nocturnally periodic.

Pathology   Adult worms cause inflammatory damage to the lymphatics.

Clinical Features   Asymptomatic microfilaremia, hydrocele, acute adenolymphangitis (ADL), and chronic lymphatic disease are the main clinical presentations. ADL is associated with high fever, lymphatic inflammation, and transient local edema. *W. bancrofti* particularly affects genital lymphatics. ADL may progress to lymphatic obstruction and elephantiasis with brawny edema, thickening of the SC tissues, and hyperkeratosis. Superinfection is a problem.

Diagnosis   Detection of the parasite is difficult, but microfilariae can be found in peripheral blood, hydrocele fluid, and occasionally other body fluids. Timing of blood collection is critical. Two assays are available to detect *W. bancrofti* circulating antigens, and a PCR has been developed to detect DNA of both *W. bancrofti* and *B. malayi* in the blood. High-frequency ultrasound of the scrotum or the female breast can identify motile adult worms. Pts have eosinophilia and elevated IgE levels. The presence of antifilarial antibody supports the diagnosis, but cross-reactivity with other helminthic infections makes interpretation difficult.

 TREATMENT

Diethylcarbamazine (DEC) given at 6 mg/kg daily for 12 days is the standard regimen, but one dose may be equally efficacious. An alternative is albendazole (400 mg bid for 21 days).

Prevention

• Mosquito control or personal protective equipment can minimize bites.
• Mass annual distribution of albendazole with DEC or ivermectin for community-based control reduces microfilaremia and interrupts transmission.

ONCHOCERCIASIS *Etiology* Onchocerciasis ("river blindness") is caused by *Onchocerca volvulus*, is the second leading cause of infectious blindness worldwide, and is transmitted by the bite of an infected blackfly. The blackfly vector breeds along free-flowing rivers and streams and restricts its flight to an area within several kilometers of these breeding sites.

Life Cycle Larvae develop into adult worms that are found in SC nodules (*onchocercomata*). After months or years, microfilariae migrate out of the nodules and concentrate in the dermis. Onchocerciasis affects primarily the skin, eyes, and lymph nodes. Microfilariae cause inflammation and fibrosis. Neovascularization and corneal scarring cause corneal opacities and blindness.

Clinical Features

• Skin: Pruritus and rash are the most common manifestations.
• Onchocercomata: palpable and/or visible, firm and nontender
• Ocular tissue: Conjunctivitis with photophobia is an early finding. Sclerosing keratitis, anterior uveitis, iridocyclitis, and secondary glaucoma due to anterior uveal tract deformity are complications.
• Lymphadenopathy: especially in the inguinal and femoral areas

Diagnosis A definitive diagnosis is based on the finding of an adult worm in an excised nodule or of microfilariae in a skin snip. Eosinophilia and elevated serum IgE levels are common. Assays to detect specific antibodies and PCR to detect onchocercal DNA in skin snips are available in some laboratories.

 TREATMENT

Nodules on the head should be excised to avoid ocular infection. Ivermectin in a single dose of 150 μg/kg given yearly or semiannually is the mainstay of treatment. Doxycycline therapy for 6 weeks may render adult female worms sterile for long periods and also may target the *Wolbachia* endosymbiont.

TREMATODES

The trematodes, or flatworms, may be classified according to the tissues invaded by the adult flukes. The life cycle involves a definitive mammalian host in whom adult worms produce eggs and an intermediate host (e.g., snails) in which larval forms multiply. Worms do not multiply within the definitive host. Human infection results from either direct penetration of intact skin or ingestion.

Schistosomiasis

Etiology Schistosomes are blood flukes that infect 200–300 million persons worldwide. Five species cause human schistosomiasis: the intestinal species *Schistosoma mansoni* (found in South America, Africa, and the Middle East), *S. japonicum* (found in China, the Philippines, and Indonesia), *S. mekongi* (found in Southeast Asia), and *S. intercalatum* (found in West and Central Africa); and the urinary species *S. haematobium* (found in Africa and the Middle East). Infection is initiated by penetration of intact skin by infective cercariae—the form of the parasite released from snails in freshwater bodies. As they mature into schistosomes, the parasites reach the portal vein, mate, then migrate to the venules of the bladder and ureters (*S. haematobium*) or the mesentery (*S. mansoni, S. japonicum, S. mekongi, S. intercalatum*) and deposit eggs. Some mature ova are extruded into the intestinal or urinary lumina, from which they may be voided and ultimately may reach water and perpetuate the life cycle. The persistence of other ova in tissues leads to a granulomatous host response and fibrosis. Factors governing disease manifestations include the intensity and duration of infection, the site of egg deposition, and the genetic characteristics of the host.

Pathogenesis In the liver, granulomata cause presinusoidal portal blockage, hemodynamic changes (including portal hypertension), and periportal fibrosis. Similar processes occur in the bladder.

Clinical Features Clinical manifestations vary by species, intensity of infection, and host factors.

- Cercarial invasion ("swimmers' itch"): An itchy maculopapular rash develops 2–3 days after parasitic invasion. This condition is most frequently caused by *S. mansoni* or *S. japonicum* but is most severe if due to avian schistosomes, which invade human skin but then die in SC tissue.
- Acute schistosomiasis (Katayama fever): A serum sickness–like illness with fever, generalized lymphadenopathy, hepatosplenomegaly, and peripheral blood eosinophilia may develop during worm maturation and at the start of oviposition. Parasite-specific antibodies may be detected before eggs are seen in excreta.
- Chronic schistosomiasis causes manifestations that depend primarily on the schistosome species.

  1. Intestinal species cause colicky abdominal pain, bloody diarrhea, malabsorption, hepatosplenomegaly, and portal hypertension. Esophageal varices with bleeding, ascites, hypoalbuminemia, and coagulation defects are late complications.
  2. Urinary species cause dysuria, frequency, hematuria, obstruction with hydroureter and hydronephrosis, fibrosis of bladder granulomas, and late development of squamous cell carcinoma of the bladder.
  3. Granulomata and fibrosis at other sites (e.g., in the lungs and the CNS) may occur.

Diagnosis Diagnosis is based on clinical presentation, blood eosinophilia, and a positive serologic assay for schistosomal antibodies. Examination of stool or urine can yield positive results. Infection may also be diagnosed by examination of tissue samples (e.g., rectal biopsies).

℞ TREATMENT

Severe acute schistosomiasis requires hospitalization and supportive measures along with a consideration of glucocorticoid treatments. After the acute critical phase has resolved, praziquantel results in parasitologic cure in ~85% of cases. The recommended doses are 20 mg/kg bid for 1 day for *S. mansoni*, *S. intercalatum*, and *S. haematobium* infections and 20 mg/kg tid for 1 day for *S. japonicum* and *S. mekongi* infections. Late established manifestations, such as fibrosis, do not improve with treatment.

Prevention Travelers should avoid contact with all freshwater bodies.

Liver (Biliary) Flukes

Stool ova and parasite (O & P) examination diagnoses infection with liver flukes.

- Clonorchiasis and opisthorchiasis occur in Southeast Asia. Infection is acquired by ingestion of contaminated raw freshwater fish. Chronic infection causes cholangitis, cholangiohepatitis, and biliary obstruction and is associated with cholangiocarcinoma. Therapy for acute infection consists of praziquantel administration (25 mg/kg tid for 1 day).

• Fascioliasis is endemic in sheep-raising countries. Infection is acquired by ingestion of contaminated aquatic plants (e.g., watercress). Acute disease causes fever, RUQ pain, hepatomegaly, and eosinophilia. Chronic infection is associated with bile duct obstruction and biliary cirrhosis. For treatment, triclabendazole is given as a single dose of 10 mg/kg.

Lung Flukes

Infection with *Paragonimus* spp. is acquired by ingestion of contaminated crayfish and freshwater crabs. Acute infection causes lung hemorrhage, necrosis with cyst formation, and parenchymal eosinophilic infiltrates. A productive cough, with brownish or bloody sputum, in association with peripheral blood eosinophilia is the usual presentation in pts with heavy infection. In chronic cases, bronchitis or bronchiectasis may predominate. CNS disease can also occur and can result in seizures. The diagnosis is made by O & P examination of sputum or stool. Praziquantel (25 mg/kg tid for 1 day) is the therapeutic agent of choice.

CESTODES

The cestodes, or tapeworms, can be classified into two groups, according to whether humans are the definitive or the intermediate hosts. The tapeworm attaches to intestinal mucosa via sucking cups or hooks located on the scolex. Proglottids (segments) form behind the scolex and constitute the bulk of the tapeworm. Eggs of the various *Taenia* species are identical; thus diagnosis to the species level relies on differences in the morphology of the scolex or proglottids.

Taeniasis Saginata

Etiology and Pathogenesis Humans are the definitive host for *Taenia saginata*, the beef tapeworm, which inhabits the upper jejunum. Eggs are excreted in feces and ingested by cattle or other herbivores; larvae encyst (cysticerci) in the striated muscles of these animals. When humans ingest raw or undercooked beef, the cysticerci mature into adult worms.

Clinical Features Pts may experience perianal discomfort, mild abdominal pain, nausea, change in appetite, weakness, and weight loss.

Diagnosis The diagnosis is made by detection of eggs or proglottids in the stool. Eggs may be found in the perianal area. Eosinophilia may develop, and IgE levels may be elevated.

 TREATMENT

Praziquantel is given in a single dose of 10 mg/kg.

Taeniasis Solium and Cysticercosis

Etiology and Pathogenesis Humans are the definitive host and pigs the intermediate host for *T. solium*, the pork tapeworm. The disease, which is due to ingestion of pork infected with cysticerci, is similar to taeniasis saginata. If humans ingest *T. solium* eggs (e.g., as a result of close contact with a tapeworm carrier or via autoinfection), they develop cysticercosis. Larvae penetrate the intestinal wall and are carried to many tissues, where cystercerci develop.

Clinical Features

• Intestinal infections: Epigastric discomfort, nausea, a sensation of hunger, weight loss, and diarrhea can occur, but most infections are asymptomatic.

- Cysticercosis: Cysticerci can be found anywhere in the body but most often are detected in the brain, skeletal muscle, SC tissue, or eye. Neurologic manifestations are most common and include seizures due to inflammation surrounding cysticerci in the brain, hydrocephalus (from obstruction of CSF flow by cysticerci and accompanying inflammation or by arachnoiditis), headache, nausea, vomiting, changes in vision, dizziness, ataxia, and confusion.

Diagnosis   Intestinal infection is diagnosed by detection of eggs or proglottids in stool. The diagnosis of cysticercosis is confirmed in pts with either one absolute criterion or a combination of two major criteria, one minor criterion, and one epidemiologic criterion (Table 116-1). Findings on neuroimaging include cystic lesions with or without enhancement, one or more nodular calcifications, or focal enhancing lesions.

℞ TREATMENT

Intestinal infections respond to a single dose of praziquantel (10 mg/kg). Neurocysticercosis can be treated with albendazole (15 mg/kg per day for 8–28 days) or praziquantel (50–60 mg/kg daily in 3 divided doses for 15 days or 100 mg/kg in 3 doses given over 1 day). Pts should be carefully monitored, given the potential for an inflammatory response to treatment. High-dose glucocorticoids can be administered during treatment, particularly if symptoms become worse during therapy; since glucocorticoids induce praziquantel metabolism, cimetidine should be given with praziquantel to inhibit this effect. Supportive measures include antiepileptic administration and treatment of hydrocephalus as indicated.

Table 116-1

Proposed Diagnostic Criteria for Human Cysticercosis, 2001

1. Absolute criteria
   a. Demonstration of cysticerci by histologic or microscopic examination of biopsy material
   b. Visualization of the parasite in the eye by funduscopy
   c. Neuroradiologic demonstration of cystic lesions containing a characteristic scolex
2. Major criteria
   a. Neuroradiologic lesions suggestive of neurocysticercosis
   b. Demonstration of antibodies to cysticerci in serum by enzyme-linked immunoelectrotransfer blot
   c. Resolution of intracranial cystic lesions spontaneously or after therapy with albendazole or praziquantel alone
3. Minor criteria
   a. Lesions compatible with neurocysticercosis detected by neuroimaging studies
   b. Clinical manifestations suggestive of neurocysticercosis
   c. Demonstration of antibodies to cysticerci or cysticercal antigen in cerebrospinal fluid by ELISA
   d. Evidence of cysticercosis outside the central nervous system (e.g., cigar-shaped soft tissue calcifications)
4. Epidemiologic criteria
   a. Residence in a cysticercosis-endemic area
   b. Frequent travel to a cysticercosis-endemic area
   c. Household contact with an individual infected with *Taenia solium*

Source: Modified from OH Del Brutto et al: Neurology 57:177, 2001.

Echinococcosis

Etiology and Pathogenesis Echinococcosis is an infection of humans that is caused by *Echinococcus* larvae. The adult worm of *E. granulosus* lives in the jejunum of dogs and releases eggs that humans may ingest. Disease is prevalent in areas where livestock is raised in association with dogs. After ingestion, embryos escape from the eggs, penetrate the intestinal mucosa, enter the portal circulation, and are carried to many organs but particularly the liver and lungs. Larvae develop into fluid-filled unilocular hydatid cysts within which daughter cysts develop, as do germinating cystic structures. Cysts expand over years. *E. multilocularis*, found in arctic or subarctic regions, is similar, but rodents are the intermediate hosts. The parasite is multilocular, and vesicles progressively invade host tissue by peripheral extension of processes from the germinal layer.

Clinical Features Expanding cysts exert the effects of space-occupying lesions, causing symptoms in the affected organ. Pts with hepatic disease most commonly present with abdominal pain or a palpable mass in the RUQ. Compression of a bile duct may cause biliary obstruction or may mimic cholelithiasis. Rupture or leakage from a hydatid cyst may cause fever, pruritus, urticaria, eosinophilia, or anaphylaxis. Pulmonary cysts may rupture into the bronchial tree or the peritoneal cavity and cause cough, chest pain, or hemoptysis. Rupture of cysts may result in multifocal dissemination. *E. multilocularis* disease may present as a hepatic tumor, with destruction of the liver and extension into vital structures.

Diagnosis Radiographic imaging is important in evaluating echinococcal cysts. Daughter cysts within a larger cyst are pathognomonic. Eggshell or mural calcification on CT is indicative of *E. granulosus* infections. Serology may be useful but can be negative in up to half of pts with lung cysts. Serology is usually positive in pts with hepatic disease. Aspiration of cysts usually is not attempted because leakage of cyst fluid can cause dissemination or anaphylactic reactions.

 TREATMENT

Ultrasound staging is recommended for *E. granulosus* infection. Therapy is based on considerations of the size, location, and manifestations of cysts and the overall health of the pt. For some uncomplicated lesions, percutaneous aspiration, infusion of scolicidal agents, and reaspiration are recommended. Albendazole (15 mg/kg daily in 2 divided doses for 4 days before the procedure and for at least 4 weeks afterward) is given for prophylaxis of secondary peritoneal echinococcosis due to inadvertent spillage of fluid during this treatment. Surgery is the treatment of choice for complicated *E. granulosus* cysts. Albendazole should also be given prophylactically, as just described. Praziquantel (50 mg/kg daily for 2 weeks) may hasten the death of protoscolices. Medical therapy alone with albendazole for 12 weeks to 6 months results in cure in ~30% of cases and in clinical improvement in another 50%. *E. multilocularis* infection is treated surgically, and albendazole is given for at least 2 years after presumptively curative surgery. If surgery is not curative, albendazole should be continued indefinitely.

Diphyllobothriasis

Diphyllobothrium latum, the longest tapeworm (up to 25 cm), attaches to the ileal and occasionally the jejunal mucosa. Humans are infected by eating raw fish. Symptoms are rare and usually mild, but infection can cause vitamin B_{12} deficiency because the tapeworm absorbs large amounts of vitamin B_{12} and interferes with ileal B_{12} absorption. Up to 2% of infected pts, especially the elderly, have megaloblastic anemia resembling pernicious anemia and can suffer neurologic sequelae due to B_{12} deficiency. The diagnosis is made by detection of eggs in the stool. Praziquantel (5–10 mg/kg once) is highly effective.

ECTOPARASITES

Ectoparasites are helminths that infest the skin of other animals, from which they derive sustenance. These organisms can incidentally inflict direct injury, elicit hypersensitivity, or inoculate toxins or pathogens.

Scabies

Etiology   Scabies is caused by the human itch mite *Sarcoptes scabiei*.

Life Cycle and Epidemiology   Gravid female mites burrow beneath the stratum corneum, deposit eggs that mature in 2 weeks, and emerge as adults to reinvade the same or another host. Scabies transmission is facilitated by intimate contact with an infested person and by crowding, uncleanliness, or contact with multiple sexual partners. The itching and rash are due to a sensitization reaction against excreta of the mite. Scratching destroys the mite, and most infestations are limited to <15 mites per person. Norwegian or crusted scabies—hyperinfestation with thousands of mites—is associated with glucocorticoid use and immunodeficiency diseases, including HIV disease.

Clinical Features   Itching is worst at night and after a hot shower. Burrows appear as dark wavy lines that end in a pearly bleb containing the female mite. Most lesions are between the fingers or on the volar wrists, elbows, and penis. Bacterial superinfection can occur.

Diagnosis   Scrapings from unroofed burrows reveal the mite, its eggs, or fecal pellets.

 TREATMENT

> Permethrin cream (5%) should be applied thinly behind the ears and from the neck down after bathing and removed 8 h later with soap and water. Alternatives include topical crotamiton cream, benzyl benzoate, and sulfur ointments. A dose of ivermectin (200 µg/kg) is also effective but is not yet approved by the FDA for scabies treatment. For crusted scabies, first a keratolytic agent (e.g., 6% salicylic acid) and then scabicides are applied to the scalp, face, and ears in addition to the rest of the body. Several doses of ivermectin may be required in pts with crusted scabies. Itching and hypersensitivity may persist for weeks or months in scabies and should be managed with symptom-based treatment. Bedding and clothing should be washed in hot water and dried in a heated dryer, and close contacts should be treated to prevent reinfestations.

Pediculosis

Etiology and Epidemiology   Nymphs and adults of human lice—*Pediculus capitis* (the head louse), *P. humanus* (the body louse), and *Pthirus pubis* (the pubic louse)—feed at least once a day and ingest human blood exclusively. The saliva of these lice produces an irritating rash in sensitized persons. Eggs are cemented firmly to hair or clothing, and empty eggs (nits) remain affixed for months after hatching. Lice are generally transmitted from person to person. Head lice are transmitted among schoolchildren, body lice are transmitted between persons who do not change their clothes often, and pubic lice are usually transmitted sexually. The tendency of the body louse to leave febrile persons or corpses may facilitate the transmission of diseases such as louse-borne typhus, relapsing fever, and trench fever.

Diagnosis The diagnosis can be suspected if nits are detected, but confirmatory measures should include the demonstration of a live louse.

 TREATMENT

If live lice are found, treatment with 1% permethrin (two 10-min applications 10 days apart) is usually adequate. If this course fails, treatment for 8–12 h with 0.5% malathion may be indicated. Ivermectin may be useful in cases resistant to permethrin and malathion. Eyelid infestations should be treated with petrolatum applied for 3–4 days or with 1% yellow oxide of mercury ointment applied 4 times daily for 2 weeks. The hair should be combed with a fine-toothed comb to remove nits. Pediculicides must be applied from head to foot to remove body lice. Clothes and bedding should be deloused by placement in a hot dryer for 30 minutes or by fumigation.

Myiasis

In this infestation, maggots invade living or necrotic tissue or body cavities and produce clinical syndromes that vary with the species of fly. In wound and body-cavity myiasis, flies are attracted to blood and pus, and newly hatched larvae enter wounds or diseased skin. Treatment consists of maggot removal and tissue debridement.

Leech Infestations

Medicinal leeches can reduce venous congestion in surgical flaps or replanted body parts. *Aeromonas hydrophila* colonizes the gullets of commercially available leeches. Prophylactic antibiotics are indicated for the prevention of human infection.

For a more detailed discussion, see Davis CE: Laboratory Diagnosis of Parasitic Infections, Chap. 192, p. 1197; Moore TA: Agents Used to Treat Infections Due to Parasites and *Pneumocystis*, Chap. 193, p. 1202; Weller PF: *Trichinella* and Other Tissue Nematodes, Chap. 200, p. 1253; Weller PF, Nutman TB: Intestinal Nematodes, Chap. 201, p. 1256; Nutman TB, Weller PF: Filarial and Related Infections, Chap. 202, p. 1260; Mahmoud AAF: Schistosomiasis and Other Trematode Infections, Chap. 203, p. 1266; White AC Jr, Weller PF: Cestodes, Chap. 204, p. 1272; and Maguire JH et al: Ectoparasite Infestations and Arthropod Bites and Stings, Chap. 379, p. 2600, in HPIM-16.

117

PHYSICAL EXAMINATION OF THE HEART

General examination of a pt with suspected heart disease should include vital signs (respiratory rate, pulse, blood pressure), skin color, clubbing, edema, evidence of decreased perfusion (cool and sweaty skin), and hypertensive changes in optic fundi. Important findings on cardiovascular examination include:

CAROTID ARTERY PULSE (Fig. 117-1)

- *Pulsus parvus*: Weak upstroke due to decreased stroke volume (hypovolemia, LV failure, aortic or mitral stenosis).
- *Pulsus tardus*: Delayed upstroke (aortic stenosis).
- *Bounding (hyperkinetic) pulse*: Hyperkinetic circulation, aortic regurgitation, patent ductus arteriosus, marked vasodilatation.
- *Pulsus bisferiens*: Double systolic pulsation in aortic regurgitation, hypertrophic cardiomyopathy.
- *Pulsus alternans*: Regular alteration in pulse pressure amplitude (severe LV dysfunction).
- *Pulsus paradoxus*: Exaggerated inspiratory fall (>10 mmHg) in systolic bp (pericardial tamponade, severe obstructive lung disease).

JUGULAR VENOUS PULSATION (JVP) Jugular venous distention develops in right-sided heart failure, constrictive pericarditis, pericardial tamponade, obstruction of superior vena cava. JVP normally falls with inspiration but may rise (Kussmaul's sign) in constrictive pericarditis. Abnormalities in examination include:

- *Large "a" wave*: Tricuspid stenosis (TS), pulmonic stenosis, AV dissociation (right atrium contracts against closed tricuspid valve).
- *Large "v" wave*: Tricuspid regurgitation, atrial septal defect.
- *Steep "y" descent*: Constrictive pericarditis.
- *Slow "y" descent*: Tricuspid stenosis.

PRECORDIAL PALPATION Cardiac apical impulse is normally localized in the fifth intercostal space, midclavicular line (Fig. 117-2). Abnormalities

A. Hypokinetic Pulse   B. Parvus et Tardus Pulse   C. Hyperkinetic Pulse

D. Bisferiens Pulse   E. Dicrotic Pulse + Alternans

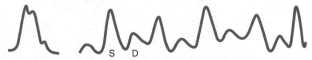

S   D

FIGURE 117-1   Carotid artery pulse patterns.

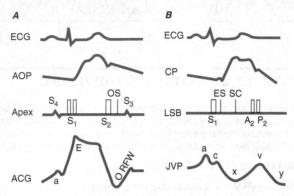

FIGURE 117-2 *A.* Schematic representation of electrocardiogram, aortic pressure pulse (AOP), phonocardiogram recorded at the apex, and apex cardiogram (ACG). On the phonocardiogram, S_1, S_2, S_3, and S_4 represent the first through fourth heart sounds; OS represents the opening snap of the mitral valve, which occurs coincident with the O point of the apex cardiogram. S_3 occurs coincident with the termination of the rapid-filling wave (RFW) of the ACG, while S_4 occurs coincident with the *a* wave of the ACG. *B.* Simultaneous recording of electrocardiogram, indirect carotid pulse (CP), phonocardiogram along the left sternal border (LSB), and indirect jugular venous pulse (JVP). ES, ejection sound; SC, systolic click.

include:

- *Forceful apical thrust*: Left ventricular hypertrophy.
- *Lateral and downward displacement of apex impulse*: Left ventricular dilatation.
- *Prominent presystolic impulse*: Hypertension, aortic stenosis, hypertrophic cardiomyopathy.
- *Double systolic apical impulse*: Hypertrophic cardiomyopathy.
- *Sustained "lift" at lower left sternal border*: Right ventricular hypertrophy.
- *Dyskinetic (outward bulge) impulse*: Ventricular aneurysm, large dyskinetic area post MI, cardiomyopathy.

AUSCULTATION

HEART SOUNDS (Fig. 117-2) *S_1* *Loud*: Mitral stenosis, short PR interval, hyperkinetic heart, thin chest wall. *Soft*: Long PR interval, heart failure, mitral regurgitation, thick chest wall, pulmonary emphysema.

S_2 Normally A_2 precedes P_2 and splitting increases with inspiration; abnormalities include:

- *Widened* splitting: Right bundle branch block, pulmonic stenosis, mitral regurgitation.
- *Fixed* splitting (no respiratory change in splitting): Atrial septal defect.
- *Narrow* splitting: Pulmonary hypertension.
- *Paradoxical* splitting (splitting narrows with inspiration): Aortic stenosis, left bundle branch block, CHF.
- *Loud* A_2: Systemic hypertension.
- *Soft* A_2: Aortic stenosis (AS).
- *Loud* P_2: Pulmonary arterial hypertension.
- *Soft* P_2: Pulmonic stenosis (PS).

S_3 Low-pitched, heard best with bell of stethoscope at apex, following S_2; normal in children; after age 30–35, indicates LV failure or volume overload.

S_4 Low-pitched, heard best with bell at apex, preceding S_1; reflects atrial contraction into a noncompliant ventricle; found in AS, hypertension, hypertrophic cardiomyopathy, and CAD.

Opening Snap (OS) High-pitched; follows S_2 (by 0.06–0.12 s), heard at lower left sternal border and apex in mitral stenosis (MS); the more severe the MS, the shorter the S_2–OS interval.

Ejection Clicks High-pitched sounds following S_1; observed in dilatation of aortic root or pulmonary artery, congenital AS (loudest at apex) or PS (upper left sternal border); the latter decreases with inspiration.

Midsystolic Clicks At lower left sternal border and apex, often followed by late systolic murmur in mitral valve prolapse.

HEART MURMURS (Table 117-1, Fig. 117-3) *Systolic Murmurs* May be "crescendo-decrescendo" ejection type, pansystolic, or late systolic; right-sided murmurs (e.g., tricuspid regurgitation) typically increase with inspiration.

Diastolic Murmurs

• *Early diastolic murmurs*: Begin immediately after S_2, are high-pitched, and are usually caused by aortic or pulmonary regurgitation.
• *Mid-to-late diastolic murmurs*: Low-pitched, heard best with bell of stethoscope; observed in MS or TS; less commonly due to atrial myxoma.
• *Continuous murmurs*: Present in systole and diastole (envelops S_2); found in patent ductus arteriosus and sometimes in coarctation of aorta; less common

Table 117-1

Heart Murmurs

SYSTOLIC MURMURS	
Ejection-type	Aortic outflow tract
	Aortic valve stenosis
	Hypertrophic obstructive cardiomyopathy
	Aortic flow murmur
	Pulmonary outflow tract
	Pulmonic valve stenosis
	Pulmonic flow murmur
Holosystolic	Mitral regurgitation
	Tricuspid regurgitation
	Ventricular septal defect
Late-systolic	Mitral or tricuspid valve prolapse
DIASTOLIC MURMURS	
Early diastolic	Aortic valve regurgitation
	Pulmonic valve regurgitation
Mid-to-late diastolic	Mitral or tricuspid stenosis
	Flow murmur across mitral or tricuspid valves
Continuous	Patent ductus arteriosus
	Coronary AV fistula
	Ruptured sinus of Valsalva aneurysm

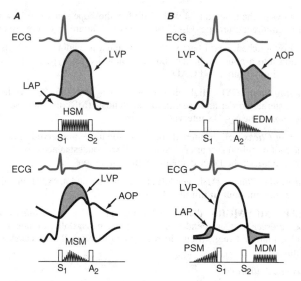

FIGURE 117-3   *A.* Schematic representation of ECG, aortic pressure (AOP), left ventricular pressure (LVP), and left atrial pressure (LAP). The hatched areas indicated a transvalvular pressure difference during systole. HSM, holosystolic murmur; MSM, midsystolic murmur. *B.* Graphic representation of ECG, aortic pressure (AOP), left ventricular pressure (LVP), and left atrial pressure (LAP) with hatched areas indicating transvalvular diastolic pressure difference. EDM, early diastolic murmur; PSM, presystolic murmur; MDM, middiastolic murmur.

causes are systemic or coronary AV fistula, aortopulmonary septal defect, ruptured aneurysm of sinus of Valsalva.

For a more detailed discussion, see O'Rourke RA, Braunwald E: Physical Examination of the Cardiovascular System, Chap. 209, p. 1304, in HPIM-16.

118

ELECTROCARDIOGRAPHY AND ECHOCARDIOGRAPHY

STANDARD APPROACH TO THE ECG
Normally, standardization is 1.0 mV per 10 mm, and paper speed is 25 mm/s (each horizontal small box = 0.04 s).

   HEART RATE   Beats/min = 300 divided by the number of *large* boxes (each 5 mm apart) between consecutive QRS complexes. For faster heart rates, divide 1500 by number of *small* boxes (1 mm apart) between each QRS.

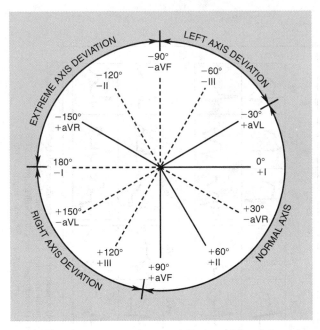

FIGURE 118-1 Electrocardiographic lead systems: The hexaxial frontal plane reference system to estimate electrical axis. Determine leads in which QRS deflections are maximum and minimum. For example, a maximum positive QRS in I which is isoelectric in aVF is oriented to 0°. Normal axis ranges from −30° to +90°. An axis > + 90° is right axis deviation and < −30° is left axis deviation.

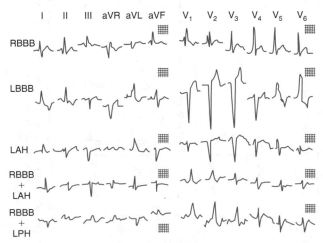

FIGURE 118-2 Intraventricular conduction abnormalities. Illustrated are right bundle branch block (RBBB); left bundle branch block (LBBB); left anterior hemiblock (LAH); right bundle branch block with left anterior hemiblock (RBBB + LAH); and right bundle branch block with left posterior hemiblock (RBBB + LPH). (*Reproduced from RJ Myerburg: HPIM-12.*)

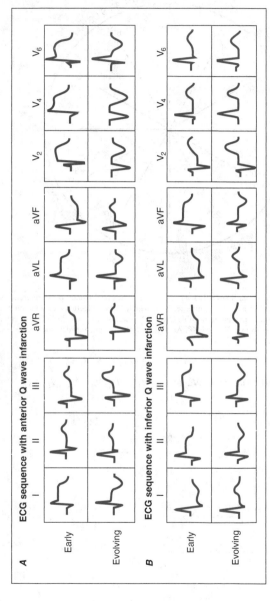

FIGURE 118-3 Sequence of depolarization and repolarization changes with (*A*) acute anterior and (*B*) acute inferior wall Q-wave infarctions. With anterior infarcts, ST elevation in leads I, aVL, and the precordial leads may be accompanied by reciprocal ST depressions in leads II, III, and aVF. Conversely, acute inferior (or posterior) infarcts may be associated with reciprocal ST depressions in leads V_1 to V_3. (*After AL Goldberger, E Goldberger: Clinical Electrocardiography: A Simplified Approach, 6th ed. St. Louis, Mosby-Year Book, 1999.*)

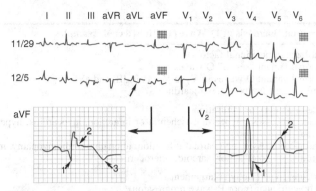

FIGURE 118-4   Acute inferior wall myocardial infarction. The ECG of 11/29 shows minor nonspecific ST-segment and T-wave changes. On 12/5 an acute myocardial infarction occurred. There are pathologic Q waves (1), ST-segment elevation (2), and terminal T-wave inversion (3) in leads II, III, and aVF indicating the location of the infarct on the inferior wall. Reciprocal changes in aVL (small arrow). Increasing R-wave voltage with ST depression and increased voltage of the T wave in V_2 are characteristic of true posterior wall extension of the inferior infarction. (*Reproduced from RJ Myerburg: HPIM-12.*)

RHYTHM   *Sinus rhythm* is present if every P wave is followed by a QRS, PR interval ≥ 0.12 s, every QRS is preceded by a P wave, and the P wave is upright in leads I, II, and III. Arrhythmias are discussed in Chap. 125.

MEAN AXIS   If QRS is primarily positive in limb leads I and II, then axis is *normal*. Otherwise, find limb lead in which QRS is most isoelectric (R = S). The mean axis is perpendicular to that lead (Fig. 118-1). If the QRS complex is *positive* in that perpendicular lead, then mean axis is in the direction of that lead; if *negative*, then mean axis points directly away from that lead.

Left-axis deviation (more negative than $-30°$) occurs in diffuse left ventricular disease, inferior MI; also in left anterior hemiblock (small R, deep S in leads II, III, and aVF).

Right-axis deviation ($>90°$) occurs in right ventricular hypertrophy (R > S in V_1) and left posterior hemiblock (small Q and tall R in leads II, III, and aVF). Mild right-axis deviation is seen in thin, healthy individuals (up to $110°$).

INTERVALS (Normal values in parentheses)   *PR* (0.12–0.20 s)

- *Short:* (1) preexcitation syndrome (look for slurred QRS upstroke due to "delta" wave), (2) nodal rhythm (inverted P in aVF).
- *Long:* first-degree AV block (Chap. 125).

Table 118-1

Leads with Abnormal Q Waves in MI

Leads with Abnormal Q Waves	Site of Infarction
V_1–V_2	Anteroseptal
V_3–V_4	Apical
I, aVL, V_5–V_6	Anterolateral
II, III, aVF	Inferior
V_1–V_2 (tall R, *not* deep Q)	True posterior

Table 118-2

Differential Diagnosis of Q Waves (with Selected Examples)

Physiologic or positional factors
1. Normal variant "septal" Q waves
2. Normal variant Q waves in V_1 to V_2, aVL, III, and aVF
3. Left pneumothorax or dextrocardia

Myocardial injury or infiltration
1. Acute processes: myocardial ischemia or infarction, myocarditis, hyperkalemia
2. Chronic processes: myocardial infarction, idiopathic cardiomyopathy, myocarditis, amyloid, tumor, sarcoid, scleroderma

Ventricular hypertrophy/enlargement
1. Left ventricular (poor R-wave progression)[a]
2. Right ventricular (reversed R-wave progression)
3. Hypertrophic cardiomyopathy

Conduction abnormalities
1. Left bundle branch block
2. Wolff-Parkinson-White patterns

---

[a] Small or absent R waves in the right to midprecordial leads.
Source: After AL Goldberger: *Myocardial Infarction: Electrocardiographic Differential Diagnosis*, 4th ed. St. Louis, Mosby-Year Book, 1991.

QRS (0.06–0.10 s) *Widened:* (1) ventricular premature beats, (2) bundle branch blocks: *right* (RsR′ in V_1, deep S in V_6) and *left* [RR′ in V_6 (Fig. 118-2)], (3) toxic levels of certain drugs (e.g., quinidine), (4) severe hypokalemia.

QT (≤0.43 s; <50% of RR interval) *Prolonged:* congenital, hypokalemia, hypocalcemia, drugs (quinidine, procainamide, tricyclics).

HYPERTROPHY

- *Right atrium:* P wave ≥ 2.5 mm in lead II.
- *Left atrium:* P biphasic (positive, then negative) in V_1, with terminal negative force wider than 0.04 s.

Table 118-3

Clinical Uses of Echocardiography

2-D echo
  Cardiac chambers:
    size, hypertrophy,
    wall motion abnormalities
  Valves: morphology and motion
  Pericardium: effusion, tamponade
  Aorta: Aneurysm, dissection
  Assess intracardiac masses
Doppler echocardiography
  Valvular stenosis and regurgitation
  Intracardiac shunts
  Diastolic filling/dysfunction
  Approximate intracardiac pressures

Transesophageal echocardiography
  Superior to 2-D echo to identify:
    Infective endocarditis
    Cardiac source of embolism
    Prosthetic valve dysfunction
    Aortic dissection
Stress echocardiography
  Assess myocardial ischemia and
    viability

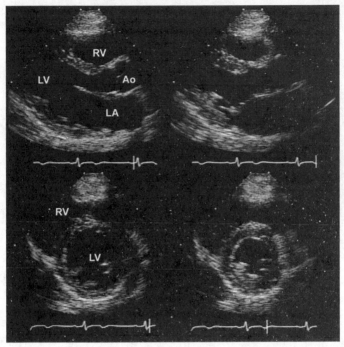

FIGURE 118-5 Two-dimensional echocardiographic still-frame images from a normal patient with a normal heart. *Upper*: Parasternal long axis view during systole and diastole (*left*) and systole (*right*). During systole, there is thickening of the myocardium and reduction in the size of the left ventricle (LV). The valve leaflets ate thin and open widely. *Lower*: Parasternal short axis view during diastole (*left*) and systole (*right*) demonstrating a decrease in the left ventricular cavity size during systole as well as an increase in wall thickening. LA, left atrium; RV, right ventricle; Ao, aorta. (*Reproduced from RJ Myerburg in HPIM-12.*)

- *Right ventricle:* R > S in V_1 and R in V_1 > 5 mm; deep S in V_6; right-axis deviation.
- *Left ventricle:* S in V_1 plus R in V_5 or V_6 ≥ 35 mm or R in aVL > 11 mm.

INFARCTION (Figs. 118-3 and 118-4) *Q-wave MI:* Pathologic Q waves (≥0.04 s and ≥25% of total QRS height) in leads shown in Table 118-1; acute *non-Q-wave MI* shows ST-T changes in these leads without Q wave development. A number of conditions (other than acute MI) can cause Q waves (Table 118-2).

ST-T WAVES

- *ST elevation*: Acute MI, coronary spasm, pericarditis (concave upward) (see Fig 121-1 and Table 121-2), LV aneurysm.
- *ST depression*: Digitalis effect, strain (due to ventricular hypertrophy), ischemia, or nontransmural MI.
- *Tall peaked T*: Hyperkalemia; acute MI ("hyperacute T").
- *Inverted T*: Non-Q-wave MI, ventricular "strain" pattern, drug effect (e.g., digitalis), hypokalemia, hypocalcemia, increased intracranial pressure (e.g., subarachnoid bleed).

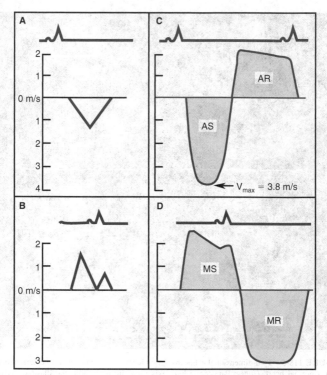

FIGURE 118-6 Schematic presentation of normal Doppler flow across the aortic (*A*) and mitral valves (*B*). Abnormal continuous wave Doppler profiles are depicted in *C*. Aortic stenosis (AS) [peak transaortic gradient = $4 \times V_{max}^2 = 4 \times (3.8)^2 = 58$ mmHg] and regurgitation (AR). *D*. Mitral stenosis (MS) and regurgitation (MR).

INDICATIONS FOR ECHOCARDIOGRAPHY
(Table 118-3 and Fig. 118-5)

VALVULAR STENOSIS Both native and artificial valvular stenosis can be evaluated, and severity can be determined by Doppler [peak gradient = $4 \times$ (peak velocity)^2].

VALVULAR REGURGITATION Structural lesions (e.g., flail leaflet, vegetation) resulting in regurgitation may be identified. Echo can demonstrate whether ventricular function is normal; Doppler (Fig. 118-6) can identify and estimate severity of regurgitation through each valve.

VENTRICULAR PERFORMANCE Global and regional wall motion abnormalities of both ventricles can be assessed; ventricular hypertrophy/infiltration may be visualized; evidence of pulmonary hypertension may be obtained.

CARDIAC SOURCE OF EMBOLISM May visualize atrial or ventricular thrombus, intracardiac tumors, and valvular vegetations. Yield of identifying cardiac source of embolism is *low* in absence of cardiac history or physical findings. Transesophageal echocardiography is more sensitive than standard transthoracic study for this purpose.

ENDOCARDITIS Vegetation visualized in more than half of pts (transesophageal echo has much higher sensitivity), but management is generally based on clinical findings, not echo. Complications of endocarditis (e.g., valvular regurgitation) may be evaluated.

CONGENITAL HEART DISEASE Echo, Doppler, and contrast echo (rapid IV injection of saline) are noninvasive procedures of choice in identifying congenital lesions.

AORTIC ROOT Aneurysm and dissection of the aorta may be evaluated and complications (aortic regurgitation, tamponade) assessed (Chap. 127).

HYPERTROPHIC CARDIOMYOPATHY, MITRAL VALVE PROLAPSE, PERICARDIAC EFFUSION Echo is the diagnostic technique of choice for identifying these conditions.

For a more detailed discussion, see Goldberger AL: Electrocardiography, Chap. 210, p. 1311; Nishimura RA, Gibbons RJ, Glockner JF, Tajik AJ: Noninvasive Cardiac Imaging: Echocardiography, Nuclear Cardiology, and MRI/CT Imaging, Chap. 211, p. 1320, in HPIM-16.

119

VALVULAR HEART DISEASE

MITRAL STENOSIS (MS)

ETIOLOGY Most commonly rheumatic, although history of acute rheumatic fever is now uncommon; congenital MS is an uncommon cause, observed primarily in infants.

HISTORY Symptoms most commonly begin in the fourth decade, but MS often causes severe disability by age 20 in economically deprived areas. Principal symptoms are dyspnea and pulmonary edema precipitated by exertion, excitement, fever, anemia, paroxysmal tachycardia, pregnancy, sexual intercourse, etc.

PHYSICAL EXAMINATION Right ventricular lift; palpable S_1; opening snap (OS) follows A_2 by 0.06 to 0.12 s; OS–A_2 interval inversely proportional to severity of obstruction. Diastolic rumbling murmur with presystolic accentuation in sinus rhythm. Duration of murmur correlates with severity of obstruction.

COMPLICATIONS Hemoptysis, pulmonary embolism, pulmonary infection, systemic embolization; endocarditis is *uncommon* in pure MS.

LABORATORY *ECG* Typically shows atrial fibrillation (AF) or left atrial (LA) enlargement when sinus rhythm is present. Right-axis deviation and RV hypertrophy in the presence of pulmonary hypertension.

CXR Shows LA and RV enlargement and Kerley B lines.

ECHOCARDIOGRAM Most useful noninvasive test; shows inadequate separation, calcification and thickening of valve leaflets, and LA enlargement.

Doppler echocardiogram allows estimation of transvalvular gradient and mitral valve area (Chap. 118).

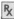 **TREATMENT** See Fig. 119-1.

Pts should receive prophylaxis for rheumatic fever (penicillin) and infective endocarditis (Chap. 85). In the presence of dyspnea, medical therapy for heart failure; digitalis, beta blockers, or rate-limiting calcium channel antagonists (i.e., verapamil or diltiazem) to slow ventricular rate in AF; diuretics and sodium restriction. Warfarin (with target INR 2.0–3.0) for pts with AF and/or history of systemic and pulmonic emboli. Mitral valvotomy in the presence of symptoms and mitral orifice ≤ ~1.7 cm². In uncomplicated MS, percutaneous balloon valvuloplasty is the procedure of choice; if not feasible, then open surgical valvotomy.

MITRAL REGURGITATION (MR)

ETIOLOGY Rheumatic heart disease in ~33%. Other causes: mitral valve prolapse, ischemic heart disease with papillary muscle dysfunction, LV dilatation of any cause, mitral annular calcification, hypertrophic cardiomyopathy, infective endocarditis, congenital.

CLINICAL MANIFESTATIONS Fatigue, weakness, and exertional dyspnea. Physical examination: sharp upstroke of arterial pulse, LV lift, S_1 diminished: wide splitting of S_2; S_3; loud holosystolic murmur and often a brief early-mid-diastolic murmur.

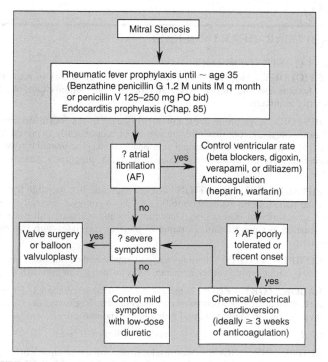

FIGURE 119-1 Management of mitral stenosis.

ECHOCARDIOGRAM Enlarged LA, hyperdynamic LV; Doppler echocardiogram helpful in diagnosing and assessing severity of MR.

Ⓡₓ **TREATMENT** See Fig. 119-2.

For severe/decompensated MR, treat as for heart failure (Chap. 126), including diuretics and digoxin. Afterload reduction (ACE inhibitors, hydralazine, or IV nitroprusside) decreases the degree of regurgitation, increases forward cardiac output, and improves symptomatology. Endocarditis prophylaxis is indicated, as is anticoagulation in the presence of atrial fibrillation. Surgical treatment, either valve repair or replacement, is indicated in the presence of symptoms or evidence of progressive LV dysfunction (LVEF < 60% or end-systolic LV diameter by echo >45 mm). Operation should be carried out *before* development of severe chronic heart failure.

MITRAL VALVE PROLAPSE (MVP)

ETIOLOGY Most commonly idiopathic; ?familial; may accompany rheumatic fever, ischemic heart disease, atrial septal defect, the Marfan syndrome.

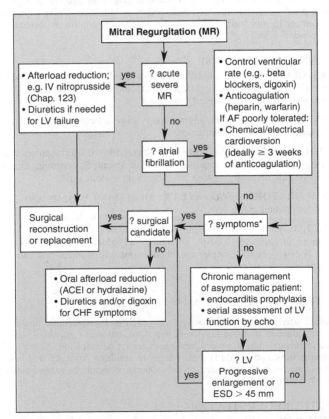

FIGURE 119-2 Management of advanced mitral regurgitation. *Including class II; ACEI, angiotensin-converting enzyme inhibitors; ESD, end-systolic diameter.

PATHOLOGY   Redundant mitral valve tissue with myxedematous degeneration and elongated chordae tendineae.

CLINICAL MANIFESTATIONS   More common in females. Most pts are asymptomatic and remain so. Most common symptoms are atypical chest pain and a variety of supraventricular and ventricular arrhythmias. Most important complication is severe MR resulting in LV failure. Rarely, systemic emboli from platelet-fibrin deposits on valve. Sudden death is a *very rare* complication.

PHYSICAL EXAMINATION   Mid or late systolic click(s) followed by late systolic murmur; exaggeration by Valsalva maneuver, reduced by squatting and isometric exercise (Chap. 117).

ECHOCARDIOGRAM   Shows posterior displacement of one or both mitral leaflets late in systole.

 TREATMENT

Asymptomatic pts should be reassured, but if systolic murmur and/or typical echocardiographic findings with thickened leaflets are present, or significant MR, prophylaxis for infective endocarditis is indicated. Valve repair or replacement for pts with severe mitral regurgitation; aspirin or anticoagulants for pts with history of TIA or embolization.

AORTIC STENOSIS (AS)

ETIOLOGY   Often congenital; rheumatic AS is usually associated with rheumatic mitral valve disease. Idiopathic, calcific AS is a degenerative disorder common in the elderly and usually mild.

SYMPTOMS   Dyspnea, angina, and syncope are cardinal symptoms; they occur late, after years of obstruction.

PHYSICAL EXAMINATION   Weak and delayed arterial pulses with carotid thrill. Double apical impulse; A_2 soft or absent; S_4 common. Diamond-shaped systolic murmur $\geq$ grade 3/6, often with systolic thrill.

LABORATORY   *ECG and CXR*   Often show LV hypertrophy, but not useful for predicting gradient.

ECHOCARDIOGRAM   Shows thickening of LV wall, calcification and thickening of aortic valve cusps. Dilatation and reduced contraction of LV indicate poor prognosis. Doppler useful for estimating gradient and calculating valve area.

 TREATMENT   See Fig. 119-3.

Avoid strenuous activity in severe AS, even in asymptomatic phase. Treat heart failure in standard fashion (Chap. 126), but *avoid afterload reduction.* Statin therapy may slow progression of leaflet calcification. Valve replacement is indicated in adults with symptoms resulting from AS and hemodynamic evidence of severe obstruction. Operation should be carried out *before* frank failure has developed.

AORTIC REGURGITATION (AR)

ETIOLOGY   Rheumatic etiology is common, especially if rheumatic mitral disease present; may also be due to infective endocarditis, syphilis, aortic

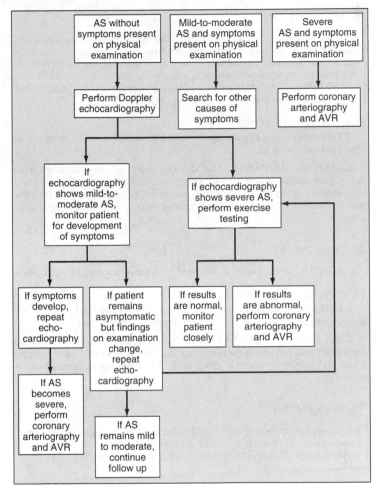

FIGURE 119-3 Algorithm for the management of aortic stenosis (AS). AVR, aortic valve replacement. (*From BA Carabello: N Engl J Med 346:677, 2002.*)

dissection, or aortic dilatation due to cystic medial necrosis; three-fourths of pts are males.

CLINICAL MANIFESTATIONS Exertional dyspnea and awareness of heartbeat, angina pectoris, and signs of LV failure. Wide pulse pressure, waterhammer pulse, capillary pulsations (Quincke's sign), A_2 soft or absent, S_3 common. Blowing, decrescendo diastolic murmur along left sternal border (along right sternal border with aortic dilatation). May be accompanied by systolic murmur of augmented blood flow.

LABORATORY *ECG and CXR* LV enlargement.

ECHOCARDIOGRAM Increased excursion of posterior LV wall, LA enlargement, LV enlargement, high-frequency diastolic fluttering of mitral valve. Doppler studies useful in detection and quantification of AR.

TREATMENT

Standard therapy for LV failure (Chap. 126). Vasodilators (long-acting nifedipine or ACE inhibitors) may delay need for operation. Surgical valve replacement should be carried out in pts with severe AR when symptoms develop or in asymptomatic pts with LV dysfunction (LV ejection fraction < 55%, LV end-systolic volume > 55 mL/m² , or end-systolic diameter > 55 mm) by echocardiography.

TRICUSPID STENOSIS (TS)

ETIOLOGY Usually rheumatic; most common in females; almost invariably associated with MS.

CLINICAL MANIFESTATIONS Hepatomegaly, ascites, edema, jaundice, jugular venous distention with slow y descent (Chap. 117). Diastolic rumbling murmur along left sternal border increased by inspiration with loud presystolic component. Right atrial and superior vena caval enlargement on chest x-ray.

 TREATMENT

In severe TS, surgical relief is indicated, with valvular repair or replacement.

TRICUSPID REGURGITATION (TR)

ETIOLOGY Usually functional and secondary to marked RV dilatation of any cause and often associated with pulmonary hypertension.

CLINICAL MANIFESTATIONS Severe RV failure, with edema, hepatomegaly, and prominent v waves in jugular venous pulse with rapid y descent (Chap. 117). Systolic murmur along lower left sternal edge is increased by inspiration.

 TREATMENT

Intensive diuretic therapy when right-sided heart failure signs are present. In severe cases (in absence of severe pulmonary hypertension), surgical treatment consists of tricuspid annuloplasty or valve replacement.

For a more detailed discussion, see Braunwald E: Valvular Heart Disease, Chap. 219, p. 1390, in HPIM-16.

120

CARDIOMYOPATHIES AND MYOCARDITIS

Table 120-1 summarizes distinguishing features of the cardiomyopathies.

DILATED CARDIOMYOPATHY (CMP)

Symmetrically dilated left ventricle (LV), with poor systolic contractile function; right ventricle (RV) commonly involved.

ETIOLOGY Previous myocarditis or "idiopathic" most common; also toxins (ethanol, doxorubicin), connective tissue disorders, muscular dystrophies, "peripartum." Severe coronary disease/infarctions or chronic aortic/mitral regurgitation may behave similarly.

SYMPTOMS Congestive heart failure (Chap. 126); tachyarrhythmias and peripheral emboli from LV mural thrombus occur.

PHYSICAL EXAMINATION Jugular venous distention (JVD), rales, diffuse and dyskinetic LV apex, S_3, hepatomegaly, peripheral edema; murmurs of mitral and tricuspid regurgitation are common.

LABORATORY *ECG* Left bundle branch block and ST-T-wave abnormalities common.

CXR Cardiomegaly, pulmonary vascular redistribution, pulmonary effusions common.

Echocardiogram LV and RV enlargement with globally impaired contraction. *Regional* wall motion abnormalities suggest coronary artery disease rather than primary cardiomyopathy.

Brain Natriuretic Peptide (BNP) Level elevated in heart failure/cardiomyopathy but not in patients with dyspnea due to lung disease.

℞ TREATMENT

Standard therapy of CHF (Chap. 126); vasodilator therapy with ACE inhibitor (preferred), angiotensin receptor blocker or hydralazine-nitrate combination shown to improve longevity. Add beta blocker in most pts (Chap. 126). Add spironolactone for patients with advanced heart failure. Chronic anticoagulation with warfarin, recommended for very low ejection fraction (<25%), if no contraindications. Antiarrhythmic drugs (Chap. 125), e.g., amiodarone, indicated only for symptomatic or sustained arrhythmias as they may cause proarrhythmic side effects; implanted internal defibrillator is often a better alternative. Consider biventricular pacing for persistently symptomatic patients with widened (≥130 ms) QRS complex. Possible trial of immunosuppressive drugs, if active myocarditis present on RV biopsy (controversial as long-term efficacy has not been demonstrated). In selected pts, consider cardiac transplantation.

RESTRICTIVE CARDIOMYOPATHY

Increased myocardial "stiffness" impairs ventricular relaxation; diastolic ventricular pressures are elevated. Etiologies include infiltrative disease (amyloid, sarcoid, hemochromatosis, eosinophilic disorders), myocardial fibrosis, Fabry's disease, and fibroelastosis.

SYMPTOMS Are of CHF, although right-sided heart failure often predominates, with peripheral edema and ascites.

Table 120-1

Laboratory Evaluation of the Cardiomyopathies

	Dilated	Restrictive	Hypertrophic
Chest roentgenogram	Moderate to marked cardiac silhouette enlargement Pulmonary venous hypertension	Mild cardiac silhouette enlargement	Mild to moderate cardiac silhouette enlargement
Electrocardiogram	ST-segment and T-wave abnormalities	Low voltage, conduction defects	ST-segment and T-wave abnormalities Left ventricular hypertrophy Abnormal Q waves
Echocardiogram	Left ventricular dilatation and dysfunction	Increased left ventricular wall thickness Normal or mildly reduced systolic function	Asymmetric septal hypertrophy (ASH) Systolic anterior motion (SAM) of the mitral valve
Radionuclide studies	Left ventricular dilatation and dysfunction (RVG)	Normal or mildly reduced systolic function (RVG)	Vigorous systolic function (RVG) Perfusion defect (^{201}Tl)
Cardiac catheterization	Left ventricular dilatation and dysfunction Elevated left- and often right-sided filling pressures Diminished cardiac output	Normal or mildly reduced systolic function Elevated left- and right-sided filling pressures	Vigorous systolic function Dynamic left ventricular outflow obstruction Elevated left- and right-sided filling pressures

Note: RVG, radionuclide ventriculogram; ^{201}Tl, thallium 201.
Source: J Wynne, E Braunwald, Table 221-3 in HPIM-16.

PHYSICAL EXAMINATION   Signs of right-sided heart failure: JVD, hepatomegaly, peripheral edema, murmur of tricuspid regurgitation. Left-sided signs may also be present.

LABORATORY   *ECG*   Low limb lead voltage, sinus tachycardia, ST-T-wave abnormalities.

CXR   Mild LV enlargement.

Echocardiogram   Bilateral atrial enlargement; increased ventricular thickness ("speckled pattern") in infiltrative disease, especially amyloidosis. Systolic function is usually normal but may be mildly reduced.

Cardiac Catheterization   Increased LV and RV diastolic pressures with "dip and plateau" pattern; RV biopsy useful in detecting infiltrative disease (rectal or fat pad biopsy useful in diagnosis of amyloidosis).

Note: Must distinguish restrictive cardiomyopathy from constrictive pericarditis, which is surgically correctable. Thickening of pericardium in pericarditis usually apparent in CT or MRI.

 TREATMENT

Salt restriction and diuretics ameliorate pulmonary and systemic congestion; digitalis is not indicated unless systolic function impaired or atrial arrhythmias present. *Note*: Increased sensitivity to digitalis in amyloidosis. Anticoagulation often indicated, particularly in pts with eosinophilic endomyocarditis. For specific therapy of hemochromatosis and sarcoidosis, see Chaps. 336 and 309, respectively, in HPIM-16.

HYPERTROPHIC OBSTRUCTIVE CARDIOMYOPATHY (HOCM)
Marked LV hypertrophy; often asymmetric, without underlying cause. Systolic function is normal; increased LV stiffness results in elevated diastolic filling pressures.

SYMPTOMS   Secondary to elevated diastolic pressure, dynamic LV outflow obstruction, and arrhythmias; dyspnea on exertion, angina, and presyncope; sudden death may occur.

PHYSICAL EXAMINATION   Brisk carotid upstroke with pulsus bisferiens; S_4, harsh systolic murmur along left sternal border, blowing murmur of mitral regurgitation at apex; murmur changes with Valsalva and other maneuvers (Chap. 117).

LABORATORY   *ECG*   LV hypertrophy with prominent "septal" Q waves in leads I, aVL, V_{5-6}. Periods of atrial fibrillation or ventricular tachycardia are often detected by Holter monitor.

Echocardiogram   LV hypertrophy, often with asymmetric septal hypertrophy (ASH) and $\geq 1.3 \times$ thickness of LV posterior wall; LV contractile function excellent with small end-systolic volume. If LV outflow tract obstruction is present, systolic anterior motion (SAM) of mitral valve and midsystolic partial closure of aortic valve are present. Doppler shows early systolic accelerated blood flow through LV outflow tract.

TREATMENT

Strenuous exercise should be avoided. Beta blockers, verapamil, diltiazem, or disopyramide used individually to reduce symptoms. Digoxin, other inotropes, diuretics, and vasodilators are generally *contraindicated*. Endocarditis antibiotic prophylaxis (Chap. 85) is necessary when outflow obstruction or mitral regurgitation is present. Antiarrhythmic agents, especially amiodarone, may suppress atrial and ventricular arrhythmias. In selected pts, LV outflow gradient can be reduced by dual-chamber permanent pacemaker or controlled septal infarction by ethanol injection into the septal artery. Consider implantable automatic defibrillator for pts with high-risk profile, e.g., history of syncope or sudden cardiac death, ventricular tachycardia, marked LVH (>3 cm), family history of sudden death. Surgical myectomy may be useful in pts refractory to medical therapy.

MYOCARDITIS

Inflammation of the myocardium most commonly due to acute viral infection; may progress to chronic dilated cardiomyopathy. Myocarditis may develop in pts with HIV infection or Lyme disease.

HISTORY   Fever, fatigue, palpitations; if LV dysfunction is present, then symptoms of CHF are present. Viral myocarditis may be preceded by URI.

PHYSICAL EXAMINATION   Fever, tachycardia, soft S_1; S_3 common.

LABORATORY   CK-MB isoenzyme and cardiac troponins may be elevated in absence of MI. Convalescent antiviral antibody titers may rise.

ECG   Transient ST-T-wave abnormalities.

CXR   Cardiomegaly

Echocardiogram   Depressed LV function; pericardial effusion present if accompanying pericarditis present.

 TREATMENT

Rest; treat as CHF (Chap. 126); immunosuppressive therapy (steroids and azathioprine) may be considered if RV biopsy shows active inflammation, but long-term efficacy has not been demonstrated.

For a more detailed discussion, see Wynne J, Braunwald E: Cardiomyopathy and Myocarditis, Chap. 221, p. 1408, in HPIM-16.

121

PERICARDIAL DISEASE

ACUTE PERICARDITIS
CAUSES   See Table 121-1

HISTORY   Chest pain, which may be intense, mimicking acute MI, but characteristically sharp, pleuritic, and positional (relieved by leaning forward); fever and palpitations are common.

Table 121-1

Most Common Causes of Pericarditis

Idiopathic
Infections (particularly viral)
Acute myocardial infarction
Metastatic neoplasm
Radiation therapy for tumor (up to 20 years earlier)
Chronic renal failure
Connective tissue disease (rheumatoid arthritis, SLE)
Drug reaction (e.g., procainamide, hydralazine)
"Autoimmune" following heart surgery or myocardial infarction (several weeks/ months later)

PHYSICAL EXAMINATION   Rapid or irregular pulse, coarse pericardial friction rub, which may vary in intensity and is loudest with pt sitting forward.

LABORATORY   *ECG*   (See Table 121-2 and Fig. 121-1)   Diffuse ST elevation (concave upward) usually present in all leads except aVR and V_1; PR-segment depression may be present; *days* later (unlike acute MI), ST returns to baseline and T-wave inversion develops. Atrial premature beats and atrial fibrillation may appear. Differentiate from ECG of early repolarization variant (ERV) (ST-T ratio <0.25 in ERV, but >0.25 in pericarditis).

CXR   Increased size of cardiac silhouette if large (>250 mL) pericardial effusion is present, with "water bottle" configuration.

Echocardiogram   Most sensitive test for detection of pericardial effusion, which commonly accompanies acute pericarditis.

℞ TREATMENT

Aspirin 650–975 mg qid or NSAIDs (e.g., indomethacin 25–75 mg qid); for *severe*, *refractory* pain, prednisone 40–80 mg/d is used and tapered over

Table 121-2

ECG in Acute Pericarditis vs. Acute (Q-Wave) MI

ST-Segment Elevation	ECG Lead Involvement	Evolution of ST and T Waves	PR-Segment Depression
PERICARDITIS			
Concave upward	All leads involved except aVR and V_1	ST remains elevated for several days; after ST returns to baseline, T waves invert	Yes, in majority
ACUTE MI			
Convex upward	ST elevation over infarcted region only; reciprocal ST depression in opposite leads	T waves invert within hours, while ST still elevated; followed by Q wave development	No

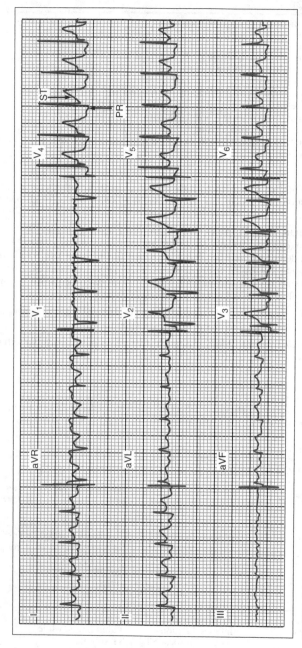

FIGURE 121-1 Electrocardiogram in acute pericarditis. Note diffuse ST-segment elevation and PR-segment depression.

several weeks or months. Intractable, prolonged pain or frequently recurrent episodes may require pericardiectomy. Anticoagulants are relatively contra-indicated in acute pericarditis because of risk of pericardial hemorrhage.

CARDIAC TAMPONADE

Life-threatening emergency resulting from accumulation of pericardial fluid under pressure; impaired filling of cardiac chambers and decreased cardiac output.

ETIOLOGY Previous pericarditis (most commonly metastatic tumor, uremia, acute MI, viral or idiopathic pericarditis), cardiac trauma, or myocardial perforation during catheter or pacemaker placement.

HISTORY Hypotension may develop suddenly; subacute symptoms include dyspnea, weakness, confusion.

PHYSICAL EXAMINATION Tachycardia, hypotension, pulsus paradoxus (inspiratory fall in systolic blood pressure >10 mmHg), jugular venous distention with preserved x descent, but loss of y descent; heart sounds distant. If tamponade develops subacutely, peripheral edema, hepatomegaly, and ascites are frequently present.

LABORATORY *ECG* Low limb lead voltage; large effusions may cause electrical alternans (alternating size of QRS complex due to swinging of heart).

CXR Enlarged cardiac silhouette if large (>250 mL) effusion present.

Echocardiogram Swinging motion of heart within large effusion; prominent respiratory alteration of RV dimension with RA and RV collapse during diastole.

Cardiac Catheterization Confirms diagnosis; shows equalization of diastolic pressures in all four chambers; pericardial = RA pressure.

 TREATMENT

Immediate pericardiocentesis and IV volume expansion.

CONSTRICTIVE PERICARDITIS

Rigid pericardium leads to impaired cardiac filling, elevation of systemic and pulmonary venous pressures, and decreased cardiac output. Results from healing and scar formation in some pts with previous pericarditis. Viral, tuberculosis, previous cardiac surgery, uremia, neoplastic pericarditis are most common causes.

HISTORY Gradual onset of dyspnea, fatigue, pedal edema, abdominal swelling; symptoms of LV failure uncommon.

PHYSICAL EXAMINATION Tachycardia, jugular venous distention (prominent y descent), which increases further on inspiration (Kussmaul's sign); hepatomegaly, ascites, peripheral edema are common; sharp diastolic sound, "pericardial knock" following S_2 sometimes present.

LABORATORY *ECG* Low limb lead voltage; atrial arrhythmias are common.

CXR Rim of pericardial calcification in up to 50% of pts.

Echocardiogram Thickened pericardium, normal ventricular contraction; abrupt halt in ventricular filling in early diastole.

CT or MRI More precise than echocardiogram in demonstrating thickened pericardium.

Cardiac Catheterization Equalization of diastolic pressures in all chambers; ventricular pressure tracings show "dip and plateau" appearance. Pts with constrictive pericarditis should be investigated for tuberculosis (Chap. 102).

℞ TREATMENT

Surgical stripping of the pericardium. Progressive improvement ensues over several months.

─────────────── *Approach to the Patient* ───────────────

With Asymptomatic Pericardial Effusion of Unknown Cause

If careful history and physical exam do not suggest etiology, the following may lead to diagnosis:

- Skin test and cultures for tuberculosis (Chap. 102)
- Serum albumin and urine protein measurement (nephrotic syndrome)
- Serum creatinine and BUN (renal failure)
- Thyroid function tests (myxedema)
- ANA (SLE and other collagen-vascular disease)
- Search for a primary tumor (especially lung and breast)

For a more detailed discussion, see Braunwald E: Pericardial Disease, Chap. 222, p. 1414, in HPIM-16.

122

HYPERTENSION

DEFINITION Chronic elevation in bp >140/90; etiology unknown in 90–95% of pts ("essential hypertension"). Always consider a secondary correctable form of hypertension, especially in pts under age 30 or those who become hypertensive after 55. Isolated systolic hypertension (systolic > 160, diastolic < 90) most common in elderly pts, due to reduced vascular compliance.

SECONDARY HYPERTENSION

RENAL ARTERY STENOSIS Due either to atherosclerosis (older men) or fibromuscular dysplasia (young women). Presents with sudden onset of hypertension, refractory to usual antihypertensive therapy. Abdominal bruit often audible; mild hypokalemia due to activation of the renin-angiotensin-aldosterone system may be present.

RENAL PARENCHYMAL DISEASE Elevated serum creatinine and/or abnormal urinalysis, containing protein, cells, or casts.

COARCTATION OF AORTA Presents in children or young adults; constriction is usually present in aorta at origin of left subclavian artery. Exam shows diminished, delayed femoral pulsations; late systolic murmur loudest over the midback. CXR shows indentation of the aorta at the level of the coarctation and rib notching (due to development of collateral arterial flow).

PHEOCHROMOCYTOMA A catecholamine-secreting tumor, typically of the adrenal medulla, that presents as paroxysmal or sustained hypertension in young to middle-aged pts. Sudden episodes of headache, palpitations, and profuse diaphoresis are common. Associated findings include chronic weight loss, orthostatic *hypotension*, and impaired glucose tolerance. Pheochromocytomas may be localized to the bladder wall and may present with micturition-associated symptoms of catecholamine excess. Diagnosis is suggested by elevated plasma metanephrine level or urinary catecholamine metabolites in a 24-h urine collection (see below); the tumor is then localized by CT scan or angiography.

HYPERALDOSTERONISM Due to aldosterone-secreting adenoma or bilateral adrenal hyperplasia. Should be suspected when hypokalemia is present in a hypertensive pt off diuretics (Chap. 174).

OTHER CAUSES Oral contraceptive usage, Cushing's and adrenogenital syndromes (Chap. 174), thyroid disease (Chap. 173), hyperparathyroidism (Chap. 179), and acromegaly (Chap. 171).

_____ *Approach to the Patient* _____

History

Most pts are asymptomatic. Severe hypertension may lead to headache, epistaxis, or blurred vision.
Clues to Specific Forms of Secondary Hypertension Use of birth control pills or glucocorticoids; paroxysms of headache, sweating, or tachycardia (pheochromocytoma); history of renal disease or abdominal traumas (renal hypertension).

Physical Examination

Measure bp with appropriate-sized cuff (large cuff for large arm). Measure bp in both arms as well as a leg (to evaluate for coarctation). Signs of hypertension include retinal arteriolar changes (narrowing/nicking); left ventricular lift, loud A_2, S_4. Clues to secondary forms of hypertension include cushingoid appearance, thyromegaly, abdominal bruit (renal artery stenosis), delayed femoral pulses (coarctation of aorta).

Laboratory Workup

Screening Tests for Secondary Hypertension Should be carried out on all pts with documented hypertension: (1) serum creatinine, BUN, and urinalysis (renal parenchymal disease); (2) serum K measured off diuretics (hypokalemia prompts workup for hyperaldosteronism or renal artery stenosis); (3) CXR (rib notching or indentation of distal aortic arch in coarctation of the aorta); (4) ECG (LV hypertrophy suggests chronicity of hypertension); (5) other useful screening blood tests include CBC, glucose, cholesterol, triglycerides, calcium, uric acid.
Further Workup Indicated for specific diagnoses if screening tests are abnormal or bp is refractory to antihypertensive therapy: (1) renal artery ste-

nosis: magnetic resonance angiography, captopril renogram, renal duplex ultrasound, digital subtraction angiography, renal arteriography, and measurement of renal vein renin; (2) Cushing's syndrome: dexamethasone suppression test (Chap. 174); (3) pheochromocytoma: 24-h urine collection for catecholamines, metanephrines, and vanillylmandelic acid or measurement of plasma metanephrine; (4) primary hyperaldosteronism: depressed plasma renin activity and hypersecretion of aldosterone, both of which fail to change with volume expansion; (5) renal parenchymal disease (Chaps. 139, 149).

℞ TREATMENT

Drug Therapy of Essential Hypertension (See Figs. 122-1 and 122-2)

Goal is to control hypertension with minimal side effects using a single drug if possible. First-line agents include diuretics, beta blockers, ACE inhibitors, angiotensin receptor antagonists, and calcium antagonists.

Diuretics (See Table 47-1) Should be cornerstone of most antihypertensive regimes. Thiazides preferred over loop diuretics because of longer duration of action; however, the latter are more potent when GFR < 25 mL/min. Major side effects include hypokalemia, hyperglycemia, and hyperuricemia, which can be minimized by using low dosage (e.g., hydrochlorothia-

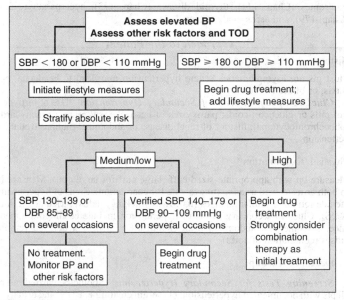

FIGURE 122-1 Initiation of treatment in patients with hypertension. See Table 122-1 for listing of classes of agents to use initially. In the initial evaluation, patients are stratified for cardiovascular risk using: level of blood pressure; the presence of risk factors—smoking, obesity, male gender, etc.—which vary from 0 factors (low risk) to three or more factors (high risk equivalent to having diabetes mellitus), target organ damage (TOD, i.e., clinical cardiovascular or renal disease) or diabetes (both high risk if present regardless of other risk factors). SBP, systolic blood pressure; DBP, diastolic blood pressure. (*From NDL Fisher, GH Williams, Fig. 230-1 in HPIM-16.*)

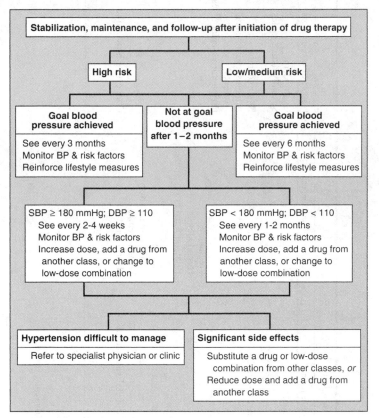

FIGURE 122-2 Approach to the hypertensive patient after initiating antihypertensive drug treatment. See Fig. 122-1 for initial steps and definition of risk and Table 122-1 for initial choice of agents. (*From NDL Fisher, GH Williams, Fig. 230-2 in HPIM-16.*)

zide 12.5–50 mg qd). Diuretics are particularly effective in elderly and black pts. Prevention of hypokalemia is especially important in pts on digitalis glycosides.

    Beta Blockers   Particularly effective in young pts with "hyperkinetic" circulation. Begin with low dosage (e.g., atenolol 25 mg qd). Relative contraindications: bronchospasm, CHF, AV block, bradycardia, and "brittle" insulin-dependent diabetes.

    ACE Inhibitors   Well tolerated with low frequency of side effects. May be used as monotherapy or in combination with beta blockers, calcium antagonists, or diuretics. Side effects are uncommon and include rash, angioedema, proteinuria, or leukopenia, particularly in pts with elevated serum creatinine. A nonproductive cough may develop in the course of therapy in up to 10% of patients, requiring an alternative regimen. Note that renal function may deteriorate as a result of ACE inhibitors in pts with bilateral renal artery stenosis.

    Potassium supplements and potassium-sparing diuretics should be used cautiously with ACE inhibitors to prevent hyperkalemia. If pt is intravascu-

Table 122-1

Guidelines for Selecting Initial Drug Treatment of Hypertension

Class of Drug	Compelling Indications	Possible Indications	Compelling Contraindications	Possible Contraindications
Diuretics	Heart failure Elderly patients Systolic hypertension	Diabetes	Gout	Dyslipidemia Sexually active males
β-Blockers	Angina After myocardial infarct Tachyarrhythmias	Heart failure Pregnancy Diabetes	Asthma and COPD Heart block[a]	Dyslipidemia Athletes and physically active patients Peripheral vascular disease
ACE inhibitors	Heart failure Left ventricular dysfunction After myocardial infarct Diabetic nephropathy		Pregnancy Hyperkalemia Bilateral renal artery stenosis	
Angiotensin receptor blockers	ACE inhibitor cough	Heart failure	Pregnancy Bilateral renal artery stenosis Hyperkalemia	
Calcium channel blocker	Angina Elderly patients Systolic hypertension	Peripheral vascular disease	Heart block[b]	Congestive heart failure[c]

[a] Grade 2 or 3 atrioventricular block.

[b] Grade 2 or 3 atrioventricular block with verapamil or diltiazem.

[c] Verapamil or diltiazem.

Note: COPD, chronic obstructive pulmonary disease; ACE, angiotensin-converting enzyme.

Source: Adapted with permission from 1999 WHO.

larly volume depleted, hold diuretics for 2–3 days prior to initiation of ACE inhibitor, which should then be administered at very low dosage (e.g., captopril, 6.25 mg bid).

For pts who do not tolerate ACE inhibitors because of cough or angioedema, consider angiotensin receptor antagonists instead.

Calcium Antagonists Direct arteriolar vasodilators; all have negative inotropic effects (particularly verapamil) and should be used cautiously if LV dysfunction is present. Verapamil, and to a lesser extent diltiazem, can result in bradycardia and AV block, so combination with beta blockers is generally avoided. Use sustained-release formulations, as short-acting dihydropyridine calcium channel blockers may increase incidence of coronary events.

If bp proves refractory to drug therapy, workup for secondary forms of hypertension, especially renal artery stenosis and pheochromocytoma.

Table 122-1 lists guidelines for initial drug treatment. (See HPIM-16, Table 230-8, p. 1473, for detailed list of antihypertensives.)

Special Circumstances

Pregnancy Safest antihypertensives include methyldopa (250–1000 mg PO bid-tid) and hydralazine (10–150 mg PO bid-tid). Calcium channel blockers also appear to be safe in pregnancy. Beta blockers need to be used cautiously—fetal hypoglycemia and low birth weights have been reported. ACE inhibitors and angiotensin receptor antagonists are contraindicated in pregnancy.

Renal Disease Standard thiazide diuretics may not be effective. Consider metolazone, furosemide, or bumetanide, alone or in combination.

Diabetes Goal bp < 130/85. Consider ACE inhibitors and angiotensin receptor blockers as first-line therapy to control bp and slow renal deterioration.

Malignant Hypertension Diastolic bp > 120 mmHg is a medical emergency. Immediate therapy is mandatory if there is evidence of cardiac decompensation (CHF, angina), encephalopathy (headache, seizures, visual disturbances), or deteriorating renal function. Drugs to treat hypertensive crisis include IV labetolol, 10- to 80-mg bolus, or nitroglycerine, 5–100 μg/min. Replace with PO antihypertensive as pt becomes asymptomatic and diastolic bp improves.

For a more detailed discussion, see Fisher NDL, Williams GH: Hypertensive Vascular Disease, Chap. 230, p. 1463, in HPIM-16.

123

ST-SEGMENT ELEVATION MYOCARDIAL INFARCTION (STEMI)

Early recognition and immediate treatment of acute MI are essential; diagnosis is based on characteristic history, ECG, and serum cardiac markers.

SYMPTOMS Chest pain similar to angina (Chap. 32) but more intense and persistent; not fully relieved by rest or nitroglycerin, often accompanied by nausea, sweating, apprehension. However, ~25% of MIs are clinically silent.

PHYSICAL EXAMINATION Pallor, diaphoresis, tachycardia, S_4, dyskinetic cardiac impulse may be present. If CHF exists, rales and S_3 are present. Jugular venous distention is common in right ventricular infarction.

ECG ST elevation, followed by T-wave inversion, then Q-wave development over several hours (see Figs. 118-3 and 118-4.

Non-Q-Wave MI (Also termed *non-ST elevation MI,* or NSTEMI) ST depression followed by persistent ST-T-wave changes *without* Q-wave development. Comparison with old ECG helpful (see Chap. 124).

CARDIAC BIOMARKERS Time course is diagnostically useful; creatine phosphokinase (CK) level rises within 4–8 h, peaks at 24 h, returns to normal by 48–72 h. CK-MB isoenzyme is more specific for MI but may also be elevated with myocarditis or after electrical cardioversion. Total CK (but not CK-MB) rises (two- to threefold) after IM injection, vigorous exercise, or other skeletal muscle trauma. A ratio of CK-MB mass:CK activity $\geq$ 2.5 suggests acute MI. CK-MB peaks earlier (about 8 h) following acute reperfusion therapy (see below). Cardiac-specific troponin T and troponin I are highly specific for myocardial injury and are the preferred biochemical markers for diagnosis of acute MI. They remain elevated for 7–10 days. Serum cardiac markers should be measured at presentation, 6–9 h later, then at 12–24 h.

NONINVASIVE IMAGING TECHNIQUES Useful when diagnosis of MI is not clear. *Echocardiography* detects infarct-associated regional wall motion abnormalities (but cannot distinguish acute MI from a previous myocardial scar). Echo is also useful in detecting RV infarction, LV aneurysm, and LV thrombus. *Myocardial perfusion imaging* (thallium 201 or technetium 99m-sestamibi) is sensitive for regions of decreased perfusion but is not specific for acute MI.

℞ TREATMENT

Initial Therapy

Initial goals are to: (1) quickly identify if patient is candidate for reperfusion therapy, (2) relieve pain, and (3) prevent/treat arrhythmias and mechanical complications.

- Aspirin should be administered immediately (162–325 mg chewed at presentation, then 162–325 mg PO qd), unless pt is aspirin-intolerant.
- Perform targeted history, exam, and ECG to identify STEMI (>1 mm ST elevation in two contiguous leads or new LBBB) and appropriateness of reperfusion therapy [percutaneous coronary intervention (PCI) or intravenous fibrinolytic agent], which reduces infarct size, LV dysfunction, and mortality.
- Primary PCI is generally more effective than fibrinolysis and is preferred at experienced centers capable of performing procedure rapidly (Fig. 123-1), especially when diagnosis is in doubt, cardiogenic shock is present, bleeding risk is increased, or if symptoms have been present for >3 h.
- Proceed with IV fibrinolysis if PCI is not available or if logistics would delay PCI >1 h longer than fibrinolysis could be initiated (Fig. 123-1). Door-to-needle time should be < 30 min for maximum benefit. Ensure absence of contraindications (Fig. 123-2) before administering fibrinolytic agent. Those treated within 1–3 h benefit most; can still be useful up to 12 h if chest pain is persistent or ST remains elevated in leads that have not developed new Q

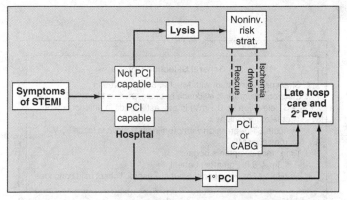

FIGURE 123-1 Reperfusion choices in STEMI. If hospital is capable, percutaneous coronary intervention (PCI) is undertaken. Otherwise, patient is considered for fibrinolytic therapy (Fig. 123-2). Patients who receive fibrinolytic therapy undergo noninvasive risk stratification (Noninv. risk strat). Those with continued chest pain or failure to resolve ST-segment elevation by 90 min after fibrinolysis should be considered for rescue PCI. Later in hospitalization, spontaneous recurrent ischemia or provoked ischemia on noninvasive testing should lead to coronary angiography and consideration of PCI or coronary artery bypass graft (CABG) surgery. (*Adapted from PW Armstrong, D Collen, EM Antman. Circulation 107:2533, 2003.*)

waves. Complications include bleeding, reperfusion arrhythmias, and, in case of streptokinase (SK), allergic reactions. Heparin [60 U/kg (maximum 4000 U), then 12 (U/kg)/h (maximum 1000 U/h)] should be initiated with fibrinolytic agents other than SK (Fig. 123-2); maintain aPTTT at 1.5–2.0 × control (~50–70 s).
• If chest pain or ST elevation persists >90 min after fibrinolysis, consider referral for rescue PCI. Later coronary angiography after fibrinolysis generally reserved for pts with recurrent angina or positive stress test.

The initial management of NSTEMI (non-Q MI) is different (see Chap. 124). In particular, fibrinolytic therapy should not be administered.

Additional Standard Treatment

(Whether or not reperfusion therapy is undertaken):

• *Hospitalize in CCU* with continuous ECG monitoring.
• *IV line* for emergency arrhythmia treatment.
• *Pain control*: (1) Morphine sulfate 2–4 mg IV q5–10min until pain is relieved or side effects develop [nausea, vomiting, respiratory depression (treat with naloxone 0.4–1.2 mg IV), hypotension (if bradycardic, treat with atropine 0.5 mg IV; otherwise use careful volume infusion)]; (2) nitroglycerin 0.3 mg SL if systolic bp > 100 mmHg; for refractory pain: IV nitroglycerin (begin at 10 μg/min, titrate upward to maximum of 200 μg/min, monitoring bp closely); do not administer nitrates within 24 h of sildenafil or within 48 h of tadalafil (used for erectile dysfunction); (3) β-adrenergic antagonists (see below).
• *Oxygen* 2–4 L/min by nasal cannula (maintain O_2 saturation > 90%).
• Mild *sedation* (e.g., diazepam 5 mg PO qid).
• *Soft diet* and stool softeners (e.g., docusate sodium 100–200 mg/d).
• *β-Adrenergic blockers* (Chap. 122) reduce myocardial O_2 consumption, limit infarct size, and reduce mortality. Especially useful in pts with hypertension, tachycardia, or persistent ischemic pain; contraindications include active CHF, systolic bp < 95 mmHg, heart rate < 50 beats/min, AV block,

General Selection Criteria

1. Chest pain consistent with MI of ≥ 30 min duration
2. Electrocardiographic evidence of acute Q-wave MI:
   - ST elevation (≥ 0.1 mV) in at least 2 leads in anterior, inferior, or lateral locations
   - Acute ST depression with prominent R wave in leads V_1-V_2 (posterior MI)
3. Time since symptoms began:
   ≤ 3h: < 6 h: greatest benefit
   up to >12h: less benefit, but still useful if chest pain continues

Check for Contraindications

- Major surgery or trauma in preceeding 2 weeks
- Active internal bleeding or hemorrhagic retinopathy
- Acute pericarditis or aortic dissection
- Cardiopulmonary resuscitation for > 10 min
- Intracranial tumor or previous intracranial surgery
- Cerebrovascular accident within previous year, or *any* history of cerebrovascular hemorrhage
- Marked hypertension (> 180/110 mmHg)
- Known bleeding diathesis or INR ≥ 2.0

Fibrinolytic drug	Intravenous Dosage
Streptokinase	1.5 million Units over one hour
tPA	15-mg bolus, then 50 mg over 30 min, then 35 mg over next hour
rPA	10-U bolus × 2 with 30-min interval

Concurrent with fibrinolytic therapy, administer

1. Aspirin 160–325 mg PO qd
2. If tPA, rPA, or TNK used: heparin to maintain a PTT = 1.5–2 × control for 48 h

Subsequent coronary arteriography reserved for

- Spontaneous recurrent ischemia during hospitalization
- Positive exercise test prior to or soon after discharge

FIGURE 123-2   Approach to fibrinolytic therapy of pts with acute MI.

or history of bronchospasm. Administer IV (e.g., metoprolol 5 mg q5–10min to total dose of 15 mg), followed by PO regimen (e.g., metoprolol 25–100 mg bid).

• *Anticoagulation/antiplatelet agents:* Pts who receive fibrinolytic therapy are begun on heparin and aspirin as indicated above. In absence of fibrinolytic therapy, administer aspirin, 160–325 mg qd, and low-dose heparin (5000 U SC q12h for DVT prevention). Full-dose IV heparin (PTT 2 × control) or low-molecular-weight heparin (e.g., enoxaparin 1 mg/kg SC q12h) followed by oral anticoagulants is recommended for pts with severe CHF, presence of ventricular thrombus by echocardiogram, or large dyskinetic region in anterior MI. Oral anticoagulants are continued for 3 to 6 months, then replaced by aspirin.

• *ACE inhibitors* reduce mortality in pts following acute MI and should be prescribed within 24 h of hospitalization for pts with STEMI—e.g., captopril (6.25 mg PO test dose) advanced to 50 mg PO tid. ACE inhibitors should be continued indefinitely after discharge in pts with CHF or those with asymptomatic LV dysfunction [ejection fraction (EF) ≤ 40%]; if ACE inhibitor intolerant, use angiotensin receptor blocker (e.g., valsartan or candesartan).

• *Serum magnesium* level should be measured and repleted if necessary to reduce risk of arrhythmias.

COMPLICATIONS (For arrhythmias, see also Chap. 125)

VENTRICULAR ARRHYTHMIAS Isolated ventricular premature beats (VPBs) occur frequently. Precipitating factors should be corrected [hypoxemia, acidosis, hypokalemia (maintain serum K^+ ~4.5 mmol/L), hypercalcemia, hypomagnesemia, CHF, arrhythmogenic drugs]. Routine beta-blocker administration (see above) diminishes ventricular ectopy. Other in-hospital antiarrhythmic therapy should be reserved for pts with sustained ventricular arrhythmias.

VENTRICULAR TACHYCARDIA If hemodynamically unstable, perform immediate electrical countershock (unsynchronized discharge of 200–300 J). If hemodynamically tolerated, use IV lidocaine [bolus of 1.0–1.5 mg/kg, infusion of 20–50 (μg/kg)/min; use lower infusion rate (~1 mg/min) in pts of advanced age or those with CHF or liver disease], IV procainamide (bolus of 15 mg/kg over 20–30 min; infusion of 1–4 mg/min), or IV amiodarone (bolus of 75–150 mg over 10–15 min; infusion of 1.0 mg/min for 6 h, then 0.5 mg/min).

VENTRICULAR FIBRILLATION VF requires immediate defibrillation (200–400 J). If unsuccessful, initiate CPR and standard resuscitative measures (Chap. 13). Ventricular arrhythmias that appear several days or weeks following MI often reflect pump failure and may warrant invasive electrophysiologic study and ICD implantation.

ACCELERATED IDIOVENTRICULAR RHYTHM Wide QRS complex, regular rhythm, rate 60–100 beats/min, is common and usually benign; if it causes hypotension, treat with atropine 0.6 mg IV.

SUPRAVENTRICULAR ARRHYTHMIAS *Sinus tachycardia* may result from CHF, hypoxemia, pain, fever, pericarditis, hypovolemia, administered drugs. If no cause is identified, may treat with beta blocker. For persistent sinus tachycardia (>120), use Swan-Ganz catheter to differentiate CHF from decreased intravascular volume. Other *supraventricular arrhythmias* (paroxysmal supraventricular tachycardia, atrial flutter, and fibrillation) are often secondary to CHF, in which digoxin (Chap. 126) is treatment of choice. In absence of

CHF, may also use verapamil or beta blocker (Chap. 125). If hemodynamically unstable, proceed with electrical cardioversion.

BRADYARRHYTHMIAS AND AV BLOCK (See Chap. 125) In *inferior MI*, usually represent heightened vagal tone or discrete AV nodal ischemia. If hemodynamically compromised (CHF, hypotension, emergence of ventricular arrhythmias), treat with atropine 0.5 mg IV q5min (up to 2 mg). If no response, use temporary external or transvenous pacemaker. Isoproterenol should be avoided. In *anterior MI*, AV conduction defects usually reflect extensive tissue necrosis. Consider temporary external or transvenous pacemaker for (1) complete heart block, (2) Mobitz type II block (Chap. 125), (3) new bifascicular block (LBBB, RBBB + left anterior hemiblock, RBBB + left posterior hemiblock), (4) any bradyarrhythmia associated with hypotension or CHF.

CONGESTIVE HEART FAILURE CHF may result from systolic "pump" dysfunction, increased LV diastolic "stiffness," and/or acute mechanical complications.

Symptoms Dyspnea, orthopnea, tachycardia.

Examination Jugular venous distention, S_3 and S_4 gallop, pulmonary rales; systolic murmur if acute mitral regurgitation or ventricular septal defect (VSD) has developed.

℞ TREATMENT (See Chaps. 16 and 126)

Initial therapy includes diuretics (begin with furosemide 10–20 mg IV), inhaled O_2, and vasodilators, particularly nitrates [PO, topical, or IV (Chap. 126) unless pt is hypotensive (systolic bp < 100 mmHg)]; digitalis is usually of little benefit in acute MI unless supraventricular arrhythmias are present. Diuretic, vasodilator, and inotropic therapy (Table 123-1) best guided by invasive hemodynamic monitoring (Swan-Ganz pulmonary artery catheter, arterial line), particularly in pts with accompanying hypotension (Table 123-2; Fig. 123-3). In acute MI, optimal pulmonary capillary wedge pressure (PCW) is 15–20 mmHg; in the absence of hypotension, PCW > 20 mmHg is treated with diuretic plus vasodilator therapy [IV nitroglycerin (begin at 10 μg/min) or nitroprusside (begin at 0.5 μg/kg per min)] and titrated to optimize bp, PCW, and systemic vascular resistance (SVR).

$$SVR = \frac{(\text{mean arterial pressure} - \text{mean RA pressure}) \times 80}{\text{cardiac output}}$$

Normal SVR = 900 – 1350 dyn·s/cm^5. If PCW > 20 mmHg and pt is hypotensive (Table 123-2 and Fig. 123-3), evaluate for VSD or acute mitral regurgitation, add dobutamine [begin at 1–2 (μg/kg)/min], titrate upward to maximum of 10 (μg/kg)/min; beware of drug-induced tachycardia or ventricular ectopy.

If CHF improves on parenteral vasodilator therapy, oral therapy follows with ACE inhibitor (e.g., captopril, enalapril, or lisinopril, an angiotensin receptor blocker) or the combination of nitrates plus hydralazine (Chap. 126).

CARDIOGENIC SHOCK (See Chap. 14) Severe LV failure with hypotension (bp < 80 mmHg) *and* elevated PCW (>20 mmHg), accompanied by oliguria (<20 mL/h), peripheral vasoconstriction, dulled sensorium, and metabolic acidosis.

Table 123-1

Intravenous Vasodilators and Inotropic Drugs Used in Acute MI

Drug	Usual Dosage Range	Comment
Nitroglycerin	5–100 μg/min	May improve coronary blood flow to ischemic myocardium
Nitroprusside	0.5–10 (μg/kg)/min	More potent vasodilator, but improves coronary blood flow less than nitroglycerin With therapy >24 h or in renal failure, watch for thiocyanate toxicity (blurred vision, tinnitus, delirium)
Dobutamine	2–20 (μg/kg)/min	Results in ↑ cardiac output, ↓ PCW, but does not raise bp

Dopamine	2–10 (μg/kg)/min (sometimes higher)	More appropriate than dobutamine if hypotensive
		Hemodynamic effect depends on dose:
		(μg/kg)/min
		  <5:↑ renal blood flow
		  2.5–10:positive inotrope
		  >10:vasoconstriction

Amrinone	0.75-mg/kg bolus, then 5–15 (μg/kg)/min	Positive inotrope and vasodilator Can combine with dopamine or dobutamine May result in thrombocytopenia
Milrinone	50-mg/kg bolus, then 0.375–0.75 (μg/kg)/min	Ventricular arrhythmias may result

℞ TREATMENT

Swan-Ganz catheter and intraarterial bp monitoring are essential; aim for mean PCW of 18–20 mmHg with adjustment of volume (diuretics or infusion) as needed. Intraaortic balloon counterpulsation may be necessary to maintain bp and reduce PCW. Administer high concentration of O_2 by mask; if pulmonary edema coexists, consider intubation and mechanical ventilation. Acute mechanical complications (see below) should be sought and promptly treated.

If cardiogenic shock develops within 4 h of first MI symptoms, acute reperfusion by PCI may markedly improve LV function.

HYPOTENSION May also result from *RV MI*, which should be suspected in inferior or posterior MI, if jugular venous distention and elevation of right-heart pressures predominate (rales are typically absent and PCW may be normal); right-sided ECG leads typically show ST elevation, and echocardiography may confirm diagnosis. *Treatment* consists of volume infusion, gauged by PCW and arterial pressure. Noncardiac causes of hypotension should be considered: hypovolemia, acute arrhythmia, or sepsis.

ACUTE MECHANICAL COMPLICATIONS Ventricular septal rupture and acute mitral regurgitation due to papillary muscle ischemia/infarct de-

Table 123-2

Hemodynamic Complications in Acute MI

Condition	Cardiac Index, (L/min)/m²	PCW, mmHg	Systolic bp, mmHg	Treatment
Uncomplicated	>2.5	≤18	>100	—
Hypovolemia	<2.5	<15	<100	Successive boluses of normal saline In setting of inferior wall MI, consider RV infarction (esp. if RA pressure >10)
Volume overload	>2.5	>20	>100	Diuretic (e.g., furosemide 10–20 mg IV) Nitroglycerin, topical paste or IV (Table 123-1)
LV failure	<2.5	>20	>100	Diuretic (e.g., furosemide 10–20 mg IV) IV nitroglycerin (or if hypertensive, use IV nitroprusside)
Severe LV failure	<2.5	>20	<100	If bp ≥90: IV dobutamine ± IV nitroglycerin or sodium nitroprusside If bp <90: IV dopamine If accompanied by pulmonary edema: attempt diuresis with IV furosemide; may be limited by hypotension If new systolic murmur present, consider acute VSD or mitral regurgitation
Cardiogenic shock	<1.8	>20	<90 with oliguria and confusion	IV dopamine Intraaortic balloon pump Coronary angiography may be life-saving

Note: PCW, pulmonary artery wedge pressure; RV, right ventricle; LV, left ventricle; VSD, ventricular septal defect.

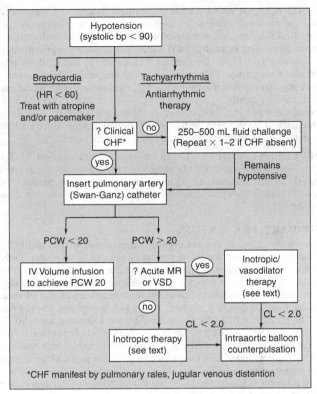

FIGURE 123-3 Approach to hypotension in pts with acute myocardial infarction; PCW, pulmonary capillary wedge pressure.

velop during the first week following MI and are characterized by sudden onset of CHF and new systolic murmur. Echocardiography with Doppler can confirm presence of these complications. PCW tracings may show large *v* waves in either condition, but an oxygen "step-up" as the catheter is advanced from RA to RV suggests septal rupture.

Acute medical therapy of these conditions includes vasodilator therapy (IV nitroprusside: begin at 10 μg/min and titrate to maintain systolic bp $\approx$100 mmHg); intraaortic balloon pump may be required to maintain cardiac output. Surgical correction is postponed for 4–6 weeks after acute MI if pt is stable; surgery should not be deferred if pt is unstable. Acute ventricular free-wall rupture presents with sudden loss of bp, pulse, and consciousness, while ECG shows an intact rhythm; emergent surgical repair is crucial, and mortality is high.

PERICARDITIS Characterized by *pleuritic, positional* pain and pericardial rub (Chap. 121); atrial arrhythmias are common; must be distinguished from recurrent angina. Often responds to aspirin, 650 mg PO qid. Anticoagulants should be withheld when pericarditis is suspected to avoid development of tamponade.

VENTRICULAR ANEURYSM   Localized "bulge" of LV chamber due to infarcted myocardium. *True aneurysms* consist of scar tissue and do not rupture. However, complications include CHF, ventricular arrhythmias, and thrombus formation. Typically, ECG shows persistent ST-segment elevation, >2 weeks after initial infarct; aneurysm is confirmed by echocardiography and by left ventriculography. The presence of thrombus within the aneurysm, or a large aneurysmal segment due to anterior MI, warrants oral anticoagulation with warfarin for 3–6 months.

Pseudoaneurysm is a form of cardiac rupture contained by a local area of pericardium and organized thrombus; direct communication with the LV cavity is present; surgical repair usually necessary to prevent rupture.

RECURRENT ANGINA   Usually associated with transient ST-T wave changes; signals high incidence of reinfarction; when it occurs in early post-MI period (<2 weeks), proceed directly to coronary arteriography, to identify those who would benefit from percutaneous coronary intervention or coronary artery bypass surgery.

SECONDARY PREVENTION

For pts who have not already undergone coronary angiography and PCI, sub-maximal exercise testing should be performed prior to or soon after discharge. A positive test in certain subgroups (angina at a low workload, a large region of provocable ischemia, or provocable ischemia with a reduced LVEF) suggests need for cardiac catheterization to evaluate myocardium at risk of recurrent infarction. *Beta blockers* (e.g., timolol, 10 mg bid; metoprolol, 25–100 mg bid) should be prescribed routinely for at least 2 years following acute MI (Table 122-1), unless contraindications present (asthma, CHF, bradycardia, "brittle" diabetes). Aspirin (80–325 mg/d) is administered to reduce incidence of subsequent infarction, unless contraindicated (e.g., active peptic ulcer, allergy). In aspirin-intolerant pts, use clopidogrel (75 mg/d) instead. If the LVEF ≤ 40%, an ACE inhibitor (e.g., captopril 6.25 mg PO tid, advanced to target dose of 50 mg PO tid) should be used indefinitely.

Modification of cardiac risk factors must be encouraged: discontinue smoking; control hypertension, diabetes, and serum lipids [target LDL ≤ 2.6 mmol/L (≤100 mg/dL)] (Chap. 181); and pursue graduated exercise.

For a more detailed discussion, see Antman EM, Braunwald E: ST-Segment Elevation Myocardial Infarction, Chap. 228, p. 1448, in HPIM-16.

124

CHRONIC STABLE ANGINA, UNSTABLE ANGINA, AND NON-ST-ELEVATION MYOCARDIAL INFARCTION

CHRONIC STABLE ANGINA

Angina pectoris, the most common clinical manifestation of CAD, results from an imbalance between myocardial O_2 supply and demand, most commonly resulting from atherosclerotic coronary artery obstruction. Other major conditions that upset this balance and result in angina include aortic valve disease (Chap. 119), hypertrophic cardiomyopathy (Chap. 120), and coronary artery spasm (see below).

SYMPTOMS   Angina is typically associated with extension or emotional upset; relieved quickly by rest or nitroglycerin (Chap. 32). Major risk factors are cigarette smoking, hypertension, hypercholesterolemia ($\uparrow$LDL fraction; $\downarrow$ HDL), diabetes, and family history of CAD below age 55.

PHYSICAL EXAMINATION   Often normal; arterial bruits or retinal vascular abnormalities suggest generalized atherosclerosis; S_4 is common. During acute anginal episode, other signs may appear: loud S_3 or S_4, diaphoresis, rales, and a transient murmur of mitral regurgitation due to papillary muscle ischemia.

LABORATORY   ECG   May be normal between anginal episodes or show old infarction (Chap. 118). During angina, ST- and T-wave abnormalities typically appear (ST-segment depression reflects subendocardial ischemia; ST-segment elevation may reflect acute infarction or transient coronary artery spasm). Ventricular arrhythmias frequently accompany acute ischemia.

Stress Testing   Enhances diagnosis of CAD (Fig. 124-1). Exercise is performed on treadmill or bicycle until target heart rate is achieved or pt becomes symptomatic (chest pain, light-headedness, hypotension, marked dyspnea, ventricular tachycardia) or develops diagnostic ST-segment changes. useful information includes duration of exercise achieved; peak heart rate and bp; depth, morphology, and persistence of ST-segment depression; and whether and at which level of exercise pain, hypotension, or ventricular arrhythmias develop. *Thallium 201* (or 99m-technetium sestamibi) imaging increases sensitivity and specificity and is particularly useful if baseline ECG abnormalities prevent interpretation of test (e.g., LBBB). *Note:* Exercise testing should not be performed in pts with acute MI, unstable angina, or severe aortic stenosis. If the pt is unable to exercise, intravenous dipyridamole (or adenosine) testing can be performed in conjunction with thallium or sestamibi imaging or a dobutamine echocardiographic study can be obtained (Table 124-1).

Some pts do not experience chest pain during ischemic episodes with exertion ("silent ischemia") but are identifed by transient ST-T-wave abnormalities during stress testing or Holter monitoring (see below).

Coronary Arteriography   The definitive test for assessing severity of CAD; major indications are (1) angina refractory to medical therapy, (2) markedly positive exercise test ($\geq$2-mm ST-segment depression or hypotension with exercise) suggestive of left main or three-vessel disease, (3) recurrent angina or positive exercise test after MI, (4) to assess for coronary artery spasm, and (5) to evaluate pts with perplexing chest pain in whom nonivasive tests are not diagnostic.

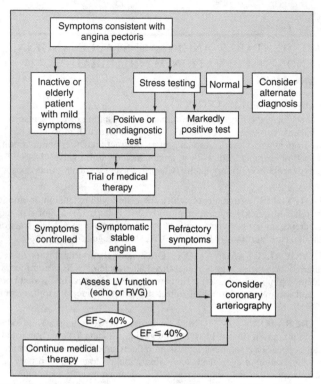

FIGURE 124-1 Role of exercise testing in management of CAD, RVG, radionuclide ventriculogram; EF, left ventricular ejection fraction. [*Modified from LS Lilly, in Textbook of Primary Care Medicine, J Nobel (ed.) St. Louis Mosby, 1996, p. 224.*]

℞ TREATMENT

General

• Identify and treat risk factors: mandatory cessation of smoking; treatment of diabetes, hypertension, and lipid disorders (Chap. 181).
• Correct exacerbating factors contributing to angina: marked obesity, CHF, anemia, hyperthyroidism.
• Reassurance and pt education.

Drug Therapy

Sublingual nitroglycerin (TNG 0.3–0.6 mg); may be repeated at 5-min intervals; warn pts of possible headache or light-headedness; teach prophylactic use of TNG prior to activity that regularly evokes angina. If chest pain persists for more than 10 min despite 2–3 TNG, pt should report promptly to nearest medical facility for evaluation of possible unstable angina or acute MI.

Long-Term Angina Suppresion

Three classes of drugs are used, frequently in combination:
Long-Acting Nitrates May be administered by many routes (Table 124-2); start at the lowest dose and frequency to limit tolerance and side effects of headache, light-headedness, tachycardia.

Table 124-1

Stress Testing Recommendations

Subgroup	Recommended Study
Patient able to exercise	
If baseline ST-T on ECG is iso-electric	Standard exercise test (treadmill, bicycle, or arm ergometry)
If baseline ST-T impairs test interpretation (e.g., LBBB, LVH with strain, digoxin)	Standard exercise test (above) combined with *either* Perfusion scintigraphy (thallium 201 or Tc99m-sestamibi) *or* Echocardiography
Patient *not* able to exercise (regardless of baseline ST-T abnormality)	Pharmacologic stress test (IV dobutamine, dipyridamole, or adenosine combined with *either* Perfusion scintigraphy (thallium 201 or Tc99m-sestamibi) *or* Echocardiography
Alternative choice (if baseline ST-T normal)	Ambulatory ECG monitor

Beta Blockers (See Table 122-1) All have antianginal properties; β_1-selective agents are less likely to exacerbate airway or peripheral vascular disease. Dosage should be titrated to resting heart rate of 50–60 beats/min. *Contraindications* to beta blockers include CHF, AV block, bronchospasm, "brittle" diabetes. Side effects include fatigue, bronchospasm, depressed LV function, impotence, depression, and masking of hypoglycemia in diabetics.

Calcium Antagonists (See Table 122-4) Useful for stable and unstable angina, as well coronary vasospasm. Combination with other antianginal

Table 124-2

Examples of Commonly Used Nitrates

	Usual Dose	Recommended Dosing Frequency
SHORT-ACTING AGENTS		
Sublingual TNG	0.3–0.6 mg	As needed
Aerosol TNG	0.4 mg (1 inhalation)	As needed
Sublingual ISDN	2.5–10 mg	As needed
LONG-ACTING AGENTS		
ISDN		
Oral	5–30 mg	tid
Sustained-action	40 mg	bid (once in A.M., then 7 h later)
TNG ointment (2%)	0.5–2	qid (with one 7- to 10-h nitrate-free interval)
TNG skin patches	0.1–0.6 mg/h	Apply in morning, remove at bedtime
ISMO		
Oral	20–40 mg	bid (once in A.M., then 7 h later)
Sustained-action	30–240 mg	qd

Note: TNG, nitroglycerin; ISDN, isosorbide dinitrate; ISMO, isosorbide mononitrate.

agents is beneficial, but verapamil should be administered very cautiously or not at all to pts on beta blockers or disopyramide (additive effects on LV dysfunction). Use sustained-release, not short-acting, calcium antagonists; the latter increase coronary mortality.

Aspirin 80–325 mg/d reduces the incidence of MI in chronic stable angina, following MI, and in asymptomatic men. It is recommended in pts with CAD in the absence of contraindications (GI bleeding or allergy). Consider clopidogrel (75 mg/d) for aspirin-intolerant individuals.

Mechanical Revascularization

Percutaneous Coronary Intervention (PCI) Includes percutaneous transluminal angioplasty (PTCA) and/or stenting. Performed on anatomically suitable stenoses of native vessels and bypass grafts; more effective than medical therapy for relief of angina. Has not been shown to reduce risk of MI or death; should not be performed on asymptomatic or only mildly symptomatic individuals. With PCI initial relief of angina occurs in 95% of pts; however, with PTCA stenosis recurs in 30–45% within 6 months (more commonly in pts with initial unstable angina, incomplete dilation, diabetes, or stenoses containing thrombi). Restenosis is reduced to 5–10% with drug-eluting stents. If restenosis occurs, PTCA can be repeated with success and risks like original procedure. Potential complications include dissection or thrombosis of the vessel and uncontrolled ischemia or CHF. Complications are most likely to occur in pts with CHF, long eccentric stenoses, calcified plaque, female gender, and dilation of an artery that perfuses a large segment of myocardium with inadequate collaterals. Placement of an intracoronary stent in suitable pts reduces the restenosis rate to 10–30% at 6 months. PCI has also been successful in some pts with recent *total* coronary occlusion (<3 months).

Table 124-3

Comparison of Revascularization Procedures in Multivessel Disease

Procedure	Advantages	Disadvantages
Percutaneous coronary revascularization (angioplasty and/or stenting)	Less invasive Shorter hospital stay Lower initial cost Easily repeated Effective in relieving symptoms	Restenosis High incidence of incomplete revascularization Unknown outcomes in pts with severe left ventricular dysfunction Limited to specific anatomic subsets Poor outcome in diabetics with 2–3 vessel coronary disease
Coronary artery bypass grafting	Effective in relieving symptoms Improved survival in certain subsets, including diabetics Ability to achieve complete revascularization	Cost Increased risk of a repeat procedure due to late graft closure Morbidity and mortality of major surgery

Source: Modified from DP Faxon, in GA Beller (ed), *Chronic Ischemic Heart Disease*, in E Braunwald (series ed), *Atlas of Heart Disease*, Philadelphia, Current Medicine, 1994.

Coronary Artery Bypass Surgery (CABG)   For angina refractory to medical therapy or when the latter is not tolerated (and when lesions are not amenable to PCI) or if severe CAD is present (left main, three-vessel disease with impaired LV function). CABG is preferred over PTCA in diabetics with CAD in ≥2 vessels because of better survival.

The relative advantages of PCD and CABG are summarized in Table 124-3.

UNSTABLE ANGINA AND NON-ST-ELEVATION MYOCARDIAL INFARCTION

Unstable angina (UA) and non-ST-elevation MI (NSTEMI) are acute coronary syndromes with similar mechanisms, clinical presentations, and treatment strategies.

CLINICAL PRESENTATION   UA includes (1) new onset of severe angina, (2) angina at rest or with minimal activity, and (3) recent increase in frequency and intensity of chronic angina. NSTEMI is diagnosed when symptoms of UA are accompanied by evidence of myocardial necrosis (e.g., elevated cardiac biomarkers). Some patients with NSTEMI present with symptoms identical to STEMI—the two are differentiated by distinct ECG abnormalities (see Chap. 123).

PHYSICAL EXAMINATION   May be normal or include diaphoresis, pale cool skin, tachycardia, S_4, basilar rales; if large region of ischemia, may demonstrate S_3, hypotension.

ELECTROCARDIOGRAM   Most commonly ST depression and/or T-wave inversion; no Q-wave development.

CARDIAC BIOMARKERS   CK-MB and/or cardiac-specific troponins are elevated in NSTEMI. Small troponin elevations may also occur in pts with CHF, myocarditis, or pulmonary embolism.

 TREATMENT

First step is appropriate triage based on likelihood of coronary artery disease and acute coronary syndrome (Fig. 124-2) and identification of high-risk pts (Table 124-4). Therapy of UA/NSTEMI is directed as follows: (1) against the inciting intracoronary thrombus, and (2) toward restoration of balance between myocardial oxygen supply and demand.

Antithrombotic Therapy

- Aspirin (162–325 mg, then 75–325 mg/d)
- Clopidogrel (300 mg PO load, then 75 mg/d) unless excessive risk of bleeding or immediate coronary artery bypass grafting (CABG) likely
- Unfractionated heparin [60 U/kg then 12 (U/kg)/h (maximum 1000 U/h)] to achieve aPTT 1.5–2.5 × control, *or* low-molecular-weight heparin (e.g., enoxaparin 1 mg/kg SC q12h)
- Add intravenous GP IIb/IIIa antagonist for high-risk pts for whom invasive management is planned [e.g., tirofiban, 0.4 (μg/kg)/min × 30 min, then 0.1 (μg/kg)/min for 48–96 h, or eptifibatide, 180-μg/kg bolus, then 2.0 (μg/kg)/min for 72–96 h].
- Do not administer fibrinolytic therapy to pts with UA/NSTEMI.

Anti-Ischemic Therapy

- Nitroglycerin 0.3–0.6 mg sublingually or by buccal spray. If chest discomfort persists after three doses given 5 min apart, consider IV nitroglycerin

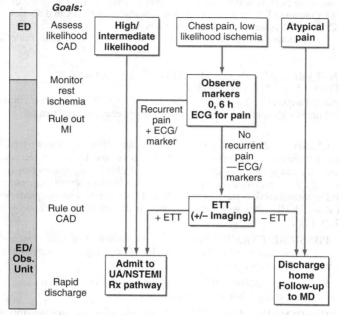

Critical Pathway for ED Evaluation of Chest Pain/ "Rule Out MI"

FIGURE 124-2 Diagnostic evaluation of patients presenting with suspected UA/NSTEMI. The first step is to assess the likelihood of coronary artery disease. Patients at high or intermediate likelihood are admitted to the hospital. Those with clearly atypical chest pain are discharged home. Patients with a *low* likelihood of ischemia enter the pathway and are observed in a monitored bed in the emergency department (ED) or observation unit over a period of 6 h and 12-lead electrocardiograms are performed if the patient has recurrent chest discomfort. A panel of cardiac markers (e.g., troponin and CK-MB) are drawn at baseline and 6 h later. If the patient develops recurrent pain, has ST-segment or T-wave changes, or had positive cardiac markers, he/she is admitted to the hospital and treated for UA/NSTEMI. If the patient has negative markers and no recurrence of pain, he/she is sent for exercise treadmill testing, with imaging reserved for patients with abnormal baseline electrocardiograms (e.g., left bundle branch block or left ventricular hypertrophy). If positive, the patient is admitted; if negative, the patient is discharged home with follow-up to his/her primary physician. (CAD, coronary artery disease; ECG, electrocardiogram; ED, emergency department; ETT, exercise tolerance test; MI, myocardial infarction; OBS, observation unit.) [*Adapted from CP Cannon, E Braunwald, in E Braunwald et al (eds): Heart Disease: A Textbook of Cardiovascular Medicine, 6th ed. Philadelphia, Saunders, 2001.*]

(5–10 μg/min, then increase by 10 μg/min every 3–5 min until symptoms relieved or systolic bp < 100 mmHg). Do not use nitrates in pts with recent use of phosphodiesterase inhibitors for erectile dysfunction (i.e., not within 24 h of sildenafil or within 48 h of tadalafil).
  • Beta blockers (e.g., metoprolol 5 mg IV q5–10min to total dose of 15 mg, then 25–50 mg PO q6h) targeted to a heart rate of 50–60 beats/min. In pts with contraindications to beta blockers (e.g., bronchospasm), consider long-acting verapamil or diltiazem (Table 122-4).

Additional Recommendations
  • Admit to unit with continuous ECG monitoring, initially with bed rest.

Table 124-4

High-Risk Features in UA/NSTEMI

Recurrent angina/ischemia at rest or minimal exertion despite anti-ischemic therapy
Elevated cardiac TnI or TnT
New ST-segment depression on presentation
Recurrent ischemia with CHF or worsening mitral regurgitation
Positive stress test
LVEF < 0.40
Hemodynamic instability or angina at rest with hypotension
Sustained ventricular tachycardia
PCI within previous 6 months or prior CABG

Note: TnI, troponin I; TnT, troponin T; LVEF, left ventricular ejection fraction; PCI, percutaneous coronary intervention; CABG, coronary artery bypass grafting.

- Consider morphine sulfate 2–5 mg IV q5–30min for refractory chest discomfort (see Chap. 123).
- For long-term secondary prevention add ACE inhibitor and HMG-CoA reductase inhibitor (see Chap. 123).

Invasive vs. Conservative Strategy

In high-risk pts (Table 124-4), an early invasive strategy (coronary arteriography within ~48 h followed by percutaneous intervention or CABG) improves outcomes. In lower-risk pts, angiography can be deferred but should be pursued if myocardial ischemia recurs spontaneously (angina or ST deviations at rest or with minimal activity) or is provoked by stress testing.

PRINZMETAL'S VARIANT ANGINA (CORONARY VASOSPASM)

Intermittent focal spasm of coronary artery; often associated with atherosclerotic lesion near site of spasm. Chest discomfort is similar to angina but more severe and occurs typically at rest, with transient ST-segment elevation. Acute infarction or malignant arrhythmias may develop during spasm-induced ischemia. Evaluation includes observation of ECG (or ambulatory Holter monitor) for transient ST elevation; diagnosis confirmed at coronary angiography using provocative (e.g., IV acetylcholine) testing. Primary treatment consists of long-acting nitrates and calcium antagonists. Prognosis is better in pts with anatomically normal coronary arteries than those with fixed coronary stenoses.

For a more detailed discussion, see Selwyn AP, Braunwald E: Ischemic Heart Disease, Chap. 226, p. 1434; and Cannon CP, Braunwald E: Unstable Angina and Non-ST-Elevation Myocardial Infarction, Chap. 227, p. 1444, in HPIM-16.

125

ARRHYTHMIAS

Arrhythmias may appear in the presence or absence of structural heart disease; they are more serious in the former. Conditions that provoke arrhythmias include (1) myocardial ischemia, (2) CHF, (3) hypoxemia, (4) hypercapnia, (5) hypotension, (6) electrolyte disturbances (especially involving K, Ca, and Mg), (7) drug toxicity (digoxin, pharmacologic agents that prolong QT interval), (8) caffeine, (9) ethanol.

DIAGNOSIS   Examine ECG for evidence of ischemic changes (Chap. 118), prolonged QT interval, and characteristics of Wolff-Parkinson-White (WPW) syndrome (see below). See Fig. 125-1 for diagnosis of tachyarrhythmias; always identify atrial activity and relationship between P waves and QRS complexes. To aid the diagnosis:

• Obtain long rhythm strip of lead II, aVF, or V_1. Double the ECG voltage and increase paper speed to 50 mm/s to help identify P waves.
• Place accessory ECG leads (right-sided chest, esophageal, right-atrial) to help identify P waves. Record ECG during carotid sinus massage (Table 125-1) for 5 s. Note: Do not massage both carotids simultaneously.

Tachyarrhythmias with wide QRS complex beats may represent ventricular tachycardia or supraventricular tachycardia with aberrant conduction. Factors favoring ventricular tachycardia include (1) AV dissociation, (2) QRS > 0.14 s, (3) LAD, (4) no response to carotid sinus massage, (5) morphology of QRS similar to that of previous ventricular premature beats (Table 125-2).

℞ TREATMENT

Tachyarrhythmias   (Tables 125-1 and 125-3) Precipitating causes (listed above) should be corrected. If pt is hemodynamically compromised (angina, hypotension, CHF), proceed to immediate cardioversion.

Do not cardiovert sinus tachycardia; exercise caution if digitalis toxicity is suspected. Initiate drugs as indicated in the tables; follow drug levels and ECG intervals (esp. QRS and QT). Reduce dosage for pts with hepatic or renal dysfunction as indicated in Table 125-3. Drug efficacy is confirmed by ECG (or Holter) monitoring, stress testing, and, in special circumstances, invasive electrophysiologic study.

Antiarrhythmic agents all have potential toxic side effects, including provocation of ventricular arrhythmias, esp. in pts with LV dysfunction or history of sustained ventricular arrhythmias. Drug-induced QT prolongation and associated torsades de pointes ventricular tachycardia (Table 125-1) is most common with group IA and III agents; the drug should be discontinued if the QTc interval (QT divided by square root of RR interval) increases by >25%. Antiarrhythmic drugs should be avoided in pts with asymptomatic ventricular arrhythmias after MI, since mortality risk increases.

Chronic Atrial Fibrillation   Evaluate potential underlying cause (e.g., thyrotoxicosis, mitral stenosis, excessive ethanol consumption, pulmonary embolism). Pts with risk factors for stroke [e.g., valvular heart disease, hypertension, coronary artery disease (CAD), CHF, age >75] should receive warfarin anticoagulation (INR 2.0–3.0; use caution to keep INR < 3.0 in pts >age 75). Substitute aspirin, 325 mg/d, for pts without these risk factors or if contraindication to warfarin exists.

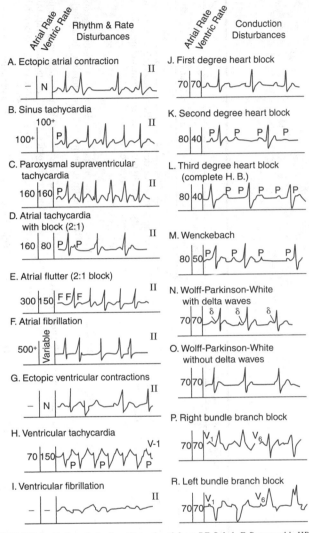

FIGURE 125-1 Tachyarrhythmias. (*Reproduced from BE Sobel, E Braunwald: HPIM-9, p. 1052.*)

Control ventricular rate (60–80 beats/min at rest, <100 beats/min with mild exercise) with beta blocker, digoxin, or calcium channel blocker (verapamil, diltiazem).

Consider cardioversion (after ≥3 weeks therapeutic anticoagulation or if no evidence of left atrial thrombus by transesophageal echo), especially if symptomatic despite rate control: use group IC, III, or IA agent (usually initiate with inpatient monitoring), followed, within a few days, by electrical cardioversion (usually 100–200 J). Type IC (Table 125-3) drugs are preferred in pts without structural heart disease and type III drugs are recommended in

Table 125-1

Clinical and Electrocardiographic Features of Common Arrhythmias

Rhythm	Example (Fig. 125-1)	Atrial Rate	Features	Carotid Sinus Massage	Precipitating Conditions	Initial Treatment
NARROW QRS COMPLEX						
Atrial premature beats	A	—	P wave abnormal; QRS width normal	—	Can be normal; or due to anxiety, CHF, hypoxia, caffeine, abnormal electrolytes (K^+, Ca^{2+}, Mg^{2+})	Remove precipitating cause; if symptomatic: beta blocker
Sinus tachycardia	B	100–160	Normal P wave	Rate gradually slows	Fever, dehydration, pain, CHF, hyperthyroidism, COPD	Remove precipitating cause; if symptomatic: beta blocker
Paroxysmal SVTs (reentrant)	C	140–250	Absent or retrograde P wave	Abruptly converts to sinus rhythm (or no effect)	Healthy individuals; preexcitation syndromes (see text)	Vagal maneuvers; if unsuccessful: adenosine, verapamil, beta blocker, cardioversion (150 J)
Atrial tachycardia with block	D	130–250	Upright "peaked" P; 2:1, 3:1, 4:1 block	No effect on atrial rate; block may ↑	Digitalis toxicity	Hold digoxin, correct [K^+]

		Rate	ECG features	Carotid massage	Associated conditions	Treatment
Atrial flutter	E	250–350	"Sawtooth" flutter waves; 2:1, 4:1 block	↑ Block; ventricular rate ↓	Mitral valve disease, hypertension, pulmonary embolism, pericarditis, postcardiac surgery, hyperthyroidism; obstructive lung disease, EtOH, idiopathic	1. Slow the ventricular rate: beta blocker, verapamil, diltiazem, or digoxin 2. Convert to NSR (after anticoagulation if chronic) with IV Ibutilide or orally with group IC, III, or IA[a] agent; may require electrical cardioversion (flutter: 50 J; fib: 100–200 J). Atrial flutter may respond to rapid atrial pacing, and radio frequency ablation highly effective to prevent recurrences
Atrial fibrillation	F	>350	No discrete P; irregularly spaced QRS	Ventricular rate ↓		
Multifocal atrial tachycardia		100–220	More than 3 different P wave shapes with varying PR intervals	No effect	Severe respiratory insufficiency	Treat underlying lung disease; verapamil may be used to slow ventricular rate

(continued)

641

Table 125-1 (Continued)

Clinical and Electrocardiographic Features of Common Arrhythmias

Rhythm	Example (Fig. 125-1)	Atrial Rate	Features	Carotid Sinus Massage	Precipitating Conditions	Initial Treatment
WIDE QRS COMPLEX						
Ventricular premature beats	G		Fully compensatory pause between normal beats	No effect	Coronary artery disease, myocardial infarction, CHF, hypoxia, hypokalemia, digitalis toxicity, prolonged QT interval (congenital or drugs: quinidine and other antiarrhythmics, tricyclics, phenothiazines)	May not require therapy; [a] use beta blocker or same drugs as ventricular tachycardia.
Ventricular tachycardia	H		QRS rate 100–250; slightly irregular rate	No effect		If unstable: electrical conversion (100 J); otherwise: Acute (IV): procainamide, amiodarone, lidocaine; chronic management: group IA, IB, IC, III drugs[a] or ICD. Patients without structural heart disease may respond to beta blockers or verapamil.
Ventricular fibrillation	I		Erratic electrical activity only	No effect		Immediate defibrillation (200–400 J)

642

Torsades de pointes	Ventricular tachycardia with sinusoidal oscillations of QRS height	No effect	Prolonged QT interval (congenital or drugs: quinidine and other antiarrhythmics, tricyclics, phenothiazines)	IV magnesium (1–2 g bolus); overdrive pacing; lidocaine; isoproterenol (unless CAD present); lidocaine. Drugs that prolong QT interval (e.g., quinidine) are contraindicated.
Supraventricular tachycardias with aberrant ventricular conduction	P wave typical of the supraventricular rhythm; wide QRS complex due to conduction through partially refractory pathways		Etiologies of the respective supraventricular rhythms listed above; atrial fibrillation with rapid, wide QRS may be due to preexcitation (WPW)	Same as treatment of respective supraventricular rhythm; if ventricular rate rapid (>200), treat as WPW (see text)

[a] Antiarrhythmic drug groups listed in Table 125-3.
[b] Indications for treating VPCs in acute MI listed in Chap. 123.

Table 125-2

Wide Complex Tachycardia

ECG CRITERIA THAT FAVOR VENTRICULAR TACHYCARDIA

1. AV dissociation
2. QRS width: >0.14 s with RBBB configuration
                 >0.16 s with LBBB configuration
3. QRS axis: Left axis deviation with RBBB morphology
             Extreme left axis deviation (northwest axis) with LBBB morphology
4. Concordance of QRS in precordial leads
5. Morphologic patterns of the QRS complex
     RBBB: Mono- or biphasic complex in V_1
           RS (*only with left axis deviation*) or QS in V_6

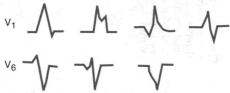

     LBBB: Broad R wave in V_1 or V_2 ≥0.04 s
           Onset of QRS to nadir of S wave in V_1 or V_2 of ≥0.07 s
           Notched downslope of S wave in V_1 or V_2
           Q wave in V_6

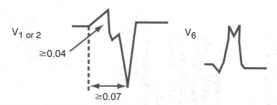

Note: AV, atrioventricular; BBB, bundle branch block.

presence of left ventricular dysfunction or CAD (Fig. 125-2). Anticoagulation should be continued for an additional 3 weeks after successful cardioversion.

Preexcitation Syndrome (WPW)

Conduction occurs through an accessory pathway between atria and ventricles. Baseline ECG typically shows a short PR interval and slurred upstroke of the QRS ("delta" wave) (Fig. 125-1*N*). Associated tachyarrhythmias are of two types:

• Narrow QRS complex tachycardia (antegrade conduction through AV node): usually paroxysmal supraventricular tachycardia. Treat cautiously with IV adenosine or beta blocker (Table 125-2).
• Wide QRS complex tachycardia (antegrade conduction through accessory pathway): often associated with AF with a very rapid (>250/min) ventricular rate (which may degenerate into VF). If hemodynamically compromised, im-

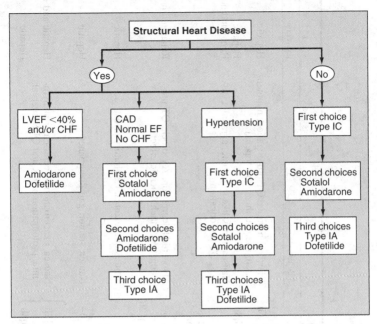

FIGURE 125-2   Recommendations for the selection of antiarrhythmic medications to prevent the recurrence of atrial fibrillation. See Table 125-3 for definition of types IA and IC drugs. An atrioventricular nodal blocking agent (i.e., beta blocker, calcium channel blocker, or digoxin) should be added to all type IC and IA agents as well as to dofetilide. LVEF, left ventricular ejection fraction; CHF, congestive heart failure; CAD, coronary artery disease; EF, ejection fraction.

mediate cardioversion is indicated; otherwise, treat with IV procainamide, not digoxin, beta blocker, or verapamil.

AV Block

FIRST DEGREE   (see Fig. 125-1*J*)   Prolonged, constant PR interval (>0.20 s). May be normal or secondary to increased vagal tone or digitalis; no treatment required.

SECOND DEGREE   *Mobitz I (Wenckebach)*   (See Fig. 125-1*M*)   Narrow QRS, progressive increase in PR interval until a ventricular beat is dropped, then sequence is repeated. Seen with drug intoxication (digitalis, beta blockers), increased vagal tone, inferior MI. Usually transient, no therapy required; if symptomatic, use atropine (0.6 mg IV, repeated × 3–4) or temporary pacemaker.

Mobitz II   (See Fig. 125-1*K*)   Fixed PR interval with occasional dropped beats, in 2:1, 3:1, or 4:1 pattern; the QRS complex is usually wide. Seen with MI or degenerative conduction system disease; a dangerous rhythm—may progress suddenly to complete AV block; pacemaker is indicated.

THIRD DEGREE (COMPLETE AV BLOCK)   (See Fig. 125-1*L*)   Atrial activity is not transmitted to ventricles; atria and ventricles contract independently. Seen with MI, digitalis toxicity, or degenerative conduction system

Table 125-3

Antiarrhythmic Drugs

Drug	Loading Dose	Maintenance Dose	Side Effects	Excretion
Group IA				
Quinidine sulfate		PO: 200–400 mg q6h	Diarrhea, tinnitus, QT prolongation, hypotension, anemia, thrombocytopenia	Hepatic
Quinidine gluconate		PO: 324–628 mg q8h		Hepatic
Procainamide	IV: 500–1000 mg	IV: 2–5 mg/min	Nausea, lupus-like syndrome, agranulocytosis, QT prolongation	Renal and hepatic
		PO: 500–1000 mg q4h		
Sustained-release:		PO: 1000–2500 mg q12h		
Disopyramide		PO: 100–300 mg q6–8h	Myocardial depression, AV block, QT prolongation anticholinergic effects	Renal and hepatic
Sustained-release:		PO: 200–400 mg q12h		
Group IB				
Lidocaine	IV: 1 mg/kg bolus followed by 0.5 mg/kg bolus q8–10 min to total 3 mg/kg	IV: 1–4 mg/min	Confusion, seizures, respiratory arrest	Hepatic
Mexiletine		PO: 100–300 mg q6–8h	Nausea, tremor, gait disturbance	Hepatic
Group IC				
Flecainide		PO: 50–100 mg q12h	Nausea, exacerbation of ventricular arrhythmia, prolongation of PR and QRS intervals	Hepatic and renal
Propafenone		PO: 150–300 mg q8h		Hepatic

646

Drug	Loading / IV dose	Maintenance dose	Adverse effects	Elimination
Group II				
Metoprolol	IV: 5–10 mg q5min × 3	PO: 25–100 mg bid	CHF, bradycardia, AV block, bronchospasm	Hepatic
Group III				
Amiodarone	PO: 800–1600 mg qd × 1–2 weeks, then 400–600 mg/d × 3 weeks	PO: 200–400 mg qd	Thyroid abnormalities, pulmonary fibrosis, hepatitis, corneal microdeposits, bluish skin, QT prolongation	Hepatic
	IV: 150 mg over 10 min	IV: 1 mg/min × 6 h, then 0.5 mg/min	—	—
Ibutilide	IV (≥60 kg): 1 mg over 10 min, can repeat after 10 min	—	Torsades de pointes, hypotension, nausea	Hepatic
Dofetilide		PO: 125–500 μg bid	Torsades de pointes, headache, dizziness	Renal
Bretylium	IV: 5–10 mg/kg	IV: 0.5–2.0 mg/min	Hypertension, orthostatic hypotension, nausea, parotid pain	Renal
Sotalol		PO: 80–320 mg q12h	Fatigue, bradycardia, exacerbation of ventricular arrhythmia	Renal
Group IV				
Verapamil	IV: 2.5–10 mg	PO: 120–480 mg qd	AV block, CHF, hypotension, constipation	Hepatic
Diltiazem	IV: 0.25 mg/kg over 2 min; can repeat with 0.35 mg/kg after 15 min	IV: 5–15 mg/h; PO: 120–360 mg/d	—	—
Other				
Digoxin	IV, PO: 0.75–1.5 mg over 24 h	IV, PO: 0.125–0.25 mg qd	Nausea, AV block, ventricular and supraventricular arrhythmias	Renal
Adenosine	IV: 6-mg bolus; if no effect then 12-mg bolus	—	Transient hypotension or atrial standstill	—

disease. Permanent pacemaker is indicated, except when associated transiently with inferior MI or in asymptomatic congenital heart block.

For a more detailed discussion, see Josephson ME, Zimetbaum P: The Bradyarrhythmias, Chap. 213, p. 1333; and The Tachyarrhythmias, Chap. 214, p. 1342, in HPIM-16.

126

CONGESTIVE HEART FAILURE AND COR PULMONALE

HEART FAILURE

DEFINITION   Condition in which heart is unable to pump sufficient blood for metabolizing tissues or can do so only from an abnormally elevated filling pressure. It is important to identify the *underlying* nature of the cardiac disease and the factors that precipitate acute CHF.

UNDERLYING CARDIAC DISEASE   Includes states that depress ventricular function (coronary artery disease, hypertension, dilated cardiomyopathy, valvular disease, congenital heart disease) and states that restrict ventricular filling (mitral stenosis, restrictive cardiomyopathy, pericardial disease).

ACUTE PRECIPITATING FACTORS   Include (1) increased Na intake, (2) noncompliance with anti-CHF medications, (3) acute MI (may be silent), (4) exacerbation of hypertension, (5) acute arrhythmias, (6) infections and/or fever, (7) pulmonary embolism, (8) anemia, (9) thyrotoxicosis, (10) pregnancy, and (11) acute myocarditis or infective endocarditis.

SYMPTOMS   Due to inadequate perfusion of peripheral tissues (fatigue, dyspnea) and elevated intracardiac filling pressures (orthopnea, paroxysmal nocturnal dyspnea, peripheral edema).

PHYSICAL EXAMINATION   Jugular venous distention, S_3, pulmonary congestion (rales, dullness over pleural effusion, peripheral edema, hepatomegaly, and ascites).

LABORATORY   CXR can reveal cardiomegaly, pulmonary vascular redistribution, Kerley B lines, pleural effusions. Left ventricular contraction and diastolic dysfunction can be assessed by *echocardiography*. In addition, echo can identify underlying valvular, pericardial, or congenital heart disease, as well as regional wall motion abnormalities typical of coronary artery disease. Measurement of brain natriuretic peptide (BNP) differentiates cardiac from pulmonary causes of dyspnea (>100 pg/mL in heart failure).

CONDITIONS THAT MIMIC CHF   *Pulmonary Disease*   Chronic bronchitis, emphysema, and asthma (Chaps. 131 and 133); look for sputum production and abnormalities on CXR and pulmonary function tests.

Other Causes of Peripheral Edema   Liver disease, varicose veins, and cyclic edema, none of which results in jugular venous distention. Edema due to renal dysfunction is often accompanied by elevated serum creatinine and abnormal urinalysis (Chap. 47).

℞ TREATMENT

Aimed at symptomatic relief, removal of precipitating factors, and control of underlying cardiac disease. Overview of treatment shown in Table 126-1; notably, ACE inhibitor should be begun early, even in pts with asymptomatic LV dysfunction. Once symptoms develop:

• *Decrease cardiac workload*: Reduce physical activity; include periods of bed rest. Prevent deep venous thrombosis of immobile pts with heparin, 5000 U SC bid, or enoxaparin, 40 mg SC qd.

• *Control excess fluid retention*: (1) *Dietary sodium restriction* (eliminate salty foods, e.g., potato chips, canned soups, bacon, salt added at table); more stringent requirements (<2 g NaCl/d) in advanced CHF. If dilutional hyponatremia present, restrict fluid intake (<1000 mL/d). (2) *Diuretics* (see Chap. 47): *Loop diuretics* (e.g., furosemide 20–120 mg/d PO or IV) are most potent and unlike thiazides remain effective when GFR < 25 mL/min. Combine loop diuretic with thiazide or metolazone for augmented effect. Potassium-

Table 126-1

Therapy for Heart Failure

1. General measures
   a. Restrict salt intake
   b. Avoid antiarrhythmics for asymptomatic arrhythmias
   c. Avoid NSAIDs
   d. Immunize against influenza and pneumococcal pneumonia
2. Diuretics
   a. Use in volume-overloaded pts to achieve normal JVP and relief of edema
   b. Weigh daily to adjust dose
   c. For diuretic resistance, administer IV or use 2 diuretics in combination (e.g., furosemide plus metolazone)
   d. Low-dose dopamine to enhance renal flow
3. ACE inhibitors
   a. For all patients with LV systolic heart failure or asymptomatic LV dysfunction
   b. Contraindications: Serum K^+ > 5.5, advanced renal failure (e.g., creatinine > 3 mg/dL), bilateral renal artery stenosis, pregnancy
4. Beta blockers
   a. For patients with class II–III heart failure, combined with ACE inhibitor and diuretics
   b. Contraindications: Bronchospasm, symptomatic bradycardia or advanced heart block, unstable heart failure or class IV symptoms
5. Digitalis
   a. For persistently symptomatic pts with systolic heart failure (especially if atrial fibrillation present) added to ACE inhibitor, diuretics, beta blocker
6. Other measures
   a. Consider angiotensin receptor blocker if not tolerant of ACE inhibitor
   b. Consider spironolactone in class III–IV heart failure
   c. Consider ventricular resynchronization in pts with class III or IV heart failure and QRS > 120 ms
   d. Consider implantable cardioverter-defibrillator in pts with class III heart failure and ejection fraction <30%

Source: Modified from E Braunwald: HPIM-15, p. 1318.

sparing diuretics are useful adjunct to reduce potassium loss; should be used cautiously when combined with ACE inhibitor to avoid hyperkalemia.

During diuresis, obtain daily weights, aiming for loss of 1–1.5 kg/d.

• *ACE inhibitors*: Recommended as standard initial CHF therapy. ACE inhibitors are mixed (arterial and venous) dilators and are particularly effective and well tolerated. They have been shown to prolong life in pts with symptomatic CHF. ACE inhibitors have also been shown to delay the onset of CHF in pts with asymptomatic LV dysfunction and to lower mortality when begun soon after acute MI. ACE inhibitors may result in significant hypotension in pts who are volume depleted, so start at lowest dosage (e.g., captopril 6.25 mg PO tid); pt should remain supine for 2–4 h after the initial doses. Angiotensin receptor blocker (e.g., losartan 50 or 100 mg/d) may be substituted if pt is intolerant of ACE inhibitor (e.g., cough, angioedema).

• *Beta blockers* administered in gradually augmented dosage improve symptoms and prolong survival in patients with moderate (NYHA class II–III) heart failure. After patient stabilized on ACE inhibitor and diuretic, begin at low dosage and increase gradually [e.g., carvedilol 3.125 mg bid, double q2weeks as tolerated to maximum of 25 mg bid (for weight < 85 kg) or 50 mg bid (weight > 85 kg)].

• *Digoxin* is useful in heart failure due to (1) marked systolic dysfunction (LV dilatation, low ejection fraction, S_3) and (2) heart failure associated with atrial fibrillation and rapid ventricular rate. Unlike ACE inhibitors and beta blockers, digoxin does not prolong survival in heart failure pts but reduces hospitalizations. Not indicated in CHF due to pericardial disease, restrictive cardiomyopathy, or mitral stenosis (unless atrial fibrillation is present). Digoxin is contraindicated in hypertrophic cardiomyopathy and in pts with AV conduction blocks.

Digoxin loading dose is administered over 24 h (0.5 mg PO/IV, followed by 0.25 mg q6h to achieve total of 1.0–1.5 mg). Subsequent dose (0.125–0.25 mg qd) depends on age, weight, and renal function and is guided by measurement of serum digoxin level.

Digitalis toxicity may be precipitated by hypokalemia, hypoxemia, hypercalcemia, hypomagnesemia, hypothyroidism, or myocardial ischemia. Early signs of toxicity include anorexia, nausea, and lethargy. *Cardiac toxicity* includes ventricular extrasystoles and ventricular tachycardia and fibrillation; atrial tachycardia with block; sinus arrest and sinoatrial block; all degrees of AV block. *Chronic* digitalis intoxication may cause cachexia, gynecomastia, "yellow" vision, or confusion. At first sign of digitalis toxicity, discontinue the drug; maintain serum K concentration between 4.0 and 5.0 mmol/L. Bradyarrhythmias and AV block may respond to atropine (0.6 mg IV); otherwise, a temporary pacemaker may be required. Digitalis-induced ventricular arrhythmias are usually treated with lidocaine (Chap. 125). Antidigoxin antibodies are available for massive overdose.

• Aldosterone antagonists, e.g., *spironolactone*, 25 mg/d, added to standard therapy in patients with advanced heart failure have been shown to reduce mortality. Its diuretic properties may also be beneficial, and it should be considered in patients with class III/IV heart failure symptoms.

• In sicker, hospitalized patients, IV vasodilator therapy (Table 126-2) is monitored by placement of a pulmonary artery catheter and indwelling arterial line. Nitroprusside is a potent mixed vasodilator for pts with markedly elevated systemic vascular resistance. It is metabolized to thiocyanate, then excreted via the kidneys. To avoid thiocyanate toxicity (seizures, altered mental status, nausea), follow thiocyanate levels in pts with renal dysfunction or if administered for more than 2 days. The combination of the oral vasodilators hydralazine and isosorbide dinitrate may be of benefit for chronic adminis-

Table 126-2

Vasodilators for Treatment of CHF

Drug and Site of Action[a]	Dose	Adverse Effects
IV AGENTS		
Nitroprusside, V = A	0.5–10 (μg/kg)/min	Thiocyanate toxicity (blurred vision, tinnitus, delirium) can occur during prolonged therapy or in renal failure
Nitroglycerin, V > A	10 μg/min–10 (μg/kg)/min	May cause hypotension if LV filling pressure is low
Nesiritide, A > V	2 μg/kg bolus followed by 0.01 (μg/kg)/min	Hypotension, renal dysfunction
ORAL AGENTS		
ACE inhibitors, V = A		Angioedema, cough, hyperkalemia, leukopenia. Reduce diuretic dosage to prevent azotemia
Captopril	6.25–50 mg tid	
Enalapril	2.5–10 mg bid	
Lisinopril	5–40 mg tid	
Hydralazine,[b] A	50–200 mg tid	May cause drug-induced lupus or angina due to reflex tachycardia
Nitrates,[b] V (e.g., isosorbide dinitrate)	10–40 mg tid	Drug tolerance may develop with more frequent administration

[a] V, venous; A, arterial.
[b] Hydralazine and nitrates are often used together to achieve combined venous and arterial effect.

tration in patients intolerant of ACE inhibitors and angiotensin receptor blockers.

IV *nesiritide* (Table 126-2), a purified preparation of BNP, is a useful vasodilator for reducing pulmonary capillary wedge pressure and dyspnea in patients with acutely decompensated CHF.

• *IV sympathomimetic amines* (see Table 14-3) are administered to hospitalized pts for refractory symptoms or acute exacerbation of CHF. They are contraindicated in hypertrophic cardiomyopathy. *Dobutamine* [2.5–10 (μg/kg)/min], the preferred agent, augments cardiac output without significant peripheral vasoconstriction or tachycardia. *Dopamine* at low dosage [1–5 (μg/kg)/min] facilitates diuresis; at higher dosage [5–10 (μg/kg)/min] positive inotropic effects predominate; peripheral vasoconstriction is greatest at dosage >10 (μg/kg)/min. *Amrinone* [5–10 (μg/kg)/min after a 0.75-mg/kg bolus] and milrinone [0.375 (μg/kg)/min after 50-μg/kg loading dose] are nonsympathetic positive inotropes and vasodilators. Vasodilators and inotropic agents may be used together for additive effect.

Patients with refractory CHF and QRS > 120 ms may be candidates for ventricular resynchronization. Pts with severe disease and <6 months expected survival, who meet stringent criteria, may be candidates for a ventricular assist device or cardiac transplantation.

• Patients with predominantly diastolic heart failure are treated with salt restriction and diuretics. Beta blockers and nondihydropyridine calcium blockers may be of benefit.

COR PULMONALE

RV enlargement resulting from *primary* lung disease; leads to RV hypertrophy and eventually to RV failure. Etiologies include:

- *Pulmonary parenchymal or airway disease.* Chronic obstructive lung disease (COPD), interstitial lung diseases, bronchiectasis, cystic fibrosis (Chaps. 133 and 136).
- *Pulmonary vascular disease.* Recurrent pulmonary emboli, primary pulmonary hypertension (PHT) (Chap. 129), vasculitis, sickle cell anemia.
- *Inadequate mechanical ventilation.* Kyphoscoliosis, neuromuscular disorders, marked obesity, sleep apnea.

SYMPTOMS Depend on underlying disorder but include dyspnea, cough, fatigue, and sputum production (in parenchymal diseases).

PHYSICAL EXAMINATION Tachypnea, cyanosis, clubbing are common. RV impulse along left sternal border, loud P_2, right-sided S_4. If RV failure develops, elevated jugular venous pressure, hepatomegaly with ascites, pedal edema.

LABORATORY *ECG* RV hypertrophy and RA enlargement (Chap. 118); tachyarrhythmias are common.

CXR RV and pulmonary artery enlargement; if PHT present, tapering of the pulmonary artery branches. Pulmonary function tests and ABGs characterize intrinsic pulmonary disease.

Echocardiogram RV hypertrophy; LV function typically normal. RV systolic pressure can be estimated from Doppler measurement of tricuspid regurgitant flow. If imaging is difficult because of air in distended lungs, RV volume and wall thickness can be evaluated by MRI. If pulmonary emboli suspected, obtain high-resolution chest CT or radionuclide lung scan.

 TREATMENT

Aimed at underlying pulmonary disease and may include bronchodilators, antibiotics, and oxygen administration. If RV failure is present, treat as CHF, instituting low-sodium diet and diuretics; digoxin must be administered cautiously (toxicity increased due to hypoxemia, hypercapnia, acidosis). Loop diuretics must also be used with care to prevent significant metabolic alkalosis that blunts respiratory drive. Supraventricular tachyarrhythmias are common and treated with digoxin or verapamil (*not* beta blockers). Chronic anticoagulation with warfarin is indicated when pulmonary hypertension is accompanied by RV failure. In selected pts, inhalation of nitric oxide and infusion of prostacyclin reduce pulmonary hypertension and are undergoing evaluation for this purpose (see Chap. 129).

For a more detailed discussion, see Braunwald E: Heart Failure and Cor Pulmonale, Chap. 216, p. 1367, in HPIM-16.

127

DISEASES OF THE AORTA

AORTIC ANEURYSM

Abnormal widening of the abdominal or thoracic aorta; in ascending aorta most commonly secondary to cystic medial necrosis or atherosclerosis; aneurysms of descending thoracic and abdominal aorta are primarily atherosclerotic.

HISTORY   May be clinically silent, but thoracic aortic aneurysms often result in deep, diffuse chest pain, dysphagia, hoarseness, hemoptysis, dry cough; abdominal aneurysms result in abdominal pain or thromboemboli to the lower extremities.

PHYSICAL EXAMINATION   Abdominal aneurysms are often palpable, most commonly in periumbilical area. Pts with ascending thoracic aneurysms may show features of the Marfan syndrome (HPIM-16, Chap. 342).

LABORATORY   Suspect thoracic aneurysm by abnormal *CXR* (enlarged aortic silhouette) and confirm by *echocardiography, contrast CT,* or *MRI*. Confirm abdominal aneurysm by *abdominal plain film* (rim of calcification), *ultrasound, CT scan,* or *MRI*. Contrast aortography is often performed preoperatively. If clinically suspected, obtain serologic test for syphilis, especially if ascending thoracic aneurysm shows thin shell of calcification.

 TREATMENT

Control of hypertension (Chap. 122) is essential. Surgical resection of thoracic aortic aneurysms >6 cm in diameter (abdominal aortic aneurysms >5.5 cm), for persistent pain despite bp control, or for evidence of rapid expansion. In pts with the Marfan syndrome, thoracic aortic aneurysms >5 cm usually warrant repair.

AORTIC DISSECTION   (Fig. 127-1)

Potentially life-threatening condition in which disruption of aortic intima allows dissection of blood into vessel wall; may involve ascending aorta (type II), descending aorta (type III), or both (type I). Alternative classification: Type A—dissection involves ascending aorta; type B—limited to descending aorta. Involvement of the ascending aorta is most lethal form.

ETIOLOGY   Ascending aortic dissection associated with hypertension, cystic medial necrosis, the Marfan syndrome; descending dissections commonly associated with atherosclerosis or hypertension. Incidence is increased in pts with coarctation of aorta, bicuspid aortic valve, and rarely in third trimester of pregnancy in otherwise normal women.

SYMPTOMS   Sudden onset of severe anterior or posterior chest pain, with "ripping" quality; maximal pain may travel if dissection propagates. Additional symptoms relate to obstruction of aortic branches (stroke, MI), dyspnea (acute aortic regurgitation), or symptoms of low cardiac output due to cardiac tamponade (dissection into pericardial sac).

PHYSICAL EXAMINATION   Sinus tachycardia common; if cardiac tamponade develops, hypotension, pulsus paradoxus, and pericardial rub appear. Asymmetry of carotid or brachial pulses, aortic regurgitation, and neurologic abnormalities associated with interruption of carotid artery flow are common findings.

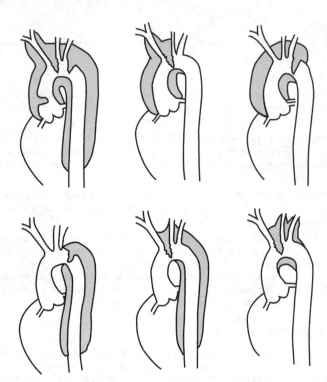

FIGURE 127-1 Classification of aortic dissections. Stanford classification: Top panels illustrate type A dissections that involve the ascending aorta independent of site of tear and distal extension; type B dissections (bottom panels) involve transverse and/or descending aorta without involvement of the ascending aorta. DeBakey classification: Type I dissection involves ascending to descending aorta (top left); type II dissection is limited to ascending or transverse aorta, without descending aorta (top center + top right); type III dissection involves descending aorta only (bottom left). [*From DC Miller, in RM Doroghazi, EE Slater (eds.), Aortic Dissection. New York, McGraw-Hill, 1983, with permission.*]

LABORATORY *CXR*: Widening of mediastinum; dissection can be confirmed by *CT scan, MRI,* or *ultrasound* (esp. transesophageal echocardiography). Aortography recommended if results of these imaging techniques are not definitive.

℞ **TREATMENT**

Reduce cardiac contractility and treat hypertension to maintain systolic bp between 100 and 120 mmHg using IV agents (Table 127-1), e.g., sodium nitroprusside accompanied by a beta blocker (aiming for heart rate of 60 beats per min), followed by oral therapy. If beta blocker contraindicated, consider IV verapamil or diltiazem (Table 125-3). Direct vasodilators (hydralazine, diazoxide) are contraindicated because they may increase shear stress. Ascending aortic dissection (type A) requires surgical repair emergently or, if pt can be stabilized with medications, semielectively. Descending aortic dissections are stabilized medically (maintain systolic bp between 110 and 120 mmHg) with oral antihypertensive agents (esp. beta blockers); immediate sur-

Table 127-1

Treatment of Aortic Dissection

Preferred Regimen	Dose
Sodium nitroprusside *plus* a beta blocker:	20–400 μg/min IV
Propranolol *or*	0.5 mg IV; then 1 mg q5min, to total of 0.15 mg/kg
Esmolol *or*	500 μg/kg IV over 1 min; then 50–200 (μg/kg)/min
Labetalol	20 mg IV over 2 min, then 40–80 mg q10–15min to max of 300 mg

gical repair is not necessary unless continued pain or extension of dissection is observed (serial MRI or CT scans).

OTHER ABNORMALITIES OF THE AORTA
ATHEROSCLEROTIC OCCLUSIVE DISEASE OF ABDOMINAL AORTA Particularly common in presence of diabetes mellitus or cigarette smoking. Symptoms include intermittent claudication of the buttocks and thighs and impotence (Leriche syndrome); femoral and other distal pulses are absent. Diagnosis is established by noninvasive leg pressure measurements and Doppler velocity analysis, and confirmed by MRI, CT, or aortography. Aortic-femoral bypass surgery is required for symptomatic treatment.

TAKAYASU'S ("PULSELESS") DISEASE Arteritis of aorta and major branches in young women. Anorexia, weight loss, fever, and night sweats occur. Localized symptoms relate to occlusion of aortic branches (cerebral ischemia, claudication, and loss of pulses in arms). ESR is increased; diagnosis confirmed by aortography. Glucocorticoid and immunosuppressive therapy may be beneficial, but mortality is high.

For a more detailed discussion, see Dzau VJ, Creager MA: Diseases of the Aorta, Chap. 231, p. 1481, in HPIM-16.

128

PERIPHERAL VASCULAR DISEASE

Occlusive or inflammatory disease that develops within the peripheral arteries, veins, or lymphatics.

ARTERIOSCLEROSIS OF PERIPHERAL ARTERIES
History *Intermittent claudication* is muscular cramping with exercise; quickly relieved by rest. Pain in buttocks and thighs suggests aortoiliac disease;

calf muscle pain implies femoral or popliteal artery disease. More advanced arteriosclerotic obstruction results in pain at rest; painful ulcers of the feet (painless in diabetics) may result.

Physical Examination Decreased peripheral pulses, blanching of affected limb with elevation, dependent rubor (redness). Ischemic ulcers or gangrene of toes may be present.

Laboratory Doppler ultrasound of peripheral pulses before and during exercise localizes stenoses; magnetic resonance angiography or contrast arteriography performed only if reconstructive surgery or angioplasty is considered.

 TREATMENT

Most pts can be managed medically with daily exercise program, careful foot care (esp. in diabetics), treatment of hypercholesterolemia, and local debridement of ulcerations. Abstinence from cigarettes is mandatory. Some, but not all, pts note symptomatic improvement with drug therapy (pentoxifylline or cilostazol). Pts with severe claudication, rest pain, or gangrene are candidates for arterial reconstructive surgery; percutaneous transluminal angioplasty or stent placement can be performed in selected pts.

Other Conditions that Impair Peripheral Arterial Flow

ARTERIAL EMBOLISM Due to thrombus or vegetation within the heart or aorta or paradoxically from a venous thrombus through a right-to-left intracardiac shunt.

History Sudden pain or numbness in an extremity in absence of previous history of claudication.

Physical Exam Absent pulse, pallor, and decreased temperature of limb distal to the occlusion. Lesion is identified by angiography.

 TREATMENT

Intravenous heparin to prevent propagation of clot. For acute severe ischemia, immediate endovascular or surgical embolectomy is indicated. Thrombolytic therapy (e.g., tPA, streptokinase, urokinase) may be effective for thrombus within atherosclerotic vessel or arterial bypass graft.

VASOSPASTIC DISORDERS Manifest by Raynaud's phenomenon in which cold exposure results in triphasic color response: blanching of the fingers, followed by cyanosis, then redness. Usually a benign disorder. However, suspect an underlying disease (e.g., scleroderma) if tissue necrosis occurs, if disease is unilateral, or if it develops after age 50.

 TREATMENT

Keep extremities warm; calcium channel blockers (nifedipine XL 30–90 mg PO qd or α-adrenergic antagonists (e.g., prazocin 1–5 mg tid) may be effective.

THROMBOANGIITIS OBLITERANS (BUERGER'S DISEASE) Occurs in young men who are heavy smokers and involves both upper and lower extremities; nonatheromatous inflammatory reaction develops in veins and small arteries leading to superficial thrombophlebitis and arterial obstruction with ulceration or gangrene of digits. Abstinence from tobacco is essential.

VENOUS DISEASE

SUPERFICIAL THROMBOPHLEBITIS   Benign disorder characterized by erythema, tenderness, and edema along involved vein. Conservative therapy includes local heat, elevation, and anti-inflammatory drugs such as aspirin. More serious conditions such as cellulitis or lymphangitis may mimic this, but these are associated with fever, chills, lymphadenopathy, and red superficial streaks along inflamed lymphatic channels.

DEEP VENOUS THROMBOSIS (DVT)   More serious condition that may lead to pulmonary embolism (Chap. 135). Particularly common in pts on prolonged bed rest, those with chronic debilitating disease, and those with malignancies (Table 128-1).

History   Pain or tenderness in calf or thigh, usually unilateral; may be asymptomatic, with pulmonary embolism as primary presentation.

Physical Exam   Often normal; local swelling or tenderness to deep palpation may be present over affected vein.

Laboratory   D-Dimer testing is sensitive but not specific for diagnosis. Most helpful noninvasive testing is ultrasound imaging of the deep veins with Doppler interrogation. These noninvasive studies are most sensitive for proximal (upper leg) DVT, less sensitive for calf DVT. Invasive venography is used when diagnosis not clear. MRI may be useful for diagnosis of proximal DVT and DVT within the pelvic veins or in the superior or inferior vena cavae.

 TREATMENT

Systemic anticoagulation with heparin (7500- to 10,000-U bolus, followed by continuous IV infusion to maintain a PTT at 2 × normal) or low-molecular-weight heparin (e.g., enoxaperin 1 mg/kg SC bid), followed by warfarin PO

Table 128-1

Conditions Associated with an Increased Risk for Development of Venous Thrombosis

Surgery
   Orthopedic, thoracic, abdominal, and genitourinary procedures
Neoplasms
   Pancreas, lung, ovary, testes, urinary tract, breast, stomach
Trauma
   Fractures of spine, pelvis, femur, tibia
Immobilization
   Acute MI, CHF, stroke, postoperative convalescence
Pregnancy
   Estrogen use (for replacement or contraception)
Hypercoagulable states
   Resistance to activated protein C; deficiencies of antithrombin III, protein C, or protein S; antiphospholipid antibodies; myeloproliferative disease; dysfibrinogenemia; DIC
Venulitis
   Thromboangiitis obliterans, Behçet's disease, homocysteinuria
Previous deep vein thrombosis

(overlap with heparin for at least 4–5 days and continue for at least 3 months if proximal deep veins involved). Adjust warfarin dose to maintain prothrombin time at INR 2.0–3.0.

DVT can be prevented by early ambulation following surgery or with low-dose unfractionated heparin during prolonged bed rest (5000 U SC bid-tid), supplemented by pneumatic compression boots. Following knee or hip surgery, warfarin (INR 2.0–3.0) is an effective regimen. Low-molecular-weight heparins are also effective in preventing DVT after general or orthopedic surgery.

LYMPHEDEMA

Chronic, painless edema, usually of the lower extremities; may be primary (inherited) or secondary to lymphatic damage or obstruction (e.g., recurrent lymphangitis, tumor, filariasis).

Physical Exam Marked pitting edema in early stages; limb becomes indurated with *non*pitting edema chronically. Differentiate from chronic *venous* insufficiency, which displays hyperpigmentation, stasis dermatitis, and superficial venous varicosities.

Laboratory Abdominal and pelvic ultrasound or CT or MRI to identify obstructing lesions. Lymphangiography or lymphoscintigraphy (rarely done) to confirm diagnosis. If *unilateral* edema, differentiate from DVT by noninvasive venous studies (above).

R̲x̲ TREATMENT

(1) Meticulous foot hygiene to prevent infection, (2) leg elevation, (3) compression stockings and/or pneumatic compression boots. Diuretics should be *avoided* to prevent intravascular volume depletion.

For a more detailed discussion, see Creager MA, Dzau VJ: Vascular Diseases of the Extremities, Chap. 232, p. 1486, in HPIM-16.

129

PULMONARY HYPERTENSION

DEFINITION Elevation of pulmonary artery (PA) pressure due to pulmonary vascular or parenchymal disease, increased left heart filling pressure, or a combination. Table 129-1 lists most common etiologies. Pulmonary hypertension is most common cause of cor pulmonale (Chap. 126).

SYMPTOMS Exertional dyspnea, fatigue angina (due to RV ischemia), syncope, peripheral edema.

PHYSICAL EXAMINATION Jugular venous distention, RV lift, increased P_2, right-sided S_4. Tricuspid regurgitation appears in advanced stages.

Table 129-1

Causes of Pulmonary Hypertension

Pulmonary Arterial Hypertension
   Primary pulmonary hypertension
   Collagen vascular diseases (e.g., CREST, scleroderma, SLE, RA)
   Congenital systemic to pulmonary shunts (e.g., ventricular septal defect, patent ductus arteriosus, atrial septal defect)
   Portal hypertension
   HIV infection
   Anorexigen use (e.g., fenfluramines)
Pulmonary Venous Hypertension
   LV diastolic dysfunction (e.g., LV hypertrophy, coronary artery disease)
   Mitral stenosis or regurgitation
Lung Disease and Hypoxemia
   Chronic obstructive lung disease
   Interstitial lung disease
   Sleep apnea
   Chronic hypoventilation
Pulmonary Thromboembolic Disease
   Acute pulmonary embolism (Chap. 135)
   Chronic pulmonary embolism

Note: CREST, calcinosis, Raynaud's phenomenon, esophageal involvement, sclerodactyly, and telangiectasia (syndrome).

LABORATORY   *CXR* shows enlarged central PA. *ECG* may demonstrate RV hypertrophy and RA enlargement. *Echocardiogram* shows RV and RA enlargement; RV systolic pressure can be estimated from Doppler recording of tricuspid regurgitation (Chap. 118). *Pulmonary function tests* identify underlying obstructive or restrictive lung disease; impaired CO diffusion capacity is common. *V/Q nuclear scan* or contrast-enhanced *high-resolution chest CT* can identify thromboembolic pulmonary vascular disease. *ANA titer* is elevated in collagen vascular diseases. *HIV testing* should be performed in individuals at risk. *Cardiac catheterization* accurately measures PA pressures, cardiac output, identifies underlying congenital vascular shunts; during procedure, response to short-acting vasodilators can be assessed.

Figure 129-1 summarizes laboratory approach for patients with unexplained pulmonary hypertension.

PRIMARY PULMONARY HYPERTENSION
Uncommon (2 cases/million), very serious form of pulmonary hypertension. Most pts present in 4th and 5th decades, female $\gg$ male predominance; up to 20% of cases are familial. Major symptom is dyspnea, often with insidious onset. Mean survival < 3 years in absence of therapy.

PHYSICAL EXAMINATION   Prominent *a* wave in jugular venous pulse, right ventricular heave, narrowly split S_2 with accentuated P_2. Terminal course is characterized by signs of right-sided heart failure. CXR: RV and central pulmonary arterial prominence. Pulmonary arteries taper sharply. PFT: usually normal or mild restrictive defect. ECG: RV enlargement, right axis deviation, and RV hypertrophy. Echocardiogram: RA and RV enlargement and tricuspid regurgitation.

DIFFERENTIAL DIAGNOSIS   Other disorders of heart, lungs, and pulmonary vasculature must be excluded. Lung function studies will identify

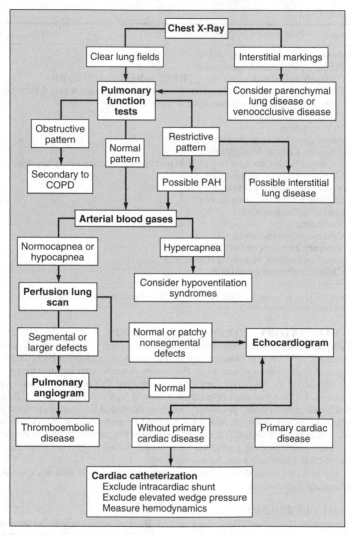

FIGURE 129-1 An algorithm for the workup of a patient with unexplained pulmonary hypertension. (*Adapted with permission from Rich S: HPIM-16.*)

chronic pulmonary disease causing pulmonary hypertension and cor pulmonale. Interstitial diseases (PFTs, CT scan) and hypoxic pulmonary hypertension (ABGs, Sa_{O_2}) should be excluded. Perfusion lung scan should be performed to exclude chronic PE. Spiral CT scan, pulmonary arteriogram, and even open-lung biopsy may be required to distinguish PE from PPH. Rarely, pulmonary hypertension is due to parasitic disease (schistosomiasis, filariasis). Cardiac disorders to be excluded include pulmonary artery and pulmonic valve stenosis. Pulmonary artery and ventricular and atrial shunts with pulmonary vascular disease (Eisenmenger reaction) should be sought. Silent mitral stenosis should be excluded by echocardiography.

℞ TREATMENT

Limit physical activities, use diuretics for peripheral edema, O_2 supplementation if PO_2 reduced, and chronic warfarin anticoagulation (target INR = 2.0–3.0).

If short-acting vasodilators are beneficial during acute testing in catheter laboratory, pt may benefit from high-dose *calcium channel blocker* (e.g., nifedipine, up to 240 mg/d), but must monitor for hypotension or worsening of right heart failure.

For patients with advanced refractory symptoms, options to improve symptoms and functional class include prostaglandins [*epoprostenol* (which has been shown to increase survival) via continuous central IV access, or *treprostinil* via continuous subcutaneous infusion pump] and the orally active endothelin receptor antagonist *bosentan*.

For selected patients with persistent right heart failure, lung transplantation can be considered.

For a more detailed discussion, see Rich S: Pulmonary Hypertension, Chap. 220, p. 1403, in HPIM-16.

130

RESPIRATORY FUNCTION AND PULMONARY DIAGNOSTIC PROCEDURES

RESPIRATORY FUNCTION

The respiratory system includes not only the lungs but also the CNS, chest wall (diaphragm, abdomen, intercostal muscles), and pulmonary circulation. Prime function of the system is to exchange gas between inspired air and venous blood.

DISTURBANCES IN VENTILATORY FUNCTION (Figs. 130-1 and 130-2) Ventilation is the process whereby lungs deliver fresh air to alveoli. Measurements of ventilatory function consist of quantification of air in the lungs [total lung capacity (TLC), residual volume (RV)] and the rate at which air can be expelled from the lungs [forced vital capacity (FVC), forced expiratory volume in 1 s (FEV_1)] during a forced exhalation from TLC. Expiratory flow rates may be plotted against lung volumes yielding a flow-volume curve (HPIM-16, Fig. 234-4).

Two major patterns of abnormal ventilatory function are restrictive and obstructive patterns (Tables 130-1 and 130-2).

In obstructive pattern:

- Hallmark is decrease in expiratory flow rate, i.e., FEV_1.
- Ratio FEV_1/FVC is reduced.
- TLC is normal or increased.
- RV is elevated due to trapping of air during expiration.

In restrictive disease:

- Hallmark is decrease in TLC.
- May be caused by pulmonary parenchymal disease or extraparenchymal (neuromuscular such as myasthenia gravis or chest wall such as kyphoscoliosis).
- Pulmonary parenchymal disease usually occurs with a reduced RV, but extraparenchymal disease (with expiratory dysfunction) occurs with an increased RV. Coexisting restrictive and obstructive disease may mimic extraparenchymal disease with ↓TLC and preserved or relatively ↑RV.

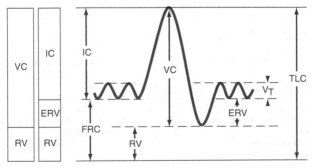

FIGURE 130-1 Lung volumes, shown by block diagrams (*left*) and by a spirographic tracing (*right*). TLC, total lung capacity; VC, vital capacity; RV, residual volume; IC, inspiratory capacity; ERV, expiratory reserve volume; FRC, functional residual capacity; V_T, tidal volume. (*From SE Weinberger, JM Drazen: HPIM-16, p. 1498.*)

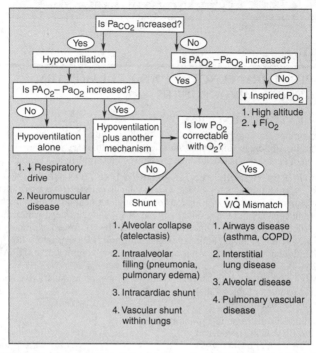

FIGURE 130-2 Flow diagram outlining the diagnostic approach to the pt with hypoxemia (Pa_{O_2} < 80 mmHg). $PA_{O_2} - Pa_{O_2}$ is usually <15 mmHg for subjects ≤ 30 years old, and increases ~3 mmHg per decade after age 30.

Table 130-1

Common Respiratory Diseases by Diagnostic Categories

OBSTRUCTIVE

Asthma	Bronchiectasis
Chronic obstructive lung disease (chronic bronchitis, emphysema)	Cystic fibrosis
	Bronchiolitis

RESTRICTIVE—PARENCHYMAL

Sarcoidosis	Pneumoconiosis
Idiopathic pulmonary fibrosis	Drug- or radiation-induced interstitial lung disease

RESTRICTIVE—EXTRAPARENCHYMAL

Neuromuscular	Chest wall
Diaphragmatic weakness/ paralysis	Kyphoscoliosis
Myasthenia gravis[a]	Obesity
Guillain-Barré syndrome[a]	Ankylosing spondylitis[a]
Muscular dystrophies[a]	
Cervical spine injury[a]	

[a] Can have inspiratory and expiratory limitation (see text).

Table 130-2

Alterations in Ventilatory Function

	TLC	RV	VC	FEV$_1$/FVC
Obstructive	N to ↑	↑	↓	↓
Restrictive				
Pulmonary parenchymal	↓	↓	↓	N to ↑
Extraparenchymal—inspiratory	↓	N to ↓	↓	N
Extraparenchymal—inspiratory + expiratory	↓	↑	↓	Variable

Note: N, normal; for other abbreviations, see text.
Source: Adapted from SE Weinberger, JM Drazen: HPIM-16, p. 1500.

DISTURBANCES IN PULMONARY CIRCULATION Pulmonary vasculature transmits the RV output, ~5 L/min at a low pressure. Perfusion of lung greatest in dependent portion. Assessment requires measuring pulmonary vascular pressures and cardiac output to derive pulmonary vascular resistance. Pulmonary vascular resistance rises with hypoxia, intraluminal thrombi, scarring, or loss of alveolar beds.

All diseases of the respiratory system causing hypoxia are capable of causing pulmonary hypertension. However, pts with hypoxemia due to chronic obstructive lung disease, interstitial lung disease, chest wall disease, and obesity-hypoventilation–sleep apnea are particularly likely to develop pulmonary hypertension.

DISTURBANCES IN GAS EXCHANGE Primary functions of the respiratory system are to remove CO_2 and provide O_2. Normal tidal volume is ~500 mL, and normal frequency is 15 breaths/min for a total ventilation of 7.5 L/min. Because of dead space, alveolar ventilation is 5 L/min.

Partial pressure of CO_2 in arterial blood (Pa_{CO_2}) is directly proportional to amount of CO_2 produced each minute ($\dot{V}_{CO_2}$) and inversely proportional to alveolar ventilation ($\dot{V}A$).

$$Pa_{CO_2} = 0.863 \times \dot{V}_{CO_2}/\dot{V}A$$

Gas exchange is critically dependent on proper matching of ventilation and perfusion.

Assessment of gas exchange requires measurement of ABGs. The actual content of O_2 in blood is determined by both P_{O_2} and hemoglobin.

Arterial P_{O_2} can be used to measure alveolar-arterial O_2 difference (A − a gradient). Increased A − a gradient (normal <15 mmHg, rising by 3 mmHg each decade after age 30) indicates impaired gas exchange.

In order to calculate A − a gradient, the alveolar P_{O_2} (PA_{O_2}) must be calculated:

$$PA_{O_2} = FI_{O_2} \times (PB - P_{H_2O}) - Pa_{CO_2}/R$$

where FI_{O_2} = fractional concentration of inspired O_2 (0.21 breathing room air), PB = barometric pressure (760 mmHg at sea level), P_{H_2O} = water vapor pressure (47 mmHg when air is saturated at 37°C), and R = respiratory quotient (the ratio of CO_2 production to O_2 consumption, usually assumed to be 0.8).

Adequacy of CO_2 removal is reflected in the partial pressure of CO_2 in arterial blood.

Because measurement of ABGs necessitates arterial puncture, noninvasive techniques may be useful, particularly to determine trends in gas exchange over time. The pulse oximeter measures oxygen saturation, Sa_{O_2}, rather than Pa_{O_2}. While widely used, clinicians must be aware that (1) the relationship between Sa_{O_2} and Pa_{O_2} is curvilinear, flattening above a Pa_{O_2} of 60 mmHg; (2) poor peripheral perfusion may interfere with the oximeter's function; and (3) the oximeter provides no information about P_{CO_2}.

Ability of gas to diffuse across the alveolar-capillary membrane is assessed by the diffusing capacity of the lung (DL_{CO}). Carried out with low concentration of carbon monoxide during a single 10-s breath-holding period or during 1 min of steady breathing. Value depends on alveolar-capillary surface area, pulmonary capillary blood volume, degree of ventilation-perfusion ($\dot{V}/\dot{Q}$) mismatching, and thickness of alveolar-capillary membrane.

MECHANISMS OF ABNORMAL FUNCTION Four basic mechanisms of hypoxemia are (1) ↓ inspired P_{O_2}, (2) hypoventilation, (3) shunt, and (4) $\dot{V}/\dot{Q}$ mismatch. Diffusion block contributes to hypoxemia only under selected circumstances. Approach to the hypoxemic pt is shown in Fig. 130-2.

The essential mechanism underlying all cases of hypercapnia is inadequate alveolar ventilation. Potential contributing factors include (1) increased CO_2 production, (2) decreased ventilatory drive, (3) malfunction of the respiratory pump or increased airways resistance, and (4) inefficiency of gas exchange (increased dead space or $\dot{V}/\dot{Q}$ mismatch) necessitating a compensatory increase in overall minute ventilation.

DIAGNOSTIC PROCEDURES

NONINVASIVE PROCEDURES *Radiography* No CXR pattern is sufficiently specific to *establish* a diagnosis; instead, the CXR serves to *detect* disease, assess magnitude, and guide further diagnostic investigation. Thoracic CT is now routine in evaluation of pts with pulmonary nodules and masses. CT is especially helpful in the assessment of pleural lesions. Contrast enhancement also makes thoracic CT useful in differentiating tissue masses from vascular structures. High-resolution CT has largely replaced bronchography in the evaluation of surgical bronchiectasis and is useful in evaluation of pts with interstitial lung disease. Spiral or helical CT is the preferred first test in most pts in whom the diagnosis of pulmonary thromboembolism is suspected. MRI is generally less useful than CT but is preferred in evaluation of abnormalities at the lung apex, adjacent to the spine, and at the thoracoabdominal junction.

Skin Tests Specific skin test antigens are available for tuberculosis, histoplasmosis, coccidioidomycosis, blastomycosis, trichinosis, toxoplasmosis, and aspergillosis. A positive delayed reaction (type IV) to a tuberculin test indicates only prior infection, not active disease. Immediate (type I) and late (type III) dermal hypersensitivity to *Aspergillus* antigen supports diagnosis of allergic bronchopulmonary aspergillosis in pts with a compatible clinical illness.

Sputum Exam Sputum is distinguished from saliva by presence of bronchial epithelial cells and alveolar macrophages. Sputum exam should include gross inspection for blood, color, and odor, as well as microscopic inspection of carefully stained smears. Culture of expectorated sputum may be misleading owing to contamination with oropharyngeal flora. Sputum samples induced by inhalation of nebulized, warm, hypertonic saline can be stained using immunofluorescent techniques for the presence of *Pneumocystis carinii*.

Pulmonary Function Tests May indicate abnormalities of airway function, alterations of lung volume, and disturbances of gas exchange. Specific patterns of pulmonary function may assist in differential diagnosis. PFTs may also provide objective measures of therapeutic response, e.g., to bronchodilators.

Pulmonary Scintigraphy Scans of pulmonary ventilation and perfusion aid in the diagnosis of pulmonary embolism. Quantitative ventilation-perfusion scans are also used to assess surgical resectability of lung cancer in pts with diminished respiratory function. PET scanning (positron emission tomography) is now standard in the evaluation and staging of patients with bronchogenic carcinoma.

INVASIVE PROCEDURES *Bronchoscopy* Permits visualization of airways, identification of endobronchial abnormalities, and collection of diagnostic specimens by lavage, brushing, or biopsy. The fiberoptic bronchoscope permits exam of smaller, more peripheral airways than the rigid bronchoscope, but the latter permits greater control of the airways and provides more effective suctioning. These features make rigid bronchoscopy particularly useful in pts with central obstructing tumors, foreign bodies, or massive hemoptysis. The fiberoptic bronchoscope increases the diagnostic potential of bronchoscopy, permitting biopsy of peripheral nodules and diffuse infiltrative diseases as well as aspiration and lavage of airways and airspaces. Fibcroptic biopsy is particularly useful in diagnosing diffuse infectious processes, lymphangitic spread of cancer, and granulomatous diseases.

Video-Assisted Thoracic Surgery Now commonly used for diagnosis of pleural lesions as well as peripheral parenchymal infiltrates and nodules. Has largely replaced "open biopsy"; may be used therapeutically.

Percutaneous Needle Aspiration of the Lung Usually performed under CT guidance to obtain cytologic or microbiologic specimens from local pulmonary lesions.

Bronchoalveolar Lavage (BAL) An adjunct to fiberoptic bronchoscopy permitting collection of cells and liquid from distal air spaces. Useful in diagnosis of *P. carinii* pneumonia, other infections, and some interstitial diseases.

Thoracentesis and Pleural Biopsy Thoracentesis should be performed as an early step in the evaluation of any pleural effusion of uncertain etiology. Analysis of pleural fluid helps differentiate transudate from exudate (Chap. 133). (Exudate: pleural fluid LDH > 200 IU, pleural fluid/serum protein > 0.5, pleural fluid/serum LDH > 0.6.) Pleural fluid pH < 7.2 suggests that an exudate associated with an infection is an empyema and will almost certainly require drainage. WBC count and differential; glucose, P_{CO_2}, amylase, Gram stain, culture, and cytologic exam should be performed on all specimens. Rheumatoid factor and complement may also be useful. Closed pleural biopsy can also be done when a pleural effusion is present, but has largely been replaced by video-assisted thoracoscopy.

Pulmonary Angiography The definitive test for pulmonary embolism; may also reveal AV malformations.

Mediastinoscopy Diagnostic procedure of choice in pts with disease involving mediastinal lymph nodes. However, lymph nodes in left superior mediastinum must be approached via *mediastinotomy*.

For a more detailed discussion, see Weinberger SE, Drazen JM: Disturbances of Respiratory Function, Chap. 234, p. 1498, and Diagnostic Procedures in Respiratory Diseases, Chap. 235, p. 1505, in HPIM-16.

131

ASTHMA AND HYPERSENSITIVITY PNEUMONITIS

ASTHMA

DEFINITION Increased responsiveness of lower airways to multiple stimuli; episodic, and with reversible obstruction; may range in severity from mild without limitation of pt's activity to severe and life-threatening. Severe obstruction persisting for days or weeks is known as *status asthmaticus*.

EPIDEMIOLOGY AND ETIOLOGY Some 4–5% of adults and up to 10% of children are estimated to experience episodes of asthma. Basic abnormality is airway hyperresponsiveness to both specific and nonspecific stimuli. All pts demonstrate enhanced bronchoconstriction in response to inhalation of methacholine or histamine (nonspecific bronchoconstrictor agents).

Some pts may be classified as having *allergic asthma*; these experience worsening of symptoms on exposure to pollens or other allergens. They characteristically give personal and/or family history of other allergic diseases, such as rhinitis, urticaria, and eczema. Skin tests to allergens are positive; serum IgE may be ↑. Bronchoprovocation studies may demonstrate positive responses to inhalation of specific allergens.

A significant number of asthmatic pts have negative allergic histories and do not react to skin or bronchoprovocation testing with specific allergens. Many of these develop bronchospasm after a URI. These pts are said to have *idiosyncratic asthma*.

Some pts experience worsening of symptoms on exercise or exposure to cold air or occupational stimuli. Many note increased wheezing following viral URI or in response to emotional stress.

PATHOGENESIS Common denominator underlying the asthmatic diathesis is nonspecific hyperirritability of the tracheobronchial tree. The etiology of airway hyperresponsiveness in asthma is unknown, but airway inflammation is believed to play a fundamental role. Airway reactivity may fluctuate, and fluctuations correlate with clinical symptoms. Airway reactivity may be increased by a number of factors: allergenic, pharmacologic, environmental, occupational, infectious, exercise-related, and emotional. Among the more common are airborne allergens, aspirin, β-adrenergic blocking agents (e.g., propranolol, timolol), sulfites in food, air pollution (ozone, nitrogen dioxide), and respiratory infections.

─────────────── *Approach to the Patient* ───────────────

History Symptoms: wheezing, dyspnea, cough, fever, sputum production, other allergic disorders. Possible precipitating factors (allergens, infection, etc.);

asthma attacks often occur at night. Response to medications. Course of previous attacks (e.g., need for hospitalization, steroid treatment).

Physical Exam General: tachypnea, tachycardia, use of accessory respiratory muscles, cyanosis, pulsus paradoxus (accessory muscle use and pulsus paradoxus correlate with severity of obstruction). Lungs: adequacy of aeration, symmetry of breath sounds, wheezing, prolongation of expiratory phase, hyperinflation. Heart: evidence for CHF. ENT/skin: evidence of allergic nasal, sinus, or skin disease.

Laboratory While PFT findings are not diagnostic, they are very helpful in judging severity of airway obstruction and in following response to therapy in both chronic and acute situations. Forced vital capacity (FVC), FEV_1, maximum mid- and peak expiratory flow rate (MMEFR, PEFR), FEV_1/FVC are decreased; residual volume and TLC increased during episodes of obstruction; DL_{CO} usually normal or slightly increased. Reduction of FEV_1 to <25% predicted or <0.75 L after administration of a bronchodilator indicates severe disease.

CBC may show eosinophilia. IgE may show mild elevations; marked elevations may suggest evidence of allergic bronchopulmonary aspergillosis (ABPA). Sputum examination: eosinophilia, Curschmann's spirals (casts of small airways), Charcot-Leyden crystals; presence of large numbers of neutrophils suggests bronchial infection.

ABGs: uniformly show hypoxemia during attacks; usually hypocarbia and respiratory alkalosis present; normal or elevated P_{CO_2} worrisome as it may suggest severe respiratory muscle fatigue and airways obstruction. CXR not always necessary: may show hyperinflation, patchy infiltrates due to atelectasis behind plugged airways; important when complicating infection is a consideration.

Differential Diagnosis "All that wheezes is not asthma": CHF; chronic bronchitis/emphysema; upper airway obstruction due to foreign body, tumor, laryngeal edema; carcinoid tumors (usually associated with stridor, not wheezing); recurrent pulmonary emboli; eosinophilic pneumonia; vocal cord dysfunction; systemic vasculitis with pulmonary involvement.

℞ TREATMENT

Removal of inciting agent, if possible, is most successful treatment. Desensitization or immunotherapy, although popular, has limited scientific support and minimal clinical effectiveness.

Pharmacologic agents for treating asthma (Table 131-1) can be divided into two general categories: (1) drugs that inhibit smooth-muscle contraction, "quick relief medications" (β-adrenergic agonists, methylxanthines, and anticholinergics); and (2) agents that prevent or reverse inflammation, "long-term control medications" (glucocorticoids, leukotriene inhibitors and receptor antagonists, and mast cell–stabilizing agents). Pts who require quick relief medication more than two or three times weekly should start an anti-inflammatory agent.

1. *β-Adrenergic agonists*: Inhaled route provides most rapid effect and best therapeutic index; resorcinols (metaproterenol, terbutaline, fenoterol), saligenins (albuterol), and catecholamines (isoproterenol, isoetharine) may be given by nebulizer or metered-dose inhaler. Epinephrine, 0.3 mL of 1:1000 solution SC (for use in acute situations in absence of cardiac history). Catecholamines have rapid onset but are short acting (30–90 min). Salmeterol, a very long acting congener of albuterol, is not recommended for acute attacks but may be helpful for nocturnal or exercise-induced asthma. IV administra-

Table 131-1

Usual Dosages of Drugs for Long-Term-Control of Asthma

Medication	Dosage Form	Adult Dose
Inhaled glucocorticoids	*(See Table 236-2 in HPIM-16)*	
Systemic glucocorticoids	*(Applies to all three formulations)*	
Methylprednisolone	2-, 4-, 8-, 16-, 32-mg tablets	7.5–60 mg daily in a single dose in A.M. or qod as needed for control
Prednisolone	5-mg tablets, 5 mg/5 mL, 15 mg/5 mL	Short-course "burst" to achieve control: 40–60 mg/d as single or 2 divided doses for 3–10 days
Prednisone	1, 2.5, 5, 10, 20, 50 mg tablets; 5 mg/mL, 5 mg/5 mL	
Long-acting inhaled β_2-agonists	*(Should not be used for symptom relief or for exacerbations. Use with inhaled glucocorticoids.)*	
Salmeterol	MDI 21 μg/puff; DPI 50 μg/blister	2 puffs q 12 h / 1 blister q 12 h
Formoterol	DPI 12 μg/single-use capsule	1 capsule q 12 h
Combined medication		
Fluticasone/salmeterol	DPI 100, 250, or 500 μg/50 μg	1 inhalation bid; dose depends on severity of asthma
Cromolyn and nedocromil		
Cromolyn	MDI 1 mg/puff; Nebulizer 20 mg/ampule	2–4 puffs tid-qid / 1 ampule tid-qid
Nedocromil	MDI 1.75 mg/puff	2–4 puffs bid-qid
Leukotriene modifiers		
Montelukast	4- or 5-mg chewable tablet, 10-mg tablet	10 mg qhs
Zafirlukast	10- or 20-mg tablet	40 mg daily (20-mg tablet bid)
Zileuton	300- or 600-mg tablet	2400 mg daily (given tablets qid)
Methylxanthines	*(Serum monitoring is important to attain a serum concentration of 5–15 μg/mL at steady state).*	
Theophylline	Liquids, sustained-release tablets, and capsules	Starting dose 10 mg/kg per day up to 300 mg max; usual max, 800 mg/d

Note: MDI, metered-dose inhaler; DPI, daily permissible intake.

tion of β-adrenergic agents for severe asthma is not considered justified due to the risk of toxicity.

2. *Methylxanthines*: Theophylline and various salts; adjust dose to maintain blood level between 5 and 15 $\mu g/mL$; may be given PO or IV (as aminophylline). Theophylline clearance varies widely and is reduced with age, hepatic dysfunction, cardiac decompensation, cor pulmonale, febrile illness. Many drugs also alter theophylline clearance (decrease half-life: cigarettes, phenobarbital, phenytoin; increase half-life: erythromycin, allopurinol, cimetidine, propranolol).

For acute therapy, IV administration is used. In children and young-adult smokers, a loading dose of 6 mg/kg is given, followed by an infusion of 1.0 (mg/kg)/h for 12 h, after which the infusion is reduced to 0.8(mg/kg)/h. In other pts not on theophylline, the loading dose remains the same, but the infusion rate is reduced to 0.1–0.5 (mg/kg)/h. In pts already taking theophylline, the loading dose is withheld or reduced. Theophylline compounds have lost favor in asthma therapy due to narrow toxic-therapeutic margin and add little to management when optimal dosing of β-adrenergic agents has been implemented.

3. *Anticholinergics*: Aerosolized atropine and related compounds, such as ipratropium, a nonabsorbable quaternary ammonium. May enhance the bronchodilation achieved by sympathomimetics but is slow acting (60–90 min to peak bronchodilation). Ipratropium may be given by metered-dose inhaler, 2 puffs up to every 6 h. Expectorants and mucolytic agents add little to the management of acute or chronic asthma.

4. *Glucocorticoids*: Systemic or oral administration are most beneficial for severe or refractory asthma. For hospitalized patients, methylprednisolone 120–180 mg q6h IV is recommended. Prednisone 60 mg q6h orally is recommended. Lower doses (prednisolone 30-40 mg qd) may be equally effective with fewer side effects. Steroids in acute asthma require ≥ 6 h to have an effect.

For exacerbations of asthma in the outpatient setting, prednisone 40–60 mg PO daily, followed by tapering schedule of 50% reduction every 3–5 days with discontinuation after 10–12 days, after transition to inhaled steroids.

Inhaled glucocorticoid preparations are important adjuncts to chronic therapy but not useful in acute attacks. Effects of inhaled steroids are dose-dependent. Inhaled steroids are a mainstay of outpatient management and should be started in any pt not easily controlled with occasional use of inhaled adrenergic agents.

Agents available include beclamethasone, budesonide, flunisolide, fluticasone proprinate, and triamcinolone acetonide. Dosing should be adjusted to disease activity, with frequent attempts to taper to low maintenance (1–2 puffs, 1–2 times/day). In addition to local symptoms (dysphonia, thrush), systemic effects may occur (e.g., adrenal suppression, cataracts, bone loss).

Combination of an inhaled steroid (fluticasone) and β_2 agonist (salmeterol) is gaining widespread use (Table 131-1).

5. *Cromolyn sodium and nedocromil sodium*: Not bronchodilators; useful in chronic therapy for prevention, not useful during acute attacks; administered as metered-dose inhaler or nebulized powder, 2 puffs daily. A trial of 4–6 weeks is often necessary to determine effectiveness in chronic asthma. Because the drugs may block acute bronchoconstriction when administered 15–20 min before exposure to antigens, chemicals, or exercise, they may be of use in selected pts who have predictable attacks of extrinsic asthma.

7. *Leukotriene modifiers*: The 5-lipoxygenase inhibitor, zileuton, and the LTD_4 receptor antagonists, zafirlukast and monteleukast, are recent additions to anti-inflammatory therapy of asthma. The LTD_4 receptor antagonists are long acting, permitting qd or bid dosing.

Effective in fewer than one-half of pts. If no improvement after 1 month, should be discontinued. Modest bronchodilators with action against exercise-induced asthma. May reduce nocturnal symptoms.

Framework for Management

Emergencies Aerosolized β_2 agonists are the primary therapy of acute episodes of asthma. Give every 20 min for 3 doses, then every 2 h until attack subsides. Aminophylline may speed resolution after first hour in 5–10% of pts. Paradoxical pulse, accessory muscle use, and marked hyperinflation indicate severe disease and mandate ABG measurement and monitoring of PEFR or FEV_1. PEFR $\geq$ 20% predicted on presentation with failure to double after 60 min of treatment suggests addition of steroid therapy. Failure of PEFR to improve to $\geq$ 70% of baseline with emergency treatment suggests need for hospitalization, with final decision made on individual factors (symptoms, past history, etc.). PEFR $\geq$ 40% after emergency treatment mandates admission.

Chronic Treatment First-line therapy for intermittent asthma consists of β_2 agonists. Persistence of symptoms should prompt addition of an anti-inflammatory agent (glucocorticoids or a mast cell–stabilizing agent). Medication adjustments should be based on objective measurement of lung function (PEFR, FEV_1), and pts should monitor PEFR regularly.

HYPERSENSITIVITY PNEUMONITIS

DEFINITION Hypersensitivity pneumonitis (HP), or extrinsic allergic alveolitis, is an immunologically mediated inflammation of lung parenchyma involving alveolar walls and terminal airways secondary to repeated inhalation of a variety of organic dusts by a susceptible host.

ETIOLOGY A number of inhaled substances have been implicated (Table 237-1, p. 1517, in HPIM-16). These *substances* are usually organic antigens, particularly thermophilic actinomycetes, but may include inorganic compounds such as isocyanates.

CLINICAL MANIFESTATIONS Symptoms may be acute, subacute, or chronic depending on the frequency and intensity of exposure to the causative agent; in acute form, cough, fever, chills, dyspnea appear 6–8 h after exposure to antigen; in subacute and chronic forms, temporal relationship to antigenic exposure may be lost, and insidiously increasing dyspnea may be predominant symptom.

DIAGNOSIS *History* Occupational history and history of possible exposures and relationship to symptoms are very important.

Physical Exam Nonspecific; may reveal rales in lung fields, cyanosis in advanced cases.

Laboratory Serum precipitins to offending antigen may be present but are not specific. After acute exposure to antigen, neutrophilia and lymphopenia are common, as are increased nonspecific tests of inflammation (C-reactive protein, rheumatoid factor, serum immunoglobulins).

CXR: nonspecific changes in interstitial structures; pleural changes or hilar adenopathy rare. High-resolution chest CT may show characteristic constellation of findings: (1) global lung involvement with ↑ lung density, (2) prominence of medium-sized bronchial walls, (3) patchy airspace consolidation, and (4) absence of lymphadenopathy. *PFTs and ABGs*: restrictive pattern possibly associated with airway obstruction; diffusing capacity decreased; hypoxemia at rest or with exercise. Bronchoalveolar lavage may show increased lymphocytes of suppressor-cytotoxic phenotype. Lung biopsy may be necessary in some pts who do not have sufficient other criteria; transbronchial biopsy may suffice, but video-assisted thoracoscopic lung biopsy is frequently necessary.

DIFFERENTIAL DIAGNOSIS Other interstitial lung diseases, including sarcoidosis, idiopathic pulmonary fibrosis, lung disease associated with collagen-vascular diseases, drug-induced lung disease; eosinophilic pneumonia; allergic bronchopulmonary aspergillosis; silo-fillers' disease; "pulmonary mycotoxicosis" or "atypical" farmer's lung; infection.

 TREATMENT

Avoidance of offending antigen is essential. Chronic form may be partially irreversible at the time of diagnosis. Prednisone 1(mg/kg)/d for 7–14 days, followed by tapering schedule over 2–4 weeks to lowest possible dose. Subacute form may have severe physiologic impairment and may progress for several days in hospital. Prednisone therapy is used at the same initial dose, tapered after 7–14 days over 5–6 weeks at a rate dictated by Sx. Pts with acute form usually recover without glucocorticoids, with withdrawal of the offending agent.

For a more detailed discussion, see McFadden ER, Jr: Asthma, Chap. 236, p. 1508; and Kline JN, Hunninghake GW: Hypersensitivity Pneumonitis and Pulmonary Infiltrates with Eosinophilia, Chap. 237, p. 1516, in HPIM-16.

132

ENVIRONMENTAL LUNG DISEASES

_____ *Approach to the Patient* _____

Ask about workplace and work history in detail: Specific contaminants? Availability and use of protective devices? Ventilation? Do co-workers have similar complaints? Ask about every job; short-term exposures may be significant. CXR is very valuable but may over- or underestimate functional impact of pneumoconioses. PFTs may both quantify impairment and suggest the nature of exposure.

An individual's dose of an environmental agent is influenced by intensity as well as by physiologic factors (ventilation rate and depth).

OCCUPATIONAL EXPOSURES AND PULMONARY DISEASE

INORGANIC DUSTS *Asbestosis* Exposures may occur in mining, milling, and manufacture of asbestos products; construction trades (pipefitting, boilermaking); and manufacture of safety garments, filler for plastic material, and friction materials (brake and clutch linings). Major health effects of asbestos include pulmonary fibrosis (asbestosis) and cancers of the respiratory tract, pleura, and peritoneum.

Asbestosis is a diffuse interstitial fibrosing disease of the lung that is directly related to intensity and duration of exposure, usually requiring ≥10 years of moderate to severe exposure. PFTs show a restrictive pattern. CXR reveals irregular or linear opacities, greatest in lower lung fields. High-resolution CT may show distinct changes of subpleural curvilinear line 5–10 cm in length. *Pleural plaques* indicate past exposure. Excess frequency of *lung cancer* occurs 15 to 20 years after first asbestos exposure. Smoking substantially increases risk of lung cancer after asbestos exposure but does not alter risk of *mesotheliomas*, which peaks 30 to 50 years after (an often brief) initial exposure.

Silicosis Exposure to free silica (crystalline quartz) occurs in mining, stone cutting, abrasive industries, blasting, quarrying. Short-term, high-intensity exposures (as brief as 10 months) may produce acute silicosis—rapidly fatal pulmonary fibrosis with radiographic picture of profuse miliary infiltration or consolidation. Longer-term, less-intense exposures are associated with upper lobe fibrosis and hilar adenopathy ≥15 years after exposure. Fibrosis is nodular and may lead to pulmonary restriction and airflow obstruction. Pts with silicosis are at higher than normal risk for tuberculosis, and pts with chronic silicosis and a positive PPD warrant antituberculous treatment.

Coal Worker's Pneumoconiosis (CWP) Symptoms of simple CWP are additive to the effects of cigarette smoking on chronic bronchitis and obstructive lung disease. X-ray signs of simple CWP are small, irregular opacities (reticular pattern) that may progress to small, rounded opacities (nodular pattern). Complicated CWP is indicated by roentgenographic appearance of nodules >1 cm in diameter in upper lung fields; DL_{CO} is reduced.

Berylliosis Beryllium exposure may produce acute pneumonitis or chronic interstitial pneumonitis. Histology is indistinguishable from sarcoidosis (noncaseating granulomas).

ORGANIC DUSTS ***Cotton Dust (Byssinosis)*** Exposures occur in production of yarns for cotton, linen, and rope making. (Flax, hemp, and jute produce a similar syndrome.) Chest tightness occurs typically on first day of work week. In 10–25% of workers, disease may be progressive with chest tightness persisting throughout the work week. After 10 years, recurrent symptoms are associated with irreversible airflow obstruction. Therapy includes bronchodilators, antihistamines, and elimination of exposure.

Grain Dust Farmers and grain elevator operators are at risk. Symptoms are those of cigarette smokers—cough, mucus production, wheezing, and airflow obstruction.

Farmer's Lung Persons exposed to moldy hay with spores of thermophilic actinomycetes may develop a hypersensitivity pneumonitis. Acute farmer's lung causes fever, chills, malaise, cough, and dyspnea 4–8 h after exposure. Chronic low-intensity exposure causes interstitial fibrosis.

TOXIC CHEMICALS Many toxic chemicals can affect the lung in the form of vapor and gases.

Smoke inhalation kills more fire victims than does thermal injury. Severe cases may develop pulmonary edema. CO poisoning causing O_2 desaturation may be fatal. Early endoscopy may distinguish thermal upper airway injury from diffuse lower airway damage due to toxic constituents of inhaled smoke.

Agents used in the manufacture of synthetic materials may produce sensitizaton to isocyanates, aromatic amines, and aldehydes. Repeated exposure causes some workers to develop productive cough, asthma, or low-grade fever and malaise.

Fluorocarbons, transmitted from a worker's hands to cigarettes, may be volatilized. The inhaled agent causes fever, chills, malaise, and sometimes wheezing. Occurring in plastic workers, the syndrome is termed *polymer fume fever*.

℞ TREATMENT

Treatment of environmental lung diseases almost invariably involves avoidance of toxic substance. Inorganic dust inhalation produces fibrosis without inflammation, unresponsive to pharmacologic treatment. Acute organic dust exposures may respond to glucocorticoids.

GENERAL ENVIRONMENTAL EXPOSURES

Air Pollution Difficult to relate specific health effects to any single pollutant. Symptoms and diseases of air pollution are also the nononcogenic conditions associated with cigarette smoking (respiratory infections, airway irritation).

Passive Cigarette Smoking Increased respiratory illness and reduced lung function have been found in children of smoking parents. Meta analyses suggest ~25% in lung cancer, cardiac and respiratory disease with household exposure.

Radon Risk factor for lung cancer, exacerbated by cigarette smoke.

PRINCIPLES OF MANAGEMENT

With many environmental agents, lung disease occurs years after exposure. If exposure continues, inciting agent must be eliminated, usually by removing pt from workplace. Pulmonary fibrosis (e.g., asbestosis, CWP) is not responsive to glucocorticoids. Therapy of occupational asthma follows usual guidelines (Chap. 131). Lung cancer screening has not yet proven effective, even in high-risk occupations.

For a more detailed discussion, see Speizer FE: Environmental Lung Diseases, Chap. 238, p. 1521, in HPIM-16.

133

CHRONIC BRONCHITIS, EMPHYSEMA, AND ACUTE OR CHRONIC RESPIRATORY FAILURE

Natural History

Chronic obstructive pulmonary disease (COPD) is a progressive disorder even when contributing factors are eliminated and aggressive therapy is instituted. Progression is inevitable, since loss of elastic tissue is a normal part of the aging process. In normal individuals, forced expiratory volume in 1 s (FEV_1) reaches lifetime peak around 25 years and declines on average ~35 mL/year thereafter. Annual loss among susceptible individuals with COPD is 50–100 mL. Greater rates of decline are associated with mucus hypersecretion (men) and with airway hyperreactivity.

Symptoms occur only in association with moderate or severe COPD. Typically, dyspnea occurs when FEV_1 falls below ~40% of predicted. Hypercarbia is most common after FEV_1 has fallen to <25% of predicted. Some pts whose symptoms are out of proportion to the decrease in FEV_1 have marked reductions in diffusing capacity for carbon monoxide.

Clinical Manifestations

HISTORY   Pts with COPD usually have exposure to tobacco of ≥20 pack years. Onset is typically in the fifth decade or later. Early age of onset should precipitate screening for α_1 antitrypsin deficiency and other inherited obstructive diseases such as cystic fibrosis, particularly if there is a minimal smoking history. Exertional dyspnea and productive cough are typical early symptoms. Functional limitation may correlate poorly with reduction in FEV_1. Sputum volume is usually small; production of >60 mL/d should prompt investigation for bronchiectasis. Weight loss is common in advanced disease. Hypoxemia and hypercarbia may result in fluid retention, morning headaches, sleep disruption, erythrocytosis, and cyanosis.

Exacerbations are more frequent as disease progresses and are most often triggered by respiratory infections, often with a bacterial component. They may also be precipitated by left ventricular failure, cardiac arrhythmia, pneumothorax, pneumonia, and pulmonary thromboembolism.

PHYSICAL FINDINGS   These correlate poorly with disease severity. Exam may be normal early. As disease progresses, signs of hyperinflation become more prominent. Mid-inspiratory crackles may reflect disease of moderate-size airways. Pursed-lip breathing may reduce dyspnea and dynamic hyperinflation. Wheezing is an inconstant finding and does not predict degree of obstruction or response to therapy.

RADIOGRAPHIC FINDINGS   Plain CXR may show hyperinflation, emphysema, and pulmonary hypertension. Local radiolucencies (>1 cm) may indicate bullae. CT scan has greater sensitivity for emphysema but is not necessary for diagnosis.

PULMONARY FUNCTION TESTS   Objective documentation of airflow obstruction is essential for diagnosis of COPD. Forced vital capacity (FVC) is typically decreased, but FEV_1 is decreased more so that the ratio of FEV_1/FVC is reduced. Exhalation may be incomplete even after a 10-s forced attempt. The American Thoracic Society grades COPD by FEV_1: stage I, mild disease, $FEV_1 \geq 50\%$ predicted; stage II, moderate disease, FEV_1 35–49% predicted; stage III, severe disease, $FEV_1 < 35\%$ predicted. Reversibility of obstruction is determined by a trial of inhaled bronchodilators.

 TREATMENT

    Smoking Cessation   Elimination of tobacco has been convincingly shown to prolong survival in patients with COPD. Although lost lung function is not regained, the rate of decline in FEV_1 reverts rapidly to that of nonsmokers. Use of nicotine replacement therapy (patch, gum, inhaler) can increase rates of cessation in motivated pts. Oral bupropion (150 mg bid) also produces significant benefit. Pharmacologic therapy should be used combined with traditional supportive therapies.

Bronchodilators (Table 133-1)   These do not influence longevity in pts with COPD but may significantly reduce symptoms. Short- and long-acting β-adrenergic agonists, anticholinergics, and theophylline derivatives may all be used. Although oral medications are associated with greater rates of adherence, inhaled medications generally have fewer side effects.

Pts with mild disease can usually be managed with an inhaled short-acting β agonist such as albuterol. Anticholinergic therapy, e.g., inhaled ipatroprium, may be added to more symptomatic pts with moderate disease. Long-acting β agents, e.g., inhaled salmeterol, should be added in pts with severe disease. The narrow toxic-therapeutic ratio of theophylline compounds limits their use.

Glucocorticoids   Long-term parenteral steroid therapy is not recommended in pts with COPD due to their unfavorable risk-benefit ratio. Inhaled steroids do not reduce the rate of decline of lung function in COPD pts, but some evidence suggests they may reduce the frequency of exacerbations by 25–30%. A trial of inhaled steroids should be undertaken in pts with 2 or more exacerbations per year.

Oxygen   Long-term domicilary O_2 therapy has been shown to reduce symptoms and improve survival in pts who are chronically hypoxemic, if they have stopped smoking. Documentation of the need for O_2 requires a measurement of Pa_{O_2} or oxygen saturation (Sa_{O_2}) after a period of stability. Pts with a $Pa_{O_2} \leq 55$ mmHg or $Sa_{O_2} \leq 88\%$ should receive O_2 to raise the $Sa_{O_2} \geq 90\%$. O_2 is also indicated for pts with Pa_{O_2} of 56–59 mmHg or $Sa_{O_2} \leq 89\%$ if associated with signs and symptoms of pulmonary hypertension or cor pulmonale. O_2 may also be prescribed for selected pts who desaturate with exercise or during sleep.

Transplantation   Lung transplantation should be considered for pts with severe COPD whose FEV_1 is <25% predicted despite maximal therapy, particularly if associated with hypoxemia and cor pulmonale.

Lung Volume Reduction Surgery   Surgery to decrease lung volume has both symptom and mortality benefit in highly selected pts with upper lobe–predominant emphysema and a low post-rehabilitation exercise capacity predicting a successful outcome.

Mild Exacerbations

These may be managed with bronchodilators, antibiotics, and short courses of systemic glucocorticoids. Short-acting β-adrenergic agonists such as albuterol may be used up to every 1–2 h by metered dose inhaler (MDI). Anticholinergics such as ipatroprium by MDI should not be used more frequently than every 4–6 h, however. With increased sputum volume or change in character, antibiotic therapy should be administered. Trimethoprim-sulfa-

Table 133-1

Recommended Bronchodilator Therapy for Chronic Obstructive Pulmonary Disease

Stage	FEV_1, % Predicted	Treatment
I	> 50	β_2-Agonist prn
II	35–49	Combined anticholinergic and β_2-agonist
III	<35	Above plus long-acting β_2-agonist and/or sustained release theophylline
		Consider oral glucocorticoid trial

Source: B Celli et al: Am J Respir Crit Care Med 152: S77, 1995; M Pearson et al: Thorax 52(Suppl5):S1, 1997.

methoxazole, doxycycline, and amoxicillin are all acceptable choices. Evidence for effectiveness of systemic glucocorticoids in outpatient management of exacerbations is lacking, but usual practice is to administer 20–40 mg of prednisone daily for 7–10 days.

Acute Respiratory Failure

Diagnosis is made on the basis of decrease in Pa_{O_2} by 10–15 mmHg from baseline or increase in Pa_{CO_2} associated with a pH ≤ 7.30.

 TREATMENT

Precipitating factors should be sought, especially the presence of left ventricular failure. Clinical signs of CHF are often difficult to identify, so empirical therapy with a diuretic (furosemide 10–60 mg IV) is appropriate if peripheral edema is present.

Bronchodilators Administer short-acting β-adrenergic agonists by inhalation (e.g., albuterol q1–2h; may be administered as frequently as q20min initially). Because absorption is unpredictable when pts are in distress, dosing should be dictated by side effects. Addition of anticholinergics is likely of benefit (ipatroprium q4–6h).

Glucocorticoids Evidence is convincing that systemic steroids may hasten resolution of symptoms and reduces relapses and subsequent exacerbations for 6 months. Dosing is not well worked out, but 30–40 mg of prednisolone daily (or IV equivalent) is standard, with a total course of 10–14 days.

Oxygen Supplemental O_2 should be administered to maintain Sa_{O_2} ≥ 90%. Delivery systems include nasal prongs, 1–2 L/min, or 24% Venturi mask.

Ventilatory Support Numerous studies suggest noninvasive mask ventilation can improve outcomes in acute exacerbations with respiratory failure (Pa_{CO_2} > 45 mmHg). Pts with marked respiratory distress (respiratory rate > 30 breaths/min) should have a trial of mask ventilation. Success is indicated by a reduction in respiratory rate to <25 breaths/min after 30–60 min. Progressive hypercarbia, refractory hypoxemia, or alteration in mental status that compromises ability to comply with therapy may necessitate endotracheal intubation.

For a more detailed discussion, see Reilly JJ Jr., Silverman EK, Shapiro SD: Chronic Obstructive Pulmonary Disease, Chap. 242, p. 1547, in HPIM-16; and Lilly C, Ingenito EP, Shapiro S: Respiratory Failure, Chap. 250, p. 1588, in HPIM-16.

134

PNEUMONIA AND LUNG ABSCESS

DEFINITIONS

Pneumonia is an infection of the alveoli, distal airways, and interstitium of the lungs.

- *Lobar pneumonia*: involvement of an entire lung lobe
- *Bronchopneumonia*: patchy consolidation in one or several lobes, usually in dependent lower or posterior portions centered around bronchi and bronchioles
- *Interstitial pneumonia*: inflammation of the interstitium, including the alveolar walls and connective tissue around the bronchovascular tree
- *Miliary pneumonia*: numerous discrete lesions due to hematogenous spread

ROUTES OF INFECTION

- *Microaspiration* of oropharyngeal secretions colonized with pathogenic microorganisms (e.g., *Streptococcus pneumoniae*, *Haemophilus influenzae*) is the most common route.
- *Gross aspiration* occurs in pts with CNS disorders that affect swallowing (e.g., stroke or seizures), in those with impaired consciousness (e.g., alcoholic pts or IV drug users), or during anesthesia or intubation. Pathogens include anaerobic organisms and gram-negative bacilli.
- *Aerosolization* (e.g., of *Mycobacterium tuberculosis*, *Legionella*)
- *Hematogenous route* (e.g., seeding of the lungs by *Staphylococcus aureus* during endocarditis)
- *Contiguous spread* from another site

COMMUNITY-ACQUIRED PNEUMONIA (CAP)

EPIDEMIOLOGY AND ETIOLOGY CAP affects ~4 million adults each year in the United States. Pneumonia is more common among pts with severe underlying illness, those with defects in phagocytosis or ciliary function, and those with anatomical defects such as bronchiectasis. Many factors influence the types of pathogens that should be considered in identifying the etiologic agent of pneumonia: alcoholism, asthma, asplenia, immunosuppression, age >70 years, travel history, exposure to pets, exposure to sick contacts, occupation, age, presence or absence of teeth, season of the year, geographic location, smoking status, and HIV status. Most cases of pneumonia are caused by a few common respiratory pathogens, including *S. pneumoniae* (which causes ~50% of cases requiring hospital admission), *H. influenzae*, *S. aureus*, *Mycoplasma pneumoniae*, *Chlamydia pneumoniae*, *Moraxella catarrhalis*, *Legionella* spp., aerobic gram-negative bacteria, influenza viruses, adenoviruses, and respiratory syncytial virus.

CLINICAL FEATURES

- Most typical symptoms: fever, cough (either nonproductive or productive of purulent sputum), pleuritic chest pain, chills or rigors, and dyspnea
- Frequent symptoms: headache, nausea, vomiting, diarrhea, fatigue, and confusion
- Physical examination: tachypnea, dullness to percussion, increased tactile and vocal fremitus, egophony, whispering pectoriloquy, crackles, and pleural friction rub. A respiratory rate of >30/min is the most useful sign of severe pneumonia in a person without underlying lung disease.

Table 134-1

Initial Empirical Antibiotic Therapy for Community-Acquired Pneumonia

Treatment Setting; Patient's Condition	Regimen[a]
Outpatient; no cardiopulmonary disease, no risk factors for DRSP infection[b]	Macrolide (e.g., clarithromycin 500 mg bid PO × 10 days; or azithromycin 500 mg PO once, then 250 mg/d × 4 days) *or* Doxycycline 100 mg bid PO × 10 days
Outpatient; cardiopulmonary disease and/or (1) risk factors for DRSP infection or (2) high DRSP prevalence in community	Quinolone with enhanced activity against *Streptococcus pneumoniae*—e.g., levofloxacin 500 mg/d PO (or, with $C_{cr} < 50$ mL/min, 250 mg/d), moxifloxacin 400 mg/d PO, or gatifloxacin 400 mg/d PO *or* β-Lactam (cefpodoxime 200 mg bid, cefuroxime axetil 750 mg tid, or amoxicillin 1000 mg tid, PO; amoxicillin/clavulanic acid 875/175 mg tid) plus macrolide or doxycycline *or* Telithromycin 800 mg q24h × 10 days
Hospital ward	Cefuroxime 750 mg q8h IV or ceftriaxone 1 g/d IV or cefotaxime 2 g q6h IV or ampicillin/sulbactam 1.5–3 g q6h IV *plus* Azithromycin 1 g/d IV followed by 500 mg/d IV *or* Quinolone with enhanced activity against *S. pneumoniae* (see above)[c]
Intensive care unit; no risk factors for *Pseudomonas aeruginosa* infection	Azithromycin 1 g IV, then start 500 mg IV 24 h later *plus* Ceftriaxone 1 g q12h IV *or* Cefotaxime 2 g q6h IV *or* Quinolone IV
Intensive care unit; risk factors for *P. aeruginosa*[b]	Imipenem (or meropenem) 500 mg q6h IV *or* Piperacillin/tazobactam 3.375 g q6h IV *plus* Ciprofloxacin 750 mg q8h IV
Nursing home[d]	Amoxicillin/clavulanic acid 875/125 mg tid PO *plus* Macrolide PO (see above) *or* Quinolone PO with enhanced activity against *S. pneumoniae* (see above) *or* Ceftriaxone 500–1000 mg/d IM or cefotaxime 500 mg IM q12h *plus* Macrolide (see above)

(continued)

Table 134-1 *(Continued)*

Initial Empirical Antibiotic Therapy for Community-Acquired Pneumonia

Treatment Setting; Patient's Condition	Regimen[a]
Aspiration pneumonitis (presumed to be due to effects of gastric acid or other irritants)	Wait 24 h; if symptoms persist, give antibiotic therapy delineated below for aspiration pneumonia.
Aspiration pneumonia; poor dental hygiene or putrid sputum, alcoholism (anaerobic infection suspected)	Metronidazole 500 mg q12h PO[e] *or* Piperacillin/tazobactam 3.375 g q6h IV *or* Imipenem 500 mg q6h IV *plus* One of the following: levofloxacin 500 mg/d IV or PO, moxifloxacin 400 mg/d PO, gatifloxacin 400 mg/d IV or PO, ceftriaxone, or cefotaxime
Aspiration pneumonia; community-acquired	Levofloxacin, moxifloxacin, gatifloxacin, ceftriaxone, or cefotaxime (see above)
Concomitant meningitis (suspected pneumococcal)	Vancomycin 1 g q12h IV *plus* Ceftriaxone 2 g q12h IV

[a] The optimal duration of therapy for CAP is unknown. With the exception of azithromycin (which has a long half-life), a 7- to 10-day course is usually recommended. Pneumonia due to *Legionella* spp., *P. aeruginosa*, or Enterobacteriaceae usually requires therapy of longer duration (often up to 21 days).

[b] Risk factors: (1) For penicillin-resistant *S. pneumoniae*: Previous use (within 3 months) of β-lactam antibiotics, alcoholism, age <5 years or >65 years, and (in some areas) residence in a nursing home. (2) For macrolide-resistant *S. pneumoniae*: Age <5 years or nosocomial acquisition of infection. (3) For quinolone-resistant *S. pneumoniae*: Older age, nursing home residence, chronic obstructive pulmonary disease, previous exposure to quinolones (especially ciprofloxacin in patients with chronic obstructive pulmonary disease) in the past 3 months, multiple hospitalizations, and β-lactam use. (4) For *P. aeruginosa*: Bronchiectasis, malnutrition, treatment with >10 mg of prednisone/d, previously undiagnosed HIV infection, and broad-spectrum antibiotic therapy for >7 days in the past month.

[c] Some authorities suggest that a β-lactam be added if a quinolone is chosen as empirical therapy until it is clear that quinolone-resistant pneumococci are not involved.

[d] For nursing home residents transferred to the hospital for treatment, see appropriate hospital/intensive care unit recommendations.

[e] Clindamycin could be used, but, because of the increased rate of *Clostridium difficile*–associated diarrhea associated with this drug, metronidazole is preferred.

Note: DRSP, drug-resistant *S. pneumoniae*.

- Mortality is highest for *Pseudomonas aeruginosa* pneumonia (>50%); death rates are next highest for *Klebsiella* spp., *Escherichia coli*, *S. aureus*, *S. pneumoniae* serotype 3, and group A *Streptococcus*.

COMPLICATIONS

- Pleural effusion develops in 40% of pts with pneumonia. If the size is >1 cm on lateral decubitus CXR, the fluid should be sampled. If the fluid has a pH < 7, a glucose level < 2.2 mmol/L, and a lactate dehydrogenase content > 1000 U and yields a positive result on Gram's stain or culture, then a chest tube should be placed and intrapleural lytic agents injected. Thoracotomy and decortication may be needed.
- *Lung abscess* is defined as localized parenchymal destruction that is manifest on CXR as a cavity with an air-fluid level. Most abscesses are aspiration-as-

Table 134-2

Empirical Antibiotic Therapy for Hospital-Acquired Pneumonia (HAP)

Treatment Setting; Patient's Condition	Risk Factor/Usual Pathogen(s)	Regimen
Hospital ward; mild to moderate HAP, no risk factors for specific pathogens	—	Second-generation cephalosporin (cefuroxime 750 mg q8h IV) *or* Nonpseudomonal third-generation cephalosporin (ceftriaxone 1 g/d IV) *or* β-Lactam/β-lactamase inhibitor combination (piperacillin/tazobactam 3.375 g q6h IV) *or* Penicillin allergy: Respiratory quinolone (levofloxacin 500 mg/d IV, moxifloxacin 400 mg/d IV, or gatifloxacin 400 mg/d IV) *or* Clindamycin plus aztreonam
Hospital ward; mild to moderate HAP with specific risk factors	—	Treat for usual pathogens (enteric gram-negative bacilli, *Staphylococcus aureus*, *Streptococcus pneumoniae*, *Haemophilus influenzae*) with cefuroxime, ceftriaxone, or piperacillin/tazobactam (see above) *plus* Treat for other pathogens related to risk factors (see below)
	Witnessed aspiration, recent abdominal surgery/anaerobes	Standard treatment (see above) *plus* Clindamycin 450–900 mg q8h IV *or* β-Lactam/β-lactamase inhibitor combination (piperacillin/tazobactam 3.375 g q6h IV)
	Coma, head trauma, diabetes mellitus, renal failure/*S. aureus*, risk for MRSA	Standard treatment (see above) *plus* Vancomycin 1 g q12h IV

682

Clinical Setting	Usual Pathogen(s)	Treatment
	High-dose glucocorticoids/*Legionella*	Standard treatment (see above) *plus* Macrolide (azithromycin 500 mg/d IV) *or* Respiratory quinolone (see above)
Intensive care unit; severe HAP, early onset, no specific risk factors	—	Second-generation cephalosporin, nonpseudomonal third-generation cephalosporin, or β-lactam/β-lactamase inhibitor combination (see above) Penicillin allergy: Respiratory quinolone (see above)
Intensive care unit; severe HAP, late onset or specific risk factors	—	Treat for usual pathogens (enteric gram-negative bacilli; *S. aureus, S. pneumoniae, H. influenzae*) with cefuroxime, ceftriaxone, or piperacillin/tazobactam (see above) *plus* Treat for other pathogens related to risk factors (see below)
	Malnutrition, structural lung disease, glucocorticoid therapy/*Pseudomonas aeruginosa*; neurosurgery, head trauma, ARDS, aspiration/*Acinetobacter* spp.	Standard treatment (see above) *plus* Aminoglycoside or ciprofloxacin 500 mg q12h IV plus one of the following: antipseudomonal penicillin (piperacillin 4 g q6h IV or piperacillin/tazobactam 4.5 g q6h IV) or cefepime 1–2 g q12h IV or imipenem (or meropenem) 500 mg q8h IV
	Prior antibiotic therapy (especially with quinolones or macrolides), previous hospitalization, enteral feeding/MRSA	Standard treatment (see above) *plus* Vancomycin 1 g q12h IV

Note: ARDS, adult respiratory distress syndrome; MRSA, methicillin-resistant *S. aureus*.

sociated and are due to aerobic and anaerobic bacteria. Presentation is usually indolent, with weight loss, malaise, night sweats, fever, and productive cough. Anaerobic lung abscesses are associated with foul-smelling and foul-tasting sputum. Spontaneous drainage of the abscess into the bronchi is accompanied by copious amounts of sputum. Treatment is prolonged, usually lasting 6–8 weeks. Medical treatment alone is successful in 90% of pts.

SPECIAL CONSIDERATIONS

- CAP in long-term care facilities: *S. aureus*, aerobic gram-negative bacilli, *S. pneumoniae*, and *M. tuberculosis* are common etiologic agents.
- *Severe CAP* is defined as CAP requiring ICU admission. The most common etiologic agents, ranked in order, include *S. pneumoniae*, *S. aureus*, viruses, gram-negative bacilli, *Legionella* spp., *M. pneumoniae*, *Pneumocystis*, and *H. influenzae*.
- Aspiration occurs in the posterior segments of the upper lobes and the superior segments of the lower lobes. Aspiration of gastric contents causes chemical pneumonitis that can be severe. Aspiration of oropharyngeal flora causes bacterial pneumonia. In the elderly, common causes of aspiration pneumonia are Enterobacteriaceae, *S. aureus*, *S. pneumoniae*, and *H. influenzae*.

DIAGNOSIS

- Radiographic studies: CXR is usually adequate for diagnosis, but CT of the chest may be required in some pts. Some patterns suggest an etiology (e.g., cavitation suggests tuberculosis, pneumatoceles suggest *S. aureus*).
- Blood cultures should precede antibiotic therapy and are positive in 6–20% of cases, most commonly yielding *S. pneumoniae* (~60%), *S. aureus*, or *E. coli*.
- Sputum stains and culture: The presence of >25 WBCs and <10 squamous epithelial cells per high-power field suggests that a sample is appropriate for culture; a single, predominant organism on Gram's stain suggests the etiology. Other stains should be used as indicated (e.g., acid-fast stains for *M. tuberculosis*, special stains for fungi, or monoclonal antibody stains for *Pneumocystis*).
- Urine antigen tests for *S. pneumoniae* and *Legionella pneumophila* type 1 can be helpful.
- Serology: The presence of IgM or a fourfold rise in antibody titer can assist in the diagnosis of pneumonia due to some pathogens (e.g., *M. pneumoniae*, *C. pneumoniae*, *Chlamydia psittaci*, *Legionella* spp., *Coxiella burnetii*, adenovirus, parainfluenza viruses, and influenza A virus).

℞ TREATMENT

Site of Care In general, older adults (especially nursing home residents) should be hospitalized for pneumonia treatment. Adults with any of the following should also be hospitalized for this purpose: respiratory rate > 28/min, systolic blood pressure < 90 mmHg or 30 mmHg below baseline, altered mental status, hypoxemia, unstable comorbid illness, multilobar pneumonia, or pleural effusion that is >1 cm on lateral decubitus CXR and has the characteristics of a complicated parapneumonic effusion on pleural fluid analysis. If a pt is not admitted, the physician should call within 48 h to check on clinical status and treatment response.

Antibiotic Therapy See Table 134-1. A retrospective review of pts >65 years of age suggests that treatment with a macrolide plus a second-generation or nonpseudomonal third-generation cephalosporin lowers the mortality rate, as does the use of a fluoroquinolone alone. Addition of an aminoglycoside is associated with an increased mortality rate. Other factors that lower the mortality rate include antibiotic administration within 8 h of arrival in the emergency room and use of two or more agents in bacteremic pneumococcal pneumonia. IV antibiotics can be switched to oral agents when the WBC count is returning toward normal, two temperature readings 16 h apart are normal, and the pt is clinically improved.

HOSPITAL-ACQUIRED (NOSOCOMIAL) PNEUMONIA (HAP)

HAP is defined as pneumonia developing at least 48 h after hospital admission. Approximately 300,000 cases of HAP occur each year in the United States. HAP occurs most frequently in ICU pts on mechanical ventilation. It carries the highest morbidity and mortality rates of all nosocomial infections, adds 7–9 days to hospital stays, and increases costs by $2 billion annually. Crude mortality rates range from 30 to 70% and are highest in bacteremic pneumonia, in pneumonia due to high-risk pathogens (e.g., *P. aeruginosa*), and in ICU pts. HAP is defined as a new or progressive infiltrate on CXR plus at least two of the following: fever of >37.8°C, leukocytosis with >10,000 WBCs/μL, and production of purulent sputum. Dyspnea, hypoxemia, and pleuritic chest pain may occur. Bronchoscopic samples are often needed to determine the etiology. See Table 134-2 for suggested antibiotic treatment regimens. See Chap. 92 for further discussion.

For a more detailed discussion, see Marrie TJ et al: Pneumonia, Chap. 239, p. 1528, in HPIM-16.

135

PULMONARY THROMBOEMBOLISM

PULMONARY EMBOLISM (PE) (See Fig. 135-1)

NATURAL HISTORY Immediate result is obstruction of pulmonary blood flow to the distal lung. Respiratory consequences include (1) wasted ventilation (lung ventilated but not perfused), (2) atelectasis that occurs 2–24 h following PE, and (3) widened alveolar-arterial P_{O_2} gradient, usually with arterial hypoxemia. Hemodynamic consequences may include (1) pulmonary hypertension, (2) acute RV failure, and (3) decline in cardiac output. These occur only when significant fraction of pulmonary vasculature is obstructed. Infarction of lung tissue is uncommon, occurring only with underlying cardiac or pulmonary disease.

SYMPTOMS Sudden onset of dyspnea most common; chest pain, hemoptysis accompany infarction; syncope may indicate massive embolism.

PHYSICAL EXAMINATION Tachypnea and tachycardia common; RV gallop; loud P_2 and prominent jugular *a* waves suggest RV failure; temperature >39°C uncommon. Hypotension suggests massive PE.

LABORATORY FINDINGS Routine studies contribute little to diagnosis; normal D-dimer level (<500 μg/mL by ELISA) essentially rules out PE, particularly in younger, ambulatory pts, but normal CXR does not exclude PE. Impedance plethysmography and femoral ultrasonography are sensitive tests for

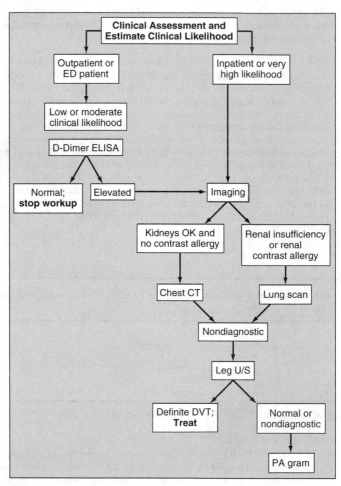

FIGURE 135-1   Diagnosis strategy for pulmonary thromboembolism: An integrated diagnostic approach. ED, emergency department; ELISA, enzyme-linked immunosorbent assay; CT, computed tomography; U/S, ultrasound; DVT, deep vein thrombosis; PA gram, pulmonary arteriogram. (From Goldhaber SZ: HPIM-16, p. 1563.)

deep venous thrombosis (DVT) only when the pt has local symptoms. Likelihood of PE with ventilation-perfusion scan is dependent on clinical suspicion. Spiral or helical CT has superseded lung scan in pts without renal insufficiency. Modern CT scanners have sensitivity >90% compared to pulmonary angiography and have ready availability. Angiography generally reserved for pts with high clinical suspicion of PE who have nondiagnostic scan (see Fig. 135-1).

R⃞ **TREATMENT**   (See Fig. 135-2)

IV heparin [18 (U/kg)/h] by continuous infusion is therapy for most pts after an initial bolus of 80 U/kg. Documentation of effectiveness (activated PTT

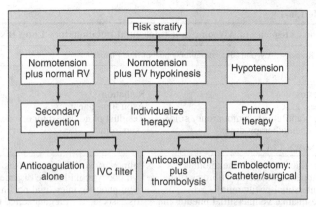

FIGURE 135-2 Acute management of pulmonary thromboembolism: RV, right ventricular; IVC, inferior vena cava. (From Goldhaber SZ: HPIM-16, p. 1564.)

1.5–2.0 × control) is essential as delay in reaching therapeutic level increases risk of recurrence. Heparin is continued 7 to 10 days for DVT and 10 days for thromboembolism. Low-molecular-weight heparin (enoxaparin 1 mg/kg q12h) may be an alternative for DVT and in pts with minimally symptomatic PE. Most pts receive minimum of 3 months of oral warfarin therapy after PE.

Fibrinolytic therapy hastens resolution of venous thrombi and is probably indicated for pts with massive embolism and systemic hypotension.

• Surgical therapy is rarely employed for DVT or acute PE.
• IVC interruption (clip or filter) is used in pts with recurrent PE despite anticoagulants and in those who cannot tolerate anticoagulants. Surgical extraction of old emboli may be helpful in pts with chronic pulmonary hypertension due to repeated PE without spontaneous resolution.

For a more detailed discussion, see Goldhaber SZ: Pulmonary Thromboembolism, Chap. 244, p. 1561, in HPIM-16.

136

INTERSTITIAL LUNG DISEASE (ILD)

Chronic, nonmalignant, noninfectious diseases of the lower respiratory tract characterized by inflammation and derangement of the alveolar walls; >200 separate diseases of known and unknown cause. Classified into two major groups: (1) Diseases associated with predominant inflammation and fibrosis, and (2) diseases with predominantly granulomatous reaction in interstitial or vascular areas (Table 136-1).

Table 136-1

Major Categories of Alveolar and Interstitial Inflammatory Lung Disease

Lung Response: Alveolitis, Interstitial Inflammation, and Fibrosis

KNOWN CAUSE

Asbestos	Radiation
Fumes, gases	Aspiration pneumonia
Drugs (antibiotics, amiodarone, gold) and chemotherapy drugs	Residual of adult respiratory distress syndrome

UNKNOWN CAUSE

Idiopathic interstitial pneumonias
  Idiopathic pulmonary fibrosis (usual interstitial pneumonia)
  Desquamative interstitial pneumonia
  Respiratory bronchiolitis-associated interstitial lung disease
  Acute interstitial pneumonia (diffuse alveolar damage)
  Cryptogenic organizing pneumonia (bronchiolitis obliterans with organizing pneumonia)
  Nonspecific interstitial pneumonia
Connective tissue diseases
  Systemic lupus erythematosus, rheumatoid arthritis, ankylosing spondylitis, systemic sclerosis, Sjögren's syndrome, polymyositis-dermatomyositis
Pulmonary hemorrhage syndromes
  Goodpasture's syndrome, idiopathic pulmonary hemosiderosis, isolated pulmonary capillaritis

Pulmonary alveolar proteinosis
Lymphocytic infiltrative disorders (lymphocytic interstitial pneumonitis associated with connective tissue disease)
Eosinophilic pneumonias
Lymphangioleiomyomatosis
Amyloidosis
Inherited diseases
  Tuberous sclerosis, neurofibromatosis, Niemann-Pick disease, Gaucher's disease, Hermansky-Pudlak syndrome
Gastrointestinal or liver diseases (Crohn's disease, primary biliary cirrhosis, chronic active hepatitis, ulcerative colitis)
Graft-vs.-host disease (bone marrow transplantation; solid organ transplantation)

Lung Response: Granulomatous

KNOWN CAUSE

Hypersensitivity pneumonitis (organic dusts)	Inorganic dusts: beryllium silica

UNKNOWN CAUSE

Sarcoidosis
Langerhans cell granulomatosis (eosinophilic granuloma of the lung)
Granulomatous vasculitides
Wegener's granulomatosis, allergic granulomatosis of Churg-Strauss

Bronchocentric granulomatosis
Lymphomatoid granulomatosis

INITIAL EVALUATION   *History*   Most pts come to medical attention for dyspnea or persistent cough. Acute presentation (days to weeks) suggests allergy (drugs, fungi, helminths), acute idiopathic interstitial pneumonia, eosinophilic pneumonia, or hypersensitivity. Pts with pulmonary Langerhans cell histiocytosis, desquamative interstitial pneumonitis, Goodpasture's syndrome, and respiratory bronchiolitis are almost invariably current or former smokers.

A careful occupational history is essential. Familial associations have been identified with tuberculous sclerosis and neurofibromatosis, and family clusters are seen with sarcoidosis and familial pulmonary fibrosis. Most pts with idiopathic pulmonary fibrosis (IPF) are >50 years.

Physical Examination Usually reveals tachypnea and end-inspiratory crackles.

Chest Imaging X-ray most commonly reveals bibasilar reticular pattern. Extensive disease on CXR out of proportion to symptoms suggests sarcoidosis, silicosis, pulmonary Langerhans cell histiocystosis, hypersensitivity pneumonitis, or lymphangitic carcinomatosis. Honeycombing portends a poor prognosis. High-resolution CT may be sufficiently specific to avoid a need for histologic examination (sarcoidosis, hypersensitivity pneumonitis, lymphangitic carcinoma, asbestosis, pulmonary Langerhans cell histiocytosis).

Tissue and Cellular Examination Rarely, clinical syndrome can be related to a causative agent, but histologic exam is usually necessary. With exception of sarcoidosis, which can often be diagnosed by transbronchial biopsy, most infiltrative diseases require open-lung biopsy for diagnosis unless contraindicated by honeycombing or other evidence of end-stage lung disease.

INDIVIDUAL ILDS
IDIOPATHIC PULMONARY FIBROSIS/USUAL INTERSTITIAL PNEUMONIA *History* Average age of 50 at presentation; sometimes familial. First manifestations are dyspnea, effort intolerance, and dry cough. Dyspnea and coughing often accompanied by constitutional symptoms (fatigue, anorexia, weight loss). One-third of pts date symptoms to aftermath of viral respiratory infection. Smoking history is common.

Physical Exam Late inspiratory crackles at posterior lung bases. Signs of pulmonary hypertension and clubbing occur late in course.

Laboratory Findings ESR may be elevated. Hypoxemia is common, but polycythemia is rare. Circulating immune-complex titers and serum immunoglobulin levels may be elevated.

Imaging Studies CXR usually reveals patchy, predominantly peripheral reticulonodular markings, prominent in lower lung zones. About 14% of biopsy-proven cases have normal CXR. High-resolution CT may show abnormalities when CXR is normal, such as ground glass opacities with traction bronchiectasis or honeycombing.

PFTs Typically restrictive pattern (Chap. 130) with reduced total lung capacity. DL_{CO} often decreased; mild hypoxemia, which worsens with exercise.

Histologic Findings Surgical biopsy usually required. Evidence of usual interstitial pneumonia (UIP) required. Characteristic is heterogeneous appearance of normal lung, interstitial inflammation, fibrosis, and honeycomb change.

Prognosis 5-year survival from diagnosis is 30–50%. No compelling evidence any therapy alters outcome, although glucocorticoids [prednisone 0.5–1.0 (mg/kg)/d] may provide symptomatic benefit. If after 4–12 weeks there is a response, the dose is tapered. If deterioration occurs on prednisone, a second agent is often added (cyclophosphamide, azathioprine).

DESQUAMATIVE INTERSTITIAL PNEUMONIA (DIP) Rare. Found exclusively in smokers in fourth and fifth decades. Better prognosis than idiopathic pulmonary fibrosis (10-year survival ∼ 70%). Treatment with glucocorticoids and smoking cessation.

ILD ASSOCIATED WITH COLLAGEN VASCULAR DISORDERS

Usually follows development of collagen-vascular disorder; typically mild but occasionally fatal.

Rheumatoid Arthritis (RA)   50% of pts with RA have abnormal lung function, 25% have abnormal CXR. Rarely causes symptoms. Males more commonly affected than females.

Progressive Systemic Sclerosis   Fibrosis with little inflammation; poor prognosis. Must be distinguished from pulmonary vascular disease.

SLE   Uncommon complication. When it occurs, it is most often an acute, inflammatory patchy process.

LANGERHANS CELL PULMONARY HISTIOCYTOSIS (EOSINO-PHILIC GRANULOMA, OR HISTIOCYTOSIS X)   Disorder of the dendritic cell system, related to Letterer-Siwe and Hand-Schuller-Christian disease. Develops between 20 and 40 years of age; 90% are present or former smokers. Complicated frequently by pneumothorax. No therapy available.

CHRONIC EOSINOPHILIC PNEUMONIA   Affects females predominantly; often a history of chronic asthma. Symptoms include weight loss, fever, chills, fatigue, dyspnea. CXR shows "photonegative pulmonary edema" pattern with central sparing. Very responsive to glucocorticoids.

IDIOPATHIC PULMONARY HEMOSIDEROSIS   Characterized by recurrent pulmonary hemorrhage; may be life-threatening. Not associated with renal disease.

GOODPASTURE'S SYNDROME   Relapsing pulmonary hemorrhage, anemia, and renal failure. Adult male smokers or ex-smokers most commonly affected. Circulating anti-basement membrane antibodies. Plasmapheresis thought to be effective.

INHERITED DISORDERS   ILD may be associated with tuberous sclerosis, neurofibromatosis, Gaucher's disease, Hermansky-Pudlak syndrome, and Niemann-Pick disease.

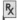 **TREATMENT**

Most important is removal of causative agent.

With exception of pneumoconioses, which are generally not treated except for discontinuation of further exposure and some other specific disorders, therapy is directed toward suppressing the inflammatory process, usually with glucocorticoids.

After diagnosis, pts are given oral prednisone, 1 (mg/kg)/d, for 8–12 weeks. Response is assessed by symptoms and PFTs.

For IPF and some other disorders, consider immunosuppressive therapy with cyclophosphamide, 1.0 (mg/kg)/d, added to prednisone, 0.25 (mg/kg)/d.

Smoking cessation, supplemental oxygen (when $Pa_{O_2} < 55$ mmHg), and therapy for right-sided heart failure and bronchospasm may all improve symptoms.

For a more detailed discussion, see King TE Jr: Interstitial Lung Diseases, Chap. 243, p. 1554, in HPIM-16.

137

DISEASES OF THE PLEURA, MEDIASTINUM, AND DIAPHRAGM

PLEURAL DISEASE

PLEURITIS Inflammation of pleura may occur with pneumonia, tuberculosis, pulmonary infarction, and neoplasm. Pleuritic pain without physical and x-ray findings suggests epidemic pleurodynia (viral inflammation of intercostal muscles); hemoptysis and parenchymal involvement on CXR suggest infection or infarction. Pleural effusion without parenchymal disease suggests postprimary tuberculosis, subdiaphragmatic abscess, mesothelioma, connective tissue disease, or primary bacterial infection of pleural space.

PLEURAL EFFUSION May or may not be associated with pleuritis. In general, effusions due to pleural disease resemble plasma (exudates); effusions with normal pleura are ultrafiltrates of plasma (transudates).

Exudates have at least one of the following criteria: high total fluid/serum protein ratio (>0.5), pleural fluid LDH greater than two-thirds of the normal upper limit, or pleural/serum LDH activity ratio >0.6.

Leading causes of transudative pleural effusions in the United States are left ventricular failure, pulmonary embolism, and cirrhosis. Leading causes of exudative effusions are bacterial pneumonia, malignancy, viral infection, and pulmonary embolism. With empyema, pH < 7.2, WBCs ↑ (>1000/mL), and glucose ↓. If neoplasm or tuberculosis is considered, closed pleural biopsy or thoracoscopic biopsy should be performed (Tables 137-1 and 137-2; and Fig. 137-1). Despite full evaluation, no cause for effusion will be found in 25% of pts.

POSTPRIMARY TUBERCULOSIS EFFUSIONS Fluid is exudative with predominant lymphocytosis; bacilli are rarely seen on smear, and fluid culture is positive in <20%; tuberculin test may be nonreactive early in illness; closed orthoracoscopic biopsy required for diagnosis.

NEOPLASTIC EFFUSIONS Most often lung cancer, breast cancer, or lymphoma. Fluid is exudative; fluid cytology and pleural biopsy will confirm diagnosis in 60%; pleural sclerosis with tetracycline or talc may be required for management (Table 137-2).

RHEUMATOID ARTHRITIS (RA) Exudative effusions may precede articular symptoms; very low glucose and pH; usually males.

PANCREATITIS Typically left-sided; up to 15% of pts with pancreatitis; high pleural fluid amylase is suggestive but may also occur with effusions due to neoplasms, infection, and esophageal rupture.

EOSINOPHILIC EFFUSION Defined as >10% eosinophils; nonspecific finding may occur with viral, bacterial, traumatic, and pancreatic effusions and may follow prior thoracentesis.

HEMOTHORAX Most commonly follows blunt or penetrating trauma. Pts with bleeding disorders may develop hemothorax following trauma or invasive procedures on pleura. Adequate drainage mandatory to avoid fibrothorax and "trapped" lung.

PARAPNEUMONIC EFFUSION/EMPYEMA An effusion associated with contiguous infection. The term *complicated parapneumonic effusion* refers

Table 137-1

Differential Diagnoses of Pleural Effusions

TRANSUDATIVE PLEURAL EFFUSIONS

1. Congestive heart failure	5. Peritoneal dialysis
2. Cirrhosis	6. Superior vena cava obstruction
3. Pulmonary embolization	7. Myxedema
4. Nephrotic syndrome	8. Urinothorax

EXUDATIVE PLEURAL EFFUSIONS

1. Neoplastic diseases	6. Post-coronary artery bypass
a. Metastatic disease	surgery
b. Mesothelioma	7. Asbestos exposure
2. Infectious diseases	8. Sarcoidosis
a. Bacterial infections	9. Uremia
b. Tuberculosis	10. Meigs' syndrome
c. Fungal infections	11. Yellow nail syndrome
d. Viral infections	12. Drug-induced pleural disease
e. Parasitic infections	a. Nitrofurantoin
3. Pulmonary embolization	b. Dantrolene
4. Gastrointestinal disease	c. Methysergide
a. Esophageal perforation	d. Bromocriptine
b. Pancreatic disease	e. Procarbazine
c. Intraabdominal abscesses	f. Amiodarone
d. Diaphragmatic hernia	13. Trapped lung
e. After abdominal surgery	14. Radiation therapy
f. Endoscopic variceal sclero-therapy	15. Post-cardiac injury syndrome
g. After liver transplant	16. Hemothorax
5. Collagen-vascular diseases	17. Iatrogenic injury
a. Rheumatoid diseases	18. Ovarian hyperstimulation syndrome
b. Systemic lupus erythematosus	19. Pericardial disease
c. Drug-induced lupus	20. Chylothorax
d. Immunoblastic lymphadenopathy	
e. Sjögren's syndrome	
f. Wegener's granulomatosis	
g. Churg-Strauss syndrome	

to effusions that require tube thoracostomy for their resolution. Empyema is pus in the pleural space with positive Gram's stain.

Tube thoracostomy of parapneumonic effusions is likely indicated if any of the following applies (descending order of importance): (1) gross pus is present, (2) organisms are visible on Gram's stain of pleural fluid, (3) pleural fluid glucose is <3.3 mmol/L (<60 mg/dL), (4) pleural fluid pH is <7.20 and 0.15 units less than arterial pH, or (5) there is loculated pleural fluid.

If closed drainage does not result in complete removal of fluid, streptokinase, 250,000 units, can be instilled through the tube. If fluid persists, open drainage is indicated, usually accomplished through a videoscope.

PNEUMOTHORAX (PNTX) Spontaneous PNTX most commonly occurs between 20 and 40 years of age; causes sudden, sharp chest pain and dyspnea. Treatment depends on size—if small, observation is sufficient; if large, closed drainage with chest tube is necessary. 50% suffer recurrence, and pleural

Table 137-2

Special Tests for Pleural Effusions

	Transudate	Exudate
RBC	<10,000/mL	>100,00/mL suggests neoplasm, infarction, trauma; >10,000 to <100,000/mL is indetermine
WBC	<100/mL	Usually >1000/mL
Differential WBC	Usually >50% lymphocytes or mononuclear cells	>50% lymphocytes (tuberculosis, neoplasm) >50% polymorphonuclear (acute inflammation)
pH	>7.3	>7.3 (inflammatory)
Glucose	Same as blood (±)	Low (infection) Extremely low (rheumatoid arthritis, occasionally neoplasm)
Amylase		>500 units/mL (pancreatitis; occasionally neoplasm, infection)
Specific proteins		Low C3, C4 components of complement (SLE, rheumatoid arthritis) Rheumatoid factor Antinuclear factor

Source: From Ingram RH Jr, HPIM-11, p. 1125.

abrasion by thoracotomy or thoracostomy may be required so that surfaces become adherent (pleurodesis).

Complications include hemothorax, cardiovascular compromise secondary to tension PNTX, and bronchopleural fistula. Many interstitial and obstructive lung diseases may predispose to PNTX.

MEDIASTINAL DISEASE

MEDIASTINITIS   Usually infectious. Routes of infection include esophageal perforation or tracheal disruption (trauma, instrumentation, eroding carcinoma). Radiographic hallmarks include mediastinal widening, air in mediastinum, pneumo- or hydropneumothorax. Therapy usually involves surgical drainage and antibiotics.

TUMORS AND CYSTS   Most common mediastinal masses in adults are metastatic carcinomas and lymphomas. Sarcoidosis, infectious mononucleosis, and AIDS may produce mediastinal lymphadenopathy. Neurogenic tumors, teratodermoids, thymomas, and bronchogenic cysts account for two-thirds of remaining mediastinal masses. Specific locations for specific etiologies (Table 137-3). Evaluation includes CXR, CT, and, when diagnosis remains in doubt, mediastinoscopy and biopsy.

Neurogenic Tumors   Most common primary mediastinal neoplasms; majority are benign; vague chest pain and cough.

Teratodermoids   Anterior mediastinum; 10–20% undergo malignant transformation.

Thymomas   10% primary mediastinal neoplasms; one-quarter are malignant; myasthenia gravis occurs in half.

SUPERIOR VENA CAVA SYNDROME   Dilation of veins of upper thorax and neck, plethora, facial and conjunctival edema, headache, visual distur-

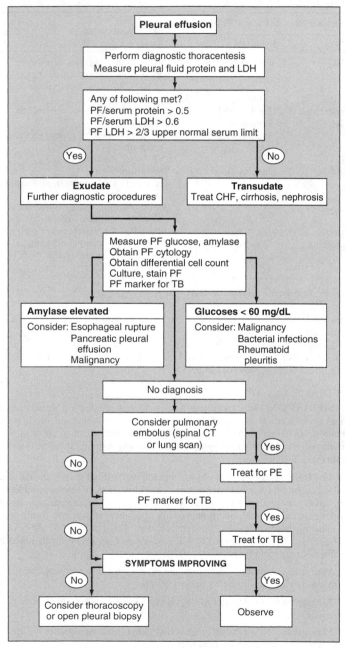

FIGURE 137-1 Approach to the diagnosis of pleural effusions. The special tests are summarized in Table 137-2. PF, pleural fluid; PE, pulmonary embolism. (*From RW Light: HPIM-16.*)

Table 137-3

Nature of Masses in Various Locations in Mediastinum

Superior	Anterior and Middle	Posterior
Lymphoma	Lymphoma	Neurogenic tumors
Thymoma	Metastatic carcinoma	Lymphoma
Retrosternal thyroid	Teratodermoid	Hernia (Bochdalek)
Metastatic carcinoma	Bronchogenic cyst	Aortic aneurysm
Parathyroid tumors	Aortic aneurysm	
Zenker's diverticulum	Pericardial cyst	
Aortic aneurysm		

bances, and reduced state of consciousness; most often due to malignant disease—75% bronchogenic carcinoma, most others lymphoma.

DISORDERS OF DIAPHRAGM

DIAPHRAGMATIC PARALYSIS   *Unilateral Paralysis*   Usually caused by phrenic nerve injury due to trauma or mediastinal tumor, but nearly half are unexplained; usually asymptomatic; suggested by CXR, confirmed by fluoroscopy.

Bilateral Paralysis   May be due to high cervical cord injury, motor neuron disease, poliomyelitis, polyneuropathies, bilateral phrenic involvement by mediastinal lesions, after cardiac surgery, dyspnea; paradoxical abdominal motion should be sought in supine pts.

For a more detailed discussion, see Light RW: Disorders of the Pleura, Mediastinum, Diaphragm and Chest Wall, Chap. 245, p. 1565, in HPIM-16.

138

DISORDERS OF VENTILATION, INCLUDING SLEEP APNEA

ALVEOLAR HYPOVENTILATION   Exists when arterial P_{CO_2} increases above the normal 37–43 mmHg. In most clinically important chronic hypoventilation syndromes, Pa_{CO_2} is 50–80 mmHg.

Cause   Alveolar hypoventilation is always (1) a defect in the metabolic respiratory control system, (2) a defect in the respiratory neuromuscular system, or (3) a defect in the ventilatory apparatus (Table 138-1).

Disorders associated with impaired respiratory drive, defects in respiratory neuromuscular system, and upper airway obstruction produce an increase in Pa_{CO_2}, despite normal lungs, because of a decrease in overall minute ventilation.

Table 138-1

Chronic Hypoventilation Syndromes

Mechanism	Site of Defect	Disorder
Impaired respiratory drive	Peripheral and central chemoreceptors	Carotid body dysfunction, trauma
	Brainstem respiratory neurons	Prolonged hypoxia
		Metabolic alkalosis
		Bulbar poliomyelitis, encephalitis
		Brainstem infarction, hemorrhage, trauma
		Brainstem demyelination, degeneration
		Chronic drug administration
		Primary alveolar hypoventilation syndrome
Defective respiratory neuromuscular system	Spinal cord and peripheral nerves	High cervical trauma
		Poliomyelitis
		Motor neuron disease
		Peripheral neuropathy
	Respiratory muscles	Myasthenia gravis
		Muscular dystrophy
		Chronic myopathy
Impaired ventilatory apparatus	Chest wall	Kyphoscoliosis
		Fibrothorax
		Thoracoplasty
		Ankylosing spondylitis
		Obesity-hypoventilation
	Airways and lungs	Laryngeal and tracheal stenosis
		Obstructive sleep apnea
		Cystic fibrosis
		Chronic obstructive pulmonary disease

Source: EA Phillipson: HPIM-16, p. 1570.

Disorders of chest wall, lower airways, and lungs produce an increase in Pa_{CO_2}, despite a normal or increased minute ventilation.

Increased Pa_{CO_2} leads to respiratory acidosis, compensatory increase in HCO_3^-, and decrease in Pa_{O_2}.

Hypoxemia may induce secondary polycythemia, pulmonary hypertension, right heart failure. Gas exchange worsens during sleep, resulting in morning headache, impaired sleep quality, fatigue, daytime somnolence, mental confusion.

HYPOVENTILATION SYNDROMES
PRIMARY ALVEOLAR   Cause unknown; rare; thought to arise from defect in metabolic respiratory control system; key diagnostic finding is chronic respiratory acidosis without respiratory muscle weakness or impaired ventilatory mechanics. Some pts respond to respiratory stimulants and supplemental O_2.

NEUROMUSCULAR Several primary neuromuscular disorders produce chronic hypoventilation (Table 138-1). Hypoventilation usually develops gradually, but acute, superimposed respiratory loads (e.g., viral bronchitis with airways obstruction) may precipitate respiratory failure. Diaphragm weakness is a common feature, with orthopnea and paradoxical abdominal movement in supine posture. Testing reveals low maximum voluntary ventilation and reduced maximal inspiratory and expiratory pressures. Therapy involves treatment of underlying condition. Many pts benefit from mechanical ventilatory assistance at night (often through nasal mask) or the entire day (typically through tracheostomy).

OBESITY-HYPOVENTILATION Massive obesity imposes a mechanical load on the respiratory system. Small percentage of morbidly obese pts develop hypercapnia, hypoxemia, and ultimately polycythemia, pulmonary hypertension, and right heart failure. Most pts have mild to moderate airflow obstruction. Treatment includes weight loss, smoking cessation, and pharmacologic respiratory stimulants such as progesterone. Nocturnal mask ventilation may minimize nocturnal hypoxemia and treats coexisting sleep-disordered breathing.

SLEEP APNEA

By convention, apnea is defined as cessation of airflow for >10 s. Hypopnea is defined as reduction in airflow resulting in arousal from sleep or oxygen desaturation. Minimum number of events per night for diagnosis is uncertain, but most pts have at least 10–15/h of sleep. Prevalence estimates vary depending on threshold for diagnosis (events/h) and on definition of hypopnea (degree of desaturation required), but conservative figures are 10% of working-age men and 4% of women.

Some pts have *central apnea* with transient loss of neural drive to respiratory muscles during sleep. Vast majority have primarily *obstructive apnea* with occlusion in the upper airway. Sleep plays a permissive role in collapse of upper airway. Alcohol and sedatives exacerbate the condition. Most pts have structural narrowing of upper airway. Obesity is frequent, but many pts have normal body habitus. Most pts have obstruction at nasal or palatal level. Mandibular deformities (retrognathia) also predispose. Symptoms include snoring, excessive daytime sleepiness, memory loss, and impotence. Sleepiness increases risk of automobile accidents. Nocturnal hypoxia, a consequence of apnea, may contribute to systemic hypertension, arrhythmias, and right ventricular hypertrophy. Sleep apnea, in the absence of co-morbidity causing daytime hypoxia, is not a cause of substantial pulmonary hypertension (present in >50% of pts) or right heart failure.

Diagnosis This requires overnight observation of the pt. The definitive test for obstructive sleep apnea is overnight polysomnography, including sleep staging and respiratory monitoring.

℞ **TREATMENT** (See Table 138-2)

Therapy is directed at increasing upper airway size, increasing upper airway tone, and minimizing upper airway collapsing pressures. Weight loss often reduces disease severity but infrequently obviates the need for other therapy. Majority of pts with severe sleep apnea require nasal continuous positive airway pressure (nasal C-PAP). Mandibular positioning device (dental) may treat pts with mild or moderate disease. Surgery (uvulopalatopharyngoplasty)

Table 138-2

Management of Obstructive Sleep Apnea (OSA)		
Mechanism	Mild to Moderate OSA	Moderate to Severe OSA
↑ Upper airway muscle tone	Avoidance of alcohol, sedatives	
↑ Upper airway lumen size	Weight reduction	Uvulopalatopharyngoplasty
	Avoidance of supine posture	
	Oral prosthesis	
↓ Upper airway subatmospheric pressure	Improved nasal patency	Nasal continuous positive airway pressure
Bypass occlusion		Tracheostomy

Source: EA Phillipson: HPIM-16, p. 1575.

is usually reserved for pts who fail other therapies, as failure rate is high (>50%).

HYPERVENTILATION

Increased ventilation, causing $Pa_{CO_2} < 37$ mmHg. Causes include lesions of the CNS, metabolic acidosis, anxiety, drugs (e.g., salicylates), hypoxemia, hypoglycemia, hepatic coma, and sepsis. Hyperventilation may also occur with some types of lung disease, particularly interstitial disease and pulmonary edema.

For a more detailed discussion, see Phillipson EA: Disorders of Ventilation, Chap. 246, p. 1569, and Sleep Apnea, Chap. 247, p. 1573, in HPIM-16.

139

APPROACH TO THE PATIENT WITH RENAL DISEASE

The approach to renal disease begins with recognition of particular syndromes on the basis of findings such as presence or absence of azotemia, proteinuria, hypertension, edema, abnormal urinalysis, electrolyte disorders, abnormal urine volumes, or infection (Table 139-1).

Acute Renal Failure (See Chap. 140)

Clinical syndrome is characterized by a rapid, severe decrease in GFR (rise in serum creatinine and BUN), usually with reduced urine output. Extracellular fluid expansion leads to edema, hypertension, and occasionally to CHF. Hyperkalemia, hyponatremia, and acidosis are common. Etiologies include ischemia; nephrotoxic injury due to drugs, toxins, or endogenous pigments; sepsis; severe renovascular disease; or conditions related to pregnancy. Prerenal and postrenal failure are potentially reversible causes.

RAPIDLY PROGRESSIVE GLOMERULONEPHRITIS Loss of renal function occurs over weeks to months. Pts are initially nonoliguric and may have recent flulike symptoms; later, oliguric renal failure with uremic symptoms supervenes. Hypertension is common. Pulmonary manifestations range from asymptomatic infiltrates to life-threatening hemoptysis. Urinalysis typically shows hematuria, proteinuria, and RBC casts.

ACUTE GLOMERULONEPHRITIS (See Chap. 144) An acute illness with sudden onset of hematuria, edema, hypertension, oliguria, and elevated BUN and creatinine. Mild pulmonary congestion may be present. An antecedent or concurrent infection or multisystem disease may be causative, or glomerular disease may exist alone. Hematuria, proteinuria, and pyuria are usually present, and RBC casts confirm the diagnosis. Serum complement may be decreased in certain conditions.

Chronic Renal Failure (See Chap. 141)

Progressive permanent loss of renal function over months to years does not cause symptoms of uremia until GFR is reduced to about 10–15% of normal. Hypertension may occur early. Later, manifestations include anorexia, nausea, vomiting, insomnia, weight loss, weakness, paresthesia, bleeding, serositis, anemia, acidosis, and hyperkalemia. Causes include diabetes mellitus, severe hypertension, glomerular disease, urinary tract obstruction, vascular disease, polycystic kidney disease, and interstitial nephritis. Indications of chronicity include long-standing azotemia, anemia, hyperphosphatemia, hypocalcemia, shrunken kidneys, renal osteodystrophy by x-ray, or findings on renal biopsy.

Nephrotic Syndrome (See Chap. 144)

Defined as heavy albuminuria (>3.5 g/d in the adult) with or without edema, hypoalbuminemia, hyperlipidemia, and varying degrees of renal insufficiency. Can be idiopathic or due to drugs, infections, neoplasms, multisystem or hereditary diseases. Complications include severe edema, thromboembolic events, infection, and protein malnutrition.

Table 139-1

Initial Clinical and Laboratory Data Base for Defining Major Syndromes in Nephrology

Syndromes	Important Clues to Diagnosis	Common Findings
Acute or rapidly progressive renal failure	Anuria Oliguria Documented recent decline in GFR	Hypertension, hematuria Proteinuria, pyuria Casts, edema
Acute nephritis	Hematuria, RBC casts Azotemia, oliguria Edema, hypertension	Proteinuria Pyuria Circulatory congestion
Chronic renal failure	Azotemia for >3 months Prolonged symptoms or signs of uremia Symptoms or signs of renal osteodystrophy Kidneys reduced in size bilaterally Broad casts in urinary sediment	Hematuria, proteinuria Casts, oliguria Polyuria, nocturia Edema, hypertension Electrolyte disorders
Nephrotic syndrome	Proteinuria >3.5 g per 1.73 m^2 per 24 h Hypoalbuminemia Hyperlipidemia Lipiduria	Casts Edema
Asymptomatic urinary abnormalities	Hematuria Proteinuria (below nephrotic range) Sterile pyuria, casts	
Urinary tract infection	Bacteriuria >10^5 colonies per milliliter Other infectious agent documented in urine Pyuria, leukocyte casts Frequency, urgency Bladder tenderness, flank tenderness	Hematuria Mild azotemia Mild proteinuria Fever
Renal tubule defects	Electrolyte disorders Polyuria, nocturia Symptoms or signs of renal osteodystrophy Large kidneys Renal transport defects	Hematuria "Tubular" proteinuria Enuresis
Hypertension	Systolic/diastolic hypertension	Proteinuria Casts Azotemia
Nephrolithiasis	Previous history of stone passage or removal Previous history of stone seen by x-ray Renal colic	Hematuria Pyuria Frequency, urgency

(continued)

Table 139-1 *(Continued)*

Initial Clinical and Laboratory Data Base for Defining Major Syndromes in Nephrology

Syndromes	Important Clues to Diagnosis	Common Findings
Urinary tract obstruction	Azotemia, oliguria, anuria Polyuria, nocturia, urinary retention Slowing of urinary stream Large prostate, large kidneys Flank tenderness, full bladder after voiding	Hematuria Pyuria Enuresis, dysuria

Source: Modified from FL Coe, BM Brenner: HPIM-14.

Asymptomatic Urinary Abnormalities

Hematuria may be due to neoplasms, stones, infection at any level of the urinary tract, sickle cell disease, or analgesic abuse. Renal parenchymal causes are suggested by RBC casts, proteinuria, or dysmorphic RBCs in urine. Pattern of gross hematuria may be helpful in localizing site. Hematuria with low-grade proteinuria may be due to benign recurrent hematuria or IgA nephropathy. Modest *proteinuria* may be an isolated finding due to fever, exertion, CHF, or upright posture. Renal causes include diabetes mellitus, amyloidosis, or other causes of glomerular disease. *Pyuria* can be caused by UTI, interstitial nephritis, glomerulonephritis, or renal transplant rejection. "Sterile" pyuria is associated with UTI treated with antibiotics, glucocorticoid therapy, acute febrile episodes, cyclophosphamide therapy, pregnancy, renal transplant rejection, genitourinary trauma, prostatitis, cystourethritis, tuberculosis and other mycobacterial infections, fungal infection, *Haemophilus influenzae*, anaerobic infection, fastidious bacteria, and bacterial L forms.

Urinary Tract Infection   (See Chap. 146)

Generally defined as $>10^5$ bacteria per mL of urine. Levels between 10^2 and 10^5/mL may indicate infection but are usually due to poor sample collection, especially if mixed flora are present. Adults at risk are sexually active women or anyone with urinary tract obstruction, vesicoureteral reflux, bladder catheterization, neurogenic bladder (associated with diabetes mellitus), or primary neurologic diseases. Prostatitis, urethritis, and vaginitis may be distinguished by quantitative urine culture. Flank pain, nausea, vomiting, fever, and chills indicate kidney infection. UTI is a common cause of sepsis, especially in the elderly and institutionalized.

Renal Tubular Defects   (See Chap. 145)

Generally inherited, they include anatomic defects (polycystic kidneys, medullary cystic disease, medullary sponge kidney) detected in the evaluation of hematuria, flank pain, infection, or renal failure of unknown cause and disorders of tubular transport that cause glucosuria, aminoaciduria, stones, or rickets. Fanconi syndrome is a generalized tubular defect that can be hereditary or acquired, due to drugs, heavy metals, multiple myeloma, amyloidosis, or renal transplantation. Nephrogenic diabetes insipidus (polyuria, polydypsia, hypernatremia, hypernatremic dehydration) and renal tubular acidosis are additional causes.

Hypertension (See Chap. 122)

Blood pressure > 140/90 mmHg affects 20% of the U.S. adult population; when inadequately controlled, it is an important cause of cerebrovascular accident, MI, and CHF and can contribute to the development of renal failure. Hypertension is usually asymptomatic until cardiac, renal, or neurologic symptoms appear. In most cases hypertension is idiopathic and becomes evident between ages 25 and 45.

Nephrolithiasis (See Chap. 148)

Causes colicky pain, UTI, hematuria, dysuria, or unexplained pyuria. Stones may be found on routine x-ray. Most are radiopaque Ca stones and are associated with high levels of urinary Ca, and/or oxalate excretion, and/or low levels of urinary citrate excretion. Staghorn calculi are large, branching radiopaque stones within the renal pelvis due to recurrent infection. Uric acid stones are radiolucent. Urinalysis may reveal hematuria, pyuria, or pathologic crystals.

Urinary Tract Obstruction (See Chap. 149)

Causes variable symptoms depending on whether it is acute or chronic, unilateral or bilateral, complete or partial, and on underlying etiology. It is an important reversible cause of unexplained renal failure. Upper tract obstruction may be silent or produce flank pain, hematuria, and renal infection. Bladder symptoms may be present in lower tract obstruction. Functional consequences include polyuria, anuria, nocturia, acidosis, hyperkalemia, and hypertension. A flank or suprapubic mass may be found on physical exam.

For a more detailed discussion, see Part 11: Disorders of the Kidney and Urinary Tract, pp. 1639-1724, in HPIM-16; and Coe, FL, and Brenner, BM: Approach to the Patient with Disease of the Kidneys and Urinary Tract, p. 1495, in HPIM-14.

140

ACUTE RENAL FAILURE

Definition

Acute renal failure (ARF), defined as a measurable increase in the serum creatinine (Cr) concentration [usually relative increase of 50% or absolute increase by 44 to 88 μmol/L (0.5 to 1.0 mg/dL)], occurs in ~5–7% of hospitalized pts. It is associated with a substantial increase in in-hospital mortality and morbidity. ARF can be anticipated in some clinical circumstances (e.g., after radiocontrast exposure or major surgery), and there are no specific pharmacologic therapies proven helpful at preventing or reversing the condition. Maintaining optimal renal perfusion and intravascular volume appears to be important in most clinical circumstances.

Differential Diagnosis

The separation into three broad categories (prerenal, intrinsic renal, and post-renal failure) is of great clinical utility (Table 140-1). *Prerenal failure* is most common among hospitalized pts. It may result from true volume depletion (e.g., diarrhea, vomiting, GI or other hemorrhage) or "effective circulatory volume" depletion, i.e., reduced renal perfusion in the setting of adequate or excess blood volume. Reduced renal perfusion may be seen in CHF (due to reduced cardiac output and/or potent vasodilator therapy), hepatic cirrhosis (due most likely to arteriovenous shunting), nephrotic syndrome and other states of severe hypo-proteinemia [total serum protein <54 g/L (<5.4 g/dL)], and renovascular disease (because of fixed stenosis at the level of the main renal artery or large branch vessels). Several drugs can reduce renal perfusion, most notably NSAIDs. ACE inhibitors and angiotensin II receptor antagonists may reduce GFR but do not tend to reduce renal perfusion.

Causes of *intrinsic renal failure* depend on the clinical setting. Among hospitalized pts, especially on surgical services or in intensive care units, acute tubular necrosis (ATN) is the most common diagnosis. Allergic interstitial nephritis, usually due to antibiotics (e.g., penicillins, cephalosporins, sulfa drugs, quinolones, and rifampin), may also be responsible. These conditions are relatively uncommon in the outpatient setting. There, intrinsic disease due to glomerulonephritis or pyelonephritis predominates.

Postrenal failure is due to urinary tract obstruction, which is also more common among ambulatory rather than hospitalized pts. More common in men than women, it is most often caused by ureteral or urethral blockade. Occasionally, stones or sloughed renal papillae may cause more proximal obstruction.

Characteristic Findings and Diagnostic Workup

All pts with ARF manifest some degree of azotemia (increased BUN and Cr). Other clinical features depend on the etiology of renal disease. Pts with *prerenal azotemia* due to volume depletion usually demonstrate orthostatic hypotension, tachycardia, low JVP, and dry mucous membranes. Pts with prerenal azotemia and CHF may show jugular venous distention, an S_3 gallop, and peripheral and pulmonary edema. Therefore, the physical exam is critical in the workup of pts with prerenal ARF. In general, the BUN/Cr ratio tends to be high (>20:1), more so with volume depletion and CHF than with cirrhosis. The uric acid may also be disproportionately elevated in noncirrhotic prerenal states (due to increased proximal tubular absorption). Urine chemistries tend to show low urine [Na^+] (<10–20 mmol/L, ≪10 with hepatorenal syndrome) and a fractional excretion of sodium (FE_{Na}) ≪ 1% (Table 140-2). The UA typically shows hyaline and a few granular casts, without cells or cellular casts. Renal ultrasonography is usually normal.

Pts with *intrinsic renal disease* present with varying complaints. Glomerulonephritis (GN) is often accompanied by hypertension and mild to moderate edema (associated with Na retention and proteinuria, and sometimes with hematuria). The urine chemistries may be indistinguishable from those in pts with prerenal failure; in fact, some pts with GN have renal hypoperfusion (due to glomerular inflammation and ischemia) with resultant hyperreninemia leading to hypertension. The urine sediment is most helpful in these cases. RBC, WBC, and cellular casts are characteristic of GN; RBC casts are rarely seen in other conditions (i.e., high specificity). In the setting of inflammatory nephritis (GN or interstitial nephritis, see below), there may be increased renal echogenicity on ultrasonography. Unlike pts with GN, pts with interstitial diseases are less likely to have hypertension or proteinuria. Hematuria and pyuria may present

Table 140-1

Common Causes of Acute Renal Failure

PRERENAL

Volume depletion
Blood loss
GI fluid loss (e.g., vomiting, diarrhea)
Overzealous diuretic use
Volume overload with reduced renal perfusion
Congestive heart failure
Low-output with systolic dysfunction
"High-output" (e.g., anemia, thyrotoxicosis)
Hepatic cirrhosis
Severe hypoproteinemia
Renovascular disease
Drugs
NSAIDs, cyclosporine, amphotericin B
Other
Hypercalcemia, "third spacing" (e.g., pancreatitis, systemic inflammatory response), hepatorenal syndrome

INTRINSIC

Acute tubular necrosis (ATN)
Hypotension or shock, prolonged prerenal azotemia, post-operative sepsis syndrome, rhabdomyolysis, hemolysis, drugs
Radiocontrast, aminoglycosides, cisplatin
Other tubulointerstitial disease
Allergic interstitial nephritis
Pyelonephritis (bilateral, or unilateral in single functional kidney)
Heavy metal poisoning
Atheroembolic disease
Glomerulonephritis
"Rapidly progressive"
Wegener's granulomatosis
Anti-GBM disease (Goodpasture's syndrome)
PAN and other pauci-immune GN
Immune complex-mediated
Subacute bacterial endocarditis, SLE, cryoglobulinemia (with or without hepatitis C infection), postinfectious GN
Other
IgA nephropathy (Henoch-Schönlein purpura), preeclampsia

POSTRENAL (URINARY TRACT OBSTRUCTION)

Bladder neck obstruction, bladder calculi
Prostatic hypertrophy
Ureteral obstruction due to compression
Pelvic or abdominal malignancy, retroperitoneal fibrosis
Nephrolithiasis
Papillary necrosis with obstruction

Note: GBM, glomerular basement membrane; PAN, polyarteritis nodosa.

Table 140-2

Urine Diagnostic Indices in Differentiation of Prerenal versus Intrinsic Renal Azotemia

	Typical Findings	
Diagnostic Index	Prerenal Azotemia	Intrinsic Renal Azotemia
Fractional excretion of sodium (%)[a] $$\frac{U_{Na} \times P_{Cr}}{P_{Na} \times U_{Cr}} \times 100$$	<1	>1
Urine sodium concentration (mmol/L)	<10	>20
Urine creatinine to plasma creatinine ratio	>40	>20
Urine urea nitrogen to plasma urea nitrogen ratio	>8	<3
Urine specific gravity	>1.018	<1.015
Urine osmolality (mosmol/kg H_2O)	>500	<300
Plasma BUN/creatinine ratio	>20	<10–15
Renal failure index $$\frac{U_{Na}}{U_{Cr}/P_{Cr}}$$	<1	>1
Urinary sediment	Hyaline casts	Muddy brown granular casts

[a] Most sensitive indices.
Note: U_{Na}, urine sodium concentration; P_{Cr}, plasma creatinine concentration; P_{Na}, plasma sodium concentration; U_{Cr}, urine creatinine concentration.

on UA; the classic sediment finding in allergic interstitial nephritis is a predominance (>10%) of urinary eosinophils with Wright's or Hansel's stain. WBC casts may also be seen, particularly in cases of pyelonephritis.

Pts with *postrenal ARF* due to urinary tract obstruction are usually less severely ill than pts with prerenal or intrinsic renal disease, and their presentation may be delayed until azotemia is markedly advanced [BUN > 54 μmol/ L (150 mg/dL), Cr > 1060–1325 μmol/L (12–15 mg/dL)]. An associated impairment of urinary concentrating ability often "protects" the pt from complications of volume overload. Urinary electrolytes typically show a FE_{Na} > 1%, and microscopic examination of the urinary sediment is usually bland. Ultrasonography is the key diagnostic tool. More than 90% of pts with postrenal ARF show obstruction of the urinary collection system on ultrasound (e.g., dilated ureter, calyces); false negatives include hyperacute obstruction and encasement of the ureter and/or kidney by tumor, functionally obstructing urinary outflow without structural dilatation.

 TREATMENT

This should focus on providing etiology-specific supportive care. For example, pts with prerenal failure due to GI fluid loss may experience relatively rapid correction of ARF after the administration of IV fluid to expand volume. The same treatment in prerenal pts with CHF would be counterproductive; in this case, treatment of the underlying disease with vasodilators and/or inotropic agents would more likely be of benefit.

There are relatively few intrinsic renal causes of ARF for which there is safe and effective therapy. ARF associated with vasculitis may respond to high-dose glucocorticoids and cytotoxic agents (e.g., cyclophosphamide); plasmapheresis and plasma exchange may be useful in other selected circumstances [e.g., Goodpasture's syndrome and hemolytic-uremic syndrome/ thrombotic thrombocytopenic purpura (HUS/TTP), respectively]. Antibiotic therapy may be sufficient for the treatment of ARF associated with pyelonephritis or endocarditis. There are conflicting data regarding the utility of glucocorticoids in allergic interstitial nephritis. Many practitioners advocate their use with clinical evidence of progressive renal insufficiency despite discontinuation of the offending drug, or with biopsy evidence of potentially reversible, severe disease.

The treatment of urinary tract obstruction often involves consultation with a urologist. Interventions as simple as Foley catheter placement or as complicated as multiple ureteral stents and/or nephrostomy tubes may be required.

Dialysis for ARF and Recovery of Renal Function   Most cases of community- and hospital-acquired ARF resolve with conservative supportive measures, time, and patience. If nonprerenal ARF continues to progress, dialysis must be considered. The traditional indications for dialysis — volume overload refractory to diuretic agents; hyperkalemia; encephalopathy not otherwise explained; pericarditis, pleuritis, or other inflammatory serositis; and severe metabolic acidosis, compromising respiratory or circulatory function — can seriously compromise recovery from acute nonrenal illness. Therefore, dialysis should generally be provided in advance of these complications. The inability to provide requisite fluids for antibiotics, inotropes and other drugs, and/or nutrition should also be considered an indication for dialysis.

Dialytic options for ARF include (1) intermittent hemodialysis (IHD), (2) peritoneal dialysis (PD), and (3) continuous renal replacement therapy (CRRT, i.e., continuous arteriovenous or venovenous hemodiafiltration). Most pts are treated with IHD. It is unknown whether conventional thrice weekly hemodialysis is sufficient or more frequent treatments are required. Few centers rely on PD for management of ARF (risks include infection associated with intraperitoneal catheter insertion and respiratory compromise due to abdominal distention). At some centers, CRRT is prescribed only in pts intolerant of IHD, usually because of hypotension; other centers use it as the modality of choice for pts in intensive care units. Hybrid hemodialysis techniques, such as slow low efficiency dialysis (SLED), may be used in centers less familiar with CRRT.

For a more detailed discussion, see Brady HR, Brenner BM: Acute Renal Failure, Chap. 260, p. 1644, in HPIM-16.

141

CHRONIC KIDNEY DISEASE (CKD) AND UREMIA

Epidemiology

The prevalence of CKD, generally defined as a long-standing, irreversible impairment of kidney function, is substantially greater than the number of pts with end-stage renal disease (ESRD), now $\geq 300,000$ in the United States. There is a spectrum of disease related to decrements in renal function; clinical and therapeutic issues differ greatly depending on whether the GFR reduction is moderate (e.g., 30–59 mL/min per 1.73 m^2), severe (15–29 mL/min per 1.73 m^2), or near "end-stage" (<15 mL/min per 1.73 m^2). Dialysis is usually required to control symptoms of uremia with GFR < 10 mL/min per 1.73 m^2. Common causes of CKD are outlined in Table 141-1.

Differential Diagnosis

The first step in the differential diagnosis of CKD is establishing its chronicity, i.e., disproving a major acute component. The two most common means of determining disease chronicity are the history (if available) and the renal ultrasound, which is used to measure kidney size. In general, kidneys that have shrunk (<10–11.5 cm, depending on body size) are more likely affected by chronic disease. While reasonably specific (few false positives), reduced kidney size is only a moderately sensitive marker for CKD, i.e., there are several relatively common conditions in which kidney disease may be chronic, without any reduction in renal size. Diabetic nephropathy, HIV-associated nephropathy, and infiltrative diseases such as multiple myeloma may be associated with relatively large kidneys despite chronicity. Renal biopsy is a more reliable means of proving chronicity; a predominance of glomerulosclerosis or interstitial fibrosis argues strongly for chronic disease. Hyperphosphatemia and other metabolic derangements are not reliable indicators in distinguishing acute from chronic disease.

Once chronicity has been established, clues from the physical exam, laboratory panel, and urine sediment evaluation can be used to determine etiology. A detailed Hx will identify important comorbid conditions, such as diabetes, HIV seropositivity, or peripheral vascular disease. The family Hx is paramount in the workup of autosomal dominant polycystic kidney disease or hereditary nephritis (Alport's syndrome). An occupational Hx may reveal exposure to en-

Table 141-1

Common Causes of Chronic Renal Failure

Diabetic nephropathy
Hypertensive nephrosclerosis[a]
Glomerulonephritis
Renovascular disease (ischemic nephropathy)
Polycystic kidney disease
Reflux nephropathy and other congenital renal diseases
Interstitial nephritis, including analgesic nephropathy
HIV-associated nephropathy
Transplant allograft failure ("chronic rejection")

[a] Often diagnosis of exclusion; very few pts undergo renal biopsy; may be occult renal disease with hypertension.

vironmental toxins or culprit drugs (including over-the-counter agents, such as analgesics or Chinese herbs).

Physical exam may demonstrate abdominal masses (i.e., polycystic kidneys), diminished pulses (i.e., atherosclerotic peripheral vascular disease), or an abdominal bruit (i.e., renovascular disease). The Hx and exam may also yield important data regarding severity of disease. The presence of foreshortened fingers (due to resorption of the distal phalangeal tufts) and/or subcutaneous nodules may be seen with advanced CKD and secondary hyperparathyroidism. Excoriations (uremic pruritus), pallor (anemia), muscle wasting, and a nitrogenous fetor are all signs of advanced CKD, as are pericarditis, pleuritis, and asterixis, complications of particular concern that usually prompt the initiation of dialysis.

LABORATORY FINDINGS Serum and urine laboratory findings typically provide additional information useful in determining the etiology and severity of CKD. Heavy proteinuria (>3.5 g/d), hypoalbuminemia, hypercholesterolemia, and edema suggest nephrotic syndrome (see Chap. 144). Diabetic nephropathy, membranous nephropathy, focal segmental glomerulosclerosis, minimal change disease, amyloid, and HIV-associated nephropathy are principal causes. Proteinuria may decrease slightly with decreasing GFR but rarely to normal levels. Hyperkalemia and metabolic acidosis may complicate all forms of CKD eventually but are more prominent in pts with interstitial renal diseases.

The Uremic Syndrome

The culprit toxin(s) responsible for the uremic syndrome remain elusive. The serum creatinine (Cr) is the most common laboratory surrogate of renal function. The creatinine clearance (Cr_{Cl}) is calculated as the urine concentration divided by serum concentration multiplied by the urine flow rate; it approximates the GFR and is a more reliable indicator of renal function than the serum Cr alone. Uremic symptoms tend to develop with serum Cr > 530–710 μmol/L (> 6–8 mg/dL) or Cr_{Cl} < 10 mL/min, although these values vary widely.

Symptoms of advanced uremia include anorexia, weight loss, dyspnea, fatigue, pruritus, sleep and taste disturbance, and confusion and other forms of encephalopathy. Key findings on physical exam include hypertension, jugular venous distention, pericardial and/or pleural friction rub, muscle wasting, asterixis, excoriations, and ecchymoses. Laboratory abnormalities may include: hyperkalemia, hyperphosphatemia, metabolic acidosis, hypocalcemia, hyperuricemia, anemia, and hypoalbuminemia. Most of these abnormalities eventually resolve with initiation of dialysis or renal transplantation (Chaps. 142, 143).

 TREATMENT

Hypertension complicates many forms of CKD and warrants aggressive treatment to reduce the risk of stroke and potentially to slow the progression of CKD (see below). Volume overload contributes to hypertension in many cases, and potent diuretic agents are frequently required. Anemia can be reversed with recombinant human erythropoetin (rHuEPO); 2000–6000 units subcutaneously once or twice weekly can increase Hb concentrations toward the normal range in most pts.

Hyperphosphatemia can be controlled with judicious restriction of dietary phosphorus and the use of postprandial phosphate binders, either calcium-based salts (calcium carbonate or acetate) or nonabsorbed agents (e.g., sevelamer). Hyperkalemia should be controlled with dietary potassium restriction. Sodium polystyrene sulfonate (Kayexalate) can be used in refractory cases, although dialysis should be considered if the potassium > 6 mmol/L on repeated occasions. If these conditions cannot be conservatively controlled, dialysis should be instituted (Chap. 142). It is also advisable to begin dialysis if severe anorexia, weight loss, and/or hypoalbuminemia develop, as it has been definitively shown that outcomes for dialysis pts with malnutrition are particularly poor.

Slowing Progression of Renal Disease Prospective clinical trials have explored the roles of blood pressure control and dietary protein restriction on the rate of progression of renal failure. Control of hypertension is of benefit, although ACE inhibitors and angiotensin receptor blockers (ARBs) may exert unique beneficial effects, most likely due to their effects on intrarenal hemodynamics. The effects of ACE inhibitors and ARBs are most pronounced in pts with diabetic nephropathy and in those without diabetes but with significant proteinuria (>1 g/d). Diuretics and other antihypertensive agents are often required, in addition to ACE inhibitors and ARBs, to optimize hypertension control and attenuate disease progression. Dietary protein restriction may offer an additional benefit, particularly in these same subgroups.

For a more detailed discussion, see Skorecki K, Green J, Brenner BM: Chronic Renal Failure, Chap. 261, p. 1653, in HPIM-16.

142

DIALYSIS

Overview

Initiation of dialysis usually depends on a combination of the pt's symptoms, comorbid conditions, and laboratory parameters. Unless a living donor is identified, transplantation is deferred by necessity, due to the scarcity of cadaveric donor organs (median waiting time 3–6 years at most transplant centers). Dialytic options include hemodialysis and peritoneal dialysis (PD). Roughly 85% of U.S. pts are started on hemodialysis.

Absolute indications for dialysis include: severe volume overload refractory to diuretic agents, severe hyperkalemia and/or acidosis, encephalopathy not otherwise explained, and pericarditis or other serositis. Additional indications for dialysis include symptomatic uremia (Chap. 141) (e.g., intractable fatigue, anorexia, nausea, vomiting, pruritus, difficulty maintaining attention and concentration) and protein-energy malnutrition/failure to thrive without other overt cause. No absolute serum creatinine, BUN, creatinine or urea clearance, or glomerular filtration rate (GFR) is used as an absolute cut-off for requiring dialysis, although most individuals experience, or will soon develop, symptoms and complications when the GFR is below $\sim$10 mL/min.

Hemodialysis

This requires direct access to the circulation, either via a native arteriovenous fistula (the preferred method of vascular access), usually at the wrist (a "Brescia-Cimino" fistula); an arteriovenous graft, usually made of polytetrafluoroethyl-

Table 142-1

Complications of Hemodialysis	
Hypotension	Dialysis-related amyloidosis
Accelerated vascular disease	Protein-calorie malnutrition
Rapid loss of residual renal function	Hemorrhage
Access thrombosis	Dyspnea/hypoxemia[a]
Access or catheter sepsis	Leukopenia[a]

[a] Particularly with first use of conventional modified cellulosic dialyzer.

ene; a large-bore intravenous catheter; or a subcutaneous device attached to intravascular catheters. Blood is pumped though hollow fibers of an artificial kidney (the "dialyzer") and bathed with a solution of favorable chemical composition (isotonic, free of urea and other nitrogenous compounds, and generally low in potassium). Most pts undergo dialysis thrice weekly, usually for 3–4 h. The efficiency of dialysis is largely dependent on the duration of dialysis, the blood flow rate, dialysate flow rate, and surface area of the dialyzer.

Complications of hemodialysis are outlined in Table 142-1. Many of these relate to the process of hemodialysis as an intense, intermittent therapy. In contrast to the native kidney or to PD, both major dialytic functions (i.e., clearance of solutes and fluid removal, or "ultrafiltration") are accomplished over relatively short time periods. The rapid flux of fluid can cause hypotension, even without a pt reaching "dry weight." Hemodialysis-related hypotension is common in diabetic pts whose neuropathy prevents the compensatory responses (vasoconstriction and tachycardia) to intravascular volume depletion. Occasionally, confusion or other CNS symptoms will occur. The dialysis "disequilibrium syndrome" refers to the development of headache, confusion, and rarely seizures, in association with rapid solute removal early in the pt's dialysis history, before adaptation to the procedure.

Peritoneal Dialysis

This does not require direct access to the circulation; rather, it obligates placement of a peritoneal catheter that allows infusion of a dialysate solution into the abdominal cavity, which allows transfer of solutes (i.e., urea, potassium, other uremic molecules) across the peritoneal membrane, which serves as the "artificial kidney." This solution is similar to that used for hemodialysis, except that it must be sterile, and uses lactate, rather than bicarbonate, to provide base equivalents. PD is far less efficient at cleansing the bloodstream than hemodialysis and therefore requires a much longer duration of therapy. Pts generally have the choice of performing their own "exchanges" (2–3 L of dialysate, 4–5 times during daytime hours) or using an automated device at night. Compared

Table 142-2

Complications of Peritoneal Dialysis	
Peritonitis	Dialysis-related amyloidosis
Hyperglycemia	Insufficient clearance due to vascular disease or
Hypertriglyceridemia	other factors
Obesity	Uremia secondary to loss of residual renal function
Hypoproteinemia	

with hemodialysis, PD offers the major advantages of (1) independence and flexibility, and (2) a more gentle hemodynamic profile.

Complications are outlined in Table 142-2. Peritonitis is the most important complication. In addition to the ill effects of the systemic inflammatory response, protein loss is magnified severalfold during the peritonitis episode. If severe or prolonged, an episode of peritonitis may prompt removal of the peritoneal catheter or even discontinuation of the modality (i.e., switch to hemodialysis). Gram-positive organisms (especially *Staphylococcus aureus* and other *Staph* spp.) predominate; *Pseudomonas* or fungal (usually *Candida*) infections tend to be more resistant to medical therapy and typically obligate catheter removal. Antibiotic administration may be intravenous or intraperitoneal when intensive therapy is required.

For a more detailed discussion, see Singh AK, Brenner BM: Dialysis in the Treatment of Renal Failure: Chap. 262, p. 1663, in HPIM-16.

143

RENAL TRANSPLANTATION

With the advent of more potent and well-tolerated immunosuppressive regimens and further improvements in short-term graft survival, renal transplantation remains the treatment of choice for most pts with end-stage renal disease. Results are best with living-related transplantation, in part because of optimized tissue matching and in part because waiting time can be minimized. Many centers now perform living-unrelated donor (e.g., spousal) transplants. Graft survival in these cases is far superior to that observed with cadaveric transplants, although less favorable than with living-related transplants. Factors that influence graft survival are outlined in Table 143-1. Contraindications to renal transplantation are outlined in Table 143-2.

Rejection

Immunologic rejection is the major hazard to the short-term success of renal transplantation. Rejection may be (1) hyperacute (immediate graft dysfunction due to presensitization) or (2) acute (sudden change in renal function occurring within weeks to months). Rejection is characterized by a rise in serum creatinine, hypertension, fever, reduced urine output, and occasionally graft tenderness. A percutaneous renal transplant biopsy confirms the diagnosis. Treatment usually consists of a "pulse" of methylprednisolone (500–1000 mg/d for 3 days). In refractory or particularly severe cases, 7–10 days of a monoclonal antibody directed at human T lymphocytes may be given.

Immunosuppression

Maintenance immunosuppressive therapy usually consists of a three-drug regimen, with each drug targeted at a different stage in the immune response. The

Table 143-1

Some Factors That Influence Graft Survival in Renal Transplantation

---

HLA mismatch	↓
Presensitization (preformed antibodies)	↓
Pretransplant blood transfusion	↑
Very young or older donor age	↓
Female donor sex	↓
African-American donor race (compared with Caucasian)	↓
Older recipient age	↑
African-American recipient race (compared with Caucasian)	↓
Prolonged cold ischemia time	↓
Large recipient body size	↓

---

calcineurin inhibitors cyclosporine and tacrolimus are the cornerstones of immunosuppressive therapy. The most potent of orally available agents, calcineurin inhibitors have vastly improved short-term graft survival. Side effects of cyclosporine include hypertension, hyperkalemia, resting tremor, hirsutism, gingival hypertrophy, hyperlipidemia, hyperuricemia, and a slowly progressive loss of renal function with characteristic histopathologic patterns (also seen in exposed recipients of heart and liver transplants). While the side effect profile of tacrolimus is generally similar to cyclosporine, there is a higher risk of hyperglycemia, a lower risk of hypertension, and occasional hair loss rather than hirsutism.

Prednisone is frequently used in conjunction with cyclosporine, at least for the first several months following successful graft function. Side effects of pred-

Table 143-2

Contraindications to Renal Transplantation

ABSOLUTE CONTRAINDICATIONS

Active glomerulonephritis
Active bacterial or other infection
Active or very recent malignancy
HIV infection
Hepatitis B surface antigenemia
Severe degrees of comorbidity (e.g., advanced atherosclerotic vascular
  disease)

RELATIVE CONTRAINDICATIONS

Age > 70 years
Severe psychiatric disease
Moderately severe degrees of comorbidity
Hepatitis C infection with chronic hepatitis or cirrhosis
Noncompliance with dialysis or other medical therapy
Primary renal diseases
  Primary focal sclerosis with prior recurrence in transplant
  Multiple myeloma
  Amyloid
  Oxalosis

---

nisone include hypertension, glucose intolerance, Cushingoid features, osteoporosis, hyperlipidemia, acne, and depression and other mood disturbances.

Mycophenolate mofetil has proved more effective than azathioprine in combination therapy with calcineurin inhibitors and prednisone. The major side effects of mycophenolate mofetil are gastrointestinal (diarrhea is most common), and leukopenia (and thrombocytopenia to a lesser extent) develops in a fraction of patients.

Sirolimus is a newer immunosuppressive agent often used in combination with other drugs, particularly when calcineurin inhibitors are reduced or eliminated. Side effects include hyperlipidemia and oral ulcers.

Other Complications

Infection and neoplasia are important complications of renal transplantation. Infection is common in the heavily immunosuppressed host (e.g., cadaveric transplant recipient with multiple episodes of rejection requiring steroid pulses or monoclonal antibody treatment). The culprit organism depends in part on characteristics of the donor and recipient and timing following transplantation. In the first month, bacterial organisms predominate. After 1 month, there is a significant risk of systemic infection with CMV, particularly in recipients without prior exposure whose donor was CMV positive. Prophylactic use of ganciclovir or valacyclovir can reduce the risk of disease. Later on, there is a substantial risk of fungal and related infections, especially in pts who are unable to taper prednisone to <20–30 mg/d. Daily low-dose trimethoprim-sulfamethoxazole is effective at reducing the risk of *Pneumocystis carinii* infection.

EBV-associated lymphoproliferative disease is the most important neoplastic complication of renal transplantation, especially in pts who receive polyclonal (antilymphocyte globulin, used at some centers for induction of immunosuppression) or monoclonal antibody therapy. Non-Hodgkin's lymphoma and squamous cell carcinoma of the skin are also more common in this population.

For a more detailed discussion, see Carpenter CB, Milford EL, Sayegh MH: Transplantation in the Treatment of Renal Failure, Chap. 263, p. 1668, in HPIM-16.

144

GLOMERULAR DISEASES

ACUTE GLOMERULONEPHRITIS (GN)

Characterized by development, over days, of azotemia, hypertension, edema, hematuria, proteinuria, and sometimes oliguria. Salt and water retention are due to reduced GFR and may result in circulatory congestion. RBC casts on UA confirm Dx. Proteinuria usually <3 g/d. Most forms of acute GN are mediated by humoral immune mechanisms. Clinical course depends on underlying lesion (Table 144-1).

Table 144-1

Causes of Acute Glomerulonephritis

I. Infectious diseases
   A. Poststreptococcal glomerulonephritis[a]
   B. Nonstreptococcal postinfectious glomerulonephritis
      1. Bacterial: infective endocarditis, "shunt nephritis," sepsis, pneumococcal pneumonia, typhoid fever, secondary syphilis, meningococcemia
      2. Viral: hepatitis B, infectious mononucleosis, mumps, measles, varicella, vaccinia, echovirus, and coxsackievirus
      3. Parasitic: malaria, toxoplasmosis
II. Multisystem diseases: SLE, vasculitis, Henoch-Schönlein purpura, Goodpasture's syndrome
III. Primary glomerular diseases: mesangiocapillary glomerulonephritis, Berger's disease (IgA nephropathy), "pure" mesangial proliferative glomerulonephritis
IV. Miscellaneous: Guillain-Barré syndrome, irradiation of Wilm's tumor, self-administered diptheria-pertussis-tetanus vaccine, serum sickness

[a] Most common causes.
Source: RJ Glassock, BM Brenner: HPIM-13.

ACUTE POSTSTREPTOCOCCAL GN The prototype and most common cause in childhood. Nephritis develops 1–3 weeks after pharyngeal or cutaneous infection with "nephritogenic" strains of group A β-hemolytic streptococci. Dx depends on a positive pharyngeal or skin culture, rising antibody titers, and hypocomplementemia. Renal biopsy reveals diffuse proliferative GN. Treatment consists of correction of fluid and electrolyte imbalance. In most cases the disease is self-limited, although the prognosis is less favorable and urinary abnormalities are more likely to persist in adults.

POSTINFECTIOUS GN May follow other bacterial, viral, and parasitic infections. Examples are bacterial endocarditis, sepsis, hepatitis B, and pneumococcal pneumonia. Features are milder than with poststreptococcal GN. Control of primary infection usually produces resolution of GN.

SLE (LUPUS) Renal involvement is due to deposition of circulating immune complexes. Clinical features of SLE with or without renal involvement include arthralgias, "butterfly" skin rash, serositis, alopecia (hair loss), and CNS disease. Nephrotic syndrome with renal insufficiency is common. Renal biopsy reveals mesangial, focal, or diffuse GN and/or membranous nephropathy. Diffuse GN, the most common finding, is characterized by an active sediment, severe proteinuria, and progressive renal insufficiency and may have an ominous prognosis. Pts have a positive ANA, anti-dsDNA, and complement. Treatment includes glucocorticoids and cytotoxic agents. Oral or IV monthly cyclophosphamide is most commonly employed, typically for a period of 6 months. Mycophenolate mofetil or azathioprine may be used for longer-term therapy.

GOODPASTURE'S SYNDROME Characterized by lung hemorrhage, GN, and circulating antibody to basement membrane, usually in young men. Hemoptysis may precede nephritis. Rapidly progressive renal failure is typical. Circulating antiglomerular basement membrane (GBM) antibody and linear immunofluorescence on renal biopsy establish Dx. Linear IgG is also present on lung biopsy. Plasma exchange may produce remission. Severe lung hemorrhage is treated with IV glucocorticoids (e.g., 1 g/d × 3 days). Disease isolated to the kidney ("anti-GBM disease") may also occur.

HENOCH-SCHÖNLEIN PURPURA A generalized vasculitis causing GN, purpura, arthralgias, and abdominal pain; occurs mainly in children. Renal involvement is manifested by hematuria and proteinuria. Serum IgA is increased in half of pts. Renal biopsy is useful for prognosis. Treatment is symptomatic.

VASCULITIS Polyarteritis nodosa causes hypertension, arthralgias, neuropathy, and renal failure. Similar features plus palpable purpura and asthma are common in hypersensitivity angiitis. Wegener's granulomatosis involves upper respiratory tract and kidney and responds well to IV or oral cyclophosphamide.

RAPIDLY PROGRESSIVE GLOMERULONEPHRITIS
Characterized by gradual onset of hematuria, proteinuria, and renal failure, which progresses over a period of weeks to months. Crescentic GN is usually found on renal biopsy. The causes are outlined in Table 144-2. Prognosis for

Table 144-2

Causes of Rapidly Progressive Glomerulonephritis

I. Infectious diseases
   A. Poststreptococcal glomerulonephritis[a]
   B. Infective endocarditis
   C. Occult visceral sepsis
   D. Hepatitis B infection (with vasculitis and/or cryoglobulinemia)
   E. HIV infection (?)
II. Multisystem diseases
   A. Systemic lupus erythematosus
   B. Henoch-Schönlein purpura
   C. Systemic necrotizing vasculitis (including Wegener's granulomatosis)
   D. Goodpasture's syndrome
   E. Essential mixed (IgG/IgM) cryoglobulinemia
   F. Malignancy
   G. Relapsing polychondritis
   H. Rheumatoid arthritis (with vasculitis)
III. Drugs
   A. Penicillamine
   B. Hydralazine
   C. Allopurinol (with vasculitis)
   D. Rifampin
IV. Idiopathic or primary glomerular disease
   A. Idiopathic crescentic glomerulonephritis
     1. Type I—with linear deposits of Ig (anti-GBM antibody-mediated)
     2. Type II—with granular deposits of Ig (immune complex-mediated)
     3. Type III—with few or no immune deposits of Ig ("pauci-immune")
     4. Antineutrophil cytoplasmic antibody-induced, ? forme fruste of vasculitis
   B. Superimposed on another primary glomerular disease
     1. Mesangiocapillary (membranoproliferative glomerulonephritis) (especially type II)
     2. Membranous glomerulonephritis Berger's disease (IgA nephropathy)

[a] Most common causes.
Source: RJ Glassock, BM Brenner: HPIM-13.

preservation of renal function is poor. Some 50% of pts require dialysis within 6 months of diagnosis. Combinations of glucocorticoids in pulsed doses, cyclophosphamide, and intensive plasma exchange may be useful, although few prospective clinical trial data are available.

NEPHROTIC SYNDROME (NS)

Characterized by albuminuria (>3.5 g/d) and hypoalbuminemia (<30 g/L) and accompanied by edema, hyperlipidemia, and lipiduria. Complications include renal vein thrombosis and other thromboembolic events, infection, vitamin D deficiency, protein malnutrition, and drug toxicities due to decreased protein binding.

In adults, a minority of cases are secondary to diabetes mellitus, SLE, amyloidosis, drugs, neoplasia, or other disorders (Table 144-3). By exclusion, the remainder are idiopathic. Renal biopsy is required to make the diagnosis and determine therapy in idiopathic NS.

MINIMAL CHANGE DISEASE Causes about 10–15% of idiopathic NS in adults. Blood pressure is normal; GFR is normal or slightly reduced; urinary sediment is benign or may show few RBCs. Protein selectivity is variable in adults. Recent URI, allergies, or immunizations are present in some cases. ARF may rarely occur, particularly among elderly persons. Renal biopsy shows only foot process fusion on electron microscopy. Remission of proteinuria with glucocorticoids carries a good prognosis; cytotoxic therapy may be required for relapse. Progression to renal failure is uncommon. Focal sclerosis has been suspected in some cases refractory to steroid therapy.

MEMBRANOUS GN Characterized by subepithelial IgG deposits; accounts for ~45% of adult NS. Pts present with edema and nephrotic proteinuria. Blood pressure, GFR, and urine sediment are usually normal at initial presentation. Hypertension, mild renal insufficiency, and abnormal urine sediment develop later. Renal vein thrombosis is relatively common, more so than with other forms of nephrotic syndrome. Underlying diseases such as SLE, hepatitis B, and solid tumors and exposure to such drugs as high-dose captopril or penicillamine should be sought. Some pts progress to end-stage renal disease (ESRD); men and persons with very heavy proteinuria are at highest risk. Glu-

Table 144-3

Causes of Nephrotic Syndrome (NS)

Systemic Causes (25%)	Glomerular Disease (75%)
Diabetes mellitus, SLE, amyloidosis, HIV-associated nephropathy	Membranous (40%)
Drugs: gold, penicillamine, probenecid, street heroin, captopril, NSAIDs	Minimal change disease (15%)
	Focal glomerulosclerosis (15%)
Infections: bacterial endocarditis, hepatitis B, shunt infections, syphilis, malaria, hepatic schistosomiasis	Membranoproliferative GN (7%)
	Mesangioproliferative GN (5%)
Malignancy: Multiple myeloma, light-chain deposition disease, Hodgkin's and other lymphomas, leukemia, carcinoma of breast, GI tract	

Source: Modified from RJ Glassock, BM Brenner: HPIM-13.

cocorticoids are frequently prescribed but are rarely effective. Cytotoxic agents may promote complete or partial remission in some pts. There is less experience, but some positive reports, using cyclosporine.

FOCAL GLOMERULOSCLEROSIS (FGS) Can be primary or secondary. Primary tends to be more acute, similar to minimal change disease in abruptness of nephrotic syndrome, but with added features of hypertension, renal insufficiency, and hematuria. Involves fibrosis of portions of some (primarily juxtamedullary) glomeruli and is found in 15% of pts with NS. African Americans are disproportionately affected. HIV-associated nephropathy (HIVAN) and collapsing nephropathy have similar pathologic features; both tend to be more rapidly progressive than typical cases. The frequency of HIVAN has decreased with highly active antiretroviral therapy (HAART). Fewer than half of pts with primary FGS undergo remission with glucocorticoids; half progress to renal failure in 10 years. FGS may recur in a renal transplant. Presence of azotemia or hypertension reflects poor prognosis.

Secondary FGS can occur in the late stages of any form of kidney disease associated with nephron loss (e.g., remote GN, pyelonephritis, vesicoureteral reflux). Typically responds to ACE inhibition and blood pressure control. No benefit of glucocorticoids in secondary FGS. Clinical history, kidney size, and associated conditions usually allow differentiation of primary vs. secondary causes.

MEMBRANOPROLIFERATIVE GLOMERULONEPHRITIS (MPGN) Mesangial expansion and proliferation extend into the capillary loop. Two ultrastructural variants exist. In MPGN I, subendothelial electron-dense deposits are present, C3 is deposited in a granular pattern indicative of immune-complex pathogenesis, and IgG and the early components of complement may or may not be present. In MPGN II, the lamina densa of the GBM is transformed into an electron-dense character, as is the basement membrane in Bowman's capsule and tubules. C3 is found irregularly in the GBM. Small amounts of Ig (usually IgM) are present, but early components of complement are absent. Serum complement levels are decreased. MPGN affects young adults. Blood pressure and GFR are abnormal, and the urine sediment is active. Some have acute nephritis or hematuria. Similar lesions occur in SLE and hemolytic-uremic syndrome. Infection with hepatitis C virus has been linked to MPGN. Treatment with interferon α and ribavirin has resulted in remission of renal disease in some cases, depending on HCV serotype. Glucocorticoids, cytotoxic agents, antiplatelet agents, and plasmapheresis have been used with limited success. MPGN may recur in allografts.

DIABETIC NEPHROPATHY Common cause of NS. Pathologic changes include diffuse and/or nodular glomerulosclerosis, nephrosclerosis, chronic pyelonephritis, and papillary necrosis. Clinical features include proteinuria, hypertension, azotemia, and bacteriuria. Although prior duration of diabetes mellitus (DM) is variable, proteinuria may develop 10–15 years after onset, progress to NS, and then lead to renal failure over 3–5 years. Other complications of DM are common; retinopathy is nearly universal. Treatment with ACE inhibitors delays the onset of nephropathy and should be instituted in all pts tolerant to that class of drug.

If a cough develops in a pt treated with an ACE inhibitor, an angiotensin (AII) receptor antagonist is the next best choice. If hyperkalemia develops and cannot be controlled with (1) optimizing glucose control, (2) loop diuretics, or (3) occasional polystyrene sulfonate (Kayexalate), then tight control of blood pressure with alternative agents is warranted. The combination of ACE inhibitor

Table 144-4

Evaluation of Nephrotic Syndrome

24-h urine for protein; creatinine clearance
Serum albumin, cholesterol, complement
Urine protein electrophoresis
Rule out SLE, diabetes mellitus
Review drug exposure
Renal biopsy
Consider malignancy (in elderly pt with membranous GN or minimal change disease)
Consider renal vein thrombosis (if membranous GN or symptoms of pulmonary embolism are present)

and AII receptor antagonist may be more effective than either agent alone, especially if there is an additive effect on blood pressure. Modest restriction of dietary protein may also slow decline of renal function.

Evaluation of NS is shown in Table 144-4.

ASYMPTOMATIC URINARY ABNORMALITIES

Proteinuria in the nonnephrotic range and/or hematuria unaccompanied by edema, reduced GFR, or hypertension can be due to multiple causes (Table 144-5).

Table 144-5

Glomerular Causes of Asymptomatic Urinary Abnormalities

I. Hematuria with or without proteinuria
  A. Primary glomerular diseases
    1. Berger's disease (IgA nephropathy)[a]
    2. Mesangiocapillary glomerulonephritis
    3. Other primary glomerular hematurias accompanied by "pure" mesangial proliferation, focal and segmental proliferative glomerulonephritis, or other lesions
    4. "Thin basement membrane" disease (? forme fruste of Alport's syndrome)
  B. Associated with multisystem or hereditary diseases
    1. Alport's syndrome and other "benign" familial hematurias
    2. Fabry's disease
    3. Sickle cell disease
  C. Associated with infections
    1. Resolving poststreptococcal glomerulonephritis
    2. Other postinfectious glomerulonephritides
II. Isolated nonnephrotic proteinuria
  A. Primary glomerular diseases
    1. "Orthostatic" proteinuria
    2. Focal and segmental glomerulosclerosis
    3. Membranous glomerulonephritis
  B. Associated with multisystem or heredofamilial diseases
    1. Diabetes mellitus
    2. Amyloidosis
    3. Nail-patella syndrome

[a] Most common.
Source: RJ Glassock, BM Brenner: HPIM-13.

Table 144-6

Serologic Findings in Selected Multisystem Diseases Causing Glomerular Disease

Disease	C3	Ig	FANA	Anti-dsDNA	Anti-GBM	Cryo-Ig	CIC	ANCA
SLE	↓↓	↑IgG	+++	++	−	++	+++	±
Goodpasture's syndrome	−	−	−	−	+++	−	±	−
Henoch-Schönlein purpura	−	↑ IgA	−	−	−	±	++	−
Polyarteritis	↓↑	↑ IgG	+	±	−	++	+++	++
Wegener's granulomatosis	→	↑ IgA, IgE	−	−	−	±	++	+++
Cryoglobulinemia	→	↓↑ IgG IgA, IgD,	−	−	−	+++	++	−
Multiple myeloma	−	IgE	−			+	−	−
Waldenström's macroglobulinemia	−	↑ IgM	−			−	−	−
Amyloidosis	−	± Ig	−			−	−	−

Note: C3, C3 component; Ig, immunoglobulin levels; FANA, fluorescent antinuclear antibody assay; anti-dsDNA, antibody to double-stranded (native) DNA; anti-GBM, antibody to glomerular basement membrane antigens; cryo-Ig, cryoimmunoglobulin; CIC, circulating immune complexes; ANCA, antineutrophil cytoplasmic antibody; −, normal; +, occasionally slightly abnormal; ++, often abnormal; +++, severely abnormal.
Source: RJ Glassock, BM Brenner: HPIM-13.

BERGER'S DISEASE, IGA NEPHROPATHY The most common cause of recurrent hematuria of glomerular origin; is most frequent in young men. Episodes of macroscropic hematuria are present with flulike symptoms, without skin rash, abdominal pain, or arthritis. Renal biopsy shows diffuse mesangial deposition of IgA, often with lesser amounts of IgG, nearly always by C3 and properdin but not by C1q or C4. Prognosis is variable; 50% develop ESRD within 25 years; men with hypertension and heavy proteinuria are at highest risk. Glucocorticoids and other immunosuppressive agents have not proved successful. A randomized clinical trial of fish oil supplementation suggested a modest therapeutic benefit. Rarely recurs in allografts.

CHRONIC GLOMERULONEPHRITIS Characterized by persistent urinary abnormalities, slow progressive impairment of renal function, symmetrically contracted kidneys, moderate to heavy proteinuria, abnormal urinary sediment (especially RBC casts), and x-ray evidence of normal pyelocalyceal systems. The time to progression to ESRD is variable, hastened by uncontrolled hypertension and infections. Control of blood pressure is of paramount importance and is the most important factor influencing the pace of progression. While ACE inhibitors and ARBs may be the most effective agents, additional agents should be added if blood pressure is not optimally controlled with ACE inhibitors alone. Diuretics, non-dihydropyridine calcium antagonists, and β-adrenergic blockers have been successfully used in a variety of clinical settings.

GLOMERULOPATHIES ASSOCIATED WITH MULTISYSTEM DISEASE (See Table 144-6)

For a more detailed discussion, see Brady HR, O'Meara YM, Brenner BM: Glomerular Diseases, Chap. 264, p. 1674, in HPIM-16.

145

RENAL TUBULAR DISEASE

Tubulointerstitial diseases constitute a diverse group of acute and chronic, hereditary and acquired disorders involving renal tubules and supporting structures (Table 145-1). Functionally, they may result in nephrogenic diabetes insipidus (DI) with polyuria, nocturia, non-anion-gap metabolic acidosis, salt-wasting, and hypo- or hyperkalemia. Azotemia is common, owing to associated glomerular fibrosis and/or ischemia. Compared with glomerulopathies, proteinuria and hematuria are less dramatic, and hypertension is less common. Functional consequences of tubular dysfunction are outlined in Table 145-2.

ACUTE (ALLERGIC) INTERSTITIAL NEPHRITIS (AIN)
Drugs are a leading cause of this type of renal failure, usually identified by a gradual rise in the serum creatinine at least several days after the institution of therapy, occasionally accompanied by fever, eosinophilia, rash, and arthralgias.

Table 145-1

Principal Causes of Tubulointerstitial Disease of the Kidney

TOXINS

Endogenous toxins
  Analgesic nephropathy[a]
  Lead nephropathy
  Miscellaneous nephrotoxins (e.g., antibiotics, cyclosporine, radiographic
    contrast media, heavy metals)[a,b]
Metabolic toxins
  Acute uric acid nephropathy
  Gouty nephropathy[a]
  Hypercalcemic nephropathy
  Hypokalemic nephropathy
  Miscellaneous metabolic toxins (e.g., hyperoxaluria, cystinosis, Fabry's
    disease

NEOPLASIA

Lymphoma	Multiple myeloma
Leukemia	

IMMUNE DISORDERS

Hypersensitivity nephropathy[a,b]	Transplant rejection
Sjögren's syndrome	HIV-associated nephropathy
Amyloidosis	

VASCULAR DISORDERS

Arteriolar nephrosclerosis[a]	Medullary cystic disease
Atheroembolic disease	Medullary sponge kidney
Sickle cell nephropathy	Polycystic kidney disease
Acute tubular necrosis[a,b]	

HEREDITARY RENAL DISEASES

Hereditary nephritis (Alport's syndrome)

INFECTIOUS INJURY

Acute pyelonephritis[a,b]	Chronic pyelonephritis

MISCELLANEOUS DISORDERS

Chronic urinary tract obstruction[a]	Radiation nephritis
Vesicoureteral reflux[a]	

[a] Common.
[b] Typically acute.

In addition to azotemia, there may be evidence of tubular dysfunction (e.g., hyperkalemia, metabolic acidosis). Drugs that commonly cause AIN include: anti-staphyloccal (i.e., methicillin, oxacillin, or nafcillin) and other penicillins, cephalosporins, sulfonamides, quinolones, rifampin, allopurinol, and cimetidine; NSAIDs may cause AIN with or without nephrotic syndrome. UA shows hematuria, pyuria, and eosinophiluria on Hansel's or Wright's stain.

Renal dysfunction usually improves after withdrawal of the offending drug, but complete recovery may be delayed and incomplete. In uncontrolled studies, glucocorticoids have been shown to promote earlier recovery of renal function. Other than kidney biopsy, no specific diagnostic tests are available. Acute py-

Table 145-2

Transport Dysfunction of Tubulointerstitial Disease

Defect	Cause(s)
Reduced GFR[a]	Obliteration of microvasculature and obstruction of tubules
Fanconi syndrome	Damage to proximal tubular reabsorption of glucose, amino acids, phosphate, and bicarbonate
Hyperchloremic acidosis[a]	1. Reduced ammonia production 2. Inability to acidify the collecting duct fluid (distal renal tubular acidosis) 3. Proximal bicarbonate wasting
Tubular or small-molecular-weight proteinuria[a]	Failure of proximal tubule protein reabsorption
Polyuria, isothenuria[a]	Damage to medullary tubules and vasculature
Hyperkalemia[a]	Potassium secretory defects including aldosterone resistance
Salt wasting	Distal tubular damage with impaired sodium reabsorption

[a] Common.

elonephritis may also cause AIN, although it is rarely associated with renal failure, unless bilateral (or present in a single functioning kidney) or complicated by urinary tract obstruction, sepsis syndrome, or volume depletion.

CHRONIC INTERSTITIAL NEPHRITIS (IN)

Analgesic nephropathy is an important cause of chronic kidney disease that results from the cumulative (in quantity and duration) effects of combination analgesic agents, usually phenacetin and aspirin. It is thought to be a more common cause of end-stage renal disease in Australia/New Zealand than elsewhere owing to the larger per capita ingestion of analgesic agents in that region of the world. Transitional cell carcinoma may develop. Analgesic nephropathy should be suspected in pts with a history of chronic headache or back pain with chronic kidney disease (CKD) that is otherwise unexplained. Manifestations include papillary necrosis, calculi, sterile pyuria, and azotemia. Metabolic causes of chronic IN include: hypercalcemia (with nephrocalcinosis), oxalosis (primary or secondary, e.g., with intestinal malabsorption, leading to nephrocalcinosis), hypokalemia, and hyperuricemia or hyperuricosuria. Chronic IN can occur in association with several systemic diseases, including sarcoidosis, Sjögren's syndrome, and tuberculosis, and following radiation or chemotherapy exposure (e.g., ifosfamide, cisplatin).

POLYCYSTIC KIDNEY DISEASE

Autosomal dominant polycystic kidney disease (ADPKD) is the most important hereditary renal disease (except perhaps for "essential" hypertension). It is characterized clinically by episodic flank pain, hematuria (often gross), hypertension, and/or urinary infection in the third or fourth decade. The kidneys are often palpable and occasionally of very large size. Hepatic cysts and intracranial Berry aneurysms may also be present.

The expression of ADPKD is variable. Some persons discover the disease incidentally in late adult life, having had mild to moderate hypertension earlier.

More often, azotemia is progressive and unfortunately does not appear to respond as favorably to ACE inhibition or to the restriction of dietary protein intake as other causes of renal disease. The diagnosis is usually made by ultrasonography. Renal cysts are common (50% of persons >50 years have at least one cyst), and multiple renal cysts do not necessarily indicate the presence of ADPKD.

RENAL TUBULAR ACIDOSIS (RTA)

This describes a number of pathophysiologically distinct entities of tubular function whose common feature is the presence of a non-anion-gap metabolic acidosis. Diarrhea and RTA together constitute the vast majority of cases of non-anion-gap metabolic acidosis.

DISTAL (TYPE 1) RTA   Pts are unable to acidify the urine despite acidosis; it may be inherited (autosomal dominant) or acquired due to autoimmune and inflammatory diseases (e.g., Sjögren's syndrome, sarcoidosis), urinary tract obstruction, or amphotericin B therapy. Type I RTA may be associated with hypokalemia, hypercalciuria, and osteomalacia.

PROXIMAL (TYPE II) RTA   There is a defect in bicarbonate reabsorption, usually associated with glycosuria, aminoaciduria, phosphaturia, and uricosuria (indicating proximal tubular dysfunction); it may be inherited or acquired due to myeloma, renal transplantation, or drugs (e.g., ifosfamide, L-lysine). Treatment requires large doses of bicarbonate, which may aggravate hypokalemia, and repletion of phosphorus to prevent bone disease.

TYPE IV RTA   Due to a defect in ammonium excretion, acidosis is accompanied by hyperkalemia and usually with low renin and aldosterone levels (and minimal response to exogenous mineralocorticoid). It is associated with diabetes, other forms of glomerulosclerosis, and many forms of advanced CKD (especially with tubulointerstitial component).

℞ TREATMENT

Tubulointerstitial diseases associated with exogenous toxins (e.g., analgesic nephropathy, lead and other heavy metal nephropathy) should be treated by withdrawal of the offending toxin. Primary oxalosis may require liver (or combined liver-kidney) transplantation, but secondary oxalosis can be improved with a low-oxalate diet, generous fluid intake, and supplemental calcium salts (calcium carbonate or calcium citrate) with meals to bind intestinal oxalate and prevent hyperoxalemia/hyperoxaluria. Calcium citrate affords additional protection against nephrolithiasis (correcting hypocitraturia). Hypercalcemia due to multiple causes (e.g., primary hyperparathyroidism, vitamin D excess, thiazide therapy, milk-alkali syndrome) can usually be corrected once recognized. Pts with pyelonephritis due to reflux or recurrent UTI with ADPKD may benefit from suppressive antibiotic therapy. The treatment of RTA depends on type but focuses on correction of the acidosis and prevention of nephrolithiasis (type I), vitamin D deficiency and other metabolic complications (type II), and severe hyperkalemia (type IV).

For a more detailed discussion, see Yu ASL, Brenner BM: Tubulointerstitial Diseases of the Kidney, Chap. 266, p. 1702, in HPIM-16.

146

URINARY TRACT INFECTIONS

ACUTE URINARY TRACT INFECTIONS: URETHRITIS, CYSTITIS, AND PYELONEPHRITIS

EPIDEMIOLOGY   Urinary tract infections (UTIs) are classified epidemiologically as catheter-associated (nosocomial) and non-catheter-associated (community-acquired). Community-acquired UTIs result in >7 million office visits annually in the United States. Most cases involve sexually active young women. UTIs are rare among men <50 years of age. Asymptomatic bacteriuria is common among young women but is most frequently documented in elderly men and women, with rates up to 50% in some studies.

ETIOLOGY   Uncomplicated community-acquired UTIs—defined as those not associated with calculi, obstruction, or urologic manipulation—are caused by *Escherichia coli* in ~80% of cases; other gram-negative rods, including *Proteus*, *Klebsiella*, and occasionally *Enterobacter*, cause smaller proportions of cases. Gram-positive etiologic agents of UTI include *Staphylococcus saprophyticus*, which causes 10–15% of acute UTIs in young women, and enterococci. *E. coli*, *Proteus*, *Klebsiella*, *Enterobacter*, *Serratia*, and *Pseudomonas* cause recurrent infections and UTIs associated with urologic manipulation, calculi, or obstruction. *Proteus* and *Klebsiella* predispose to stone formation and are isolated more often from pts with calculi.

PATHOGENESIS   Most UTIs result when bacteria gain access to the bladder via the urethra. Some strains of bacteria (e.g., *E. coli*, *Proteus*) are uropathogenic. These strains have virulence genes that increase the likelihood of UTI (e.g., genes encoding fimbriae that mediate attachment to uroepithelial cells). Upper tract disease occurs when bacteria ascend from the bladder. Women prone to infections are colonized with enteric gram-negative bacilli in the periurethral area and distal urethra prior to bacteriuria. Alterations of the normal vaginal flora (e.g., due to antibiotic treatment, other genital infections, or contraceptive use) all contribute to UTIs. Other risk factors include female gender, sexual activity, pregnancy, genitourinary obstruction, neurogenic bladder dysfunction, and vesiculoureteral reflux. Hematogenous infection of the kidney is less common and occurs most often in debilitated pts or in the setting of staphylococcal bacteremia or candidemia.

CLINICAL PRESENTATIONS

• Cystitis: Pts have dysuria, frequency, urgency, and suprapubic pain. Urine is cloudy, malodorous, and sometimes bloody. Systemic signs are usually absent. Approximately one-third of pts may have silent upper tract disease.
• Acute pyelonephritis: Symptoms develop quickly over hours to a day. Pts are febrile with shaking chills and can have nausea, vomiting, and diarrhea. Symptoms of cystitis may be absent. Marked tenderness may be evident on deep pressure in one or both costovertebral angles or on deep abdominal palpation.
• Urethritis: Women with dysuria, frequency, and pyuria but insignificant or no growth on bacterial urine cultures may have urethritis due to sexually transmitted pathogens such as *Chlamydia trachomatis*, *Neisseria gonorrhoeae*, or herpes simplex virus (Chap. 88). Pts with hematuria, suprapubic pain, an abrupt onset of illness, an illness duration of <3 days, and a history of UTIs along with a urine culture yielding low counts of *E. coli* usually have cystitis.

• Catheter-associated UTIs (Chap. 92): Most of these infections cause minimal symptoms and no fever; they often resolve after catheter removal. Treatment without catheter removal usually fails. Bacteriuria should be ignored unless the pt develops symptoms or is at high risk for bacteremia.

DIAGNOSIS

• Urine cultures should be performed for all pts with suspected upper tract infections, for those with complicating factors, and when the diagnosis of cystitis is in question. Most symptomatic pts have $\geq 10^5$ bacteria/mL of urine. Asymptomatic pts should be treated if a single bacterial species is identified at counts of $\geq 10^5$/mL in two consecutive urine cultures. Bacteriuria from suprapubic aspirates or $\geq 10^2$ bacteria/mL of urine obtained via catheterization is significant.
• The presence of bacteria in Gram-stained uncentrifuged urine indicates infection and correlates with $\geq 10^5$ bacteria/mL in urine cultures.
• Urinalysis: Pyuria is a highly sensitive indicator of infection. Leukocyte esterase "dipstick" positivity is useful when microscopy is not available. Pyuria without bacteriuria may indicate infection with unusual organisms such as *C. trachomatis* or *Mycobacterium tuberculosis* or may be due to noninfectious causes such as calculi. Leukocyte casts are pathognomonic of acute pyelonephritis.

 TREATMENT

Underlying Principles

• Except in acute uncomplicated cystitis in women, a quantitative urine culture should precede empirical treatment, and susceptibility testing should be performed.
• Factors predisposing to infection should be identified and corrected if possible.
• Each course of treatment should be classified as a cure or a failure, and recurrent infections should be classified as early (developing within 2 weeks of the end of therapy) or late and as same-strain or different-strain. Relief of clinical symptoms does not always indicate bacteriologic cure.
• Lower-tract infections usually require only short courses of treatment. Early recurrences may be due to upper-tract foci of infection, while late infections usually represent reinfection.
• Most community-acquired infections are due to antibiotic-sensitive strains, despite increasing antibiotic resistance.
• Antibiotic-resistant infections should be suspected in pts with recurrent infections, instrumentation, or recent hospitalization.

Specific Recommendations
See Table 146-1 for antibiotic choices. Asymptomatic bacteriuria in noncatheterized pts should not be treated unless the pt is pregnant or has other medical conditions such as neutropenia, renal transplantation, obstruction, or other complicating factors. Urologic evaluation should be considered in pts with relapsing infection, a history of childhood infection, stones, or painless hematuria and in women with recurrent pyelonephritis. Most men with UTIs should have a urologic evaluation. Anyone with signs or symptoms of obstruction or stones should undergo prompt urologic evaluation.

PROGNOSIS Repeated symptomatic UTIs with obstructive uropathy, neurogenic bladder, structural renal disease, or diabetes progress to chronic renal disease with high frequency.

Table 146-1

Treatment Regimens for Bacterial Urinary Tract Infections

Condition	Characteristic Pathogens	Mitigating Circumstances	Recommended Empirical Treatment[a]
Acute uncomplicated cystitis in women	Escherichia coli, Staphylococcus saprophyticus, Proteus mirabilis, Klebsiella pneumoniae	None	3-Day regimens: oral TMP-SMX, TMP, quinolone; 7-day regimen: macrocrystalline nitrofurantoin[b]
		Diabetes, symptoms for >7 d, recent UTI, use of diaphragm, age >65 years	Consider 7-day regimen: oral TMP-SMX, TMP, quinolone[b]
		Pregnancy	Consider 7-day regimen: oral amoxicillin, macrocrystalline nitrofurantoin, cefpodoxime proxetil, or TMP-SMX[b]
Acute uncomplicated pyelonephritis in women	E. coli, P. mirabilis, S. saprophyticus	Mild to moderate illness, no nausea or vomiting; outpatient therapy	Oral[c] quinolone for 7–14 d (initial dose given IV if desired); or single-dose ceftriaxone (1 g) or gentamicin (3–5 mg/kg) IV followed by oral TMP-SMX[b] for 14 d
		Severe illness or possible urosepsis: hospitalization required	Parenteral[d] quinolone, gentamicin (± ampicillin), ceftriaxone, or aztreonam until defervescence; then oral[c] quinolone, cephalosporin, or TMP-SMX for 14 d
Complicated UTI in men and women	E. coli, Proteus, Klebsiella, Pseudomonas, Serratia, enterococci, staphylococci	Mild to moderate illness, no nausea or vomiting; outpatient therapy	Oral[c] quinolone for 10–14 d
		Severe illness or possible urosepsis: hospitalization required	Parenteral[d] ampicillin and gentamicin, quinolone, ceftriaxone, aztreonam, ticarcillin/clavulanate, or imipenem-cilastatin until defervescence; then oral[c] quinolone or TMP-SMX for 10–21 d

[a] Treatments listed are those to be prescribed before the etiologic agent is known; Gram's staining can be helpful in the selection of empirical therapy. Such therapy can be modified once the infecting agent has been identified. Fluoroquinolones should not be used in pregnancy. TMP-SMX, although not approved for use in pregnancy, has been widely used. Gentamicin should be used with caution in pregnancy because of its possible toxicity to eighth-nerve development in the fetus.

[b] Multiday oral regimens for cystitis are as follows: TMP-SMX, 160/800 mg q12h; TMP, 100 mg q12h; norfloxacin, 400 mg q12h; ciprofloxacin, 250 mg q12h; ofloxacin, 200 mg q12h; levofloxacin, 250 mg/d; gatifloxacin, 200 or 400 mg/d; moxifloxacin, 400 mg/d; enoxacin, 400 mg q12h; macrocrystalline nitrofurantoin, 100 mg qid; amoxicillin, 250 mg q8h; cefpodoxime proxetil, 100 mg q12h.

[c] Oral regimens for pyelonephritis and complicated UTI are as follows: TMP-SMX, 160/800 mg q12h; ciprofloxacin, 500 mg q12h; ofloxacin, 200–300 mg q12h; lomefloxacin, 400 mg/d; enoxacin, 400 mg q12h; gatifloxacin, 400 mg/d; levofloxacin, 250 mg/d; amoxicillin, 500 mg q8h; cefpodoxime proxetil, 200 mg q12h.

[d] Parenteral regimens are as follows: ciprofloxacin, 400 mg q12h; ofloxacin, 400 mg q12h; gatifloxacin, 400 mg/d; levofloxacin, 500 mg/d; gentamicin, 1 mg/kg q8h; ceftriaxone, 1–2 g/d; ampicillin, 1 g q6h; imipenem-cilastatin, 250–500 mg q6–8h; ticarcillin/clavulanate, 3.2 g q8h; aztreonam, 1 g q8–12h.

PREVENTION Women experiencing symptomatic UTIs ≥3 times a year are candidates for long-term administration of low-dose antibiotics. These women should avoid spermicide use and should void after intercourse. Trimethoprim-sulfamethoxazole (TMP-SMX; 80/400 mg), trimethoprim (100 mg), or nitrofurantoin (50 mg) daily or thrice weekly is effective. Alternatively, if UTIs are temporally related to sexual intercourse, the same regimens prevent infection if given only after intercourse.

PAPILLARY NECROSIS

* Papillary necrosis is an infection of the renal pyramids in association with vascular disease of the kidney or urinary tract obstruction. Acute renal failure with oliguria or anuria can occur.
* Risk factors include diabetes, sickle cell disease, alcoholism, and vascular disease.
* Hematuria, flank or abdominal pain, chills, and fever are common symptoms.

EMPHYSEMATOUS PYELONEPHRITIS

* Emphysematous pyelonephritis is seen in diabetic pts in concert with urinary obstruction and chronic infection.
* This disease is characterized by a rapidly progressive course, fever, leukocytosis, renal parenchymal necrosis, and the accumulation of fermentative gases in kidney and perinephric tissues.
* *E. coli* is the most common etiologic agent, but other members of the Enterobacteriaceae can also cause the syndrome.

PROSTATITIS
Acute Bacterial Prostatitis

Acute bacterial prostatitis occurs spontaneously in young men but is associated with indwelling catheters in older men. Pts have fever, chills, dysuria, and a tense or boggy, tender prostate. Prostatic massage can cause bacteremia and should be avoided. Gram's staining and culture of urine identify the etiologic agent. *E. coli* or *Klebsiella* causes most non-catheter-associated cases, while catheter-associated cases are caused by a broader spectrum of pathogens. Third-generation cephalosporins, fluoroquinolones, or aminoglycosides are efficacious.

Chronic Bacterial Prostatitis

Chronic bacterial prostatitis is an uncommon entity. The diagnosis is suggested by a pattern of relapsing UTI in middle-aged men. Symptoms are lacking between episodes, and the prostate feels normal on examination. Some pts have obstructive symptoms or perineal pain. *E. coli*, *Klebsiella*, *Proteus*, or other uropathogenic bacteria can be cultured from expressed prostatic secretions or postmassage urine. Antibiotics relieve acute symptoms, but antibiotic penetration into an uninflamed prostate is poor, and relapse is common. Fluoroquinolones are the most effective agents but must be given for at least 12 weeks. Prolonged courses with low-dose antimicrobial agents may suppress symptoms and keep bladder urine sterile.

Chronic Pelvic Pain Syndrome

Chronic pelvic pain syndrome is characterized by the symptoms of prostatitis with few clinical signs and no bacterial growth in cultures. In sexually active young men, a sexually transmitted disease is likely. Some pts improve with

4–6 weeks of treatment with erythromycin, doxycycline, TMP-SMX, or a fluor-oquinolone, but controlled trials are lacking.

For a more detailed discussion, see Stamm WE: Urinary Tract Infections and Pyelonephritis, Chap. 269, p. 1715, in HPIM-16.

147

RENOVASCULAR DISEASE

Ischemic injury to the kidney depends on the rate, site, severity, and duration of vascular compromise. Manifestations range from painful infarction to acute renal failure (ARF), impaired GFR, hematuria, or tubular dysfunction. Renal ischemia of any etiology may cause renin-mediated hypertension.

Acute Occlusion of a Renal Artery

Can be due to thrombosis or embolism (from valvular disease, endocarditis, mural thrombi, or atrial arrhythmias).

Thrombosis of Renal Arteries Large renal infarcts cause pain, vomiting, nausea, hypertension, fever, proteinuria, hematuria, and elevated LDH and AST. In unilateral lesion, renal functional loss depends on contralateral function. IVP or radionuclide scan shows unilateral hypofunction; ultrasound is typically normal until scarring develops. Renal arteriography establishes diagnosis. With occlusions of large arteries, surgery may be the initial therapy; anticoagulation should be used for occlusions of small arteries.

Renal Atheroembolism Usually arises when aortic angiography or surgery causes cholesterol embolization of small renal vessels. Renal insufficiency may develop suddenly or gradually. Pace may be progressive or "stuttering." Associated findings are GI or retinal ischemia with cholesterol emboli visible on funduscopic examination, pancreatitis, neurologic deficits (especially confusion), livedo reticularis, toe gangrene, and hypertension. Skin or renal biopsy may be necessary for diagnosis. Heparin and other anticoagulants are contraindicated. Should be suspected when renal function does not improve >1 week after radiocontrast exposure with presumed contrast nephropathy.

Renal Vein Thrombosis

This occurs in a variety of settings, including pregnancy, oral contraceptive use, trauma, nephrotic syndrome (especially membranous nephropathy, see Chap. 144), dehydration (in infants), extrinsic compression of the renal vein (lymph nodes, aortic aneurysm, tumor), and invasion of the renal vein by renal cell carcinoma. Definitive Dx is established by selective renal renography. Thrombolytic therapy may be effective. Oral anticoagulants (warfarin) usually prescribed for longer term.

Renal Artery Stenosis (See Table 147-1)

Main cause of renovascular hypertension; due to (1) atherosclerosis (two-thirds of cases; usually men aged >60 years, advanced retinopathy) or (2) fibromuscular dysplasia (a third of cases; usually white women aged <45 years, brief history of hypertension). Renal hypoperfusion activates renin-angiotensin-aldosterone (RAA) axis. Suggestive clinical features include onset of hypertension <30 or >50 years of age, abdominal or femoral bruits, hypokalemic alkalosis, moderate to severe retinopathy, acute onset of hypertension or malignant hypertension, and hypertension resistant to medical therapy. Malignant hypertension (Chap. 122) may also be caused by renal vascular occlusion. Nitroprusside, labetalol, or calcium antagonists are generally effective in lowering bp acutely, although inhibitors of the RAA axis [e.g., ACE inhibitors, angiotensin II receptor blockers (ARBs)] are most effective long-term treatment, if disease is not bilateral.

The "gold standard" in diagnosis of renal artery stenosis is conventional arteriography. Magnetic resonance angiography (MRA) is used in many centers, especially among pts with renal insufficiency at higher risk for contrast nephropathy. MRA may overestimate the severity of stenosis relative to angiography. In pts with normal renal function and hypertension, the captopril (or enalaprilat) renogram may be used. Lateralization of renal function [accentuation of the difference between affected and unaffected (or "less affected") sides] is suggestive of significant vascular disease. Test results may be falsely negative in the presence of bilateral disease.

Surgical revascularization appears to be superior for ostial lesions characteristic of atherosclerosis. The relative efficacy of surgery compared with angioplasty (especially with stenting) for fibromuscular dysplasia or for nonocclusive, nonostial atherosclerotic disease is unclear. Angioplasty (with or without stenting) tends to be most effective for mid-vessel or more distal lesions. No studies have adequately compared revascularization with medical therapy.

Table 147-1

Clinical Findings Associated with Renal Artery Stenosis

Hypertension
  Abrupt onset of hypertension before the age of 50 years (suggestive of fibromuscular dysplasia)
  Abrupt onset of hypertension at or after the age of 50 years (suggestive of atherosclerotic renal artery stenosis)
  Accelerated or malignant hypertension
  Refractory hypertension (not responsive to therapy with ≥3 drugs)
Renal abnormalities
  Unexplained azotemia (suggestive of atherosclerotic renal artery stenosis)
  Azotemia induced by treatment with an angiotensin-converting enzyme inhibitor
  Unilateral small kidney
  Unexplained hypokalemia
Other findings
  Abdominal bruit, flank bruit, or both
  Severe retinopathy
  Carotid, coronary, or peripheral vascular disease
  Unexplained congestive heart failure or acute pulmonary edema

Source: From RD Safian, SC Textor: Am J Kidney Dis 36:1089, 2000, reprinted with permission.

ACE inhibitors or ARBs are ideal agents for hypertension associated with renal artery stenosis, except in pts with bilateral disease (see "Ischemic Nephropathy," below) or disease in a solitary kidney (including an allograft).

Ischemic Nephropathy

In addition to the association between renal artery stenosis and hypertension, there is an important (and less well recognized) association between renal artery stenosis and progressive chronic kidney disease (CKD). Because most pts do not undergo either kidney biopsy or angiography prior to the initiation of dialysis, it is difficult to estimate the incidence of renovascular disease as a primary cause of end-stage renal disease (ESRD) (some have suggested up to 15–20%, even greater among elderly pts). Indeed, many individuals diagnosed with ESRD due to hypertension or diabetes suffer from ischemic nephropathy, with diabetes being a secondary cause and hypertension a consequence, rather than a cause.

The presence of widespread atherosclerotic vascular disease, asymmetric kidney size and function, and hypertension suggest renovascular disease; episodic "flash" pulmonary edema, renal insufficiency, and ARF in response to a trial of ACE inhibitors suggests that the disease may be severe and bilateral.

Revascularization with the goal of preservation of renal function is sometimes entertained. Angioplasty is less often successful than for fibromuscular dysplasia, although stenting may offer the potential for better "noninvasive" results. Whether with surgical or angiographic intervention, it appears that kidneys <8 cm in size are unlikely to recover substantial renal function. The use of aspirin and lipid-lowering agents is advisable in pts with evidence of renovascular disease, regardless of revascularization options.

Scleroderma

May cause sudden oliguric renal failure and severe hypertension due to small-vessel occlusion in previously stable pts. Aggressive control of bp with ACE inhibitors and dialysis, if necessary, improve survival and may restore renal function.

Arteriolar Nephrosclerosis

Persistent hypertension causes arteriosclerosis of the renal arterioles and loss of renal function (nephrosclerosis). "Benign" nephrosclerosis is associated with loss of cortical kidney mass and thickened afferent arterioles and mild to moderate impairment of renal function. Malignant nephrosclerosis is characterized by accelerated rise in bp and the clinical features of malignant hypertension, including renal failure (Chap. 122). Malignant nephrosclerosis may be seen in association with cocaine use. Agressive control of the bp can usually halt or reverse the deterioration of renal function, and some pts have a return of renal function to near normal.

Hemolytic-Uremic Syndrome

Characterized by ARF, microangiopathic hemolytic anemia, and thrombocytopenia; increasingly recognized in adults; may be preceded by a prodrome of bloody diarrhea and abdominal pain. Fibrin deposition leads to small-vessel occlusion. Lack of fever or CNS involvement helps to distinguish it from thrombotic thrombocytopenic purpura. Plasmapheresis may be of benefit; prognosis for recovery of renal function is generally poor.

Toxemias of Pregnancy

Preeclampsia is characterized by hypertension, proteinuria, edema, consumptive coagulopathy, sodium retention, hyperuricemia, and hyperreflexia; eclampsia is the further development of seizures. Glomerular swelling and/or ischemia causes renal insufficiency. Coagulation abnormalities and ARF may occur. Treatment consists of bed rest, sedation, control of neurologic manifestations with magnesium sulfate, control of hypertension with vasodilators and other antihypertensive agents proved safe in pregnancy, and delivery of the infant.

Vasculitis

Renal complications are frequent and severe in polyarteritis nodosa, hypersensitivity angiitis, Wegener's granulomatosis, and other forms of vasculitis (Chap. 162). Therapy is directed toward the underlying disease.

Sickle Cell Nephropathy

The hypertonic and relatively hypoxic renal medulla coupled with slow blood flow in the vasa recta favors sickling. Papillary necrosis, cortical infarcts, functional tubule abnormalities (nephrogenic diabetes insipidus), glomerulopathy, nephrotic syndrome, and, rarely, ESRD may be complications.

For a more detailed discussion, see Badr KF, Brenner BM: Vascular Injury to the Kidney, Chap. 267, p. 1706, in HPIM-16.

148

NEPHROLITHIASIS

Renal calculi are common, affecting ~1% of the population, and recurrent in more than half of pts. Stone formation begins when urine becomes supersaturated with insoluble components due to (1) low volume, (2) excessive excretion of selected compounds, or (3) other factors (e.g., urinary pH) that diminish solubility. Approximately 75% of stones are Ca-based (the majority are Ca oxalate; also Ca phosphate and other mixed stones), 15% struvite (magnesium-ammonium-phosphate), 5% uric acid, and 1% cystine, depending on the metabolic disturbance(s) from which they arise.

Signs and Symptoms

Stones in the renal pelvis may be asymptomatic or cause hematuria alone; with passage, obstruction may occur at any site along the collecting system. Obstruction related to the passing of a stone leads to severe pain, often radiating to the groin, sometimes accompanied by intense visceral symptoms (i.e., nausea, vomiting, diaphoresis, light-headedness), hematuria, pyuria, UTI, and, rarely, hydronephrosis. Staghorn calculi are associated with recurrent UTI with urea-splitting organisms (*Proteus, Klebsiella, Providencia, Morganella*, and others).

Stone Composition

Most stones are composed of Ca oxalate. These may be associated with hypercalciuria or hyperoxaluria. Hypercalciuria can be seen in association with a very high Na diet, loop diuretic therapy, distal (type I) renal tubular acidosis (RTA), sarcoidosis, Cushing's syndrome, conditions associated with hypercalcemia (e.g., primary hyperparathyroidism, vitamin D excess, milk-alkali syndrome), or may be idiopathic.

Hyperoxaluria may be seen with intestinal (especially ileal) malabsorption syndromes (e.g., inflammatory bowel disease, pancreatitis), due to the binding of intestinal Ca by fatty acids within the bowel lumen to form soaps, allowing free oxalate to be absorbed (and then excreted via the urinary tract). Ca oxalate stones may also form due to (1) a deficiency of urinary citrate, an inhibitor of stone formation that is underexcreted with metabolic acidosis; and (2) hyperuricosuria (see below). Ca phosphate stones are much less common and tend to occur in the setting of an abnormally high urinary pH (7–8), usually in association with a complete or partial distal (type I) RTA.

Struvite stones form in the collecting system when infection with urea-splitting organisms is present. Struvite is the most common component of staghorn calculi and obstruction. Risk factors include previous UTI, nonstruvite stone disease, urinary catheters, neurogenic bladder (e.g., with diabetes or multiple sclerosis), and instrumentation.

Uric acid stones develop when the urine is saturated with uric acid in the presence of dehydration and an acid urine pH. Pts with myeloproliferative disorders (esp. after treatment with chemotherapy), gout, acute and chronic renal failure, and following cyclosporine therapy often develop hyperuricemia and hyperuricosuria and are at risk for stones if the urine volume diminishes. Hyperuricosuria without hyperuricemia may be seen in association with certain drugs (e.g., probenecid, high-dose salicylates).

Cystine stones are the result of a rare inherited defect of renal and intestinal transport resulting in overexcretion of cystine. Stones begin in childhood and are a rare cause of staghorn calculi; they occasionally lead to end-stage renal disease. Stones are more likely to form in acidic urinary pH.

Workup

Although some have advocated a complete workup after a first stone episode, others would defer that evaluation until there has been evidence of recurrence or if there is no obvious cause (e.g., low fluid intake during the summer months with obvious dehydration). Table 148-1 outlines a reasonable workup for an outpatient with an uncomplicated kidney stone.

Table 148-1

Workup for an Outpatient with a Renal Stone

1. Dietary and fluid intake history
2. Careful medical history and physical examination, focusing on systemic diseases
3. Abdominal flat plate examination
4. Serum chemistries: BUN, creatinine (Cr), uric acid, calcium, phosphate, chloride, bicarbonate
5. Timed urine collections (at least one day during week, one day on weekend): Cr, Na, K, urea nitrogen, uric acid, calcium, phosphate, oxalate, citrate, magnesium

Table 148-2

Specific Therapies for Nephrolithiasis

Stone Type	Dietary Modifications	Other
Calcium oxalate	Increase fluid intake Moderate sodium intake Moderate oxalate intake Moderate protein intake Moderate fat intake	Citrate supplementation (calcium or potassium salts > sodium) Cholestyramine or other therapy for fat malabsorption Thiazides if hypercalciuric Allopurinol if hyperuricosuric
Calcium phosphate	Increase fluid intake Moderate sodium intake	Thiazides if hypercalciuric
Struvite	Increase fluid intake; same as calcium oxalate if evidence of calcium oxalate nidus for struvite	Mandelamine and vitamin C or daily suppressive antibiotic therapy (e.g., trimethoprim-sulfamethoxazole)
Uric acid	Increase fluid intake Moderate dietary protein intake	Allopurinol
Cystine	Increase fluid intake	Alkali therapy Penicillamine

Note: Sodium excretion correlates with calcium excretion.

℞ TREATMENT

Treatment of renal calculi is often empirical, based on odds (Ca oxalate most common stones) or clinical Hx. Sometimes a stone is recovered and can be analyzed for content. Stone analysis is advisable, especially for pts with more complex presentations or recurrent disease. An increase in fluid intake to at least 2.5–3 L/d is advisable, regardless of the type of stone. Conservative recommendations for pts with Ca oxalate stones (i.e., low-salt, low-fat, moderate-protein diet) are thought to be healthful in general and therefore advisable in pts whose condition is otherwise uncomplicated. In contrast to prior assumptions, dietary calcium intake does not contribute to stone risk; rather, dietary calcium may help to reduce oxalate absorption and reduce stone risk. Table 148-2 outlines stone-specific therapies for pts with complex or recurrent nephrolithiasis.

For a more detailed discussion, see Asplin JR, Coe FL, Favus MJ: Nephrolithiasis, Chap. 268, p. 1710, in HPIM-16

149

URINARY TRACT OBSTRUCTION

Urinary tract obstruction (UTO), a potentially reversible cause of renal failure (RF), should be considered in all cases of acute or abrupt worsening of chronic RF. Consequences depend on duration and severity and whether the obstruction is unilateral or bilateral. UTO may occur at any level from collecting tubule to urethra. It is preponderant in women (pelvic tumors), elderly men (prostatic disease), diabetic pts (papillary necrosis), pts with neurologic diseases (spinal cord injury or multiple sclerosis, with neurogenic bladder), or in individuals with retroperitoneal lymphadenopathy or fibrosis, vesicoureteral reflux, nephrolithiasis, or other causes of functional urinary retention (e.g., anticholinergic drugs).

Clinical Manifestations

Pain can occur in some settings (obstruction due to stones) but is not common. In men, there is frequently a history of prostatism. Physical exam may reveal an enlarged bladder by percussion over the lower abdominal wall. Other findings depend on the clinical scenario. Prostatic hypertrophy can be determined by digital rectal examination. A bimanual examination in women may show a pelvic or rectal mass. The workup of pts with RF suspected of having UTO is shown in Fig. 149-1. Laboratory studies may show marked elevations of BUN and creatinine; if the obstruction has been of sufficient duration, there may be evidence of tubulointerstitial disease (e.g., hyperkalemia, non-anion-gap metabolic acidosis, mild hypernatremia). Urinalysis is most often benign or with a small number of cells; heavy proteinuria is rare. An opaque (all but uric acid) stone may be visualized on abdominal radiography.

Ultrasonography can be used to assess the degree of hydronephrosis and the integrity of the renal parenchyma; CT or intravenous urography may be required to localize the level of obstruction. Calyceal dilation is commonly seen; it may be absent with hyperacute obstruction, upper tract encasement by tumor or retroperitoneal fibrosis, or indwelling staghorn calculi. Kidney size may indicate the duration of obstruction. It should be noted that unilateral obstruction may be prolonged and severe (ultimately leading to loss of renal function in the obstructed kidney), with no hint of abnormality on physical exam and laboratory survey.

 TREATMENT

Management of acute RF associated with UTO is dictated by (1) the level of obstruction (upper vs. lower tract), and (2) the acuity of the obstruction and its clinical consequences, including renal dysfunction and infection. Benign causes of UTO, including bladder outlet obstruction and nephrolithiasis, should be ruled out as conservative management, including Foley catheter placement and IV fluids, respectively, will usually relieve the obstruction in most cases.

Among more seriously ill pts, ureteral obstruction due to tumor is the most common and concerning cause of UTO. If technically feasible, ureteral obstruction due to tumor is best managed by cystoscopic placement of a ureteral stent. Otherwise, the placement of nephrostomy tubes with external drainage may be required. IV antibiotics should also be given if there are signs of pyelonephritis or urosepsis. Fluid and electrolyte status should be carefully

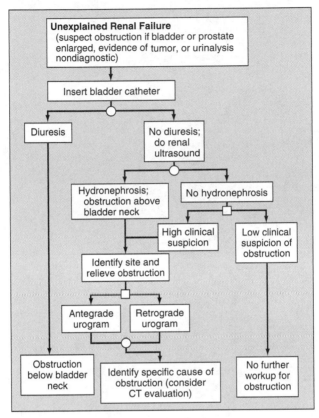

FIGURE 149-1 Diagnostic approach for urinary tract obstruction in unexplained renal failure. Circles represent diagnostic procedures and squares indicate clinical decisions based on available data. CT, computed tomography.

monitored after obstruction is relieved. There may be a physiologic natriuresis/diuresis related to volume overload. However, there may be an "inappropriate" natriuresis/diuresis related to (1) elevated urea nitrogen, leading to an osmotic diuresis; and (2) acquired nephrogenic diabetes insipidus. Hypernatremia, sometimes of a severe degree, may develop.

For a more detailed discussion, see Seifter JL, Brenner BM: Urinary Tract Obstruction, Chap. 270, p. 1722, in HPIM-16.

GASTROINTESTINAL DISEASES

150

PEPTIC ULCER AND RELATED DISORDERS

PEPTIC ULCER DISEASE (PUD)

PUD occurs most commonly in duodenal bulb (duodenal ulcer—DU) and stomach (gastric ulcer—GU). It may also occur in esophagus, pyloric channel, duodenal loop, jejunum, Meckel's diverticulum. PUD results when "aggressive" factors (gastric acid, pepsin) overwhelm "defensive" factors involved in mucosal resistance (gastric mucus, bicarbonate, microcirculation, prostaglandins, mucosal "barrier"), and from effects of *Helicobacter pylori*.

CAUSES AND RISK FACTORS *General* Major role for *H. pylori*, spiral urease-producing organism that colonizes gastric antral mucosa in up to 100% of persons with DU and 80% with GU. Also found in normals (increasing prevalence with age) and those of low socioeconomic status. Invariably associated with histologic evidence of active chronic gastritis, which over years can lead to atrophic gastritis and gastric cancer. Other major cause of ulcers is NSAIDs (those not due to *H. pylori*). Fewer than 1% are due to gastrinoma (Zollinger-Ellison syndrome). Other risk factors and associations: hereditary (? increased parietal cell number), smoking, hypercalcemia, mastocytosis, blood group O (antigens may bind *H. pylori*). Unproven: stress, coffee, alcohol.

DU Mild gastric acid hypersecretion resulting from (1) increased release of gastrin, presumably due to (a) stimulation of antral G cells by cytokines released by inflammatory cells and (b) diminished production of somatostatin by D cells, both resulting from *H. pylori* infection; and (2) an exaggerated acid response to gastrin due to an increased parietal cell mass resulting from gastrin stimulation. These abnormalities reverse rapidly with eradication of *H. pylori*. However, a mildly elevated maximum gastric acid output in response to exogenous gastrin persists in some pts long after eradication of *H. pylori*, suggesting that gastric acid hypersecretion may be, in part, genetically determined. *H. pylori* may also result in elevated serum pepsinogen levels. Mucosal defense in duodenum is compromised by toxic effects of *H. pylori* infection on patches of gastric metaplasia that result from gastric acid hypersecretion or rapid gastric emptying. Other risk factors include glucocorticoids, NSAIDs, chronic renal failure, renal transplantation, cirrhosis, chronic lung disease.

GU *H. pylori* is also principal cause. Gastric acid secretory rates usually normal or reduced, possibly reflecting earlier age of infection by *H. pylori* than in DU pts. Gastritis due to reflux of duodenal contents (including bile) may play a role. Chronic salicylate or NSAID use may account for 15–30% of GUs and increase risk of associated bleeding, perforation.

CLINICAL FEATURES *DU* Burning epigastric pain 90 min to 3 h after meals, often nocturnal, relieved by food.

GU Burning epigastric pain made worse by or unrelated to food; anorexia, food aversion, weight loss (in 40%). Great individual variation. Similar symptoms may occur in persons without demonstrated peptic ulcers ("nonulcer dyspepsia"); less responsive to standard therapy.

COMPLICATIONS Bleeding, obstruction, penetration causing acute pancreatitis, perforation, intractability.

Table 150-1

Tests for Detection of *H. pylori*

Test	Sensitivity/Specificity, %	Comments
INVASIVE (ENDOSCOPY/BIOPSY REQUIRED)		
Rapid urease	80–95/95–100	Simple; false negative with recent use of PPIs, antibiotics, or bismuth compounds
Histology	80–90/>95	Requires pathology processing and staining; provides histologic information
Culture	—/—	Time-consuming, expensive, dependent on experience; allows determination of antibiotic susceptibility
NONINVASIVE		
Serology	>80/>90	Inexpensive, convenient; not useful for early follow-up
Urea breath test	>90/>90	Simple, rapid; useful for early follow-up; false negative with recent therapy (see rapid urease test)

Note: PPI, proton pump inhibitor.

DIAGNOSIS   *DU*   Upper endoscopy or upper GI barium radiography.

GU   Upper endoscopy preferable to exclude possibility that ulcer is malignant (brush cytology, ≥6 pinch biopsies of ulcer margin). Radiographic features suggesting malignancy: ulcer within a mass, folds that do not radiate from ulcer margin, a large ulcer (>2.5–3 cm).

DETECTION OF *H. pylori*   Detection of antibodies in serum (inexpensive, preferred when endoscopy is not required); rapid urease test of antral biopsy (when endoscopy is required). Urea breath test generally used to confirm eradication of *H. pylori*, if necessary (Table 150-1).

 TREATMENT

Medical

Objectives: pain relief, healing, prevention of complications, prevention of recurrences. For GU, exclude malignancy (follow endoscopically to healing). Dietary restriction unnecessary with contemporary drugs; discontinue NSAIDs; smoking may prevent healing and should be stopped. Eradication of *H. pylori* markedly reduces rate of ulcer relapse and is indicated for all DUs and GUs associated with *H. pylori* (Table 150-2). Acid suppression is generally included in regimen. Standard drugs (H_2-receptor blockers, sucralfate, antacids) heal 80–90% of DUs and 60% of GUs in 6 weeks; healing is more rapid with omeprazole (20 mg/d).

Surgery

For complications (persistent or recurrent bleeding, obstruction, perforation) or, uncommonly, intractability (first screen for surreptitious NSAID use and gastrinoma). For DU, see Table 150-3. For GU, perform subtotal gastrectomy.

Table 150-2

Regimens Recommended for Eradication of *H. pylori* Infection

Drug	Dose
TRIPLE THERAPY	
1. Bismuth subsalicylate *plus*	2 tablets qid
Metronidazole *plus*	250 mg qid
Tetracycline[a]	500 mg qid
2. Ranitidine bismuth citrate *plus*	400 mg bid
Tetracycline *plus*	500 mg bid
Clarithromycin *or* metronidazole	500 mg bid
3. Omeprazole (lansoprazole) *plus*	20 mg bid (30 mg bid)
Clarithromycin *plus*	250 or 500 mg bid
Metronidazole[b] *or*	500 mg bid
Amoxicillin[c]	1 g bid
QUADRUPLE THERAPY	
Omeprazole (lansoprazole)	20 mg (30 mg) daily
Bismuth subsalicylate	2 tablets qid
Metronidazole	250 mg qid
Tetracycline	500 mg qid

[a] Alternative: use prepacked Helidac.
[b] Alternative: use prepacked Prevpac.
[c] Use either metronidazole or amoxicillin, but not both.

Complications of Surgery (1) Obstructed afferent loop (Billroth II), (2) bile reflux gastritis, (3) dumping syndrome (rapid gastric emptying with abdominal distress + postprandial vasomotor symptoms), (4) postvagotomy diarrhea, (5) bezoar, (6) anemia (iron, B_{12}, folate malabsorption), (7) malabsorption (poor mixing of gastric contents, pancreatic juices, bile; bacterial overgrowth), (8) osteomalacia and osteoporosis (vitamin D and Ca malabsorption), (9) gastric remnant carcinoma.

—————————— *Approach to the Patient* ——————————

Optimal approach is uncertain. Serologic testing for *H. pylori* and treating, if present, may be cost-effective. Other options include trial of acid-suppressive therapy, endoscopy only in treatment failures, or initial endoscopy in all cases.

Table 150-3

Surgical Treatment of Duodenal Ulcer

Operation	Recurrence Rate	Complication Rate
Vagotomy + antrectomy (Billroth I or II)[a]	1%	Highest
Vagotomy and pyloroplasty	10%	Intermediate
Parietal cell (proximal gastric, superselective) vagotomy	≥10%	Lowest

[a] Billroth I, gastroduodenostomy; Billroth II, gastrojejunostomy.

GASTROPATHIES

EROSIVE GASTROPATHIES Hemorrhagic gastritis, multiple gastric erosions. Caused by aspirin and other NSAIDs (lower risk with newer agents, e.g., nabumetone and etodolac, which do not inhibit gastric mucosal prostaglandins) or severe stress (burns, sepsis, trauma, surgery, shock, or respiratory, renal, or liver failure). May be asymptomatic or associated with epigastric discomfort, nausea, hematemesis, or melena. Diagnosis by upper endoscopy.

$\boxed{\text{R}\!x}$ TREATMENT

Removal of offending agent and maintenance of O_2 and blood volume as required. For prevention of stress ulcers in critically ill pts, hourly oral administration of liquid antacids (e.g., Maalox 30 mL), IV H_2-receptor antagonist (e.g., cimetidine, 300-mg bolus + 37.5–50 mg/h IV), or both is recommended to maintain gastric pH > 4. Alternatively, sucralfate slurry, 1 g PO q6h, can be given; does not raise gastric pH and may thus avoid increased risk of aspiration pneumonia associated with liquid antacids. Misoprostol, 200 μg PO qid, or profound acid suppression (e.g., famotidine, 40 mg PO bid) can be used with NSAIDs to prevent NSAID-induced ulcers.

CHRONIC GASTRITIS Identified histologically by an inflammatory cell infiltrate dominated by lymphocytes and plasma cells with scant neutrophils. In its early stage, the changes are limited to the lamina propria (*superficial gastritis*). When the disease progresses to destroy glands, it becomes *atrophic gastritis*. The final stage is *gastric atrophy*, in which the mucosa is thin and the infiltrate sparse. Chronic gastritis can be classified based on predominant site of involvement.

Type A Gastritis This is the body-predominant and less common form. Generally asymptomatic, common in elderly; autoimmune mechanism may be associated with achlorhydria, pernicious anemia, and increased risk of gastric cancer (value of screening endoscopy uncertain). Antibodies to parietal cells present in >90%.

Type B Gastritis This is antral-predominant disease and caused by *H. pylori*. Often asymptomatic but may be associated with dyspepsia. May also lead to atrophic gastritis, gastric atrophy, gastric lymphoid follicles, and low-grade gastric B cell lymphomas. Infection early in life or in setting of malnutrition or low gastric acid output is associated with gastritis of entire stomach (including body) and increased risk of gastric cancer. Eradication of *H. pylori* (Table 150-2) not routinely recommended unless PUD or low-grade MALT lymphoma is present.

SPECIFIC TYPES OF GASTROPATHY OR GASTRITIS Alcoholic gastropathy (submucosal hemorrhages), Ménétrier's disease (hypertrophic gastropathy), eosinophilic gastritis, granulomatous gastritis, Crohn's disease, sarcoidosis, infections (tuberculosis, syphilis, fungi, viruses, parasites), pseudolymphoma, radiation, corrosive gastritis.

ZOLLINGER-ELLISON (Z-E) SYNDROME (GASTRINOMA)

Consider when ulcer disease is severe, refractory to therapy, associated with ulcers in atypical locations, or associated with diarrhea. Tumors usually pancreatic or in duodenum (submucosal, often small), may be multiple, slowly growing; >60% malignant; 25% associated with MEN 1, i.e., multiple endocrine neoplasia type 1 (gastrinoma, hyperparathyroidism, pituitary neoplasm),

Table 150-4

Differential Diagnostic Tests

Condition	Fasting Gastrin	Gastrin Response to	
		IV Secretin	Food
DU	N (≤150 ng/L)	NC	Slight ↑
Z-E	↑↑↑	↑↑↑	NC
Antral G (gastrin) cell hyperplasia	↑	↑, NC	↑↑↑

Note: N, normal; NC, no change.

often duodenal, small, multicentric, less likely to metastasize to liver than pancreatic gastrinomas but often metastasize to local lymph nodes.

DIAGNOSIS *Suggestive* Basal acid output > 15 mmol/h; basal/maximal acid output > 60%; large mucosal folds on endoscopy or upper GI radiograph.

Confirmatory Serum gastrin > 1000 ng/L or rise in gastrin of 200 ng/L following IV secretin and, if necessary, rise of 400 ng/L following IV calcium (Table 150-4).

DIFFERENTIAL DIAGNOSIS *Increased Gastric Acid Secretion* Z-E syndrome, antral G cell hyperplasia or hyperfunction (? due to *H. pylori*), postgastrectomy retained antrum, renal failure, massive small bowel resection, chronic gastric outlet obstruction.

Normal or Decreased Gastric Acid Secretion Pernicious anemia, chronic gastritis, gastric cancer, vagotomy, pheochromocytoma.

℞ TREATMENT

Omeprazole, beginning at 60 mg PO qA.M. and increasing until maximal gastric acid output is <10 mmol/h before next dose, is drug of choice during evaluation and in pts who are not surgical candidates; dose can often be reduced over time. Radiolabeled octreotide scanning has emerged as the most sensitive test for detecting primary tumors and metastases; may be supplemented by endoscopic ultrasonography. Exploratory laparotomy with resection of primary tumor and solitary metastases when possible. In pts with MEN 1, tumor is often multifocal and unresectable; treat hyperparathyroidism first (hypergastrinemia may improve). For unresectable tumors, parietal cell vagotomy may enhance control of ulcer disease by drugs. Chemotherapy for metastatic tumor to control symptoms (e.g., streptozocin, 5-fluorouracil, doxorubicin, or interferon α); 40% partial response rate.

For a more detailed discussion, see Del Valle J: Peptic Ulcer Disease and Related Disorders, Chap. 274, p. 1746, in HPIM-16.

151

INFLAMMATORY BOWEL DISEASES

Inflammatory bowel diseases (IBD) are chronic inflammatory disorders of unknown etiology involving the GI tract. Peak occurrence between ages 15 and 30 and between ages 60 and 80, but onset may occur at any age. Pathogenesis of IBD involves activation of immune cells by unknown inciting agent (?microorganism, dietary component, bacterial or self-antigen) leading to release of cytokines and inflammatory mediators. Genetic component suggested by increased risk in first-degree relatives of pts with IBD and concurrence of type of IBD, location of Crohn's disease, and clinical course. Reported associations include HLA-DR2 in Japanese patients with ulcerative colitis and a Crohn's disease–related gene called *NOD2* on chromosome 16. Other potential pathogenic factors include serum antineutrophil cytoplasmic antibodies (ANCA) in 70% of pts with ulcerative colitis and granulomatous angiitis (vasculitis) in Crohn's disease. Acute flares may be precipitated by infections, NSAIDs, stress. Onset of ulcerative colitis often follows cessation of smoking.

ULCERATIVE COLITIS (UC)

PATHOLOGY　Colonic mucosal inflammation; rectum almost always involved, with inflammation extending continuously (no skip areas) proximally for a variable extent; histologic features include epithelial damage, inflammation, crypt abscesses, loss of goblet cells.

CLINICAL MANIFESTATIONS　Bloody diarrhea, mucus, fever, abdominal pain, tenesmus, weight loss; spectrum of severity (majority of cases are mild, limited to rectosigmoid). In severe cases dehydration, anemia, hypokalemia, hypoalbuminemia.

COMPLICATIONS　Toxic megacolon, colonic perforation; cancer risk related to extent and duration of colitis; often preceded by or coincident with dysplasia, which may be detected on surveillance colonoscopic biopsies.

DIAGNOSIS　Sigmoidoscopy/colonoscopy: mucosal erythema, granularity, friability, exudate, hemorrhage, ulcers, inflammatory polyps (pseudopolyps). Barium enema: loss of haustrations, mucosal irregularity, ulcerations.

CROHN'S DISEASE (CD)

PATHOLOGY　Any part of GI tract, usually terminal ileum and/or colon; transmural inflammation, bowel wall thickening, linear ulcerations, and submucosal thickening leading to cobblestone pattern; discontinuous (skip areas); histologic features include transmural inflammation, granulomas (often absent), fissures, fistulas.

CLINICAL MANIFESTATIONS　Fever, abdominal pain, diarrhea (often without blood), fatigue, weight loss, growth retardation in children; acute ileitis mimicking appendicitis; anorectal fissures, fistulas, abscesses. Clinical course falls into three broad patterns: (1) inflammatory, (2) stricturing, and (3) fistulizing.

COMPLICATIONS　Intestinal obstruction (edema vs. fibrosis); rarely toxic megacolon or perforation; intestinal fistulas to bowel, bladder, vagina, skin, soft tissue, often with abscess formation; bile salt malabsorption leading to cholesterol gallstones and/or oxalate kidney stones; intestinal malignancy; amyloidosis.

DIAGNOSIS   Sigmoidoscopy/colonoscopy, barium enema, upper GI and small-bowel series: nodularity, rigidity, ulcers that may be deep or longitudinal, cobblestoning, skip areas, strictures, fistulas. CT may show thickened, matted bowel loops or an abscess.

DIFFERENTIAL DIAGNOSIS

INFECTIOUS ENTEROCOLITIS   *Shigella, Salmonella, Campylobacter, Yersinia* (acute ileitis), *Plesiomonas shigelloides, Aeromonas hydrophilia, Escherichia coli* serotype O157:H7, *Gonorrhea, Lymphogranuloma venereum, Clostridium difficile* (pseudomembranous colitis), tuberculosis, amebiasis, cytomegalovirus, AIDS.

OTHERS   Ischemic bowel disease, appendicitis, diverticulitis, radiation enterocolitis, bile salt–induced diarrhea (ileal resection), drug-induced colitis (e.g., NSAIDs), bleeding colonic lesion (e.g., neoplasm), irritable bowel syndrome (no bleeding), microscopic (lymphocytic) or collagenous colitis (chronic watery diarrhea)—normal colonoscopy, but biopsies show superficial colonic epithelial inflammation and, in collagenous colitis, a thick subepithelial layer of collagen; response to aminosalicylates and glucocorticoids variable.

EXTRAINTESTINAL MANIFESTATIONS   (UC and CD)

1. *Joint*: Peripheral arthritis—parallels activity of bowel disease; ankylosing spondylitis and sacroiliitis (associated with HLA-B27)—activity independent of bowel disease.
2. *Skin*: Erythema nodosum, aphthous ulcers, pyoderma gangrenosum, cutaneous Crohn's disease.
3. *Eye*: Episcleritis, iritis, uveitis.
4. *Liver*: Fatty liver, "pericholangitis" (intrahepatic sclerosing cholangitis), primary sclerosing cholangitis, cholangiocarcinoma, chronic hepatitis.
5. *Others*: Autoimmune hemolytic anemia, phlebitis, pulmonary embolus (hypercoagulable state).

[Rx] **TREATMENT**   (See Table 151-1)

  Supportive   Antidiarrheal agents (diphenoxylate and atropine, loperamide) in mild disease; IV hydration and blood transfusions in severe disease; parenteral nutrition or defined enteral formulas—effective as primary therapy in CD, although high relapse rate when oral feeding is resumed; should not replace drug therapy; important role in preoperative preparation of malnourished pt; emotional support.

  Sulfasalazine and Aminosalicylates   Active component of sulfasalazine is 5-aminosalicylic acid (5-ASA) linked to sulfapyridine carrier; useful in colonic disease of mild to moderate severity (1–1.5 g PO qid); efficacy in maintaining remission demonstrated only for UC (500 mg PO qid). Toxicity (generally due to sulfapyridine component): dose-related—nausea, headache, rarely hemolytic anemia—may resolve when drug dose is lowered; idiosyncratic—fever, rash, neutropenia, pancreatitis, hepatitis, etc.; miscellaneous—oligospermia. Newer aminosalicylates are as effective as sulfasalazine but with fewer side effects. Enemas containing 4 g of 5-ASA (mesalamine) may be used in distal UC, 1 nightly retained qhs until remission, then q2hs or q3hs. Suppositories containing 500 mg of 5-ASA may be used in proctitis.

Table 151-1

Medical Management of IBD

ULCERATIVE COLITIS: ACTIVE DISEASE

	Mild
Distal	5-ASA oral and/or enema
Extensive	5-ASA oral or enema

ULCERATIVE COLITIS: MAINTENANCE THERAPY

Distal	5-ASA oral and/or enema 6-MP or azathioprine
Extensive	5-ASA oral and/or enema 6-MP or azathioprine

CROHN'S DISEASE: ACTIVE DISEASE

Mild–Moderate	Severe
5-ASA oral or enema	5-ASA oral or enema
Metronidazole and/or ciprofloxacin	Metronidazole and/or ciprofloxacin
Oral glucocorticoids	Oral or IV glucocorticoids
Azathioprine or 6-MP	Azathioprine or 6-MP
Infliximab	Infliximab
	TPN or elemental diet
	Intravenous cyclosporine

CROHN'S DISEASE: MAINTENANCE THERAPY

Inflammatory	Perianal or Fistulizing Disease
5-ASA oral or enema	Metronidazole and/or ciprofloxacin
Metronidazole and/or ciprofloxacin	Azathioprine or 6-MP
Azathioprine or 6-MP	

Note: CSA, cyclosporine; 6-MP, 6-mercaptopurine; TPN, total parenteral nutrition.

Glucocorticoids Useful in severe disease and ileal or ileocolonic CD. Prednisone, 40–60 mg PO qd, then taper; IV hydrocortisone, 100 mg tid or equivalent, in hospitalized pts; IV ACTH drip (120 U qd) may be preferable in first attacks of UC. Nightly hydrocortisone retention enemas in proctosigmoiditis. Numerous side effects make long-term use problematic.

Immunosuppressive Agents Azathioprine, 6-mercaptopurine—50 mg PO qd up to 2.0 or 1.5 mg/kg qd, respectively. Useful as steroid-sparing agents and in intractable or fistulous CD (may require 2- to 6-month trial before efficacy seen). Toxicity—immunosuppression, pancreatitis, ? carcinogenicity. Avoid in pregnancy.

Metronidazole Appears effective in colonic CD (500 mg PO bid) and refractory perineal CD (10–20 mg/kg PO qd). Toxicity—peripheral neurop-

Moderate	Severe	Fulminant
5-ASA oral and/or enema	5-ASA oral and/or enema	Intravenous glucocorticoid
Glucocorticoid enema	Glucocorticoid enema	Intravenous CSA
Oral glucocorticoid	Oral or IV glucocorticoid	
5-ASA oral and/or enema	5-ASA oral and/or enema	Intravenous glucocorticoid
Glucocorticoid enema	Glucocorticoid enema	Intravenous CSA
Oral glucocorticoid	Oral or IV glucocorticoid	

Perianal or Fistulizing Disease
Metronidazolc and/or ciprofloxacin
Azathioprine or 6-MP
Infliximab
Intravenous CSA

athy, metallic taste, ?carcinogenicity. Avoid in pregnancy. Other antibiotics (e.g., ciprofloxacin 500 mg PO bid) may be of value in terminal ileal and perianal CD, and broad-spectrum IV antibiotics are indicated for fulminant colitis and abscesses.

Others Cyclosporine [potential value in a dose of 4 (mg/kg)/d IV for 7–14 days in severe UC and possibly intractable Crohn's fistulas]; experimental—methotrexate, chloroquine, fish oil, nicotine, others.

Surgery UC: Colectomy (curative) for intractability, toxic megacolon (if no improvement with aggressive medical therapy in 24–48 h), cancer, dysplasia. Ileal pouch—anal anastomosis is operation of choice in UC but contraindicated in CD and in elderly. CD: Resection for fixed obstruction (or stricturoplasty), abscesses, persistent symptomatic fistulas, intractability.

For a more detailed discussion, see Friedman S, Blumberg RS: Inflammatory Bowel Disease, Chap. 276, p. 1776, in HPIM-16.

152

COLONIC AND ANORECTAL DISEASES

IRRITABLE BOWEL SYNDROME (IBS)

Characterized by altered bowel habits, abdominal pain, and absence of detectable organic pathology. Most common GI disease in clinical practice. Three types of clinical presentations: (1) spastic colon (chronic abdominal pain and constipation), (2) alternating constipation and diarrhea, or (3) chronic, painless diarrhea.

PATHOPHYSIOLOGY   Visceral hyperalgesia to mechanoreceptor stimuli is common. Reported abnormalities include altered colonic motility at rest and in response to stress, cholinergic drugs, cholecystokinin; altered small-intestinal motility; enhanced visceral sensation (lower pain threshold in response to gut distention); and abnormal extrinsic innervation of the gut. Patients presenting with IBS to a physician have an increased frequency of psychological disturbances—depression, hysteria, obsessive-compulsive disorder. Specific food intolerances and malabsorption of bile acids by the terminal ileum may account for a few cases.

CLINICAL MANIFESTATIONS   Onset often before age 30; females: males = 2:1. Abdominal pain and irregular bowel habits. Additional symptoms often include abdominal distention, relief of abdominal pain with bowel movement, increased frequency of stools with pain, loose stools with pain, mucus in stools, and sense of incomplete evacuation. Associated findings include pasty stools, ribbony or pencil-thin stools, heartburn, bloating, back pain, weakness, faintness, palpitations, urinary frequency.

DIAGNOSIS   IBS is a diagnosis of exclusion. Rome criteria for diagnosis are shown in Table 152-1. Consider sigmoidoscopy and barium radiographs to exclude inflammatory bowel disease or malignancy; consider excluding giardiasis, intestinal lactase deficiency, hyperthyroidism.

 TREATMENT

Reassurance and supportive physician-patient relationship, avoidance of stress or precipitating factors, dietary bulk (fiber, psyllium extract, e.g., Metamucil 1 tbsp daily or bid); for diarrhea, trials of loperamide (2 PO qA.M. then 1 PO after each loose stool to a maximum of 8/d, then titrate), diphenoxylate (Lomotil) (up to 2 PO qid), or cholestyramine (up to 1 packet mixed in water PO qid); for pain, anticholinergics (e.g., dicyclomine HCl 10–40 mg PO qid) or hyoscyamine as Levsin 1–2 PO q4h prn. Amitryptiline 25–50 mg PO qhs or other antidepressants in low doses may relieve pain. Selective serotonin reuptake inhibitors such as paroxetine are being evaluated in constipation-dominant patients, and seratonin receptor antagonists such as alosetron are being evaluated in diarrhea-dominant patients. Prokinetic 5HT4

Table 152-1

Rome II Criteria for the Diagnosis of IBS

At least 12 weeks, which need not be consecutive, in the preceding 12 months of abdominal discomfort or pain that has two of following three features:
1. Relieved by defecation
2. Onset associated with changes in stool frequency
3. Onset associated with changes in stool form

receptor agonist, tegaserod, is approved for use in constipation-dominant patients. Psychotherapy, hypnotherapy of possible benefit in severe refractory cases.

DIVERTICULAR DISEASE

Herniations or saclike protrusions of the mucosa through the muscularis at points of nutrient artery penetration; possibly due to increased intraluminal pressure, low-fiber diet; most common in sigmoid colon.

CLINICAL PRESENTATION

1. *Asymptomatic* (detected by barium enema or colonoscopy).
2. *Pain*: Recurrent left lower quadrant pain relieved by defecation; alternating constipation and diarrhea. Diagnosis by barium enema.
3. *Diverticulitis*: Pain, fever, altered bowel habits, tender colon, leukocytosis. Best confirmed and staged by CT after opacification of bowel. (In pts who recover with medical therapy, perform elective barium enema or colonoscopy in 4–6 weeks to exclude cancer.) Complications: pericolic abscess, perforation, fistula (to bladder, vagina, skin, soft tissue), liver abscess, stricture. Frequently require surgery or, for abscesses, percutaneous drainage.
4. *Hemorrhage*: Usually in absence of diverticulitis, often from ascending colon and self-limited. If persistent, manage with mesenteric arteriography and intraarterial infusion of vasopressin, or surgery (Chap. 53).

 TREATMENT

Pain High-fiber diet, psyllium extract (e.g., Metamucil 1 tbsp PO qd or bid), anticholinergics (e.g., dicyclomine HCl 10–40 mg PO qid).

Diverticulitis NPO, IV fluids, antibiotics (e.g., cefoxitin 2 g IV q6h or imipenem 500 mg IV q6–8h); for ambulatory pts, ampicillin or tetracycline 500 mg PO qid (clear liquid diet); surgical resection in refractory or frequently recurrent cases, young persons (<age 50), immunosuppressed pts, or when there is inability to exclude cancer.

Patients who have had at least two documented episodes and those who respond slowly to medical therapy should be offered surgical options to achieve removal of the diseased colonic segment, controlling sepsis, eliminating obstructions or fistulas, and restoring intestinal continuity.

INTESTINAL PSEUDOOBSTRUCTION

Recurrent attacks of nausea, vomiting, and abdominal pain and distention mimicking mechanical obstruction; may be complicated by steatorrhea due to bacterial overgrowth.

CAUSES *Primary*: Familial visceral neuropathy, familial visceral myopathy, idiopathic. *Secondary*: Scleroderma, amyloidosis, diabetes, celiac disease, parkinsonism, muscular dystrophy, drugs, electrolyte imbalance, postsurgical.

TREATMENT

For acute attacks: intestinal decompression with long tube. Oral antibiotics for bacterial overgrowth (e.g., metronidazole 250 mg PO tid, tetracycline 500 mg PO qid, or ciprofloxacin 500 mg bid 1 week out of each month, usually in an alternating rotation of at least two antibiotics). Avoid surgery. In refractory cases, consider long-term parenteral hyperalimentation.

VASCULAR DISORDERS (SMALL AND LARGE INTESTINE)

MECHANISMS OF MESENTERIC ISCHEMIA   (1) Occlusive: embolus (atrial fibrillation, valvular heart disease); arterial thrombus (atherosclerosis); venous thrombosis (trauma, neoplasm, infection, cirrhosis, oral contraceptives, antithrombin-III deficiency, protein S or C deficiency, lupus anticoagulant, factor V Leiden mutation, idiopathic); vasculitis (SLE, polyarteritis, rheumatoid arthritis, Henoch-Schönlein purpura); (2) nonocclusive: hypotension, heart failure, arrhythmia, digitalis (vasoconstrictor).

ACUTE MESENTERIC ISCHEMIA   Periumbilical pain out of proportion to tenderness; nausea, vomiting, distention, GI bleeding, altered bowel habits. Abdominal x-ray shows bowel distention, air-fluid levels, thumbprinting (submucosal edema) but may be normal early in course. Peritoneal signs indicate infarcted bowel requiring surgical resection. Early celiac and mesenteric arteriography is recommended in all cases following hemodynamic resuscitation (avoid vasopressors, digitalis). Intraarterial vasodilators (e.g., papaverine) can be administered to reverse vasoconstriction. Laparotomy indicated to restore intestinal blood flow obstructed by embolus or thrombosis or to resect necrotic bowel. Postoperative anticoagulation indicated in mesenteric venous thrombosis, controversial in arterial occlusion.

CHRONIC MESENTERIC INSUFFICIENCY   "Abdominal angina": dull, crampy periumbilical pain 15–30 min after a meal and lasting for several hours; weight loss; occasionally diarrhea. Evaluate with mesenteric arteriography for possible bypass graft surgery.

ISCHEMIC COLITIS   Usually due to nonocclusive disease in pt with atherosclerosis. Severe lower abdominal pain, rectal bleeding, hypotension. Abdominal x-ray shows colonic dilatation, thumbprinting. Sigmoidoscopy shows submucosal hemorrhage, friability, ulcerations; rectum often spared. Conservative management (NPO, IV fluids); surgical resection for infarction or postischemic stricture.

COLONIC ANGIODYSPLASIA

In persons over age 60, vascular ectasias, usually in right colon, account for up to 40% of cases of chronic or recurrent lower GI bleeding. May be associated with aortic stenosis. Diagnosis is by arteriography (clusters of small vessels, early and prolonged opacification of draining vein) or colonoscopy (flat, bright red, fernlike lesions). For bleeding, treat by colonoscopic electro- or laser coagulation, band ligation, arteriographic embolization, or, if necessary, right hemicolectomy (Chap. 53).

ANORECTAL DISEASES

HEMORRHOIDS   Due to increased hydrostatic pressure in hemorrhoidal venous plexus (associated with straining at stool, pregnancy). May be external, internal, thrombosed, acute (prolapsed or strangulated), or bleeding. Treat pain with bulk laxative and stool softeners (psyllium extract, dioctyl sodium sulfosuccinate 100–200 mg/d), sitz baths 1–4 per day, witch hazel compresses, analgesics as needed. Bleeding may require rubber band ligation or injection sclerotherapy. Operative hemorrhoidectomy in severe or refractory cases.

ANAL FISSURES   Medical therapy as for hemorrhoids. Relaxation of the anal canal with nitroglycerin ointment (0.2%) applied tid or botulinum toxin type A up to 20 U injected into the internal sphincter on each side of the fissure. Internal anal sphincterotomy in refractory cases.

PRURITUS ANI   Often of unclear cause; may be due to poor hygiene, fungal or parasitic infection. Treat with thorough cleansing after bowel movement, topical glucocorticoid, antifungal agent if indicated.

ANAL CONDYLOMAS (GENITAL WARTS)   Wartlike papillomas due to sexually transmitted papillomavirus. Treat with cautious application of liquid nitrogen or podophyllotoxin or with intralesional interferon-α. Tend to recur.

For a more detailed discussion, see Owyang C: Irritable Bowel Syndrome, **Chap. 277, p. 1789**; and Gearhart SL, Bulkley G: Common Diseases of the Colon and Anorectum and Mesenteric Vascular Insufficiency, **Chap. 279, p. 1795**, in HPIM-16.

153

CHOLELITHIASIS, CHOLECYSTITIS, AND CHOLANGITIS

CHOLELITHIASIS

There are two major types of gallstones: cholesterol and pigment stones. Cholesterol gallstones contain >50% cholesterol monohydrate. Pigment stones have <20% cholesterol and are composed primarily of calcium bilirubinate. In the United States, 80% of stones are cholesterol and 20% pigment.

EPIDEMIOLOGY   One million new cases of cholelithiasis per year in the United States. Predisposing factors include demographic/genetics (increased prevalence in North American Indians), obesity, weight loss, female sex hormones, age, ileal disease, pregnancy, type IV hyperlipidemia, and cirrhosis.

SYMPTOMS AND SIGNS   Many gallstones are "silent," i.e., present in asymptomatic pts. Symptoms occur when stones produce inflammation or obstruction of the cystic or common bile ducts. Major symptoms: (1) biliary colic—a severe steady ache in the RUQ or epigastrium that begins suddenly; often occurs 30–90 min after meals, lasts for several hours, and occasionally radiates to the right scapula or back; (2) nausea, vomiting. Physical exam may be normal or show epigastric or RUQ tenderness.

LABORATORY   Occasionally, mild and transient elevations in bilirubin [<85 μmol/L (<5 mg/dL)] accompany biliary colic.

Table 153-1

Radiologic and Imaging Modalities for Biliary Tract Disease

Plain films of abdomen	Rarely useful for diagnosis of gallstones
	Can exclude other causes of abdominal pain (intestinal obstruction, perforated ulcer)
Ultrasound	High sensitivity/specificity for detecting gallstones
	Dilated ducts suggest ductal obstruction
	Intramural gas, pericholecystic fluid suggest gallbladder inflammation or infection
	Cannot definitively exclude choledocholithiasis
Scintigraphy (HIDA)	High sensitivity/specificity for acute cholecystitis
Oral cholecystogram	Seldom used for diagnosis of gallstone disease
	Can help select pts for nonsurgical therapy
CT scan	Useful if suspicion of cancer is high
Endoscopic retrograde cholangiopancreatography	Delineates lower limit of common bile duct (CBD) obstruction
	Therapeutic intervention possible
Percutaneous transhepatic cholangiography	Delineates upper limit of CBD obstruction
MR cholangiography	Useful for visualizing pancreatic and biliary ducts
Endoscopic ultrasound	Most sensitive method to detect ampullary stones

IMAGING   Only 10% of cholesterol gallstones are radiopaque. Ultrasonography is best diagnostic test. The oral cholecystogram has been largely replaced by ultrasound but may be used to assess the patency of the cystic duct and gallbladder emptying function (Table 153-1).

DIFFERENTIAL DIAGNOSIS   Includes peptic ulcer disease (PUD), gastroesophageal reflux, irritable bowel syndrome, and hepatitis.

COMPLICATIONS   Cholecystitis, pancreatitis, cholangitis.

 TREATMENT

In asymptomatic pts, risk of developing complications requiring surgery is small. Elective cholecystectomy should be reserved for: (1) symptomatic pts (i.e., biliary colic despite low-fat diet); (2) persons with previous complications of cholelithiasis (see below); and (3) presence of an underlying condition predisposing to an increased risk of complications (calcified or porcelain gallbladder). Pts with gallstones >3 cm or with an anomalous gallbladder containing stones should also be considered for surgery. Laparoscopic cholecystectomy is minimally invasive and is the procedure of choice for most pts undergoing elective cholecystectomy. Oral dissolution agents (ursodeoxycholic acid) partially or completely dissolve small radiolucent stones in 50% of selected pts within 6–24 months. Extracorporeal shockwave lithotripsy followed by medical litholytic therapy is effective in selected pts with solitary radiolucent gallstones. Because of the frequency of stone recurrence and the effectiveness of laparoscopic surgery, the role of oral dissolution therapy and lithotripsy has been reduced to selected patients who are not candidates for elective cholecystectomy.

ACUTE CHOLECYSTITIS

Acute inflammation of the gallbladder usually caused by cystic duct obstruction by an impacted stone.

ETIOLOGY 90% calculous; 10% acalculous. Acalculous cholecystitis associated with higher complication rate and associated with acute illness (i.e., burns, trauma, major surgery), fasting, hyperalimentation leading to gallbladder stasis, vasculitis, carcinoma of gallbladder or common bile duct, some gallbladder infections (*Leptospira, Streptococcus*, parasitic, etc.), but in >50% of cases an underlying explanation is not found.

SYMPTOMS AND SIGNS (1) Attack of biliary colic (RUQ or epigastric pain) that progressively worsens; (2) nausea, vomiting, anorexia; and (3) fever. Examination typically reveals RUQ tenderness; palpable RUQ mass found in 20% of pts. *Murphy's sign* is present when deep inspiration or cough during palpation of the RUQ produces increased pain or inspiratory arrest.

LABORATORY Mild leukocytosis; serum bilirubin, alkaline phosphatase, and AST may be mildly elevated.

IMAGING Ultrasonography is useful for demonstrating gallstones and occasionally a phlegmonous mass surrounding the gallbladder. Radionuclide scans (HIDA, DIDA, DISIDA, etc.) may identify cystic duct obstruction.

DIFFERENTIAL DIAGNOSIS Includes acute pancreatitis, appendicitis, pyelonephritis, PUD, hepatitis, and hepatic abscess.

COMPLICATIONS Empyema, hydrops, gangrene, perforation, fistulization, gallstone ileus, porcelain gallbladder.

℞ TREATMENT

No oral intake, nasogastric suction, IV fluids and electrolytes, analgesia (meperidine or NSAIDS), and antibiotics (ureidopenicillins, ampicillin sulbactam, third-generation cephalosporins; anaerobic coverage should be added if gangrenous or emphysematous cholecystitis is suspected; consider combination with aminoglycosides in diabetic pt or others with signs of gram-negative sepsis). Acute symptoms will resolve in 70% of pts. Optimal timing of surgery depends on patient stabilization and should be performed as soon as feasible. Urgent cholecystectomy is appropriate in most patients with a suspected or confirmed complication. Delayed surgery is reserved for pts with high risk of emergent surgery and where the diagnosis is in doubt.

CHRONIC CHOLECYSTITIS

ETIOLOGY Chronic inflammation of the gallbladder; almost always associated with gallstones. Results from repeated acute/subacute cholecystitis or prolonged mechanical irritation of gallbladder wall.

SYMPTOMS AND SIGNS May be asymptomatic for years, may progress to symptomatic gallbladder disease or to acute cholecystitis, or present with complications.

LABORATORY Tests are usually normal.

IMAGING Ultrasonography preferred; usually shows gallstones within a contracted gallbladder (Table 153-1).

DIFFERENTIAL DIAGNOSIS PUD, esophagitis, irritable bowel syndrome.

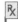 TREATMENT

Surgery indicated if pt is symptomatic.

CHOLEDOCHOLITHIASIS/CHOLANGITIS

ETIOLOGY In pts with cholelithiasis, passage of gallstones into common bile duct occurs in 10–15%; increases with age. At cholecystectomy, undetected stones are left behind in 1–5% of pts.

SYMPTOMS AND SIGNS Choledocholithiasis may present as an incidental finding, biliary colic, obstructive jaundice, cholangitis, or pancreatitis. Cholangitis usually presents as fever, RUQ pain, and jaundice (*Charcot's triad*).

LABORATORY Elevations in serum bilirubin, alkaline phosphatase, and aminotransferases. Leukocytosis usually accompanies cholangitis; blood cultures are frequently positive. Amylase is elevated in 15% of cases.

IMAGING Diagnosis usually made by cholangiography either preoperatively by endoscopic retrograde cholangiopancreatography (ERCP) or intraoperatively at the time of cholecystectomy. Ultrasonography may reveal dilated bile ducts but is not sensitive for detecting common duct stones (Table 153-1).

DIFFERENTIAL DIAGNOSIS Acute cholecystitis, renal colic, perforated viscus, pancreatitis.

COMPLICATIONS Cholangitis, obstructive jaundice, gallstone-induced pancreatitis, and secondary biliary cirrhosis.

 TREATMENT

Laparoscopic cholecystectomy and ERCP have decreased the need for choledocholithotomy and T-tube drainage of the bile ducts. Endoscopic biliary sphincterotomy followed by spontaneous passage or stone extraction is the treatment of choice in the management of pts with common duct stones, especially in elderly or high-risk pts. Preoperative ERCP is indicated in gallstone pts with (1) history of jaundice or pancreatitis, (2) abnormal LFT, and (3) ultrasound evidence of a dilated common bile duct or stones in the duct. Cholangitis treated like acute cholecystitis; no oral intake, hydration, and analgesia are the mainstays; stones should be removed surgically or endoscopically.

PRIMARY SCLEROSING CHOLANGITIS (PSC)

PSC is a sclerosing inflammatory process involving the biliary tree.

ETIOLOGY Associations: inflammatory bowel disease (ulcerative colitis—70% of cases of PSC), AIDS, rarely retroperitoneal fibrosis.

SYMPTOMS AND SIGNS Pruritus, RUQ pain, jaundice, fever, weight loss, and malaise. May progress to cirrhosis with portal hypertension.

LABORATORY Evidence of cholestasis (elevated bilirubin and alkaline phosphatase) common.

RADIOLOGY/ENDOSCOPY Transhepatic or endoscopic cholangiograms reveal stenosis and dilation of the intra- and extrahepatic bile ducts.

DIFFERENTIAL DIAGNOSIS Cholangiocarcinoma, Caroli's disease (cystic dilation of bile ducts), *Fasciola hepatica* infection, echinococcosis, and ascariasis.

℞ TREATMENT

No satisfactory therapy. Cholangitis should be treated as outlined above. Cholestyramine may control pruritus. Supplemental vitamin D and calcium may retard bone loss. Glucocorticoids, methotrexate, and cyclosporine have not been shown to be effective. Urodeoxycholic acid improves liver tests but has not been shown to affect survival. Surgical relief of biliary obstruction may be appropriate but has a high complication rate. Liver transplantation should be considered in pts with end-stage cirrhosis. Median survival: 9–12 years after diagnosis, with age, bilirubin level, histologic stage, and splenomegaly being predictors of survival.

For a more detailed discussion, see Greenberger NJ, Paumgartner G: Diseases of the Gallbladder and Bile Ducts, Chap. 292, p. 1880, in HPIM-16.

154

PANCREATITIS

ACUTE PANCREATITIS

The pathologic spectrum of acute pancreatitis varies from *edematous pancreatitis*, which is usually a mild and self-limited disorder, to *necrotizing pancreatitis*, in which the degree of pancreatic necrosis correlates with the severity of the attack and its systemic manifestations.

ETIOLOGY Most common causes in the United States are cholelithiasis and alcohol. Others include abdominal trauma; postoperative or postendoscopic retrograde cholangiopancreatography (ERCP); metabolic (e.g., hypertriglyceridemia, hypercalcemia, renal failure); hereditary pancreatitis; infection (e.g., mumps, viral hepatitis, coxsackievirus, ascariasis, *Mycoplasma*); opportunistic infections (CMV, *Cryptococcus, Candida*, TB); medications (e.g., azathioprine, sulfonamides, thiazides, furosemide, estrogens, tetracycline, valproic acid, pentamidine, dideoxyinosine); connective tissue diseases/vasculitis (e.g., lupus, thrombotic thrombocytopenic purpura); penetrating peptic ulcer; obstruction of the ampulla of Vater (e.g., regional enteritis); pancreas divisum.

CLINICAL FEATURES Can vary from mild abdominal pain to shock. *Common symptoms*: (1) steady, boring midepigastric pain radiating to the back that is frequently increased in the supine position; (2) nausea, vomiting.

Physical exam: (1) low-grade fever, tachycardia, hypotension; (2) erythematous skin nodules due to subcutaneous fat necrosis; (3) basilar rales, pleural effusion (often on the left); (4) abdominal tenderness and rigidity, diminished bowel sounds, palpable upper abdominal mass; (5) Cullen's sign: blue discoloration in the periumbilical area due to hemoperitoneum; (6) Turner's sign: blue-red-purple or green-brown discoloration of the flanks due to tissue catabolism of hemoglobin.

LABORATORY

1. *Serum amylase*: Large elevations (>3 × normal) virtually assure the diagnosis if salivary gland disease and intestinal perforation/infarction are excluded. However, normal serum amylase does not exclude the diagnosis of acute pancreatitis, and the degree of elevation does not predict severity of pancreatitis. Amylase levels typically return to normal in 48–72 h.

2. *Urinary amylase–creatinine clearance ratio*: no more sensitive or specific than blood amylase levels.

3. *Serum lipase* level: increases in parallel with amylase level and measurement of both tests increases the diagnostic yield.

4. *Other tests*: *Hypocalcemia* occurs in ~25% of pts. *Leukocytosis* (15,000–20,000/µL) occurs frequently. *Hypertriglyceridemia* occurs in 15–20% of cases and can cause a spuriously normal serum amylase level. *Hyperglycemia* is common. *Serum bilirubin, alkaline phosphatase*, and *aspartame aminotransferase* can be transiently elevated. *Hypoalbuminemia* and marked elevations of *serum lactic dehydrogenase* (LDH) are associated with an increased mortality rate. *Hypoxemia* is present in 25% of pts. Arterial pH < 7.32 may spuriously elevate serum amylase.

IMAGING

1. *Abdominal radiographs* are abnormal in 30–50% of pts but are not specific for pancreatitis. Common findings include total or partial ileus ("sentinel loop") and the "colon cut-off sign," which results from isolated distention of the transverse colon. Useful for excluding diagnoses such as intestinal perforation with free air.

2. *Ultrasound* often fails to visualize the pancreas because of overlying intestinal gas but may detect gallstones, pseudocysts, mass lesions, or edema or enlargement of the pancreas.

3. *CT* can confirm diagnosis of pancreatitis (edematous pancreas) and is useful for predicting and identifying late complications. Contrast-enhanced dynamic CT is indicated for clinical deterioration, the presence of risk factors that adversely affect survival (Table 154-1), or other features of serious illness.

DIFFERENTIAL DIAGNOSIS Intestinal perforation (especially peptic ulcer), cholecystitis, acute intestinal obstruction, mesenteric ischemia, renal colic, myocardial ischemia, aortic dissection, connective tissue disorders, pneumonia, and diabetic ketoacidosis.

℞ TREATMENT

Most (90%) cases subside over a period of 3–7 days. Conventional measures: (1) analgesics, such as meperidine; (2) IV fluids and colloids; (3) no oral alimentation; (4) treatment of hypocalcemia, if symptomatic; (5) antibiotics, if there is established infection or prophylactically in acute necrotizing pancreatitis. Current recommendation is use of an antibiotic such as imipenem-cilastatin, 500 mg tid for 2 weeks. Not effective: cimetidine (or related agents), H_2 blockers, protease inhibitors, glucocorticoids, nasogastric suction, glucagon, peritoneal lavage, and anticholinergic medications. Precipitating factors (alcohol, medications) must be eliminated. In mild or moderate pancreatitis, a clear liquid diet can usually be started after 3–6 days. Pts with severe gallstone-induced pancreatitis often benefit from early (<3 days) papillotomy.

COMPLICATIONS It is important to identify pts who are at risk of poor outcome. Key indicators of a severe attack of pancreatitis are listed in Table

Table 154-1

Risk Factors that Adversely Affect Survival in Acute Pancreatitis

1. Organ failure[a]
   a. Cardiovascular: hypotension (systolic blood pressure < 90 mmHg) or tachycardia > 130 beats/min
   b. Pulmonary: P_{O_2} < 60 mmHg
   c. Renal: oliguria (<50 mL/h) or increasing BUN or creatinine
   d. Gastrointestinal bleeding
2. Pancreatic necrosis[a] (see Table 294-4, HPIM-16)
3. Obesity[a] (BMI > 29); age > 70
4. Hemoconcentration[a] (hematocrit > 44%)
5. C-reactive protein > 150 mg/L
6. Trypsinogen activation peptide
   a. >3 Ranson criteria (not fully utilizable until 48 h)[b]
   b. Apache II score > 8 (cumbersome)[b]

[a] Most useful.
[b] Often cited, but less useful.
Note: BUN, blood urea nitrogen; BMI, body mass index.

154-1. Fulminant pancreatitis requires aggressive fluid support and meticulous management. Mortality is largely due to infection.

Systemic   Shock, GI bleeding, common duct obstruction, ileus, splenic infarction or rupture, DIC, subcutaneous fat necrosis, ARDS, pleural effusion, acute renal failure, sudden blindness.

Local

1. Sterile or infected *pancreatic necrosis*—necrosis may become secondarily infected in 40–60% of pts, typically within 1–2 weeks after the onset of pancreatitis. Most frequent organisms: gram-negative bacteria of alimentary origin, but intraabdominal *Candida* infection increasing in frequency. Necrosis can be visualized by contrast-enhanced dynamic CT, with infection diagnosed by CT-guided needle aspiration. Laparotomy with removal of necrotic material and adequate drainage should be considered for pts with sterile acute necrotic pancreatitis if pt continues to deteriorate despite conventional therapy. Infected pancreatic necrosis requires aggressive surgical debridement and antibiotics.

2. *Pancreatic pseudocysts* develop over 1–4 weeks in 15% of pts. Abdominal pain is the usual complaint, and a tender upper abdominal mass may be present. Can be detected by abdominal ultrasound or CT. In pts who are stable and uncomplicated, treatment is supportive; pseudocysts that are >5 cm in diameter and persist for >6 weeks should be considered for drainage. In pts with an expanding pseudocyst or one complicated by hemorrhage, rupture, or abscess, surgery should be performed.

3. *Pancreatic abscess*—ill-defined liquid collection of pus that evolves over 4–6 weeks. Can be treated surgically or in selected cases by percutaneous drainage.

4. *Pancreatic ascites* and *pleural effusions* are usually due to disruption of the main pancreatic duct. Treatment involves nasogastric suction and parenteral alimentation for 2–3 weeks. If medical management fails, pancreatography followed by surgery should be performed.

CHRONIC PANCREATITIS
Chronic pancreatitis may occur as recurrent episodes of acute inflammation superimposed upon a previously injured pancreas or as chronic damage with pain and malabsorption.

ETIOLOGY   Chronic alcoholism most frequent cause of pancreatic exocrine insufficiency in U.S. adults; also hypertriglyceridemia, hypercalcemia, hereditary pancreatitis, hemochromatosis. Cystic fibrosis most frequent cause in children. In 25% of adults, etiology is unknown.

SYMPTOMS AND SIGNS   *Pain* is cardinal symptom. Weight loss, steatorrhea, and other signs and symptoms of malabsorption common. Physical exam often unremarkable.

LABORATORY   No specific laboratory test for chronic pancreatitis. Serum amylase and lipase levels are often normal. Serum bilirubin and alkaline phosphatase may be elevated. Steatorrhea (fecal fat concentration $\geq 9.5\%$) late in the course. The bentiromide test, a simple, effective test of pancreatic exocrine function, may be helpful. D-Xylose urinary excretion test is usually normal. Impaired glucose tolerance is present in $>50\%$ of pts. Secretin stimulation test is a relatively sensitive test for pancreatic exocrine deficiency.

IMAGING   *Plain films of the abdomen* reveal pancreatic calcifications in 30–60%. *Ultrasound* and *CT scans* may show dilation of the pancreatic duct. *ERCP* and endoscopic ultrasound (*EUS*) provide information about the main pancreatic and smaller ducts.

DIFFERENTIAL DIAGNOSIS   Important to distinguish from pancreatic carcinoma; may require radiographically guided biopsy.

 TREATMENT

Aimed at controlling pain and malabsorption. Intermittent attacks treated like acute pancreatitis. Alcohol and large, fatty meals must be avoided. Narcotics for severe pain, but subsequent addiction is common. Pts unable to maintain adequate hydration should be hospitalized, while those with milder symptoms can be managed on an ambulatory basis. Surgery may control pain if there is a ductal stricture. Subtotal pancreatectomy may also control pain but at the cost of exocrine insufficiency and diabetes. Malabsorption is managed with a low-fat diet and pancreatic enzyme replacement (8 conventional tablets or 3 enteric-coated tablets with meals). Because pancreatic enzymes are inactivated by acid, agents that reduce acid production (e.g., omeprazole or sodium bicarbonate) may improve their efficacy (but should not be given with enteric-coated preparations). Insulin may be necessary to control serum glucose.

COMPLICATIONS   Vitamin B_{12} malabsorption in 40% of alcohol-induced and all cystic fibrosis cases. Impaired glucose tolerance. Nondiabetic retinopathy due to vitamin A and/or zinc deficiency. GI bleeding, icterus, effusions, subcutaneous fat necrosis, and bone pain occasionally occur. Increased risk for pancreatic carcinoma. Narcotic addiction common.

For a more detailed discussion, see Greenberger NJ, Toskes PP: Acute and Chronic Pancreatitis, Chap. 294, p. 1895; Toskes PP, Greenberger NJ: Approach to the Patient with Pancreatic Disease, Chap. 293, p. 1891, in HPIM-16.

155

ACUTE HEPATITIS

VIRAL HEPATITIS

Clinically characterized by malaise, nausea, vomiting, diarrhea, and low-grade fever followed by dark urine, jaundice, and tender hepatomegaly; may be subclinical and detected on basis of elevated aspartate and alanine aminotransferase (AST and ALT) levels. Hepatitis B may be associated with immune-complex phenomena, including arthritis, serum-sickness–like illness, glomerulonephritis, and polyarteritis nodosa. Hepatitis-like illnesses may be caused not only by hepatotropic viruses (A, B, C, D, E) but also by other viruses (Epstein-Barr, CMV, coxsackievirus, etc.), alcohol, drugs, hypotension and ischemia, and biliary tract disease (Table 155-1).

HEPATITIS A (HAV)   27-nm picornavirus (hepatovirus) with single-stranded RNA genome.

Clinical Course   See Fig. 155-1.

Outcome   Recovery within 6–12 months, occasionally after one or two apparent clinical and serologic relapses; in some cases, pronounced cholestasis suggesting biliary obstruction may occur; rare fatalities (fulminant hepatitis), no chronic carrier state.

Diagnosis   IgM anti-HAV in acute or early convalescent serum sample.

Epidemiology   Fecal-oral transmission; endemic in underdeveloped countries; food-borne and waterborne epidemics; outbreaks in day-care centers, residential institutions.

Prevention   *After exposure*: immune globulin 0.02 mL/kg IM within 2 weeks to household and institutional contacts (not casual contacts at work). *Before exposure*: inactivated HAV vaccine 1 mL IM (unit dose depends on formulation); half dose to children; repeat at 6–12 months; target travelers, military recruits, animal handlers, day-care personnel.

HEPATITIS B (HBV)   42-nm hepadnavirus with outer surface coat (HBsAg), inner nucleocapsid core (HBcAg), DNA polymerase, and partially double-stranded DNA genome of 3200 nucleotides. Circulating form of HBcAg is HBeAg, a marker of viral replication and infectivity. Multiple serotypes and genetic heterogeneity.

Clinical Course See Fig. 155-2.

Outcome   Recovery >90%, fulminant hepatitis (<1%), chronic hepatitis or carrier state (only 1–2% of immunocompetent adults; higher in neonates, elderly, immunocompromised), cirrhosis, and hepatocellular carcinoma (especially following chronic infection beginning in infancy or early childhood) (see Chap. 157).

Diagnosis   HBsAg in serum (acute or chronic infection); IgM anti-HBc (early anti-HBc indicative of acute or recent infection). Most sensitive test is detection of HBV DNA in serum; not generally required for routine diagnosis.

Epidemiology   Percutaneous (needle stick), sexual, or perinatal transmission. Endemic in sub-Saharan Africa and Southeast Asia, where up to 20% of population acquire infection, usually early in life.

Table 155-1

The Hepatitis Viruses

	HAV	HBV	HCV	HDV	HEV
Viral Properties					
Size, nm	27	42	~55	~36	~32
Nucleic acid	RNA	DNA	RNA	RNA	RNA
Genome length, kb	7.5	3.2	9.4	1.7	7.5
Classification	Picornavirus	Hepadnavirus	Flavivirus-like	—	Calicivirus-like or alpha-virus-like
Incubation, days	15–45	30–180	15–160	21–140	14–63
Transmission					
Fecal-oral	+++	—	—	—	+++
Percutaneous	Rare	+++	+++	+++	—
Sexual	?	++	Uncommon	++	—
Perinatal	—	+++	Uncommon	+	—
Clinical Features					
Severity	Usually mild	Moderate	Mild	May be severe	Usually mild
Chronic infection	No	1–10%; up to 90% in neonates	80–90%	Common	No
Carrier state	No	Yes	Yes	Yes	No
Fulminant hepatitis	0.1%	1%	Rare	Up to 20% in super-infection	10–20% in pregnant women
Hepatocellular carcinoma	No	Yes	Yes	?	No
Prophylaxis	Ig; vaccine	HBIg; vaccine	None	None (HBV vaccine for susceptibles)	None

Note: HAV, hepatitis A virus; HBV, hepatitis B virus; HCV, hepatitis C virus; HDV, hepatitis D virus; HEV, hepatitis E virus; Ig, immune globulin; +, sometimes; + +, often; ?, possibly.

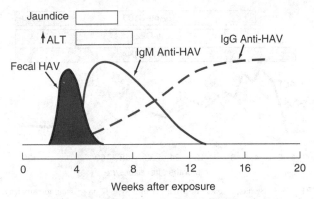

FIGURE 155-1 Scheme of typical clinical and laboratory features of HAV. (*Reproduced from Dienstag JL, Isselbacher KJ, HPIM-16, p. 1822.*)

Prevention   *After exposure*: hepatitis B immune globulin (HBIg) 0.06 mL/ kg IM immediately after needle stick, within 14 days of sexual exposure, or at birth (HbsAg+ mother) in combination with vaccine series. *Before exposure*: recombinant hepatitis B vaccine 10–20µg IM (dose depends on formulation); half dose to children, 40-µg dose for hemodialysis patients and immunocompromised adults; at 0, 1, and 6 months; deltoid, not gluteal injection. Has been targeted to high-risk groups (e.g., health workers, gay men, IV drug users, hemodialysis pts, hemophiliacs, household and sexual contacts of HBsAg carriers, all neonates in endemic areas, or high-risk neonates in lower-risk areas). Universal vaccination of all children is now recommended in the U.S.

HEPATITIS C (HCV)   Caused by flavi-like virus with RNA genome of >9000 nucleotides (similar to yellow fever virus, dengue virus); some genetic heterogeneity. Incubation period 7–8 weeks.

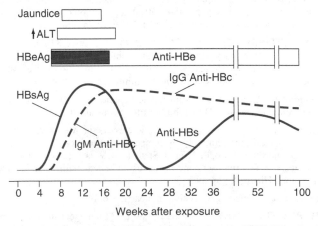

FIGURE 155-2 Scheme of typical clinical and laboratory features of HBV. (*Reproduced from Dienstag JL, Isselbacher KJ, HPIM-16, p. 1825.*)

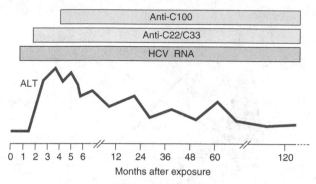

FIGURE 155-3 Serologic course of acute hepatitis type C progressing to chronicity. HCV RNA is detectable before the ALT elevation. Antibody to C22 and anti-C33 appears during acute hepatitis C, whereas antibody to C100 appears 1 to 3 months later. (*Reproduced from Dienstag JL, Isselbacher KJ, HPIM-16, p. 1827.*)

Clinical Course   Often clinically mild and marked by fluctuating elevations of serum aminotransferase levels; >50% likelihood of chronicity, leading to cirrhosis in >20%.

Diagnosis   Anti-HCV in serum. Current second- and third-generation enzyme immunoassay detects antibody to epitopes designated C200, C33c, C22-3; may appear after acute illness but generally present by 3–5 months after exposure. A positive enzyme immunoassay can be confirmed by recombinant immunoblot assay (RIBA) or by detection of HCV RNA in serum (Fig. 155-3).

Epidemiology   Percutaneous transmission accounts for >90% of transfusion-associated hepatitis cases. IV drug use accounts >50% of reported cases. Little evidence for frequent sexual or perinatal transmission.

Prevention   Exclusion of paid blood donors, testing of donated blood for anti-HCV. Anti-HCV detected by enzyme immunoassay in blood donors with normal ALT is often falsely positive (30%); result should be confirmed with RIBA, which correlates with presence of HCV RNA in serum.

HEPATITIS D (HDV, DELTA AGENT)   Defective 37-nm RNA virus that requires HBV for its replication; either co-infects with HBV or superinfects a chronic HBV carrier. Enhances severity of HBV infection (acceleration of chronic hepatitis to cirrhosis, occasionally fulminant acute hepatitis).

Diagnosis   Anti-HDV in serum (acute hepatitis D—often in low titer, is transient; chronic hepatitis D—in higher titer, is sustained).

Epidemiology   Endemic among HBV carriers in Mediterranean Basin, where it is spread predominantly by nonpercutaneous means. In nonendemic areas (e.g., northern Europe, United States) HDV is spread percutaneously among HbsAg+ IV drug users or by transfusion in hemophiliacs and to a lesser extent among HbsAg+ gay men.

Prevention   Hepatitis B vaccine (noncarriers only).

HEPATITIS E (HEV)   Caused by 29- to 32-nm agent thought to be related to caliciviruses. Enterically transmitted and responsible for waterborne epidemics of hepatitis in India, parts of Asia and Africa, and Central America. Self-limited illness with high (10–20%) mortality rate in pregnant women.

℞ TREATMENT

Activity as tolerated, high-calorie diet (often tolerated best in morning), IV hydration for severe vomiting, cholestyramine up to 4 g PO qid for severe pruritus, avoid hepatically metabolized drugs; no role for glucocorticoids. Liver transplantation for fulminant hepatic failure and grades III–IV encephalopathy. Meta-analysis of small clinical trials suggests that treatment of acute HCV infection with α-interferon may be effective at reducing the rate of chronicity. Based on these data, many experts feel that acute HCV infection should be treated with the best available regimens currently used to treat chronic HCV infection (see Chap. 156).

TOXIC AND DRUG-INDUCED HEPATITIS

DOSE-DEPENDENT (DIRECT HEPATOTOXINS) Onset is within 48 h, predictable, necrosis around terminal hepatic venule—e.g., carbon tetrachloride, benzene derivatives, mushroom poisoning, acetaminophen, or microvesicular steatosis (e.g., tetracyclines, valproic acid).

IDIOSYNCRATIC Variable dose and time of onset; small number of exposed persons affected; may be associated with fever, rash, arthralgias, eosinophilia. In many cases, mechanism may actually involve toxic metabolite, possibly determined on genetic basis—e.g., isoniazid, halothane, phenytoin, methyldopa, carbamazepine, diclofenac, oxacillin, sulfonamides.

℞ TREATMENT

Supportive as for viral hepatitis; withdraw suspected agent. Liver transplantation if necessary. In acetaminophen overdose, more specific therapy is available in the form of sulfhydryl compounds (e.g., N-acetylcysteine). These agents appear to act by providing a reservoir of sulfhydryl groups to bind the toxic metabolites or by stimulating synthesis of hepatic glutathione. Therapy should be begun within 8 h of ingestion but may be effective even if given as late as 24–36 h after overdose.

ACUTE HEPATIC FAILURE

Massive hepatic necrosis with impaired consciousness occurring within 8 weeks of the onset of illness.

CAUSES Infections [viral, including HAV, HBV, HCV (rarely), HDV, HEV; bacterial, rickettsial, parasitic], drugs and toxins, ischemia (shock), Budd-Chiari syndrome, idiopathic chronic active hepatitis, acute Wilson's disease, microvesicular fat syndromes (Reye's syndrome, acute fatty liver of pregnancy).

CLINICAL MANIFESTATIONS Neuropsychiatric changes—delirium, personality change, stupor, coma; cerebral edema—suggested by profuse sweating, hemodynamic instability, tachyarrhythmias, tachypnea, fever, papilledema, decerebrate rigidity (though all may be absent); deep jaundice, coagulopathy, bleeding, renal failure, acid-base disturbance, hypoglycemia, acute pancreatitis, cardiorespiratory failure, infections (bacterial, fungal).

ADVERSE PROGNOSTIC INDICATORS Age <10 or >40, certain causes (e.g., halothane, hepatitis C), duration of jaundice >7 d before onset of encephalopathy, serum bilirubin > 300 μmol/L (>18 mg/dL), coma (survival <20%), rapid reduction in liver size, respiratory failure, marked prolongation of PT, factor V level < 20%. In acetaminophen overdose, adverse prognosis is suggested by blood pH < 7.30, serum creatinine > 266 μmol/L (>3 mg/dL), markedly prolonged PT.

TREATMENT

Endotracheal intubation often required. Monitor serum glucose—IV D10 or D20 as necessary. Prevent gastrointestinal bleeding with H_2-receptor antagonists and antacids (maintain gastric pH $\geq$ 3.5). In many centers intracranial pressure is monitored—more sensitive than CT in detecting cerebral edema. Value of dexamethasone for cerebral edema unclear; IV mannitol may be beneficial. Liver transplantation should be considered in pts with grades III–IV encephalopathy and other adverse prognostic indicators.

For a more detailed discussion, see Dienstag JL, Isselbacher KJ: Acute Viral Hepatitis, Chap. 285, p. 1822, and Dienstag JL, Isselbacher KJ: Toxic and Drug-Induced Hepatitis, Chap. 286, p. 1838, in HPIM-16.

156

CHRONIC HEPATITIS

A group of disorders characterized by a chronic inflammatory reaction in the liver for at least 6 months.

OVERVIEW

ETIOLOGY   Hepatitis B virus (HBV), hepatitis C virus (HCV), hepatitis D virus (HDV, delta agent), drugs (methyldopa, nitrofurantoin, isoniazid, dantrolene), autoimmune hepatitis, Wilson's disease, hemochromatosis, α_1-antitrypsin deficiency.

HISTOLOGIC CLASSIFICATION   Chronic hepatitis can be classified by *grade* and *stage*. The grade is a histologic assessment of necrosis and inflammatory activity and is based on examination of the liver biopsy. The stage of chronic hepatitis reflects the level of disease progression and is based on the degree of fibrosis (see Table 287-2, p. 1845, HPIM-16).

PRESENTATION   Wide clinical spectrum ranging from asymptomatic serum aminotransferase elevations to apparently acute, even fulminant, hepatitis. Common symptoms include fatigue, malaise, anorexia, low-grade fever; jaundice is frequent in severe disease. Some pts may present with complications of cirrhosis: ascites, variceal bleeding, encephalopathy, coagulopathy, and hypersplenism. In chronic hepatitis B or C and autoimmune hepatitis, extrahepatic features may predominate.

CHRONIC HEPATITIS B

Follows up to 1–2% of cases of acute hepatitis B in immunocompetent hosts; more frequent in immunocompromised hosts. Spectrum of disease: asymptomatic antigenemia, chronic hepatitis, cirrhosis, hepatocellular cancer; early phase often associated with continued symptoms of hepatitis, elevated aminotransferase levels, presence in serum of HBeAg and HBV DNA, and presence in liver of replicative form of HBV; later phase in some pts may be associated with clinical and biochemical improvement, disappearance of HBeAg and HBV DNA and appearance of anti-HBeAg in serum, and integration of HBV DNA into host hepatocyte genome. In Mediterranean and European countries as well as in Asia, a frequent variant is characterized by readily detectable HBV DNA, but without HBeAg (anti-HBeAg-reactive). Most of these cases are due to a mutation in the pre-C region of the HBV genome that prevents HBeAg synthesis (may appear during course of chronic wild-type HBV infection as a result of immune pressure and may also account for some cases of fulminant hepatitis B). Chronic hepatitis B ultimately leads to cirrhosis in 25–40% of cases (particularly in pts with HDV superinfection or the pre-C mutation) and hepatocellular carcinoma in many of these pts (particularly when chronic infection is acquired early in life).

EXTRAHEPATIC MANIFESTATIONS (IMMUNE-COMPLEX– MEDIATED) Rash, urticaria, arthritis, polyarteritis, polyneuropathy, glomerulonephritis.

℞ TREATMENT

Interferon-α 5 million units qd or 10 million units three times per week for 4 months for serum HBeAg/HBV-DNA-positive pts with symptoms, elevated aminotransferase levels, and biopsy evidence of chronic hepatitis. Results in anti-HBe seroconversion with clinical, biochemical, and histologic improvement in ~30% of cases. Best predictors of response are lower levels of HBV DNA and substantial elevations of aminotransferases. Poor responders: pts positive for anti-HDV or HIV, adult carriers infected in childhood, immunocompromised pts, persons infected with HBeAg-negative "pre-core" mutant. Side effects: flulike reactions (common), bone marrow depression, precipitation of autoimmune diseases including thyroid disease, CNS symptoms, anorexia, sleep disturbance. Avoid interferon in pts with decompensated cirrhosis (e.g., ascites, jaundice, coagulopathy, encephalopathy). The nucleoside analogue *lamivudine* (3TC) is approved by the FDA for the treatment of chronic HBV. Treatment with lamivudine (100 mg/d) for 12 months results in significant biochemical and histologic improvement in >50% of pts and anti-HBeAg seroconversion in 16–20%. Lamivudine is associated with minimal side effects in HBV-infected pts. Flares of HBV, which can potentially lead to decompensation of liver disease, can occur on stopping lamivudine, with development of lamivudine resistance mutations, and with seroconversion. Lamivudine should be considered as first-line therapy in pts with evidence of active hepatitis and viral replication who fall into one of the following groups: contraindications to interferon (especially decompensated cirrhosis); pts with pre-core mutations; pts with chronic immunosuppression; or pts not responsive to interferon. The nucleotide analogue *adefovir* has recently been approved by the FDA for the treatment of chronic HBV. At an oral daily dose of 10 mg, a 48-week course of adefovir results in biochemical and histologic improvement in ~50% of cases; anti-HBeAg seroconversion in 12%. Adefovir is well tolerated but has the potential to be nephrotoxic; for pts with underlying renal insufficiency, dose reductions are necessary. Table 156-1 summarizes indications for antiviral therapy in pts with chronic HBV.

CHRONIC HEPATITIS C
Follows 50–70% of cases of transfusion-associated and sporadic hepatitis C. Clinically mild, often waxing and waning aminotransferase elevations; mild chronic hepatitis on liver biopsy. Extrahepatic manifestations include essential mixed cryoglobulinemia, porphyria cutanea tarda, membranoproliferative glo-

Table 156-1

Patients with Chronic Hepatitis B Who Are Candidates for Antiviral Therapy

Clinical Feature	Interferon	Lamivudine	Adefovir
Detectable markers of HBV replication	Yes	Yes	Yes
Normal ALT activity	No	No	No
ALT <2 × upper limit of normal	No	No	No
ALT >2 × upper limit of normal	Yes	Yes	Yes
Immunocompetent	Yes	Yes	Yes
Immunocompromised	No	Yes	Yes
Adult acquisition (western)	Yes	Yes	Yes
Childhood acquisition (Asian)	No	Yes	Yes
Compensated liver disease	Yes	Yes	Yes
Decompensated liver disease	No	Yes	Yes
"Wild-type" HBeAg-reactive	Yes	Yes	Yes
HBeAg-negative chronic hepatitis	Yes	Yes	Yes
Interferon-refractory	No	Yes	Yes

Note: HBV, hepatitis B virus; ALT, alanine aminotransferase; HBeAg, hepatitis B e antigen.

merulonephritis, and lymphocytic sialadenitis. Diagnosis confirmed by detecting anti-HCV in serum. May lead to cirrhosis in ≥20% of cases after 20 years.

 TREATMENT

Therapy should be considered in pts with aminotransferase elevations, biopsy evidence of moderate or severe chronic hepatitis, HCV RNA in serum. The current therapy of choice for treatment of chronic HCV infection is a combination of pegylated interferon-α and the guanosine nucleoside analogue ribavirin. The dosage and duration of therapy depends on the preparation of pegylated interferon-α and viral genotype (see Table 156-2). Monitoring of HCV plasma RNA is useful in assessing response to therapy. The failure to achieve a 2-log drop in HCV RNA by week 12 of therapy ("early virologic response") makes it unlikely that further therapy will result in a sustained virologic response. Thus, it is recommended that HCV RNA be measured at baseline and after 12 weeks of therapy. The current consensus view is that therapy can be stopped if an early virologic response is not achieved; however, some experts feel that histologic benefit may occur even in the absence of a virologic response.

AUTOIMMUNE HEPATITIS

CLASSIFICATION   *Type I*: classic autoimmune hepatitis, anti-smooth-muscle and/or antinuclear antibodies. *Type II*: associated with anti-liver/kidney microsomal (anti-LKM) antibodies, which are directed against cytochrome P450IID6 (seen primarily in southern Europe). *Type III* patients lack antinuclear antibodies and anti-LKM, have antibodies reactive with hepatocyte cytokeratins; clinically similar to type I.

CLINICAL MANIFESTATIONS   Classic autoimmune hepatitis (type I): 80% women, third to fifth decades. Abrupt onset (acute hepatitis) in a third. Insidious onset in two-thirds: progressive jaundice, anorexia, hepatomegaly, abdominal pain, epistaxis, fever, fatigue, amenorrhea. Leads to cirrhosis; >50% 5-year mortality if untreated.

Table 156-2

Comparison of Pegylated Interferon-α2a and -α2b for Chronic Hepatitis C[a]

	PEG IFN-α2b	PEG IFN-α2a
PEG size	12 kDa linear	40 kDa branched
Mean terminal half-life	40 h	80 h
Mean clearance	94 mL/h per kg	22 mL/h per kg
Best-dose monotherapy	1.0 μg/kg (weight-based)	180 μg
Best-dose combination therapy	1.5 μg/kg (weight-based)	180 μg
Storage	Room temperature	Refrigerated
Ribavirin		
Genotype 1	800 mg[b]	1000–1200 mg[c]
Genotype 2/3	800 mg	800 mg
Duration of therapy		
Genotype 1	48 weeks	48 weeks
Genotype 2/3	48 weeks[d]	24 weeks
Efficacy of combination Rx	54%	56%
Genotype 1	42%	46–51%
Genotype 2/3	82%	76–78%
Side effects of pegylated interferon/ribavirin vs standard interferon/ribavirin[e]		
Fever	46% vs 33%	43% vs 56%
Myalgias	56% vs 50%	42% vs 50%
Rigors	48% vs 41%	24% vs 35%
Depression	31% vs 34%	22% vs 30%
Irritability	35% vs 34%	24% vs 28%

[a] These comparisons are based upon data on each drug tested individually versus other regimens in registration trials; because these comparisons are not based on head-to-head comparisons between the two drugs, and because the populations tested are not entirely analogous, relative advantages and disadvantages should be interpreted with caution.

[b] In the registration trial for pegylated IFN-α2b plus ribavirin, the optimal regimen was 1.5 μg of pegylated IFN plus 800 mg of ribavirin; however, a post hoc analysis of this study as well as data from other studies suggest that 1000 (for pts < 75 kg)–1200 (for pts ≥ 75 kg) mg of ribavirin might be better, certainly for genotype 1, and many clinicians prescribe the higher ribavirin doses.

[c] 1000 mg for pts < 75 kg; 1200 mg for pts ≥ 75 kg.

[d] In the registration trial for pegylated IFN-α2b plus ribavirin, all pts were treated for 48 weeks; however, data from other trials of standard IFNs and the other pegylated IFN suggest that 24 weeks should suffice for pts with genotypes 2 and 3.

[e] These comparisons show the frequency in registration trials of the listed side effects for the respective pegylated IFN plus ribavirin as compared to the listed side effects in comparative groups who received standard IFN-α2b plus ribavirin. As noted above, these comparisons do not represent head-to-head tests of the two pegylated IFNs.

Note: PEG, polyethylene glycol; IFN, interferon.

EXTRAHEPATIC MANIFESTATIONS Rash, arthralgias, keratoconjunctivitis sicca, thyroiditis, hemolytic anemia, nephritis.

SEROLOGIC ABNORMALITIES Hypergammaglobulinemia, positive rheumatoid factor, smooth-muscle antibody (40–80%), ANA (20–50%), antimitochondrial antibody (10–20%), false-positive anti-HCV enzyme immunoassay but usually not recombinant immunoblot assay (RIBA). Type II: anti-LKM antibody.

℞ TREATMENT

Indicated for symptomatic disease with biopsy evidence of severe chronic hepatitis (bridging necrosis), marked aminotransferase elevations (5- to 10- fold), and hypergammaglobulinemia. Prednisone or prednisolone 30–60 mg PO qd tapered to 10–15 mg qd over several weeks; often azathioprine 50 mg PO qd is also administered to permit lower glucocorticoid doses and avoid steroid side effects. Monitor LFTs monthly. Symptoms may improve rapidly, but biochemical improvement may take weeks or months and subsequent histologic improvement (to lesion of mild chronic hepatitis or normal biopsy) up to 18–24 months. Therapy should be continued for at least 12–18 months. Relapse occurs in at least 50% of cases (re-treat). For frequent relapses, consider maintenance therapy with low-dose glucocorticoids or azathioprine 2(mg/kg)/d.

Although hepatitis A rarely causes fulminant hepatic failure, it may do so more frequently in pts with chronic liver disease—especially those with chronic hepatitis B or C. The hepatitis A vaccine is immunogenic and well tolerated in pts with chronic hepatitis. Thus, pts with chronic liver disease, especially those with chronic hepatitis B or C, should be vaccinated against hepatitis A.

For a more detailed discussion, see Dienstag JL, Isselbacher KJ: **Chronic Hepatitis,** Chap. 287, p. 1844, in HPIM-16.

157

CIRRHOSIS AND ALCOHOLIC LIVER DISEASE

CIRRHOSIS

Chronic disease of the liver characterized by fibrosis, disorganization of the lobular and vascular architecture, and regenerating nodules of hepatocytes.

CAUSES Alcohol, viral hepatitis (B, C, D), primary or secondary biliary cirrhosis, hemochromatosis, Wilson's disease, α_1-antitrypsin deficiency, autoimmune hepatitis, Budd-Chiari syndrome, chronic CHF (cardiac cirrhosis), drugs and toxins, schistosomiasis, cryptogenic.

CLINICAL MANIFESTATIONS May be absent.

Symptoms Anorexia, nausea, vomiting, diarrhea, fatigue, weakness, fever, jaundice, amenorrhea, impotence, infertility.

Signs Spider telangiectases, palmar erythema, parotid and lacrimal gland enlargement, nail changes (Muehrcke lines, Terry's nails), clubbing, Dupuytren's contracture, gynecomastia, testicular atrophy, hepatosplenomegaly, ascites, gastrointestinal bleeding (e.g., varices), hepatic encephalopathy.

Laboratory Findings Anemia (microcytic due to blood loss, macrocytic due to folate deficiency), pancytopenia (hypersplenism), prolonged PT, rarely overt DIC; hyponatremia, hypokalemic alkalosis, glucose disturbances, hypoalbuminemia, hypoxemia (hepatopulmonary syndrome).

Other Associations Gastritis, duodenal ulcer, gallstones. Altered drug metabolism because of decreased drug clearance, metabolism (e.g., by cytochrome P450), and elimination; hypoalbuminemia; and portosystemic shunting.

DIAGNOSTIC STUDIES Depend on clinical setting. Serum: HBsAg, anti-HBc, anti-HBs, anti-HCV, anti-HDV, Fe, total iron-binding capacity, ferritin, antimitochondrial antibody (AMA), smooth-muscle antibody (SMA), anti-liver/kidney microsomal (anti-LKM) antibody, ANA, ceruloplasmin, α_1-antitrypsin (and pi typing); abdominal ultrasound with doppler study, CT or MRI (may show cirrhotic liver, splenomegaly, collaterals, venous thrombosis), portal venography, and wedged hepatic vein pressure measurement. Definitive diagnosis often depends on liver biopsy (percutaneous, transjugular, or open).

ALCOHOLIC LIVER DISEASE

Three forms: fatty liver, alcoholic hepatitis, cirrhosis; may coexist. History of excessive alcohol use often denied. Severe forms (hepatitis, cirrhosis) associated with ingestion of 160 g/d for >5–10 years; women more susceptible than men due to poorly understood differences in the gastric and hepatic metabolism of alcohol and hormonal factors. Hepatitis B and C may be cofactors in the development of liver disease. Malnutrition may contribute to development of cirrhosis.

FATTY LIVER May follow even brief periods of ethanol use. Often presents as asymptomatic hepatomegaly and mild elevations in biochemical liver tests. Reverses on withdrawal of ethanol; does not lead to cirrhosis.

ALCOHOLIC HEPATITIS Clinical presentation ranges from asymptomatic to severe liver failure with jaundice, ascites, GI bleeding, and encephalopathy. Typically anorexia, nausea, vomiting, fever, jaundice, tender hepatomegaly. Occasional cholestatic picture mimicking biliary obstruction. Aspartate aminotransferase (AST) usually <300 U and more than twofold higher than alanine aminotransferase (ALT). Bilirubin may be >170 μmol/L (>10 mg/dL). WBC may be as high as 20,000/μL. Diagnosis defined by liver biopsy findings: hepatocyte swelling, alcoholic hyaline (Mallory bodies), infiltration of PMNs, necrosis of hepatocytes, pericentral venular fibrosis.

Other Metabolic Consequences of Alcoholism Increased NADH/NAD ratio leads to lactic acidemia, ketoacidosis, hyperuricemia, hypoglycemia. Hypomagnesemia, hypophosphatemia. Also mitochondrial dysfunction, induction of microsomal enzymes resulting in altered drug metabolism, lipid peroxidation leading to membrane damage, hypermetabolic state; many features of alcoholic hepatitis are attributable to toxic effects of acetaldehyde and cytokines (IL-1, IL-6, and TNF, released because of impaired detoxification of endotoxin).

Adverse Prognostic Factors *Short-term*: PT > 5 s above control, bilirubin > 137 μmmol/L (>8 mg/dL), encephalopathy, hypoalbuminemia, azotemia. A discriminant function can be calculated as 4.6 × (patient's PT in seconds) − (control PT in seconds) + serum bilirubin (mg/dL). Values ≥ 32 are associated with poor prognosis.

Long-term: severe hepatic necrosis and fibrosis, portal hypertension, continued alcohol consumption.

 TREATMENT

Abstinence is essential; 8500–12,500 kJ (2000–3000 kcal) diet with 1 g/kg protein (less if encephalopathy). Daily multivitamin, thiamine 100 mg, folic acid 1 mg. Correct potassium, magnesium, and phosphate deficiencies. Transfusions of packed red cells, plasma as necessary. Monitor glucose (hypoglycemia in severe liver disease). Prednisone 40 mg or prednisolone 32 mg PO qd for 1 month may be beneficial in severe alcoholic hepatitis with encephalopathy (in absence of GI bleeding, renal failure, infection). New evidence that proinflammatory cytokines may play an important role in alcoholic liver injury and emerging experience with pharmacologic inhibition of TNF by pentoxifylline have led to the recent inclusion of this agent as an alternative to glucocorticoids in the treatment of severe alcoholic hepatitis. Liver transplantation may be an option in carefully selected pts who have been abstinent >6 months.

PRIMARY BILIARY CIRRHOSIS

Progressive nonsuppurative destructive intrahepatic cholangitis. Affects middle-age women. Presents as asymptomatic elevation in alkaline phosphatase (better prognosis) or with pruritus, progressive jaundice, consequences of impaired bile excretion, and ultimately cirrhosis and liver failure.

CLINICAL MANIFESTATIONS Pruritus, jaundice, xanthelasma, xanthomata, osteoporosis, steatorrhea, skin pigmentation, hepatosplenomegaly, portal hypertension; elevations in serum alkaline phosphatase, bilirubin, cholesterol, and IgM levels.

ASSOCIATED DISEASES Sjögren's syndrome, collagen vascular diseases, thyroiditis, glomerulonephritis, pernicious anemia, renal tubular acidosis.

DIAGNOSIS Antimitochondrial antibodies (AMA) in >90–95% (directed against the E_2 component of pyruvate dehydrogenase and other 2-oxo-acid dehydrogenase mitochondrial enzymes). Liver biopsy: stage 1—destruction of interlobular bile ducts, granulomas; stage 2—ductular proliferation; stage 3—fibrosis; stage 4—cirrhosis.

PROGNOSIS Correlates with age, serum bilirubin, serum albumin, prothrombin time, edema.

 TREATMENT

Cholestyramine 4 g PO with meals for pruritus; in refractory cases consider rifampin, phototherapy with UVB light, naloxone infusion, plasmapheresis. Vitamin K 10 mg IM qd X 3 (then once a month) for elevated PT due to intestinal bile-salt deficiency. Vitamin D 100,000 U IM q 4 weeks plus oral calcium 1 g qd for osteoporosis (often unresponsive). Vitamin A 25,000–50,000 U PO qd or 100,000 U IM q 4 weeks and zinc 220 mg PO qd may help night blindness. Vitamin E 10 mg IM or PO qd. Substituting medium-chain triglycerides (MCTs) for dietary fat may reduce steatorrhea. Glucocorticoids, D-penicillamine, azathioprine, chlorambucil, cyclosporine of no value. Most widely used agent is ursodeoxycholic acid 10–15(mg/kg)/d PO in 2 divided doses—improves symptoms and LFTs and slows progression, delaying need for liver transplantation. Colchicine less effective, and methotrexate requires more study. Liver transplantation for end-stage disease.

LIVER TRANSPLANTATION

Consider for chronic, irreversible, progressive liver disease or fulminant hepatic failure when no alternative therapy is available. (Also indicated to correct certain congenital enzyme deficiencies and inborn errors of metabolism.)

CONTRAINDICATIONS *Absolute* Uncontrolled extrahepatobiliary infection or malignancy, active sepsis, severe cardiopulmonary disease, preexisting advanced cardiovascular or pulmonary disease, active alcoholism or drug abuse, metastatic malignancy to the liver, AIDS.

Relative Age >70, HIV infection, extensive previous abdominal surgery, portal and superior mesenteric vein thrombosis, renal failure, severe obesity, lack of pt understanding.

INDICATIONS Ideally, transplantation should be considered in pts with end-stage liver disease who are experiencing or have experienced a life-threatening complication of hepatic decompensation, whose quality of life has deteriorated to unacceptable levels, or whose liver disease will result predictably in irreversible damage to the CNS (for specific guidelines, see Table 291-3, p. 1875, in HPIM-16).

SELECTION OF DONOR Matched for ABO blood group compatibility and liver size (reduced-size grafts may be used, esp. in children). Should be negative for HIV, HBV, and HCV.

IMMUNOSUPPRESSION Various combinations of tacrolimus or cyclosporine and glucocorticoids, sirolimus, mycophenolate mofetil, azathioprine, or OKT3 (monoclonal antithymocyte globulin).

MEDICAL COMPLICATIONS AFTER TRANSPLANTATION Liver graft dysfunction (primary nonfunction, acute or chronic rejection, ischemia, hepatic artery thrombosis, biliary obstruction or leak, recurrent hepatitis B or C); infections (bacterial, viral, fungal, opportunistic); renal dysfunction; neuropsychiatric disorders.

SUCCESS RATE Currently, 5-year survival rates exceed 60%; less for certain conditions (e.g., chronic hepatitis B, hepatocellular carcinoma).

For a more detailed discussion, see Chung RT, Podolsky DK: Cirrhosis and Its Complications, Chap. 289, p. 1858; Mailliard ME, Sorrell MF: Alcoholic Liver Disease, Chap. 288, p. 1855; Dienstag JL: Liver Transplantation, Chap. 291, p. 1873, in HPIM-16.

158

PORTAL HYPERTENSION

Portal hypertension is defined as an increase in portal vein pressure (>10 mmHg) due to anatomic or functional obstruction to blood flow in the portal venous system. Normal portal vein pressure is 5–10 mmHg.

CLASSIFICATION See Table 158-1.

CONSEQUENCES (1) Increased collateral circulation between high-pressure portal venous system and low-pressure systemic venous system: lower

Table 158-1

Pathophysiologic Classification of Portal Hypertension

Site of obstruction	Pressure		Examples
	Portal	Corrected wedged hepatic vein[a]	
Presinu-soidal	↑	Normal	Splenic AV fistula, portal or splenic vein thrombosis, schistosomiasis
Sinusoidal	↑	↑	Cirrhosis, hepatitis
Postsinu-soidal	↑	↑ (May be un-measurable due to hepatic vein occlusion)	Budd-Chiari syndrome, veno-occlusive disease

[a] Wedged hepatic vein minus inferior vena cava pressure.

esophagus/upper stomach (varices, portal hypertensive gastropathy), rectum (varices, portal hypertensive colopathy), anterior abdominal wall (caput medusae; flow away from umbilicus), parietal peritoneum, splenorenal; (2) increased lymphatic flow; (3) increased plasma volume; (4) ascites; (5) splenomegaly, possible hypersplenism; (6) portosystemic shunting (including hepatic encephalopathy).

ESOPHAGOGASTRIC VARICES

Bleeding is major life-threatening complication; risk correlates with variceal size and the degree of portal hypertension (portal venous pressure >12 mmHg). Mortality correlates with severity of underlying liver disease (hepatic reserve), e.g., Child-Turcotte classification (Table 158-2).

DIAGNOSIS *Esophagogastroscopy*: procedure of choice for evaluation of upper gastrointestinal hemorrhage in pts with known or suspected portal hypertension. *Celiac* and *mesenteric arteriography* is an alternative when massive bleeding prevents endoscopy and to evaluate portal vein patency (portal vein may also be studied by ultrasound with doppler and MRI).

Table 158-2

Classification of Cirrhosis According to Child and Turcotte

	Class		
	A	B	C
Serum bilirubin, μmol/L (mg/dL)	<34 (<2)	34–51 (2–3)	>51 (>3)
Serum albumin, g/L (g/dL)	>35 (>3.5)	30–35 (3.0–3.5)	<30 (<3.0)
Ascites	None	Easily controlled	Poorly controlled
Encephalopathy	None	Mild	Advanced
Nutrition	Excellent	Good	Poor
Prognosis	Good	Fair	Poor

℞ TREATMENT

See Chap. 53 for general measures to treat GI bleeding.

Control of Acute Bleeding   Choice of approach depends on clinical setting and availability.

1.   Endoscopic band ligation or sclerotherapy—procedure of choice (not always suitable for gastric varices); band ligation is now preferred because of lower complication rate and possibly greater efficacy—application of bands around "pseudopolyp" of varix created by endoscopic suction; sclerotherapy involves direct injection of sclerosant into varix; >90% success rate in controlling acute bleeding; complications (less frequent with band ligation than sclerotherapy)—esophageal ulceration and stricture, fever, chest pain, mediastinitis, pleural effusions, aspiration.

2.   Intravenous vasopressin up to 0.1–0.4 U/min until bleeding is controlled for 12–24 h (50–80% success rate, but no effect on mortality), then discontinue or taper (0.1 U/min q6–12h); add nitroglycerin up to 0.6 mg SL q 30 min, 40–400 μg/min IV, or by transdermal patch 10 mg/24 h to prevent coronary and renal vasoconstriction. Maintain systolic BP >90 mmHg. Somatostatin and its analogue octreotide are direct splanchnic vasoconstrictors. Somatostatin (initial bolus of 250 μg followed by a constant infusion of 250 μg/h) or octreotide (50–100 μg/h) appear to be as effective as vasopressin with fewer serious complications.

3.   Blakemore-Sengstaken balloon tamponade; can be inflated for up to 24–48 h; complications—obstruction of pharynx, asphyxiation, aspiration, esophageal ulceration. Due to risk of aspiration, endotracheal intubation should be performed prior to placing Blakemore-Sengstaken tube. Generally reserved for massive bleeding, failure of vasopressin and/or endoscopic therapy.

4.   Transjugular intrahepatic portosystemic shunt (TIPS)— portacaval shunt placed by interventional radiologic technique, reserved for failure of other approaches; risk of hepatic encephalopathy (20–30%), shunt stenosis or occlusion (30–60%), infection.

Prevention of Recurrent Bleeding

1.   Repeated endoscopic band ligation or sclerotherapy (e.g., q2–4 weeks) until obliteration of varices. Decreases but does not eliminate risk of recurrent bleeding; effect on overall survival uncertain but compares favorably to shunt surgery.

2.   Propranolol or nadolol—nonselective beta blockers that act as portal venous antihypertensives; most effective in well-compensated cirrhotics; generally given in doses that reduce heart rate by 25%.

3.   Splenectomy (for splenic vein thrombosis).

4.   TIPS—regarded as useful "bridge" to liver transplantation in pt awaiting a donor liver who has failed on pharmacologic therapy.

5.   Portosystemic shunt surgery: portacaval (total decompression) or distal splenorenal (Warren) (selective; contraindicated in ascites; ? lower incidence of hepatic encephalopathy). Alternative procedure—devascularization of lower esophagus and upper stomach (Sugiura). Surgery is now generally reserved for pts with compensated cirrhosis (Child's class A) who fail nonsurgical therapy (e.g., band ligation). Liver transplantation should be considered in appropriate candidates. (A previous portosystemic shunt does not preclude subsequent liver transplantation, though best to avoid portacaval shunts in transplant candidates.)

Prevention of Initial Bleed   Recommended for pts at high risk of variceal bleeding—large varices, "red wales." Beta blockers appear to be more effective than sclerotherapy; role of band ligation uncertain.

PROGNOSIS (AND SURGICAL RISK)   Correlated with Child and Turcotte classification (see Table 158-2).

HEPATIC ENCEPHALOPATHY

A state of disordered CNS function associated with severe acute or chronic liver disease; may be acute and reversible or chronic and progressive.

CLINICAL FEATURES   *Stage 1*: euphoria or depression, mild confusion, slurred speech, disordered sleep, asterixis (flapping tremor). *Stage 2*: lethargy, moderate confusion. *Stage 3*: marked confusion, sleeping but arousable, inarticulate speech. *Stage 4*: coma; initially responsive to noxious stimuli, later unresponsive. Characteristic EEG abnormalities.

PATHOPHYSIOLOGY   Failure of liver to detoxify agents noxious to CNS, i.e., ammonia, mercaptans, fatty acids, γ-aminobutyric acid (GABA), due to decreased hepatic function and portosystemic shunting. Ammonia may deplete brain of glutamate, an excitatory neurotransmitter, to form glutamine. False neurotransmitters may also enter CNS due to increased aromatic and decreased branched-chain amino acid levels in blood. Endogenous benzodiazepine agonists may play a role. Blood ammonia most readily measured marker, although may not always correlate with clinical status.

PRECIPITANTS   GI bleeding (100 mL = 14–20 g of protein), azotemia, constipation, high-protein meal, hypokalemic alkalosis, CNS depressant drugs (e.g., benzodiazepines and barbiturates), hypoxia, hypercarbia, sepsis.

 TREATMENT

Remove precipitants; reduce blood ammonia by decreasing protein intake (20–30 g/d initially, then 60–80 g/d, vegetable sources); enemas/cathartics to clear gut. Lactulose (converts NH_3 to unabsorbed NH_4^+, produces diarrhea, alters bowel flora) 30–60 mL PO qh until diarrhea, then 15–30 mL tid-qid prn titrated to produce 3–4 loose stools/day. In coma, give as enema (300 mL in 700 mL H_2O). Lactilol, a second-generation disaccharide that is less sweet than lactulose and can be dispensed as a powder, is not yet available in the United States. In refractory cases, add neomycin 0.5–1 g PO bid, metronidazole 250 mg PO tid, or vancomycin 1 g PO bid. Unproven: IV branched-chain amino acids, levodopa, bromocriptine, keto-analogues of essential amino acids. Flumazenil, a short-acting benzodiazepine receptor antagonist, may have a role in management of hepatic encephalopathy precipitated by benzodiazepine use. Liver transplantation when otherwise indicated.

For a more detailed discussion, see Chung RT, Podolsky DK: Cirrhosis and Its Complications, Chap. 289, p.1858; in HPIM-16.

159

DISEASES OF IMMEDIATE TYPE HYPERSENSITIVITY

DEFINITION   These diseases result from IgE-dependent release of mediators from sensitized basophils and mast cells on contact with appropriate antigen (allergen). Associated disorders include anaphylaxis, allergic rhinitis, urticaria, asthma, and eczematous (atopic) dermatitis. Atopic allergy implies a familial tendency to the development of these disorders singly or in combination.

PATHOPHYSIOLOGY   IgE binds to surface of mast cells and basophils through a high-affinity receptor. Cross-linking of this IgE by antigen causes cellular activation with the subsequent release of preformed and newly synthesized mediators. These include histamine, prostaglandins, leukotrienes (including C_4, D_4, and E_4, collectively known as *slow-reacting substance of anaphylaxis*—SRS-A), acid hydrolases, neutral proteases, proteoglycans, and cytokines (Fig. 298-2, p.1949, HPIM-16). The mediators have been implicated in many pathophysiologic events associated with immediate type hypersensitivity, such as vasodilatation, increased vasopermeability, smooth-muscle contraction, and chemotactic attraction of neutrophils and other inflammatory cells. The clinical manifestations of each allergic reaction depend largely on the anatomic site(s) and time course of mediator release.

URTICARIA AND ANGIOEDEMA

DEFINITION   May occur together or separately. *Urticaria* involves superficial dermis and presents as circumscribed wheals with raised serpiginous borders and blanched centers; wheals may coalesce. *Angioedema* involves deeper layers of skin and may include subcutaneous tissue. These disorders may be classified as (1) IgE-dependent, including atopic, secondary to specific allergens, and physical stimuli, especially cold; (2) bradykinin-mediated (including hereditary angioedema and angiotension-converting enzyme inhibitors); (3) complement-mediated (including necrotizing vasculitis, serum sickness, and reactions to blood products); (4) nonimmunologic due to direct mast cell–releasing agents or drugs that influence mediator release; and (5) idiopathic.

PATHOPHYSIOLOGY   Characterized by massive edema formation in the dermis (and subcutaneous tissue in angioedema). Presumably the edema is due to increased vasopermeability caused by mediator release from mast cells or other cell populations.

DIAGNOSIS   History, with special attention to possible offending exposures and/or ingestion as well as the duration of lesions. Vasculitic urticaria typically persists >72 h, whereas conventional urticaria often has a duration <48 h.

- Skin testing to food and/or inhalant antigens.
- Physical provocation, e.g., challenge with vibratory or cold stimuli.
- Laboratory exam: complement levels, ESR (neither an elevated ESR nor hypocomplementemia is observed in IgE-mediated urticaria or angioedema);

C1-esterase inhibitor levels if history suggests hereditary angioedema; cryoglobulins, hepatitis B antigen, and antibody studies; autoantibody screen.
- Skin biopsy may be necessary.

DIFFERENTIAL DIAGNOSIS Atopic dermatitis, contact sensitivity, cutaneous mastocytosis (urticaria pigmentosa), systemic mastocytosis.

PREVENTION Identification and avoidance of offending agent(s), if possible.

 TREATMENT

- H_1 and H_2 antihistamines may be helpful: e.g., ranitidine 150 mg PO bid; diphenhydramine 25–50 mg PO qid; hydroxyzine 25–50 mg PO qid.
- Cyproheptadine 4 mg PO tid may be helpful.
- Sympathomimetic agents are occasionally useful.
- Topical glucocorticoids are of no value in the management of urticaria and/or angioedema. Because of their long-term toxicity, systemic glucocorticoids should not be used in the treatment of idiopathic, allergen-induced, or physical urticaria.

ALLERGIC RHINITIS

DEFINITION An inflammatory condition of the nose characterized by sneezing, rhinorrhea, and obstruction of nasal passages; may be associated with conjunctival and pharyngeal itching, lacrimation, and sinusitis. Seasonal allergic rhinitis is commonly caused by exposure to pollens, especially from grasses, trees, weeds, and molds. Perennial allergic rhinitis is frequently due to contact with house dust (containing dust mite antigens) and animal danders.

PATHOPHYSIOLOGY Impingement of pollens and other allergens on nasal mucosa of sensitized individuals results in IgE-dependent triggering of mast cells with subsequent release of mediators that cause development of mucosal hyperemia, swelling, and fluid transudation. Inflammation of nasal mucosal surface probably allows penetration of allergens deeper into tissue, where they contact perivenular mast cells. Obstruction of sinus ostia may result in development of secondary sinusitis, with or without bacterial infection.

DIAGNOSIS Accurate history of symptoms correlated with time of pollenation of plants in a given locale; special attention must be paid to other potentially sensitizing antigens such as pets.
- Physical examination: nasal mucosa may be boggy or erythematous; nasal polyps may be present; conjunctivae may be inflamed or edematous; manifestations of other allergic conditions (e.g., asthma, eczema) may be present.
- Skin tests to inhalant and/or food antigens.
- Nasal smear may reveal large numbers of eosinophils; presence of neutrophils may suggest infection.
- Total and specific serum IgE (as assessed by immunoassay) may be elevated.

DIFFERENTIAL DIAGNOSIS Vasomotor rhinitis, URI, irritant exposure, pregnancy with nasal mucosal edema, rhinitis medicamentosa, nonallergic rhinitis with eosinophilia, rhinitis due to use of α-adrenergic agents.

PREVENTION Identification and avoidance of offending antigen(s).

 TREATMENT

- Older antihistamines (e.g., chlorpheniramine, diphenhydramine) are effective but cause sedation and psychomotor impairment including reduced hand-

eye coordination and impaired automobile driving skills. Newer antihistamines (e.g., fexofenadine, loratadine, desloradine, cetirizine, and azelastine) are equally effective but are less sedating and more H_1 specific.
• Oral sympathomimetics, e.g., pseudoephedrine 30–60 mg PO qid; may aggravate hypertension; combination antihistamine/decongestant preparations may balance side effects and provide improved pt convenience.
• Topical vasoconstrictors—should be used sparingly due to rebound congestion and chronic rhinitis associated with prolonged use.
• Topical nasal glucocorticoids, e.g., beclomethasone, 2 sprays in each nostril bid, or fluticasone, 2 sprays in each nostril once daily.
• Topical nasal cromolyn sodium, 1–2 sprays in each nostril qid.
• Hyposensitization therapy if more conservative therapy is unsuccessful.

SYSTEMIC MASTOCYTOSIS

DEFINITION   A systemic disorder characterized by mast cell hyperplasia; generally recognized in bone marrow, skin, GI mucosa, liver, and spleen. Classified as (1) indolent, (2) associated with concomitant hematologic disorder, (3) aggressive, (4) mastocytic leukemia, and (5) mast cell sarcoma.

PATHOPHYSIOLOGY AND CLINICAL MANIFESTATIONS   The clinical manifestations of systemic mastocytosis are due to tissue occupancy by the mast cell mass, the tissue response to that mass (fibrosis), and the release of bioactive substances acting both locally (urticaria pigmentosa, crampy abdominal pain, gastritis, peptic ulcer) and at distal sites (headache, pruritus, flushing, vascular collapse). Clinical manifestations may be aggravated by alcohol, use of narcotics (e.g., codeine), ingestion of NSAIDs.

DIAGNOSIS   Although the diagnosis of mastocytosis may be suspected on the basis of clinical and laboratory findings, it can be established only by tissue biopsy (usually bone marrow biopsy). The diagnostic criteria for systemic mastocytosis are shown in Table 159-1. Laboratory studies that can help support a diagnosis of systemic mastocytosis include measurement of urinary or blood levels of mast cell products such as histamine, histamine metabolites, prostaglandin D_2 (PGD_2) metabolites, or mast cell tryptase. Other studies including bone scan, skeletal survey, GI contrast studies may be helpful. Other flushing disorders (e.g., carcinoid syndrome, pheochromocytoma) should be excluded.

Table 159-1

Diagnostic Criteria for Systemic Mastocytosis[a]

Major: Multifocal dense infiltrates of mast cells in bone marrow or other extracutaneous tissues with confirmation by immunodetection of tryptase or metachromasia

Minor: Abnormal mast cell morphology with a spindle shape and/or multilobed or eccentric nucleus
    Aberrant mast cell surface phenotype with expression of CD25 and CD2 (IL-2 receptor) in addition to C117 (c-*kit*)
    Detection of codon 816 mutation in peripheral blood cells, bone marrow cells, or lesional tissue
    Total serum tryptase (mostly alpha) >20 ng/mL

[a] Diagnosis requires either major and one minor or three minor criteria.

Ⓡ TREATMENT

- H_1 and H_2 antihistamines.
- Proton pump inhibitor for gastric hypersecretion.
- Oral cromolyn sodium for diarrhea and abdominal pain.
- NSAIDs (in nonsensitive pts) may help by blocking PGD2 production.
- Systemic glucocorticoids may help but frequently are associated with complications.
- Chemotherapy for frank leukemias.

For a more detailed discussion, see Austen KF: Allergies, Anaphylaxis, and Systemic Mastocytosis, Chap. 298, p. 1947, in HPIM-16.

PRIMARY IMMUNODEFICIENCY DISEASES

DEFINITION

Disorders involving the cell-mediated (T cell) or antibody-mediated (B cell) pathways of the immune system; some disorders may manifest abnormalities of both pathways. Pts are prone to development of recurrent infections and, in certain disorders, lymphoproliferative neoplasms. *Primary disorders* may be congenital or acquired; some are familial in nature. *Secondary disorders* are not caused by intrinsic abnormalities of immune cells but may be due to infection (such as in AIDS; see HPIM-16, Chap. 173), treatment with cytotoxic drugs, radiation therapy, or lymphoreticular malignancies. Pts with disorders of antibody formation are chiefly prone to infection with encapsulated bacterial pathogens (e.g., streptococci, *Haemophilus*, meningococcus) and *Giardia*. Individuals with T cell defects are generally susceptible to infections with viruses, fungi, and protozoa.

DIAGNOSIS See Table 160-1

CLASSIFICATION
Severe Combined Immunodeficiency (SCID)

Congenital (autosomal recessive or X-linked); affected infants rarely survive beyond 1 year without treatment. Dysfunction of both cellular and humoral immunity.

1. *Swiss-type*: Autosomal recessive; severe lymphopenia involving B and T cells. Some cases due to mutations in the *RAG-1* or *RAG-2* genes, the combined activities of which are needed for V(D)J recombination of the T and B cell antigen receptors.

2. *Adenosine deaminase (ADA) deficiency*: Autosomal recessive; has been treated with gene therapy.

3. *X-linked SCID*: Characterized by an absence of peripheral T cells and natural killer (NK) cells. B lymphocytes are present in normal numbers but are functionally defective. These pts have a mutation in the gene that encodes the gamma chain common to the interleukin (IL) -2, -4, -7, -9, -15 receptors, thus

disrupting the action of these important cytokines. The same phenotype seen in X-linked SCID can be inherited as an autosomal recessive disease due to mutations in the JAK3 protein kinase gene. This enzyme associates with the common gamma chain of the receptors for IL-2, -4, -9, and -15 and is a key element in the signal transduction pathways used by these receptors.

 TREATMENT

Bone marrow transplantation is useful in some SCID pts.

T Cell Immunodeficiency

1. *DiGeorge's syndrome*: Maldevelopment of organs derived embryologically from third and fourth pharyngeal pouches (including thymus); associated with congenital cardiac defects, parathyroid hypoplasia with hypocalcemic tetany, abnormal facies, thymic aplasia; serum Ig levels may be normal, but specific IgG and IgA antibody responses are impaired.

2. *T cell receptor (TCR) complex deficiency*: Immunodeficiencies due to inherited mutations of the CD3γ and CD3ε components of the TCR complex have been identified. CD3γ mutations result in a selective defect in CD8 T cells, whereas CD3ε mutations lead to a preferential reduction in CD4 T cells.

3. *MHC class II deficiency*: Antigen-presenting cells from pts with this rare disorder fail to express the class II molecules DP, DQ, and DR on their surface, which results in limited development of CD4+ T cells in the thymus and defective interaction of CD4 T cells and antigen-presenting cells in the periphery. Affected pts experience recurrent bronchopulmonary infections, chronic diarrhea, and severe viral infections.

4. *Inherited deficiency of purine nucleoside phosphorylase*: Functions in same salvage pathway as ADA; cellular dysfunction may be related to intracellular accumulation of purine metabolites.

5. *Ataxia-telangiectasia*: Autosomal recessive disorder caused by mutation in the *ATM* gene (gene product involved in DNA repair). Clinical manifestations include cerebellar ataxia, oculocutaneous telangiectasia, immunodeficiency; not all pts have immunodeficiency; lymphomas common; IgG subclasses may be abnormal.

6. *The nude syndrome*: This is the counterpart to the *nude* mouse and is caused by a mutation in the *whn* gene resulting in impairment of hair follicle and epithelial thymic development. The phenotype is characterized by congenital baldness, nail dystrophy, and severe T cell immunodeficiency.

7. *Zap70 kinase deficiency*: This tyrosine kinase is a pivotal component of the T cell receptor complex. Mutations in this gene result in a T cell immunodeficiency manifested by recurrent opportunistic infections that begin in the first year of life.

 TREATMENT

Treatment for T cell disorders is complex and largely investigational. Live vaccines and blood transfusions containing viable T cells should be assiduously avoided. Preventive therapy for *Pneumocystis carinii* pneumonia should be considered in selected pts with severe T cell deficiency.

Immunoglobulin Deficiency Syndromes

1. *X-linked agammaglobulinemia*: Due to a mutation in the *Bruton's tyrosine kinase (Btk)* gene. Marked deficiency of circulating B lymphocytes; all Ig classes low; recurrent sinopulmonary infections and chronic enteroviral encephalitis, including vaccine-acquired poliomyelitis infection, are common

complications. A similar phenotype, but with an autosomal recessive pattern of inheritance, can be seen with mutations in a variety of genes required for normal B cell development.

2. *Transient hypogammaglobulinemia of infancy*: This occurs between 3 and 6 months of age as maternally derived IgG levels decline.

3. *Isolated IgA deficiency*: Most common immunodeficiency; the majority of affected individuals do not have increased infections; antibodies against IgA may lead to anaphylaxis during transfusion of blood or plasma; may be associated with deficiencies of IgG subclasses; often familial.

4. *IgG subclass deficiencies*: Total serum IgG may be normal, yet some individuals may be prone to recurrent sinopulmonary infections due to selective deficiencies of certain IgG subclasses.

Table 160-1

Laboratory Work-Up for Primary Immunodeficiency

INITIAL SCREENING ASSAYS[a]

Complete blood count with differential smear.
Serum immunoglobulin levels: IgM, IgG, IgA, IgD, IgE

OTHER READILY AVAILABLE ASSAYS

Quantification of blood mononuclear cell populations by immunofluorescence assays employing monoclonal antibody markers[b]

    T cells: CD3, CD4, CD8, TCRα/β, TCRγ/δ
    B cells: CD19, CD20, CD21, Ig(μ, δ, γ, α, κ, λ), Ig-associated molecules
           (α, β)
    NK cells: CD16/CD56
    Monocytes: CD15
    Activation markers: HLA-DR, CD25, CD80 (B cells)
T cell functional evaluation

    1. Delayed hypersensitivity skin tests (PPD, *Candida, histoplasmin*, tetanus toxoid)
    2. Proliferative response to mitogens (anti-CD3 antibody, phytohemagglutinin, concanavalin A) and allogeneic cells (mixed lymphocyte response)
    3. Cytokine production
B cell functional evaluation

    1. Natural or commonly acquired antibodies: isohemagglutinins; antibodies to common viruses (influenza, rubella, rubeola) and bacterial toxins (diphtheria, tetanus)
    2. Response to immunization with protein (tetanus toxoid) and carbohydrate (pneumococcal vaccine) antigens
    3. Quantitative IgG subclass determinations
Complement

    1. CH50 assays (classic and alternative pathways)
    2. C3, C4, and other components
Phagocyte function

    1. Reduction of nitroblue tetrazolium
    2. Chemotaxis assays
    3. Bactericidal activity

[a] Together with a history and physical examination, these tests will identify more than 95 percent of pts with primary immunodeficiencies.
[b] The menu of monoclonal antibody markers may be expanded or contracted to focus on particular clinical questions.

5. *Common variable immunodeficiency*: Heterogeneous group of syndromes characterized by panhypogammaglobulinemia, deficiency of IgG and IgA, or selective IgG deficiency and recurrent sinopulmonary infections; associated conditions include chronic giardiasis, intestinal malabsorption, atrophic gastritis with pernicious anemia, benign lymphoid hyperplasia, lymphoreticular neoplasms, arthritis, and autoimmune diseases.

6. *X-linked immunodeficiency with increased IgM*: In most pts this syndrome results from genetic mutation in the gene encoding CD40 ligand, a transmembrane protein expressed by activated T cells and necessary for normal T and B cell cooperation, germinal center formation, and immunoglobulin isotype switching. Pts exhibit normal or increased serum IgM with low or absent IgG and IgA and recurrent sinopulmonary infections; pts also exhibit T lymphocyte abnormalities with increased susceptibility to infection with opportunistic pathogens (*P. carinii, Cryptosporidium*). Associated conditions include neutropenia and hepatobiliary tract disease.

 TREATMENT

Intravenous immunoglobulin administration (only for pts who have recurrent bacterial infections and are deficient in IgG):

- Starting dose 400–500 mg/kg given every 3–4 weeks
- Adjust dose to keep trough IgG level > 500 mg/dL
- Usually done in outpatient setting
- Decision to treat based on severity of clinical symptoms and response to antigenic challenge

MISCELLANEOUS IMMUNODEFICIENCY SYNDROMES

- Mucocutaneous candidiasis
- X-linked lymphoproliferative syndrome
- Immunodeficiency with thymoma
- Wiskott-Aldrich syndrome
- Hyper-IgE syndrome
- Metabolic abnormalities associated with immunodeficiency

For a more detailed discussion, see Cooper MD, Schroeder HW Jr: Primary Immune Deficiency Diseases, Chap. 297, p. 1939, in HPIM-16.

161

SLE, RA, AND OTHER CONNECTIVE TISSUE DISEASES

CONNECTIVE TISSUE DISEASE
   DEFINITION Heterogeneous disorders that share certain common features, including inflammation of skin, joints, and other structures rich in con-

nective tissue, as well as altered patterns of immunoregulation, including production of autoantibodies and abnormalities of cell-mediated immunity. While certain distinct clinical entities may be defined, manifestations may vary considerably from one pt to the next, and overlap of clinical features between and among specific diseases is common.

SYSTEMIC LUPUS ERYTHEMATOSUS (SLE)

DEFINITION AND PATHOGENESIS Disease of unknown etiology in which tissues and cells are damaged by deposition of pathogenic autoantibodies and immune complexes. Genetic, environmental, and sex hormonal factors are likely of pathogenic importance. T and B cell hyperactivity, production of autoantibodies with specificity for nuclear antigenic determinants, and abnormalities of T cell function occur.

CLINICAL MANIFESTATIONS 90% of pts are women, usually of child-bearing age; more common in blacks than whites. Course of disease is often one of periods of exacerbation and relative quiescence. May involve virtually any organ system and have a wide range of disease severity. Common features include:

- *Constitutional*—fatigue, fever, malaise, weight loss
- *Cutaneous*—rashes (especially malar "butterfly" rash), photosensitivity, vasculitis, alopecia, oral ulcers
- *Arthritis*—inflammatory, symmetric, nonerosive
- *Hematologic*—anemia (may be hemolytic), neutropenia, thrombocytopenia, lymphadenopathy, splenomegaly, venous or arterial thrombosis
- *Cardiopulmonary*—pleuritis, pericarditis, myocarditis, endocarditis
- *Nephritis*
- *GI*—peritonitis, vasculitis
- *Neurologic*—organic brain syndromes, seizures, psychosis, cerebritis

Drug-Induced Lupus A clinical and immunologic picture similar to spontaneous SLE may be induced by drugs; in particular: procainamide, hydralazine, isoniazid, chlorpromazine, methyldopa. Features are predominantly constitutional, joint, and pleuropericardial; CNS and renal disease are rare. All pts have antinuclear antibodies (ANA); antihistone antibodies may be present, but antibodies to dsDNA and hypocomplementemia are uncommon. Most pts improve following withdrawal of offending drug.

EVALUATION

- Hx and physical exam
- Presence of ANA is a cardinal feature, but a (+) ANA is not specific for SLE. Laboratory assessment should include: CBC, ESR, ANA and subtypes (antibodies to dsDNA, ssDNA, Sm, Ro, La, histone), complement levels (C3, C4, CH50), serum immunoglobulins, VDRL, PT, PTT, anticardiolipin antibody, lupus anticoagulant, UA.
- Appropriate radiographic studies
- ECG
- Consideration of renal biopsy if evidence of glomerulonephritis

DIAGNOSIS Made in the presence of four or more published criteria (Table 300-2, p. 1962, in HPIM-16).

℞ TREATMENT

Choice of therapy is based on type and severity of disease manifestations. Goals are to control acute, severe flares and to develop maintenance strategies where symptoms are suppressed to an acceptable level. Treatment choices depend on (1) whether disease is life-threatening or likely to cause organ damage; (2) whether manifestations are reversible; and (3) the best approach to prevent complications of disease and treatment (see Fig. 300-1, p. 1962, and Table 300-4, p. 1965, in HPIM-16).

Conservative Therapies for Non-Life-Threatening Disease

• *NSAIDs* (e.g., ibuprofen 400–800 mg tid–qid).
• *Antimalarials* (hydroxychloroquine 400 mg/d)—may improve constitutional, cutaneous, articular manifestations. Ophthalmologic evaluation required before and during Rx to rule out ocular toxicity.

Treatments for Life-Threatening SLE

• *Systemic glucocorticoids.*
• *Cytotoxic agents*—beneficial in active glomerulonephritis; may be required for severe disease not successfully controlled by acceptable doses of steroids.

1. Cyclophosphamide—considered the standard drug for controlling life-threatening active lupus nephritis. Administered as IV pulse 7–25 mg/ kg every 4 weeks. Daily oral dosing 1.5–2.5 mg/kg per day can also be used but has a greater risk of urinary bladder toxicity.
2. Mycophenolate mofetil—short-term studies suggest efficacy in some patients with SLE.
3. Azathioprine—indicated in pts who cannot take cyclophosphamide.

• *Anticoagulation*—may be indicated in pts with thrombotic complications.

RHEUMATOID ARTHRITIS (RA)

DEFINITION AND PATHOGENESIS   A chronic multisystem disease of unknown etiology characterized by persistent inflammatory synovitis, usually involving peripheral joints in a symmetric fashion. Although cartilaginous destruction, bony erosions, and joint deformity are hallmarks, the course of RA can be variable. An association with HLA-DR4 has been noted; both genetic and environmental factors may play a role in initiating disease. The propagation of RA is an immunologically mediated event in which joint injury occurs from synovial hyperplasia; lymphocytic infiltration of synovium; and local production of cytokines and chemokines by activated lymphocytes, macrophages, and fibroblasts.

CLINICAL MANIFESTATIONS   RA occurs in ~0.8% of the population; women affected 3 times more often than men; prevalence increases with age, onset most frequent in fourth and fifth decades.
Articular manifestations—typically a symmetric polyarthritis of peripheral joints with pain, tenderness, and swelling of affected joints; morning stiffness is common; PIP and MCP joints frequently involved; joint deformities may develop after persistent inflammation.
Extraarticular manifestations:

Cutaneous—rheumatoid nodules, vasculitis
Pulmonary—nodules, interstitial disease, bronchiolitis obliterans–organizing pneumonia (BOOP), pleural disease, Caplan's syndrome [sero (+) RA associated with pneumoconiosis]
Ocular—keratoconjunctivitis sicca, episcleritis, scleritis
Hematologic—anemia, Felty's syndrome (splenomegaly and neutropenia)
Cardiac—pericarditis, myocarditis
Neurologic—myelopathies secondary to cervical spine disease, entrapment, vasculitis.

EVALUATION

- Hx and physical exam with careful examination of all joints.
- Rheumatoid factor is present in 85% of pts; its presence correlates with severe disease, nodules, extraarticular features.
- Other laboratories: CBC, ESR.
- Synovial fluid analysis—useful to rule out crystalline disease, infection.
- Radiographs—juxtaarticular osteopenia, joint space narrowing, marginal erosions. CXR should be obtained.

DIAGNOSIS   Not difficult in pts with typical established disease. May be confusing early. Classification criteria were developed for investigational purposes but may be useful (Table 301-1, p. 1973, in HPIM-16).

Differential Diagnosis   Gout, SLE, psoriatic arthritis, infectious arthritis, osteoarthritis, sarcoid.

℞ TREATMENT

Goals: lessen pain, reduce inflammation, improve/maintain function, prevent long-term joint damage, control of systemic involvement. Increasing trend to treat RA more aggressively earlier in disease course (Fig. 161-1).

- Pt education on disease, joint protection

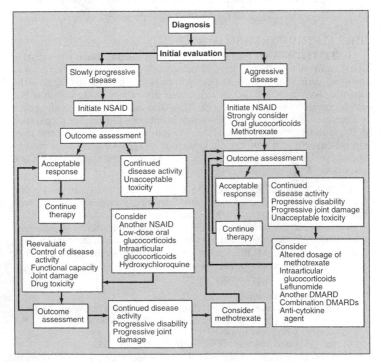

FIGURE 161-1   Algorithm for the medical management of rheumatoid arthritis. NSAID, nonsteroidal anti-inflammatory drug; DMARD, disease-modifying antirheumatic drug.

- Physical and occupational therapy—strengthen periarticular muscles, consider assistive devices.
- Aspirin or NSAIDs.
- Intra-articular glucocorticoids.
- Systemic glucocorticoids.
- Disease-modifying antirheumatic drugs (DMARDs)—e.g., methotrexate; IM gold compounds; hydroxychloroquine; sulfasalazine; D-penicillamine. Each agent has individual toxicities—pt education and monitoring required. Have been used in combination but with increased toxicity.
- Anti-cytokine therapy—TNF modulatory agents (etanercept, infliximab, adalimumab) effective at controlling RA in many patients and can slow the rate of progression of radiographic joint damage and decrease disability; carries potential for serious infection and individual toxicities. IL-1 receptor antagonist (anakinra) can improve the signs and symptoms of RA.
- Immunosuppressive therapy—e.g., azathioprine, leflunomide, cyclosporine, and cyclophosphamide. Generally reserved for pts who have failed DMARDs.
- Surgery—may be considered for severe functional impairment due to deformity.

SYSTEMIC SCLEROSIS (SCLERODERMA, SSC)

DEFINITION AND PATHOGENESIS Multisystem disorder characterized by inflammatory, vascular, and fibrotic changes of skin and various internal organ systems (chiefly GI tract, lungs, heart, and kidney). Pathogenesis unclear; involves immunologic mechanisms leading to vascular endothelial damage and activation of fibroblasts.

CLINICAL MANIFESTATIONS

- *Cutaneous*—edema followed by fibrosis of the skin (chiefly extremities, face, trunk); telangiectasis; calcinosis; Raynaud's phenomenon
- *Arthralgias and/or arthritis*
- *GI*—esophageal hypomotility; intestinal hypofunction
- *Pulmonary*—fibrosis, pulmonary hypertension, alveolitis
- *Cardiac*—pericarditis, cardiomyopathy, conduction abnormalities
- *Renal*—hypertension; renal crisis/failure (leading cause of death)

Two main subsets can be identified:

1. *Diffuse cutaneous scleroderma*—rapid development of symmetric skin thickening of proximal and distal extremity, face, and trunk. At high risk for development of visceral disease early in course.
2. *Limited cutaneous scleroderma*—skin involvement limited to face and extremity distal to elbows; associated with better prognosis; frequently has features of *CREST syndrome* (calcinosis, Raynaud's, esophageal dysmotility, sclerodactyly, telangiectasias).

EVALUATION

- Hx and physical exam with particular attention to blood pressure (heralding feature of renal disease).
- Laboratories: ESR, ANA (anticentromere pattern associated with CREST), specific antibodies may include antitopoisomerase I (Scl-70), UA
- Radiographs: CXR, barium swallow if indicated, hand x-rays may show distal tuft resorption and calcinosis.
- Additional studies: ECG, consider skin biopsy.

TREATMENT

- Education regarding warm clothing, smoking cessation, antireflux measures
- Calcium channel blockers (e.g., nifedipine) useful for Raynaud's phenomenon. Other agents with potential benefit include sildenafil, losartan, ketanserin, fluoxetine.
- ACE inhibitors—particularly important for controlling hypertension and limiting progression of renal disease.
- Antacids, H2 antagonists, omeprazole, and metoclopramide may be useful for esophageal reflux.
- D-Penicillamine—controversial benefit to reduce skin thickening and prevent organ involvement; no advantages to using doses >125 mg every other day.
- Glucocorticoids—no efficacy in slowing progression of SSc; indicated for inflammatory myositis or pericarditis; high doses early in disease may be associated with development of renal crisis.
- Cyclophosphamide—improves lung function outcomes and survival in pts with alveolitis.
- Epoprostenol (prostacyclin) and bosentan (endothelin-1 receptor antagonist)—may improve cardiopulmonary hemodynamics in pts with pulmonary hypertension.

MIXED CONNECTIVE TISSUE DISEASE (MCTD)

DEFINITION   Syndrome characterized by a combination of clinical features similar to those of SLE, SSc, polymyositis, and RA; unusually high titers of circulating antibodies to a nuclear ribonucleoprotein (RNP) are found.

CLINICAL MANIFESTATIONS   Raynaud's phenomenon, polyarthritis, swollen hands or sclerodactyly, esophageal dysfunction, pulmonary fibrosis, inflammatory myopathy. Renal involvement occurs in about 25%. Laboratory abnormalities include high-titer ANAs, very high titers of antibody to RNP, positive rheumatoid factor in 50% of pts.

EVALUATION   Similar to that for SLE and SSc.

 TREATMENT

Little published data. Treat based upon manifestations with similar approach to that used if feature occurred in SLE/SSc/polymyositis/RA.

SJÖGREN'S SYNDROME

DEFINITION   An immunologic disorder characterized by progressive lymphocytic destruction of exocrine glands most frequently resulting in symptomatic eye and mouth dryness; can be associated with extraglandular manifestations; predominantly affects middle-age females; may be primary or secondary when it occurs in association with other autoimmune diseases.

CLINICAL MANIFESTATIONS

- *Constitutional*—fatigue
- *Sicca symptoms*—keratoconjunctivitis sicca (KCS) and xerostomia
- *Dryness of other surfaces*—nose, vagina, trachea, skin
- *Extraglandular features*—arthralgia/arthritis, Raynaud's, lymphadenopathy, interstitial pneumonitis, vasculitis (usually cutaneous), nephritis, lymphoma.

EVALUATION

- Hx and physical exam—with special attention to oral, ocular, lymphatic exam and presence of other autoimmune disorders.
- Presence of autoantibodies is a hallmark of disease (ANA, RF, anti-Ro, anti-La)
- Other laboratories—ESR; CBC; renal, liver, and thyroid function tests; serum protein electrophoresis (SPEP) (hypergammaglobulinemia or monoclonal gammopathy common); UA.
- Ocular studies—to diagnose and quantitate KCS; Schirmer's test, Rose bengal staining.
- Oral exam—unstimulated salivary flow, dental exam.
- Labial salivary gland biopsy—demonstrates lymphocytic infiltration and destruction of glandular tissue.

DIAGNOSIS Criteria often include: KCS, xerostomia, (+) serologic features of autoimmunity. Positive lip biopsy considered necessary in some series—should be performed in setting of objective KCS/xerostomia with negative serologies.

℞ TREATMENT

- Regular follow-up with dentist and ophthalmologist.
- Symptomatic relief of dryness with artificial tears, ophthalmic lubricating ointments, nasal saline sprays, frequent sips of water, sugarless candy, moisturizing skin lotions.
- Pilocarpine or cevimeline—may help sicca manifestations.
- Hydroxychloroquine—may help arthralgias.
- Glucocorticoids—not effective for sicca Sx but may have role in treatment of extraglandular manifestations.

For a more detailed discussion, see Hahn BH: Systemic Lupus Erythematosus, Chap. 300, p. 1960; Lipsky PE: Rheumatoid Arthritis, Chap. 301, p. 1968; Gilliland BC: Systemic Sclerosis (Scleroderma) and Related Disorders, Chap. 303, p. 1979; Moutsopoulos HM: Sjögren's Syndrome, Chap. 304, p. 1990, in HPIM-16.

162

VASCULITIS

Definition and Pathogenesis

A clinicopathologic process characterized by inflammation of and damage to blood vessels, compromise of vessel lumen, and resulting ischemia. Clinical manifestations depend on size and location of affected vessel. Most vasculitic syndromes appear to be mediated in whole or in part by immune mechanisms. May be primary or sole manifestation of a disease or secondary to another disease process. Unique vasculitic syndromes can be identified that can differ greatly with regards to clinical features, disease severity, histology, and treatment.

Primary Vasculitis Syndromes

WEGENER'S GRANULOMATOSIS Granulomatous vasculitis of upper and lower respiratory tracts together with glomerulonephritis; upper airway lesions affecting the nose and sinuses can cause purulent or bloody nasal discharge, mucosal ulceration, septal perforation, and cartilaginous destruction (saddlenose deformity). Lung involvement may be asymptomatic or cause cough, hemoptysis, dyspnea; eye involvement may occur; renal involvement accounts for most deaths.

CHURG-STRAUSS SYNDROME (ALLERGIC ANGIITIS AND GRANULOMATOSIS) Granulomatous vasculitis of multiple organ systems, particularly the lung; characterized by asthma, peripheral eosinophilia, eosinophilic tissue infiltration; glomerulonephritis can occur.

POLYARTERITIS NODOSA (PAN) Medium-sized muscular arteries involved; frequently associated with arteriographic aneurysms; commonly affects renal arteries, liver, GI tract, peripheral nerves, skin, heart; can be associated with hepatitis B.

MICROSCOPIC POLYANGIITIS Small-vessel vasculitis that can affect the glomerulus and lungs; medium-sized vessels may also be affected.

GIANT CELL ARTERITIS (TEMPORAL ARTERITIS) Inflammation of medium- and large-sized arteries; primarily involves temporal artery but systemic involvement may occur; symptoms include headache, jaw/tongue claudication, scalp tenderness, fever, musculoskeletal symptoms (polymyalgia rheumatica); sudden blindness from involvement of optic vessels is a dreaded complication.

TAKAYASU'S ARTERITIS Vasculitis of the large arteries with strong predilection for aortic arch and its branches; most common in young women; presents with inflammatory or ischemic symptoms in arms and neck, systemic inflammatory symptoms, aortic regurgitation.

HENOCH-SCHÖNLEIN PURPURA Characterized by involvement of skin, GI tract, kidneys; more common in children; may recur after initial remission.

ESSENTIAL MIXED CRYOGLOBULINEMIA Majority of cases are associated with hepatitis C where an aberrant immune response leads to formation of cryoglobulin; characterized by cutaneous vasculitis, arthritis, peripheral neuropathy, and glomerulonephritis.

POLYANGIITIS OVERLAP SYNDROME Primary systemic vasculitis that does not precisely fit into a single diagnostic category.

CUTANEOUS VASCULITIS (HYPERSENSITIVITY VASCULITIS) Heterogeneous group of disorders; common feature is small-vessel involvement; skin disease usually predominates.

MISCELLANEOUS VASCULITIC SYNDROMES

- Kawasaki disease (mucocutaneous lymph node syndrome)
- Isolated vasculitis of the central nervous system
- Behçet's syndrome
- Cogan's syndrome

Secondary Vasculitis Syndromes

- Drug-induced vasculitis
- Serum sickness
- Vasculitis associated with infection, malignancy, rheumatic disease

Evaluation (See Fig. 162-1)

- Thorough Hx and physical exam—special reference to ischemic manifestations and systemic inflammatory signs/symptoms.
- Laboratories—important in assessing organ involvement: CBC with differential, ESR, renal function tests, UA. Should also be obtained to rule out other diseases: ANA, rheumatoid factor, anti-GBM, hepatitis B/C serologies, HIV.
- Antineutrophil cytoplasmic autoantibodies (ANCA)—cytoplasmic pattern associated with Wegener's granulomatosis; presence of ANCA is adjunctive and should not be used in place of biopsy as a means of diagnosis.
- Radiographs—CXR should be performed even in the absence of symptoms.
- Diagnosis—can usually be made only by arteriogram or biopsy of affected organ(s).

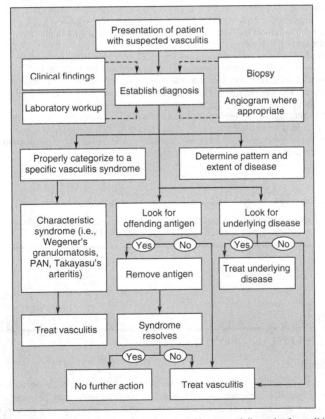

FIGURE 162-1 Algorithm for the approach to a pt with suspected diagnosis of vasculitis.

Differential Diagnosis

Guided by organ manifestations. In many instances includes infections and neoplasms, which must be ruled out prior to beginning immunosuppressive therapy.

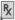 **TREATMENT**

Therapy is based on the specific vasculitic syndrome and its manifestations. Immunosuppressive therapy should be avoided in disease that rarely results in irreversible organ system dysfunction or that usually does not respond to such agents (e.g., isolated cutaneous vasculitis). Antiviral agents play an important role in treating vasculitis occurring with hepatitis B or C. Glucocorticoids alone may control giant cell arteritis and Takayasu's arteritis. Cytotoxic agents are particularly important in syndromes with life-threatening organ system involvement, especially active glomerulonephritis. Frequently used agents:

- Prednisone 1 (mg/kg)/d initially, then tapered; convert to alternate-day regimen and discontinue.
- Cyclophosphamide 2 (mg/kg)/d, adjusted to avoid severe leukopenia. Morning administration with a large amount of fluid is important in minimizing bladder toxicity. Pulsed intravenous cyclophosphamide (1 g/m^2 per month) is less effective but may be considered in selected pts who cannot tolerate daily dosing.
- Methotrexate in weekly doses up to 25 mg/week may be used to induce remission in Wegener's granulomatosis pts who do not have immediately life-threatening disease or cannot tolerate cyclophosphamide. It may also be considered for maintaining remission after induction with cyclophosphamide. Cannot be used in renal insufficiency or chronic liver disease.
- Azathioprine 2 (mg/kg)/d. Less effective in treating active disease but useful in maintaining remission after induction with cyclophosphamide.
- Plasmapheresis may have an adjunctive role in management if manifestations not controlled by above measures.

For a more detailed discussion, see Sneller MC, Langford CA, Fauci AS: The Vasculitis Syndromes, Chap. 306 p. 2002, in HPIM-16.

163

ANKYLOSING SPONDYLITIS

Definition

Chronic and progressive inflammatory disease of the axial skeleton with sacroiliitis (usually bilateral) as its hallmark. Peripheral joints and extraarticular structures may also be affected. Most frequently presents in young men in second or third decade; strong association with histocompatibility antigen HLA-B27. In Europe, also known as *Marie-Strumpell* or *Bechterew's disease*.

Clinical Manifestations

• *Back pain and stiffness*—not relieved by lying down, often present at night forcing pt to leave bed, worse in the morning, improves with activity, insidious onset, duration >3 months (often called symptoms of "inflammatory" back pain).

• *Extraaxial arthritis*—hip and shoulders 25–35%, other peripheral joint involvement up to 30%, usually asymmetric.

• *Chest pain*—from involvement of thoracic skeleton and muscular insertions.

• *Extra/juxtaarticular pain*—due to "enthesitis": inflammation at insertion of tendons and ligaments into bone; frequently affects greater trochanter, iliac crests, ischial tuberosities, tibial tubercles, heels.

• *Extraarticular findings*—include acute anterior uveitis in about 20% of pts, aortitis, aortic insufficiency, GI inflammation, cardiac conduction defects, amyloidosis, bilateral upper lobe pulmonary fibrosis.

• *Constitutional symptoms*—fever, fatigue, weight loss may occur.

• *Neurologic complications*—related to spinal fracture/dislocation (can occur with even minor trauma), atlantoaxial subluxation, cauda equina syndrome.

Physical Examination

• Tenderness over involved joints
• Diminished chest expansion
• Diminished anterior flexion of lumbar spine (Schober test)

Evaluation

• ESR and C-reactive protein elevated in majority.
• Mild anemia.
• Rheumatoid factor and ANA negative.
• HLA-B27 may be helpful in pts with inflammatory back Sx but negative x-rays.
• Radiographs: early may be normal. Sacroiliac joints: usually symmetric; bony erosions with "pseudowidening" followed by fibrosis and ankylosis. Spine: squaring of vertebrae; syndesmophytes; ossification of annulus fibrosis and anterior longitudinal ligament causing "bamboo spine." Sites of enthesitis may ossify and be visible on x-ray. MRI is procedure of choice when plain radiographs do not reveal sacroiliac abnormalities and can show early intraarticular inflammation, cartilage changes, and bone marrow edema.

Diagnosis

Modified New York criteria widely used: radiographic evidence of sacroiliitis plus one of: (1) Hx of inflammatory back pain symptoms, (2) lumbar motion limitation, (3) limited chest expansion.

DIFFERENTIAL DIAGNOSIS Spondyloarthropathy associated with reactive arthritis, psoriatic arthritis, enteropathic arthritis (Fig. 163-1). Diffuse idiopathic skeletal hyperostosis.

R_x TREATMENT

• Exercise program to maintain posture and mobility is important.
• TNF modulatory agents (etanercept, infliximab) have been found to suppress disease activity and improve function.
• NSAIDs (e.g., indomethacin 75 mg slow-release qd or bid) useful in most pts.

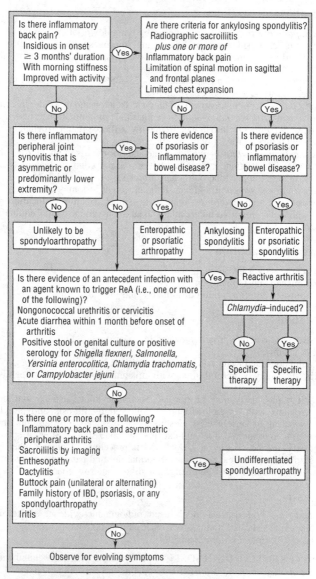

FIGURE 163-1 Algorithm for diagnosis of the spondyloarthritides.

- Sulfasalazine 2–3 g/d and methotrexate 10–25 mg/week may be useful.
- No therapeutic role for systemic glucocorticoids or other immunosuppressive has been documented in ankylosing spondylitis.
- Adjunctive therapy includes intraarticular glucocorticoids for persistent enthesitis or peripheral synovitis; ocular glucocorticoids for uveitis; surgery for severely affected or deformed joints.

For a more detailed discussion, see Taurog JD: The Spondyloarthritides, Chap. 305, p. 1993, in HPIM-16.

164

PSORIATIC ARTHRITIS

Definition

Psoriatic arthritis is a chronic inflammatory arthritis that affects 5–30% of persons with psoriasis. Some pts, especially those with spondylitis, will carry the HLA-B27 histocompatibility antigen. Onset of psoriasis usually precedes development of joint disease; approximately 15–20% of pts develop arthritis prior to onset of skin disease. Nail changes are seen in 90% of patients with psoriatic arthritis.

Patterns of Joint Involvement

- Asymmetric oligoarthritis: often involves distal interphalangeal/proximal interphalangeal (DIP/PIP) joints of hands and feet, knees, wrists, ankles; "sausage digits" may be present, reflecting tendon sheath inflammation.
- Symmetric polyarthritis (40%) resembles rheumatoid arthritis except rheumatoid factor is negative, absence of rheumatoid nodules.
- Predominantly DIP joint involvement (15%): high frequency of association with psoriatic nail changes.
- "Arthritis mutilans" (3–5%): aggressive, destructive form of arthritis with severe joint deformities and bony dissolution.
- Spondylitis and/or sacroiliitis: axial involvement is present in 20–40% of pts with psoriatic arthritis; may occur in absence of peripheral arthritis.

Evaluation

- Negative tests for rheumatoid factor.
- Hypoproliferative anemia, elevated ESR.
- Hyperuricemia may be present.
- HIV should be suspected in fulminant disease.
- Inflammatory synovial fluid and biopsy without specific findings.
- Radiographic features include erosion at joint margin, bony ankylosis, tuft resorption of terminal phalanges, "pencil-in-cup" deformity (bone proliferation at base of distal phalanx with tapering of proximal phalanx), axial skeleton with asymmetric sacroiliitis, asymmetric nonmarginal syndesmophytes.

Diagnosis

Suggested by: pattern of arthritis and inflammatory nature, absence of rheumatoid factor, radiographic characteristics, presence of skin and nail changes of psoriasis (see Fig. 163-1).

℞ TREATMENT

- Coordinated therapy is directed at the skin and joints.
- Pt education, physical and occupational therapy.

- TNF modulatory agents (etanercept, infliximab) can improve skin and joint disease.
- NSAIDs.
- Intraarticular steroid injections—useful in some settings. Systemic glucocorticoids should rarely be used as may induce rebound flare of skin disease upon tapering.
- Efficacy of gold salts and antimalarials controversial.
- Methotrexate 15–25 mg/week and sulfasalazine 2–3 g/d have clinical efficacy but do not halt joint erosion.

For a more detailed discussion, see Taurog JD: The Spondyloarthritides, Chap. 305, p. 1993, in HPIM-16.

165

REACTIVE ARTHRITIS AND REITER'S SYNDROME

Definition

Reactive arthritis refers to acute nonpurulent arthritis complicating an infection elsewhere in the body. The term has been used primarily to refer to spondyloarthritides following enteric or urogenital infections occurring predominantly in HLA-B27-positive individuals. *Reiter's syndrome* describes the triad of arthritis, conjunctivitis, and nongonococcal urethritis. This term is largely of historic interest and is now considered to be part of the spectrum of reactive arthritis.

Pathogenesis

Up to 85% of pts possess the HLA-B27 alloantigen. It is thought that in individuals with appropriate genetic background, reactive arthritis may be triggered by an enteric infection with any of several *Shigella*, *Salmonella*, *Yersinia*, and *Campylobacter* species; by genitourinary infection with *Chlamydia trachomatis*; and possibly by other agents.

Clinical Manifestations

The sex ratio following enteric infection is 1:1, but genitourinary acquired reactive arthritis is predominantly seen in young males. In a majority of cases Hx will elicit Sx of genitourinary or enteric infection 1–4 weeks prior to onset of other features.

Constitutional—fatigue, malaise, fever, weight loss.
Arthritis—usually acute, asymmetric, oligoarticular, involving predominantly lower extremities; sacroiliitis may occur.
Enthesitis—inflammation at insertion of tendons and ligaments into bone; dactylitis or "sausage digit," plantar fasciitis, and Achilles tendinitis common.
Ocular features—conjunctivitis, usually minimal; uveitis, keratitis, and optic neuritis rarely present.

Urethritis—discharge intermittent and may be asymptomatic.

Other urogenital manifestations—prostatitis, cervicitis, salpingitis.

Mucocutaneous lesions—painless lesions on glans penis (*circinate balanitis*) and oral mucosa in approximately a third of pts; *keratoderma blenorrhagica*: cutaneous vesicles that become hyperkerotic, most common on soles and palms.

Uncommon manifestations—pleuropericarditis, aortic regurgitation, neurologic manifestations, secondary amyloidosis.

Reactive arthritis is associated with and may be the presenting Sx of HIV.

Evaluation

• Pursuit of triggering infection by culture, serology, or molecular methods as clinically suggested.

• Rheumatoid factor and ANA negative.

• Mild anemia, leukocytosis, elevated ESR may be seen.

• HLA-B27 may be helpful in atypical cases.

• HIV screening should be performed in all pts.

• Synovial fluid analysis—often very inflammatory; negative for crystals or infection.

• Radiographs—erosions may be seen with new periosteal bone formation, ossification of entheses, sacroiliitis (often unilateral).

Differential Diagnosis

Includes septic arthritis (gram +/−), gonococcal arthritis, crystalline arthritis, psoriatic arthritis (see Fig. 163-1).

℞ TREATMENT

• Controlled trials have failed to demonstrate any benefit of antibiotics in reactive arthritis. Prompt antibiotic treatment of acute chlamydial urethritis may prevent subsequent reactive arthritis.

• NSAIDs (e.g., indomethacin 25–50 mg PO tid) benefit most pts.

• Intraarticular glucocorticoids.

• Sulfasalazine up to 3 g/d in divided doses may help some pts with persistent arthritis.

• Cytotoxic therapy, such as azathioprine [1–2 (mg/kg)/d] or methotrexate (7.5–15 mg/week) may be considered for debilitating disease refractory to other modalities; contraindicated in HIV disease.

• Uveitis may require therapy with ocular or systemic glucocorticoids

Outcome

Prognosis is variable; 30–60% will have recurrent or sustained disease, with 15–25% developing permanent disability.

For a more detailed discussion, see Taurog JD: The Spondyloarthritides, Chap. 305, p. 1993, in HPIM-16.

166

OSTEOARTHRITIS

Definition

Osteoarthritis (OA), also called degenerative joint disease, is a disorder characterized by progressive deterioration and loss of articular cartilage accompanied by proliferation of new bone and soft tissue in and around involved joint.

Primary (idiopathic) OA—no underlying cause is apparent.

Secondary OA—a predisposing factor is present such as trauma, repetitive stress (occupation, sports), congenital abnormality, metabolic disorder, or other bone/joint disease.

Erosive OA—term often applied to pts who have distal and/or proximal interphalangeal (DIP/PIP) OA of the hands associated with synovitis and radiographic central erosions of the articular surface.

Generalized OA—characterized by involvement of ≥3 joints or groups of joints.

Epidemiology

OA is the most common form of joint disease. Risk factors include age, female sex, race, genetic factors, joint trauma, repetitive stress, obesity, congenital defects, prior inflammatory disease, and metabolic/endocrine disorders.

Pathogenesis

Initial changes begin in cartilage, with change in arrangement and size of collagen fibers. Proteases lead to loss of cartilage matrix. Proteoglycan synthesis initially undergoes a compensatory increase but eventually falls off, leading to full-thickness cartilage loss.

Clinical Manifestations

OA can affect almost any joint, but usually occurs in weight-bearing and frequently used joints such as the knee, hip, spine, and hands. The hand joints that are typically affected are the DIP, PIP, or first carpometacarpal (thumb base); metacarpophalangeal joint involvement is rare.

SYMPTOMS

- Use-related pain affecting one or a few joints (rest and nocturnal pain less common)
- Stiffness after rest or in morning may occur but usually brief (< 30 min)
- Loss of joint movement or functional limitation
- Joint instability
- Joint deformity
- Joint crepitation ("crackling")

PHYSICAL EXAMINATION

- Chronic monarthritis or asymmetric oligo/polyarthritis
- Firm or "bony" swellings of the joint margins, e.g., Heberden's nodes (hand DIP) or Bouchard's nodes (hand PIP)
- Mild synovitis with a cool effusion can occur but is uncommon
- Crepitance—audible creaking or crackling of joint on passive or active movement

• Deformity, e.g., OA of knee may involve medial, lateral, or patellofemoral compartments resulting in varus or valgus deformities
• Restriction of movement, e.g., limitation of internal rotation of hip
• Objective neurologic abnormalities may be seen with spine involvement (may affect intervertebral disks, apophyseal joints, and paraspinal ligaments)

Evaluation

• Routine lab work usually normal.
• ESR usually normal but may be elevated in pts who have synovitis.
• Rheumatoid factor, ANA studies negative.
• Joint fluid is straw-colored with good viscosity; fluid WBCs < 2000/μL; of value in ruling out crystal-induced arthritis or infection.
• Radiographs may be normal at first but as disease progresses may show joint space narrowing, subchondral bone sclerosis, subchondral cysts, and osteophytes. Erosions are distinct from those of rheumatoid and psoriatic arthritis as they occur subchondrally along the central portion of the joint surface.

Diagnosis

Usually established on basis of pattern of joint involvement, radiographic features, normal laboratory tests, and synovial fluid findings.

DIFFERENTIAL DIAGNOSIS Osteonecrosis, Charcot joint, rheumatoid arthritis, psoriatic arthritis, crystal-induced arthritides.

 TREATMENT

• Pt education, weight reduction, appropriate use of cane and other supports, isometric exercises to strengthen muscles around affected joints.
• Topical capsaicin cream may help relieve hand or knee pain.
• Acetaminophen, salicylates, or NSAIDs.
• Tramadol—may be considered in pts whose symptoms are inadequately controlled with NSAIDs; as it is a synthetic opioid agonist, habituation is a potential concern.
• Intraarticular glucocorticoids—may provide symptomatic relief but should be performed infrequently as cartilage breakdown may be accelerated if performed too often.
• Intraarticular hyaluronin—indicated in pts who have not responded to nonpharmacologic therapy and analgesics; consider when NSAIDs contraindicated or ineffective.
• Tidal irrigation—although patients have perceived a benefit in some instances, results from a randomized trial concluded this to be attributable to the placebo effect.
• Glucosamine and chondroitin—although widely sold, not FDA approved for use in OA. Several studies have suggested a moderate symptomatic benefit relative to placebo. Proof of efficacy from large placebo-controlled trials has not been established.
• Systemic glucocorticoids have no place in the treatment of OA.
• Arthroscopic debridement and lavage—can be helpful in the subgroup of pts with knee OA in whom loose bodies, cartilage flaps, or disruption of the meniscus cause mechanical symptoms such as locking or giving way. In pts who do not have mechanical symptoms, this modality appears to be of no greater benefit than placebo.

• Joint replacement surgery may be considered in pts with advanced OA who have intractable pain and loss of function in whom aggressive medical management has failed.

For a more detailed discussion, see Brandt KD: Osteoarthritis, Chap. 312, p. 2036, in HPIM-16.

167

GOUT, PSEUDOGOUT, AND RELATED DISEASES

GOUT
Definition

The term *gout* is applied to a spectrum of manifestations that may occur singly or in combination. Hyperuricemia is the biologic hallmark of gout. When present, plasma and extracellular fluids become supersaturated with uric acid, which, under the right conditions, may crystallize and result in clinical gout.

Pathogenesis

Uric acid is the end product of purine nucleotide degradation; its production is closely linked to pathways of purine metabolism, with the intracellular concentration of 5-phosphoribosyl-1-pyrophosphate (PRPP) being the major determinant of the rate of uric acid biosynthesis. Uric acid is excreted primarily by the kidney through mechanisms of glomerular filtration, tubular secretion, and reabsorption. Hyperuricemia may thus arise in a wide range of settings that cause overproduction or reduced excretion of uric acid or a combination of the two (Table 338-1, p. 2309; HPIM-16).

ACUTE GOUTY ARTHRITIS Monosodium urate (MSU) crystals present in the joint are phagocytosed by leukocytes; release of inflammatory mediators and lysosomal enzymes leads to recruitment of additional phagocytes into the joint and to synovial inflammation.

Clinical Manifestations

Acute inflammatory arthritis—usually an exquisitely painful monarthritis but may be polyarticular and accompanied by fever; *podagra* (attack in the great toe) is the site of first attack in half and may occur eventually in 90%. Attack will generally subside spontaneously after days to weeks. Although some pts may have a single attack, 75% have a second attack within 2 years. Differential diagnosis includes septic arthritis, reactive arthritis, calcium pyrophosphate deposition (CPPD) disease, rheumatoid arthritis.
Tenosynovitis
Chronic tophaceous arthritis—*tophi*: aggregates of MSU crystals surrounded by a giant cell inflammatory reaction. Occurs in the setting of long-standing gout.
Extraarticular tophi—often occur in olecranon bursa, helix and antihelix of ears, ulnar surface of forearm, Achilles tendon.

Urate nephrosis—deposition of MSU crystals in interstitium and pyramids. Can cause chronic renal insufficiency.

Acute uric acid nephropathy—reversible cause of acute renal failure due to precipitation of urate in the tubules; pts receiving cytotoxic treatment for neoplastic disease are at risk.

Uric acid nephrolithiasis—responsible for 10% of renal stones in the United States.

Evaluation

• Synovial fluid analysis—only definitive method of diagnosing gouty arthritis is joint aspiration and demonstration of characteristic needle-shaped negatively birefringent MSU crystals by polarizing microscopy. Gram stain and culture should be performed on all fluid to rule out infection.

• Serum uric acid—normal levels do not rule out gout.

• Urine uric acid—excretion of >800 mg/d on regular diet in the absence of drugs suggests overproduction.

• Screening for risk factors or sequelae—urinalysis; serum creatinine, glucose and lipids; complete blood counts.

• If overproduction is suspected, measurement of erythrocyte hypoxanthine guanine phosphoribosyl transferase (HGPRT) and PRPP levels may be indicated.

• Joint x-rays—may demonstrate erosions late in disease.

• If renal stones suggested, abdominal flat plate (stones often radiolucent), possibly IVP.

• Chemical analysis of renal stones.

℞ TREATMENT

Asymptomatic Hyperuricemia As only ~5% of hyperuricemic pts develop gout, treatment of asymptomatic hyperuricemia is not indicated. Exceptions are pts about to receive cytotoxic therapy for neoplasms.

Acute Gouty Arthritis Treatment is given for symptomatic relief only as attack is self-limited and will resolve spontaneously. Toxicity of therapy must be considered in each pt.

• Analgesia

• NSAIDs—Rx of choice when not contraindicated.

• Colchicine—generally only effective within first 24 h of attack; overdose has potentially life-threatening side effects; use is contraindicated in pts with renal insufficiency, cytopenias, LFTs > 2× normal, sepsis. PO—0.6 mg qh until pt improves, has GI side effects, or maximal dose of 5 mg is reached. IV—dangerous and best avoided; if used, give no more than 2 mg over 24 h and no further drug for 7 days following; IV must never be given in a pt who has received PO colchicine.

• Intraarticular glucocorticoids—septic arthritis must be ruled out prior to injection.

• Systemic glucocorticoids—brief taper may be considered in pts with a polyarticular gouty attack for whom other modalities are contraindicated and where articular or systemic infection has been ruled out.

Uric Acid–Lowering Agents Indications for initiating uric acid–lowering therapy include recurrent frequent acute gouty arthritis, polyarticular gouty arthritis, tophaceous gout, renal stones, cytotoxic therapy prophylaxis. Should not start during an attack. Initiation can precipitate an acute flare; consider concomitant PO colchicine 0.6 mg qd until uric acid <5.0 mg/dL, then discontinue.

1. *Allopurinol*: Decreases uric acid synthesis by inhibiting xanthine oxidase. Must be dose-reduced in renal insufficiency. Has significant side effects and drug interactions.

2. *Uricosuric drugs* (probenecid, sulfinpyrazone): Increases uric acid excretion by inhibiting its tubular reabsorption; ineffective in renal insufficiency; should not be used in these settings: age >60, renal stones, tophi, increased urinary uric acid excretion, cytotoxic therapy prophylaxis.

CPPD DEPOSITION DISEASE (PSEUDOGOUT)
Definition and Pathogenesis

CPPD disease is characterized by acute and chronic inflammatory joint disease, usually affecting older individuals. The knee and other large joints most commonly affected. Calcium deposits in articular cartilage (*chondrocalcinosis*) may be seen radiographically; these are not always associated with symptoms.

CPPD may be hereditary; idiopathic, associated chiefly with aging; or occur secondary to hyperparathyroidism, hemochromatosis, hypophosphatasia, hypomagnesemia, hypothyroidism, gout, ochronosis, joint trauma, severe medical illness, or surgery.

Crystals are thought not to form in synovial fluid but are probably shed from articular cartilage into joint space, where they are phagocytosed by neutrophils and incite an inflammatory response.

Clinical Manifestations

- *Acute "pseudogout"* —occurs in ~25% of pts with CPPD disease; knee is most frequently involved, but other joints may be affected; involved joint is erythematous, swollen, warm, and painful; most pts have evidence of chondrocalcinosis. A minority will have involvement of multiple joints.
- *Chronic arthropathy*—progressive degenerative changes in multiple joints. Joint distribution may suggest CPPD with common sites including knee, wrist, MCP, hips, and shoulders.
- *Symmetric proliferative synovitis*—seen in familial forms with early onset
- *Intervertebral disk and ligament calcification*
- *Spinal stenosis*

Diagnosis

- Made by demonstration of calcium pyrophosphate dihydrate crystals (appearing as short blunt rods, rhomboids, and cuboids with weak positive birefringence) in synovial fluid.
- Radiographs may demonstrate chondrocalcinosis and degenerative changes (joint space narrowing, subchondral sclerosis/cysts).
- Secondary causes of CPPD should be considered in pts <50 years.

DIFFERENTIAL DIAGNOSIS   OA, RA, gout, septic arthritis.

℞ **TREATMENT**

- NSAIDs
- Intraarticular injection of glucocorticoids
- Colchicine is variably effective.

HYDROXYAPATITE ARTHROPATHY

Calcium hydroxyapatite (HA) deposition can cause a calcific bursitis or tendinitis and arthropathy primarily affecting the shoulder and knee. Abnormal HA accumulation can occur idiopathically or secondary to tissue damage, hypercalcemia, hyperparathyroidism, or chronic renal failure. HA is an important factor in *Milwaukee shoulder*, a destructive arthropathy of the elderly that occurs in the shoulders and knees. HA crystals are small; clumps may stain purplish on Wright's stain and bright red with alizarin red S. Definitive identification requires electron microscopy or x-ray diffraction studies. Radiographic appearance resembles CPPD disease. *Treatment*: NSAIDs, repeated aspiration, and rest of affected joint.

CALCIUM OXALATE DEPOSITION DISEASE

CaOx crystals may be deposited in joints in primary oxalosis (rare) or secondary oxalosis (a complication of end-stage renal disease). Clinical syndrome similar to gout and CPPD disease. *Treatment*: marginally effective.

For a more detailed discussion, see Wortmann RL: Disorders of Purine and Pyrimidine Metabolism, Chap. 338, p. 2308; and Reginato AJ: Gout and Other Crystal Arthropathies, Chap. 313, p. 2046, in HPIM-16.

168

OTHER ARTHRITIDES

ENTEROPATHIC ARTHRITIS

Both peripheral and axial arthritis may be associated with ulcerative colitis or Crohn's disease. The arthritis can occur after or before the onset of intestinal symptoms. Peripheral arthritis is episodic, asymmetric, and most frequently affects knee and ankle. Attacks usually subside within several weeks and characteristically resolve completely without residual joint damage. Enthesitis (inflammation at insertion of tendons and ligaments into bone) can occur with manifestations of "sausage digit," Achilles tendinitis, plantar fasciitis. Axial involvement can manifest as spondylitis and/or sacroiliitis (often symmetric). Laboratory findings are nonspecific; rheumatoid factor (RF) absent; radiographs of peripheral joints usually normal; axial involvement is often indistinguishable from ankylosing spondylitis (see Fig. 163-1).

℞ TREATMENT

Directed at underlying inflammatory bowel disease; NSAIDs may alleviate joint symptoms; sulfasalazine may benefit peripheral arthritis; anecdotal reports indicate treatment of Crohn's disease with infliximab has improved arthritis.

WHIPPLE'S DISEASE Characterized by arthritis in up to 75% of pts that usually precedes appearance of other symptoms. Usually oligo- or polyarticular, symmetric, transient but may become chronic. Joint manifestations respond to antibiotic therapy.

NEUROPATHIC JOINT DISEASE

Also known as *Charcot's joint*, this is a severe destructive arthropathy that occurs in joints deprived of pain and position sense; may occur in diabetic neuropathy, tabes dorsalis, syringomyelia, amyloidosis, spinal cord or peripheral nerve injury. Distribution depends on the underlying joint disease. Joint effusions are usually noninflammatory but can be hemorrhagic. Radiographs can reveal either bone resorption or new bone formation with bone dislocation and fragmentation.

 TREATMENT

Stabilization of joint; surgical fusion may improve function.

RELAPSING POLYCHONDRITIS

An idiopathic disorder characterized by recurrent inflammation of cartilaginous structures. Cardinal manifestations include ear and nose involvement with floppy ear and saddlenose deformities, inflammation and collapse of tracheal and bronchial cartilaginous rings, asymmetric episodic nondeforming polyarthritis. Other features can include scleritis, conjunctivitis, iritis, keratitis, aortic regurgitation, glomerulonephritis, and other features of systemic vasculitis. Onset is frequently abrupt, with the appearance of 1–2 sites of cartilaginous inflammation. Diagnosis is made clinically and may be confirmed by biopsy of affected cartilage.

 TREATMENT

Glucocorticoids (prednisone 40–60 mg/d with subsequent taper) may suppress acute features and reduce the severity/frequency of recurrences. Cytotoxic agents should be reserved for unresponsive disease or for pts who require high glucocorticoid doses. When airway obstruction is severe, tracheostomy is required.

HYPERTROPHIC OSTEOARTHROPATHY

Syndrome consisting of periosteal new bone formation, digital clubbing, and arthritis. Most commonly seen in association with lung carcinoma but also occurs with chronic lung or liver disease; congenital heart, lung, or liver disease in children; and idiopathic and familial forms. Symptoms include burning and aching pain most pronounced in distal extremities. Radiographs show periosteal thickening with new bone formation of distal ends of long bones.

 TREATMENT

Identify and treat associated disorder; aspirin, NSAIDs, other analgesics, vagotomy or percutaneous nerve block may help to relieve symptoms.

FIBROMYALGIA

A common disorder characterized by pain, aching, stiffness of trunk and extremities, and presence of a number of specific tender points. More common in women than men. Frequently associated with sleep disorders. Diagnosis is made clinically; evaluation reveals soft tissue tender points but no objective joint abnormalities by exam, laboratory, or radiograph.

TREATMENT

Benzodiazepines or tricyclics for sleep disorder, local measures (heat, massage, injection of tender points), NSAIDs.

REFLEX SYMPATHETIC DYSTROPHY SYNDROME (RSDS)

A syndrome of pain and tenderness, usually of a hand or foot, associated with vasomotor instability, trophic skin changes, and rapid development of bony demineralization. Frequently, development will follow a precipitating event (local trauma, myocardial infarction, stroke, or peripheral nerve injury). Early recognition and treatment can be effective in preventing disability.

 TREATMENT

Options include pain control, application of heat or cold, exercise, sympathetic nerve block, and short courses of high-dose prednisone in conjunction with physical therapy.

POLYMYALGIA RHEUMATICA (PMR)

Clinical syndrome characterized by aching and morning stiffness in the shoulder girdle, hip girdle, or neck for >1 month, elevated ESR, and rapid response to low-dose prednisone (15 mg qd). Rarely occurs before age 50. PMR can occur in association with giant cell (temporal) arteritis, which requires treatment with higher doses of prednisone. Evaluation should include a careful history to elicit Sx suggestive of giant cell arteritis (Chap. 162); ESR; labs to rule out other processes usually include RF, ANA, CBC, CPK, serum protein electrophoresis; and renal, hepatic, and thyroid function tests.

 TREATMENT

Pts rapidly improve on prednisone, 10–20 mg qd, but may require treatment over months to years.

OSTEONECROSIS (AVASCULAR NECROSIS)

Caused by death of cellular elements of bone, believed to be due to impairment in blood supply. Frequent associations include glucocorticoid treatment, connective tissue disease, trauma, sickle cell disease, embolization, alcohol use. Commonly involved sites include femoral and humeral heads, femoral condyles, proximal tibia. Hip disease is bilateral in >50% of cases. Clinical presentation is usually the abrupt onset of articular pain. Early changes are not visible on plain radiograph and are best seen by MRI; later stages demonstrate bone collapse ("crescent sign"), flattening of articular surface with joint space loss.

 TREATMENT

Limited weight-bearing of unclear benefit; NSAIDs for Sx. Surgical procedures to enhance blood flow may be considered in early-stage disease but are of controversial efficacy; joint replacement may be necessary in late-stage disease for pain unresponsive to other measures.

PERIARTICULAR DISORDERS

BURSITIS Inflammation of the thin-walled bursal sac surrounding tendons and muscles over bony prominences. The subacromial and greater trochanteric bursae are most commonly involved.

TREATMENT

Prevention of aggravating conditions, rest, NSAIDs, and local glucocorticoid injections.

TENDINITIS May involve virtually any tendon but frequently affects tendons of the rotator cuff around shoulder, especially the supraspinatus. Pain is dull and aching but becomes acute and sharp when tendon is squeezed below acromion.

 TREATMENT

NSAIDs, glucocorticoid injection, and physical therapy may be beneficial. The rotator cuff tendons or biceps tendon may rupture acutely, frequently requiring surgical repair.

CALCIFIC TENDINITIS Results from deposition of calcium salts in tendon, usually supraspinatus. The resulting pain may be sudden and severe.

ADHESIVE CAPSULITIS ("Frozen Shoulder") Results from conditions that enforce prolonged immobility of shoulder joint. Shoulder is painful and tender to palpation, and both active and passive range of motion is restricted.

 TREATMENT

Spontaneous improvement may occur; NSAIDs, local injections of glucocorticoids, and physical therapy may be helpful.

For a more detailed discussion, see Taurog JD: The Spondyloarthritides, Chap. 305, p. 1993; Gilliland BC: Fibromyalgia, Arthritis Associated with Systemic Disease, and Other Arthritides, Chap. 315, p. 2055; Gilliland BC: Periarticular Disorders of the Extremities, Chap. 316, p. 2064; and Gilliland BC: Relapsing Polychondritis, Chap. 308, p. 2015, in HPIM-16.

169

SARCOIDOSIS

Definition

A systemic granulomatous disease of unknown etiology. Affected organs are characterized by an accumulation of T lymphocytes and mononuclear phagocytes, noncaseating epithelioid granulomas, and derangements of normal tissue architecture.

Pathophysiology

Mononuclear cells, mostly T helper lymphocytes and mononuclear phagocytes, accumulate in affected organs followed by formation of granulomas. It does not appear that this process injures parenchyma by releasing mediators; rather, organ dysfunction results from the accumulated inflammatory cells distorting the architecture of the affected tissue. Severe damage of parenchyma can lead to irreversible fibrosis.

Clinical Manifestations

In 10–20% of cases, sarcoidosis may first be detected as asymptomatic hilar adenopathy. Sarcoid manifests clinically in organs where it affects function or where it is readily observed. Onset may be acute or insidious.

1. Acute sarcoid: 20–40% of cases.
   a. Lofgren's syndrome: hilar adenopathy, erythema nodosum, acute arthritis presenting in one or both ankles spreading to involve other joints.
   b. Heerfordt-Waldenström syndrome: parotid enlargement, fever, anterior uveitis, facial nerve palsy.
2. Insidious onset: 40–70% of cases. Respiratory Sx most common presenting feature with constitutional or extrathoracic Sx less frequent.

Disease manifestations of sarcoid include:

• *Constitutional symptoms*—fever, weight loss, anorexia, fatigue.
• *Lung*—most commonly involved organ; 90% with sarcoidosis will have abnormal CXR some time during course. Features include: hilar adenopathy, alveolitis, interstitial pneumonitis; airways may be involved and cause obstruction to airflow; pleural disease and hemoptysis are uncommon.
• *Lymph nodes*—intrathoracic nodes enlarged in 75–90% of pts.
• *Skin*—25% will have skin involvement; lesions include erythema nodosum, plaques, maculopapular eruptions, subcutaneous nodules, and lupus pernio (indurated blue-purple shiny lesions on face, fingers, and knees).
• *Eye*—uveitis in ~25%; may progress to blindness.
• *Upper respiratory tract*—nasal mucosa involved in up to 20%, larynx 5%.
• *Bone marrow and spleen*—mild anemia and thrombocytopenia may occur.
• *Liver*—involved on biopsy in 60–90%; rarely important clinically.
• *Kidney*—parenchymal disease, nephrolithiasis secondary to abnormalities of calcium metabolism.
• *Nervous system*—cranial/peripheral neuropathy, chronic meningitis, pituitary involvement, space-occupying lesions, seizures.
• *Heart*—disturbances of rhythm and/or contractility, pericarditis.
• *Musculoskeletal*—bone lesions involving cortical bone seen in 3–13%, consisting of cysts in areas of expanded bone or lattice-like changes; dactylitis; joint involvement occurs in 25–50% with chronic mono- or oligoarthritis of knee, ankle, proximal interphalangeal joints.
• *Other organ systems*—endocrine/reproductive, exocrine glands, GI.

Evaluation

• Hx and physical exam to rule out exposures and other causes of interstitial lung disease.
• CBC, Ca^{2+}, LFTs, ACE, PPD and control skin tests.
• CXR, ECG, PFTs.
• Biopsy of lung or other affected organ.

- Bronchoalveolar lavage and gallium scan of lungs may help decide when treatment is indicated and may help to follow therapy; however, these are not uniformly accepted.

Diagnosis

Made on basis of clinical, radiographic, and histologic findings. Biopsy of lung or other affected organ is mandatory to establish diagnosis before starting therapy. Transbronchial lung biopsy usually adequate to make diagnosis. No blood findings are diagnostic. Differential includes neoplasms, infections, HIV, other granulomatous processes.

TREATMENT

Many cases remit spontaneously; therefore, deciding when treatment is necessary is difficult and controversial. Significant involvement of the eye, heart, or CNS or progressive lung disease is the main indication for treatment. Glucocorticoids are mainstay of therapy. Usual therapy is prednisone 1 (mg/kg)/d for 4–6 weeks followed by taper over 2–3 months. Methotrexate is usually the second-line medication. Other immunomodulatory agents have been used in refractory cases, but data consist of only anecdotal, uncontrolled reports.

Outcome

Most pts with acute disease are left with no significant sequelae. Overall, 50% of pts with sarcoid have some permanent organ dysfunction; in 15–20% disease remains active or recurrent; death directly due to disease occurs in 10% of cases. Respiratory tract abnormalities cause most of the morbidity and mortality related to sarcoid.

For a more detailed discussion, see Crystal RG: Sarcoidossis, Chap. 309, p. 2017, in HPIM-16.

#

AMYLOIDOSIS

Definition

Amyloidosis results from a sequence of changes in protein folding that leads to the deposition of insoluble amyloid fibrils, mainly in the extracellular spaces of organs and tissues. Clinical manifestations depend on anatomic distribution and intensity of amyloid protein deposition and range from local deposition with little significance to involvement of virtually any organ system with consequent severe pathophysiologic changes.

Classification

The amyloidoses are classified according to the identity of the fibril-forming protein and have biochemical and clinical differences (see Table 310-1, p. 2024, in HPIM-16):

• Light chain amyloidosis (AL): most common form of systemic amyloidosis seen in clinical practice; occurs in primary idiopathic amyloidosis and amyloid associated with multiple myeloma.
• Amyloid A amyloidosis (AA): occurs in secondary amyloidosis as a complication of chronic inflammatory disease and the hereditary periodic fever syndromes.
• Heredofamilial amyloidoses: number of different types that are dominantly transmitted in association with a mutation that enhances protein misfolding and fibril formation.
• $A\beta_2M$: Chronic hemodialysis-related amyloid; identical to β_2 microglobulin.
• Localized or organ-limited amyloidoses: includes $A\beta$: found in neuritic plaques and cerebrovascular walls of pts with Alzheimer's disease and Down's syndrome.

Clinical Manifestations

Clinical features are varied and depend entirely on biochemical nature of the fibril protein. Frequent sites of involvement:

• *Kidney*—seen with AA and AL; proteinuria, nephrosis, azotemia.
• *Liver*—occurs in AA, AL, and heredofamilial; hepatomegaly.
• *Skin*—characteristic of AL but can be seen in AA; raised waxy papules.
• *Heart*—common in AL and heredofamilial; CHF, cardiomegaly, arrhythmias.
• *GI*—common in all types; GI obstruction or ulceration, hemorrhage, protein loss, diarrhea, macroglossia, disordered esophageal motility.
• *Joints*—usually AL, frequently with myeloma; periarticular amyloid deposits, "shoulder pad sign": firm amyloid deposits in soft tissue around the shoulder, symmetric arthritis of shoulders, wrists, knees, hands.
• *Nervous system*—prominent in heredofamilial; peripheral neuropathy, postural hypotension, dementia. Carpal tunnel syndrome may occur in AL and $A\beta_2M$.
• *Respiratory*—lower airways can be affected in AL; localized amyloid can cause obstruction along upper airways.
• *Hematologic*—selective clotting factor deficiency.
• *Endocrine*—may infiltrate the thyroid or other glands but rarely causes dysfunction.

Diagnosis

Requires demonstration of amyloid in a biopsy of affected tissue using appropriate stains (e.g., Congo red). Aspiration of abdominal fat pad or biopsy of rectal mucosa may demonstrate amyloid fibrils. Electrophoresis and immuno-electrophoresis of serum and urine may assist in detecting paraproteins.

Prognosis

Outcome is variable and depends on type of amyloidosis and organ involvement. Average survival of AL amyloid is ~12 months; prognosis is poor when associated with myeloma. Renal failure and heart disease are the major causes of death.

℞ TREATMENT

AL amyloidosis may respond to regimens incorporating prednisone and alkylating agents, presumably because of the effects of these agents on synthesis of the AL amyloid protein. Stem cell transplantation and immunosuppressive drugs have brought about long-term remissions in some patients, but serious complications and death can occur. Iododoxyrubicin (IDOX) can bind to and promote resorption of AL amyloid and a subset of patients responded transiently in preliminary studies. Renal transplantation may be effective in selected pts. Treatment of AA amyloidosis is directed towards controlling the underlying inflammatory condition. Colchicine (1–2 mg/d) may prevent acute attacks in FMF and thus may block amyloid deposition. In certain of the heredofamilial amyloidoses, genetic counseling is important and liver transplantation has been successful.

For a more detailed discussion, see Sipe JD, Cohen AS: Amyloidosis, Chap. 310, p. 2024, in HPIM-16.

171

DISORDERS OF THE ANTERIOR PITUITARY AND HYPOTHALAMUS

The anterior pituitary is often referred to as the "master gland" because, together with the hypothalamus, it orchestrates the complex regulatory functions of multiple other glands (Fig. 171-1). The anterior pituitary produces six major hormones: (1) prolactin (PRL); (2) growth hormone (GH); (3) adrenocorticotropin hormone (ACTH); (4) luteinizing hormone (LH); (5) follicle-stimulating hormone (FSH); and (6) thyroid-stimulating hormone (TSH). Pituitary hormones are secreted in a pulsatile manner, reflecting intermittent stimulation by specific hypothalamic-releasing factors. Each of these pituitary hormones elicits specific responses in peripheral target glands. The hormonal products of these peripheral glands, in turn, exert feedback control at the level of the hypothalamus and pituitary to modulate pituitary function. Disorders of the pituitary include neoplasms that lead to mass effects and clinical syndromes due to excess or deficiency of one or more pituitary hormones.

PITUITARY TUMORS

Pituitary adenomas are benign monoclonal tumors that arise from one of the five anterior pituitary cell types and may cause clinical effects from either overproduction of a pituitary hormone or compressive effects on surrounding structures, including the hypothalamus, pituitary, or both. Tumors secreting prolactin are most common and have a greater prevalence in women than in men. GH- and ACTH-secreting tumors each account for about 10–15% of pituitary tumors. About one-third of all adenomas are clinically nonfunctioning and produce no distinct clinical hypersecretory syndrome. Adenomas are classified as microadenomas (<10 mm) or macroadenomas (≥10 mm). Other entities that can present as a sellar mass include craniopharyngiomas, Rathke's cleft cysts, sella chordomas, meningiomas, pituitary metastases, and gliomas.

Clinical Features Symptoms from mass effects include headache; visual loss through compression of the optic chiasm superiorly (classically a bitemporal hemianopsia); and diplopia, ptosis, ophthalmoplegia, and decreased facial sensation from cranial nerve compression laterally. Pituitary stalk compression from the tumor may also result in mild hyperprolactinemia. Symptoms of hypopituitarism or hormonal excess may be present as well (see below).

Pituitary apoplexy is an endocrine emergency that typically presents with features that include severe headache, bilateral visual changes, ophthalmoplegia, and, in severe cases, cardiovascular collapse and loss of consciousness. It may result in hypotension, severe hypoglycemia, CNS hemorrhage, and death. Patients with no evident visual loss or impaired consciousness can usually be observed and managed conservatively with high-dose glucocorticoids; surgical decompression should be considered when these features are present.

Diagnosis Sagittal and coronal T1-weighted MRI images with specific pituitary cuts should be obtained before and after administration of gadolinium. In patients with lesions close to the optic chiasm, visual field assessment that uses perimetry techniques should be performed. Initial hormonal evaluation is listed in Table 171-1.

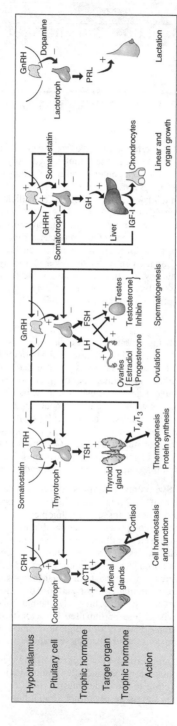

FIGURE 171-1 Diagram of pituitary axes. Hypothalamic hormones regulate anterior pituitary tropic hormones that, in turn, determine target gland secretion. Peripheral hormones feed back to regulate hypothalamic and pituitary hormones. TRH, thyrotropin-releasing hormone; for other abbreviations, see text.

Table 171-1

Initial Hormonal Evaluation of Pituitary Adenomas

Pituitary Hormone	Test for Hyperfunction	Test for Deficiency
Prolactin	Prolactin	
Growth hormone	Insulin-like growth factor I (IGF-I)	GH stimulation tests
ACTH	24-h urinary free cortisol *or* 1-mg overnight dexamethasone suppression test	8 A.M. serum cortisol *or* ACTH stimulation test
Gonadotropins	FSH, LH	Testosterone in men Menstrual history in women
TSH	TSH, free T_4	TSH, free T_4
Other	α-subunit	

In pituitary apoplexy, CT or MRI of the pituitary may reveal signs of sellar hemorrhage, with deviation of the pituitary stalk and compression of pituitary tissue.

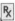 TREATMENT

Pituitary surgery is indicated for mass lesions that impinge on surrounding structures or to correct hormonal hypersecretion (see below). Transsphenoidal surgery, rather than transfrontal resection, is the desired surgical approach for most patients. The goal is selective resection of the pituitary mass lesion without damage to the normal pituitary tissue, to decrease the likelihood of hypopituitarism. Transient or permanent diabetes insipidus, hypopituitarism, CSF rhinorrhea, visual loss, and oculomotor palsy may occur postoperatively. Tumor invasion outside of the sella is rarely amenable to surgical cure, but debulking procedures may relieve tumor mass effects and reduce hormonal hypersecretion. Radiation may be used as an adjunct to surgery, but >50% of patients develop hormonal deficiencies within 10 years, usually due to hypothalamic damage. Prolactin-, GH-, and TSH-secreting tumors may also be amenable to medical therapy.

PITUITARY HORMONE HYPERSECRETION SYNDROMES
Hyperprolactinemia

Prolactin is unique among the pituitary hormones in that the predominant central control mechanism is inhibitory, reflecting dopamine-mediated suppression of prolactin release. Prolactin acts to induce and maintain lactation and decrease reproductive function and drive [via suppression of gonadotropin-releasing hormone (GnRH), gonadotropins, and gonadal steroidogenesis].

Etiology Physiologic elevation of prolactin occurs in pregnancy and lactation. Otherwise, prolactin-secreting pituitary adenomas (prolactinomas) are the most common cause of prolactin levels > 100 μg/L. Less pronounced hyperprolactinemia is commonly caused by medications [chlorpromazine, perphenazine, haloperidol, metoclopramide, opiates, H_2 antagonists, amitriptyline, selective serotonin reuptake inhibitors (SSRIs), calcium channel blockers, estrogens], pituitary stalk damage (tumors, lymphocytic hypophysitis, granulomas, trauma, irradiation), primary hypothyroidism, or renal failure. Nipple stimulation may also cause acute prolactin increases.

Clinical Features   In women, amenorrhea, galactorrhea, and infertility are the hallmarks of hyperprolactinemia. In men, symptoms of hypogonadism (Chap. 177) or mass effects are the usual presenting symptoms, and galactorrhea is uncommon.

Diagnosis   Fasting, morning prolactin levels should be measured; when clinical suspicion is high, measurement of levels on several different occasions may be required. If hyperprolactinemia is present, non-neoplastic causes should be excluded (e.g., pregnancy test, hypothyroidism, medications).

 TREATMENT

If the patient is taking a medication that is known to cause hyperprolactinemia, the drug should be withdrawn, if possible. A pituitary MRI should be performed if the underlying cause of prolactin elevation is unknown. Resection of hypothalamic or sellar mass lesions can reverse hyperprolactinemia due to stalk compression. Medical therapy with a dopamine agonist is indicated in microprolactinomas for control of symptomatic galactorrhea, restoration of gonadal function, or when fertility is desired. Alternatively, estrogen replacement may be indicated if fertility is not desired. Dopamine agonist therapy for macroprolactinomas generally results in both adenoma shrinkage and reduction of prolactin levels. Cabergoline (initial dose 0.5 mg q week, usual dose 0.5–1 mg twice a week) or bromocriptine (initial dose 1.25 mg qhs, usual dose 2.5–5 mg PO tid) are the two most frequently used dopamine agonists. These medications should initially be taken at bedtime with food, followed by gradual dose increases, to reduce the side effects of nausea and postural hypotension. Other side effects include constipation, nasal stuffiness, dry mouth, nightmares, insomnia, or vertigo; decreasing the dose usually alleviates these symptoms. Dopamine agonists may also precipitate or worsen underlying psychiatric conditions. Spontaneous remission of microadenomas, presumably caused by infarction, occurs in up to 30% of patients. Surgical debulking may be required for macroprolactinomas that do not respond to medical therapy.

Women with microprolactinomas who become pregnant should discontinue bromocriptine therapy, as the risk for significant tumor growth during pregnancy is low. In those with macroprolactinomas, visual field testing should be performed at each trimester. A pituitary MRI should be performed if severe headache and/or visual defects occur.

Acromegaly

Etiology   GH hypersecretion is usually the result of pituitary adenomas, but can rarely be due to extrapituitary production of GH or hypothalamic or peripheral growth hormone–releasing hormone (GHRH) secreting tumors.

Clinical Features   In children, GH hypersecretion prior to long bone epiphyseal closure results in gigantism. The presentation of acromegaly in adults is usually indolent. Patients may note a change in facial features, widened teeth spacing, deepening of the voice, snoring, increased shoe or glove size, ring tightening, hyperhidrosis, oily skin, arthropathy, and carpal tunnel syndrome. Frontal bossing, mandibular enlargement with prognathism, macroglossia, an enlarged thyroid, skin tags, thick heel pads, and hypertension may be present on examination. Associated conditions include cardiomyopathy, left ventricular hypertrophy, diastolic dysfunction, sleep apnea, diabetes mellitus, colon polyps, and colonic malignancy. Overall mortality is increased approximately threefold.

Diagnosis   IGF-I levels are a useful screening measure, with elevation suggesting acromegaly. Due to the pulsatility of GH, measurement of a single random GH level is not useful for screening. The diagnosis of acromegaly is confirmed by demonstrating the failure of GH suppression to <1 μg/L within 1–2 h of a 75-g oral glucose load.

 TREATMENT

> GH levels are not normalized by surgery alone in many patients with macroadenomas; somatostatin analogues provide adjunctive medical therapy that suppresses GH secretion with modest effects on tumor size. Octreotide (50 μg SC tid) is used for initial therapy. Once tolerance of side effects (nausea, abdominal discomfort, diarrhea, flatulence) is established, patients may be changed to long-acting depot formulations (20–30 mg IM q2–4 weeks). Pituitary irradiation may also be required as adjuvant therapy but has a high rate of late hypopituitarism.

Cushing's Disease See Chap. 174.

Nonfunctioning and Gonadotropin-Producing Adenomas

These tumors usually present with symptoms of one or more hormonal deficiencies or mass effect. They typically produce small amounts of intact gonadotropins (usually FSH) as well as uncombined α and LHβ and FSHβ subunits. Surgery is indicated for mass effects or hypopituitarism; asymptomatic small adenomas may be followed with regular MRI and visual field testing. Diagnosis is based on immunohistochemical analysis of resected tumor tissue.

TSH-Secreting Adenomas

TSH-producing adenomas are rare but often large and locally invasive when they occur. Patients present with goiter and hyperthyroidism, and/or sella mass effects. Diagnosis is based on elevated serum free T_4 levels in the setting of inappropriately normal or high TSH secretion and MRI evidence of pituitary adenoma. Surgery is indicated and is usually followed by somatostatin analogue therapy to treat residual tumor. Thyroid ablation or antithyroid drugs can be used to reduce thyroid hormone levels.

HYPOPITUITARISM

Etiology A variety of disorders may cause deficiencies of one or more pituitary hormones. These disorders may be congenital, traumatic (pituitary surgery, cranial irradiation, head injury), neoplastic (large pituitary adenoma, parasellar mass, craniopharyngioma, metastases, meningioma), infiltrative (hemochromatosis, lymphocytic hypophysitis, sarcoidosis, histiocytosis X), vascular (pituitary apoplexy, postpartum necrosis, sickle cell disease), or infectious (tuberculous, fungal, parasitic).

Clinical Features Hormonal abnormalities after cranial irradiation may occur 5 to 15 years later, with GH deficiency occurring first, followed sequentially by gonadotropin, TSH, and ACTH deficiency.

Each hormone deficiency is associated with specific findings:

- GH: growth disorders in children; increased intraabdominal fat, reduced lean body mass, hyperlipidemia, reduced bone mineral density, and social isolation in adults
- FSH/LH: menstrual disorders and infertility in women (Chap. 178); hypogonadism in men (Chap. 177)
- ACTH: features of hypocortisolism (Chap. 174) without mineralocorticoid deficiency

- TSH: growth retardation in children, features of hypothyroidism in children and adults (Chap. 173)

Diagnosis Biochemical diagnosis of pituitary insufficiency is made by demonstrating low or inappropriately normal levels of pituitary hormones in the setting of low target hormone levels. Initial testing should include an 8 A.M. cortisol level, TSH and free T$_4$, IGF-I, testosterone in men, and assessment of menstrual cycles in women. Provocative tests may be required to assess pituitary reserve for individual hormones. Adult GH deficiency is diagnosed by demonstrating a subnormal GH response to a standard provocative test (insulin tolerance test, L-dopa, arginine, GHRH). Acute ACTH deficiency may be diagnosed by a subnormal response in an insulin tolerance test, metyrapone test, or corticotropin-releasing hormone (CRH) stimulation test. Standard ACTH (cosyntropin) stimulation tests may be normal in acute ACTH deficiency; with adrenal atrophy, the cortisol response to cosyntropin is blunted.

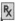 **TREATMENT**

> Hormonal replacement should aim to mimic physiologic hormone production. Effective dose schedules are outlined in Table 171-2. GH therapy, particularly when excessive, may be associated with fluid retention, joint pain, and carpal tunnel syndrome. Glucocorticoid replacement should always precede levothyroxine therapy to avoid precipitation of adrenal crisis. Patients requiring glucocorticoid replacement should wear a medical alert bracelet and should be instructed to take additional doses during stressful events such as acute illness, dental procedures, trauma, and acute hospitalization.

Table 171-2

Hormone Replacement Therapy for Adult Hypopituitarism[a]

Trophic Hormone Deficit	Hormone Replacement
ACTH	Hydrocortisone (10–20 mg A.M.; 10 mg P.M.)
	Cortisone acetate (25 mg A.M.; 12.5 mg P.M.)
	Prednisone (5 mg A.M.; 2.5 mg P.M.)
TSH	L-Thyroxine (0.075–0.15 mg daily)
FSH/LH	Males
	Testosterone enanthate (200 mg IM every 2 weeks)
	Testosterone skin patch (5 mg/d)
	Testosterone gel (5–10 g/d)
	Females
	Conjugated estrogen (0.65–1.25 mg qd for 25 days)
	Progesterone (5–10 mg qd) on days 16–25
	Estradiol skin patch (0.5 mg, every other day)
	For fertility: Menopausal gonadotropins, human chorionic gonadotropins
GH	Adults: Somatotropin (0.3–1.0 mg SC qd)
	Children: Somatotropin [0.02–0.05 (mg/kg per day)]
Vasopressin	Intranasal desmopressin (5–20 μg twice daily)
	Oral 300–600 μg qd

[a] All doses shown should be individualized for specific patients and should be reassessed during stress, surgery, or pregnancy. Male and female fertility requirements should be managed as discussed in Chaps. 177 and 178.
Note: For abbreviations, see text.

For a more detailed discussion, see Melmed S, Jameson JL: Disorders of the Anterior Pituitary and Hypothalamus, Chap. 318, p. 2076, in HPIM-16.

172

DISORDERS OF THE POSTERIOR PITUITARY

The neurohypophysis, or posterior pituitary gland, produces two hormones: (1) arginine vasopressin (AVP), also known as antidiuretic hormone (ADH), and (2) oxytocin. AVP acts on the renal tubules to induce water retention, leading to concentration of the urine. Oxytocin stimulates postpartum milk letdown in response to suckling. Clinical syndromes may result from deficiency or excess of AVP. There are no known clinical disorders associated with oxytocin deficiency or excess.

DIABETES INSIPIDUS

ETIOLOGY Diabetes insipidus (DI) results from abnormalities of AVP production from the hypothalamus or AVP action in the kidney. AVP deficiency is characterized by production of large amounts of dilute urine. In *central DI*, insufficient AVP is released in response to physiologic stimuli. Causes include acquired (head trauma; neoplastic or inflammatory conditions affecting the posterior pituitary), congenital, and genetic disorders, but almost half of cases are idiopathic. In gestational DI, increased metabolism of plasma AVP by an aminopeptidase produced by the placenta leads to a deficiency of AVP during pregnancy. *Primary polydipsia* results in secondary insufficiencies of AVP due to inhibition of AVP secretion by excessive fluid intake. *Nephrogenic DI* can be genetic or acquired from drug exposure (lithium, demeclocycline, amphotericin B), metabolic conditions (hypercalcemia), or renal damage.

CLINICAL FEATURES Symptoms include polyuria, excessive thirst, and polydipsia, with a 24-h urine output of >50 (mL/kg)/day and a urine osmolality that is less than that of serum (<300 mosmol/kg; specific gravity <1.010). Clinical or laboratory signs of dehydration, including hypernatremia, occur only if the pt simultaneously has a thirst defect or does not have access to water. Other etiologies of hypernatremia are described in Chap. 3.

DIAGNOSIS DI must be differentiated from other etiologies of polyuria (Chap. 56). Unless an inappropriately dilute urine is present in the setting of serum hyperosmolality, a fluid deprivation test is used to make the diagnosis of DI. This test should be started in the morning, and body weight, plasma osmolality, sodium concentration, and urine volume and osmolality should be measured hourly. The test should be stopped when body weight decreases by 5% or plasma osmolality/sodium exceed the upper limit of normal. If the urine osmolality is <300 mosmol/kg with serum hyperosmolality, desmopressin (0.03 μg/kg SC) should be administered with repeat measurement of urine osmolality 1–2 h later. An increase of >50% indicates severe pituitary DI, whereas a smaller or absent response suggests nephrogenic DI. Measurement of AVP levels before and after fluid deprivation may be required to diagnose partial DI.

Occasionally, hypertonic saline infusion may be required if fluid deprivation does not achieve the requisite level of hypertonic dehydration.

 TREATMENT

Pituitary DI can be treated with desmopressin (DDAVP) subcutaneously (1–2 μg qd-bid), via nasal spray (10–20 μg bid-tid), or orally (100–400 μg bid-tid), with recommendations to drink to thirst. Chlorpropamide has also been used, though caution must be used to avoid hypoglycemia and a disulfuram-like reaction to ethanol. Symptoms of nephrogenic DI may be ameliorated by treatment with a thiazide diuretic and/or amiloride in conjunction with a low-sodium diet, or with prostaglandin synthesis inhibitors (e.g., indomethacin).

SYNDROME OF INAPPROPRIATE ANTIDIURETIC HORMONE (SIADH)

ETIOLOGY   Excessive or inappropriate production of AVP predisposes to hyponatremia, reflecting water retention. The evaluation of hyponatremia is described in Chap. 3. Etiologies of SIADH include neoplasms, lung infections, CNS disorders, and drugs (Table 172-1).

Table 172-1

Causes of Syndrome of Inappropriate Antidiuretic Hormone (SIADH)

Neoplasms	Neurologic
Carcinomas	Guillain-Barré syndrome
Lung	Multiple sclerosis
Duodenum	Delerium tremens
Pancreas	Amyotrophic lateral sclerosis
Ovary	Hydrocephalus
Bladder, ureter	Psychosis
Other neoplasms	Peripheral neuropathy
Thymoma	Congenital malformations
Mesothelioma	Agenesis corpus callosum
Bronchial adenoma	Cleft lip/palate
Carcinoid	Other midline defects
Gangliocytoma	Metabolic
Ewing's sarcoma	Acute intermittent porphyria
Head trauma	Pulmonary
Infections	Asthma
Pneumonia, bacterial or viral	Pneumothorax
Abscess, lung or brain	Positive-pressure respiration
Cavitation (aspergillosis)	Drugs
Tuberculosis, lung or brain	Vasopressin or DDAVP
Meningitis, bacterial or viral	Chlorpropamide
Encephalitis	Oxytocin, high dose
AIDS	Vincristine
Vascular	Carbamazepine
Cerebrovascular occlusions,	Nicotine
hemorrhage	Phenothiazines
Cavernous sinus thrombosis	Cyclophosphamide
	Tricyclic antidepressants
	Monoamine oxidase inhibitors
	Serotonin reuptake inhibitors

CLINICAL FEATURES   If hyponatremia develops gradually, it may be asymptomatic. However, if it develops acutely, symptoms of water intoxication may include mild headache, confusion, anorexia, nausea, vomiting, coma, and convulsions. Laboratory findings include low BUN, creatinine, uric acid, and albumin; serum Na < 130 mmol/L and plasma osmolality < 270 mmol/kg; urine is almost always hypertonic to plasma, and urinary Na^+ is usually >20 mmol/L.

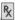 **TREATMENT**

Fluid intake should be restricted to 500 mL less than urinary output. In patients with severe symptoms or signs, hypertonic (3%) saline can be infused at ≤0.05 mL/kg body weight IV per minute, with hourly sodium levels measured until Na increases by 12 mmol/L or to 130 mmol/L, whichever occurs first. However, if the hyponatremia has been present for more than 24–48 h and is corrected too rapidly, saline infusion has the potential to produce central pontine myelinolysis. Demeclocycline (150–300 mg PO tid-qid) or fludrocortisone (0.05–0.2 mg PO bid) may be required to manage chronic SIADH.

For a more detailed discussion, see Robertson GL: Disorders of the Neurohypophysis, Chap. 319, p. 2097, in HPIM-16.

173

DISORDERS OF THE THYROID

Disorders of the thyroid gland result primarily from autoimmune processes that stimulate the overproduction of thyroid hormones (*thyrotoxicosis*) or cause glandular destruction and underproduction of thyroid hormones (*hypothyroidism*). *Neoplastic processes* in the thyroid gland can lead to benign nodules or thyroid cancer.

The hypothalamus releases thyrotropin-releasing hormone (TRH), which stimulates release of thyroid-stimulating hormone (TSH) from the anterior pituitary. TSH is secreted into the circulation and binds to receptors in the thyroid gland, where it controls production and release of thyroxine (T_4) and triiodothyronine (T_3), which in turn inhibit further release of TSH from the pituitary. Some T_3 is secreted by the thyroid, but most is produced by deiodination of T_4 in peripheral tissues. Both T_4 and T_3 are bound to carrier proteins [thyroid-binding globulin (TBG), transthyretin, and albumin] in the circulation. Increased levels of total T_4 and T_3 with normal free levels are seen in states of increased carrier proteins (pregnancy, estrogens, cirrhosis, hepatitis, and inherited disorders). Conversely, decreased total T_4 and T_3 levels with normal free levels are seen in severe systemic illness, chronic liver disease, and nephrosis.

HYPOTHYROIDISM

ETIOLOGY   Deficient thyroid hormone secretion can be due to thyroid failure (primary hypothyroidism) or pituitary or hypothalamic disease (secondary hypothyroidism) (Table 173-1). Transient hypothyroidism may occur in silent or subacute thyroiditis. *Subclinical* (or *mild*) *hypothyroidism* is a state of normal thyroid hormone levels and mild elevation of TSH; despite the name, some pts may have minor symptoms. With higher TSH levels and low free T_4 levels, symptoms become more readily apparent in *clinical* (or *overt*) *hypothyroidism*. In areas of iodine sufficiency, autoimmune disease and iatrogenic causes are most common.

CLINICAL FEATURES   Symptoms of hypothyroidism include lethargy, dry hair and skin, cold intolerance, hair loss, difficulty concentrating, poor memory, constipation, mild weight gain with poor appetite, dyspnea, hoarse voice, muscle cramping, and menorrhagia. Cardinal features on examination include bradycardia, mild diastolic hypertension, prolongation of the relaxation phase of deep tendon reflexes, and cool peripheral extremities. Goiter may be palpated, or the thyroid may be atrophic and nonpalpable. Carpal tunnel syndrome may be present. Cardiomegaly may be present due to pericardial effusion. The most extreme presentation is a dull, expressionless face, sparse hair, periorbital puffiness, large tongue, and pale, doughy, cool skin. The condition may progress into a hypothermic, stuporous state (*myxedema coma*) with respiratory depression. Factors that predispose to myxedema coma include cold exposure, trauma, infection, and administration of narcotics.

DIAGNOSIS   Decreased serum T_4 is common to all varieties of hypothyroidism. An elevated TSH is a sensitive marker of primary hypothyroidism. A summary of the investigations used to determine the existence and cause of hypothyroidism is provided in Fig. 173-1. Thyroid peroxidase (TPO) antibodies

Table 173-1

Causes of Hypothyroidism

Primary
  Autoimmune hypothyroidism: Hashimoto's thyroiditis, atrophic thyroiditis
  Iatrogenic: ^{131}I treatment, subtotal or total thyroidectomy, external irradiation
    of neck for lymphoma or cancer
  Drugs: iodine excess (including iodine-containing contrast media and amiodarone), lithium, antithyroid drugs, *p*-aminosalicyclic acid, interferon-α and
    other cytokines, aminoglutethimide
  Congenital hypothyroidism: absent or ectopic thyroid gland, dyshormonogenesis, TSH-R mutation
  Iodine deficiency
  Infiltrative disorders: amyloidosis, sarcoidosis, hemochromatosis, scleroderma, cystinosis, Riedel's thyroiditis
Transient
  Silent thyroiditis, including postpartum thyroiditis
  Subacute thyroiditis
  Withdrawal of thyroxine treatment in individuals with an intact thyroid
  After ^{131}I treatment or subtotal thyroidectomy for Graves' disease
Secondary
  Hypopituitarism: tumors, pituitary surgery or irradiation, infiltrative disorders, Sheehan's syndrome, trauma, genetic forms of combined pituitary hormone deficiencies
  Isolated TSH deficiency or inactivity
  Bexarotene treatment
  Hypothalamic disease: tumors, trauma, infiltrative disorders, idiopathic

Note: TSH, thyroid-stimulating hormone; TSH-R, TSH receptor.

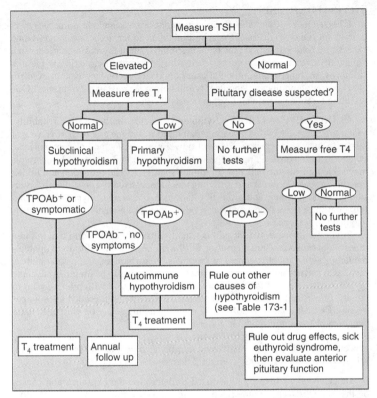

FIGURE 173-1 Evaluation of hypothyroidism, TPOAb+, thyroid peroxidase antibodies present: TPOAb-, thyroid peroxidase antibodies not present.

are increased in 90–95% of pts with autoimmune-mediated hypothyroidism. Elevated cholesterol, increased creatine phosphokinase, and anemia may be present; bradycardia, low-amplitude QRS complexes, and flattened or inverted T waves may be present on ECG.

℞ TREATMENT

Adult pts <60 years without evidence of heart disease may be started on 50–100 μg of levothyroxine (T_4) daily. In the elderly or in pts with known coronary artery disease, the starting dose of levothyroxine is 12.5–25 μg/d. The dose should be adjusted in 12.5- to 25-μg increments every 6–8 weeks on the basis of TSH levels, until a normal TSH level is achieved. The usual daily replacement dose is 1.6 (μg/kg)/d. Women on levothyroxine replacement should have a TSH level checked as soon as pregnancy is diagnosed, as the replacement dose typically increases by 30–50% during pregnancy. Failure to recognize and treat maternal hypothyroidism may adversely affect fetal neural development. Therapy for myxedema coma should include levothyroxine (200 μg) and liothyroinine (25 μg) as a single IV bolus followed by daily treatment with levothyroxine (50–100 μg/d) and liothyronine (10 μg q8h), along with hydrocortisone (50 mg q6h) for impaired adrenal reserve, ventilatory support, space blankets, and therapy of precipitating factors.

THYROTOXICOSIS

ETIOLOGY Causes of thyroid hormone excess include primary hyperthyroidism (Graves' disease, toxic multinodular goiter, toxic adenoma, iodine excess); thyroid destruction (subacute thyroiditis, silent thyroiditis, amiodarone, radiation); extrathyroidal sources of thyroid hormone (thyrotoxicosis factitia, struma ovarii, functioning follicular carcinoma); and secondary hyperthyroidism (TSH-secreting pituitary adenoma, thyroid hormone resistance syndrome, hCG-secreting tumors, gestational thyrotoxicosis).

CLINICAL FEATURES Symptoms include nervousness, irritability, heat intolerance, excessive sweating, palpitations, fatigue and weakness, weight loss with increased appetite, frequent bowel movements, and oligomenorrhea. Pts are anxious, restless, and fidgety. Skin is warm and moist, and fingernails may separate from the nail bed (Plummer's nails). Eyelid retraction and lid lag may be present. Cardiovascular findings include tachycardia, systolic hypertension, systolic murmur, and atrial fibrillation. A fine tremor, hyperreflexia, and proximal muscle weakness may also be present. Long-standing thyrotoxicosis may lead to osteopenia.

In Graves' disease, the thyroid is usually diffusely enlarged to two to three times its normal size, and a bruit or thrill may be present. Infiltrative ophthalmopathy (with variable degrees of proptosis, periorbital swelling, and ophthalmoplegia) and dermopathy (pretibial myxedema) may also be found. In subacute thyroiditis, the thyroid is exquisitely tender and enlarged with referred pain to the jaw or ear, and sometimes accompanied by fever and preceded by an upper respiratory tract infection. Solitary or multiple nodules may be present in toxic adenoma or toxic multinodular goiter.

Thyrotoxic crisis, or thyroid storm, is rare, presents as a life-threatening exacerbation of hyperthyroidism, and can be accompanied by fever, delirium, seizures, arrhythmias, coma, vomiting, diarrhea, and jaundice.

DIAGNOSIS Investigations used to determine the existence and causes of thyrotoxicosis are summarized in Fig. 173-2. Serum TSH is a sensitive marker of thyrotoxicosis caused by Graves' disease, autonomous thyroid nodules, thyroiditis, and exogenous levothyroxine treatment. Associated laboratory abnormalities include elevation of bilirubin, liver enzymes, and ferritin. Radionuclide uptake may be required to distinguish the various etiologies: high uptake in Graves' disease and nodular disease vs. low uptake in thyroid destruction, iodine excess, and extrathyroidal sources of thyroid hormone. The ESR is elevated in subacute thyroiditis.

 TREATMENT

Graves' disease may be treated with antithyroid drugs or radioiodine; subtotal thyroidectomy is rarely indicated. The main antithyroid drugs are carbimazole or methimazole (10–20 mg bid-tid initially, titrated to 2.5–10 mg qd) and propylthiouracil (100–200 mg q8h initially, titrated to 50 mg qd-bid). Thyroid function tests should be checked 3–4 weeks after initiation of treatment, with adjustments to maintain a normal free T_4 level. The common side effects are rash, urticaria, fever, and arthralgia (1–5% of pts). Rare but major side effects include hepatitis, an SLE-like syndrome, and agranulocytosis (<1%). All pts should be given written instructions regarding the symptoms of possible agranulocytosis (sore throat, fever, mouth ulcers) and the need to stop treatment pending a complete blood count to confirm that agranulocytosis is not present. Propranolol (20–40 mg q6h) or longer acting beta blockers such as atenolol (50 mg qd) may be useful to control adrenergic symptoms. Antico-

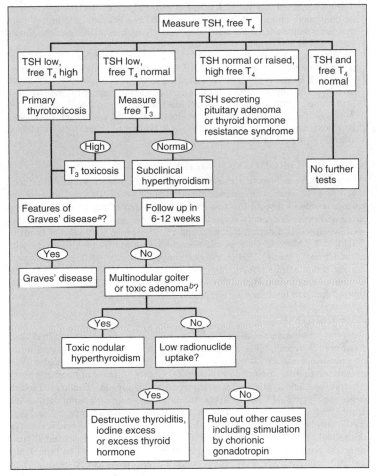

FIGURE 173-2 Evaluation of thyrotoxicosis. [a]Diffuse goiter, positive TPO antibodies, ophthalmopathy, dermopathy; [b]can be confirmed by radionuclide scan.

agulation with warfarin should be considered in all pts with atrial fibrillation. Radioiodine can also be used as initial treatment or in pts who do not undergo remission after a 1- to 2-year trial of antithyroid drugs. Antecedent treatment with antithyroid drugs should be considered in elderly pts and those with cardiac problems, with cessation of antithyroid drugs 3–5 days prior to radioiodine administration. Radioiodine treatment is contraindicated in pregnancy; instead, symptoms should be controlled with the lowest effective dose of propylthiouracil (PTU). Corneal drying may be relieved with artificial tears and taping the eyelids shut during sleep. Progressive exophthalmos with chemosis, ophthalmoplegia, or vision loss is treated with large doses of prednisone (40–80 mg qd) and ophthalmologic referral; orbital decompression may be required.

In thyroid storm, large doses of PTU (600-mg loading dose) should be administered orally, per nasogastric tube, or per rectum, followed 1 h later by

5 drops saturated solution of KI (SSKI) q6h. PTU (200–300 mg q6h) should be continued, along with propranolol (40–60 mg PO q4h or 2 mg IV q4h) and dexamethasone (2 mg q6h). Any underlying precipitating cause should be identified and treated.

Radioiodine is the treatment of choice for toxic nodules. Subacute thyroiditis should be treated with NSAIDs and beta blockade to control symptoms, with monitoring of the TSH and free T_4 levels every 4 weeks. Transient levothyroxine replacement (50–100 μg qd) may be required if the hypothyroid phase is prolonged. Silent thyroiditis (or postpartum thyroiditis if within 3–6 months of delivery) should be treated with beta blockade during the thyrotoxic phase and levothyroxine in the hypothyroid phase, with withdrawal after 6–9 months to assess recovery.

SICK EUTHYROID SYNDROME

Any acute, severe illness can cause abnormalities of circulating thyroid hormone levels or TSH, even in the absence of underlying thyroid disease. Therefore, the routine testing of thyroid function should be avoided in acutely ill pts unless a thyroid disorder is strongly suspected. The most common pattern in sick euthyroid syndrome is a decrease in total and free T_3 levels, with normal levels of TSH and T_4. More ill pts may additionally have a fall in total T_4 levels, with normal free T_4 levels. TSH levels may range from <0.1 to >20 mU/L, with normalization after recovery from illness. Unless there is historic or clinical evidence of hypothyroidism, thyroid hormone should not be administered and thyroid function tests should be repeated after recovery.

AMIODARONE

Amiodarone treatment is associated with (1) acute, transient changes in thyroid function, (2) hypothyroidism, or (3) thyrotoxicosis. There are two major forms of amiodarone-induced thyrotoxicosis (AIT). Type 1 AIT is associated with an underlying thyroid abnormality (preclinical Graves' disease or nodular goiter). Thyroid hormone synthesis becomes excessive as a result of increased iodine exposure. Type 2 AIT occurs in pts with no intrinsic thyroid abnormalities and is the result of destructive thyroiditis. Differentiation between type 1 and type 2 AIT may be difficult as the high iodine load interferes with thyroid scans. The drug should be stopped, if possible, with administration of high-dose antithyroid drugs in type 1 AIT or potassium perchlorate (200 mg q6h) in type 1 and glucocorticoids in type 2 AIT. Oral contrast agents may also be useful in type 2 AIT.

NONTOXIC GOITER

Goiter refers to an enlarged thyroid gland (>20–25 g) and is more common in women than men. Biosynthetic defects, iodine deficiency, autoimmune disease, and nodular diseases can lead to goiter. If thyroid function is preserved, most goiters are asymptomatic. Substernal goiter may obstruct the thoracic inlet and should be evaluated with CT or MRI in pts with obstructive signs or symptoms (difficulty swallowing, tracheal compression, or plethora). Thyroid function tests should be performed in all pts with goiter to exclude thyrotoxicosis or hypothyroidism. Ultrasound is not generally indicated in the evaluation of diffuse goiter, unless a nodule is palpable on physical exam.

Iodine or thyroid hormone replacement induces variable regression of goiter in iodine deficiency. For other causes of nontoxic diffuse goiter, levothyroxine can be used in an attempt to reduce goiter size. Significant regression is usually seen within 3 to 6 months of treatment; after this time it is unlikely to occur.

Suppressive therapy is rarely effective for nontoxic multinodular goiters. Radioiodine reduces goiter size by about 50% in the majority of pts. Surgery is rarely indicated for diffuse goiter but may be required to alleviate compression in pts with nontoxic multinodular goiter.

TOXIC MULTINODULAR GOITER AND TOXIC ADENOMA
Toxic Multinodular Goiter (MNG)

In addition to features of goiter, the clinical presentation of toxic MNG includes subclinical hyperthyroidism or mild thyrotoxicosis. The pt is usually elderly and may present with atrial fibrillation or palpitations, tachycardia, nervousness, tremor, or weight loss. Recent exposure to iodine, from contrast dyes or other sources, may precipitate or exacerbate thyrotoxicosis. The TSH level is low. T_4 may be normal or minimally increased; T_3 is often elevated to a greater degree than T_4. Thyroid scan shows heterogeneous uptake with multiple regions of increased and decreased uptake; 24-h uptake of radioiodine may not be increased and rarely induces remission. Antithyroid drugs, often in combination with beta blockers, can normalize thyroid function and improve clinical features of thyrotoxicosis but may stimulate goiter growth. A trial of radioiodine should be considered before subjecting pts, many of whom are elderly, to surgery.

Toxic Adenoma

A solitary, autonomously functioning thyroid nodule is referred to as *toxic adenoma*. A thyroid scan provides a definitive diagnostic test, demonstrating focal uptake in the hyperfunctioning nodule and diminished uptake in the remainder of the gland, as activity of the normal thyroid is suppressed. Radioiodine ablation (e.g., 10–29.9 mCi ^{131}I) is usually the treatment of choice.

THYROID NEOPLASMS

ETIOLOGY Thyroid neoplasms may be benign (adenomas) or malignant (carcinomas). Benign neoplasms include macrofollicular (colloid) and normofollicular adenomas. Microfollicular, trabecular, and Hurthle cell variants raise greater concern. Carcinomas of the follicular epithelium include papillary, follicular, and anaplastic thyroid cancer. Papillary thyroid cancer is the most common type of thyroid cancer. It tends to be multifocal and to invade locally. Follicular thyroid cancer is difficult to diagnose via fine-needle aspiration because the distinction between benign and malignant follicular neoplasms rests largely on evidence of invasion into vessels, nerves, or adjacent structures. It tends to spread hematogenously, leading to bone, lung, and CNS metastases. Anaplastic carcinoma is rare, highly malignant, and rapidly fatal. Thyroid lymphoma often arises in the background of Hashimoto's thyroiditis and occurs in the setting of a rapidly expanding thyroid mass. Medullary thyroid carcinoma arises from parafollicular (C) cells and may occur sporadically or as a familial disorder, sometimes in association with multiple endocrine neoplasia type 2.

CLINICAL FEATURES It is important to distinguish between a solitary nodule or a prominent nodule in the context of a multinodular goiter, as the incidence of malignancy is greater in solitary nodules. Features suggesting carcinoma include recent or rapid growth of a nodule or mass, history of neck irradiation, lymph node involvement, and fixation to surrounding tissues. Glandular enlargement may result in compression and displacement of the trachea or esophagus and obstructive symptoms.

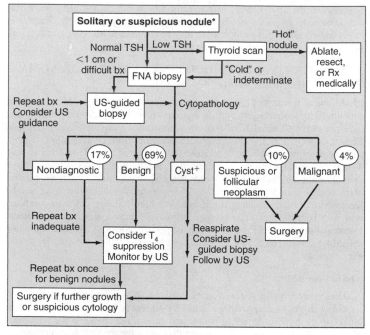

FIGURE 173-3 Approach to the patient with a thyroid nodule. *There are many exceptions to the suggested options. See Chap. 320, HPIM-16. †About one-third of nodules are cystic or mixed solid-cystic. US, ultrasound.

DIAGNOSIS An approach to the evaluation of a solitary nodule is outlined in Fig. 173-3.

℞ TREATMENT

Benign nodules should be monitored via serial examination. Surgical resection or radioiodine ablation may be required in multinodular goiters with compressive effects.

Near-total thyroidectomy with lymph node dissection is required for papillary and follicular carcinoma and should be performed by a surgeon who is highly experienced in the procedure. If risk factors and pathologic features indicate the need for radioiodine treatment, the pt should be treated for several weeks postoperatively with liothyronine (25 μg bid-tid), followed by withdrawal for an additional 2 weeks, in preparation for postsurgical radioablation of remnant tissue. A scanning dose of ^{131}I is administered when the TSH level is >50 IU/L, followed by a therapeutic dose. Subsequent levothyroxine suppression of TSH to a low, but detectable, level should be attempted in pts with a high risk of recurrence, and to 0.1–0.5 IU/L in those with a low risk of recurrence. Follow-up scans and thyroglobulin levels should be performed at regular intervals after either thyroid hormone withdrawal or administration of recombinant human TSH.

The management of medullary thyroid carcinoma is surgical, as these tumors do not take up radioiodine. Testing for the *RET* mutation should be considered. Elevated serum calcitonin provides a marker of residual or recurrent disease.

For a more detailed discussion, see Jameson JL, Weetman AP: Disorders of the Thyroid Gland, Chap. 320, p. 2104, in HPIM-16.

174

DISORDERS OF THE ADRENAL GLAND

The adrenal cortex produces three major classes of steroids: (1) glucocorticoids, (2) mineralocorticoids, and (3) adrenal androgens. Clinical syndromes may result from deficiencies or excesses of these hormones. The adrenal medulla produces catecholamines, with excess leading to pheochromocytoma (Chap. 122).

HYPERFUNCTION OF THE ADRENAL GLAND
Cushing's Syndrome

Etiology   Cushing's syndrome results from production of excess cortisol (and other steroid hormones) by the adrenal cortex. The major cause is bilateral adrenal hyperplasia secondary to hypersecretion of adrenocorticotropic hormone (ACTH) by the pituitary (Cushing's disease) or from ectopic sources such as small cell carcinoma of the lung; medullary carcinoma of the thyroid; or tumors of the thymus, pancreas, or ovary. Adenomas or carcinoma of the adrenal gland account for about 25% of Cushing's syndrome cases. Administration of glucocorticoids for therapeutic reasons may result in iatrogenic Cushing's syndrome.

Clinical Features   Some common manifestations (central obesity, hypertension, osteoporosis, psychological disturbances, acne, amenorrhea, and diabetes mellitus) are relatively nonspecific. More specific findings include easy bruising, purple striae, proximal myopathy, fat deposition in the face and interscapular areas (moon facies and buffalo hump), and virilization. Thin, brittle skin and plethoric moon facies may also be found. Hypokalemia and metabolic alkalosis are prominent, particularly with ectopic production of ACTH.

Diagnosis   The diagnosis of Cushing's syndrome requires demonstration of increased cortisol production and abnormal cortisol suppression in response to dexamethasone (Fig. 174-1). For initial screening, the 1-mg overnight dexamethasone test (8 A.M. plasma cortisol <5 μg/dL) or measurement of 24-h urinary free cortisol is appropriate. Definitive diagnosis is established by inadequate suppression of urinary (<10 μg/d) or plasma cortisol (<5 μg/dL) after 0.5 mg dexamethasone q6h for 48 h. Once the diagnosis of Cushing's syndrome is established, further biochemical testing is required to localize the source. Low levels of plasma ACTH levels suggest an adrenal adenoma or carcinoma; inappropriately normal or high plasma ACTH levels suggest a pituitary or ectopic source. In 95% of ACTH-producing pituitary microadenomas, cortisol production is suppressed by high-dose dexamethasone (2 mg q6h for 48 h), and MRI of the pituitary should be obtained. However, because up to 10% of ectopic sources of ACTH may also suppress after high-dose dexamethasone testing, inferior petrosal sinus sampling may be required to distinguish pituitary from peripheral sources of ACTH. Imaging of the chest and abdomen is required to localize the source of ectopic ACTH production. Pts with chronic alcoholism

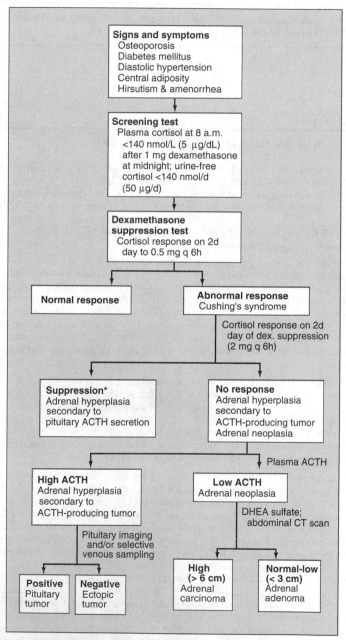

FIGURE 174-1   Diagnostic flowchart for evaluating patients suspected of having Cushing's syndrome. *This group probably includes some patients with pituitary-hypothalamic dysfunction and some with pituitary microadenomas. In some instances, a microadenoma may be visualized by pituitary MRI scanning. DHEA, dehydroepiandrosterone.

and depression may have false-positive results in testing for Cushing's syndrome. Similarly, pts with acute illness may have abnormal laboratory test results, since major stress disrupts the normal regulation of ACTH secretion.

TREATMENT

Therapy of adrenal adenoma or carcinoma requires surgical excision; stress doses of glucocorticoids must be given pre- and postoperatively. Metastatic and unresectable adrenal carcinomas are treated with mitotane in doses gradually increased to 6 g/d in three or four divided doses. Transsphenoidal surgery can be curative for pituitary microadenomas that secrete ACTH, though radiation may be used when cure is not achieved (see Chap. 171). On occasion, debulking of lung carcinoma or resection of carcinoid tumors can result in remission of ectopic Cushing's syndrome. If the source of ACTH cannot be resected, bilateral total adrenalectomy or medical management with ketoconazole (600–1200 mg/d), metyrapone (2–3 g/d), or mitotane (2–3 mg/d) may relieve manifestations of cortisol excess. Patients with unresectable pituitary adenomas who have bilateral adrenalectomy are at risk for Nelson's syndrome (pituitary adenoma enlargement).

Aldosteronism

Etiology Aldosteronism is caused by hypersecretion of the adrenal mineralocorticoid aldosterone. *Primary aldosteronism* refers to an adrenal cause and can be due to either an adrenal adenoma or bilateral adrenal hyperplasia. The term *secondary aldosteronism* is used when an extraadrenal stimulus is present, as in renal artery stenosis or diuretic therapy.

Clinical Features Most pts with primary hyperaldosteronism have headaches and diastolic hypertension. Edema is characteristically absent, unless congestive heart failure or renal disease is present. Hypokalemia, caused by urinary potassium losses, may cause muscle weakness and fatigue, though potassium levels may be normal in mild primary aldosteronism. Hypernatremia and metabolic alkalosis may also occur.

Diagnosis The diagnosis is suggested by hypertension that is associated with persistent hypokalemia in a nonedematous pt who is not receiving potassium-wasting diuretics. In pts receiving potassium-wasting diuretics, the diuretic should be discontinued and potassium supplements should be administered for 1–2 weeks. If hypokalemia persists after supplementation, screening using a serum aldosterone and plasma renin activity should be performed. A ratio of serum aldosterone (in ng/dL) to plasma renin activity (in ng/mL per hour) >30 and an absolute level of aldosterone >15 ng/dL suggest primary aldosteronism. Failure to suppress plasma aldosterone (to <5 ng/dL after 500 mL/h of normal saline × 4 h) or urinary aldosterone after saline or sodium loading (to < 10 μg/d on day 3 of 200 mmol Na PO qd + fludrocortisone 0.2 mg bid × 3 days) confirms primary hyperaldosteronism. Localization should then be undertaken with a high-resolution CT scan of the adrenal glands. If the CT scan is negative, bilateral adrenal vein sampling may be required to diagnose a unilateral aldosterone-producing adenoma. Secondary hyperaldosteronism is associated with elevated plasma renin activity.

TREATMENT

Surgery can be curative in pts with adrenal adenoma but is not effective for adrenal hyperplasia, which is managed with sodium restriction and spironolactone (25–100 mg tid) or amiloride. Secondary aldosteronism is treated with salt restriction and correction of the underlying cause.

Syndromes of Adrenal Androgen Excess

See Chap. 178 for discussion of hirsutism and virilization.

HYPOFUNCTION OF THE ADRENAL GLAND

Primary adrenal insufficiency is due to failure of the adrenal gland, whereas *secondary adrenal insufficiency* is due to failure of ACTH production or release.

Addison's Disease

Etiology Addison's disease occurs when >90% of adrenal tissue is destroyed surgically, by granulomatous disease (tuberculosis, histoplasmosis, coccidioidomycosis, cryptococcosis), or via autoimmune mechanisms (alone, or in type I or type II polyglandular autoimmune syndromes). Bilateral tumor metastases, bilateral hemorrhage, CMV, HIV, amyloidosis, sarcoidosis, and adrenoleukodystrophy are rare causes.

Clinical Features Manifestations include fatigue, weakness, anorexia, nausea and vomiting, weight loss, abdominal pain, cutaneous and mucosal pigmentation, salt craving, hypotension, and, occasionally, hypoglycemia. Routine laboratory parameters may be normal, or serum Na can be reduced and serum K increased. Extracellular fluid depletion accentuates hypotension.

Diagnosis The best screening test is the cortisol response 60 min after 250 μg ACTH (cosyntropin) IV or IM. Cortisol levels should exceed 18 μg/dL 30–60 min after the ACTH. If the response is abnormal, then primary and secondary deficiency may be distinguished by measurement of aldosterone from the same blood samples. In secondary, but not primary, adrenal insufficiency, the aldosterone increment from baseline will be normal ($\geq$5 ng/dL). Furthermore, in primary adrenal insufficiency, plasma ACTH is elevated, whereas in secondary adrenal insufficiency, plasma ACTH values are low or inappropriately normal. Pts with recent onset or partial pituitary insufficiency may have a normal response to the rapid ACTH stimulation test. In these pts, alternative testing (metyrapone test, insulin tolerance testing, or the 1-μg ACTH test) may be used for diagnosis.

℞ TREATMENT

Hydrocortisone, at 20–30 mg/d divided into 2/3 in the morning and 1/3 in the afternoon, is the mainstay of glucocorticoid replacement. Some pts benefit from doses administered three times daily, and other glucocorticoids may be given at equivalent doses. Mineralocorticoid supplementation is usually needed for primary adrenal insufficiency, with administration of 0.05–0.1 mg fludrocortisone PO qd and maintenance of adequate Na intake. Doses should be titrated to normalize Na and K levels and to maintain normal bp without postural changes. Measurement of plasma renin levels may also be useful in titrating the dose. All pts with adrenal insufficiency should be instructed in the parenteral self-administration of steroids and should be registered with a medical alert system. During periods of intercurrent illness, the dose of hydrocortisone should be doubled. During adrenal crisis, high-dose hydrocortisone (10 mg/h continuous IV or 100 mg bolus IV TID) should be administered along with normal saline.

Hypoaldosteronism

Isolated aldosterone deficiency accompanied by normal cortisol production occurs with hyporeninism, as an inherited biosynthetic defect, postoperatively following removal of aldosterone-secreting adenomas, and during protracted heparin therapy. Hyporeninemic hypoaldosteronism is seen most commonly in adults with mild renal failure and diabetes mellitus in association with disproportionate hyperkalemia. Oral fludrocortisone (0.05–0.15 mg PO qd) restores electrolyte balance if salt intake is adequate. In pts with hypertension, mild renal insufficiency, or congestive heart failure, an alternative approach is to reduce salt intake and to administer furosemide.

INCIDENTAL ADRENAL MASSES

Adrenal masses are common findings on abdominal CT or MRI scans. More than 90% of such "incidentalomas" are nonfunctional, and the probability of an adrenal carcinoma is low (<0.01%). The first step in evaluation is to determine the functional status by measuring 24-h urinary catecholamines and metabolites, obtaining a serum potassium, and performing an overnight dexamethasone-suppression test. Surgery should be considered for nonfunctional masses >4 cm and for all functional masses. If surgery is not performed, a follow-up CT scan should be obtained in 3–6 months. In a pt with a known extraadrenal malignancy, there is a 30–50% chance that the incidentaloma is a metastasis.

CLINICAL USES OF GLUCOCORTICOIDS

Glucocorticoids are pharmacologic agents used for a variety of disorders such as asthma, rheumatoid arthritis, and psoriasis. The almost certain development of complications (weight gain, hypertension, Cushingoid facies, diabetes mellitus, osteoporosis, myopathy, increased intraocular pressure, ischemic bone necrosis, infection, and hypercholesterolemia) must be weighed against the potential therapeutic benefits of glucocorticoid therapy. These side effects can be minimized by a careful choice of steroid preparations (Table 174-1), alternate-day or interrupted therapy; the use of topical steroids, i.e., inhaled, intranasal, or dermal whenever possible; the judicious use of non-steroid therapies; monitoring of caloric intake; and instituting measures to minimize bone loss. Pts should be evaluated for the risk of complications before the initiation of glucocorticoid therapy (Table 174-2). Higher doses of glucocorticoids may be re-

Table 174-1

Glucocorticoid Preparations

Generic Name	Relative Potency		Dose equivalent
	Glucocorticoid	Mineralocorticoid	
Short-acting			
Hydrocortisone	1.0	1.0	20.0
Cortisone	0.8	0.8	25.0
Intermediate-acting			
Prednisone	4.0	0.25	5.0
Methylprednisolone	5.0	0	4.0
Triamcinolone	5.0	0	4.0
Long-acting			
Dexamethasone	25.0	0	0.75
Betamethasone	25.0	0	0.6

Table 174-2

A Checklist for Use Prior to the Administration of Glucocorticoids in Pharmacologic Doses
Presence of tuberculosis or other chronic infection (chest x-ray, tuberculin test)
Evidence of glucose intolerance or history of gestational diabetes mellitus
Evidence of preexisting osteoporosis (bone density assessment in organ transplant recipients or postmenopausal patients)
History of peptic ulcer, gastritis, or esophagitis (stool guaiac test)
Evidence of hypertension or cardiovascular disease
History of psychological disorders

quired during periods of stress, since the adrenal gland may atrophy in the setting of exogenous glucocorticoids. In addition, following long-term use, glucocorticoids should be tapered with the dual goals of allowing the pituitary-adrenal axis to recover and the avoidance of underlying disease flare.

For a more detailed discussion, see Williams GH, Dluhy RG: Disorders of the Adrenal Cortex, Chap. 321, p. 2127, in HPIM-16.

175

OBESITY

Obesity is a state of excess adipose tissue mass. Obesity should not be defined by body weight alone, as muscular individuals may be overweight by arbitrary standards without having increased adiposity. The most widely used method to gauge obesity is the *body mass index* (BMI), which is equal to weight/height^2 in kg/m^2. At a similar BMI, women have more body fat than men. A BMI between 19 and 25 kg/m^2 is considered an appropriate weight for most individuals. Overweight is defined as a BMI between 25 and 30 kg/m^2, and obesity is defined as a BMI > 30 kg/m^2. Furthermore, regional fat distribution may influence the risks associated with obesity. Central obesity (high ratio of the circumference of the waist to the circumference of the hips, >0.9 in women and 1.0 in men) is associated with high triglyceride levels, low HDL cholesterol levels, and insulin resistance.

Etiology

Obesity can result from increased energy intake, decreased energy expenditure, or a combination of the two. Excess accumulation of body fat is the consequence of environmental and genetic factors; social factors and economic conditions also represent important influences. The susceptibility to obesity is polygenic in nature, and 30–50% of the variability in total fat stores is believed to be genetically determined. Monogenic causes of obesity are rare; heterozygous

Table 175-1

Drugs That Enhance Appetite and Predispose to Obesity

Phenothiazines (chlorpromazine > thioridazine ≥ trifluoperazine > mesoridazine > promazine ≥ mepazine ≥ perphenazine ≥ prochlorperazine > haloperidol ≥ loxapine)

Antidepressants (amitriptyline > imipramine = doxepine = phenelzine ≥
amoxapine = desipramine = trazodone = tranylcypromine)

Antiepileptics (valproate; carbamazepine)

Steroids (glucocorticoids; megestrol acetate)

Antihypertensives (terazosin)

Source: Bray GA: HPIM-14, p. 457.

mutations of the melanocortin receptor 4 (MC4R) are found in a few percent
of massively obese children. Secondary causes of obesity include hypothalamic
injury, hypothyroidism, Cushing's syndrome, hypogonadism, and certain drugs
(Table 175-1). Insulin-secreting tumors can cause overeating.

Clinical Features

Obesity has major adverse effects on health. Increased mortality from obesity
is primarily due to cardiovascular disease, hypertension, gall bladder disease,
diabetes mellitus, and certain forms of cancer. The incidence of endometrial
cancer and postmenopausal breast cancer, prostate cancer, and colorectal cancer
in both men and women is increased with obesity. Sleep apnea in severely obese
individuals poses serious health risks. Obesity is also associated with an increased incidence of osteoarthritis.

℞ TREATMENT

Obesity is a chronic medical condition that requires ongoing treatment and
life-style modifications. Treatment is important because of the associated
health risks but is made difficult by a limited repertoire of effective therapeutic
options. Weight regain after weight loss is common with all forms of nonsurgical therapy. The urgency and selection of treatment modalities should be
based on the BMI and a risk assessment.

    Low to Moderate Risk Behavior modification including group coun-
seling, diet diaries, and changes in eating patterns should be initiated. Food-
related behaviors should be monitored carefully (avoid cafeteria-style settings,
eat small and frequent meals, eat breakfast). A deficit of 7500 kcal will produce a weight loss of approximately 1 kg. Therefore, eating 100 kcal/d less
for a year should cause a 5-kg weight loss, and a deficit of 1000 kcal/d should
cause a loss of ~1 kg per week. Physical activity should be increased. Exercise increases energy expenditure and helps to maintain weight loss.

    High Risk Appetite-suppressing drugs such as fenfluramine and phen-
termine may result in greater weight loss than behavior modification alone;
unfortunately, these drugs are associated with development of pulmonary hypertension and valvular heart disease and are no longer FDA approved in
combination. Sibutramine is a central reuptake inhibitor of both norepinephrine and serotonin with efficacy in short-term trials, though it increases pulse
and bp in some pts. Orlistat is an inhibitor of intestinal lipase that causes
modest weight loss due to drug-induced fat malabsorption. Surgery is also an
option for those with BMI > 35 with an associated comorbidity or BMI >
40, repeated failures of other therapeutic approaches, at eligible weight for
>3 years, capable of tolerating surgery, without addictions or major psycho-

pathology. Weight regain and other medical problems are minimal with either a Roux-en-Y gastric bypass procedure or vertically banded gastroplasty (Fig. 64-8, p. 429, in HPIM-16).

For a more detailed discussion, see Flier JS, Maratos-Flier E: Obesity, Chap. 64, p. 422, in HPIM-16.

176

DIABETES MELLITUS

ETIOLOGY   Diabetes mellitus (DM) comprises a group of metabolic disorders that share the common phenotype of hyperglycemia. DM is currently classified on the basis of the pathogenic process that leads to hyperglycemia. Under this classification, the terms *type 1 DM* and *type 2 DM* have replaced insulin-dependent diabetes mellitus (IDDM) and non-insulin-dependent diabetes mellitus (NIDDM), respectively. Type 1 DM is characterized by insulin deficiency and a tendency to develop ketosis, whereas type 2 DM is a heterogeneous group of disorders characterized by variable degrees of insulin resistance, impaired insulin secretion, and excessive hepatic glucose production. Other specific types include DM caused by genetic defects [maturity-onset diabetes of the young (MODY)], diseases of the exocrine pancreas (chronic pancreatitis, cystic fibrosis, hemochromatosis), endocrinopathies (acromegaly, Cushing's syndrome, glucagonoma, pheochromocytoma, hyperthyroidism), drugs (nicotinic acid, glucocorticoids, thiazides, protease inhibitors), and pregnancy (gestational diabetes mellitus).

DIAGNOSIS   Criteria for the diagnosis of DM include one of the following:

* Fasting plasma glucose $\geq$ 7.0 mmol/L ($\geq$126 mg/dL)
* Symptoms of diabetes plus a random blood glucose concentration $\geq$ 11.1 mmol/L ($\geq$ 200 mg/dL)
* 2-h plasma glucose $\geq$ 11.1 mmol/L ($\geq$ 200 mg/dL) during a 75-g oral glucose tolerance test.

These criteria should be confirmed by repeat testing on a different day, unless unequivocal hyperglycemia with acute metabolic decompensation is present.

Two intermediate categories have also been designated:

* Impaired fasting glucose (IFG) for a fasting plasma glucose between 6.1 and 7.0 mmol/L (110 and 126 mg/dL)
* Impaired glucose tolerance (IGT) for plasma glucose levels between 7.8 and 11.1 mmol/L (140 and 200 mg/dL) 2 h after a 75-g oral glucose load

Individuals with IFG or IGT do not have DM but are at substantial risk for developing type 2 DM and cardiovascular disease in the future. The hemoglobin A_{1c} (HbA_{1c}) level is useful for monitoring responses to therapy but is not recommended for screening or diagnosis of DM.

Table 176-1

Risk Factors for Type 2 Diabetes Mellitus

- Family history of diabetes (i.e., parent or sibling with type 2 diabetes)
- Obesity (BMI ≥ 25 kg/m²)
- Habitual physical inactivity
- Race/ethnicity (e.g., African American, Hispanic American, Native American, Asian American, Pacific Islander)
- Previously identified IFG or IGT
- History of GDM or delivery of baby >4 kg (>9 lb)
- Hypertension (blood pressure ≥ 140/90 mmHg)
- HDL cholesterol level ≤ 35 mg/dL (0.90 mmol/L) and/or a triglyceride level ≥250 mg/dL (2.82 mmol/L)
- Polycystic ovary syndrome or acanthosis nigricans
- History of vascular disease

Note: BMI, body mass index; IFG, impaired fasting glucose; IGT, impaired glucose tolerance; GDM, gestational diabetes mellitus; HDL, high-density lipoprotein.
Source: Adapted from American Diabetes Association, 2004.

Screening with a fasting plasma glucose level is recommended every 3 years for individuals over the age of 45, as well as for younger individuals with additional risk factors (Table 176-1).

The *metabolic syndrome*, the *insulin resistance syndrome*, and *syndrome X* are terms used to describe a commonly found constellation of metabolic derangements that includes insulin resistance (with or without diabetes), hypertension, dyslipidemia, central or visceral obesity, and endothelial dysfunction and is associated with accelerated cardiovascular disease.

CLINICAL FEATURES   Common presenting symptoms of DM include polyuria, polydipsia, weight loss, fatigue, weakness, blurred vision, frequent superficial infections, and poor wound healing. A complete medical history should be obtained with special emphasis on weight, exercise, ethanol use, family history of DM, and risk factors for cardiovascular disease. In a patient with established DM, assessment of prior diabetes care, HbA$_{1c}$ levels, self-monitoring blood glucose results, frequency of hypoglycemia, and pt's knowledge about DM should be obtained. Special attention should be given on physical exam to retinal exam, orthostatic bp, foot exam (including vibratory sensation and monofilament testing), peripheral pulses, and insulin injection sites. Acute complications of diabetes that may be seen on presentation include diabetic ketoacidosis (DKA) and hyperglycemic hyperosmolar state (Chap. 24).

The chronic complications of DM are listed below:

- Ophthalmologic: nonproliferative or proliferative diabetic retinopathy, macular edema
- Renal: proteinuria, end-stage renal disease (ESRD), type IV renal tubular acidosis
- Neurologic: distal symmetric polyneuropathy, polyradiculopathy, mononeuropathy, autonomic neuropathy
- Gastrointestinal: gastroparesis, diarrhea, constipation
- Genitourinary: cystopathy, erectile dysfunction, female sexual dysfunction
- Cardiovascular: coronary artery disease, congestive heart failure, peripheral vascular disease, stroke
- Lower extremity: foot deformity (hammer toe, claw toe, Charcot foot), ulceration, amputation

℞ TREATMENT

Optimal treatment of diabetes requires more than plasma glucose management. Comprehensive diabetes care should also detect and manage DM-specific complications and modify risk factors for DM-associated diseases. The pt with type 1 or type 2 DM should receive education about nutrition, exercise, care of diabetes during illness, and medications to lower the plasma glucose. In general, the target HbA_{1c} level should be <7.0%, though individual considerations (age, ability to implement a complex treatment regimen, and presence of other medical conditions) should also be taken into account. Intensive therapy reduces long-term complications but is associated with more frequent and more severe hypoglycemic episodes.

In general, pts with type 1 DM require 0.5–1.0 U/kg per day of insulin divided into multiple doses. Combinations of insulin preparations with different times of onset and duration of action should be used (Table 176-2). Commonly used regimens include twice-daily injections of an intermediate insulin combined with a short-acting insulin before the morning and evening meal, injection of glargine at bedtime and preprandial lispro or insulin aspart, and continuous subcutaneous insulin using an infusion device.

Pts with type 2 DM may be managed with diet and exercise alone or in conjunction with oral glucose-lowering agents, insulin, or a combination of oral agents and insulin. The classes of oral glucose-lowering agents and dosing regimens are listed in Table 176-3. A reasonable treatment algorithm for initial therapy proposes either a sulfonlyurea or metformin as initial therapy because of their efficacy (1–2% decrease in HbA_{1c}), known side-effect profile, and relatively low cost (Fig. 176-1). Metformin has the advantage that it

Table 176-2

Pharmacokinetics of Insulin Preparations

Preparation	Time of Action		
	Onset, h	Peak, h	Effective Duration, h
Short-acting			
Lispro	<0.25	0.5–1.5	3–4
Insulin aspart	<0.2–0.3	0.67–0.83	1–3
Regular	0.5–1.0	2–3	3–6
Intermediate-acting			
NPH	2–4	6–10	10–16
Lente	3–4	6–12	12–18
Long-acting			
Ultralente	6–10	10–16	18–20
Glargine	4	—[a]	24
Combinations			
75/25–75% protamine lispro, 25% lispro	0.5–1	Dual	10–14
70/30–70% aspart protamine, 30% aspart	<0.2–0.3	2.4	1–4
70/30–70% NPH, 30% regular	0.5–1	Dual	10–16

[a] Glargine has minimal peak activity.

Source: Adapted from JS Skyler, *Therapy for Diabetes Mellitus and Related Disorders*, American Diabetes Association, Alexandria, VA, 1998.

Table 176-3

Oral Glucose-Lowering Agents

Agent	Daily Dose, mg	Doses/d	Contraindications
Sulfonylureas			Renal/liver disease
Glimepiride	1–8	1	
Glipizide	2.5–40	1–2	
Glipizide (ext. release)	5–10	1	
Glyburide	1.25–20	1–2	
Glyburide (micronized)	0.75–12	1–2	
Meglitinide			Liver disease
Repaglinide	0.5–16	1–4	
Netaglenide	180–360	1–3	
Biguanide			Cr>133 μmol/L (1.5 mg/dL) (men); >124 μmol/L (1.4 mg/dL) (women); liver disease
Metformin	500–2500	1–3	
α-Glucosidase inhibitor			IBD, liver disease, or Cr> 177 μmol/L (2.0 mg/dL)
Acarbose	25–300	1–3	
Miglitol	25–300	1–3	
Thiazolidinedione			Liver disease, CHF
Rosiglitazone	2–8	1–2	
Pioglitazone	15–45	1	

promotes mild weight loss, lowers insulin levels, improves the lipid profile slightly, and does not cause hypoglycemia when used as monotherapy, though it is contraindicated in renal insufficiency, congestive heart failure, any form of acidosis, liver disease, or severe hypoxia, and should be temporarily discontinued in pts who are seriously ill or receiving radiographic contrast material. Combinations of two oral agents may be used with additive effects, with stepwise addition of bedtime insulin or a third oral agent if adequate control is not achieved. As endogenous insulin production falls, multiple injections of intermediate-acting and short-acting insulin may be required, as in type 1 DM. Individuals who require >1 U/kg per day of intermediate-acting insulin should be considered for combination therapy with an insulin-sensitizing agent such as metformin or a thiazolidinedione.

The morbidity and mortality of DM-related complications can be greatly reduced by timely and consistent surveillance procedures (Table 176-4). A routine urinalysis may be performed as an initial screen for diabetic nephropathy. If it is positive for protein, quantification of protein on a 24-h urine collection should be performed. If the urinalysis is negative for protein, a spot collection for microalbuminuria should be performed (present if 30–300 μg/mg creatinine on two of three tests within a 3- to 6-month period). A resting ECG should be performed in adults, with more extensive cardiac testing for high-risk pts. Therapeutic goals to prevent complications of DM include management of proteinuria with ACE inhibitor therapy, bp control (<130/80 mmHg if no proteinuria, <125/75 if proteinuria), and dyslipidemia management [LDL <2.6 mmol/L (<100 mg/dL) HDL >1.1 mmol/L (>40 mg/dL) in men and >1.38 mmol/L (50 mg/dL) in women, triglycerides <1.7 mmol/L (<150 mg/dL)].

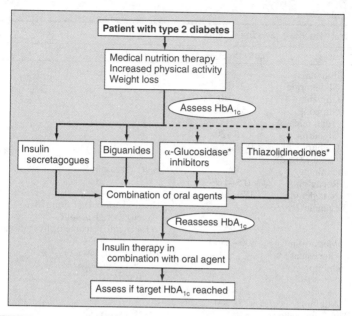

FIGURE 176-1 Glycemic management of type 2 diabetes. See text for discussion. *See text about use as monotherapy. The broken line indicates that biguanides or insulin secretagogues, but not α-glucosidase inhibitors or thiazolidinediones, are preferred for initial therapy.

Management of the Hospitalized Patient The goals of diabetes management during hospitalization are avoidance of hypoglycemia, optimization of glycemic control [5.6–9.8 mmol/L (100–175 mg/dL)], and transition back to the outpatient diabetes treatment regimen. Pts with type 1 DM undergoing general anesthesia and surgery, or with serious illness, should receive continuous insulin, either through an IV insulin infusion or by SC administration of a reduced dose of a long-acting insulin. Short-acting insulin alone is insufficient to prevent the onset of diabetic ketoacidosis. Oral hypoglycemic agents should be discontinued in pts with type 2 DM at the time of hospitalization. Either regular insulin infusion (0.05–0.15 U/kg per hour) or a reduced dose (by 30–50%) of long- or intermediate-acting insulin and short-acting

Table 176-4

Guidelines for Ongoing Medical Care for Patients with Diabetes

- Self-monitoring of blood glucose (individualized frequency)
- HbA$_{1c}$ testing (2–4 times/year)
- Patient education in diabetes management (annual)
- Medical nutrition therapy and education (annual)
- Eye examination (annual)
- Foot examination (1–2 times/year by physician; daily by patient)
- Screening for diabetic nephropathy (annual urine microalbumin)
- Blood pressure measurement (quarterly)
- Lipid profile (annual)
- Influenza/pneumococcal immunizations
- Consider aspirin therapy

insulin (held, or reduced by 30–50%), with infusion of a solution of 5% dextrose, should be administered when pts are NPO for a procedure. A regimen of intermediate- and short-acting SC insulin should be be used in type 2 pts who are eating. Those with DM undergoing radiographic procedures with contrast dye should be well hydrated before and after dye exposure, and the serum creatinine should be monitored after the procedure.

For a more detailed discussion, see Powers AC: Diabetes Mellitus, Chap. 323, p. 2152, in HPIM-16.

177

DISORDERS OF THE MALE REPRODUCTIVE SYSTEM

The testes produce sperm and testosterone. Inadequate production of sperm can occur in isolation or in the presence of androgen deficiency, which impairs spermatogenesis secondarily.

ANDROGEN DEFICIENCY

ETIOLOGY Androgen deficiency can be due to either testicular failure (*primary hypogonadism*) or hypothalamic-pituitary defects (*secondary hypogonadism*).

Primary hypogonadism is diagnosed when testosterone levels are low and gonadotropin levels [luteinizing hormone (LH) and follicle-stimulating hormone (FSH)] are high. Klinefelter's syndrome is the most common cause and is due to the presence of one or more extra X chromosomes, usually a 47, XXY karyotype. Acquired primary testicular failure usually results from viral orchitis but may be due to trauma, cryptorchidism, radiation damage, or systemic diseases such as amyloidosis, Hodgkin's disease, sickle cell disease, or granulomatous diseases. Testicular failure can occur as a part of a polyglandular autoimmune failure syndrome in which multiple primary endocrine deficiencies coexist. Malnutrition, AIDS, renal failure, liver disease, myotonic dystrophy, paraplegia, and toxins such as alcohol, marijuana, heroin, methadone, lead, and antineoplastic and chemotherapeutic agents can also cause testicular failure. Testosterone synthesis may be blocked by ketoconazole, and testosterone action may be diminished by competition at the androgen receptor by spironolactone and cimetidine.

Secondary hypogonadism is diagnosed when levels of both testosterone and gonadotropins are low (*hypogonadotropic hypogonadism*). Kallmann's syndrome is due to impairment of the synthesis and/or release of gonadotropin-releasing hormone (GnRH) and is characterized by low levels of LH and FSH, and anosmia. Other individuals present with idiopathic congenital GnRH deficiency without anosmia. Critical illness, Cushing's syndrome, adrenal hypoplasia congenita, hemochromatosis, and hyperprolactinemia (due to pituitary adenomas or drugs such as phenothiazines) are other causes of isolated hypogonadotropic hypogonadism. Destruction of the pituitary gland by tumors, infection, trauma, or metastatic disease causes hypogonadism in conjunction with disturbances in the production of other pituitary hormones (see Chap. 171).

CLINICAL FEATURES The history should focus on developmental stages such as puberty and growth spurts, as well as androgen-dependent events such as early morning erections, frequency and intensity of sexual thoughts, and frequency of masturbation or intercourse. The physical examination should focus on secondary sex characteristics such as hair growth in the face, axilla, chest, and pubic regions; gynecomastia; testicular volume; prostate; and height and body proportions. Eunuchoidal proportions are defined as an arm span >2 cm greater than height and suggest that androgen deficiency occurred prior to epiphyseal fusion. Normal testicular size ranges from 3.5–5.5 cm in length, which corresponds to a volume of 12–25 mL. The presence of varicocele should be sought by palpation of the testicular veins with the patient standing. Patients with Klinefelter syndrome have small (1–2 mL), firm testes.

A morning total testosterone level <6.93 nmol/L (<200 ng/dL), in association with symptoms, suggests testosterone deficiency. A level of >12.13 nmol/L (>350 ng/dL) makes the diagnosis of androgen deficiency unlikely. In men with testosterone levels between 6.93 and 12.13 nmol/L (200 and 350 ng/dL), the total testosterone level should be repeated and a free testosterone level should be measured. In older men and in patients with other clinical states that are associated with alterations in sex hormone binding globulin levels, a direct measurement of free testosterone by equilibrium dialysis can be useful in unmasking testosterone deficiency. Levels of LH and FSH can be used to differentiate between primary and secondary hypogonadism. In men with primary hypogonadism of unknown cause, a karyotype should be performed to exclude Klinefelter syndrome. Measurement of a prolactin level and MRI scan of the hypothalamic-pituitary region should be considered in men with secondary hypogonadism.

 TREATMENT

Treatment of hypogonadal men with androgens restores normal male secondary sexual characteristics (beard, body hair, external genitalia), male sexual drive, and masculine somatic development (hemoglobin, muscle mass). Administration of gradually increasing doses of testosterone is recommended for disorders in which hypogonadism occurred prior to puberty. Testosterone levels in the normal range may be achieved through daily application of transdermal testosterone patches (5–10 mg/d) or gel (50–100 mg/d) or parenteral administration of a long-acting testosterone ester (100–200 mg testosterone enanthate at 1- to 3-week intervals). Prostate cancer, severe symptoms of lower urinary tract obstruction, baseline hematocrit > 52%, severe sleep apnea, and class IV congestive heart failure are contraindications for androgen replacement.

MALE INFERTILITY

ETIOLOGY Male infertility plays a role in one-third of infertile couples (couples who fail to conceive after 1 year of unprotected intercourse). Known causes of male infertility include primary hypogonadism (30–40%), disorders of sperm transport (10–20%), and secondary hypogonadism (2%), with an unknown etiology in up to half of men with suspected male factor infertility (see Fig. 178-3). Impaired spermatogenesis occurs with testosterone deficiency but may also be present without testosterone deficiency. Y chromosome microdeletions and substitutions, viral orchitis, tuberculosis, STDs, radiation, chemotherapeutic agents, and environmental toxins have all been associated with isolated impaired spermatogenesis. Prolonged elevations of testicular temperature, as in varicocele, cryptorchidism, or after an acute febrile illness, may impair spermatogenesis. Ejaculatory obstruction can be a congenital (cystic fibrosis, in utero diethylstilbesterol exposure, or idiopathic) or acquired (vasectomy, accidental ligation of the vas deferens, or obstruction of the epididymis) etiology of male infertility. Androgen abuse by male athletes can lead to testicular atrophy and a low sperm count.

CLINICAL FEATURES   Evidence of hypogonadism may be present. Testicular size and consistency may be abnormal, and a varicocele may be apparent on palpation. When the seminiferous tubules are damaged prior to puberty, the testes are small (usually <12 mL) and firm, whereas postpubertal damage causes the testes to be soft (the capsule, once enlarged, does not contract to its previous size). The key diagnostic test is a *semen analysis.* Sperm counts of <13 million/mL, motility of <32%, and <9% normal morphology are associated with subfertility. Testosterone levels should be measured if the sperm count is low on repeated exam or if there is clinical evidence of hypogonadism.

 TREATMENT

Men with primary hypogonadism occasionally respond to androgen therapy if there is minimal damage to the seminiferous tubules, whereas those with secondary hypogonadism require gonadotropin therapy to achieve fertility. Fertility occurs in about half of men with varicocele who undergo surgical repair. In vitro fertilization is an option for men with mild to moderate defects in sperm quality; intracytoplasmic sperm injection (ICSI) has been a major advance for men with severe defects in sperm quality.

ERECTILE DYSFUNCTION

ETIOLOGY   Erectile dysfunction (ED) is the failure to achieve erection, ejaculation, or both. It affects 10–25% of middle-aged and elderly men. ED may result from three basic mechanisms: (1) failure to initiate (psychogenic, endocrinologic, or neurogenic); (2) failure to fill (arteriogenic); or (3) failure to store adequate blood volume within the lacunar network (venoocclusive dysfunction). Diabetic, atherosclerotic, and drug-related causes account for >80% of cases of ED in older men. Among the antihypertensive agents, the thiazide diuretics and beta blockers have been implicated most frequently. Estrogens, GnRH agonists, H_2 antagonists, and spironolactactone suppress gonadotropin production or block androgen action. Antidepressant and antipsychotic agents— particularly neuroleptics, tricyclics, and selective serotonin reuptake inhibitors—are associated with erectile, ejaculatory, orgasmic, and sexual desire difficulties. Recreational drugs, including ethanol, cocaine, and marijuana, may also cause ED. Any disorder that affects the sacral spinal cord or the autonomic fibers to the penis may lead to ED.

CLINICAL FEATURES   Men with sexual dysfunction may complain of loss of libido, inability to initiate or maintain an erection, ejaculatory failure, premature ejaculation, or inability to achieve orgasm. Initial questions should focus on the onset of symptoms, the presence and duration of partial erections, and the progression of ED. A history of nocturnal or early morning erections is useful for distinguishing physiologic from psychogenic ED. Relevant risk factors should be identified, such as diabetes mellitus, coronary artery disease, lipid disorders, hypertension, peripheral vascular disease, smoking, alcoholism, and endocrine or neurologic disorders. The patient's surgical history should be explored, with an emphasis on bowel, bladder, prostate, or vascular procedures.

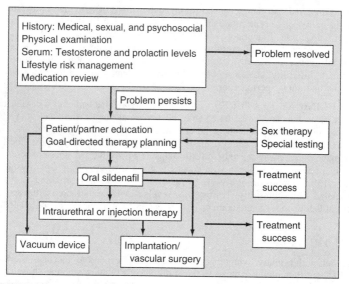

FIGURE 177-1 Algorithm for the evaluation and management of patients with ED.

Evaluation includes a detailed general as well as genital physical exam. Penile abnormalities (Peyronie's disease), testicular size, and gynecomastia should be noted. Peripheral pulses should be palpated, and bruits should be sought. Neurologic exam should assess anal sphincter tone, perineal sensation, and bulbocavernosus reflex. Serum testosterone and prolactin should be measured. Penile arteriography, electromyography, or penile Doppler ultrasound is occasionally performed.

℞ TREATMENT

An approach to the evaluation and treatment of ED is summarized in Fig. 177-1. Correction of the underlying disorders or discontinuation of responsible medications should be attempted. Oral sildenafil or related drugs enhances erections after sexual stimulation, with an onset of approximately 60–90 min. They are contraindicated in men receiving any form of nitrate therapy and should be avoided in those with congestive heart failure. Vacuum constriction devices or injection of alprostadil into the urethra or corpora cavernosa may also be effective. The insertion of penile prosthesis is rarely indicated.

For a more detailed discussion, see Bhasin S, Jameson JL: Disorders of the Testes and Male Reproductive System, Chap. 325, p. 2185; Hall JE: Infertility and Fertility Control, Chap. 45, p. 279; McVary KT: Sexual Dysfunction, Chap. 43, p. 271, in HPIM- 16.

178

DISORDERS OF THE FEMALE REPRODUCTIVE SYSTEM

The pituitary hormones, luteinizing hormone (LH) and follicle-stimulating hormone (FSH), stimulate ovarian follicular development and result in ovulation at about day 14 of the 28-day menstrual cycle.

ABNORMAL UTERINE BLEEDING

ETIOLOGY   During the reproductive years, the menstrual cycle averages 28 ± 3 days, and the mean duration of blood flow is 4 ± 2 days. A variety of descriptive terms (such as *menorrhagia, metrorrhagia*, and *menometrorrhagia*) have been used to characterize patterns of abnormal uterine bleeding, which may be associated with ovulatory cycles or with anovulatory cycles. In the premenarchal period, abnormal uterine bleeding may result from trauma, infection, or precocious puberty. In premenopausal women, abnormal uterine bleeding may also be caused by ectopic pregnancy or threatened abortion. Vaginal bleeding after menopause is frequently due to malignancy.

Menstrual bleeding associated with normal, ovulatory cycles is spontaneous, regular in onset, predictable in duration and amount of flow, and frequently associated with discomfort (*dysmenorrhea*). Deviations from the established pattern of menstrual flow can result from bleeding dyscrasias, abnormalities of the outflow tract (uterine synechiae or scarring), leiomyomas, adenomyosis, or endometrial polyps. Bleeding between cyclic ovulatory menses can be due to cervical or endometrial lesions.

Anovulatory menstrual bleeding (dysfunctional uterine bleeding) is painless, irregular in occurrence, and unpredictable in amount and duration. Transient disruption of ovulatory cycles occurs most often in the peripubertal years, during the perimenopausal period, or as the consequence of a variety of stresses and intercurrent illnesses. Persistent dysfunctional uterine bleeding in reproductive years is usually due to continuous estrogen effects on the uterus uninterrupted by cyclic fluctuations in progesterone associated with ovulation, and is most commonly due to polycystic ovarian syndrome (PCOS).

DIAGNOSIS   The approach to a pt with dysfunctional uterine bleeding begins with a careful history of menstrual patterns and prior hormonal therapy. Since not all urogenital tract bleeding is from the uterus, rectal, bladder, vaginal, and cervical sources must be excluded by physical exam. If the bleeding is from the uterus, a pregnancy-related disorder such as abortion or ectopic pregnancy must be ruled out.

 TREATMENT

During a first episode of dysfunctional bleeding the pt can be observed, provided the bleeding is not copious and there is no evidence of a bleeding dyscrasia. If bleeding is more severe, control can be achieved with relatively high-dose estrogen oral contraceptives for 3 weeks. Hospitalization, bed rest, and IM injections of estradiol valerate (10 mg) and hydroxyprogesterone caproate (500 mg) or IV or IM conjugated estrogens (25 mg) usually control severe bleeding. Uterine biopsy should be performed in women approaching the age of menopause, or those who are massively obese, to evaluate for endometrial cancer. After initial treatment, iron replacement should be instituted along with either cyclic oral contraceptives or medroxyprogesterone acetate 10 mg PO qd for 10 days every 2–3 months. Additional evaluation (endometrial biopsy, hysteroscopy, or dilatation and curettage) may be required for diagnosis and therapy.

AMENORRHEA

ETIOLOGY Pregnancy should be excluded in women of childbearing age with amenorrhea, even when history and physical exam are not suggestive.

Primary amenorrhea is defined as failure of menarche by age 15, regardless of the presence or absence of secondary sexual characteristics; *secondary amenorrhea* is failure of menstruation for 6 months in a woman with previous periodic menses. The causes of primary and secondary amenorrhea overlap, and it is generally more useful to classify the disorder according to the source of dysfunction: (1) anatomic defects, (2) ovarian failure, or (3) chronic anovulation with or without estrogen present (Fig. 178-1).

Anatomic defects of the outflow tract that prevent vaginal bleeding include absence of vagina or uterus, imperforate hymen, transverse vaginal septae, and cervical stenosis. Ovarian failure may be due to Turner's syndrome, pure gonadal dygenesis, premature ovarian failure, the resistant-ovary syndrome, and chemotherapy or radiation therapy for malignancy. The diagnosis of premature ovarian failure is applied to women who cease menstruating before age 40. Chronic anovulation with estrogen present is usually due to PCOS and is characterized by amenorrhea or oligomenorrhea, infertility, insulin resistance, and evidence of androgen excess (hirsutism, acne, male pattern balding). Features of PCOS are worsened by coexistent obesity. Additional disorders with a similar presentation include excess androgen production from adrenal or ovarian tumors, adult-onset congenital adrenal hyperplasia, and thyroid disorders. Women with chronic anovulation with absent estrogen usually have hypogonadotropic hypogonadism due to disease of either the hypothalamus or the pituitary. Hypothalamic causes include Kallmann's syndrome or Sheehan's syndrome, hypothalamic lesions (craniopharyngiomas and other tumors, tuberculosis, sarcoidosis, metastatic tumors), hypothalamic trauma or irradiation, rigorous exercise, eating disorders, stressful events, and chronic debilitating diseases (end-stage renal disease, malignancy, malabsorption). Disorders of the pituitary can lead to amenorrhea by two mechanisms: direct interference with gonadotropin secretion or inhibition of gonadotropin secretion via excess prolactin (Chap. 171).

DIAGNOSIS The initial evaluation involves careful physical exam, serum or urine human chorionic gonadotropin (hCG), serum prolactin assay, and evaluation of estrogen status (Fig. 178-1). To determine estrogen status, medroxyprogesterone acetate (10 mg PO qd-bid×5 days) or 100 mg of progesterone in oil IM should be administered. If estrogen levels are adequate and the outflow tract is intact, menstrual bleeding should occur within 1 week of ending progestin treatment. Ovarian failure is associated with a lack of withdrawal menses to progestin challenge and elevated plasma gonadotropin levels. Anatomic defects are usually diagnosed by physical exam and failure to induce menses, though hysterosalpingography or direct visual examination by hysteroscopy may be required. Chromosomal analysis should be performed when gonadal dysgenesis is suspected. The diagnosis of PCOS is based on the coexistence of chronic anovulation and androgen excess, after ruling out other etiologies for these features. The evaluation of hyperprolactinemia is described in Chap. 171. In the absence of a known etiology for hypogonadotropic hypogonadism, MRI of the pituitary-hypothalamic region should be performed when gonadotropins are low or inappropriately normal.

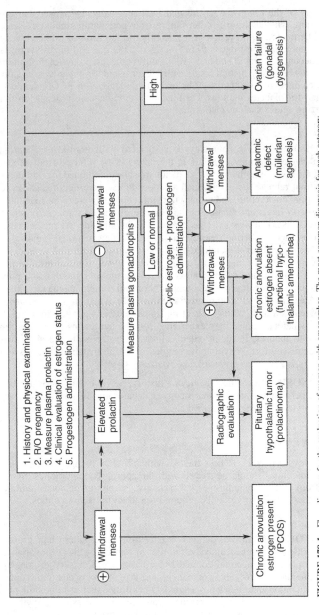

FIGURE 178-1 Flow diagram for the evaluation of women with amenorrhea. The most common diagnosis for each category is shown in parentheses. The dotted lines indicate that in some instances a correct diagnosis can be reached on the basis of history and physical exam alone. (*Reproduced from Carr BR, Bradshaw KD: HPIM-16, p. 2207.*)

TREATMENT

Disorders of the outflow tract are managed surgically. Decreased estrogen production, whether from ovarian failure or hypothalamic/pituitary disease, should be treated with cyclic estrogens, either in the form of oral contraceptives or conjugated estrogens (0.625–1.25 mg PO qd) and medroxyprogesterone acetate (2.5 mg PO qd or 5–10 mg during the last 5 days of the month). PCOS may be treated by oral contraceptive agents and weight reduction, along with treatment of hirsutism (see below). Individuals with PCOS should be screened for diabetes mellitus. Fertility may be enhanced by using insulin-sensitizing agents such as metformin.

PELVIC PAIN

ETIOLOGY Pelvic pain may be associated with normal or abnormal menstrual cycles and may originate in the pelvis or be referred from another region of the body. A high index of suspicion must be entertained for extrapelvic disorders that refer to the pelvis, such as appendicitis, diverticulitis, cholecystitis, intestinal obstruction, and urinary tract infections. Severe or incapacitating cramping with ovulatory menses in the absence of demonstrable disorders of the pelvis is termed *primary dysmenorrhea*. Pelvic pain due to organic causes may be classified as uterine (leiomyomas, adenomyosis, cervical stenosis, infections, cancer), adnexal (salpingo-oophoritis, cysts, neoplasms, torsion, endometriosis), vulvar or vaginal (*Monilia, Trichomonas, Gardnerella*, herpes, condyloma acuminatum, cysts or abscesses of Bartholin's glands), and pregnancy-associated (threatened or incomplete abortion, ectopic pregnancy). Many women experience lower abdominal discomfort with ovulation (*mittelschmerz*), characterized as a dull, aching pain at midcycle that lasts minutes to hours. In addition, ovulatory women may experience somatic symptoms during the few days prior to menses, including edema, breast engorgement, and abdominal bloating or discomfort. A symptom complex of cyclic irritability, depression, and lethargy is known as *premenstrual syndrome* (PMS).

DIAGNOSIS Evaluation includes a history, pelvic exam, hCG measurement, and pelvic ultrasound. Laparoscopy or laparotomy is indicated in some cases of pelvic pain of undetermined cause.

 TREATMENT

Primary dysmenorrhea is best treated with NSAIDs or oral contraceptive agents. Infections should be treated with the appropriate antibiotics. Symptoms from PMS may improve with selective serotonin reuptake inhibitor (SSRI) therapy. Surgery may be required for structural abnormalities.

HIRSUTISM

ETIOLOGY *Hirsutism*, defined as excessive male-pattern hair growth, affects ~10% of women. It may be familial or caused by PCOS, ovarian or adrenal neoplasms, congenital adrenal hyperplasia, Cushing's syndrome, hyperprolactinemia, acromegaly, pregnancy, and drugs (androgens, oral contraceptives containing androgenic progestins). Other drugs, such as minoxidil, phenytoin, diazoxide, and cyclosporine, can cause excessive growth of non-androgen-dependent vellus hair, leading to hypertrichosis.

CLINICAL FEATURES An objective clinical assessment of hair distribution and quantity is central to the evaluation. A commonly used method to grade hair growth is the Ferriman-Gallwey score (see Fig. 44-1, p. 276, in

HPIM-16). Associated manifestations of androgen excess include acne and male-pattern balding (androgenic alopecia). *Virilization*, on the other hand, refers to the state in which androgen levels are sufficiently high to cause deepening of the voice, breast atrophy, increased muscle bulk, clitoromegaly, and increased libido. Historic elements include menstrual history and the age of onset, rate of progression, and distribution of hair growth. Sudden development of hirsutism, rapid progression, and virilization suggest an ovarian or adrenal neoplasm.

DIAGNOSIS An approach to testing for androgen excess is depicted in Fig. 178-2. PCOS is a relatively common cause of hirsutism. The dexamethasone androgen-suppression test (0.5 mg PO q6h × 4 days, with free testosterone levels obtained before and after administration of dexamethasone) may distinguish ovarian from adrenal overproduction. Incomplete suppression suggests ovarian androgen excess. Congenital adrenal hyperplasia due to 21-hydroxylase deficiency can be excluded by a 17-hydroxyprogesterone level that is <6 nmol/L (<2 μg/L) either in the morning during the follicular phase or 1 h after administration of 250 μg of cosyntropin. CT may localize an adrenal mass, and ultrasound will identify an ovarian mass, if evaluation suggests these possibilities.

 TREATMENT

Nonpharmacologic treatments include (1) bleaching; (2) depilatory such as shaving and chemical treatments; and (3) epilatory such as plucking, waxing, electrolysis, and laser therapy. Pharmacologic therapy includes oral contraceptives with a low androgenic progestin and spironolactone (100–200 mg PO qd), often in combination. Glucocorticoids (dexamethasone, 0.25–0.5 mg qhs, or prednisone, 5–10 mg qhs) are the mainstay of treatment in pts with congenital adrenal hyperplasia. Attenuation of hair growth with pharmacologic therapy is typically not evident until 4–6 months after initiation of medical treatment and therefore should be used in conjunction with nonpharmacologic treatments.

MENOPAUSE

ETIOLOGY *Menopause* is defined as the final episode of menstrual bleeding and occurs at a median age of 50–51 years. It is the consequence of depletion of ovarian follicles or of oophorectomy. The onset of *perimenopause*, when fertility wanes and menstrual irregularity increases, precedes the final menses by 2–8 years.

CLINICAL FEATURES The most common menopausal symptoms are vasomotor instability (hot flashes and night sweats), mood changes (nervousness, anxiety, irritability, and depression), insomnia, and atrophy of the urogenital epithelium and skin. FSH levels are elevated to ≥40 IU/L.

 TREATMENT

During the perimenopause, low-dose combined oral contraceptives may be of benefit. The rational use of postmenopausal hormone therapy requires balancing the potential benefits and risks. Short-term therapy (<5 years) may be beneficial in controlling symptoms of menopause, as long as no contraindications exist. These include unexplained vaginal bleeding, active liver disease, venous thromboembolism, history of endometrial cancer (except stage I without deep invasion), or breast cancer. Hypertriglyceridemia (>400 mg/dL), active gallbladder disease, and preexisting coronary heart disease are relative

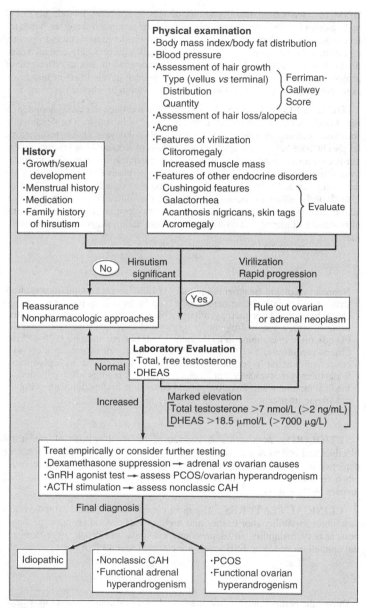

FIGURE 178-2 Algorithm for the evaluation and differential diagnosis of hirsutism. ACTH, adrenocorticotropic hormone; CAH, congenital adrenal hyperplasia; DHEAS, sulfated form of dehydroepiandrosterone; GnRH, gonadotropin-releasing hormone; PCOS, polycystic ovarian syndrome.

contraindications. Alternative therapies for symptoms include SSRIs, clonidine (0.1–0.2 mg/d), vitamin E (400–800 IU/d), or soy-based products. Long-term therapy (≥5 years) should be carefully considered, particularly in light of alternative therapies for osteoporosis (bisphosphonates, raloxifene) and of the risks of venous thromboembolism and breast cancer. Estrogens should be given in the minimal effective doses (conjugated estrogen, 0.625 mg PO qd; micronized estradiol, 1.0 mg PO qd; or transdermal estradiol, 0.05–1.0 mg once or twice a week). Women with an intact uterus should be given estrogen in combination with a progestin (medroxyprogesterone either cyclically, 5–10 mg PO qd for days 15–25 each month, or continuously, 2.5 mg PO qd) to avoid the increased risk of endometrial carcinoma seen with unopposed estrogen use.

CONTRACEPTION

The most widely used methods for fertility control include (1) rhythm and withdrawal techniques, (2) barrier methods, (3) intrauterine devices, (4) oral contraceptives, (5) long-acting progestins, (6) sterilization, and (7) abortion.

Oral contraceptive agents are widely used for both prevention of pregnancy and control of dysmenorrhea and anovulatory bleeding. Combination oral contraceptive agents contain synthetic estrogen (ethinyl estradiol or mestranol) and synthetic progestins. Low-dose norgestimate and third-generation progestins (desogestrel, gestodene, drosperinone) have a less androgenic profile; levonorgestrel appears to be the most androgenic of the progestins and should be avoided in pts with hyperandrogenic symptoms. The three major formulation types include fixed-dose estrogen-progestin, phasic estrogen-progestin, and progestin only.

Despite overall safety, oral contraceptive users are at risk for venous thromboembolism, hypertension, and cholelithiasis. Risks for myocardial infarction and stroke are increased with smoking and aging. Side effects, including breakthrough bleeding, amenorrhea, breast tenderness, and weight gain, are often responsive to a change in formulation.

Absolute contraindications to the use of oral contraceptives include previous thromboembolic disorders, cerebrovascular or coronary artery disease, carcinoma of the breasts or other estrogen-dependent neoplasia, liver disease, hypertriglyceridemia, heavy smoking with age over 35, undiagnosed genital bleeding, or known or suspected pregnancy. Relative contraindications include hypertension and anticonvulsant drug therapy.

New methods include a weekly contraceptive patch, a monthly contraceptive injection, and a monthly vaginal ring. Long term progestins may be administered in the form of Depo-Provera and Norplant.

Emergency contraceptive pills, containing progestin only or estrogen and progestin, can be used within 72 h of unprotected intercourse for prevention of pregnancy. Both Plan B and Preven are emergency contraceptive kits specifically designed for postcoital contraception. In addition, certain oral contraceptive pills may be dosed within 72 h for emergency contraception (Ovral, 2 tabs, 12 h apart; Lo/Ovral, 4 tabs, 12 h apart). Side effects include nausea, vomiting, and breast soreness.

INFERTILITY

ETIOLOGY   *Infertility* is defined as the inability to conceive after 12 months of unprotected sexual intercourse. The causes of infertility are outlined in Fig. 178-3. Male infertility is discussed in Chap. 177.

CLINICAL FEATURES   The initial evaluation includes discussion of the appropriate timing of intercourse, semen analysis in the male, confirmation of ovulation in the female, and, in the majority of situations, documentation of

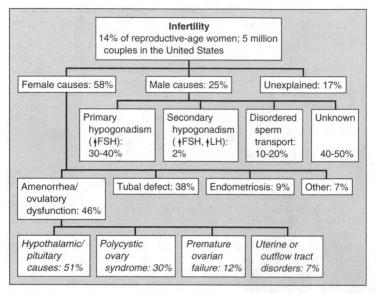

FIGURE 178-3   Causes of infertility, FSH, follicle-stimulating hormone; LH, luteinizing hormone.

tubal patency in the female. A history of regular, cyclic, predictable, spontaneous menses usually indicates ovulatory cycles, which may be confirmed by urinary ovulation predictor kits, basal body temperature graphs, or plasma progesterone measurements during the luteal phase of the cycle. An FSH level <10 IU/mL on day 3 of the cycle predicts adequate ovarian oocyte reserve. Tubal disease can be evaluated by obtaining a hysterosalpingogram or by diagnostic laparoscopy. Endometriosis may be suggested by history and exam but is often clinically silent and can only be excluded definitively by laparoscopy.

℞ TREATMENT

The treatment of infertility should be tailored to the problems unique to each couple. Treatment options include expectant management, clomiphene citrate with or without intrauterine insemination (IUI), gonadotropins with or without IUI, and in vitro fertilization (IVF). In specific situations, surgery, pulsatile GnRH therapy, intracytoplasmic sperm injection (ICSI), or assisted reproductive technologies with donor egg or sperm may be required.

For a more detailed discussion, see Ehrmann DA: Hirsutism and Virilization, Chap. 44, p. 275; Hall JE: Infertility and Fertility Control, Chap. 45, p. 279; Carr BR, Bradshaw KD: Disorders of the Ovary and Female Reproductive Tract, Chap. 326, p. 2198; and Manson JE, Bassuk SS: The Menopause Transition and Postmenopausal Hormone Therapy, Chap. 327, p. 2209, in HPIM-16.

179

HYPERCALCEMIC AND HYPOCALCEMIC DISORDERS

HYPERCALCEMIA

Hypercalcemia from any cause can result in fatigue, depression, mental confusion, anorexia, nausea, constipation, renal tubular defects, polyuria, a short QT interval, and arrhythmias. CNS and GI symptoms can occur at levels of serum calcium >2.9 mmol/L (>11.5 mg/dL), and nephrocalcinosis and impairment of renal function occur when serum calcium is 3.2 mmol/L (>13 mg/dL). Severe hypercalcemia, usually defined as >3.7 mmol/L (>15 mg/dL), can be a medical emergency, leading to coma and cardiac arrest.

ETIOLOGY   The causes of hypercalcemia are listed in Table 179-1. Hyperparathyroidism and malignancy account for 90% of cases.

Primary hyperparathyroidism is a generalized disorder of bone metabolism due to increased secretion of parathyroid hormone (PTH) by an adenoma (81%) or carcinoma (4%) in a single gland, or by parathyroid hyperplasia (15%). Familial hyperparathyroidism may be part of multiple endocrine neoplasia type 1 (MEN 1), which also includes pituitary and pancreatic islet tumors, or of MEN 2A, in which hyperparathyroidism occurs with pheochromocytoma and medullary carcinoma of the thyroid.

Hypercalcemia associated with malignancy is often severe and difficult to manage. Mechanisms for this include release of PTH-related protein (PTHrP) in lung, kidney, and squamous cell carcinoma; local bone destruction in myeloma and breast carcinoma; activation of lymphocytes leading to release of IL-

Table 179-1

Classification of Causes of Hypercalcemia

I. Parathyroid-related
   A. Primary hyperparathyroidism
      1. Solitary adenomas
      2. Multiple endocrine neoplasia
   B. Lithium therapy
   C. Familial hypocalciuric hypercalcemia
II. Malignancy-related
   A. Solid tumor with humoral mediation of hypercalcemia (lung, kidney)
   B. Solid tumor with metastases (breast)
   C. Hematologic malignancies (multiple myeloma, lymphoma, leukemia)
III. Vitamin D–related
   A. Vitamin D intoxication
   B. ↑ 1,25(OH)$_2$D; sarcoidosis and other granulomatous diseases
   C. Idiopathic hypercalcemia of infancy
IV. Associated with high bone turnover
   A. Hyperthyroidism
   B. Immobilization
   C. Thiazides
   D. Vitamin A intoxication
V. Associated with renal failure
   A. Severe secondary hyperparathyroidism
   B. Aluminum intoxication
   C. Milk-alkali syndrome

Source: Potts JT Jr: HPIM-16, p. 2252.

Table 179-2

Differential Diagnosis of Hypercalcemia: Laboratory Criteria

	Blood[a]			
	Ca	P_i	$1,25(OH)_2D$	iPTH
Primary hyperparathyroidism	↑	↓	↑↔	↑(↔)
Malignancy-associated hypercalcemia:				
Humoral hypercalcemia	↑↑	↓	↓↔	↓
Local destruction (osteolytic metastases)	↑	↔	↓↔	

[a] Symbols in parentheses refer to values rarely seen in the particular disease.
Note: P_i, inorganic phosphate; iPTH, immunoreactive parathyroid hormone.
Source: JT Potts Jr: HPIM-12, p. 1911.

1 and TNF in myeloma and lymphoma; or an increased synthesis of $1,25(OH)_2D$ in lymphoma.

Several other conditions have been associated with hypercalcemia. These include: sarcoidosis and other granulomatous diseases, which lead to increased synthesis of $1,25(OH)_2D$; vitamin D intoxication from chronic ingestion of large vitamin doses (50–100 × physiologic requirements); lithium therapy, which results in hyperfunctioning of the parathyroid glands; and familial hypocalciuric hypercalcemia (FHH) due to autosomal dominant inheritance of a mutation in the calcium-sensing receptor, which results in inappropriate secretion of PTH and enhanced renal calcium resorption. Severe secondary hyperparathyroidism may also complicate end-stage renal disease. Progression to tertiary hyperthyroidism occurs when PTH hypersecretion becomes autonomous and is no longer responsive to medical therapy.

CLINICAL FEATURES Most pts with hyperparathyroidism are asymptomatic, even when the disease involves the kidneys and the skeletal system. Pts frequently have hypercalciuria and polyuria, and calcium can be deposited in the renal parenchyma or form calcium oxalate stones. The characteristic skeletal lesion is osteopenia or, rarely, the more severe disorder osteitis fibrosa cystica. Increased bone resorption primarily involves cortical rather than trabecular bone. Hypercalcemia may be intermittent or sustained, and serum phosphate is usually low but may be normal.

DIAGNOSIS Primary hyperparathyroidism is confirmed by demonstration of an inappropriately high PTH level for the degree of hypercalcemia. Hypercalciuria helps to distinguish this disorder from FHH, in which PTH levels are usually in the normal range and the urine calcium level is low. Levels of PTH are low in hypercalcemia of malignancy (Table 179-2).

℞ TREATMENT

The type of treatment is based on the severity of the hypercalcemia and the nature of the associated symptoms. Table 179-3 shows general recommendations that apply to therapy of acute hypercalcemia from any cause.

In pts with severe primary hyperparathyroidism, surgical parathyroidectomy should be performed promptly. Asymptomatic disease may not require surgery; usual surgical indications include age <50, nephrolithiasis, urine Ca > 400 mg/d, reduced creatinine clearance, reduction in bone mass (T score < −2.5), or

Table 179-3

Therapies for Severe Hypercalcemia

Treatment	Onset of Action	Duration of Action	Advantages	Disadvantages
Hydration with saline (≤6 L/d)	Hours	During infusion	Rehydrates; rapid action	Volume overload; electrolyte disturbance
Forced diuresis (furosemide q1–2h along with aggressive hydration)	Hours	During treatment	Rapid action	Monitoring required to avoid dehydration
Pamidronate 30–90 mg IV over 4 h	1–2 days	10–14 days	High potency; prolonged action	Fever in 20% $\downarrow$ Ca, $\downarrow$ phosphate, $\downarrow$ Mg
Zolendronate 1–4 mg IV over minutes	1–2 days	>3 weeks	High potency; prolonged action; rapid infusion	Minor: Fever; rare $\downarrow$ Ca, $\downarrow$ phosphate
Calcitonin (2–8 U/kg SC 6–12 h)	Hours	1–2 days	Rapid onset	Limited effect; tachyphylaxis
Glucocorticoids (prednisone 10–25 mg PO qid)	Days	Days–weeks	Useful in myeloma, lymphoma, breast CA, sarcoid, vitamin D intox	Effects limited to certain disorders; glucocorticoid side effects
Dialysis	Hours	During use–2 days	Useful in renal failure; immediate effect	Complex procedure

serum calcium > 0.25 mmol/L (>1 mg/dL) above the normal range. A minimally invasive approach may be used if preoperative localization via sestamibi scans with SPECT demonstrates a solitary adenoma and intraoperative PTH assays are available. Otherwise, neck exploration is required. Postoperative management requires close monitoring of calcium and phosphorus. Calcium supplementation is given for symptomatic hypocalcemia.

Hypercalcemia of malignancy is managed by treating the underlying tumor. Adequate hydration and parenteral bisphosphonates can be used to reduce calcium levels.

No therapy is recommended for FHH. Secondary hyperparathyroidism should be treated with phosphate restriction, the use of nonabsorbable antacids, and calcitriol. Tertiary hyperparathyroidism requires parathyroidectomy.

HYPOCALCEMIA

Chronic hypocalcemia is less common than hypercalcemia but is usually symptomatic and requires treatment. Symptoms include peripheral and perioral paresthesia, muscle spasms, carpopedal spasm, laryngeal spasm, seizure, and respiratory arrest. Increased intracranial pressure and papilledema may occur with long-standing hypocalcemia, and other manifestations may include irritability, depression, psychosis, intestinal cramps, and chronic malabsorption. Chvostek's and Trousseau's signs are frequently positive, and the QT interval is prolonged. Both hypomagnesemia and alkalosis lower the threshold for tetany.

ETIOLOGY   Transient hypocalcemia often occurs in critically ill pts with burns, sepsis, and acute renal failure; following transfusion with citrated blood; or with medications such as protamine and heparin. Hypoalbuminemia can reduce serum calcium below normal, although ionized calcium levels remain normal. A simplified correction is sometimes used to assess whether the serum calcium concentration is abnormal when serum proteins are low. The correction is to add 0.2 mmol/L (0.8 mg/dL) to the serum calcium level for every 10 g/L (1 g/dL) by which the serum albumin level is below 40 g/L (4.0 g/dL). Alkalosis increases calcium binding to proteins, and in this setting direct measurements of ionized calcium should be used.

The causes of hypocalcemia can be divided into those in which PTH is absent (hereditary or acquired hypoparathyroidism, hypomagnesemia), PTH is ineffective (chronic renal failure, vitamin D deficiency, intestinal malabsorption, pseudohypoparathyroidism), or PTH is overwhelmed (severe, acute hyperphosphatemia in tumor lysis, acute renal failure, or rhabdomyolysis; hungry bone syndrome postparathyroidectomy). The cause of hypocalcemia associated with acute pancreatitis is unclear.

 TREATMENT

Symptomatic hypocalcemia may be treated with intravenous calcium gluconate (1 mg/mL of elemental calcium in D_5W infused 30–100 mL/h). Management of chronic hypocalcemia requires an oral calcium preparation, usually with a vitamin D preparation (Chap. 180). Hypoparathyroidism requires administration of calcium (1–3 g/d) and calcitriol (0.25–1 μg/d), adjusted according to serum calcium levels and urinary excretion. Restoration of magnesium stores may be required to reverse hypocalcemia in the setting of severe hypomagnesemia (<1.0 mg/dL).

HYPOPHOSPHATEMIA

Mild hypophosphatemia is not usually associated with clinical symptoms. In severe hypophosphatemia, pts may have muscle weakness, numbness, paresthesia, and confusion. Rhabdomyolysis may develop during rapidly progressive hypophosphatemia. Respiratory insufficiency can result from diaphragm muscle weakness.

ETIOLOGY The causes of hypophosphatemia include: decreased intestinal absorption (vitamin D deficiency, phosphorus-binding antacids, malabsorption); urinary losses (hyperparathyroidism, vitamin D deficiency, hyperglycemic states, X-linked hypophosphatemic rickets, oncogenic osteomalacia, alcoholism, or certain toxins); and shifts of phosphorus from extracellular to intracellular compartments (administration of insulin in diabetic ketoacidosis or by hyperalimentation or refeeding in a malnourished pt).

 TREATMENT

Mild hypophosphatemia can be replaced orally with milk, carbonated beverages, or Neutraphos or K-phos (up to 3 g/d in 4–6 divided doses/d). For severe hypophosphatemia (<1.5 mg/dL), IV phosphate may be administered at initial doses of 0.4–0.8 mmol/kg of elemental phosphorus over 6 h. Hypocalcemia should be corrected first, and the dose reduced 50% in hypercalcemia. Serum calcium and phosphate levels should be measured every 6–12 h; a serum calcium × phosphate level >50 must be avoided.

HYPERPHOSPHATEMIA
In adults, hyperphosphatemia is defined as a level >5.5 mg/dL. The most common causes are acute and chronic renal failure, but it may also be seen in hypoparathyroidism, vitamin D intoxication, acidosis, rhabdomyolysis, and hemolysis. In addition to treating the underlying disorder, dietary phosphorus intake should be limited. Oral aluminum phosphate binders may be used, and hemodialysis should be considered in severe cases.

HYPOMAGNESEMIA
Muscle weakness, prolonged PR and QT intervals, and cardiac arrhythmias are the most common manifestations of hypomagnesemia. Magnesium is important for effective PTH secretion as well as the renal and skeletal responsiveness to PTH. Therefore, hypomagnesemia is often associated with hypocalcemia.

ETIOLOGY Hypomagnesemia generally results from a derangement in renal or intestinal handling of magnesium and is classified as primary (hereditary) or secondary (acquired). Secondary causes are much more common, with renal losses being due to volume expansion, hypercalcemia, osmotic diuresis, loop diuretics, alcohol, aminoglycosides, cisplatin, cyclosporine, and amphotericin B, and gastrointestinal losses most commonly resulting from vomiting and diarrhea.

 TREATMENT

For mild deficiency, oral replacement in divided doses totaling 20–30 mmol/d (40–60 meq/d) is effective, though diarrhea may result. Parenteral magnesium administration is usually needed for serum levels <1.2 mg/dL, with a continuous infusion of magnesium chloride IV to deliver 50 mmol/d over a 24-h period (dose reduced by 50–75% in renal failure). Therapy may be required for several days. Patients with associated seizures or acute arrhythmias can be given 1–2 g of magnesium sulfate IV over 5–10 min.

HYPERMAGNESEMIA

Hypermagnesemia is rare but can be seen in renal failure when pts are taking magnesium-containing antacids, laxatives, enemas, or infusions, or in acute rhabdomyolysis. The most readily detectable clinical sign of hypermagnesemia is the disappearance of deep tendon reflexes, but hypotension, paralysis of respiratory muscles, complete heart block, and cardiac arrest can occur. Treatment includes stopping the preparation, dialysis against a low magnesium bath, or, if associated with life-threatening complications, 100–200 mg of elemental calcium IV over 5–10 min.

For a more detailed discussion, see Bringhurst FR, Demay MB, Krane SM, Kronenberg HM: Bone and Mineral Metabolism in Health and Disease, Chap. 331, p. 2238; and Potts JT Jr: Diseases of the Parathyroid Gland and Other Hyper- and Hypocalcemic Disorders, Chap. 332, p. 2249, in HPIM-16.

180

OSTEOPOROSIS AND OSTEOMALACIA

OSTEOPOROSIS

Osteoporosis is defined as a reduction in bone mass (or density) or the presence of fragility fracture. It is defined operationally as a bone density that falls 2.5 SD below the mean for a young normal individual (a T-score of <−2.5). Those with a T-score of <1.0 have low bone density and are at increased risk for osteoporosis. The most common sites for osteoporosis-related fractures are the vertebrae, hip, and distal radius.

ETIOLOGY Low bone density may result from low peak bone mass or increased bone loss. Risk factors for an osteoporotic fracture are listed in Table 180-1, and diseases associated with osteoporosis are listed in Table 180-2. Certain drugs, primarily glucocorticoids, cyclosporine, cytotoxic drugs, anticonvulsants, aluminum, and heparin, also have detrimental effects on the skeleton.

CLINICAL FEATURES Pts with multiple vertebral crush fractures may have height loss, kyphosis, and secondary pain from altered biomechanics of the back. Thoracic fractures can be associated with restrictive lung disease, whereas lumbar fractures are sometimes associated with abdominal symptoms or nerve compression leading to sciatica. Dual-energy x-ray absorptiometry has become the standard for measuring bone density. Criteria approved for Medicare reimbursement of bone mass measurement are summarized in Table 180-3. A general laboratory evaluation includes complete blood count, serum calcium, and a 24-h urine calcium. Further testing is based on clinical suspicion and may include thyroid-stimulating hormone (TSH), urinary free cortisol, parathyroid hormone (PTH), serum and urine electrophoresis, and testosterone levels (in

Table 180-1

Risk Factors for Osteoporosis Fracture

Nonmodifiable
  Personal history of fracture
    as an adult
  History of fracture in first-
    degree relative
  Female sex
  Advanced age
  Caucasian race
  Dementia
Potentially modifiable
  Current cigarette smoking
  Low body weight [<58 kg
    (127 lb)]
	Estrogen deficiency
	  Early menopause (<45 years) or bi-
	    lateral ovariectomy
	  Prolonged premenstrual amenorrhea
	    (>1 year)
	Low calcium intake
	Alcoholism
	Impaired eyesight despite
	  adequate correction
	Recurrent falls
	Inadequate physical activity
	Poor health/frailty

Table 180-2

Diseases Associated with an Increased Risk of Generalized Osteoporosis in Adults

Hypogonadal states
  Turner syndrome
  Klinefelter syndrome
  Anorexia nervosa
  Hypothalamic amenorrhea
  Hyperprolactinemia
  Other primary or second-
    ary hypogonadal states
Endocrine disorders
  Cushing's syndrome
  Hyperparathyroidism
  Thyrotoxicosis
  Insulin-dependent diabetes
    mellitus
  Acromegaly
  Adrenal insufficiency
Nutritional and gastrointesti-
  nal disorders
  Malnutrition
  Parenteral nutrition
  Malabsorption syndromes
  Gastrectomy
  Severe liver disease, espe-
    cially biliary cirrhosis
  Pernicious anemia
Rheumatologic disorders
  Rheumatoid arthritis
  Ankylosing spondylitis
	Hematologic disorders/malignancy
	  Multiple myeloma
	  Lymphoma and leukemia
	  Malignancy-associated parathyroid
	    hormone–related (PTHrP) production
	  Mastocytosis
	  Hemophilia
	  Thalassemia
	Selected inherited disorders
	  Osteogenesis imperfecta
	  Marfan syndrome
	  Hemochromatosis
	  Hypophosphatasia
	  Glycogen storage diseases
	  Homocystinuria
	  Ehlers-Danlos syndrome
	  Porphyria
	  Menkes' syndrome
	  Epidermolysis bullosa
	Other disorders
	  Immobilization
	  Chronic obstructive pulmonary
	    disease
	  Pregnancy and lactation
	  Scoliosis
	  Multiple sclerosis
	  Sarcoidosis
	  Amyloidosis

Table 180-3

FDA-Approved Indications for BMD Tests[a]

Estrogen-deficient women at clinical risk of osteoporosis
Vertebral abnormalities on x-ray suggestive of osteoporosis (osteopenia, vertebral fracture)
Glucocorticoid treatment equivalent to ≥ 7.5 mg of prednisone, or duration of therapy >3 months
Primary hyperparathyroidism
Monitoring response to an FDA-approved medication for osteoporosis
Repeat BMD evaluations at >23-month intervals, or more frequently, if medically justified

[a] Criteria adapted from the 1998 Bone Mass Measurement Act.
Note: BMD, bone mineral density.

men). Transglutaminase Ab testing may identify asymptomatic celiac disease. Markers of bone resorption (e.g., urine cross-linked *N*-telopeptide) may be helpful in detecting an early response to antiresorptive therapy if measured prior to and 4 to 6 months after initiating therapy.

 TREATMENT

Treatment involves the management of acute fractures, modifying risk factors, and treating any underlying disorders that lead to reduced bone mass. Treatment decisions are based on an individual's risk factors, but active treatment is generally recommended if the T-score is ≤ 2.5. Oral calcium (1–1.5 g/d of elemental calcium in divided doses), vitamin D (400–800 IU qd), exercise, and smoking cessation should be initiated in all patients with osteoporosis. Bisphosphonates (alendronate, 70 mg PO weekly; risedronate, 35 mg PO weekly) augment bone density and decrease fracture rates. Bisphosphonates are poorly absorbed and should be taken in the morning on an empty stomach with 0.25 L (8 oz) of tap water. Estrogen decreases the rate of bone reabsorption, but therapy should be considered carefully in the context of increased risks of cardiovascular disease and breast cancer. Raloxifene (60 mg PO qd), a selective estrogen receptor modulator, increases bone density and decreases total and LDL cholesterol without stimulating endometrial hyperplasia, though it may precipitate hot flashes. PTH(1-34) induces bone formation and may be administered as a daily injection for a maximum of 2 years.

OSTEOMALACIA

ETIOLOGY Defective mineralization of the organic matrix of bone results in *osteomalacia*. Osteomalacia is caused by inadequate intake or malabsorption of vitamin D (chronic pancreatic insufficiency, gastrectomy, malabsorption) and disorders of vitamin D metabolism (anticonvulsant therapy, chronic renal failure).

CLINICAL FEATURES Skeletal deformities may be overlooked until fractures occur after minimal trauma. Symptoms include diffuse skeletal pain and bony tenderness and may be subtle. Proximal muscle weakness may mimic primary muscle disorders. A decrease in bone density is usually associated with loss of trabeculae and thinning of the cortices. Characteristic x-ray findings are radiolucent bands (Looser's zones or pseudofractures) ranging from a few millimeters to several centimeters in length, usually perpendicular to the surface of the femur, pelvis, and scapula. Changes in serum calcium, phosphorus, 25(OH)D, and 1,25(OH)$_2$D levels vary depending on the cause. However, modest vitamin D deficiency leads to compensatory secondary hyperparathyroidism characterized by increased levels of PTH and alkaline phosphatase and relatively low levels of ionized calcium. 1,25-Dihydroxyvitamin D levels may be preserved, reflecting upregulation of 1α-hydroxylase activity.

℞ TREATMENT

In osteomalacia due to vitamin D deficiency [serum 25(OH)D < 37 nmol/L (<15 ng/mL)], vitamin D$_2$ (ergocalciferol) is given orally in doses of 50,000 IU weekly for 8 weeks, followed by maintenance therapy with 800 IU daily. Osteomalacia due to malabsorption requires larger doses of vitamin D (up to 100,000 IU/d or 250,000 IU IM biannually). In pts taking anticonvulsants, concurrent vitamin D should be administered in doses that maintain the serum calcium and 25(OH)D levels in the normal range. Calcitriol (0.25–1 μg PO qd or 1.0–2.5 μg IV thrice weekly) is effective in treating hypocalcemia or osteodystrophy caused by chronic renal failure. Vitamin D deficiency should always be repleted in conjunction with calcium supplementation (1.5–2.0 g of elemental calcium daily). Serum and urinary calcium measurements are efficacious for monitoring resolution of vitamin D deficiency, with a goal 24-h urinary calcium excretion of 100–250 mg/24h.

For a more detailed discussion, see Bringhurst FR, Demay MB, Krane SM, Kronenberg HM: **Bone and Mineral Metabolism in Health and Disease,** Chap. 331, p. 2238; and Lindsay R, Cosman F: Osteoporosis, Chap. 333, p. 2268, in HPIM-16.

181

DISORDERS OF LIPID METABOLISM

Hyperlipoproteinemia may be characterized by hypercholesterolemia, isolated hypertriglyceridemia, or both (Table 181-1). Diabetes mellitus, obesity, ethanol consumption, oral contraceptives, renal disease, hepatic disease, and hypothyroidism can cause secondary hyperlipoproteinemias or worsen underlying hyperlipoproteinemic states.

Standard lipoprotein analysis assesses total cholesterol, HDL, and triglycerides with a calculation of LDL levels using the equation: LDL = total cholesterol − HDL − triglycerides/5. The LDL cholesterol concentration can be estimated using this method only if triglycerides are <4.0 mmol/L (< 350 mg/dL). Both LDL and HDL cholesterol levels are temporarily decreased for several weeks after myocardial infarction or acute inflammatory states but can be accurately measured if blood is obtained within 8 h of the event.

Table 181-1

Characteristics of Common Hyperlipidemias

Lipid Phenotype	Plasma Lipid Levels, mmol/L (mg/dL)	Lipoproteins Elevated	Phenotype	Clinical Signs
ISOLATED HYPERCHOLESTEROLEMIA				
Familial hypercholesterolemia	Heterozygotes: total chol = 7–13 (275–500)	LDL	IIa	Usually develop xanthomas in adulthood and vascular disease at 30–50 years
	Homozygotes: total chol > 13 (>500)	LDL	IIa	Usually develop xanthomas and vascular disease in childhood
Familial defective apo B100	Heterozygotes: total chol = 7–13 (275–500)	LDL	IIa	Usually asymptomatic until vascular disease develops; no xanthomas
Polygenic hypercholesterolemia	Total chol = 6.5–9.0 (250–350)	LDL	IIa	
ISOLATED HYPERTRIGLYCERIDEMIA				
Familial hypertriglyceridemia	TG = 2.8–8.5 (250–750) (plasma may be cloudy)	VLDL	IV	Asymptomatic; may be associated with increased risk of vascular disease
Familial lipoprotein lipase deficiency	TG > 8.5 (>750) (plasma may be milky)	Chylomicrons	I, V	May be asymptomatic; may be associated with pancreatitis, abdominal pain, hepatosplenomegaly
Familial apo CII deficiency	TG > 8.5 (>750) (plasma may be milky)	Chylomicrons	I, V	As above
HYPERTRIGLYCERIDEMIA AND HYPERCHOLESTEROLEMIA				
Combined hyperlipidemia	TG = 2.8–8.5 (250–750) Total chol = 6.5–13.0 (250–500)	VLDL, LDL	IIb	Usually asymptomatic until vascular disease develops; familial form may also present as isolated high TG or an isolated high LDL cholesterol
Dysbetalipoproteinemia	TG = 2.8–5.6 (250–500) Total chol = 6.5–13.0 (250–500)	VLDL, IDL; LDL normal	III	Usually asymptomatic until vascular disease develops; may have palmar or tuboeruptive xanthomas

Note: Total chol, the sum of free and esterified cholesterol; LDL, low-density lipoprotein; TG, triglycerides; VLDL, very low density lipoproteins; IDL, intermediate-density lipoprotein.
Source: From HN Ginsberg, IJ Goldberg: HPIM-15, p. 2250.

ISOLATED HYPERCHOLESTEROLEMIA

Elevated levels of fasting plasma total cholesterol [>5.2 mmol/L (>200 mg/dL)] in the presence of normal levels of triglycerides are almost always associated with increased concentrations of plasma LDL cholesterol. A rare individual with markedly elevated HDL cholesterol may also have increased plasma total cholesterol levels. Elevations of LDL cholesterol can result from single-gene defects, polygenic disorders, or from the secondary effects of other disease states.

Familial Hypercholesterolemia (FH)

FH is a codominant genetic disorder that is due to mutations in the gene for the LDL receptor. Plasma LDL levels are elevated at birth and remain so throughout life. In untreated heterozygous adults, total cholesterol levels range from 7.1–12.9 mmol/ L (275–500 mg/dL). Plasma triglyceride levels are typically normal, and HDL cholesterol levels are normal or reduced. Heterozygotes, especially men, are prone to accelerated atherosclerosis and premature coronary artery disease (CAD). *Tendon xanthomas* (most commonly of the Achilles tendons and the extensor tendons of the knuckles), *tuberous xanthomas* (softer, painless nodules on the ankles and buttocks), and *xanthelasmas* (deposits on the eyelids) are common.

Familial Defective Apo B-100

This autosomal dominant disorder impairs the synthesis and/or function of apo B-100, thereby reducing the affinity for the LDL receptor, slowing LDL catabolism, and causing a phenocopy of FH.

Polygenic Hypercholesterolemia

Most moderate hypercholesterolemia [<9.1 mmol/L (<350 mg/dL)] arises from an interaction of multiple genetic defects and environmental factors such as diet, age, and exercise. Plasma HDL and triglyceride levels are normal, and xanthomas are not present.

℞ TREATMENT

An algorithm for the evaluation and treatment of hypercholesterolemia is displayed in Fig. 181-1. Therapy for all of these disorders includes restriction of dietary cholesterol, HMG-CoA reductase inhibitors, and bile acid sequestrants (Table 181-2).

ISOLATED HYPERTRIGLYCERIDEMIA

The diagnosis of hypertriglyceridemia is made by measuring plasma lipid levels after an overnight fast. Hypertriglyceridemia in adults is defined as a triglyceride level >2.3 mmol/L (>200 mg/dL). An isolated increase in plasma triglycerides indicates that chylomicrons and/or very low density lipoprotein (VLDL) are increased. Plasma is usually clear when triglyceride levels are <4.5 mmol/L (<400 mg/dL) and cloudy when levels are higher due to VLDL (and/or chylomicron) particles becoming large enough to scatter light. When chylomicrons are present, a creamy layer floats to the top of plasma after refrigeration for several hours. Tendon xanthomas and xanthelasmas do not occur with isolated hypertriglyceridemia, but *eruptive xanthomas* (small orange-red papules) can appear on the trunk and extremities and *lipemia retinalis* (orange-yellow retinal vessels) may be seen when the triglyceride levels are >11.3 mmol/L (>1000 mg/dL). Pancreatitis is associated with these high concentrations.

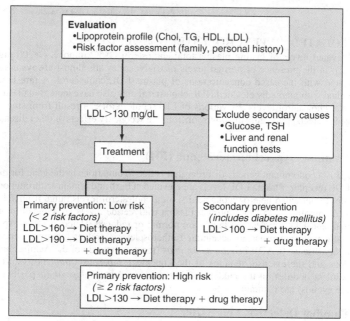

A

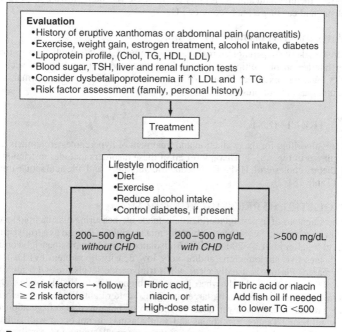
B

FIGURE 181-1 Algorithms for the evaluation and treatment of hypercholesterolemia (*A*) and hypertriglyceridemia (*B*). Statin, HMG-CoA reductase inhibitor; Chol, cholesterol; HDL, high-density lipoprotein; LDL, low-density lipoprotein; TG, triglyceride; TSH, thyroid-stimulating hormone; CHD, coronary heart disease.

Table 181-2

Hypolipidemic Drugs

Drugs	Lipoprotein Class Affected	Common Side Effects	Contraindications
HMG-CoA reductase inhibitors Lovastatin 20–80 mg/d Pravastatin 40–80 mg qhs Simvastatin 20–80 mg qhs Fluvastatin 20–80 mg qhs Atorvastatin 10–80 mg qhs Rosuvastatin 10–40 mg qhs	↓ LDL 25–55% ↓ TG 10–20% ↑ HDL 5–10%	Myalgias, arthralgias, ↑ transaminases, dyspepsia	Acute or chronic liver disease of myositis increased by impaired renal function and in combination with a fibrate
Nicotinic acid	↓ LDL 15–25% ↓ TG 25–35% ↑ HDL 15–30%	Flushing (may be relieved by aspirin), hepatic dysfunction, nausea, diarrhea, glucose intolerance, hyperuricemia	Peptic ulcer disease, hepatic disease, gout
Fish oils 3–12 g qd	↓ LDL 5–10% ↓ TG 18%	Dyspepsia, diarrhea, fishy odor to breath	
Cholesterol absorption inhibitors Ezetimibe 10 mg qd	↓ LDL 18% ↑ TG 8%	Transaminases	
Bile acid sequestrant Cholestyramine 4–32 g qd Colestipol 5–40 g qd Colesevelam 3750–4375 mg qd	↓ LDL 20–30% ↑ TG 10% ↑ HDL 5%	Constipation, gastric discomfort, nausea	Biliary tract obstruction, gastric outlet obstruction
Fibric acid derivatives Gemfibrozil 600 mg bid Fenofibrate 160 mg qd Immediate release 100 mg tid, gradual increase to 2 g tid Sustained release 250 mg–1.5 g bid Extended release 500 mg–2 g qhs	↑ or ↓ LDL ↓ TG 25–40% ↑ HDL 5–15%	↓ Absorption of other drugs ↑ Gallstones, dyspepsia, hepatic dysfunction, myalgia	Hepatic or biliary disease, renal insufficiency associated with ↑ risk of myositis

Note: LDL, low-density lipoprotein; VLDL, very low density lipoprotein; TG, triglycerides; HDL, high-density lipoprotein; LPL, lipoprotein lipase; CPK, creative phosphokinase.

Familial Hypertriglyceridemia

In this autosomal dominant disorder, increased plasma VLDL causes plasma triglyceride concentrations to range from 2.3–5.6 mmol/L (200–500 mg/dL). Obesity, hyperglycemia, and hyperinsulinemia are characteristic, and diabetes mellitus, ethanol consumption, oral contraceptives, and hypothyroidism may exacerbate the condition. The diagnosis is suggested by the triad of elevated plasma triglycerides [2.8–11.3 mmol/L (250–1000 mg/dL)], normal or only mildly increased cholesterol levels [<6.5 mmol/L (<250 mg/dL)], and reduced plasma HDL. The identification of other first-degree relatives with hypertriglyceridemia is useful in making the diagnosis. Familial dysbetalipoproteinemia and familial combined hyperlipidemia should be ruled out, as these two conditions are associated with accelerated atherosclerosis.

Lipoprotein Lipase Deficiency

This rare autosomal recessive disorder results from the absence or deficiency of lipoprotein lipase, which in turn impairs the metabolism of chylomicrons. Accumulation of chylomicrons in plasma causes recurrent bouts of pancreatitis, usually beginning in childhood, and hepatosplenomegaly is present. Accelerated atherosclerosis is not a feature.

Apo CII Deficiency

This rare autosomal recessive disorder is due to the absence of apo CII, an essential cofactor for lipoprotein lipase. As a result, chylomicrons and triglycerides accumulate and cause manifestations similar to those in lipoprotein lipase deficiency.

 TREATMENT

An algorithm for the evaluation and treatment of hypertriglyceridemia is displayed in Fig. 181-1. All pts with hypertriglyceridemia should be placed on a fat-free diet with fat-soluble vitamin supplementation. In those with familial hypertriglyceridemia, fibric acid derivatives should be administered if dietary measures fail (Table 181-2).

HYPERCHOLESTEROLEMIA AND HYPERTRIGLYCERIDEMIA

Elevations of both triglycerides and cholesterol are caused by elevations in both VLDL and LDL or in VLDL remnant particles.

Familial Combined Hyperlipidemia (FCHL)

This inherited disorder, present in 1/200 persons, can cause different lipoprotein abnormalities in affected individuals, including hypercholesterolemia (elevated LDL), hypertriglyceridemia (elevated triglycerides and VLDL), or both. Atherosclerosis is accelerated. A mixed dyslipidemia [plasma triglycerides 2.3–9.0 mmol/L (200–800 mg/dL), cholesterol levels 5.2–10.3 mmol/L (200–400 mg/dL) and HDL levels <10.3 mmol/L (<40 mg/dL)] and a family history of hyperlipidemia and/or premature cardiovascular disease suggests the diagnosis of FCHL. All pts should restrict dietary cholesterol and fat and avoid alcohol and oral contraceptives. An HMG-CoA reductase inhibitor plus niacin may be used.

Dysbetalipoproteinemia

This rare disorder is associated with homozygosity for apo E2, but the development of disease requires additional environmental and/or genetic factors.

Plasma cholesterol [6.5–13.0 mmol/L (250–500 mg/dL)] and triglycerides [2.8–5.6 mmol/L (250–500 mg/dL)] are increased due to accumulation of VLDL and chylomicron remnant particles. Patients usually present in adulthood with xanthomas and premature coronary and peripheral vascular disease. Cutaneous xanthomas are distinctive, in the form of *palmar* and *tuberoeruptive xanthomas*. Triglycerides and cholesterol are both elevated. Diagnosis is established by a ratio of VLDL (by centrifugation) to total plasma triglycerides of >0.3. If present, hypothyroidism and diabetes mellitus should be treated, and HMG-CoA reductase inhibitors, fibrates, and/or niacin may be necessary.

PREVENTION OF THE COMPLICATIONS OF ATHEROSCLEROSIS

The National Cholesterol Education Program guidelines (Fig. 181-1) are based on plasma LDL levels and estimations of other risk factors. The goal in pts with the highest risk (known coronary heart or other atherosclerotic disease, 10-year risk for coronary heart disease >20%, or diabetes mellitus) is to lower LDL cholesterol to <2.6 mmol/L (<100 mg/dL). In pts with very high risk, recent clinical trials suggest additional benefit by reducing LDL cholesterol to <1.8 mmol/L (<70 mg/dL). The goal is an LDL cholesterol <3.4 mmol/ L (<130 mg/dL) in pts with two or more risk factors for atherosclerotic heart disease. Risk factors include (1) men >age 45, women >age 55 or after menopause; (2) family history of early CAD (< 55 years in a male parent or sibling and <65 years in a female parent or sibling); (3) hypertension (even if it is controlled with medications); (4) cigarette smoking (>10 cigarettes/day); and (5) HDL cholesterol <1.0 mmol/L (<40 mg/dL). Therapy begins with a low-fat diet, but pharmacologic intervention is often required (Table 181-2).

For a more detailed discussion, see Rader DJ, Hobbs HH: Disorders of Lipoprotein Metabolism, Chap. 335, p. 2286; in HPIM-16.

182

HEMOCHROMATOSIS, PORPHYRIAS, AND WILSON'S DISEASE

HEMOCHROMATOSIS

Hemochromatosis is a disorder of iron storage that results in increased intestinal iron absorption with Fe deposition and damage to many tissues, including the liver, heart, pancreas, joints, and pituitary. Two major causes of hemochromatosis exist: hereditary (due to inheritance of mutant *HFE* genes) and secondary iron overload (usually the result of disordered erythropoiesis). Alcoholic liver disease and chronic excessive Fe ingestion may also be associated with a moderate increase in hepatic Fe and elevated body Fe stores.

CLINICAL FEATURES Early symptoms include weakness, lassitude, weight loss, a bronze pigmentation or darkening of skin, abdominal pain, and loss of libido. Hepatomegaly occurs in 95% of pts, sometimes in the presence of normal LFTs. Other signs include spider angiomas, splenomegaly, arthropathy, ascites, cardiac arrythmias, CHF, loss of body hair, palmar erythema, gynecomastia, and testicular atrophy. Diabetes mellitus occurs in about 65%, usually in pts with family history of diabetes. Adrenal insufficiency, hypothyroidism, and hypoparathyroidism rarely occur.

DIAGNOSIS   Serum Fe, percent transferrin saturation, and serum ferritin levels are increased. In an otherwise-healthy person, a fasting serum transferrin saturation > 50% is abnormal and suggests homozygosity for hemochromatosis. In most untreated pts with hemochromatosis, the serum ferritin level is also greatly increased. If either the percent transferrin saturation or the serum ferritin level is abnormal, genetic testing for hemochromatosis should be performed. All first-degree relatives of pts with hemochromatosis should be tested for the C282Y and H63D mutations. Liver biopsy may be required in affected individuals to evaluate possible cirrhosis or to quantify tissue iron. An algorithm for evaluating pts with possible hemochromatosis is shown in Fig. 182-1. Death in untreated pts results from cardiac failure (30%), cirrhosis (25%), and hepatocellular carcinoma (30%); the latter may develop despite adequate Fe removal.

 TREATMENT

Therapy involves removal of excess body Fe, usually by intermittent phlebotomy, and supportive treatment of damaged organs. Since 1 unit of blood contains ~250 mg Fe, and since ≥25 g of Fe must be removed, phlebotomy is performed weekly for 1–2 years. Less frequent phlebotomy is then used to maintain serum Fe at <27 μmol/L (<150 μg/dL). Chelating agents such as deferoxamine (infused SC using a portable pump) remove 10–20 mg iron per day, a fraction of that mobilized by weekly phlebotomy. Chelation therapy is indicated, however, when phlebotomy is inappropriate, such as with anemia or hypoproteinemia. Alcohol consumption should be eliminated.

PORPHYRIAS

The porphyrias are inherited or acquired disturbances in heme biosynthesis. Each disorder causes a unique pattern of overproduction, accumulation, and excretion of intermediates of heme synthesis. These disorders are classified as either hepatic or erythropoietic, depending on the primary site of overproduction and accumulation of the porphyrin precursor or porphyrin. The major manifestations of the hepatic porphyrias are neurologic (neuropathic abdominal pain, neuropathy, and mental disturbances), whereas the erythropoietic porphyrias characteristically cause cutaneous photosensitivity. Laboratory testing is required to confirm or exclude the various types of porphyria. However, a definite diagnosis requires demonstration of the specific enzyme deficiency or gene defect.

Acute Intermittent Porphyria

This is an autosomal dominant disorder with variable expressivity. Manifestations include colicky abdominal pain, vomiting, constipation, port-wine colored urine, and neurologic and psychiatric disturbances. Acute attacks rarely occur before puberty and may last from days to months. Photosensitivity does not occur. Clinical and biochemical manifestations may be precipitated by barbiturates, anticonvulsants, estrogens, oral contraceptives, alcohol, or low-calorie diets. Diagnosis is established by demonstrating elevation of urinary porphobilinogen (PBG) and γ-aminolevulinic acid (ALA) during an acute attack.

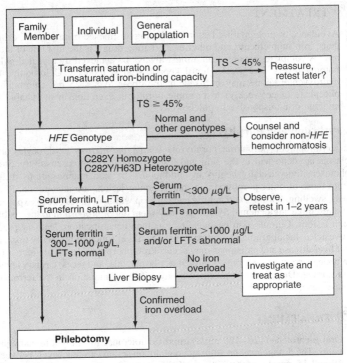

FIGURE 182-1 Algorithm for screening for *HFE*-associated hemochromatosis. LFT, liver function tests; TS, transferrin saturation. (*With permission from The Canadian Journal of Gastroenterology.*)

℞ TREATMENT

As soon as possible after the onset of an attack, 3–4 mg of heme, in the form of heme arginate, heme albumin, or hematin, should be infused daily for 4 days. Administration of IV glucose at rates up to 20 g/h or parenteral nutrition, if oral feeding is not possible for long periods, can be effective in acute attacks. Narcotic analgesics may be required during acute attacks for abdominal pain, and phenothiazines are useful for nausea, vomiting, anxiety, and restlessness. Treatment between attacks involves adequate nutritional intake, avoidance of drugs known to exacerbate the disease, and prompt treatment of other intercurrent diseases or infections.

Porphyria Cutanea Tarda

This is the most common porphyria and is characterized by cutaneous photosensitivity and, usually, hepatic disease. It is due to deficiency (inherited or acquired) of hepatic uroporphyrinogen decarboxylase. Photosensitivity causes facial pigmentation, increased fragility of skin, erythema, and vesicular and ulcerative lesions, typically involving face, forehead, and forearms. Neurologic manifestations are not observed. Contributing factors include excess alcohol, iron, and estrogens. Pts with liver disease are at risk for hepatocellular carcinoma. Plasma and urine uroporphyrin and 7-carboxylate porphyrin are increased.

TREATMENT

Avoidance of precipitating factors, including abstinence from alcohol, estrogens, iron supplements, and other exacerbating drugs, is the first line of therapy. A complete response can almost always be achieved by repeated phlebotomy (every 1–2 weeks) until hepatic iron is reduced. Chloroquine or hydroxychloroquine may be used in low doses (e.g., 125 mg chloroquine phosphate twice weekly) to promote porphyrin excretion in pts unable to undergo or unresponsive to phlebotomy.

Erythropoietic Porphyria

In erythropoietic porphyria, porphyrins from bone marrow erythrocytes and plasma are deposited in the skin and lead to cutaneous photosensitivity. Skin photosensitivity usually begins in childhood. The skin manifestations differ from those of other porphyrias, in that vesicular lesions are uncommon. Redness, swelling, burning, and itching can develop within minutes of sun exposure and resemble angioedema. Symptoms may seem out of proportion to the visible skin lesions. Chronic skin changes may include lichenification, leathery pseudovesicles, labial grooving, and nail changes. Liver function is usually normal, but liver disease and gallstones may occur. Protophorphyrin levels are increased in bone marrow, circulating erythrocytes, plasma, bile, and feces. Urinary levels are normal. Diagnosis is confirmed by identifying a mutation in the ferrochelatase gene.

 **TREATMENT**

Oral β-carotene (120–180 mg/d) improves tolerance to sunlight in many patients. The dosage may be adjusted to maintain serum carotene levels between 10 and 15 μmol/L (600–800 μg/dL). Cholestyramine or activated charcoal may promote fecal excretion of protoporphyrin. Transfusions or intravenous heme therapy may be beneficial.

WILSON'S DISEASE

Wilson's disease is an inherited disorder of copper metabolism, resulting in the toxic accumulation of copper in the liver, brain, and other organs. Individuals with Wilson's disease have mutations in the *ATP7B* gene.

CLINICAL FEATURES Hepatic disease may present as hepatitis, cirrhosis, or hepatic decompensation. In other pts, neurologic or psychiatric disturbances are the first clinical sign and are always accompanied by Kayser-Fleischer rings (corneal deposits of copper). Dystonia, incoordination, or tremor may be present, and dysarthria and dysphagia are common. Autonomic disturbances may also be present. Microscopic hematuria is common. In about 5% of pts, the first manifestation may be primary or secondary amenorrhea or repeated spontaneous abortions.

DIAGNOSIS Serum ceruloplasmin levels are often low, and urine copper levels are elevated. The "gold standard" for diagnosis is an elevated copper level on liver biopsy.

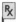 **TREATMENT**

Hepatitis or cirrhosis without decompensation should be treated with zinc (50 mg PO tid). For pts with hepatic decompensation, trientene (500 mg PO bid) plus zinc (separated by at least 1 h) is recommended, though liver transplantation should be considered for severe hepatic decompensation. For initial neurologic therapy, trientine and zinc are recommended for 8 weeks, followed by therapy with zinc alone. Tetrathiomolybdate is an alternative therapeutic option available in the future. Penicillamine is no longer first-line therapy. Zinc treatment does not require monitoring for toxicity, and 24-h urine copper can be followed for a therapeutic response. Trientine may induce bone marrow suppression and proteinuria, and free serum copper levels (adjusting total serum copper for ceruloplasmin copper) must be followed for a therapeutic response. Anticopper therapy must be lifelong.

For a more detailed discussion, see Powell LW: Hemochromatosis, Chap. 336, p. 2298; Desnick RJ: The Porphyrias, Chap. 337, p. 2303; Brewer GJ: Wilson Disease, Chap. 339, p. 2313; in HPIM-16.

183

THE NEUROLOGIC EXAMINATION

MENTAL STATUS EXAM

• *The bare minimum: During the interview, look for difficulties with communication and determine whether the pt has recall and insight into recent and past events.*

The goal of the mental status exam is to evaluate attention, orientation, memory, insight, judgment, and grasp of general information. Attention is tested by asking the pt to respond every time a specific item recurs in a list. Orientation is evaluated by asking about the day, date, and location. Memory can be tested by asking the pt to immediately recall a sequence of numbers and by testing recall of a series of objects after defined times (e.g., 5 and 15 min). More remote memory is evaluated by assessing pt's ability to provide a cogent chronologic history of his or her illness or personal life events. Recall of major historic events or dates of major current events can be used to assess knowledge. Evaluation of language function should include assessment of spontaneous speech, naming, repetition, reading, writing, and comprehension. Additional tests such as ability to draw and copy, perform calculations, inter-

Table 183-1

The Mini-Mental Status Examination

	Points
Orientation	
Name: season/date/day/month/year	5 (1 for each name)
Name: hospital/floor/town/state/country	5 (1 for each name)
Registration	
Identify three objects by name and ask patient to repeat	3 (1 for each object)
Attention and calculation	
Serial 7s; subtract from 100 (e.g., 93–86–79–72–65)	5 (1 for each subtraction)
Recall	
Recall the three objects presented earlier	3 (1 for each object)
Language	
Name pencil and watch	2 (1 for each object)
Repeat "No ifs, ands, or buts"	1
Follow a 3-step command (e.g., "Take this paper, fold it in half, and place it on the table")	3 (1 for each command)
Write "close your eyes" and ask patient to obey written command	1
Ask patient to write a sentence	1
Ask patient to copy a design (e.g., intersecting pentagons)	1
TOTAL	30

Table 183-2

Muscles That Move Joints

	Muscle	Nerve	Segmental Innervation
Shoulder	Supraspinatus	Suprascapular n.	C5,6
	Deltoid	Axillary n.	C5,6
Forearm	Biceps	Musculocutaneous n.	C5,6
	Brachioradialis	Radial n.	C5,6
	Triceps	Radial n.	C6,7,8
	Ext. carpi radialis	Radial n.	C5,6
	Ext. carpi ulnaris	P. interosseous n.	C7,8
	Ext. digitorum	P. interosseous n.	C7,8
	Supinator	P. interosseous n.	C6,7
	Flex. carpi radialis	Median n.	C6,7
	Flex. carpi ulnaris	Ulnar n.	C7,8,T1
	Pronator teres	Median n.	C6,7
Wrist	Ext. carpi ulnaris	Ulnar n.	C7,8,T1
	Flex. carpi radialis	Median n.	C6,7
Hand	Lumbricals	Median + ulnar n.	C8,T1
	Interossei	Ulnar n.	C8,T1
	Flex. digitorum	Median + A. interosseous n.	C7,C8,T1
Thumb	Opponens pollicis	Median n.	C8,T1
	Ext. pollicis	P. interosseous n.	C7,8
	Add. pollicis	Median n.	C8,T1
	Abd. pollicis	Ulnar n.	C8,T1
	Flex. pollicis br.	Ulnar n.	C8,T1
Thigh	Iliopsoas	Femoral n.	L1,2,3
	Glutei	Sup. + inf. gluteal n.	L4,L5,S1,S2
	Quadriceps	Femoral n.	L2,3,4
	Adductors	Obturator n.	L2,3,4
	Hamstrings	Sciatic n.	L5,S1,S2
Foot	Gastrocnemius	Tibial n.	S1,S2
	Tibialis ant.	Deep peroneal n.	L4,5
	Peronei	Deep peroneal n.	L5,S1
	Tibialis post.	Tibial n.	L4,5
Toes	Ext. hallucis l.	Deep peroneal n.	L5,S1

---

pret proverbs or logic problems, identify right vs. left, name and identify body parts, etc., are also important.

A useful standardized screening examination of cognitive function is the mini-mental status examination (MMSE) (Table 183-1).

CRANIAL NERVE (CN) EXAM

• *The bare minimum: Check the fundi, visual fields, pupil size and reactivity, extraocular movements, and facial movements.*

CN I Occlude each nostril sequentially and ask pt to gently sniff and correctly identify a mild test stimulus, such as soap, toothpaste, coffee, or lemon oil.

CN II Check visual acuity with and without correction using a Snellen chart (distance) and Jaeger's test type (near). Map visual fields (VFs) by confrontation testing in each quadrant of visual field for each eye individually. The best method is to sit facing pt (2–3 ft apart),

Function
Abduction of upper arm
Abduction of upper arm
Flexion of the supinated forearm
Forearm flexion with arm between pronation and supination
Extension of forearm
Extension and abduction of hand at the wrist
Extension and adduction of hand at the wrist
Extension of fingers at the MCP joints
Supination of the extended forearm
Flexion and abduction of hand at the wrist
Flexion and adduction of hand at the wrist
Pronation of the forearm
Extension/adduction at the wrist
Flexion/abduction at the wrist
Extension of fingers at PIP joint with the MCP joint extended and fixed
Abduction/adduction of the fingers
Flexion of the fingers
Touching the base of the 5th finger with thumb
Extension of the thumb
Adduction of the thumb
Abduction of the thumb
Flexion of the thumb
Flexion of the thigh
Abduction, extension, and internal rotation of the leg
Extension of the leg at the knee
Adduction of the leg
Flexion of the leg at the knee
Plantar flexion of the foot
Dorsiflexion of the foot
Eversion of the foot
Inversion of the foot
Dorsiflexion of the great toe

have pt cover one eye gently, and fix uncovered eye on examiner's nose. A small white object (e.g., a cotton-tipped applicator) is then moved slowly from periphery of field toward center until seen. Pt's VF should be mapped against examiner's for comparison. Formal perimetry and tangent screen exam are essential to identify and delineate small defects. Optic fundi should be examined with an ophthalmoscope, and the color, size, and degree of swelling or elevation of the optic disc recorded. The retinal vessels should be checked for size, regularity, AV nicking at crossing points, hemorrhage, exudates, and aneurysms. The retina, including the macula, should be examined for abnormal pigmentation and other lesions.

   CNS III, IV, VI   Describe size, regularity, and shape of pupils; reaction (direct and consensual) to light; and convergence (pt follows an object as it moves closer). Check for lid drooping, lag, or retraction. Ask pt to follow your finger as you move it horizontally to left and right and vertically with each eye first fully adducted then fully ab-

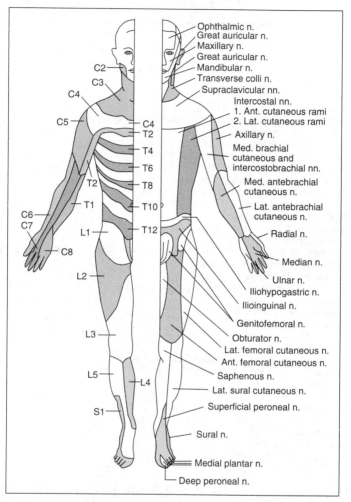

FIGURE 183-1 Anterior view of dermatomes (*left*) and cutaneous areas supplied by individual peripheral nerves (*right*). (*From HPIM-16, Fig. 22-2, p. 144.*)

ducted. Check for failure to move fully in particular directions and for presence of regular, rhythmic, involuntary oscillations of eyes (nystagmus). Test quick voluntary eye movements (saccades) as well as pursuit (e.g., follow the finger).

CN V Feel the masseter and temporalis muscles as pt bites down and test jaw opening, protrusion, and lateral motion against resistance. Examine sensation over entire face as well as response to touching each cornea lightly with a small wisp of cotton.

CN VII Look for asymmetry of face at rest and with spontaneous as well as emotion-induced (e.g., laughing) movements. Test eyebrow el-

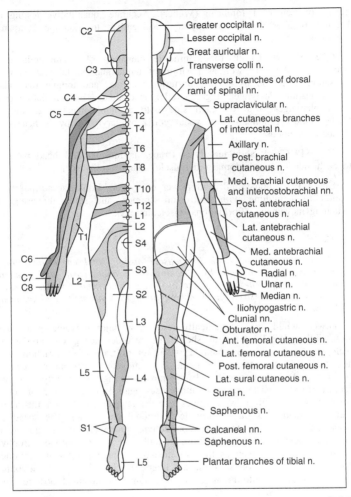

FIGURE 183-2 Posterior view of dermatomes (*left*) and cutaneous areas supplied by individual nerves (*right*). (*From HPIM-16, Fig. 22-3 p. 144.*)

evation, forehead wrinkling, eye closure, smiling, frowning; check puff, whistle, lip pursing, and chin muscle contraction. Observe for differences in strength of lower and upper facial muscles. Taste on the anterior two-thirds of tongue can be affected by lesions of the seventh CN proximal to the chorda tympani. Test taste for sweet (sugar), salt, sour (lemon), and bitter (quinine) using a cotton-tipped applicator moistened in appropriate solution and placed on lateral margin of protruded tongue halfway back from tip.

CN VIII Check ability to hear tuning fork, finger rub, watch tick, and whispered voice at specified distances with each ear. Check for air vs. mastoid bone conduction (Rinne) and lateralization of a tuning fork placed on center of forehead (Weber). Accurate, quantitative testing of hearing requires formal audiometry. Remember to examine tympanic membranes.

CNS IX, X   Check for symmetric elevation of palate-uvula with phonation ("ahh"), as well as position of uvula and palatal arch at rest. Sensation in region of tonsils, posterior pharynx, and tongue may also require testing. Pharyngeal ("gag") reflex is evaluated by stimulating posterior pharyngeal wall on each side with a blunt object (e.g., tongue blade). Direct examination of vocal cords by laryngoscopy is necessary in some situations.

CN XI   Check shoulder shrug (trapezius muscle) and head rotation to each side (sternocleidomastoid muscle) against resistance.

CN XII   Examine bulk and power of tongue. Look for atrophy, deviation from midline with protrusion, tremor, and small flickering or twitching movements (fibrillations, fasciculations).

MOTOR EXAM

• *The bare minimum: Look for muscle atrophy and check limb tone. Assess upper limb strength by checking for pronator drift and strength of wrist or finger reflexes. Tap the biceps, patellar, and Achilles reflexes. Test for lower limb strength by asking pt to walk normally and on heels and toes.*

Power should be systematically tested for major movements at each joint (Table 183-2). Strength should be recorded using a reproducible scale (e.g., 0 = no movement, 1 = flicker or trace of contraction with no associated movement at a joint, 2 = movement present but cannot be sustained against gravity, 3 = movement against gravity but not against applied resistance, 4 = movement against some degree of resistance, and 5 = full power; values can be supplemented with the addition of + and − signs to provide additional gradations). The speed of movement, the ability to relax contractions promptly, and fatigue with repetition should all be noted. Loss in bulk and size of muscle (atrophy) should be noted, as well as the presence of irregular involuntary contraction (twitching) of groups of muscle fibers (fasciculations). Any involuntary movements should be noted at rest, during maintained posture, and with voluntary action.

REFLEXES

Important muscle-stretch reflexes to test routinely and the spinal cord segments involved in their reflex arcs include biceps (**C5**, 6); brachioradialis (C5, **6**); triceps (**C7**, 8); patellar (**L3**, 4); and Achilles (**S1**, 2). A common grading scale is 0 = absent, 1 = present but diminished, 2 = normal, 3 = hyperactive, and 4 = hyperactive with clonus (repetitive rhythmic contractions with maintained stretch). The plantar reflex should be tested by using a blunt-ended object such as the point of a key to stroke the outer border of the sole of the foot from the heel toward the base of the great toe. An abnormal response (Babinski sign) is extension (dorsiflexion) of the great toe at the metatarsophalangeal joint. In some cases this may be associated with abduction (fanning) of other toes and variable degrees of flexion at ankle, knee, and hip. Normal response is plantar flexion of the toes. Abdominal, anal, and sphincteric reflexes are important in certain situations, as are additional muscle-stretch reflexes.

SENSORY EXAM

- *The bare minimum: Ask whether the pt can feel light touch and the temperature of a cool object in each distal extremity. Check double simultaneous stimulation using light touch on the hands.*

For most purposes it is sufficient to test sensation to pinprick, touch, position, and vibration in each of the four extremities (Figs. 183-1 and 183-2). Specific problems often require more thorough evaluation. Patients with cerebral lesions may have abnormalities in "discriminative sensation" such as the ability to perceive double simultaneous stimuli, to localize stimuli accurately, to identify closely approximated stimuli as separate (two-point discrimination), to identify objects by touch alone (stereognosis), or to judge weights, evaluate texture, or identify letters or numbers written on the skin surface (graphesthesia).

COORDINATION AND GAIT

- *The bare minimum: Test rapid alternating movements of the fingers and feet, and the finger-to-nose maneuver. Observe the patient while he or she is walking along a straight line.*

The ability to move the index finger accurately from the nose to the examiner's outstretched finger and the ability to slide the heel of each foot from the knee down the shin are tests of coordination. Additional tests (drawing objects in the air, following a moving finger, tapping with index finger against thumb or alternately against each individual finger) may also be useful. The ability to stand with feet together and eyes closed (Romberg test), to walk a straight line (tandem walk), and to turn should all be observed.

For a more detailed discussion, see Martin JB, Lowenstein DH, Hauser SL: Approach to the Patient with Neurologic Disease, Chap. 346, p. 2344, in HPIM-16.

184

NEUROIMAGING

The clinician caring for pts with neurologic symptoms is faced with an expanding number of imaging options. Magnetic resonance imaging (MRI) is more sensitive than computed tomography (CT) for the detection of lesions affecting the central nervous system (CNS), particularly those of the spinal cord, cranial nerves, and posterior fossa structures. Diffusion MR, a sequence that detects reduction of microscopic motion of water, is the most sensitive technique for detecting acute ischemic stroke and is useful in the detection of encephalitis, abscesses, and prion diseases. CT, however, can be quickly obtained and is

Table 184-1

Guidelines for the Use of CT, Ultrasound, and MRI

Condition	Recommended Technique
Hemorrhage	
Acute parenchymal	CT > MR
Subacute/chronic	MRI
Subarachnoid hemorrhage	CT, CTA, lumbar puncture → angiography
Aneurysm	Angiography > CTA, MRA
Ischemic infarction	
Hemorrhagic infarction	CT
Bland infarction	MRI > CT
Carotid or vertebral dissection	MRI/MRA
Vertebral basilar insufficiency	CTA, MRI/MRA
Carotid stenosis	CTA > Doppler ultrasound, MRA
Suspected mass lesion	
Neoplasm, primary or metastatic	MRI + contrast
Infection/abscess	MRI + contrast
Immunosuppression with focal findings	MRI + contrast
Vascular malformation	MRI +/− angiography
White matter disorders	MRI
Demyelinating disease	MRI +/− contrast
Dementia	MRI
Trauma	
Acute trauma	CT (noncontrast)
Shear injury/chronic hemorrhage	MRI
Headache/migraine	CT (noncontrast) / MRI
Seizure	
First time, no focal neurologic deficits	?CT as screen
Partial complex/refractory	MRI with coronal T2W imaging
Cranial neuropathy	MRI with contrast
Meningeal disease	MRI with contrast
SPINE	
Low back pain	
No neurologic deficits	MRI or CT after 4 weeks
With focal deficits	MRI > CT
Spinal stenosis	MRI or CT
Cervical spondylosis	MRI or CT myelography
Infection	MRI + contrast, CT
Myelopathy	MRI + contrast > myelography
Arteriovenous malformation	MRI, myelography/angiography

Note: CT, computed tomography; MRI, magnetic resonance imaging; MRA, MR angiography; CTA, CT angiography; T2W, T2-weighted.

widely available, making it a pragmatic choice for the initial evaluation of pts with suspected acute stroke, hemorrhage, and intracranial or spinal trauma. CT is also more sensitive than MRI for visualizing fine osseous detail and is indicated in the initial evaluation of conductive hearing loss as well as lesions affecting the skull base and calvarium. Myelography has been largely replaced by MRI and CT-myelography for diagnosis of disease of the spinal cord and canal. Conventional angiography is now reserved for patients in whom small-vessel detail is essential for diagnosis or for whom interventional therapies are planned. An increasing number of interventional neuroradiologic techniques are also available including embolization and stenting of vascular structures. Guidelines for initial selection of neuroimaging studies are shown in Table 184-1.

For a more detailed discussion, see Dillon WP: Neuroimaging in Neurologic Disorders, Chap. 347, p. 2350, in HPIM-16.

185

SEIZURES AND EPILEPSY

A seizure is a paroxysmal event due to abnormal, excessive, hypersynchronous discharges from an aggregate of CNS neurons. Epilepsy is diagnosed when there are recurrent seizures due to a chronic, underlying process.

Seizure Classification

Proper seizure classification is essential for diagnosis, therapy, and prognosis. *Partial* (or *focal*) *seizures* originate in localized area of cortex; *generalized seizures* involve diffuse regions of the brain in a bilaterally symmetric fashion. *Simple-partial seizures* do not affect consciousness and may have motor, sensory, autonomic, or psychic symptoms. *Complex-partial seizures* include alteration in consciousness coupled with automatisms (e.g., lip smacking, chewing, aimless walking, or other complex motor activities).

Generalized seizures may occur as a primary disorder or result from secondary generalization of a partial seizure. *Tonic-clonic seizures* (grand mal) cause sudden loss of consciousness, loss of postural control, tonic muscular contraction producing teeth-clenching and rigidity in extension (tonic phase), followed by rhythmic muscular jerking (clonic phase). Tongue-biting and incontinence may occur during the seizure. Recovery of consciousness is typically gradual over many minutes to hours. Headache and confusion are common postictal phenomena. In *absence seizures* (petit mal) there is sudden, brief impairment of consciousness without loss of postural control. Events rarely last longer than 5–10 s but can recur many times per day. Minor motor symptoms are common, while complex automatisms and clonic activity are not. Other types of generalized seizures include atypical absence, infantile spasms, and tonic, atonic, and myoclonic seizures.

Etiology

Seizure type and age of pt provide important clues to etiology. Causes of seizures by age group are shown in Table 185-1.

Table 185-1

The Causes of Seizures

Neonates (<1 month)	Perinatal hypoxia and ischemia Intracranial hemorrhage and trauma Acute CNS infection Metabolic disturbances (hypoglycemia, hypocal- cemia, hypomagnesemia, pyridoxine deficiency) Drug withdrawal Developmental disorders Genetic disorders
Infants and children (>1 mo and <12 years)	Febrile seizures Genetic disorders (metabolic, degenerative, primary epilepsy syndromes) CNS infection Developmental disorders Trauma Idiopathic
Adolescents (12–18 years)	Trauma Genetic disorders Infection Brain tumor Illicit drug use Idiopathic
Young adults (18–35 years)	Trauma Alcohol withdrawal Illicit drug use Brain tumor Idiopathic
Older adults (>35 years)	Cerebrovascular disease Brain tumor Alcohol withdrawal Metabolic disorders (uremia, hepatic failure, electrolyte abnormalities, hypoglycemia) Alzheimer's disease and other degenerative CNS diseases Idiopathic

Clinical Evaluation

Careful history is essential since diagnosis of seizures and epilepsy is often based solely on clinical grounds. Differential diagnosis (Table 185-2) includes syncope or psychogenic seizures (pseudoseizures). General exam includes search for infection, trauma, toxins, systemic illness, neurocutaneous abnormalities, and vascular disease. A number of drugs lower the seizure threshold (Table 185-3). Asymmetries in neurologic exam suggest brain tumor, stroke, trauma, or other focal lesions. An algorithmic approach is illustrated in Fig. 185-1.

Electroencephalography

All pts should be evaluated with an EEG, which measures electrical activity of the brain by recording from electrodes placed on the scalp. The presence of electrographic seizure activity during the clinically evident event, i.e., abnormal,

Table 185-2

The Differential Diagnosis of Seizures

Syncope	Transient ischemic attack (TIA)
Vasovagal syncope	Basilar artery TIA
Cardiac arrhythmia	Sleep disorders
Valvular heart disease	Narcolepsy/cataplexy
Cardiac failure	Benign sleep myoclonus
Orthostatic hypotension	Movement disorders
Psychological disorders	Tics
Psychogenic seizure	Nonepileptic myoclonus
Hyperventilation	Paroxysmal choreoathetosis
Panic attack	Special considerations in children
Metabolic disturbances	Breath-holding spells
Alcoholic blackouts	Migraine with recurrent abdom-
Delirium tremens	inal pain and cyclic vomiting
Hypoglycemia	Benign paroxysmal vertigo
Hypoxia	Apnea
Psychoactive drugs (e.g.,	Night terrors
hallucinogens)	Sleepwalking
Migraine	
Confusional migraine	
Basilar migraine	

repetitive, rhythmic activity having an abrupt onset and termination, establishes the diagnosis. The absence of electrographic seizure activity does not exclude a seizure disorder, however. The EEG is always abnormal during generalized tonic-clonic seizures. Continuous monitoring for prolonged periods may be required to capture the EEG abnormalities. The EEG can show abnormal discharges during the interictal period that support the diagnosis of epilepsy, and is useful for classifying seizure disorders and determining prognosis.

Table 185-3

Drugs and Other Substances That Can Cause Seizures

Antimicrobials/antivirals	Psychotropics
β-lactam and related compounds	Antidepressants
Quinolones	Antipsychotics
Acyclovir	Lithium
Isoniazid	Radiographic contrast agents
Ganciclovir	Theophylline
Anesthetics and analgesics	Sedative-hypnotic drug withdrawal
Meperidine	Alcohol
Tramadol	Barbiturates
Local anesthetics	Benzodiazepines
Class 1B agents	Drugs of abuse
Immunomodulatory drugs	Amphetamine
Cyclosporine	Cocaine
OKT3	Phencyclidine
Tacrolimus (FK-506)	Methylphenidate
Interferons	Flumazenil[a]

[a] In benzodiazepine-dependent patients.

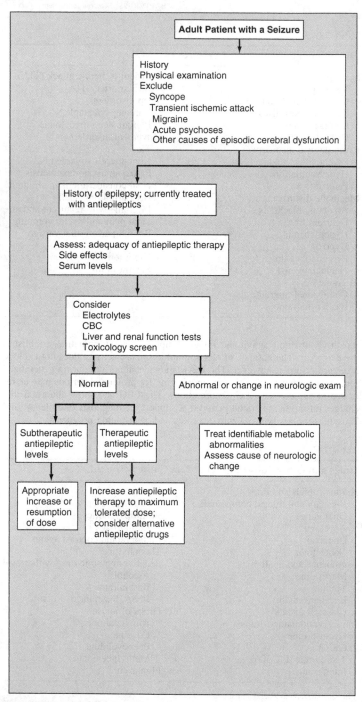

FIGURE 185-1 Evaluation of the adult pt with a seizure.

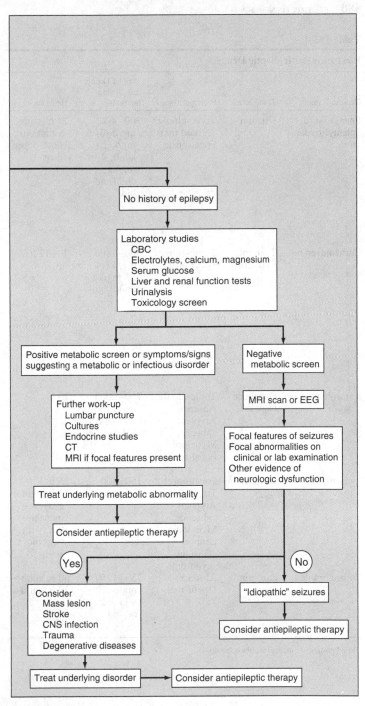

No history of epilepsy

Laboratory studies
- CBC
- Electrolytes, calcium, magnesium
- Serum glucose
- Liver and renal function tests
- Urinalysis
- Toxicology screen

Positive metabolic screen or symptoms/signs suggesting a metabolic or infectious disorder

Negative metabolic screen

Further work-up
- Lumbar puncture
- Cultures
- Endocrine studies
- CT
- MRI if focal features present

MRI scan or EEG

Treat underlying metabolic abnormality

Focal features of seizures
Focal abnormalities on clinical or lab examination
Other evidence of neurologic dysfunction

Consider antiepileptic therapy

Yes   No

Consider
- Mass lesion
- Stroke
- CNS infection
- Trauma
- Degenerative diseases

"Idiopathic" seizures

Consider antiepileptic therapy

Treat underlying disorder → Consider antiepileptic therapy

FIGURE 185-1 *(continued)*

Table 185-4

First-Line Antiepileptic Drugs

Generic Name	Trade Name	Principal Uses	Typical Dosage and Dosing Intervals	Half-Life
Phenytoin (di-phenyl-hydan-toin	Dilantin	Tonic-clonic (grand mal) Focal-onset	300–400 mg/d (3–6 mg/kg, adult; 4–8 mg/kg, child) qd-bid	24 h (wide variation, dose-depen-dent)
Carbamazepine	Tegretol Carbatrol	Tonic-clonic Focal-onset	600–1800 mg/d (15–35 mg/kg, child) bid-qid	10–17 h
Valproic acid	Depakene Depakote	Tonic-clonic Absence Atypical absence Myoclonic Focal-onset	750–2000 mg/d (20–60 mg/kg) bid-qid	15 h
Lamotrigine	Lamictal	Focal-onset Tonic-clonic Atypical absence Myoclonic Lennox-Gastaut syndrome	150–500 mg/d bid	25 h 14 h (with enzyme-inducers) 59 h (with valproic acid)
Ethosuximide	Zarontin	Absence (petit mal)	750–1250 mg/d (20–40 mg/kg) qd-bid	60 h, adult 30 h, child

[a] Phenytoin, carbamazepine, phenobarbital

Therapeutic Range	Adverse Effects		Drug Interactions
	Neurologic	Systemic	
10–20 μg/mL	Dizziness Diplopia Ataxia Incoordination Confusion	Gum hyperplasia Lymphadenopathy Hirsutism Osteomalacia Facial coarsening Skin rash	Level increased by isoniazid, sulfonamides, fluoxetine Level decreased by enzyme-inducing drugs[a] Altered folate metabolism
6–12 μg/mL	Ataxia Dizziness Diplopia Vertigo	Aplastic anemia Leukopenia Gastrointestinal irritation Hepatotoxicity Hyponatremia	Level decreased by enzyme-inducing drugs[a] Level increased by erythromycin, propoxyphene, isoniazid, cimetidine, fluoxetine
50–150 μg/mL	Ataxia Sedation Tremor	Hepatotoxicity Thrombocytopenia Gastrointestinal irritation Weight gain Transient alopecia Hyperammonemia	Level decreased by enzyme-inducing drugs[a]
Not established	Dizziness Diplopia Sedation Ataxia Headache	Skin rash Stevens-Johnson syndrome	Level decreased by enzyme-inducing drugs[a] Level increased by valproic acid
40–100 μg/mL	Ataxia Lethargy Headache	Gastrointestinal irritation Skin rash Bone marrow suppression	

Table 185-5

Selection of Antiepileptic Drugs

	Primary Generalized Tonic-Clonic	Partial[a]	Absence	Atypical Absence, Myoclonic, Atonic
First-Line	Valproic acid Lamotrigine	Carbamazepine Phenytoin Lamotrigine Valproic acid	Valproic acid Ethosuximide	Valproic acid
Alternatives	Phenytoin Carbamazepine Topiramate[b] Zonisamide[b] Felbamate Primidone Phenobarbital	Topiramate[b] Levetiracetam[b] Tiagabine[b] Zonisamide[b] Gabapentin[b] Primidone Phenobarbital	Lamotrigine Clonazepam	Lamotrigine Topiramate[b] Clonazepam Felbamate

[a] Includes simple partial, complex partial, and secondarily generalized seizures.
[b] As adjunctive therapy.

Brain Imaging

All patients with unexplained new-onset seizures should have a brain imaging study (MRI or CT) to search for an underlying structural abnormality. Newer MRI methods, such as fluid-attenuated inversion recovery (FLAIR), have increased the sensitivity for detection of abnormalities of cortical architecture, including hippocampal atrophy associated with mesial temporal sclerosis, and abnormalities of neuronal migration.

 TREATMENT

Acutely, the pt should be placed in semiprone position with head to the side to avoid aspiration. Tongue blades or other objects should not be forced between clenched teeth. Oxygen should be given via face mask. Reversible metabolic disorders (e. g., hypoglycemia, hyponatremia, hypocalcemia, drug or alcohol withdrawal) should be promptly corrected. Treatment of status epilepticus is discussed in Chap. 22.

Longer-term therapy includes treatment of underlying conditions, avoidance of precipitating factors, prophylactic therapy with antiepileptic medications or surgery, and addressing various psychological and social issues. Choice of antiepileptic drug therapy depends on a variety of factors including seizure type, dosing schedule, and potential side effects (Tables 185-4 and 185-5). Therapeutic goal is complete cessation of seizures without side effects using a single drug (monotherapy). If ineffective, medication should be increased to maximal tolerated dose based primarily on clinical response rather than serum levels. If unsuccessful, a second drug should be added, and when control is obtained, the first drug can be slowly tapered. Approximately one-third of pts will require polytherapy with two or more drugs. Pts with certain epilepsy syndromes (e.g., temporal lobe epilepsy) are often refractory to medical therapy and benefit from surgical excision of the seizure focus.

For a more detailed discussion, see Lowenstein DH: Seizures and Epilepsy, Chap. 348, p. 2357, in HPIM-16.

186

TUMORS OF THE NERVOUS SYSTEM

Approach to the Patient

Clinical Presentation Brain tumors present with (1) progressive focal neurologic deficits, (2) seizures, or (3) "nonfocal" neurologic disorders (headache, dementia, personality change, gait disorder). Nonfocal disorders due to increased intracranial pressure (ICP), hydrocephalus, or diffuse tumor spread. Elevated ICP suggested by papilledema, impaired lateral gaze, headache that intensifies with recumbency. Strokelike onset may reflect hemorrhage into tumor. Brain tumors may be large at presentation if located in clinically silent region (i.e., prefrontal) or slow-growing; diencephalic, frontal, or temporal lobe tumors may present as psychiatric disorder. Systemic symptoms (malaise, anorexia, weight loss, fever) suggest metastatic rather than primary brain tumor.

Evaluation Primary brain tumors have no serologic features of malignancy such as an elevated ESR or tumor-specific antigens, unlike metastases. Neuroimaging (CT or MRI) reveals mass effect (volume of neoplasm and surrounding edema) and contrast enhancement (breakdown of blood-brain barrier). CSF exam is limited to diagnosis of possible meningitis or meningeal metastases but may cause brain herniation if mass effect or hydrocephalus present.

TREATMENT

Symptomatic Treatment Glucocorticoids (dexamethasone 12–20 mg/d in divided doses) to temporarily reduce edema; prophylaxis with anticonvulsants (phenytoin, carbamazepine, or valproic acid) for tumors involving cortex or hippocampus. Low-dose subcutaneous heparin for immobile pts.

Primary Intracranial Tumors

Astrocytomas Most common primary intracranial neoplasm. Only known risk factors are ionizing radiation and uncommon hereditary syndromes (neurofibromatosis, tuberous sclerosis). Prognosis poor if age >65 years, poor baseline functional status, high-grade tumor. Difficult to treat; infiltration along white matter pathways prevents total resection. Imaging studies fail to indicate full tumor extent. Surgery for tissue diagnosis and to control mass effect. Mean survival ranges from 93 months for low-grade tumors to 12 months for high-grade tumors. Radiation therapy (RT) prolongs survival and improves quality of life. Systemic chemotherapy with nitrosoureas is only marginally effective, often employed as adjunct to RT for high-grade gliomas. Role of stereotaxic radiosurgery (single dose, highly focused radiation—gamma knife) unclear; most useful for tumors <4 cm in diameter. Interstitial brachytherapy (stereotaxic implantation of radioactive beads) reserved for tumor recurrence; associated with necrosis of normal brain tissue. For low-grade astrocytoma, optimal management is uncertain; resection with or without RT most often employed.

Oligodendrogliomas Supratentorial; mixture of astrocytic and oligodendroglial cells. As oligodendroglial component increases, so does long-term survival; 5-year survival >50%. Total surgical resection often possible; chemotherapy response when deletions of chromosomes 1p and 19q present.

Ependymomas Derived from ependymal cells; highly cellular. Location— spinal canal in adults. If histologically aggressive (cellular atypia, frequent mitotic figures), recurrence is certain. If total excision possible, 5-year disease-free survival >80%; postoperative RT used if complete excision not possible.

Germinomas Tumors of midline brain structures; onset in second decade. Neuroimaging—uniformly enhancing mass. Complete surgical excision results in 5-year survival >85%. Radiosensitive and chemosensitive.

Primitive Neuro-Ectodermal Tumors (PNET) Half in posterior fossa; highly cellular; derived from neural precursor cells. Treat with surgery, chemotherapy, and RT.

Primary CNS Lymphomas B cell malignancy; most occur in immunosuppressed pts (organ transplantation, AIDS). May present as a single mass lesion (immunocompetent pts) or as multiple mass lesions or meningeal disease (immunosuppressed pts). Slit-lamp exam necessary to exclude ocular involvement. Prognosis generally poor. Dramatic, transient responses occur with glucocorticoids. In immunocompetent pts, RT, chemotherapy (methotrexate and cytarabine), and RT may increase survival to ≥18 months; AIDS-related cases survive ≤3 months.

Meningiomas Extraaxial mass attached to dura; dense and uniform contrast enhancement is diagnostic. Total surgical resection of benign meningiomas is curative. With subtotal resection, local RT reduces recurrence to <10%. Small, asymptomatic meningiomas may be followed radiologically without surgery. Treat rare aggressive meningiomas with excision and RT.

Schwannomas Vestibular schwannomas present as progressive, unexplained unilateral hearing loss. MRI reveals dense, uniformly enhancing tumor at the cerebellopontine angle. Surgical excision may preserve hearing.

Tumors Metastatic to the Nervous System

Hematogenous spread most common. Skull metastases rarely invade CNS; may compress adjacent brain or cranial nerves or obstruct intracranial venous sinuses. Primary tumors that commonly metastasize to the nervous system are listed in Table 186-1. Brain metastases are well demarcated by MRI and enhance with gadolinium; triple-dose contrast is most sensitive for detection; ring enhancement is nonspecific. Differential diagnosis includes brain abscess, radiation necrosis, toxoplasmosis, granulomas, demyelinating lesions, primary brain tumors, CNS lymphoma, stroke, hemorrhage, and trauma. CSF cytology is unnecessary—intraparenchymal metastases rarely shed cells into CSF. One-third of pts presenting with brain metastasis have unknown primary (ultimately small cell lung cancer, melanoma most frequent); primary tumor never identified in 30%. Screen for occult cancer: examine skin and thyroid gland; blood carcinoembryonic antigen (CEA) and liver function tests; CT of chest, abdomen, and pelvis. Further imaging studies unhelpful if above studies negative. Biopsy of primary tumor or accessible brain metastasis is needed to plan treatment. Treatment is palliative—glucocorticoids, anticonvulsants, or RT may improve qual-

Table 186-1

Origin of Metastases to the Nervous System by Primary Tumors

Site of Primary Tumor	Brain Metastases, %	Leptomeningeal Metastases, %	Spinal Cord Compression, %
Lung	40	24	18
Breast	19	41	24
Melanoma	10	12	4
Gastrointestinal tract	7	13	6
Genitourinary tract	7		18
Other	17	10	30

ity of life. Whole-brain RT is given, because multiple microscopic tumor deposits are likely throughout the brain. If a single metastasis is found, it may be surgically excised followed by whole-brain RT. Systemic chemotherapy may produce dramatic responses in isolated cases.

Leptomeningeal Metastases Presents as headache, encephalopathy, cranial nerve or polyradicular symptoms. Diagnosis by CSF cytology, MRI (nodular meningeal tumor deposits or diffuse meningeal enhancement), or meningeal biopsy. Associated with hydrocephalus due to CSF pathway obstruction. Aggressive treatment (intrathecal methotrexate, focal external beam RT) produces sustained response (~6 months) in 20% of pts.

Spinal Cord Compression from Metastases (See Chap. 196) Expansion of vertebral body metastasis posteriorly into epidural space compresses cord. Most common is lung, breast, or prostate primary. Back pain (>90%) precedes development of weakness, sensory level, or incontinence. Medical emergency; early recognition of impending spinal cord compression essential to avoid devastating sequelae. Diagnosis is by spine MRI. Progression may be slowed by administration of glucocorticoids while awaiting surgery or RT.

Complications of Radiation Therapy

Three patterns of radiation injury after CNS RT:

1. Acute—headache, sleepiness, worse neurologic deficits during or immediately after RT. Self-limited and glucocorticoid-responsive.
2. Early delayed—somnolence (children), Lhermitte's sign; within 4 months of RT. Increased T2 signal on MRI. Also self-limited and improves with glucocorticoids.
3. Late delayed—dementia or other progressive neurologic deficits; typically >1 year after RT. White matter abnormalities on MRI; ring-enhancing mass due to radiation necrosis. Positron emission tomography (PET) distinguishes delayed necrosis from tumor recurrence. Progressive radiation necrosis is best treated palliatively with surgical resection. Endocrine dysfunction due to hypothalamus or pituitary gland injury can be due to delayed effects of RT.

For a more detailed discussion, see Sagar SM, Israel MA: Primary and Metastic Tumors of the Nervous System, Chap. 358, p. 2452, in HPIM-16.

187

ACUTE MENINGITIS AND ENCEPHALITIS

Acute infections of the nervous system include bacterial meningitis, viral meningitis, encephalitis, focal infections such as brain abscess and subdural empyema, and infectious thrombophlebitis. Key goals: emergently distinguish between these conditions, identify the pathogen, and initiate appropriate antimicrobial therapy.

_____ *Approach to the Patient* _____

(Fig. 187-1A)   First identify whether infection predominantly involves the subarachnoid space (*meningitis*) or brain tissue (*encephalitis*). Nuchal rigidity is the pathognomonic sign of meningeal irritation and is present when the neck resists passive flexion. Principles of management: (1) Initiate empirical therapy whenever bacterial meningitis is considered. (2) All pts with head trauma, immunocompromised states, known malignancies, or focal neurologic findings (including papilledema or stupor/coma) should undergo a neuroimaging study of the brain prior to LP. If bacterial meningitis is suspected, begin empirical antibiotic therapy prior to neuroimaging and LP. (3) Stupor/coma, seizures, or focal neurologic deficits only rarely occur in viral ("aseptic") meningitis; pts with these symptoms should be hospitalized and treated empirically for bacterial and viral meningoencephalitis. (4) Immunocompetent pts with a normal level of consciousness, no prior antimicrobial treatment, and a CSF profile consistent with viral meningitis (lymphocytic pleocytosis and a normal glucose concentration) can often be treated as outpatients. Failure of a pt with suspected viral meningitis to improve within 48 h should prompt a reevaluation.

_____

ACUTE BACTERIAL MENINGITIS

Pathogens most frequently involved in immunocompetent adults are *Streptococcus pneumoniae* ("pneumococcus") and *Neisseria meningitidis* ("meningococcus"). Predisposing factors for pneumococcal meningitis include infection (otitis, sinusitis, pneumonia, endocarditis), asplenia, sickle cell disease, hypogammaglobulinemia, multiple myeloma, alcoholism, cirrhosis, and head trauma with CSF leak. Pts with deficiency of complement components, including properdin, are highly susceptible to meningococcal infection, which may also occur in epidemics. *Listeria monocytogenes* is an important consideration in pregnant women, individuals >60 years, alcoholics, and immunocompromised individuals of all ages. Enteric gram-negative bacilli and group B streptococcus are increasingly common causes of meningitis in individuals with chronic medical conditions. *Staphylococcus aureus* and coagulase-negative staphylococci are important causes following invasive neurosurgical procedures.

   CLINICAL MANIFESTATIONS   Presents as an acute fulminant illness that progresses rapidly in a few hours or as a subacute infection that progressively worsens over several days. The classic clinical triad of meningitis is fever, headache, and nuchal rigidity ("stiff neck"). Each occurs in >90% of cases. Alteration in mental status occurs in >75% of pts and can vary from lethargy to coma. Nausea, vomiting, and photophobia are also common. Seizures occur in 20 to 40% of pts. Raised intracranial pressure (ICP) is the major cause of obtundation and coma. The rash of meningococcemia begins as a diffuse maculopapular rash resembling a viral exanthem but rapidly becomes petechial on trunk and lower extremities, mucous membranes and conjunctiva, and occasionally palms and soles.

LABORATORY FINDINGS The CSF profile is shown in Table 187-1. CSF bacterial cultures are positive in >80% of pts, and CSF Gram stain demonstrates organisms in >60%. The latex agglutination (LA) test for detection of bacterial antigens of *S. pneumoniae, N. meningitidis, Haemophilus influenzae* type b, group B streptococcus, and *Escherichia coli* K1 strains in the CSF is very useful for rapid diagnosis, especially in pts pretreated with antibiotics and when the CSF Gram stain and culture are negative. The Limulus amebocyte lysate assay rapidly detects gram-negative endotoxin in CSF and thus is useful in diagnosis of gram-negative bacterial meningitis; false-positives may occur. Petechial skin lesions, if present, should be biopsied. Blood cultures should always be obtained.

DIFFERENTIAL DIAGNOSIS Includes viral meningoencephalitis, especially herpes simplex virus encephalitis (see below); rickettsial diseases such as Rocky Mountain spotted fever (immunofluorescent staining of skin lesions); focal suppurative CNS infections including subdural empyema and brain abscess (see below); subarachnoid hemorrhage (Chap. 19); and the demyelinating disease acute disseminated encephalomyelitis (Chap. 189).

℞ TREATMENT

Recommendations for empirical therapy are summarized in Table 187-2. Therapy is then modified based on results of CSF culture (Table 187-3). In general, the treatment course is 7 days for meningococcus, 14 days for pneumococcus, 21 days for gram-negative meningitis, and at least 21 days for *L. monocytogenes*.

Adjunctive therapy with dexamethasone (10 mg IV), administered 15 to 20 min before the first dose of an antimicrobial agent and repeated every 6 h for 4 days, improves outcome from bacterial meningitis. Dexamethasone may decrease the penetration of vancomycin into CSF, and thus its potential benefit should be carefully weighed when vancomycin is the antibiotic of choice.

In meningococcal meningitis, all close contacts should receive prophylaxis with rifampin [600 mg in adults (10 mg/kg in children > 1 year)] q12h for 2 d; rifampin is not recommended in pregnant women. Alternatively, adults can

Table 187-1

Cerebrospinal Fluid (CSF) Abnormalities in Bacterial Meningitis

Opening pressure	>180 mmH$_2$O
White blood cells	10/μL to 10,000/μL; neutrophils predominate
Red blood cells	Absent in nontraumatic tap
Glucose	<2.2 mmol/L (<40 mg/dL)
CSF/serum glucose	<0.4
Protein	>0.45 g/L (>45 mg/dL)
Gram's stain	Positive in >60%
Culture	Positive in >80%
Latex agglutination	May be positive in patients with meningitis due to *S. pneumoniae, N. meningitidis, H. influenzae* type b, *E. coli*, group B streptococci
Limulus lysates	Positive in cases of gram-negative meningitis
PCR for bacterial DNA	Research test

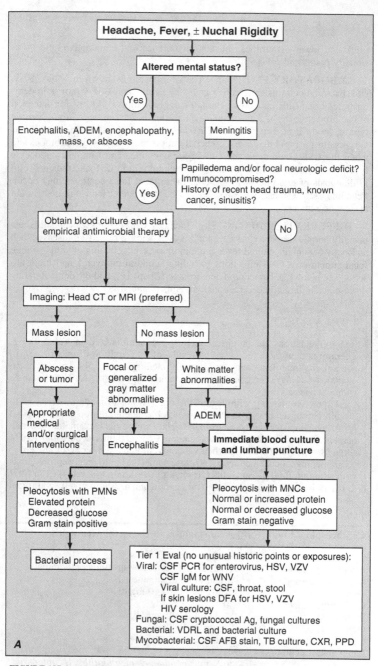

FIGURE 187-1 Algorithm for management of patients with suspected CNS infections. ADEM, acute disseminated encephalomyelitis; PMNs, polymorphonuclear leukocytes; MNCs, mononuclear cells; HSV, herpes simplex virus; VZV, varicella-zoster virus; WNV, West Nile Virus; DFA, direct fluorescent antibody; Ag, antigen; VDRL, Venereal Disease Research Laboratory; AFB, acid-fast bacillus; TB, tuberculosis; PPD, purified protein derivative; CTFV, Colorado tick fever virus; HHV, human herpesvirus; LCMV, lymphocytic choriomeningitis virus.

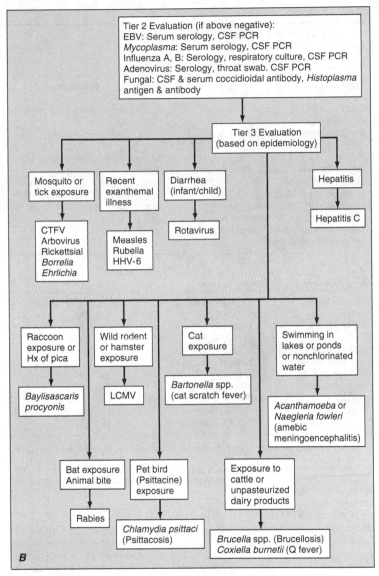

FIGURE 187-1 *(continued)*

be treated with one dose of ciprofloxacin (750 mg), one dose of azithromycin (500 mg), or one IM dose of ceftriaxone (250 mg).

PROGNOSIS Moderate or severe sequelae occur in ~25% of survivors; outcome varies with the infecting organism. Common sequelae include decreased intellectual function, memory impairment, seizures, hearing loss and dizziness, and gait disturbances.

Table 187-2

Antibiotics Used in Empirical Therapy of Bacterial Meningitis and Focal CNS Infections[a]

Indication	Antibiotic
Preterm infants to infants <1 month	Ampicillin + cefotaxime
Infants 1–3 mos	Ampicillin + cefotaxime or ceftriaxone
Immunocompetent children > 3 mos and adults <55	Cefotaxime or ceftriaxone + vancomycin
Adults > 55 and adults of any age with alcoholism or other debilitating illnesses	Ampicillin + cefotaxime or ceftriaxone + vancomycin
Hospital-acquired meningitis, posttraumatic or postneurosurgery meningitis, neutropenic patients, or patients with impaired cell-mediated immunity	Ampicillin + ceftazidime + vancomycin

Antimicrobial Agent	Total Daily Dose and Dosing Interval	
	Child (>1 month)	Adult
Ampicillin	200 (mg/kg)/d, q4h	12 g/d, q4h
Cefepime	150 (mg/kg)/d, q8h	6 g/d, q8h
Cefotaxime	200 (mg/kg)/d, q6h	12 g/d, q4h
Ceftriaxone	100 (mg/kg)/d, q12h	4 g/d, q12h
Ceftazidime	150 (mg/kg)/d, q8h	6 g/d, q8h
Gentamicin	7.5 (mg/kg)/d, q8h[b]	7.5 (mg/kg)/d, q8h
Meropenem	120 (mg/kg)/d, q8h	3 g/d, q8h
Metronidazole	30 (mg/kg)/d, q6h	1500–2000 mg/d, q6h
Nafcillin	100–200 (mg/kg)/d, q6h	9–12 g/d, q4h
Penicillin G	400,000 (U/kg)/d, q4h	20–24 million U/d, q4h
Vancomycin	60 (mg/kg)/d, q6h	2 g/d, q12h[b]

[a] All antibiotics are administered intravenously; doses indicated assume normal renal and hepatic function.

[b] Doses should be adjusted based on serum peak and trough levels: gentamicin therapeutic level: peak: 5–8 μg/mL; trough: <2 μg/mL; vancomycin therapeutic level: peak: 25–40 μg/mL; trough: 5–15 μg/mL.

VIRAL MENINGITIS

Presents as fever, headache, and meningeal irritation associated with a CSF lymphocytic pleocytosis. Fever may be accompanied by malaise, myalgia, anorexia, nausea and vomiting, abdominal pain, and/or diarrhea. A mild degree of lethargy or drowsiness may occur; however, a more profound alteration in consciousness should prompt consideration of alternative diagnoses.

ETIOLOGY Enteroviruses account for 75 to 90% of aseptic meningitis cases (Table 187-4). Viruses belonging to the *Enterovirus* genus include the coxsackieviruses, echoviruses, polioviruses, and human enteroviruses 68 to 71. Other common causes include herpes simplex virus (HSV) type 2, arboviruses, and HIV. The incidence of enteroviral and arboviral infections is greatly increased during the summer (Table 187-5). Using CSF PCR tests, culture, and serology, a specific viral cause can be found in 75 to 90% of cases of viral meningitis.

Table 187-3

Antimicrobial Therapy of CNS Bacterial Infections Based on Pathogen[a]

Organism	Antibiotic
Neisseria meningitides	
Penicillin-sensitive	Penicillin G or Ampicillin
Penicillin-resistant	Ceftriaxone or cefotaxime
Streptococcus pneumoniae	
Penicillin-sensitive	Penicillin G
Penicillin-intermediate	Ceftriaxone or cefotaxime
Penicillin-resistant	(Ceftriaxone or cefotaxime) + vancomycin
Gram-negative bacilli (except *Pseudomonas* spp.)	Ceftriaxone or cefotaxime
Pseudomonas aeruginosa	Ceftazidime
Staphylococci spp.	
Methicillin-sensitive	Nafcillin
Methicillin-resistant	Vancomycin
Listeria monocytogenes	Ampicillin + gentamicin
Haemophilus influenzae	Ceftriaxone or cefotaxime
Streptococcus agalactiae	Penicillin G or Ampicillin
Bacteroides fragilis	Metronidazole
Fusobacterium spp.	Metronidazole

[a] Doses are as indicated in Table 187-2.

Table 187-4

Viruses Causing Acute Meningitis and Acute Encephalitis

Common	Less Common	Rare
ACUTE MENINGITIS		
Enteroviruses	HSV-1	Adenoviruses
Arboviruses	LCMV	CMV
HIV	VZV	EBV
HSV-2		Influenza A, B, parainfluenza, mumps, rubella
ACUTE ENCEPHALITIS		
Arboviruses	CMV	Adenoviruses, CTFV, hepatitis C, influenza A, LCMV, parainfluenza, rabies, rotavirus, rubella
Enteroviruses	EBV	
HSV-1	HIV	
	Mumps	

Note: CTFV, Colorado tick fever virus; HSV, herpes simplex virus; LCMV, lymphocytic choriomeningitis virus; VZV, varicella-zoster virus.

Table 187-5

Seasonal Prevalence of Viruses Commonly Causing Meningitis

Summer/Early Fall	Fall/Winter	Winter/Spring	Nonseasonal
Arboviruses	LCMV	Mumps	HIV
Enteroviruses			HSV

Note: For abbreviations, see Table 187-4.

DIAGNOSIS   Most important test is examination of the CSF. The typical profile is a lymphocytic pleocytosis (25 to 500 cells/μL), a normal or slightly elevated protein concentration [0.2 to 0.8 g/L (20 to 80 mg/dL)], a normal glucose concentration, and a normal or mildly elevated opening pressure (100 to 350 mmH$_2$O). Organisms are *not* seen on Gram or acid-fast stained smears or india ink preparations of CSF. Rarely, polymorphonuclear leukocytes (PMN) predominate in the first 48 h of illness, especially with echovirus 9, West Nile virus (WNV) or Eastern equine encephalitis virus, or mumps. The total CSF cell count in viral meningitis is typically 25 to 500/μL. As a general rule, a lymphocytic pleocytosis with a low glucose concentration should suggest fungal, listerial, or tuberculous meningitis or noninfectious disorders (e.g., sarcoid, neoplastic meningitis).

CSF PCR testing is the procedure of choice for rapid, sensitive, and specific identification of enteroviruses, HSV, EBV, varicella zoster virus (VZV), and CMV. Attempts should also be made to culture virus from CSF and other sites and body fluids including blood, throat swabs, feces, and urine. Serologic studies, including those utilizing paired CSF and serum specimens, may be helpful for retrospective diagnosis; they are particularly important for diagnosis of WNV and other arbovirus etiologies.

DIFFERENTIAL DIAGNOSIS   Consider bacterial, fungal, tuberculous, spirochetal, and other infectious causes of meningitis; parameningeal infections; partially treated bacterial meningitis; neoplastic meningitis; noninfectious inflammatory diseases including sarcoid and Behçet's disease.

 TREATMENT

Supportive or symptomatic therapy is usually sufficient, and hospitalization is not required. The elderly and immunocompromised pts should be hospitalized, as should individuals in whom the diagnosis is uncertain. Severe cases of meningitis due to HSV, EBV, and VZV can be treated with IV acyclovir (10 mg/kg q8h for 7 d); for mildly affected pts, a 1-week course of oral acyclovir (800 mg five times daily), famciclovir (500 mg q8h), or valacyclovir (1000 mg q8h), may be useful. Additional supportive or symptomatic therapy can include analgesics and antipyretics. Prognosis for full recovery is excellent.

VIRAL ENCEPHALITIS

An infection of the brain parenchyma commonly associated with meningitis ("meningoencephalitis"). Clinical features are those of viral meningitis plus evidence of brain tissue involvement, commonly including altered consciousness, seizures, and focal neurologic findings such as aphasia, hemiparesis, involuntary movements, and cranial nerve deficits.

ETIOLOGY   The same organisms responsible for aseptic meningitis are also responsible for encephalitis, although relative frequencies differ. The most common causes of sporadic encephalitis in immunocompetent adults are HSV-1, VZV, and, less commonly, enteroviruses (Table 187-4). HSV encephalitis should be considered when focal findings are present and when involvement of the inferomedial frontotemporal regions of the brain is likely (olfactory hallucinations, anosmia, bizarre behavior, or memory disturbance). Epidemics of encephalitis are usually caused by arboviruses (Table 187-6). WNV has recently produced the largest epidemic of encephalitis ever recorded in the U.S.; prominent motor manifestations, including acute poliomyelitis-like paralysis, may occur with WNV. New causes of viral encephalitis are constantly appearing: a recent outbreak in Malaysia was caused by Nipah virus, a member of the Paramyxovirus family.

Table 187-6

Features of Selected Arbovirus Encephalitides

Feature	WNV	WEE	EEE	VEE	SLE	CE
Region	All	West, midwest	Atlantic and Gulf coasts	SW, W	All	East and NC
Age	Adults > 60	Infants, adults > 50	Children, adults > 60	Adults	Adults > 60	Children
Deaths	7%	3–15%	50–75%	1%	2–20%	<1%
Sequelae	?	Common	80%	Rare	20%	Rare
Vector	M	M	M	M	M	M
Animal reservoir	B	B	B	H, sm M	B	sm M

Note: WNV, West Nile virus; WEE, Western equine encephalitis (virus); EEE, Eastern equine encephalitis (virus); VEE, Venezuelan equine encephalitis (virus); SLE, St. Louis encephalitis; CE, California encephalitis (virus); B, bird; H, horse; M, mosquito; NC, north central United States; sm M, small mammal; SW, southwest; W, west.

DIAGNOSIS CSF studies are essential; typical CSF profile is similar to viral meningitis. CSF PCR tests allow for rapid and reliable diagnosis of HSV, EBV, VZV, CMV, and enteroviruses. CSF virus cultures are generally negative. Serologic studies also have a role for some viruses. In HSV encephalitis, antibodies to HSV-1 antigens can be detected in the CSF after the first week of illness, limiting utility of these tests in acute diagnosis. Demonstration of WNV IgM antibodies is diagnostic of WNV encephalitis. For VZV, CSF antibody and PCR studies are complementary.

MRI is the neuroimaging procedure of choice and demonstrates areas of increased T2 signal. Bitemporal and orbitofrontal areas of increased signal are seen in HSV encephalitis but are not diagnostic. The EEG may suggest seizures or show temporally predominant periodic spikes on a slow, low-amplitude background suggestive of HSV encephalitis.

Brain biopsy is now used only when CSF PCR studies fail to identify the cause, focal abnormalities on MRI are present, and progressive clinical deterioration occurs despite treatment with acyclovir and supportive therapy.

DIFFERENTIAL DIAGNOSIS Includes both infectious and noninfectious causes of encephalitis, including vascular diseases; abscess and empyema; fungal (*Cryptococcus* and *Mucor*), spirochetal (*Leptospira*), rickettsial, bacterial (*Listeria*), tuberculous, and mycoplasma infections; tumors; toxic encephalopathy; SLE; and acute disseminated encephalomyelitis.

 TREATMENT

All pts with suspected HSV encephalitis should be treated with IV acyclovir (10 mg/kg q8h). Pts with a PCR-confirmed diagnosis of HSV encephalitis should receive a 14-day course of therapy. Consider repeat CSF PCR after completion of acyclovir therapy; pts with a persistently positive CSF PCR for HSV after completing a standard course of acyclovir therapy should be treated for an additional 7 days, followed by a repeat CSF PCR test. Acyclovir treatment may also benefit encephalitis due to EBV and VZV. No therapy currently available for enteroviral, mumps, or measles encephalitis. Intravenous ribovarin [15–25 (mg/kg)/d given in 3 divided doses] may benefit severe arbovirus encephalitis due to California encephalitis (LaCrosse) virus. CMV encephalitis should be treated with ganciclovir, foscarnet, or a combination of the two drugs; cidofovir may provide an alternative for nonresponders. No proven therapy is available for WNV encephalitis; small groups of pts have been treated with interferon, ribavarin, and IVIg preparations of non-U.S. origin containing high titer anti-WNV antibody.

PROGNOSIS In HSV encephalitis treated with acyclovir, 81% survival in one series; neurologic sequelae were mild or absent in 46%, moderate in 12%, and severe in 42%.

BRAIN ABSCESS

A focal, suppurative infection within the brain parenchyma, typically surrounded by a vascularized capsule. The term *cerebritis* is used to describe a nonencapsulated brain abscess. Predisposing conditions include otitis media and mastoiditis, paranasal sinusitis, pyogenic infections in the chest or other body sites, head trauma or neurosurgical procedures, and dental infections. In most modern series, many brain abscesses occur in immunocompromised hosts and are caused less often by bacteria than by fungi and parasites including *Toxoplasma gondii*, *Aspergillus* spp., *Nocardia* spp., *Mycobacteria* spp., and *Cryptococcus neoformans*. In Latin America and in immigrants from Latin America, the most common cause of brain abscess is *Taenia solium* (neurocysticercosis). In India and the Far East, mycobacterial infection (tuberculoma) remains a major cause of focal CNS mass lesions.

CLINICAL PRESENTATION Brain abscess typically presents as an expanding intracranial mass lesion, rather than as an infectious process. The classic triad of headache, fever, and a focal neurologic deficit is present in <50% of cases.

DIAGNOSIS MRI is better than CT for demonstrating abscesses in the early (cerebritis) stages and is superior to CT for identifying abscesses in the posterior fossa. A mature brain abscess appears on CT as a focal area of hypodensity surrounded by ring enhancement. The CT and MRI appearance may be altered by treatment with glucocorticoids. The distinction between a brain abscess and other focal lesions such as tumors may be facilitated with diffusion-weighted imaging (DWI) sequences in which brain abscesses typically show increased signal and low apparent diffusion coefficient.

Microbiologic diagnosis best determined by Gram stain and culture of abscess material obtained by stereotactic needle aspiration. Up to 10% of patients will also have positive blood cultures. CSF analysis contributes nothing to diagnosis or therapy, and LP increases the risk of herniation.

℞ TREATMENT

Optimal therapy involves a combination of high-dose parenteral antibiotics and neurosurgical drainage. Empirical therapy of community-acquired brain abscess in an immunocompetent patient typically includes a third-generation cephalosporin (e.g., cefotaxime or ceftriaxone) and metronidazole (see Table 187-2 for antibiotic dosages). In pts with penetrating head trauma or recent neurosurgical procedures, treatment should include ceftazidime as the third-generation cephalosporin to enhance coverage of *Pseudomonas* spp. and vancomycin for coverage of staphylococci. Meropenem plus vancomycin also provides good coverage in this setting.

Aspiration and drainage essential in most cases. Empirical antibiotic coverage is modified based on the results of Gram stain and culture of the abscess contents. Medical therapy alone is reserved for pts whose abscesses are neurosurgically inaccessible and for cerebritis. All pts should receive a minimum of 6 to 8 weeks of parenteral antibiotic therapy.

PROGNOSIS   In modern series the mortality is typically <15%. Significant sequelae including seizures, persisting weakness, aphasia, or mental impairment occur in ≥20% of survivors.

PROGRESSIVE MULTIFOCAL LEUKOENCEPHALOPATHY (PML)

CLINICAL FEATURES   A progressive disorder characterized pathologically by multifocal areas of demyelination of varying size distributed throughout the CNS. In addition, there are characteristic cytologic alterations in both astrocytes and oligodendrocytes. Pts often present with visual deficits (45%), typically a homonymous hemianopia, and mental impairment (38%) (dementia, confusion, personality change). Motor weakness may not be present early but eventually occurs in 75% of cases. Almost all pts have an underlying immunosuppressive disorder. More than 60% of currently diagnosed PML cases occur in patients with AIDS; it has been estimated that nearly 1% of AIDS patients will develop PML.

DIAGNOSTIC STUDIES   MRI reveals multifocal asymmetric, coalescing white matter lesions located periventricularly, in the centrum semiovale, in the parietal-occipital region, and in the cerebellum. These lesions have increased T2 and decreased T1 signal, are generally nonenhancing or show only minimal peripheral enhancement, and are not associated with edema or mass effect. CT scans, which are less sensitive than MRI for the diagnosis of PML, often show hypodense nonenhancing white matter lesions.

The CSF is typically normal, although mild elevation in protein and/or IgG may be found. Pleocytosis occurs in <25% of cases, is predominantly mononuclear, and rarely exceeds 25 cells/μL. PCR amplification of JC virus DNA from CSF has become an important diagnostic tool. A positive CSF PCR for JC virus DNA in association with typical MRI lesions in the appropriate clinical setting is diagnostic of PML. Pts with negative CSF PCR studies may require brain biopsy for definitive diagnosis; JC virus antigen and nucleic acid can be detected by immunocytochemistry, in situ hybridization, or PCR amplification. Detection of JC virus antigen or genomic material should be considered diagnostic of PML only if accompanied by characteristic pathologic changes, since both antigen and genomic material have been found in the brains of normal pts.

℞| TREATMENT

No effective therapy is available. Some pts with HIV-associated PML have shown dramatic clinical gains associated with improvement in immune status following institution of highly active antiretroviral therapy.

For a more detailed discussion, see Roos KL, Tyler KL: Meningitis, Encephalitis, Brain Abscess, and Empyema, Chap. 360, p. 2471, in HPIM-16; and HPIM-16 chapters covering specific organisms or infections.

188

CHRONIC MENINGITIS

Chronic inflammation of the meninges (pia, arachnoid, and dura) can produce profound neurologic disability and may be fatal if not successfully treated. The causes are varied. Five categories of disease account for most cases of chronic meningitis: (1) meningeal infections, (2) malignancy, (3) noninfectious inflammatory disorders, (4) chemical meningitis, and (5) parameningeal infections. Neurologic manifestations consist of persistent headache with or without stiff neck and hydrocephalus, cranial neuropathies, radiculopathies, and cognitive or personality changes (Table 188-1). On occasion the diagnosis is made when a neuroimaging study shows contrast enhancement of the meninges. Once chronic meningitis is confirmed by CSF examination, effort is focused on identifying the cause (Tables 188-2 and 188-3) by (1) further analysis of the CSF, (2) diagnosis of an underlying systemic infection or noninfectious inflammatory condition, or (3) examination of meningeal biopsy tissue.

Two clinical forms of chronic meningitis exist. In the first, symptoms are chronic and persistent, whereas in the second there are recurrent, discrete episodes. In the latter group, likely etiologies are herpes simplex virus type 2, chemical meningitis due to leakage from a tumor, a primary inflammatory condition, or drug hypersensitivity.

Approach to the Patient

Proper analysis of the CSF is essential; if the possibility of raised intracranial pressure (ICP) exists, a brain imaging study should be performed before LP. In pts with communicating hydrocephalus caused by impaired resorption of CSF, LP is safe and may lead to temporary improvement. However, if ICP is elevated because of a mass lesion, brain swelling, or a block in ventricular CSF outflow (obstructive hydrocephalus), then LP carries the potential risk of brain hernia-

Table 188-1

Symptoms and Signs of Chronic Meningitis

Symptoms	Signs
Chronic headache	+/− Papilledema
Neck or back pain	Brudzinski's or Kernig's sign of meningeal irritation
Change in personality	Altered mental status—drowsiness, inattention, disorientation, memory loss, frontal release signs (grasp, suck, snout), perseveration
Facial weakness	Peripheral seventh CN palsy
Double vision	Palsy of CNs III, IV, VI
Visual loss	Papilledema, optic atrophy
Hearing loss	Eighth CN palsy
Arm or leg weakness	Myelopathy or radiculopathy
Numbness in arms or legs	Myelopathy or radiculopathy
Sphincter dysfunction	Myelopathy or radiculopathy
	Frontal lobe dysfunction
Clumsiness	Ataxia

Note: CN, cranial nerve.

Table 188-2

Infectious Causes of Chronic Meningitis

COMMON BACTERIAL CAUSES

Partially treated suppurative meningitis
Parameningeal infection
Mycobacterium tuberculosis
Lyme disease (Bannwarth's syndrome): *Borrelia burgdorferi*
Syphilis (secondary, tertiary): *Treponema pallidum*

UNCOMMON BACTERIAL CAUSES

Actinomyces	*Brucella*
Nocardia	Whipple's disease: *Tropherema whippelii*

RARE BACTERIAL CAUSES

Leptospirosis; *Pseudoallescheria boydii*

FUNGAL CAUSES

Cryptococcus neoformans	*Blastomyces dermatitidis*
Coccidioides immitis	*Aspergillus* sp.
Candida sp.	*Sporothrix schenckii*
Histoplasma capsulatum	

RARE FUNGAL CAUSES

Xylohypha (formerly *Cladosporium*) *trichoides* and other dark-walled (dema-teaceous) fungi such as *Curvularia, Drechslera; Mucor, Pseudoallescheria boydii*

PROTOZOAL CAUSES

Toxoplasma gondii
Trypanosomiasis *Trypanosoma gambiense, Trypanosoma rhodesiense*

RARE PROTOZOAL CAUSES

Acanthamoeba sp.

HELMINTHIC CAUSES

Cysticercosis (infection with cysts of *Taenia solium*)
Gnathostoma spinigerum
Angiostrongylus cantonensis
Baylisascaris procyonis (raccoon ascarid)

RARE HELMINTHIC CAUSES

Trichinella spiralis (trichinosis); *Echinococcus* cysts; *Schistosoma* sp.

VIRAL CAUSES

Mumps	HIV (acute retroviral syndrome)
Lymphocytic choriomeningitis	Herpes simplex (HSV)
Echovirus	

tion. Obstructive hydrocephalus usually requires direct ventricular drainage of CSF.

Contrast-enhanced MRI or CT studies of the brain and spinal cord can iden-tify meningeal enhancement, parameningeal infections (including brain ab-scess), encasement of the spinal cord (malignancy or inflammation and infec-

Table 188-3

Noninfectious Causes of Chronic Meningitis

Malignancy
Chemical compounds (may cause recurrent meningitis)
Primary inflammation
   CNS sarcoidosis
   Vogt-Koyanagi-Harada syndrome (recurrent meningitis)
   Isolated granulomatous angiitis of the nervous system
   Systemic lupus erythematosus
   Behçet's syndrome (recurrent meningitis)
   Chronic benign lymphocytic meningitis
   Mollaret's recurrent meningitis
   Drug hypersensitivity
   Wegener's granulomatosis
Other: multiple sclerosis, Sjögren's syndrome, and rarer forms of vasculitis
   (e.g., Cogan's syndrome)

tion), or nodular deposits on the meninges or nerve roots (malignancy or sarcoidosis). Imaging studies are also useful to localize areas of meningeal disease prior to meningeal biopsy. Cerebral angiography may identify arteritis.

A meningeal biopsy should be considered in pts who are disabled, who need chronic ventricular decompression, or whose illness is progressing rapidly. The diagnostic yield of meningeal biopsy can be increased dramatically by targeting regions that enhance with contrast on MRI or CT; in one series, diagnostic biopsies most often identified sarcoid (31%) or metastatic adenocarcinoma (25%).

In approximately one-third of cases, the diagnosis is not known despite careful evaluation. A number of the organisms that cause chronic meningitis may take weeks to be identified by cultures. It is prudent to wait until cultures are finalized if symptoms are mild and not progressive. In many cases progressive neurologic deterioration occurs, and rapid treatment is required. In general, empirical therapy in the United States consists of antimycobacterial agents, amphotericin for fungal infection, or glucocorticoids for noninfectious inflammatory causes (most common). It is important to direct empirical therapy of lymphocytic meningitis, particularly if the condition is associated with hypoglycorrhachia and sixth and other cranial nerve palsies, since untreated disease is fatal in 4–8 weeks. Carcinomatous or lymphomatous meningitis may be difficult to diagnose initially, but the diagnosis becomes evident with time. Important causes of chronic meningitis in AIDS include infection with *Toxoplasma*, *Cryptococcus*, *Nocardia*, *Candida*, or other fungi; syphilis; and lymphoma.

For a more detailed discussion, see Koroshetz WJ, Swartz MN: Chronic and Recurrent Meningitis, Chap. 361, p. 2490, in HPIM-16.

189

MULTIPLE SCLEROSIS (MS)

Characterized by chronic inflammation and selective destruction of CNS myelin; peripheral nervous system is spared. Pathologically, the multifocal scarred lesions of MS are termed *plaques*. Etiology is thought to be autoimmune, with susceptibility determined by genetic and environmental factors. MS affects 350,000 Americans; onset is most often in early to middle adulthood, and women are affected approximately twice as often as men.

Clinical Manifestations

Onset may be dramatic or insidious. Most common are recurrent attacks of focal neurologic dysfunction, typically lasting weeks or months, and followed by variable recovery; some pts initially present with slowly progressive neurologic deterioration. Symptoms often transiently worsen with fatigue, stress, exercise, or heat. Manifestations of MS are protean but commonly include weakness and/or sensory symptoms involving a limb, visual difficulties, abnormalities of gait and coordination, urinary urgency or frequency, and abnormal fatigue. Motor involvement can present as a heavy, stiff, weak, or clumsy limb. Localized tingling, "pins and needles," and "dead" sensations are common. Optic neuritis can result in blurring or misting of vision, especially in the central visual field, often with associated retroorbital pain accentuated by eye movement. Involvement of the brainstem may result in diplopia, nystagmus, vertigo, or facial symptoms of pain, numbness, weakness, hemispasm, or myokymia (rippling muscular contractions). Ataxia, tremor, and dysarthria may reflect disease of cerebellar pathways. Lhermitte's symptom, a momentary electric shock–like sensation evoked by neck flexion, indicates disease in the cervical spinal cord. Diagnostic criteria are listed in Table 189-1; MS mimics are summarized in Table 189-2.

Physical Examination

Abnormal signs usually more widespread than expected from the history. Check for abnormalities in visual fields, loss of visual acuity, disturbed color perception, optic pallor or papillitis, afferent pupillary defect (paradoxical dilation to direct light following constriction to consensual light), nystagmus, internuclear ophthalmoplegia (slowness or loss of adduction in one eye with nystagmus in the abducting eye on lateral gaze), facial numbness or weakness, dysarthria, weakness and spasticity, hyperreflexia, ankle clonus, upgoing toes, ataxia, sensory abnormalities.

Disease Course

Four general categories:

• *Relapsing-remitting MS* (RRMS) is characterized by recurrent attacks of neurologic dysfunction with or without recovery; between attacks, no progression of neurologic impairment is noted.
• *Secondary progressive MS* (SPMS) initially presents with a relapsing-remitting pattern but evolves to be gradually progressive.
• *Primary progressive MS* (PPMS) is characterized by gradual progression of disability from onset; 15% of cases.
• *Progressive-relapsing MS* (PRMS) is a rare form that begins with a primary progressive course, but superimposed relapses occur.

Table 189-1

Diagnostic Criteria for MS

1. Examination must reveal *objective* abnormalities of the CNS.
2. Involvement must reflect predominantly disease of white matter long tracts, usually including (a) pyramidal pathways, (b) cerebellar pathways, (c) medial longitudinal fasciculus, (d) optic nerve, and (e) posterior columns.
3. Examination or history must implicate involvement of two or more areas of the CNS.
   a. MRI may be used to document a second lesion when only one site of abnormality has been demonstrable on examination. A confirmatory MRI must have either four lesions involving the white matter or three lesions if one is periventricular in location. Acceptable lesions must be >3 mm in diameter. For patients older than 50 years, two of the following criteria must also be met: (a) lesion size >5 mm, (b) lesions adjacent to the bodies of the lateral ventricles, and (c) lesion(s) present in the posterior fossa.
   b. Evoked response testing may be used to document a second lesion not evident on clinical examination.
4. The clinical pattern must consist of (a) two or more separate episodes of worsening involving different sites of the CNS, each lasting at least 24 h and occurring at least 1 month apart, or (b) gradual or stepwise progression over at least 6 months if accompanied by increased IgG synthesis or two or more oligoclonal bands. MRI may be used to document dissemination in time if a new T2 lesion or a Gd-enhancing lesion is seen 3 or more months after a single attack.
5. The patient's neurologic condition could not be better attributed to another disease.

DIAGNOSTIC CATEGORIES

1. *Definite MS*: All five criteria fulfilled.
2. *Probable MS*: All five criteria fulfilled except (a) only one objective abnormality despite two symptomatic episodes or (b) one symptomatic episode despite two or more objective abnormalities.
3. *At risk for MS*: Criteria 1, 2, 3, and 5 fulfilled; patient has only one symptomatic episode and one objective abnormality.

Note: Gd, gadolinium.

MS is a chronic illness; 15 years after diagnosis, 20% of pts have no functional limitation; half will have progressed to SPMS and will require assistance with ambulation.

Laboratory Findings

MRI reveals multifocal bright areas on T2-weighted sequences in >95% of pts, often in periventricular location; gadolinium enhancement indicates acute lesions with disruption of blood-brain barrier. MRI also useful to exclude MS mimics. CSF findings include mild lymphocytic pleocytosis (5–75 cells in 25%), oligoclonal bands (75–90%), elevated IgG (80%), and normal total protein level. Visual, auditory, and somatosensory evoked response tests can identify lesions that are clinically silent; one or more evoked response tests abnormal in > 80% of pts. Urodynamic studies aid in management of bladder symptoms.

Table 189-2

Disorders That Can Mimic MS

Acute disseminated encephalomyelitis (ADEM)
Antiphospholipid antibody syndrome
Behçet's disease
Cerebral autosomal dominant arteriopathy, subcortical infarcts, and leukoen-
cephalopathy (CADASIL)
Congenital leukodystrophies (e.g., adrenoleukodystrophy, metachromatic leu-
kodystrophy)
HIV infection
Ischemic optic neuropathy (arteritic and nonarteritic)
Lyme disease
Mitochondrial encephalopathy with lactic acidosis and stroke (MELAS)
Neoplasms (e.g., lymphoma, glioma, meningioma)
Sarcoid
Sjögren's syndrome
Stroke and ischemic cerebrovascular disease
Syphilis
Systemic lupus erythematosus and related collagen vascular disorders
Tropical spastic paraparesis (HTLV I/II infection)
Vascular malformations (especially spinal dural AV fistulas)
Vasculitis (primary CNS or other)
Vitamin B_{12} deficiency

Note: HTLV, human T cell lymphotropic virus; AV, arteriovenous.

 TREATMENT (Fig. 189-1)

    Prophylaxis Against Relapses Four treatments are available: inter-
feron (IFN)-β1a (Avonex; 30μg IM once a week), IFN-β1a (Rebif; 44μg SC
thrice weekly), IFN-β1b (Betaseron; 250 μg SC every other day), and glatiramer acetate (Copaxone; 12 mg SC qd). Each of these therapies reduces annual exacerbation rates by ~30% and also reduces the development of new
MRI lesions. IFN preparations that are given multiple times weekly (e.g.,
Rebif or Betaseron) appear to have slightly greater efficacy compared with
once weekly agents (e.g., Avonex) but are also more likely to induce neutralizing antibodies, which may reduce the clinical benefit. Regardless of
which agent is chosen first, treatment should probably be altered in pts who
continue to have frequent attacks (Fig. 189-1).
    Side effects of IFN include flulike symptoms, local injection site reactions
(with SC dosing), and mild abnormalities on routine laboratory evaluation
(e.g., elevated liver function tests or lymphopenia). Rarely, more severe hepatotoxicity may occur. Side effects to IFN usually subside with time. Injection
site reactions also occur with glatiramer acetate but are less severe than with
IFN. Approximately 15% of pts experience one or more episodes of flushing,
chest tightness, dyspnea, palpitations, and anxiety.
    Early treatment with a disease-modifying drug is appropriate for most MS
patients. It is reasonable to delay initiating treatment in pts with (1) normal
neurologic exams, (2) a single attack or a low attack frequency, and (3) a low
"burden of disease" as assessed by brain MRI. Untreated pts need to be followed closely with periodic brain MRI scans; the need for therapy is reassessed if the scans reveal ongoing evidence of ongoing disease.
    Acute Relapses Acute relapses that produce functional impairment may
be treated with a short course of IV methylprednisolone (1 g IV qA.M. ×3)

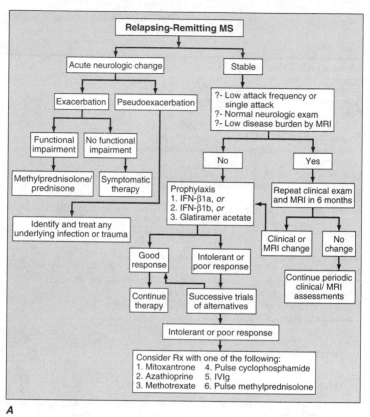

A

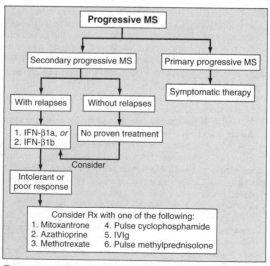

B

FIGURE 189-1 Therapeutic decision-making for MS. *A*. Relapsing-remitting MS. *B*. Progressive MS. IVIg, intravenous immunoglobulin.

followed by oral prednisone (60 mg qA.M. ×4; 40 mg qA.M. ×4; 20 mg qA.M. ×3). This regimen modestly reduces the severity and shortens the duration of attacks. Plasma exchange (7 exchanges: 54 mL/kg or 1.1 plasma volumes per exchange, every other day for 14 days) may benefit patients with fulminant attacks of demyelination (not only MS) that are unresponsive to glucocorticoids.

Progressive Symptoms For pts with secondary progressive MS who continue to experience relapses, treatment with one of the IFNs is reasonable; however, the IFNs are ineffective against purely progressive MS symptoms. The immunosuppressant/immunomodulator drug mitoxantrone (12 mg/m² by IV infusion every 3 months) is approved in the United States for treatment of secondary progressive MS; however, the evidence for efficacy is relatively weak, and dose-related cardiac toxicity is an important concern. Methotrexate (7.5–20 mg PO once each week) or azathioprine [2–3 (mg/kg)/d PO] is sometimes tried, but efficacy is modest. Pulse therapy with cyclophosphamide is employed in some centers for young adults with aggressive forms of MS. For patients with PPMS, symptomatic therapy only is recommended.

Symptomatic Therapy Spasticity may respond to baclofen (15–80 mg/d in divided doses), diazepam (2 mg bid-tid), or tizanidine (2–8 mg tid). Dysesthesia may respond to carbamazepine (100–1200 mg/d in divided doses), phenytoin (300 mg/d), or amitriptyline (50–200 mg/d). Treatment of bladder symptoms is based on the underlying pathophysiology: hyperreflexia is treated with anticholinergics such as oxybutinin (5 mg bid-tid), hyporeflexia with the cholinergic drug bethanecol (10–50 mg tid-qid), and dyssynergia with anticholinergics and intermittent catheterization. Depression should be treated aggressively.

CLINICAL VARIANTS OF MS

Neuromyelitis optica (NMO), or Devic's syndrome, consists of separate attacks of acute optic neuritis (bilateral or unilateral) and myelitis. In contrast to MS, the brain MRI is typically normal. A focal enhancing region of swelling and cavitation, extending over three or more spinal cord segments, is typically seen on spinal MRI. Acute attacks are usually treated with high-dose glucocorticoids as for MS exacerbations. Plasma exchange has also been used empirically for acute episodes that fail to respond to glucocorticoids. Immunosuppressants or IFNs are sometimes used in the hope that further relapses will be prevented.

Acute MS (Marburg's variant) is a fulminant demyelinating process that progresses to death within 1 to 2 years. No controlled trials of therapy exist; high-dose glucocorticoids, plasma exchange, and cyclophosphamide have been tried, with uncertain benefit.

ACUTE DISSEMINATED ENCEPHALOMYELITIS (ADEM)

A fulminant, often devastating, demyelinating disease that has a monophasic course and may be associated with antecedent immunization or infection. Signs of disseminated neurologic disease are consistently present (e.g., hemiparesis or quadriparesis, extensor plantar responses, lost or hyperactive tendon reflexes, sensory loss and brainstem involvement). Fever, headache, meningismus, lethargy progressing to coma, and seizures may occur. CSF pleocytosis is common. MRI may reveal extensive gadolinium enhancement of white matter in brain and spinal cord. Initial treatment is with high-dose glucocorticoids. Patients who fail to respond may benefit from a course of plasma exchange or intravenous immunoglobulin.

For a more detailed discussion, see Hauser SL, Goodin DS: **Multiple Sclerosis and Other Demyelinating Diseases, Chap. 359, p. 2461, in HPIM-16.**

190

ALZHEIMER'S DISEASE AND OTHER DEMENTIAS

DEMENTIA

Dementia is an acquired deterioration in cognitive ability that impairs the successful performance of activities of daily living. Memory is the most common cognitive ability lost with dementia; 10% of persons over age 70 and 20–40% of individuals over age 85 have clinically identifiable memory loss. In addition to memory, other mental faculties are also affected in dementia, such as language, visuospatial ability, calculation, judgment, and problem solving. Neuropsychiatric and social deficits develop in many dementia syndromes, resulting in depression, withdrawal, hallucinations, delusions, agitation, insomnia, and disinhibition. Dementia is chronic and usually progressive, whereas delirium is an acute condition associated with fluctuating altered consciousness (agitation or lethargy), often accompanied by fever, tachycardia, or tremor.

DIAGNOSIS   The mini-mental status examination is a useful screening test for dementia (Table 183-1). A score of <24 points (out of 30) indicates a need for more detailed cognitive and physical assessment.

--------------------- *Approach to the Patient* ---------------------

Differential Diagnosis

Dementia has many causes (Table 190-1). It is essential to exclude treatable etiologies, present in nearly 20% of pts; in one study, the most common potentially reversible diagnoses were depression, hydrocephalus, and alcohol dependence. The major degenerative dementias can usually be distinguished by distictive symptoms, signs, and neuroimaging features (Table 190-2).

History

A subacute onset of confusion may represent delirium and should trigger the search for intoxication, infection, or metabolic derangement. An elderly person with slowly progressive memory loss over several years is likely to have Alzheimer's disease (AD). A change in personality, disinhibition, gain of weight, or food obsession suggests frontotemporal dementia (FTD), not AD; apathy, loss of executive function, progressive abnormalities in speech, or relative sparing of memory also suggests FTD. Dementia with Lewy bodies (DLB) is suggested by the early presence of visual hallucinations, parkinsonism, delirium, or a sleep disorder.

A history of stroke suggests multi-infarct dementia, which may also occur with hypertension, atrial fibrillation, peripheral vascular disease, and diabetes. Rapid progression of dementia with myoclonus suggests a prion disease. Gait disturbance is prominent with multi-infarct dementia, Parkinson's disease, or normal-pressure hydrocephalus. Multiple sex partners or intravenous drug use should trigger a search for an infection, especially in persons with HIV. A history of head trauma could indicate chronic subdural hematoma, dementia

Table 190-1

Differential Diagnosis of Dementia

MOST COMMON CAUSES OF DEMENTIA

Alzheimer's disease
Vascular dementia[a]
   Multi-infarct
   Diffuse white matter disease
   (Binswanger's)

Alcoholism[a]
Parkinson's disease
Drug/medication intoxication[a]

LESS COMMON CAUSES OF DEMENTIA

Vitamin deficiencies
   Thiamine (B_1): Wernicke's
   encephalopathy[a]
   B_{12} (Pernicious anemia)[a]
   Nicotinic acid (pellagra)[a]
Endocrine and other organ failure
   Hypothyroidism[a]
   Adrenal insufficiency and
    Cushing's syndrome[a]
   Hypo- and hyperparathyroidism[a]
   Renal failure[a]
   Liver failure[a]
   Pulmonary failure[a]
Chronic infections
   HIV
   Neurosyphilis[a]
   Papovavirus (progressive multifo-
    cal leukoencephalopathy)
   Prion (Creutzfeldt-Jakob and
    Gerstmann-Sträussler-Scheinker
    disease)
   Tuberculosis, fungal, and proto-
    zoal[a]
   Sarcoidosis[a]
   Whipple's disease[a]
Head trauma and diffuse brain
  damage
   Dementia pugilistica
   Chronic subdural hematoma[a]
   Postanoxia
   Postencephalitis
   Normal-pressure hydrocephalus[a]
Neoplastic
   Primary brain tumor[a]
   Metastatic brain tumor[a]
   Paraneoplastic limbic encephalitis
Toxic disorders
   Drug, medication, and narcotic
    poisoning[a]
   Heavy metal intoxication[a]
   Dialysis dementia (aluminum)
   Organic toxins

Psychiatric
   Depression (peudodementia)[a]
   Schizophrenia[a]
   Conversion reaction[a]
Degenerative disorders
   Huntington's disease
   Pick's disease
   Diffuse Lewy body disease
   Progressive supranuclear palsy
    (Steel-Richardson syndrome)
   Multisystem degeneration
    (Shy-Drager syndrome)
   Hereditary ataxias (some forms)
   Motor neuron disease
    [amyotrophic lateral sclerosis
    (ALS); some forms]
   Frontotemporal dementia
   Cortical basal degeneration
   Multiple sclerosis
   Adult Down's syndrome with
    Alzheimer's
   ALS-Parkinson's-Dementia
    complex of Guam
Miscellaneous
   Vasculitis[a]
   CADASIL[a]
   Acute intermittent porphyria[a]
   Recurrent nonconvulsive
    seizures[a]
Additional conditions in children
  or adolescents
   Hallervorden-Spatz disease
   Subacute sclerosing panenceph-
    alitis
   Metabolic disorders (e.g.,
    Wilson's and Leigh's diseases,
    leukodystrophies, lipid storage
    diseases, mitochondrial
    mutations)

[a] Potentially reversible dementia.
Note: CADASIL, cerebral autosomal dominant arteriopathy, subcortical infarcts, and leukoen-cephalopathy.

Table 190-2

Clinical Differentiation of the Major Dementias

Disease	Initial Symptom	Mental Status	Neuropsychiatry	Neurology	Imaging
AD	Memory loss	Episodic memory loss	Initially normal	Initially normal	Entorhinal and hippocampal atrophy
Vascular	Often sudden; variable initial symptoms; apathy, falls, focal weakness	Frontal/executive cognitive slowing; can spare memory	Apathy, delusions, anxiety	Usually motor slowing, spasticity; can be normal	Cortical and/or subcortical infarctions, confluent white matter disease
FTD	Apathy; reduced judgment/insight/speech/language; hyperorality	Frontal/executive, language; spares drawing	Apathy, disinhibition, hyperorality, euphoria, depression	Vertical gaze palsy, axial rigidity, dystonia, alien hand (due to PSP/CBD overlap)	Frontal and/or temporal atrophy; spares posterior parietal lobe
DLB	Visual hallucinations, REM-sleep disorder, delirium, Capgras syndrome, parkinsonism	Drawing and frontal/executive; spares memory; delirium prone	Visual hallucinations, depression, sleep disorder, delusions	Parkinsonism	Posterior parietal; hippocampi larger than in AD
Prion	Dementia, mood changes, anxiety, movement disorder	Variable, frontal/executive, focal cortical, memory	Depression, anxiety	Myoclonus, rigidity, parkinsonism	Cortical ribboning and basal ganglia hyperintensities on diffusion/flare MRI

Note: AD, Alzheimer's disease; FTD, frontotemporal dementia; PSP, progressive supranuclear palsy; CBD, cortical basal degeneration; DLB, dementia with Lewy bodies.

pugilistica, or normal-pressure hydrocephalus. Alcoholism may suggest malnutrition and thiamine deficiency. A history of gastric surgery may result in loss of intrinsic factor and vitamin B_{12} deficiency. A careful review of medications, especially of sedatives and tranquilizers, may raise the issue of drug intoxication. A family history of dementia is found in Huntington's disease, familial AD, or familial FTD. Insomnia or weight loss is often seen with pseudodementia due to depression, which can also be caused by the recent death of a loved one.

Examination

It is essential to document the dementia, look for other signs of nervous system involvement, and search for clues of a systemic disease that might be responsible for the cognitive disorder. AD does not affect motor systems until late in the course. In contrast, FTD patients often develop axial rigidity, supranuclear gaze palsy, or features of amyotrophic lateral sclerosis. In DLB, initial symptoms may be the new onset of a parkinsonian syndrome (resting tremor, cogwheel rigidity, bradykinesia, and festinating gait). Unexplained falls, axial rigidity, and gaze deficits suggest progressive supranuclear palsy (PSP).

Focal neurologic deficits occur in multi-infarct dementia or brain tumor. Dementia with a myelopathy and peripheral neuropathy suggests vitamin B_{12} deficiency. A peripheral neuropathy could also indicate an underlying vitamin deficiency or metal intoxication. Dry cool skin, hair loss, and bradycardia suggest hypothyroidism. Confusion associated with repetitive stereotyped movements may indicate ongoing seizure activity. Hearing impairment or visual loss may produce confusion and disorientation misinterpreted as dementia. Such sensory deficits are common in the elderly.

Choice of Diagnostic Studies

The choice of tests in the evaluation of dementia is not straightforward. A reversible or treatable cause must not be missed, yet no single etiology is common; thus a screen must employ multiple tests, each of which has a low yield. Table 190-3 lists most screening tests for dementia. Guidelines recommend the routine measurement of thyroid function tests, a vitamin B_{12} level, and a neuroimaging study (CT or MRI). Lumbar puncture need not be done routinely but is indicated if infection is a consideration. An EEG is rarely helpful except to suggest a prion disease.

ALZHEIMER'S DISEASE (AD)

Most common cause of dementia; affects 4 million persons in the United States Cost > $50 billion/year.

CLINICAL MANIFESTATIONS Pts present with subtle recent memory loss, then develop slowly progressive dementia. Memory loss is often not recognized initially, in part due to preservation of social graces until later phases; impaired activities of daily living (keeping track of finances, appointments) draw attention of friends/family. Disorientation, poor judgment, poor concentration, aphasia, and apraxia are increasingly evident as the disease progresses. Pts may be frustrated or unaware of deficit. In end-stage AD, pts become rigid, mute, incontinent, and bedridden. Help may be needed with the simplest tasks, such as eating, dressing, and toilet function. Often, death results from malnutrition, secondary infections, pulmonary emboli, or heart disease. Typical duration, 8–10 years.

PATHOGENESIS Risk factors for AD are old age, positive family history. Pathology: neuritic plaques composed in part of $A\beta$ amyloid, derived from amyloid precursor protein (APP); neurofibrillary tangles composed of abnor-

Table 190-3

Evaluation of the Patient with Dementia

Routine Evaluation	Optional Focused Tests	Occasionally Helpful Tests
History	HIV	EEG
Physical examination	Chest x-ray	Parathyroid function
Laboratory tests	Lumbar puncture	Adrenal function
Thyroid function	Liver function	Urine heavy metals
(TSH)	Renal function	RBC sedimentation
Vitamin B_{12}	Urine toxin screen	rate
Complete blood	Psychometric testing	Angiogram
count	Apolipoprotein E	Brain biopsy
Electrolytes		SPECT
VDRL		
CT/MRI		

DIAGNOSTIC CATEGORIES

Reversible Causes	Irreversible/Degenerative Dementias	Psychiatric Disorders
Examples	Examples	Depression
Hypothyroidism	Alzheimer's	Schizophrenia
Thiamine deficiency	Frontotemporal	Conversion reaction
Vitamin B_{12} deficiency	dementia	
Normal-pressure	Huntington's	
hydrocephalus	Dementia with Lewy	
Chronic infection	bodies	
Brain tumor	Multi-infarct	
Drug intoxication	Leukoencephalopathies	
	Parkinson's	

Associated Treatable Conditions	
Depression	Agitation
Seizures	Caregiver "burnout"
Insomnia	Drug side effects

mally phosphorylated tau protein. The apolipoprotein E (apo E) gene (chromosome 19) has a role in pathogenesis; the ε4 allele accelerates age of onset of AD and is associated with sporadic and late-onset familial cases. Apo E testing is not indicated as a predictive test. Rare genetic causes of AD are Down's syndrome (trisomy 21), APP gene mutations (chromosome 21), mutations in presenilin I (chromosome 14) and presenilin II (chromosome 1) genes; all appear to increase production of Aβ amyloid. Genetic testing available for presenilin mutations.

 TREATMENT

AD cannot be cured, and no highly effective drug exists. The focus is on judicious use of cholinesterase inhibitor drugs; symptomatic management of behavioral problems; and building rapport with the pt, family members, and other caregivers.

Tacrine (tetrahydroaminoacridine), donepezil, rivastigmine, and galantamine are approved by the FDA for treatment of AD. Their action is inhibition of cholinesterase, with a resulting increase in cerebral levels of acetylcholine. These compounds are only modestly efficacious and offer little or no benefit in the late stages of AD. Donepezil (Aricept), 5–10 mg/d PO, has the advantages of few side effects and single daily dosage.

For AD of moderate severity, memantine, an NMDA receptor antagonist recently approved by the FDA, may be added to a cholinesterase inhibitor or used alone; dosing of memantine begins at 5mg qd with gradual increases (over 1 month) to 10 mg bid.

The antioxidants selegiline, α-tocopherol (vitamin E), or both slowed institutionalization and progression to death of AD in one study. Because vitamin E is less toxic than selegiline and is inexpensive, it is offered to many pts; the dose is 1000 IU bid. However, its beneficial effects are likely to be small. One trial of *Ginkgo biloba* found modest improvement in cognitive function in AD; this study requires confirmation. There is no role for hormone replacement therapy in prevention of AD in women, and no benefit has been found in the treatment of established AD with estrogen.

Depression, common in early stages of AD, may respond to antidepressant or cholinesterase inhibitors. Selective serotonin reuptake inhibitors (SSRIs) are often used due to their low anticholinergic side effects. Management of behavioral problems in conjunction with family and caregivers is essential. Mild sedation may help insomnia. Agitation is controlled with low-dose haloperidol (0.5–2 mg). Notebooks and posted daily reminders can function as memory aids in early stages. Kitchens, bathrooms, and bedrooms need evaluation for safety. Pts must eventually stop driving. Caregiver burnout is common; nursing home placement may be necessary. Local and national support groups (Alzheimer's Disease and Related Disorders Association) are valuable resources.

OTHER CAUSES OF DEMENTIA

VASCULAR DEMENTIA   Typically follows multiple strokelike episodes (multi-infarct dementia) or rarely develops in a slow progressive fashion (diffuse white matter, or Binswanger's, disease). Unlike AD, focal neurologic signs (e.g., hemiparesis) are usually apparent at presentation.

FRONTOTEMPORAL DEMENTIA   Responsible for 10% of all cases of dementia. Extremely heterogeneous; presents with combinations of disinhibition, dementia, apraxia, parkinsonism, and motor neuron disease. May be sporadic or inherited; some familial cases due to intronic mutations of tau gene on chromosome 17. Treatment is symptomatic; no therapies known to slow progression or improve cognitive symptoms. Many of the behaviors that accompany FTD such as depression, hyperorality, compulsions, and irritability can be helped with SSRIs.

DEMENTIA WITH LEWY BODIES   Characterized by visual hallucinations, parkinsonism, fluctuating alertness, and falls. Dementia can precede or follow the appearance of parkinsonism. Lewy bodies are intraneuronal cytoplasmic inclusions. Anticholinesterase compounds, exercise programs to maximize motor function, antidepressants to treat depressive syndromes, and antipsychotics in low doses to alleviate psychosis may be helpful.

NORMAL-PRESSURE HYDROCEPHALUS (NPH)   Presents as a gait disorder (ataxic or apractic), dementia, and urinary incontinence. Gait improves in 30–50% of pts following ventricular shunting; dementia and incontinence do not improve.

HUNTINGTON'S DISEASE   Chorea, behavioral disturbance, and a frontal/executive disorder. Typical onset fourth to fifth decade but can present at almost any age. Autosomal dominant inheritance due to expanded trinucleotide repeat in gene encoding the protein huntingtin. Diagnosis confirmed with genetic testing coupled with genetic counseling. Symptomatic treatment of movements and behaviors; SSRIs may help depression.

For a more detailed discussion, see Bird TD, Miller BL: Alzheimer's Disease and Other Dementias, Chap. 350, p. 2393, in HPIM-16.

PARKINSON'S DISEASE

Clinical Features

Parkinsonism consists of tremor, rigidity, bradykinesia, and characteristic abnormalities of gait and posture; may occur with many disorders. Parkinson's disease (PD) is idiopathic parkinsonism without evidence of more widespread neurologic involvement. PD afflicts >1 million individuals in the United States (~1% of those >55 years). Peak age of onset in the 60s (range is 35 to 85); course progressive over 10 to 25 years. Tremor ("pill rolling" of hands) at rest (4–6 Hz); worsens with stress. A faster (7–8 Hz) "action tremor" may also occur when the hands are held against gravity. Presentation with tremor confined to one limb or side of body is common. Other findings: rigidity ("cogwheeling"—increased ratchet-like resistance to passive limb movements), bradykinesia (slowness of voluntary movements), fixed expressionless face (facial masking) with reduced frequency of blinking, hypophonic voice, drooling, impaired rapid alternating movements, micrographia (small handwriting), reduced arm swing while walking, flexed "stooped" posture with walking, shuffling gait, difficulty initiating or stopping walking, en-bloc turning (multiple small steps required to turn), retropulsion (tendency to fall backwards). Non-motor aspects of PD include depression and anxiety, cognitive impairment, sleep disturbances, sensation of inner restlessness, loss of smell (*anosmia*), and disturbances of autonomic function. In advanced PD, intellectual and behavioral deterioration, aspiration pneumonia, and bedsores (due to immobility) common. Normal muscular strength, deep tendon reflexes, and sensory exam. Diagnosis based upon history and examination; neuroimaging, EEG, and CSF studies usually normal for age.

Etiology

Degeneration of pigmented pars compacta neurons of the substantia nigra in the midbrain resulting in lack of dopaminergic input to striatum; accumulation of eosinophilic intraneural inclusion granules (Lewy bodies). Cause of cell death is unknown, but it may result from generation of free radicals and oxidative stress. Rare genetic forms of parkinsonism exist; most common are mutations in α-synuclein or parkin genes. Early age of onset suggests a possible genetic cause of PD.

Differential Diagnosis

Features of parkinsonism may occur with: depression (paucity of vocal inflection and facial movement); essential tremor (high-frequency tremor with limbs held against gravity, head tremor, improves with alcohol); normal-pressure hydrocephalus (apraxic gait, urinary incontinence, dementia); Wilson's disease (early age of onset, Kayser-Fleischer rings, low serum copper, low ceruloplasmin); Huntington's disease (family history, chorea, dementia); multiple system atrophy (early urinary incontinence, orthostatic hypotension, dysarthria); dementia with Lewy bodies (early hallucinations, behavioral disturbances); progressive supranuclear palsy (early imbalance and falls, downgaze paresis).

℞ TREATMENT

Goals are to maintain function and avoid drug-induced complications. It is not always possible to exclude other causes of parkinsonism prior to initiating treatment for PD. Bradykinesia, tremor, rigidity, and abnormal posture respond early in illness; cognitive symptoms, hypophonia, autonomic dysfunction, and balance difficulties respond poorly.

Initiation of Therapy Dopaminomimetic therapy initiated when symptoms interfere with quality of life. In early PD, dopamine agonist monotherapy well tolerated and reduces risk of later treatment-related complications such as motor fluctuations and dyskinesias (50% of pts treated over 5 years with levodopa). *Motor fluctuations* are the exaggerated ebb and flow of parkinsonian signs between doses of medications. *Dyskinesias* refer to choreiform and dystonic movements that can occur as a peak dose effect or at the beginning or end of the dose. Dopamine agonist monotherapy requires higher doses than needed when agonist is used to supplement levodopa (Table 191-1); slow titration necessary to avoid side effects. Most pts require addition of levodopa or another agent within 1 to 3 years of initiating dopamine agonist monotherapy. Levodopa, the metabolic precurser of dopamine, remains most effective treatment for PD.

Dopamine Agonists Compared to levodopa, they are longer acting and thus provide a more uniform stimulation of dopamine receptors. They are effective as monotherapeutic agents and as adjuncts to carbidopa/levodopa therapy. They can also be used in combination with anticholinergics and amantadine. Agonists are effective against bradykinesia and gait disturbances but less effective against tremor. Side effects include nausea, postural hypotension, psychiatric symptoms, daytime sedation, and occasional sleep attacks. Table 191-1 provides a guide to the doses and uses of these agents.

Carbidopa/Levodopa Formulations Available in regular, immediate release (IR) formulations (Sinemet, Atamet and others; 10/100 mg, 25/100 mg, and 25/250 mg), controlled release (CR) formulations (Sinemet CR 25/100 mg, 50/200 mg), and more recently as Stalevo (Table 191-1). The latter combines IR carbidopa/levodopa with 200 mg of entacapone (see below). Carbidopa blocks peripheral levodopa decarboxylation into dopamine and thus symptoms of nausea and orthostasis often associated with the initiation of levodopa. Initial target doses of these medications are summarized in the table. Gradual dose escalation recommended; initiation of dosing at mealtimes will reduce nausea.

Levodopa Augmentation Selegiline is a selective and irreversible monoamine oxidase (MAO) B inhibitor with a weak symptomatic effect when used as monotherapy or as an adjunct to carbidopa/levodopa. Typically, selegiline is used as initial therapy or is added to alleviate tremor or levodopa-associated wearing off; dose is 5 mg with breakfast and lunch. A side effect is insomnia. Older individuals, and those with cardiac disease, may benefit

Table 191-1

Guide to the Use of Levodopa Formulations and Dopamine Agonists in Parkinson's Disease

	LD Dose Equivalency, mg	Available Strengths, mg	Initial Dose	Other Considerations
CARBIDOPA/LEVODOPA (TYPICAL INITIAL STRENGTH)				
Carbidopa/levodopa IR 25/100	→ 100 (anchor dose)	10/100 25/100 25/250	25/100; 0.5 tab tid	Target dose = 3–6 25/100 tabs/d
Carbidopa/levodopa CR 50/200	→ 150	25/100 50/200	50/200; one tab bid to tid	Increased bioavailability with food; splitting the tablet negates the CR property
Carbidopa/levodopa/entacapone 25/100/200	→ 120	12.5/50/200 25/100/200 37.5/150/200	25/100/200; one tab bid to tid	Do not split tablets

912

Approximate Target Doses

	DA Equivalent to LD Anchor Dose Above, mg[a]	Available Strengths, mg	Initial Dose, mg	As monotherapy, mg/d	As adjuncts to LD, mg/d	Other Considerations
DOPAMINE AGONISTS						
Non-ergot alkaloids						
Ropinirole	5	0.25, 0.5, 1, 2, 3, 4, 5	0.25 tid	12–24	6–16	Hepatic metabolism; potential drug-drug interactions; Occasionally associated with "sleep attacks"
Pramipexole	1	0.125, 0.25, 1, 1.5	0.125 tid	1.5–4.5	0.375–3.0	Renal metabolism; dose adjustments needed in renal insufficiency; Occasionally associated with "sleep attacks"
Ergot alkaloids						
Pergolide	1	0.05, 0.25, 1.0	0.05 tid	1.5–6	0.3–3	Rare reports of valvular heart disease; fewer reports of sleep attacks compared to non-ergots
Bromocriptine	2	2.5, 5.0	1.25 bid to tid	7.5–15	3.75–7.5	Rare reports of pulmonary and retroperitoneal fibrosis; Relative incidence of sleep attacks not well studied

[a] Equivalency doses are approximations based on clinical experience and may not correlate with the relative in vitro binding properties of these compounds.

Note: LD, levodopa (with carbidopa); IR, immediate release; CR, controlled release; DA, dopamine agonist. Carbidopa/levodopa/entacapone, Stalevo.

from doses as low as 2.5 mg/d. The potential role of selegiline as neuropro-tective therapy remains controversial.

The catechol *O*-methyltransferase (COMT) inhibitors entacapone and tol-capone offer yet another strategy to augment the effects of levodopa by block-ing the enzymatic degradation of levodopa and dopamine. Entacapone is pre-ferred to tolcapone (hepatic and hematologic side effects). When used with carbidopa/levodopa, these agents alleviate wearing-off symptoms and in-crease time a pt remains "on" (i.e., well medicated) during the day. Common side effects are gastrointestinal and hyperdopaminergic, including increased dyskinesias. The dose of entacapone is 200 mg coadministered with each dose of carbidopa/levodopa. The dose of tolcapone is 50 to 200 mg tid.

Anticholinergics and amantadine are useful adjuncts. Anticholinergics (tri-hexyphenidyl, 2–5 mg tid; benztropine, 0.5–2 mg tid) are particularly useful for controlling rest tremor and dystonia, and amantadine can reduce drug-induced dyskinesias by up to 70%. The mechanism of action of amantadine (100 mg bid) is unknown; it has anticholinergic, dopaminomimetic, and glu-tamate antagonist properties. In older patients, it may aggravate confusion and psychosis.

Surgical Treatments In refractory cases, surgical treatment of PD should be considered. The use of ablation (e.g., pallidotomy or thalamotomy) has decreased greatly since the introduction of deep-brain stimulation. The selection of suitable patients for surgery is most important, since in general patients with atypical Parkinson's do not have a favorable response. The in-dications for surgery are (1) a diagnosis of idiopathic PD, (2) a clear response to levodopa, (3) significant intractable symptoms of PD, and/or (4) drug-induced dyskinesias and wearing off. Contraindications to surgery include atypical PD, cognitive impairment, major psychiatric illness, substantial med-ical comorbidities, and advanced age (a relative factor). Symptoms not re-sponding to levodopa are unlikely to benefit from surgery.

For a more detailed discussion, see Delong MR, Juncos JL: Parkinson's Disease and Other Movement Disorders, Chap. 351, p. 2406, in HPIM-16.

192

ATAXIC DISORDERS

Clinical Presentation

Symptoms and signs may include gait instability, nystagmus, dysarthria (scan-ning speech), impaired limb coordination, intention tremor (i.e., with move-ment), hypotonia. *Differential diagnosis:* Unsteady gait associated with vertigo can resemble gait instability of cerebellar disease but produces a sensation of head movement, dizziness, or light-headedness. Sensory disturbances can also simulate cerebellar disease; with sensory ataxia, imbalance dramatically wors-ens when visual input is removed (Romberg sign). Bilateral proximal leg weak-ness can also rarely mimic cerebellar ataxia.

—————————— *Approach to the Patient* ——————————

Causes are best grouped by determining whether ataxia is symmetric or asymmetric and by the time course (Table 192-1). It is also important to distinguish whether ataxia is present in isolation or is part of a multisystem neurologic disorder. Acute symmetric ataxia is usually due to medications, toxins, viral infection, or a postinfectious syndrome (especially varicella). Subacute or chronic symmetric ataxia can result from hypothyroidism, vitamin deficiencies, infections (Lyme disease, tabes dorsalis, prions), alcohol, other toxins, or an inherited condition (see below). An immune-mediated progressive ataxia is associated with anti-gliadin antibodies; biopsy of the small intestine may reveal villous atrophy of gluten enteropathy. Progressive nonfamilial cerebellar ataxia after age 45 suggests a paraneoplastic syndrome, either subacute cortical cerebellar degeneration (ovarian, breast, lung, Hodgkin's) or opsoclonus-myoclonus (neuroblastoma, breast, lung)

Unilateral ataxia suggests a focal lesion in the ipsilateral cerebellar hemisphere or its connections. An important cause of acute unilateral ataxia is stroke. Mass effect from cerebellar hemorrhage or swelling from cerebellar infarction can compress brainstem structures, producing altered consciousness and ipsilateral pontine signs (small pupil, lateral gaze or sixth nerve paresis, facial weakness); limb ataxia may not be prominent. Other diseases producing asymmetric or unilateral ataxia include tumors, multiple sclerosis, progressive multifocal leukoencephalopathy (immunodeficiency states), and congenital malformations.

Inherited Ataxias

May be autosomal dominant, autosomal recessive, or mitochondrial (maternal inheritance); more than 30 disorders recognized (Table 352-2, HPIM-16). Friedreich's ataxia is most common; autosomal recessive, onset before age 25; ataxia with areflexia, upgoing toes, vibration and position sensation deficits, cardiomyopathy, hammer toes, scoliosis; linked to expanded trinucleotide repeat in the intron of "frataxin" gene; a second form of Friedreich's is associated with vitamin E deficiency. Common dominantly inherited ataxias are spinocerebellar ataxia (SCA) 1 (olivopontocerebellar degeneration; "ataxin-1" gene) and SCA 3 (Machado-Joseph disease); both may manifest as ataxia with brainstem and/or extrapyramidal signs; SCA 3 may also have dystonia and amyotrophy; genes for each disorder contain unstable trinucleotide repeats in coding region.

Evaluation

Diagnostic approach is determined by the nature of the ataxia (Table 192-1). For symmetric ataxias, drug and toxicology screens; vitamin B_1, B_{12}, and E levels; thyroid function tests; antibody tests for syphilis and Lyme infection; anti-gliadin antibodies; paraneoplastic antibodies (see Chap. 81); and CSF studies often indicated. Genetic testing is available for many inherited ataxias. For unilateral or asymmetric ataxias, brain MRI or CT scan is the initial test of choice.

 TREATMENT

Hypothyroidism, vitamin deficiency, infectious causes of ataxia are treatable. Parainfectious ataxia can be treated with glucocorticoids. Ataxia with anti-gliadin antibodies and gluten enteropathy may improve with a gluten-free diet. Paraneoplastic disorders are often refractory to therapy, but some pts improve

Table 192-1

Etiology of Cerebellar Ataxia

Symmetric and Progressive Signs			Focal and Ipsilateral Cerebellar Signs		
Acute (Hours to Days)	Subacute (Days to Weeks)	Chronic (Months to Years)	Acute (Hours to Days)	Subacute (Days to Weeks)	Chronic (Months to Years)
Intoxication: alcohol, lithium, diphenylhydantoin, barbiturates (positive history and toxicology screen) Acute viral cerebellitis (CSF supportive of acute viral infection) Postinfection syndrome	Intoxication: mercury, solvents, gasoline, glue; cytotoxic chemotherapeutic drugs Alcoholic-nutritional (vitamin B_1 and B_{12} deficiency) Lyme disease	Paraneoplastic syndrome Anti-gliadin antibody syndrome Hypothyroidism Inherited diseases Tabes dorsalis (tertiary syphilis) Phenytoin toxicity	Vascular: cerebellar infarction, hemorrhage, or subdural hematoma Infectious: cerebellar abscess (positive mass lesion on MRI/CT, positive history in support of lesion)	Neoplastic: cerebellar glioma or metastatic tumor (positive for neoplasm on MRI/CT) Demyelinating: multiple sclerosis (history, CSF, and MRI are consistent) AIDS-related multifocal leukoencephalopathy (positive HIV test and CD4+ cell count for AIDS)	Stable gliosis secondary to vascular lesion or demyelinating plaque (stable lesion on MRI/CT older than several months) Congenital lesion: Chiari or Dandy-Walker malformations (malformation noted on MRI/CT)

following removal of the tumor or immunotherapy (Chap. 81). Vitamins B_1 and B_{12} should be administered to pts with deficient levels. The deleterious effects of diphenylhydantoin and alcohol on the cerebellum are well known, and these exposures should be avoided in pts with ataxia of any cause. There is no proven therapy for any of the autosomal dominant ataxias. There is preliminary evidence that idebenone, a free-radical scavenger, can improve myocardial hypertrophy in Friedreich's ataxia; there is no evidence that it improves neurologic function. Iron chelators and antioxidant drugs are potentially harmful in Friedreich pts as they may increase heart muscle injury. Cerebellar hemorrhage and other mass lesions of the posterior fossa may require surgical treatment to prevent fatal brainstem compression.

For a more detailed discussion, see Rosenberg RN: Ataxic Disorders, Chap. 352, p. 2418, in HPIM-16.

193

ALS AND OTHER MOTOR NEURON DISEASES

Etiology

Amyotrophic lateral sclerosis (ALS) is the most important of the motor neuron diseases (Table 193-1). ALS is caused by degeneration of motor neurons at all levels of the CNS, including anterior horns of the spinal cord, brainstem motor nuclei, and motor cortex. Familial ALS (FALS) represents 5–10% of the total and is inherited as an autosomal dominant disorder.

Table 193-1

Sporadic Motor Neuron Diseases

CHRONIC

> Upper and lower motor neurons
> > Amyotrophic lateral sclerosis
> Predominantly upper motor neurons
> > Primary lateral sclerosis
> Predominantly lower motor neurons
> > Multifocal motor neuropathy with conduction block
> > Motor neuropathy with paraproteinemia or cancer
> > Motor-predominant peripheral neuropathies
> Other
> > Associated with other degenerative disorders
> > Secondary motor neuron disorders (see Table 193-2)

ACUTE

> Poliomyelitis
> Herpes zoster
> Coxsackie virus

Clinical Presentation

Onset is usually midlife, with most cases progressing to death in 3–5 years. Common initial symptoms are weakness, muscle wasting, stiffness and cramping, and twitching in muscles of hands and arms. Legs are less severely involved than arms, with complaints of leg stiffness, cramping, and weakness common. Symptoms of brainstem involvement include dysarthria and dysphagia.

Physical Examination

Lower motor neuron disease results in weakness and wasting that often first involves intrinsic hand muscles but later becomes generalized. Fasciculations occur in involved muscles, and fibrillations may be seen in the tongue. Hyperreflexia, spasticity, and upgoing toes in weak, atrophic limbs provide evidence of upper motor neuron disease. Brainstem disease produces wasting of the tongue; difficulty in articulation, phonation, and deglutition; and pseudobulbar palsy (e.g., involuntary laughter, crying). Important additional features that characterize ALS are preservation of intellect, lack of sensory abnormalities, and absence of bowel or bladder dysfunction.

Laboratory Findings

EMG provides objective evidence of extensive muscle denervation not confined to the territory of individual peripheral nerves and nerve roots. CSF is usually normal. Muscle enzymes (e.g., CK) may be elevated. Genetic testing is available for superoxide dismutase 1 (SOD1) (20% of FALS) and for rare mutations in other genes (Table 193-2). Pulmonary function studies may aid in management of ventilation.

Several types of secondary motor neuron disorders that resemble ALS are treatable (Table 193-2). All pts should have a careful search for these disorders. MRI or CT-myelography is often required to exclude compressive lesions of the foramen magnum or cervical spine. When involvement is restricted to lower motor neurons only, another important entity is multifocal motor neuropathy with conduction block (MMCB). A diffuse, lower motor axonal neuropathy mimicking ALS sometimes evolves in association with hematopoietic disorders such as lymphoma; an M-component in serum should prompt consideration of a bone marrow biopsy. Lyme disease may also cause an axonal, lower motor neuropathy. Other treatable disorders that occasionally mimic ALS are chronic lead poisoning and thyrotoxicosis.

Complications

Weakness of ventilatory muscles leads to respiratory insufficiency; dysphagia may lead to aspiration pneumonia and compromised energy intake.

 TREATMENT

There is no treatment capable of arresting ALS. The drug riluzole produces modest lengthening of survival; in one trial the survival rate at 18 months with riluzole (100 mg/d) was similar to placebo at 15 months. It may act by diminishing glutamate release and thereby decreasing excitotoxic neuronal cell death. Side effects of riluzole include nausea, dizziness, weight loss, and elevation of liver enzymes. Clinical trials of several other agents are in progress, including insulin-like growth factor (IGF-1), the COX-2 inhibitor celecoxib, and minocycline.

A variety of rehabilitative aids may substantially assist ALS patients. Foot-drop splints facilitate ambulation, and finger extension splints can potentiate

Table 193-2

Etiology and Investigation of Motor Neuron Disorders

Diagnostic Category	Investigations
Structural lesions	MRI scan of head (including foramen magnum), cervical spine[a]
Parasagittal or foramen magnum tumors	
Cervical spondylosis	
Chiari malformation or syrinx	
Spinal cord arteriovenous malformation	
Infections	CSF exam, culture[a]
Bacterial—tetanus, Lyme	Lyme antibody titer[a]
Viral—poliomyelitis, herpes zoster	Antiviral antibody titers
Retroviral myelopathy	HTLV-1 titers
Intoxications, physical agents	
Toxins—lead, aluminum, others	24-h urine for heavy metals[a]
Drugs—strychnine, phenytoin	Serum for lead level[a]
Electric shock, x-irradiation	
Immunologic mechanisms	Complete blood count[a]
Plasma cell dyscrasias	Sedimentation rate[a]
Autoimmune polyradiculoneuropathy	Protein immunoelectrophoresis[a]
Motor neuropathy with conduction block	Anti-GM1 antibodies[a]
Paraneoplastic	Anti-Hu antibody
Paracarcinomatous/lymphoma	MRI scan, bone marrow biopsy
Metabolic	
Hypoglycemia	Fasting blood sugar (FBS), routine chemistries including calcium[a]
Hyperparathyroidism	PTH, calcium, phosphate
Hyperthyroidism	Thyroid function[a]
Deficiency of folate vitamin B_{12}, vitamin E	Vitamin B_{12}, vitamin E, folate levels[a]
Malabsorption	24-h stool fat, carotene, prothrombin time
Mitochondrial dysfunction	Fasting lactate, pyruvate, ammonia
	Consider mtDNA analysis
Hereditary biochemical disorders	
Superoxide dismutase 1 gene mutation	White blood cell DNA analysis
Androgen receptor defect (Kennedy's disease)	Abnormal CAG insert in androgen receptor gene
Hexosaminidase deficiency	Lysosomal enzyme screen
Infantile (α-glucosidase deficiency/Pompe's disease)	
Hyperlipidemia	Lipid electrophoresis
Hyperglycinuria	Urine and serum amino acids
Methylcrotonylglycinuria	CSF amino acids

[a] Denotes studies that should be obtained in all cases.

Note: HTLV, human T cell lymphotropic virus; PTH, parathyroid hormone.

grip. Respiratory support may be life-sustaining. For pts electing against long-term ventilation by tracheostomy, positive-pressure ventilation by mouth or nose provides transient (several weeks) relief from hypercarbia and hypoxia. Also beneficial are respiratory devices that produce an artificial cough; these help to clear airways and prevent aspiration pneumonia. When bulbar disease prevents normal chewing and swallowing, gastrostomy is helpful. Speech synthesizers can augment speech when there is advanced bulbar palsy.

Web-based information on ALS is offered by the Muscular Dystrophy Association (www.mdausa.org) and the Amyotrophic Lateral Sclerosis Association (www.alsa.org).

For a more detailed discussion, see Brown RH Jr: Amyotrophic Lateral Sclerosis and Other Motor Neuron Diseases, Chap. 353, p. 2424, in HPIM-16.

194

TRIGEMINAL NEURALGIA, BELL'S PALSY, AND OTHER CRANIAL NERVE DISORDERS

Disorders of vision and ocular movement are discussed in Chaps. 40 and 59; dizziness and vertigo in Chap. 39; and disorders of hearing in Chap. 59.

FACIAL PAIN OR NUMBNESS [TRIGEMINAL NERVE (V)] (See Fig. 194-1)

TRIGEMINAL NEURALGIA (TIC DOULOUREUX)   Frequent, excruciating paroxysms of pain in lips, gums, cheek, or chin (rarely in ophthalmic division of fifth nerve) lasting seconds to minutes. Typically presents in middle or old age. Pain is often stimulated at trigger points. Sensory deficit cannot be demonstrated. Must be distinguished from other forms of facial pain arising from diseases of jaw, teeth, or sinuses. Rare causes are herpes zoster or a tumor. Onset in young adulthood raises the possibility of multiple sclerosis.

℞ TREATMENT

Carbamazepine is effective in 50–75% of cases. Begin at 100 mg single daily dose taken with food and advance by 100 mg every 1–2 days until substantial (50%) pain relief occurs. Most pts require 200 mg qid; doses >1200 mg daily usually provide no additional benefit. Follow CBC for rare complication of agranulocytosis. For nonresponders, phenytoin (300–400 mg qd) or baclofen (5–20 mg tid-qid) can be tried. When medications fail, surgical lesions (heat or glycerol injection) can be effective; in some centers, microvascular decompression recommended if a tortuous blood vessel found in posterior fossa near trigeminal nerve.

TRIGEMINAL NEUROPATHY   Usually presents as facial sensory loss or weakness of jaw muscles. Causes are varied (Table 194-1), including tumors

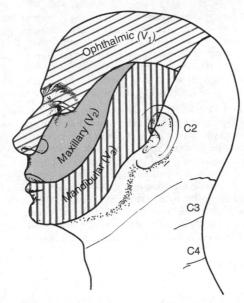

FIGURE 194-1   The three major sensory divisions of the trigeminal nerve consist of the ophthalmic, maxillary, and mandibular nerves.

of middle cranial fossa or trigeminal nerve, metastases to base of skull, or lesions in cavernous sinus (affecting first and second divisions of fifth nerve) or superior orbital fissure (affecting first division of fifth nerve).

FACIAL WEAKNESS [FACIAL NERVE (VII)]

Look for hemifacial weakness that includes muscles of forehead and orbicularis oculi. If lesion is in middle ear portion, taste is lost over the anterior two-thirds

Table 194-1

Trigeminal Nerve Disorders

Nuclear (brainstem) lesions	Peripheral nerve lesions
Multiple sclerosis	Nasopharyngeal carcinoma
Stroke	Trauma
Syringobulbia	Guillain-Barré syndrome
Glioma	Sjögren's syndrome
Lymphoma	Collagen-vascular diseases
Preganglionic lesions	Sarcoidosis
Acoustic neuroma	Leprosy
Meningioma	Drugs (stilbamidine, trichloroethylene)
Metastasis	Idiopathic trigeminal neuropathy
Chronic meningitis	
Cavernous carotid aneurysm	
Gasserian ganglion lesions	
Trigeminal neuroma	
Herpes zoster	
Infection (spread from otitis media or mastoiditis)	

of tongue and there may be hyperacusis; if lesion is at internal auditory meatus, there may be involvement of auditory and vestibular nerves; pontine lesions usually affect abducens nerve and often corticospinal tract. Peripheral nerve lesions with incomplete recovery may produce continuous contractions of affected musculature (*facial myokymia*); contraction of all facial muscles on attempts to move one group selectively (*synkinesis*); hemifacial spasms; or anomalous tears when facial muscles activated as in eating (*crocodile tears*).

BELL'S PALSY   Most common form of idiopathic facial paralysis; affects 1 in 60–70 persons over a lifetime. Association with herpes simplex virus type 1. Weakness evolves over 12–48 h, sometimes preceded by retroaural pain. Hyperacusis may be present. Full recovery within several weeks or months in 80%; incomplete paralysis in first week is a favorable prognostic sign.

Diagnosis can be made clinically in pts with (1) a typical presentation, (2) no risk factors or preexisting symptoms for other causes of facial paralysis, (3) no lesions of herpes zoster in the external ear canal, and (4) a normal neurologic examination with the exception of the facial nerve. In uncertain cases, an ESR, testing for diabetes mellitus, a Lyme titer, angiotensin-converting enzyme and chest x-ray for possible sarcoidosis, or MRI scanning may be indicated.

 TREATMENT

Protect the eye with paper tape to depress the upper eyelid during sleep. Prednisone (60–80 mg qd over 5 days, tapered off over the next 5 days) when started early appears to shorten the recovery period and modestly improve functional outcome. Treatment within 3 days of onset with both acyclovir (400 mg five times daily for 10 days) plus prednisone may improve outcome.

OTHER FACIAL NERVE DISORDERS   *Ramsay Hunt syndrome* is caused by herpes zoster infection of geniculate ganglion; distinguished from Bell's palsy by a vesicular eruption in pharynx and external auditory canal, and by frequent involvement of eighth cranial nerve. *Acoustic neuromas* often compress the seventh nerve. *Infarcts, demyelinating lesions of multiple sclerosis,* and *tumors* are common pontine causes. *Bilateral facial weakness* may occur in Guillain-Barré syndrome, sarcoidosis, Lyme disease, and leprosy. *Hemifacial spasm* may occur with Bell's palsy, irritative lesions (e.g., acoustic neuroma, basilar artery aneurysm, or aberrant vessel compressing the nerve) or as an idiopathic disorder. *Blepharospasm* consists of involuntary recurrent spasms of both eyelids, usually occurring in the elderly and sometimes with associated facial spasm. May subside spontaneously. Hemifacial spasm or blepharospasm can be treated by injection of botulinus toxin into the orbicularis oculi; spasms are relieved for 3–4 months, and injections can be repeated.

OTHER CRANIAL NERVE DISORDERS

DISORDERS OF THE SENSE OF SMELL   Olfactory nerve (I) disorders are due to interference with access of the odorant to the olfactory neuroepithelium (transport loss), injury to receptor region (sensory loss), or damage to central olfactory pathways (neural loss). The causes of olfactory disorders are summarized in Table 194-2; most common are head trauma in young adults and viral infections in older adults.

 TREATMENT

Therapy for allergic rhinitis, bacterial rhinitis and sinusitis, polyps, neoplasms, and structural abnormalities of the nasal cavities is usually successful in re-

Table 194-2

Causes of Olfactory Dysfunction

Transport Losses	Neural Losses
Allergic rhinitis	AIDS
Bacterial rhinitis and sinusitis	Alcoholism
Congenital abnormalities	Alzheimer's disease
Nasal neoplasms	Cigarette smoke
Nasal polyps	Depression
Nasal septal deviation	Diabetes mellitus
Nasal surgery	Drugs/toxins
Viral infections	Huntington's chorea
Sensory Losses	Hypothyroidism
Drugs	Kallmann syndrome
Neoplasms	Malnutrition
Radiation therapy	Neoplasms
Toxin exposure	Neurosurgery
Viral infections	Parkinson's disease
	Trauma
	Vitamin B_{12} deficiency
	Zinc deficiency

storing the sense of smell. There is no proven treatment for sensorineural olfactory losses; fortunately, spontaneous recovery often occurs. Cases due to exposure to cigarette smoke and other airborne toxic chemicals can recover if the insult is discontinued.

GLOSSOPHARYNGEAL NEURALGIA   This form of neuralgia involves the ninth (glossopharyngeal) and sometimes portions of the tenth (vagus) cranial nerves. Paroxysmal, intense pain in tonsillar fossa of throat that may be precipitated by swallowing. There is no demonstrable sensory and motor deficit. Other diseases affecting this nerve include herpes zoster or compressive neuropathy due to tumor or aneurysm in region of jugular foramen (when associated with vagus and accessory nerve palsies).

℞ TREATMENT

Medical therapy is similar to that for trigeminal neuralgia, and carbamazepine is generally the first choice. If drug therapy is unsuccessful, surgical procedures (including microvascular decompression, if vascular compression is evident, or rhizotomy of glossopharyngeal and vagal fibers in the jugular bulb) are frequently successful.

DYSPHAGIA AND DYSPHONIA   Lesions of the vagus nerve (X) may be responsible. Unilateral lesions produce drooping of soft palate, loss of gag reflex, and "curtain movement" of lateral wall of pharynx with hoarse, nasal voice. Diseases that may involve the vagus include diphtheria, neoplastic and infectious processes of the meninges, tumors and vascular lesions in the medulla, or compression of the recurrent laryngeal nerve by intrathoracic processes. Aneurysm of the aortic arch, an enlarged left atrium, and tumors of the mediastinum and bronchi are much more frequent causes of an isolated vocal cord palsy than are intracranial disorders. A substantial number of cases of recurrent laryngeal palsy remain idiopathic.

With laryngeal palsy, first determine the site of the lesion. If intramedullary, there are usually other brainstem signs. If extramedullary, the glossopharyngeal (IX) and spinal accessory (XI) nerves are frequently involved (jugular foramen syndrome). If extracranial in the retroparotid space, there may be combinations of ninth, tenth, eleventh, and twelfth cranial nerve palsies and a Horner syndrome. If there is no sensory loss over the palate and pharynx and no palatal weakness or dysphagia, lesion is below the origin of the pharyngeal branches, which leave the vagus nerve high in the cervical region; the usual site of disease is then the mediastinum.

NECK WEAKNESS   Isolated involvement of the accessory (XI) nerve can occur anywhere along its route, resulting in paralysis of the sternocleidomastoid and trapezius muscles. More commonly, involvement occurs in combination with deficits of the ninth and tenth cranial nerves in the jugular foramen or after exit from the skull. An idiopathic form of accessory neuropathy, akin to Bell's palsy, has been described; most pts recover.

TONGUE PARALYSIS   The hypoglossal (XII) nerve supplies the ipsilateral muscles of the tongue. The nucleus of the nerve or its fibers of exit may be involved by intramedullary lesions such as tumor, poliomyelitis, or most often motor neuron disease. Lesions of the basal meninges and the occipital bones (platybasia, Paget's disease) may compress the nerve in its extramedullary course or in the hypoglossal canal. Isolated lesions of unknown cause can occur. Atrophy and fasciculation of the tongue develop weeks to months after interruption of the nerve.

MULTIPLE CRANIAL NERVE PALSIES

First determine whether the process is within the brainstem or outside it. Lesions on the surface of the brainstem tend to involve adjacent cranial nerves in suc-

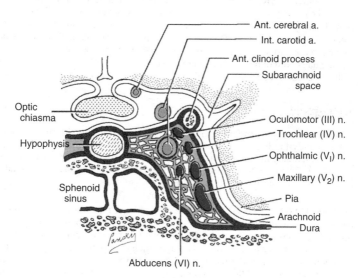

FIGURE 194-2   Anatomy of the cavernous sinus in coronal section, illustrating the location of the cranial nerves in relation to the vascular sinus, internal carotid artery (which loops anteriorly to the section), and surrounding structures.

cession with only late and slight involvement of long sensory and motor pathways. The opposite is true of processes within the brainstem. Involvement of multiple cranial nerves outside of the brainstem may be due to diabetes, trauma, infectious and noninfectious causes of meningitis; granulomatous diseases including sarcoidosis, tuberculosis, and Wegener's granulomatosis; tumors; and enlarging saccular aneurysms. A purely motor disorder raises a question of myasthenia gravis. *Facial diplegia* is common in Guillain-Barré syndrome. *Ophthalmoplegia* may occur with Guillain-Barré syndrome (Fisher variant) or Wernicke's disease.

The *cavernous sinus syndrome* (Fig. 194-2) is frequently life-threatening. It often presents as orbital or facial pain; orbital swelling and chemosis; fever; oculomotor neuropathy; and trigeminal neuropathy affecting the ophthalmic (V_1) and occasionally maxillary (V_2) divisions. Cavernous sinus thrombosis, often secondary to infection from orbital cellulitis or sinusitis, is the most frequent cause; other etiologies include aneurysm of the carotid artery, a carotid-cavernous fistula (orbital bruit may be present), meningioma, nasopharyngeal carcinoma, other tumors, or an idiopathic granulomatous disorder (Tolosa-Hunt syndrome). In infectious cases, prompt administration of broad-spectrum antibiotics, drainage of any abscess cavities, and identification of the offending organism is essential. Anticoagulant therapy may benefit cases of primary thrombosis. Repair or occlusion of the carotid artery may be required for treatment of fistulas or aneurysms. The Tolosa-Hunt syndrome generally responds to glucocorticoids.

For a more detailed discussion, see Beal MF, Hauser SL: **Trigeminal Neuralgia, Bell's Palsy, and Other Cranial Nerve Disorders, Chap. 355, p. 2434; and Lalwani AK, Snow JB Jr: Disorders of Smell, Taste, and Hearing, Chap. 26, p. 176, in HPIM-16.**

195

AUTONOMIC NERVOUS SYSTEM DISORDERS

The autonomic nervous system (ANS) (Fig. 195-1) innervates the entire neuraxis and permeates all organ systems. It regulates blood pressure (bp), heart rate, sleep, and bladder and bowel function. It operates in the background, so that its full importance becomes recognized only when ANS function is compromised, resulting in dysautonomia.

ANS Overview

Key features of the ANS are summarized in Table 195-1. Responses to sympathetic or parasympathetic activation often have opposite effects; partial activation of both systems allows for simultaneous integration of multiple body functions.

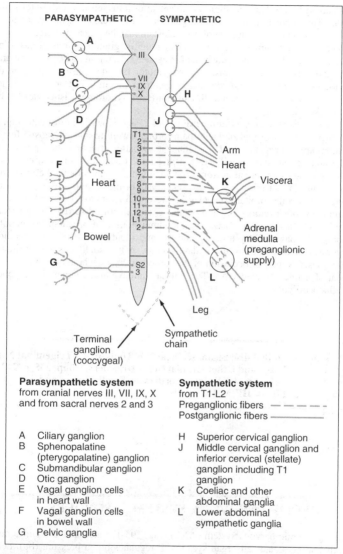

FIGURE 195-1 Schematic representation of the autonomic nervous system. (*From M. Moskowitz: Clin Endocrinol Metab 6:77, 1977.*)

Symptoms of Autonomic Dysfunction

Impotence, although not specific for autonomic failure, often heralds autonomic failure in men and may precede other symptoms by years. Bladder dysfunction may appear early in men and women, particularly in those with CNS involvement. Gastrointestinal autonomic dysfunction typically presents as severe constipation. Diarrhea occurs occasionally due to rapid transit of contents or uncoordinated small-bowel motor activity, or from bacterial overgrowth associated

Table 195-1

Functional Consequences of Normal ANS Activation

	Sympathetic	Parasympathetic
Heart rate	Increased	Decreased
Blood pressure	Increased	Mildly decreased
Bladder	Increased sphincter tone	Voiding (decreased tone)
Bowel motility	Decreased motility	Increased
Lung	Bronchodilation	Bronchoconstriction
Sweat glands	Sweating	—
Pupils	Dilation	Constriction
Adrenal glands	Catecholamine release	—
Sexual function	Ejaculation, orgasm	Erection
Lacrimal glands	—	Tearing
Parotid glands	—	Salivation

with small-bowel stasis. Impaired glandular secretory function may cause difficulty with food intake due to decreased salivation or with eye irritation due to decreased lacrimation. Occasionally, temperature elevation and vasodilation can result from anhidrosis because sweating is normally important for heat dissipation. Disorders of autonomic function need to be considered in the differential diagnosis of pts with impotence, bladder dysfunction (urinary frequency, hesitancy, or incontinence), diarrhea, constipation, or altered sweating (hyperhidrosis or hypohidrosis).

Orthostatic hypotension (OH) is perhaps the most disabling feature of autonomic dysfunction. Syncope results when the drop in bp impairs cerebral perfusion (Chap. 38). Other manifestations of impaired baroreflexes are supine hypertension, a heart rate that is fixed regardless of posture, postprandial hypotension, and an excessively high nocturnal bp. Many patients with OH have a preceding diagnosis of hypertension. The most common causes of OH are not neurologic in origin; these must be distinguished from the neurogenic causes.

_____ *Approach to the Patient* _____

The first step in the evaluation of symptomatic OH is the exclusion of treatable causes. The history should include a review of medications that may cause OH (e.g., diuretics, antihypertensives, antidepressants, phenothiazines, ethanol, narcotics, insulin, barbiturates, and calcium channel blocking agents). However, the precipitation of OH by medications may also be the first sign of an underlying autonomic disorder. The history may reveal an underlying cause for symptoms (e.g., diabetes, Parkinson's disease) or specific underlying mechanisms (e.g., cardiac pump failure, reduced intravascular volume). The relationship of symptoms to meals (splanchnic pooling), standing on awakening in the morning (intravascular volume depletion), ambient warming (vasodilatation), or exercise (muscle arteriolar vasodilatation) should be sought.

Physical exam includes measurement of supine and standing pulse and bp. OH is defined as a sustained drop in systolic ($\geq$20 mmHg) or diastolic ($\geq$10 mmHg) bp within 3 min of standing up. In nonneurogenic causes of OH (such as hypovolemia), the bp drop is accompanied by a compensatory increase in heart rate of >15 beats/min. A clue that the pt has neurogenic OH is the aggravation or precipitation of OH by autonomic stressors (such as a meal, hot tub/hot bath, and exercise). Neurologic evaluation should include a mental status exam (to exclude neurodegenerative disorders), cranial nerve exam (impaired downgaze in progressive supranuclear palsy), abnormal pupils (Horner's or Adie's pupils), motor exam (Parkinson's), and sensory exam (polyneuropathies). In pts without a clear initial diagnosis, follow-up neurologic exams and repeat laboratory evaluations over 1 to 2 years may reveal an evolution of findings that enables a specific diagnosis to be made.

Autonomic Testing

Autonomic function tests are helpful when the history and physical exam findings are inconclusive. Heart rate variation with deep breathing is a measure of vagal function. The Valsalva maneuver measures changes in heart rate and bp while a constant expiratory pressure of 40 mmHg for 15 s is maintained. The Valsalva ratio is calculated as the maximum heart rate during the maneuver divided by the minimum heart rate following the maneuver. The ratio reflects the integrity of the entire baroreceptor reflex arc and sympathetic efferents to blood vessels. Tilt-table beat-to-beat bp measurements in the supine, 80° tilt, and tilt-back positions can be used to evaluate orthostatic failure in bp control in pts with unexplained syncope.

Other tests of autonomic function include the quantitative sudomotor axon reflex test (QSART), the thermoregulatory sweat test (TST), and the cold pressor test. The QSART provides a quantitative, regional measure of sweating in response to iontophoresis of ACh. The TST provides a qualitative measure of regional sweating over the entire anterior surface of the body in response to a standardized elevation of body temperature. The cold pressor test is used to assess sympathetic efferent function. For a more complete discussion of autonomic function tests, see Chap. 354, HPIM-16.

Disorders of the Autonomic Nervous System

Autonomic disorders may occur with a large number of disorders of the central and/or peripheral nervous systems (Table 195-2). Diseases of the CNS may cause ANS dysfunction at many levels, including hypothalamus, brainstem, or spinal cord. *Multiple system atrophy* (MSA) is a progressive neurodegenerative disorder comprising autonomic failure (OH and/or a neurogenic bladder are required for diagnosis) combined with either parkinsonism (Shy-Drager syndrome) or olivopontocerebellar atrophy (Chap. 192). Dysautonomia is also common in advanced Parkinson's disease (Chap. 191).

Spinal cord injury may be accompanied by autonomic hyperreflexia affecting bowel, bladder, sexual, temperature regulation, or cardiovascular functions. Dangerous increases or decreases in body temperature may result from the inability to experience the sensory accompaniments of heat or cold exposure below the level of the injury. Markedly increased autonomic discharge (autonomic dysreflexia) can be elicited by bladder pressure or stimulation of the skin or muscles. Bladder distention from palpation, catheter insertion, catheter obstruction, or urinary infection is a common and correctable trigger of autonomic dysreflexia.

Peripheral neuropathies affecting the small myelinated and unmyelinated fibers of the sympathetic and parasympathetic nerves are the most common cause of chronic autonomic insufficiency (Chap. 197). Autonomic involvement in *diabetes mellitus* typically begins ~10 years after the onset of diabetes and slowly progresses. Diabetic enteric neuropathy may result in gastroparesis, nausea and vomiting, malnutrition, and bowel incontinence. Impotence, urinary incontinence, pupillary abnormalities, and postural hypotension may occur as well. Prolongation of the QT interval increases the risk of sudden death. Autonomic neuropathy occurs in both sporadic and familial forms of *amyloidosis*. Pts typically present with distal, painful polyneuropathy. *Alcoholic polyneurop-*

Table 195-2

Classification of Clinical Autonomic Disorders

I. Autonomic disorders with brain involvement
  A. Associated with multisystem degeneration
    1. Multisystem degeneration: autonomic failure clinically prominent
      a. Multiple system atrophy (MSA)
      b. Parkinson's disease with autonomic failure
      c. Diffuse Lewy body disease (some cases)
    2. Multisystem degeneration: autonomic failure clinically not usually prominent
      a. Parkinson's disease
      b. Other extrapyramidal disorders (inherited spinocerebellar atrophies, progressive supranuclear palsy, corticobasal degeneration, Machado-Joseph disease)
  B. Unassociated with multisystem degeneration
    1. Disorders mainly due to cerebral cortex involvement
      a. Frontal cortex lesions causing urinary/bowel incontinence
      b. Partial complex seizures
    2. Disorders of the limbic and paralimbic circuits
      a. Shapiro's syndrome (agenesis of corpus callosum, hyperhidrosis, hypothermia)
      b. Autonomic seizures
    3. Disorders of the hypothalamus
      a. Wernicke-Korsakoff syndrome
      b. Diencephalic syndrome
      c. Neuroleptic malignant syndrome
      d. Serotonin syndrome
      e. Fatal familial insomnia
      f. Antidiuretic hormone (ADH) syndromes (diabetes insipidus, inappropriate ADH)
      g. Disturbances of temperature regulation (hyperthermia, hypothermia)
      h. Disturbances of sexual function
      i. Disturbances of appetite
      j. Disturbances of bp/HR and gastric function
      k. Horner's syndrome
    4. Disorders of the brainstem and cerebellum
      a. Posterior fossa tumors
      b. Syringobulbia and Arnold-Chiari malformation
      c. Disorders of bp control (hypertension, hypotension)
      d. Cardiac arrhythmias
      e. Central sleep apnea
      f. Baroreflex failure
      g. Horner's syndrome
II. Autonomic disorders with spinal cord involvement
  A. Traumatic tetraplegia
  B. Syringomyelia
  C. Subacute combined degeneration
  D. Multiple sclerosis
  E. Amyotrophic lateral sclerosis
  F. Tetanus
  G. Stiff-man syndrome
  H. Spinal cord tumors

(continued)

Table 195-2 (Continued)

Classification of Clinical Autonomic Disorders

III. Autonomic neuropathies
  A. Acute/subacute autonomic neuropathies
    1. Subacute autoimmune autonomic neuropathy (panautonomic neuropathy, pandysautonomia)
      a. Subacute paraneoplastic autonomic neuropathy
      b. Guillain-Barré syndrome
      c. Botulism
      d. Porphyria
      e. Drug-induced autonomic neuropathies
      f. Toxic autonomic neuropathies
  B. Chronic peripheral autonomic neuropathies
    1. Distal small fiber neuropathy
    2. Combined sympathetic and parasympathetic failure
      a. Amyloid
      b. Diabetic autonomic neuropathy
      c. Autoimmune autonomic neuropathy (paraneoplastic and idiopathic)
      d. Sensory neuronopathy with autonomic failure
      e. Familial dysautonomia (Riley-Day syndrome)

Note: HR, heart rate.

athy produces symptoms of autonomic failure only when the neuropathy is severe. BP fluctuation and cardiac arrhythmias can be severe in *Guillain-Barré syndrome.* Attacks of *acute intermittent porphyria* (AIP) are associated with tachycardia, sweating, urinary retention, and hypertension. *Botulism* is associated with blurred vision, dry mouth, nausea, unreactive pupils, urinary retention, and constipation. *Autoimmune autonomic neuropathy* presents as the subacute development of autonomic failure with OH, enteric neuropathy (gastroparesis, ileus, constipation/diarrhea), loss of sweating, sicca complex, and a tonic pupil. Onset may follow a viral infection; serum antibodies to the ganglionic ACh receptor (A_3 AChR) are present, and some pts appear to respond to immunotherapy. Rare patients develop *dysautonomia* as a paraneoplastic disorder (Chap. 81) or on a hereditary basis. *Postural orthostatic tachycardia syndrome* (POTS) presents with symptoms of orthostatic intolerance, including shortness of breath, light-headedness, and exercise intolerance accompanied by an increase in heart rate but no drop in bp. *Primary hyperhidrosis* affects 0.6–1.0% of the population; the usual symptoms are excessive sweating of the palms and soles. Onset is in adolescence, and symptoms tend to improve with age. Although not dangerous, this condition is socially embarrassing.

Complex Regional Pain Syndrome (Reflex Sympathetic Dystrophy—RSD)

Complex regional pain syndrome (CRPS) type I is a regional pain syndrome that usually develops after trauma. *Allodynia* (the perception of a nonpainful stimulus as painful), *hyperpathia* (an exaggerated pain response to a painful stimulus), and *spontaneous pain* occur. The symptoms are unrelated to the severity of the initial trauma and are not confined to the distribution of a single peripheral nerve. CRPS type II is a regional pain syndrome that develops after injury to a peripheral nerve, usually a major nerve trunk. Spontaneous pain initially develops within the territory of the affected nerve but eventually may spread outside the nerve distribution.

CRPS type I (RSD) has been divided into three clinical phases: (1) pain and swelling in the distal extremity, which is warm and edematous with tender joints; increased sweating and hair growth; (2) appearance of thin, shiny, cool skin; and (3) atrophy of the skin and subcutaneous tissue plus flexion contractures.

Early mobilization with physical therapy or a brief course of glucocorticoids may be helpful for CRPS type I. Other treatments include the use of adrenergic blockers, NSAIDs, calcium channel blockers, or phenytoin. Stellate ganglion blockade is a commonly used invasive therapeutic technique that often provides temporary pain relief, but the efficacy of repetitive blocks is uncertain.

℞ TREATMENT

Of particular importance is the removal of drugs or amelioration of underlying conditions that cause or aggravate the autonomic symptom. For instance, OH can be related to angiotensin-converting enzyme inhibitors, calcium channel blocking agents, tricyclic antidepressants, levodopa, alcohol, or insulin. Nonpharmacologic approaches are summarized in Table 195-3. Adequate intake of salt and fluids to produce a voiding volume between 1.5 and 2.5 L of urine (containing >170 meq of Na^+) each 24 h is essential. Sleeping with the head of the bed elevated will minimize the effects of supine nocturnal hypertension. Prolonged recumbency should be avoided. Pts are advised to sit with legs dangling over the edge of the bed for several minutes before attempting to stand in the morning. Compressive garments such as compression stockings and abdominal binders may be helpful. Anemia should be corrected, if necessary, with erythropoietin; the increased intravascular volume that accompanies the rise in hematocrit can exacerbate supine hypertension. Postprandial OH may respond to frequent, small, low-carbohydrate meals.

If these measures are not sufficient, drug treatment might be necessary. Midodrine is a directly acting α_1 agonist that does not cross the blood-brain barrier. The dose is 5 to 10 mg orally tid, but some pts respond best to a decremental dose (e.g., 15 mg on awakening, 10 mg at noon, and 5 mg in the afternoon). Midodrine should not be taken after 6 P.M. Side effects include pruritus, uncomfortable piloerection, and supine hypertension. Pyridostigmine appears to improve OH without aggravating supine hypertension by enhancing ganglionic transmission (maximal when orthostatic, minimal supine). Fludrocortisone (0.1–0.3 mg bid orally) will reduce OH, but it aggravates supine hypertension. Susceptible patients may develop fluid overload, congestive heart failure, supine hypertension, or hypokalemia.

Table 195-3

Initial Treatment of Orthostatic Hypotension (OH)

Patient education: mechanisms and stressors of OH
High-salt diet (10–20 g/d)
High-fluid intake (2 L/d)
Elevate head of bed 10 cm (4 in.)
Maintain postural stimuli
Learn physical countermaneuvers
Compression garments
Correct anemia

For a more detailed discussion, see Low PA, Engstrom JW: Disorders of the Autonomic Nervous System, Chap. 354, p. 2428, in HPIM-16.

196

SPINAL CORD DISEASES

These can be devastating, but many are treatable if recognized early (Table 196-1). Knowledge of relevant spinal cord anatomy is often the key to correct diagnosis (Fig. 196-1).

Symptoms and Signs

Principal signs are loss of sensation below a horizontal meridian on the trunk ("sensory level"), accompanied by weakness and spasticity.

Table 196-1

Some Treatable Spinal Cord Disorders

Compressive
    Epidural, intradural, or intramedullary neoplasm
    Epidural abscess
    Epidural hemorrhage
    Cervical spondylosis
    Herniated disc
    Posttraumatic compression by fractured or displaced vertebra or hemorrhage
Vascular
    Arteriovenous malformation
    Antiphospholipid syndrome and other hypercoagulable states
Inflammatory
    Multiple sclerosis including neuromyelitis optica
    Transverse myelitis
    Sarcoidosis
    Vasculitis
Infectious
    Viral: VZV, HSV-1 and -2, CMV, HIV, HTLV-I, others
    Bacterial and mycobacterial: *Borrelia*, *Listeria*, syphilis, others
    Mycoplasma pneumoniae
    Parasitic: schistosomiasis, toxoplasmosis
Developmental
    Syringomyelia
    Meningomyelocoele
    Tethered cord syndrome
Metabolic
    Vitamin B_{12} deficiency (subacute combined degeneration)
    Adrenomyeloneuropathy

Note: VZV, varicella-zoster virus; HSV, herpes simplex virus; CMV, cytomegalovirus; HTLV, human T cell lymphotropic virus.

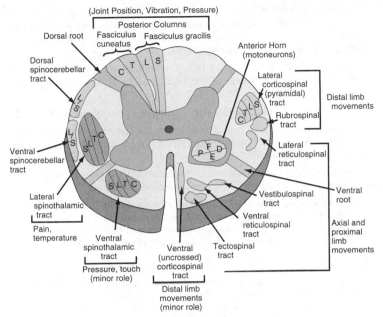

FIGURE 196-1 Transverse section through the spinal cord, composite representation, illustrating the principal ascending (*left*) and descending (*right*) pathways. The lateral and ventral spinothalamic tracts (dark green) ascend contralateral to the side of the body that is innervated. C, cervical; T, thoracic; L, lumbar; S, sacral; P, proximal; D, distal; F, flexors, E, extensors.

Sensory Symptoms   Often paresthesia; may begin in one or both feet and ascend. Sensory level to pin sensation or vibration often correlates well with location of transverse lesions. May have isolated pain/temperature sensation loss over the shoulders ("cape" or "syringomyelic" pattern) or loss of sensation to vibration/position on one side of the body and pain/temperature loss on the other (Brown-Séquard hemicord syndrome).

Motor Impairment   Disruption of corticospinal tracts causes quadriplegia or paraplegia with increased muscle tone, hyperactive deep tendon reflexes, and extensor plantar responses. With acute severe lesions there may be initial flaccidity and areflexia (spinal shock).

Segmental Signs   These are approximate indicators of level of lesion, e.g., band of hyperalgesia/hyperpathia, isolated flaccidity, atrophy, or single lost tendon reflex.

Autonomic Dysfunction   Primarily urinary retention; should raise suspicion of spinal cord disease when associated with back or neck pain, weakness, and/or a sensory level.

Pain   Midline back pain is of localizing value; interscapular pain may be first sign of midthoracic cord compression; radicular pain may mark site of more laterally placed spinal lesion; pain from lower cord (conus medullaris) lesion may be referred to low back.

Specific Signs by Spinal Cord Level

Lesions Near the Foramen Magnum   Weakness of the ipsilateral shoulder and arm, followed by weakness of ipsilateral leg, then contralateral leg, then contralateral arm, with respiratory paralysis.

Cervical Cord   Best localized by noting pattern of motor weakness and areflexia; shoulder (C5), biceps (C5-6), brachioradialis (C6), triceps/finger and wrist extensors (C7), finger flexors (C8).

Thoracic Cord   Localized by identification of a sensory level on the trunk.

Lumbar Cord   Upper lumbar cord lesions paralyze hip flexion and knee extension, whereas lower lumbar lesions affect foot and ankle movements, knee flexion, and thigh extension.

Sacral Cord (Conus Medullaris)   Saddle anesthesia, early bladder/ bowel dysfunction, impotence; muscle strength is largely preserved.

Cauda Equina (Cluster of Nerve Roots Derived from Lower Cord)   Lesions below spinal cord termination at the L1 vertebral level produce a flaccid, areflexic, asymmetric paraparesis with bladder/bowel dysfunction and sensory loss below L1; pain is common and projected to perineum or thighs.

Intramedullary and Extramedullary Syndromes

Spinal cord disorders may be intramedullary (arising from within the substance of the cord) or extramedullary (compressing the cord or its blood supply). Extramedullary lesions often produce radicular pain, early corticospinal signs, and sacral sensory loss. Intramedullary lesions produce poorly localized burning pain, less prominent corticospinal signs, and often spare perineal/sacral sensation.

Acute and Subacute Spinal Cord Diseases

——————————— *Approach to the Patient* ———————————

First priority: identify a treatable mass lesion. The common causes in this category are tumor, epidural abscess or hematoma, herniated disc, or other vertebral pathology. Epidural compression due to malignancy or abscess often causes warning signs of neck or back pain, bladder disturbances, and sensory symptoms that precede paralysis. MRI with contrast at clinically suspected level of pathology is the initial diagnostic procedure; it is often appropriate to image the entire spine to search for additional, clinically silent, lesions. Once compressive lesions have been excluded, noncompressive causes of acute myelopathy that are intrinsic to the cord are considered: primarily vascular, inflammatory, and infectious etiologies. CSF analysis useful for infectious and inflammatory processes.

1. *Neoplastic spinal cord compression*: Most are epidural in origin, resulting from metastases to the adjacent spinal bones. Almost any tumor can be responsible: breast, lung, prostate, lymphoma, and plasma cell dyscrasias most frequent. Thoracic cord most commonly involved. Initial symptom is usually back pain, worse when recumbent, with local tenderness preceding other symptoms by many weeks. Spinal cord compression due to metastases is a medical emergency; in general, therapy will not reverse paralysis of >48 h duration. Treatment consists of glucocorticoids (dexamethasone, 40 mg daily) to reduce interstitial edema, local radiotherapy initiated as early as possible to the symptomatic lesion, and specific therapy for the underlying tumor type. Intradural tumors are generally benign—meningiomas or neurofibromas; treatment is surgical resection.

2. *Spinal epidural abscess*: Triad of fever, localized spinal pain, and my-elopathy (progressive weakness and bladder symptoms); once neurologic signs appear, cord compression rapidly progresses. Two-thirds of infections spread hematogenously; one-third spread from a nearby skin infection. Impaired im-mune status and IV drug abuse are risk factors. Treatment is emergency decom-pressive laminectomy with debridement combined with long-term antibiotic therapy.

3. *Spinal epidural hematoma*: Presents as focal or radicular pain followed by variable signs of a spinal cord or cauda equina disorder. Therapeutic anti-coagulation, trauma, tumor, or blood dyscrasias are predisposing conditions; rare cases complicate LP or epidural anesthesia. Therapy is supportive, and surgical evacuation is generally not useful.

4. *Acute disk herniation*: Cervical and thoracic disk herniations are less common than lumbar.

5. *Spinal cord infarction*: Anterior spinal artery infarction produces para-plegia or quadriplegia, sensory loss affecting pain/temperature but sparing vi-bration/position sensations (supplied by posterior spinal arteries), and loss of sphincter control. Onset sudden or evolving over minutes or a few hours. As-sociated conditions: aortic atherosclerosis, dissecting aortic aneurysm, hypoten-sion. Therapy is directed at the predisposing condition.

6. *Immune-mediated myelopathies*: Acute transverse myelopathy (ATM) occurs in 1% of pts with SLE; associated with antiphospholipid antibodies. Sjögren's and Behçet's syndromes, mixed connective tissue disease, and p-ANCA vasculitis are other causes. Sarcoid can produce ATM with large edem-atous swelling of the spinal cord. Demyelinating diseases, either neuromyelitis optica or multiple sclerosis (especially in Asians), can also present as ATM; glucocorticoids, consisting of IV methylprednisolone followed by oral predni-sone, are indicated for moderate to severe symptoms and refractory cases may respond to plasma exchange (Chap. 189). Other cases of ATM are idio-pathic.

7. *Infectious myelopathies*: Herpes zoster is the most common viral agent; schistosomiasis is an important cause worldwide.

Chronic Myelopathies

1. *Spondylitic myelopathies*: One of the most common causes of gait dif-ficulty in the elderly. Presents as neck and shoulder pain, radicular arm pain, and progressive spastic paraparesis with paresthesia and loss of vibration sense; in advanced cases, urinary incontinence may occur. A tendon reflex in the arms is often diminished at some level. Diagnosis is best made by MRI. Treatment is surgical (Chap. 35).

2. *Vascular malformations*: An important treatable cause of progressive or episodic myelopathy. May occur at any level; diagnosis is made by contrast-enhanced MRI, confirmed by selective spinal angiography. Treatment is em-bolization with occlusion of the major feeding vessels.

3. *Retrovirus-associated myelopathies*: Infection with HTLV-I may pro-duce a slowly progressive spastic paraparesis with variable pain, sensory loss, and bladder disturbance; diagnosis is made by demonstration of specific serum antibody. Treatment is symptomatic. A progressive vacuolar myelopathy may also occur in AIDS.

4. *Syringomyelia*: Cavitary expansion of the spinal cord resulting in pro-gressive myelopathy; may be an isolated finding or associated with protrusion of cerebellar tonsils into cervical spinal canal (Chiari type 1). Classic presen-tation is loss of pain/temperature sensation in the neck, shoulders, forearms, or hands with areflexic weakness in the upper limbs and progressive spastic par-

aparesis; cough headache, facial numbness, or thoracic kyphoscoliosis may occur. Diagnosis is made by MRI; treatment is surgical and often unsatisfactory.

5. *Multiple sclerosis*: Spinal cord involvement is common, and is major cause of disability in progressive forms of MS (Chap. 189).

6. *Subacute combined degeneration (vitamin B$_{12}$ deficiency)*: Paresthesia in hands and feet, early loss of vibration/position sense, progressive spastic/ataxic weakness, and areflexia due to associated peripheral neuropathy; mental changes ("megaloblastic madness") and optic atrophy may be present. Diagnosis is confirmed by a low serum B$_{12}$ level, elevated levels of homocysteine and methylmalonic acid, and a positive Schilling test. Treatment is vitamin replacement.

7. *Tabes dorsalis (tertiary syphilis)*: May present as lancinating pains, gait ataxia, bladder disturbances, and visceral crises. Cardinal signs are areflexia in the legs, impaired vibration/position sense, Romberg sign, and Argyll Robertson pupils, which fail to constrict to light but react to accommodation.

8. *Familial spastic paraplegia*: Progressive spasticity and weakness in the legs occurring on a familial basis; may be autosomal dominant, recessive, or X-linked.

Complications

Bladder dysfunction with risk of urinary tract infection; bowel dysmotility; pressure sores; in high cervical cord lesions, mechanical respiratory failure; paroxysmal hypertension or hypotension with volume changes; severe hypertension and bradycardia in response to noxious stimuli or bladder or bowel distention; venous thrombosis and pulmonary embolism.

For a more detailed discussion, see Hauser SL, Ropper AH: Diseases of the Spinal Cord, Chap. 356, p. 2438, in HPIM-16.

197

PERIPHERAL NEUROPATHIES INCLUDING GUILLAIN-BARRÉ SYNDROME

Peripheral neuropathy (PN) refers to a peripheral nerve disorder of any cause. Nerve involvement may be single (mononeuropathy) or multiple (polyneuropathy); pathology may be axonal or demyelinating. An approach to pts with suspected neuropathy appears in Fig. 197-1.

POLYNEUROPATHY

CLINICAL FEATURES   The typical axonal polyneuropathy begins with sensory symptoms (tingling or burning) distally in the toes or feet. Symptoms spread proximally to the ankles, then involve the calves. Ankle reflexes are lost. Once sensory loss reaches the knees, proximal spread extends into the thighs and numbness of fingers appears. This pattern results in a "stocking-glove" distribution of sensory and motor findings. Further progression results in loss

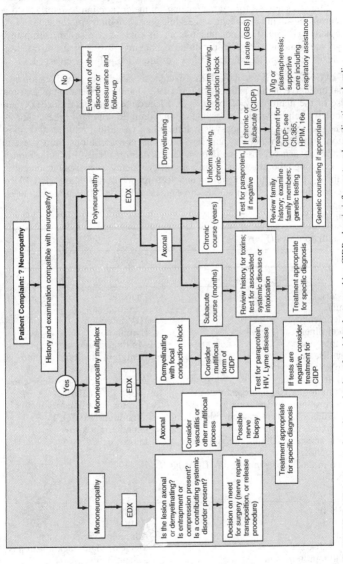

FIGURE 197-1 Approach to the evaluation of peripheral neuropathies. CIDP, chronic inflammatory demyelinating polyradiculoneuropathy; EDX, electrodiagnostic studies; GBS, Guillain-Barré syndrome; IVIg, intravenous immunoglobulin.

of knee reflexes. Light touch may be perceived as uncomfortable (allodynia) or pinprick as excessively painful (hyperpathia). Weakness and atrophy evolve from distal to proximal—initial toe dorsiflexion weakness may progress to bilateral foot drop, intrinsic hand muscle weakness, or (in extreme cases) impairment of muscles needed for ventilation and sphincter function. A family history for neuropathy should be sought, since adult-onset hereditary motor and sensory neuropathy (HMSN II) is not uncommon. In contrast to axonal neuropathy, demyelinating neuropathy does not produce stocking-glove deficits; diffuse loss of reflexes and strength is usual, and nerves are often palpably enlarged.

DIAGNOSTIC EVALUATION   Diagnosis is aided by classification into axonal or demyelinating pathology (Table 197-1) and consideration of the time course of the neuropathy (Table 197-2). Electrodiagnostic studies (EDX) are particularly helpful when history and examination do not clarify the diagnosis (see below). Sural nerve biopsy is helpful when vasculitis, multifocal demyelination, amyloidosis, leprosy, and sarcoidosis are considerations; biopsy results in lateral foot sensory loss, and rarely a painful neuroma may form at the biopsy site. Screening laboratory studies in a distal, symmetric axonal polyneuropathy are Hb A_{1C}, ESR, serum protein/immunoelectrophoresis, and vitamin B_{12}, BUN, and creatinine levels. Other studies are suggested by the differential diagnosis;

Table 197-1

Polyneuropathies (PN)[a]

Axonal	Demyelinative
ACQUIRED	
Diabetes	Diabetes
Uremia	Carcinoma
B_{12} deficiency	HIV infection
Critical illness	Lymphoma
HIV infection	Multiple myeloma
Lyme disease	Benign monoclonal gammo-
Lymphoma	pathy (IgM)
Multiple myeloma	Acute inflammatory demyelin-
Acute motor axonal neuropathy	ating PN (AIDP)
Drugs: cisplatin, hydralazine, isoniazid,	Chronic inflammatory demye-
metronidazole, nitrofurantoin, phenytoin,	linating PN (CIDP)
pyridoxine, vincristine	Diphtheria toxin
Toxins: arsenic, thallium, inorganic lead,	Idiopathic
organophosphates	
Benign monoclonal gammopathy (IgA, IgG)	
Idiopathic	
HEREDITARY	
HMSN II[b]	HMSN I
Amyloid	HMSN III
Porphyria	Adrenomyeloneuropathy
Fabry's disease	Metachromatic leukodystrophy
Abetalipoproteinemia	Refsum's disease
Friedreich's ataxia	Hereditary liability to pressure
Adrenomyeloneuropathy	palsies
Ataxia telangiectasia	

[a] Does not include rare causes.
[b] Hereditary motor and sensory neuropathy

Table 197-2
___

Diagnostic Considerations in Polyneuropathy

Type of Polyneuropathy	Time Course	Causes
AXONAL		
Acute	Days to weeks	Massive intoxications (arsenic; inhalants); porphyria; Guillain-Barré syndrome
Subacute	Weeks to months	Usually toxic or metabolic; eliminate toxins and treat underlying systemic disorder
Chronic	Months to years	<5 years, consider toxic or metabolic; >5 years, hereditary, diabetic, dysproteinemic causes
DEMYELINATIVE		
Acute	Days to weeks	Guillain-Barré syndrome; rarely diptheria or buckthorn berry intoxication
Subacute	Weeks to months	CIDP; rarely toxins listed above plus auro-thioglucose or taxol
Chronic	Months to years	Many possibilities including hereditary; inflammatory; dysproteinemias; other metabolic or toxic causes

Note: CIDP, chronic inflammatory demyelinating polyneuropathy.

it is important to recall that many systemic diseases, drugs, and toxins can produce neuropathy.

Electrodiagnosis   The EDX examination ordinarily comprises electromyography (EMG) and nerve conduction studies (NCSs). EMG involves recording for electrical potentials from a needle electrode in muscle at rest and during voluntary contraction. EMG is most useful for distinguishing between and among myopathic and neuropathic disorders. Myopathic disorders are marked by small, short-duration, polyphasic muscle action potentials; by contrast, neuropathic disorders are characterized by muscle denervation. Denervation features a decrease in the number of motor units (e.g., an anterior horn cell, its axon, and the motor end plates and muscle fibers it innervates). In long-standing muscle denervation, motor unit potentials become large and polyphasic. This occurs as a result of collateral reinnervation of denervated muscle fibers by axonal sprouts from surviving motor axons. Other EMG features that favor denervation include fibrillations (random, unregulated firing of individual denervated muscle fibers) and fasciculations (random, spontaneous firing of motor units). NCSs are carried out by stimulating motor or sensory nerves electrically at two or more sites. EDX features of demyelination are slowing of nerve conduction velocity (NCV), dispersion of evoked compound action potentials, conduction block (major decrease in amplitude of muscle compound action potentials on proximal stimulation of the nerve, as compared to distal stimulation), and marked prolongation of distal latencies. In contrast, axonal neuropathies are characterized by a reduced amplitude of evoked compound action potentials with relative preservation of NCV.

SPECIFIC POLYNEUROPATHIES

1. *Acute inflammatory demyelinating polyneuropathy (AIDP) or Guillain-Barré syndrome (GBS)*: an ascending, usually demyelinating, motor > sensory

Table 197-3

Common Mononeuropathies—Findings and Treatment

	Median	Ulnar	Common Peroneal
Site	Wrist—carpal tunnel	Elbow—cubital tunnel or condylar groove	Knee—fibular head
Sensory loss	Lateral palm: 1st–3rd finger ± 4th finger	Medial palm: 5th ± 4th finger	Dorsal foot Lateral calf
Motor weakness	Thumb abduction Thumb opposition	Index finger abduction 5th finger abduction	Foot dorsiflexion Foot eversion
Conservative Rx	Wrist splint, NSAIDs	Elbow pad Avoid elbow trauma	Avoid direct compression
Surgical Rx	Transverse carpal ligament section	Cubital tunnel release; ulnar nerve transposition	—

polyneuropathy accompanied by areflexia, motor paralysis, and elevated CSF total protein without pleocytosis. Over two-thirds are preceded by infection with EBV or other herpesviruses, *Campylobacter jejuni* gastroenteritis, HIV, other viruses, or *Mycoplasma*. Maximum weakness is usually reached within 2 weeks; demyelination by EMG. Most pts are hospitalized; one-third require ventilatory assistance. 85% make a complete or near-complete recovery with supportive care. Intravenous immune globulin (IVIg) (2 g/kg given over 5 days) or plasmapheresis (40–50 mL/kg daily for 4–5 days) significantly shortens the course. Glucocorticoids are ineffective. Variants of GBS include Fisher syndrome (ophthalmoparesis, facial diplegia, ataxia, areflexia; associated with antibodies to ganglioside GQ1b) and acute motor axonal neuropathy (more severe course than demyelinating GBS; antibodies to GM_1 in some cases).

2. *Chronic inflammatory demyelinating polyneuropathy (CIDP)*: a slowly progressive or relapsing polyneuropathy characterized by diffuse hyporeflexia or areflexia, diffuse weakness, elevated CSF protein without pleocytosis, and demyelination by EMG. Begin treatment when progression is rapid or walking is compromised. Initial treatment is usually IVIg; most pts require periodic retreatment at 6-week intervals. Other treatment options include plasmapheresis or glucocorticoids; immunosuppressants (azathioprine, methotrexate, cyclophosphamide) used in refractory cases.

3. *Diabetic neuropathy*: typically a distal symmetric, sensorimotor, axonal polyneuropathy, but many variations occur. A mixture of demyelination and axonal loss is frequent. Isolated sixth or third cranial nerve palsies, asymmetric proximal motor neuropathy in the legs, truncal neuropathy, autonomic neuropathy, and an increased frequency of entrapment neuropathy (see below).

4. *Mononeuropathy multiplex (MM)*: defined as involvement of multiple noncontiguous nerves. One-third of adults with MM have an acquired demyelinating disorder that is treatable. The remainder have an axonal disorder; 50% of these have vasculitis—usually due to a connective tissue disorder. In this latter group, immunosuppressive treatment of the underlying disease (usually with glucocorticoids and cyclophosphamide) is indicated.

MONONEUROPATHY

CLINICAL FEATURES Mononeuropathies are usually caused by trauma, compression, or entrapment. Sensory and motor symptoms are in the distribution of a single nerve—most commonly ulnar or median nerves in the arms or peroneal nerve in the leg. Clinical features favoring conservative management of median neuropathy at the wrist (carpal tunnel syndrome) or ulnar neuropathy at the elbow include sudden onset, no motor deficit, few or no sensory findings (pain or paresthesia may be present), and no evidence of axonal loss by EMG. Surgical decompression considered if chronic course (lack of response to conservative treatment), motor deficit, and electrodiagnostic evidence of axonal loss. Patterns of weakness, sensory loss, and conservative/surgical treatment options are listed in Table 197-3.

For a more detailed discussion, see Asbury AK: Approach to the Patient with Peripheral Neuropathy, Chap. 363, p. 2500; and Hauser SL, Asbury AK: Guillain-Barré Syndrome and Other Immune-Mediated Neuropathies, Chap. 365, p. 2513, in HPIM-16.

198

MYASTHENIA GRAVIS (MG)

An autoimmune neuromuscular disorder resulting in weakness and fatigability of skeletal muscles, due to autoantibodies directed against acetylcholine receptors (AChRs) at neuromuscular junctions (NMJs).

Clinical Features

May present at any age. Symptoms fluctuate throughout the day and are provoked by exertion. Characteristic distribution: cranial muscles (lids, extraocular muscles, facial weakness, "nasal" or slurred speech, dysphagia); in 85%, limb muscles (often proximal and asymmetric) become involved. Reflexes and sensation normal. May be limited to extraocular muscles only—particularly in elderly. Complications: aspiration pneumonia (weak bulbar muscles), respiratory failure (weak chest wall muscles), exacerbation of myasthenia due to administration of drugs with neuromuscular junction blocking effects (tetracycline, aminoglycosides, procainamide, propranolol, phenothiazines, lithium).

Pathophysiology

Specific anti-AChR antibodies reduce the number of AChRs at the NMJ. Postsynaptic folds are flattened or "simplified," with resulting inefficient neuromuscular transmission. During repeated or sustained muscle contraction, decrease in amount of ACh released per nerve impulse (a normal occurrence), combined with disease-specific decrease in postsynaptic AChRs, results in pathologic fatigue. Thymus is abnormal in 75% of pts (65% hyperplasia, 10% thymoma). Other autoimmune diseases in 10%; Hashimoto's thyroiditis, Graves' disease, rheumatoid arthritis, lupus erythematosus, red cell aplasia.

Differential Diagnosis

1. Lambert-Eaton syndrome (autoantibodies to calcium channels in presynaptic motor nerve terminals)—reduced ACh release; associated with malignancy or idiopathic
2. Neurasthenia—weakness/fatigue without underlying organic disorder
3. Penicillamine may cause MG; resolves weeks to months after discontinuing drug
4. Hyperthyroidism
5. Botulism—toxin inhibits presynaptic ACh release
6. Diplopia from an intracranial mass lesion—compression of nerves to extraocular muscles
7. Progressive external ophthalmoplegia—seen in mitochondrial disorders

Laboratory Evaluation

• AChR antibodies—no correlation with disease severity; 80% of all MG patients positive; 50% with ocular findings only are positive; positive antibodies are diagnostic. Muscle-specific kinase (MuSK) antibodies present in 40% of AchR antibody-negative pts with generalized MG.

• Tensilon (edrophonium) test—a short-acting anticholinesterase—look for rapid and transient improvement of strength; false-positive (placebo response, motor neuron disease) and false-negative tests occur.

• EMG—low-frequency (2–4 Hz) repetitive stimulation produces decrement in amplitude of evoked motor responses.

• Chest CT/MRI—search for thymoma.

• Consider thyroid and other studies (e.g., ANA) for associated autoimmune disease.

℞ **TREATMENT**   (See Fig. 198-1)

The anticholinesterase drug pyridostigmine (Mestinon) titrated to assist pt with functional activities (chewing, swallowing, strength during exertion); usual initial dose of 60 mg 3–5 times daily; long-acting tablets help at night.

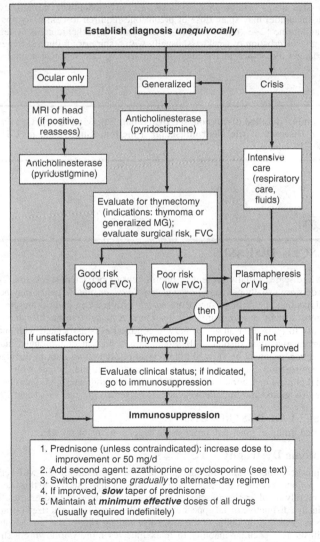

FIGURE 198-1   Algorithm for the management of myasthenia gravis. FVC, forced vital capacity; IVIg, intravenous immunoglobulin.

Muscarinic side effects (diarrhea, abdominal cramps, salivation, nausea) blocked with propantheline if required. Plasmapheresis and IV immune globulin [IVIg; 400 (mg/kg)/d for 5 days] provide temporary boost for seriously ill pts; used to improve condition prior to surgery or during myasthenic crisis (severe exacerbation of weakness). Thymectomy improves likelihood of long-term remission in adult (less consistently in elderly) pts. Glucocorticoids are a mainstay of treatment; begin prednisone at low dose (15–25 mg/d), increase by 5 mg/d q2–3 d until marked clinical improvement or dose of 50 mg/d is reached. Maintain high dose for 1–3 months, then decrease to alternate-day regimen. Long-term treatment with low-dose prednisone usual. Immunosuppressive drugs (azathioprine, cyclosporine, mycophenolate mofetil, cyclophosphamide) may spare dose of prednisone required to control symptoms; azathioprine [2–3 (mg/kg)/d] most often used. Myasthenic crisis is defined as an exacerbation of weakness, usually with respiratory failure, sufficient to endanger life; expert management in an intensive care setting essential.

For a more detailed discussion, see Drachman DB: Myasthenia Gravis and Other Diseases of the Neuromuscular Junction, Chap. 366, p. 2518, in HPIM-16.

199

MUSCLE DISEASES

Muscle diseases usually present as intermittent or persistent weakness. These disorders are usually painless; however, *myalgias*, or muscle pains, may occur. Myalgias must be distinguished from *muscle cramps*, i.e., painful muscle contractions, usually due to neurogenic disorders. A *muscle contracture* due to an inability to relax after an active muscle contraction is associated with energy failure in glycolytic disorders. *Myotonia* is a condition of prolonged muscle contraction followed by slow muscle relaxation. It is important to distinguish between true muscle weakness and a complaint of fatigue; fatigue without abnormal clinical or laboratory findings almost never indicates a true muscle disorder. An approach to muscle weakness is presented in Figs. 199-1 and 199-2.

MUSCULAR DYSTROPHIES
A varied group of inherited, progressive degenerations of muscle.

Myotonic Dystrophy
The most common adult muscular dystrophy. Autosomal dominant with genetic anticipation. Weakness typically becomes obvious in the second to third decade and initially involves the muscles of the face, neck, and distal extremities. This results in a distinctive facial appearance ("hatchet face") characterized by ptosis, temporal wasting, drooping of the lower lip, and sagging of the jaw. Myotonia manifests as a peculiar inability to relax muscles rapidly following a strong exertion (e.g., after tight hand grip), as well as by sustained contraction of muscles following percussion (e.g., of tongue or thenar eminence).

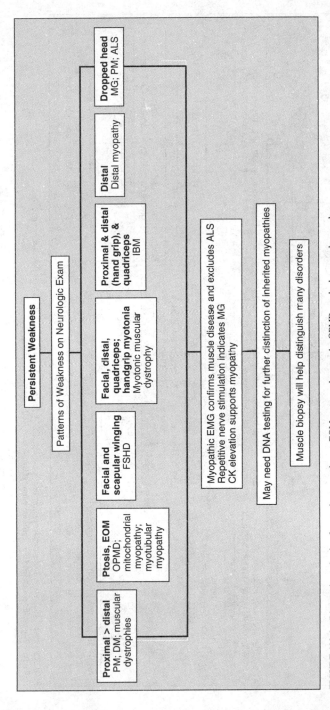

FIGURE 199-1 Diagnostic evaluation for persistent weakness. EOM, extraocular muscle; OPMD, oculopharyngeal muscular dystrophy; FSHD, facioscapulohumeral muscular dystrophy; IBM, inclusion body myositis; DM, dermatomyositis; PM, polymyositis; MG, myasthenia gravis; ALS, amyotrophic lateral sclerosis; CK, creatine kinase.

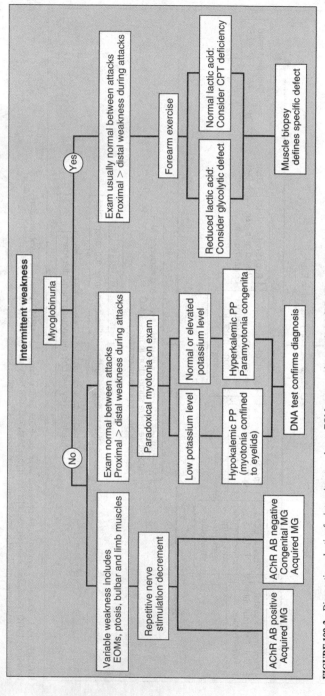

FIGURE 199-2 Diagnostic evaluation for intermittent weakness. EOMs, extraocular muscles; AChR AB, acetylcholine receptor antibody; PP, periodic paralysis; CPT, carnitine palmityl transferase; MG, myasthenia gravis.

Associated problems can include frontal baldness, posterior subcapsular cataracts, gonadal atrophy, respiratory and cardiac problems, endocrine abnormalities, intellectual impairment, and hypersomnia. Cardiac complications, including complete heart block, may be life-threatening. Respiratory function should be carefully followed, as chronic hypoxia may lead to cor pulmonale.

Laboratory Studies Normal or mildly elevated CK, characteristic myotonia and myopathic features on EMG, and a typical pattern of muscle fiber injury on biopsy, including selective type I fiber atrophy. Pts have an unstable region of DNA with an increased number of trinucleotide CTG repeats at chromosome location 19q13.3. The expanded repeat may alter expression of a nearby protein kinase gene. Genetic testing for early detection and prenatal diagnosis is possible.

 TREATMENT

Phenytoin, quinine, or procainamide may help myotonia, but they must be used carefully in pts with heart disease as they may worsen cardiac conduction. Pacemaker insertion may be required for syncope or heart block. Orthoses may control foot drop, stabilize the ankle, and decrease falling.

Facioscapulohumeral Dystrophy

An autosomal dominant, slowly progressive disorder with onset in the third to fourth decade. Weakness involves facial, shoulder girdle, and proximal arm muscles and can result in atrophy of biceps, triceps, scapular winging, and slope shoulders. Facial weakness results in inability to whistle and loss of facial expressivity. Foot drop and leg weakness may cause falls and progressive difficulty with ambulation.

Laboratory studies reveal normal or slightly elevated CK and mixed myopathic and neuropathic features on EMG and muscle biopsy. Pts have deletions at chromosome 4q35. Genetic testing available for carrier detection and prenatal diagnosis.

Limb-Girdle Dystrophy

A constellation of diseases with proximal muscle weakness involving the arms and legs as the core symptom. Age of onset, rate of progression, severity of manifestations, inheritance pattern (autosomal dominant or autosomal recessive), and associated complications (e.g., cardiac, respiratory) vary with the specific subtype of disease. *Laboratory findings* include elevated CK and myopathic features on EMG and muscle biopsy. At least eight autosomal recessive forms have been identified by molecular genetic analysis.

Duchenne Dystrophy

X-linked recessive mutation of the dystrophin gene that affects males almost exclusively. Progressive weakness in hip and shoulder girdle muscles beginning by age 5; by age 12, the majority are nonambulatory. Survival beyond age 25 is rare. Associated problems include tendon and muscle contractures, progressive kyphoscoliosis, impaired pulmonary function, cardiomyopathy, and intellectual impairment. Palpable enlargement and firmness of some muscles. Becker dystrophy is a less severe form, with a slower course and later age of onset (5–15) but similar clinical, laboratory, and genetic features. *Laboratory findings* include massive elevations (20–100 × normal) of muscle enzymes (CK, aldolase), a myopathic pattern on EMG testing, and evidence of groups of necrotic muscle fibers with regeneration, phagocytosis, and fatty replacement of muscle on biopsy. Diagnosis is established by determination of dystrophin in muscle tissue by Western blot and/or immunochemical staining. Serum CK is elevated in 50% of female carriers. Testing available for detecting carriers and prenatal diagnosis. Glucocorticoids [prednisone, 0.75 (mg/kg)/d] slow progression of disease for up to 3 years, but complications of chronic use often outweigh the benefits.

Oculopharyngeal Dystrophy (Progressive External Ophthalmoplegia)

Onset in the fifth to sixth decade of ptosis, limitation of extraocular movements, and facial and cricopharyngeal weakness. Most pts are Hispanic or of French-Canadian descent. Mutation in a poly-A RNA binding protein responsible.

INFLAMMATORY MYOPATHIES

The most common group of acquired and potentially treatable skeletal muscle disorders. Three major forms: polymyositis (PM), dermatomyositis (DM), and inclusion body myositis (IBM). Usually present as progressive and symmetric muscle weakness; extraocular muscles spared but pharyngeal weakness (dysphagia) and head drop from neck muscle weakness common. Respiratory muscles may be affected in advanced cases. IBM is characterized by early involvement of quadriceps (leading to falls) and distal muscles. Progression is over weeks or months in PM and DM, but typically over years in IBM. Skin involvement in DM may consist of a heliotrope rash (blue-purple discoloration) on the upper eyelids with edema, a flat red rash on the face and upper trunk, or erythema over knuckles. A variety of cancers, including ovarian, breast, melanoma, and colon cancer, are associated with DM. Diagnostic criteria are summarized in Table 199-1.

 TREATMENT

Often effective for PM and DM but not for IBM. Step 1: Glucocorticoids [prednisone, 1 (mg/kg)/d for 3–4 weeks, then tapered very gradually]; step 2: Azathioprine [up to 3 (mg/kg)/d] or methotrexate (7.5 mg/week gradually increasing to 25 mg/week); step 3: Intravenous immunoglobulin (2 g/kg divided over 2–5 days); step 4: Cyclosporine, chlorambucil, cyclophosphamide, or mycophenolate mofetil. IBM is generally resistant to immunosuppressive therapies; many experts recommend a short trial of glucocorticoids together with azathioprine or methotrexate.

METABOLIC MYOPATHIES

These disorders result from abnormalities in utilization by muscle of glucose or fatty acids as sources of energy. Pts present with either an acute syndrome of myalgia, myolysis, and myoglobinuria or chronic progressive muscle weakness. Definitive diagnosis requires biochemical-enzymatic studies of biopsied muscle. However, muscle enzymes, EMG, and muscle biopsy are all typically abnormal and may suggest specific disorders.

Glycogen storage disorders can mimic muscular dystrophy or polymyositis. In some types the presentation is one of episodic muscle cramps and fatigue provoked by exercise. The ischemic forearm lactate test is helpful as normal postexercise rise in serum lactic acid does not occur. In adults, progressive muscle weakness beginning in the third or fourth decade can be due to the adult form of *acid maltase deficiency*; respiratory failure is often the initial manifestation. Progressive weakness beginning after puberty occurs with *debranching enzyme deficiency*. *Glycolytic defects*, including *myophosphorylase deficiency*

Table 199-1

Criteria for Diagnosis of Inflammatory Myopathies

Criterion	Polymyositis			Dermatomyositis	Inclusion Body Myositis
	Definite	Probable			
Myopathic muscle weakness[a]	Yes	Yes		Yes[b]	Yes; slow onset, early involvement of distal muscles, frequent falls
Electromyographic findings	Myopathic	Myopathic		Myopathic	Myopathic with mixed potentials
Muscle enzymes	Elevated (up to 50-fold)	Elevated (up to 50-fold)		Elevated (up to 50-fold) or normal	Elevated (up to 10-fold) or normal
Muscle biopsy findings[c]	"Primary" inflammation with the CD8/MHC-I complex and no vacuoles	Ubiquitous MCH-I expression but minimal inflammation and no vacuoles[d]		Perifascicular, perimysial, or perivascular infiltrates, perifascicular atrophy	Primary inflammation with CD8/MHC-I complex; vacuolated fibers with β-amyloid deposits; cytochrome oxygenase–negative fibers; signs of chronic myopathy[e]
Rash or calcinosis	Absent	Absent		Present[f]	Absent

[a] Myopathic muscle weakness, affecting proximal muscles more than distal ones and sparing eye and facial muscles, is characterized by a subacute onset (weeks to months) and rapid progression in patients who have no family history of neuromuscular disease, no endocrinopathy, no exposure to myotoxic drugs or toxins, and no biochemical muscle disease (excluded on the basis of muscle-biopsy findings).

[b] In some cases with the typical rash, the muscle strength is seemingly normal (dermatomyositis sine myositis); these patients often have new onset of easy fatigue and reduced endurance. Careful muscle testing may reveal mild muscle weakness.

[c] See Chap. 369 in HPIM-16 for details.

[d] An adequate trial of prednisone or other immunosuppressive drugs is warranted in probable cases. If, in retrospect, the disease is unresponsive to therapy, another muscle biopsy should be considered to exclude other diseases or possible evolution in inclusion body myositis.

[e] If the muscle biopsy does not contain vacuolated fibers but shows chronic myopathy with hypertrophic fibers, primary inflammation with the CD8/MHC-I complex, and cytochrome oxygenase–negative fibers, the diagnosis is probable inclusion body myositis.

[f] If rash is absent but muscle biopsy findings are characteristic of dermatomyositis, the diagnosis is probable DM.

(McArdle's disease) or *phosphofructokinase deficiency*, present as exercise intolerance with myalgias, and recurrent myoglobinuria. Disorders of fatty acid metabolism present with a similar picture. In adults, the most common cause is *carnitine palmitoyltransferase deficiency*. Exercise-induced cramps, myolysis, and myoglobinuria are common. A normal rise of venous lactate distinguishes this condition from glycolytic defects. Dietary approaches (frequent meals and a low-fat high-carbohydrate diet, or a diet rich in medium-chain triglycerides) are of uncertain value.

MITOCHONDRIAL MYOPATHIES

More accurately referred to as *mitochondrial cytopathies* because multiple tissues are usually affected, these disorders result from defects in mitochondrial DNA. The clinical presentations vary greatly: muscle symptoms may include weakness, ophthalmoparesis, pain, stiffness, or may even be absent; age of onset ranges from infancy to adulthood; associated clinical presentations include ataxia, encephalopathy, seizures, strokelike episodes, and recurrent vomiting. Three groups: chronic progressive external ophthalmoplegia (CPEO), skeletal muscle–central nervous system syndromes, and pure myopathy simulating muscular dystrophy. The characteristic finding on muscle biopsy is "ragged red fibers," which are muscle fibers with accumulations of abnormal mitochondria. Genetics show a maternal pattern of inheritance because mitochondrial genes are inherited almost exclusively from the oocyte.

PERIODIC PARALYSES

Characterized by muscle stiffness due to electrical irritability of the muscle membrane (*myotonia*), usually without significant muscle weakness until late in the course. Onset is usually in childhood or adolescence. Episodes typically occur after rest or sleep, often following earlier exercise. May be due to genetic disorders of calcium [hypokalemic periodic paralysis (hypoKPP)], sodium (hyperkalemic periodic paralysis), or chloride channels. Attacks of hypoKPP are treated with potassium chloride (usually oral), and prophylaxis with acetazolamide (125–1000 mg/d in divided doses) is usually effective. Attacks of thyrotoxic periodic paralysis (usually in Asian men) resemble those of hypoKPP.

ENDOCRINE DISORDERS, DRUGS, AND TOXINS

Abnormalities of thyroid function can cause a wide array of muscle disorders. Hypothyroidism is associated with muscle cramps, pain, and stiffness, and proximal muscle weakness occurs in one-third of pts; the relaxation phase of muscle stretch reflexes is characteristically prolonged, and serum CK is often elevated (up to 10 times normal). Hyperthyroidism can produce proximal muscle weakness and atrophy; bulbar, respiratory, and even esophageal muscles are occasionally involved, causing dysphagia, dysphonia, and aspiration. Other neuromuscular disorders associated with hyperthyroidism include hypoKPP, myasthenia gravis, and a progressive ocular myopathy associated with proptosis (*Graves' ophthalmopathy*). Other endocrine conditions, including parathyroid, pituitary, and adrenal disorders, can also produce myopathy.

Drugs (including glucocorticoids, statins and other lipid-lowering agents, and zidovudine) and toxins (e.g., alcohol) are commonly associated with myopathies (Table 199-2). In most cases weakness is symmetric and involves proximal limb girdle muscles. Weakness, myalgia, and cramps are common symptoms. An elevated CK is an important indication of toxicity. Diagnosis often depends on resolution of signs and symptoms with removal of offending agent. Deficiencies of vitamins D and E are additional causes of muscle weakness.

Table 199-2

Toxic Myopathies

Drugs	Major Toxic Reaction
Lipid-lowering agents Fibric acid derivatives HMG-CoA reductase inhibitors Niacin (nicotinic acid)	Drugs belonging to all three of the major classes of lipid-lowering agents can produce a spectrum of toxicity: asymptomatic serum creatine kinase elevation, myalgias, exercised-induced pain, rhabdomyolysis, and myoglobinuria.
Glucocorticoids	Acute, high-dose glucocorticoid treatment can cause acute quadriplegic myopathy. These high doses of steroids are often combined with non-depolarizing neuromuscular blocking agents, but the weakness can occur without their use. Chronic steroid administration produces predominantly proximal weakness.
Nondepolarizing neuro-muscular blocking agents	Acute quadriplegic myopathy can occur with or without concomitant glucocorticoids.
Zidovudine	Mitochondrial myopathy with ragged red fibers.
Drugs of abuse Alcohol Amphetamines Cocaine Heroin Phencyclidine Meperidine	All drugs in this group can lead to widespread muscle breakdown, rhabdomyolysis, and myoglobinuria. Local injections cause muscle necrosis, skin induration, and limb contractures.
Autoimmune toxic myopathy D-Penicillamine	Use of D-penicillamine may cause polymyositis and myasthenia gravis.
Amphophilic cationic drugs Amiodarone Chloroquine Hydroxychloroquine	All amphophilic drugs have the potential to produce painless, proximal weakness associated with autophagic vacuoles in the muscle biopsy.
Antimicrotubular drugs Colchicine	This drug produces painless, proximal weakness especially in the setting of renal failure. Muscle biopsy shows autophagic vacuoles.

For a more detailed discussion, see Mendell JR: Approach to the Patient with Muscle Disease, Chap. 367, p. 2524; Brown RH Jr., Mendell JR: Muscular Dystrophies and Other Muscle Diseases, Chap. 368, p. 2527; Dalakas MC: Polymyositis, Dermatomyositis, and Inclusion Body Myositis, Chap. 369, p. 2540, in HPIM-16.

200

CHRONIC FATIGUE SYNDROME

Chronic fatigue syndrome (CFS) is characterized by debilitating fatigue and several associated physical, constitutional, and neuropsychological complaints (Table 200-1). The CDC has developed diagnostic criteria for CFS based upon symptoms and the exclusion of other illnesses (Table 200-2); 100–300 individuals per 100,000 population in the United States meet the CDC case definition.

Pathogenesis

The cause is uncertain; many controversial hypotheses exist about its etiology. It is often postinfectious; it is associated with minor immunologic findings of uncertain significance; and it is commonly accompanied or even preceded by neuropsychological complaints, somatic preoccupation, and/or depression. Many studies have attempted, without success, to link CFS to infection with EBV, a retrovirus, or an enterovirus. Thus, while antecedent viral infections are associated with CFS, a direct viral pathogenesis is unproven and unlikely. Depression is present in half to two-thirds of pts, and some experts believe that CFS is fundamentally a psychiatric disorder.

Clinical Manifestations

Typically, CFS arises suddenly in a previously active individual. Pts are twice as likely to be women as men and are generally 25 to 45 years old. An otherwise unremarkable flulike illness or some other acute stress leaves severe exhaustion in its wake. Other symptoms, such as headache, sore throat, tender lymph nodes, muscle and joint aches, and frequent feverishness, lead to the belief that an

Table 200-1

Specific Symptoms Reported by Patients with Chronic Fatigue Syndrome

Symptom	Percentage
Fatigue	100
Difficulty concentrating	90
Headache	90
Sore throat	85
Tender lymph nodes	80
Muscle aches	80
Joint aches	75
Feverishness	75
Difficulty sleeping	70
Psychiatric problems	65
Allergies	55
Abdominal cramps	40
Weight loss	20
Rash	10
Rapid pulse	10
Weight gain	5
Chest pain	5
Night sweats	5

Source: From SE Straus: J Infect Diseases 157:405, 1988; with permission.

Table 200-2

CDC Criteria for Diagnosis of Chronic Fatigue Syndrome

A case of chronic fatigue syndrome is defined by the presence of:

1. Clinically evaluated, unexplained, persistent or relapsing fatigue that is of new or definite onset; is not the result of ongoing exertion; is not alleviated by rest; and results in substantial reduction of previous levels of occupational, educational, social, or personal activities; and

2. Four or more of the following symptoms that persist or recur during six or more consecutive months of illness and that do not predate the fatigue:
   - Self-reported impairment in short-term memory or concentration
   - Sore throat
   - Tender cervical or axillary nodes
   - Muscle pain
   - Multijoint pain without redness or swelling
   - Headaches of a new pattern or severity
   - Unrefreshing sleep
   - Postexertional malaise lasting ≥ 24 h

Note: CDC, U.S. Centers for Disease Control and Prevention.
Source: Adapted from K Fukuda et al: Ann Intern Med 121:953, 1994; with permission.

infection persists, and medical attention is sought. Over several weeks, despite reassurances that nothing serious is wrong, the symptoms persist and other features become evident—disturbed sleep, difficulty in concentration, and depression (Table 200-1).

Most pts remain capable of meeting obligations despite their symptoms; discretionary activities are abandoned first. Some feel unable to engage in any gainful employment. A minority require help with the activities of daily living. Ultimately, isolation, frustration, and resignation can mark the protracted course of illness. Pts may become angry at physicians for failing to acknowledge or resolve their plight. Fortunately, CFS does not appear to progress. On the contrary, many pts experience gradual improvement, and a minority recover fully.

Diagnosis

A thorough history, physical examination, and judicious use of laboratory tests are required to exclude other causes of the pt's symptoms. CFS remains a diagnosis of exclusion; no laboratory test can diagnose CFS or measure its severity. Often the pt presents with features that also meet criteria for other subjective disorders such as fibromyalgia and irritable bowel syndrome.

℞ TREATMENT

Many symptoms of CFS respond to treatment. NSAIDs alleviate headache, diffuse pain, and feverishness. Antihistamines or decongestants may be helpful for symptoms of rhinitis and sinusitis. Although the pt may be averse to psychiatric diagnoses, depression and anxiety are often prominent and should be treated. Psychiatric assessment is sometimes advisable. Nonsedating antidepressants improve mood and disordered sleep and may attenuate the fatigue. Even modest improvements in symptoms can make an important difference in level of self-sufficiency and capacity to enjoy life.

Practical advice should be given regarding life-style adjustments. Consumption of heavy meals with alcohol and caffeine at night can make sleep more difficult, compounding fatigue. Total rest leads to deconditioning and the self-image of being an invalid, whereas overexertion may worsen exhaustion. A moderate, carefully graded regimen should be encouraged.

Controlled trials have established that acyclovir, fludrocortisone, and intravenous immunoglobulin, among others, are of little or no value in CFS. Low doses of hydrocortisone provide modest benefit, but they may lead to adrenal suppression. Many anecdotes circulate regarding other traditional and nontraditional therapies; pts should be advised to avoid therapeutic modalities that are toxic, expensive, or unreasonable.

For a more detailed discussion, see Straus SE: Chronic Fatigue Syndrome, Chap. 370, p 2545, in HPIM-16.

201

PSYCHIATRIC DISORDERS

Disorders of mood, thinking, and behavior may be due to a primary psychiatric diagnosis (DSM-IV* Axis I major psychiatric disorders) or a personality disorder (DSM-IV Axis II disorders) or may be secondary to metabolic abnormalities, drug toxicities, focal cerebral lesions, seizure disorders, or degenerative neurologic disease. Any pt presenting with new onset of psychiatric symptoms must be evaluated for underlying psychoactive substance abuse and/or medical or neurologic illness. Specific psychiatric medications are discussed in Chap. 202. The DSM-IV-PC (Primary Care) Manual provides a synopsis of mental disorders commonly seen in medical practice.

MAJOR PSYCHIATRIC DISORDERS (AXIS I DIAGNOSES)
Mood Disorders (Major Affective Disorders)

MAJOR DEPRESSION *Clinical Features* Affects 15% of the general population at some point in life. Diagnosis is made when a depressed/irritable mood or a lack of normal interest/pleasure exists for at least 2 weeks, in combination with four or more of the following symptoms: (1) change in appetite plus change in weight; (2) insomnia or hypersomnia; (3) fatigue or loss of energy; (4) motor agitation or retardation; (5) feelings of worthlessness, self-reproach, or guilt; (6) decreased ability to concentrate and make decisions; (7) recurrent thoughts of death or suicide. A small number of pts with major depression will have psychotic symptoms—hallucinations and delusions—with their depressed mood; many present with a "masked depression," unable to describe their psychological distress but with multiple diffuse somatic complaints.

Onset of a first depressive episode is typically in the thirties or forties, although major depression can occur at any age. Untreated episodes generally resolve spontaneously in 5–9 months; however, a sizable number of pts suffer from chronic, unremitting depression or from partial treatment response. Half of all pts experiencing a first depressive episode will go on to a recurrent course, with a second episode occurring within 2 years. Untreated or partially treated episodes put the pt at risk for future problems with mood disorder. A family history of mood disorder is common and tends to predict a recurrent course. Major depression can also be the initial presentation of bipolar disorder (manic depressive illness).

Suicide Most suicides occur in pts with a mood disorder, and many pts seek contact with a physician prior to their suicide attempt. Physicians must always inquire about suicide when evaluating a pt with depression. Features that place a pt at high risk for suicidal behavior include: (1) a formulated plan and a method, as well as an intent; (2) prior attempts; (3) concomitant alcohol

---

*Diagnostic and Statistical Manual, Fourth Edition, American Psychiatric Association

or other psychoactive substance use; (4) psychotic symptoms; (5) older age; (6) male gender; (7) Caucasian; (8) social isolation; (9) serious medical illness; (10) recent loss and/or profound hopelessness.

Depression with Medical Illness Virtually every class of *medication* can potentially induce or worsen depression. Antihypertensive drugs, anticholesterolemic agents, and antiarrhythmic agents are common triggers of depressive symptoms. Among the antihypertensive agents, β-adrenergic blockers and, to a lesser extent, calcium channel blockers are the most likely to cause depressed mood. Iatrogenic depression should also be considered in pts receiving glucocorticoids, antimicrobials, systemic analgesics, antiparkinsonian medications, and anticonvulsants.

Between 20 and 30% of cardiac pts manifest a depressive disorder. Tricyclic antidepressants (TCAs) are contraindicated in patients with bundle branch block, and TCA-induced tachycardia is an additional concern in pts with congestive heart failure. Selective serotonin reuptake inhibitors (SSRIs) appear not to induce ECG changes or adverse cardiac events and thus are reasonable first-line drugs for patients at risk for TCA-related complications. SSRIs may interfere with hepatic metabolism of anticoagulants, however, causing increased anticoagulation.

In *cancer*, the prevalence of depression is 25%, but it occurs in 50% of pts with cancers of the pancreas or oropharynx. Extreme cachexia from cancer may be misinterpreted as depression. Antidepressant medications in cancer pts improve quality of life as well as mood.

Diabetes mellitus is another consideration; the severity of the mood state correlates with the level of hyperglycemia and the presence of diabetic complications. Monoamine oxidase inhibitors (MAOIs) can induce hypoglycemia and weight gain. TCAs can produce hyperglycemia and carbohydrate craving. SSRIs, like MAOIs, may reduce fasting plasma glucose, but they are easier to use and may also improve dietary and medication compliance.

Depression may also occur with *hypothyroidism* or *hyperthyroidism*, *neurologic disorders*, in *HIV*-positive individuals, and in *chronic hepatitis C infection* (depression worsens with interferon treatment). Finally, some chronic disorders of uncertain etiology, such as *chronic fatigue syndrome* (Chap. 200) and *fibromyalgia* (Chap. 168), are strongly associated with depression.

℞ TREATMENT

Pts with suicidal ideation require treatment by a psychiatrist and may require hospitalization. Most other pts with an uncomplicated unipolar major depression (a major depression that is not part of a cyclical mood disorder, such as a bipolar disorder) can be successfully treated by a nonpsychiatric physician. Vigorous intervention and successful treatment appear to decrease the risk of future relapse. Pts who do not respond fully to standard treatment should be referred to a psychiatrist.

Antidepressant medication is the mainstay of treatment; symptoms are ameliorated after 2–6 weeks at a therapeutic dose. Once remission is achieved, antidepressants should be continued for 6–9 months. Pts must be monitored carefully after termination of treatment since relapse is common. The combination of pharmacotherapy with psychotherapy [usually cognitive-behavioral therapy (CBT) or interpersonal therapy (IPT)] produces better and longer-lasting results than drug therapy alone. Electroconvulsive therapy is generally reserved for life-threatening depression unresponsive to medication or for pts in whom the use of antidepressants is medically contraindicated.

BIPOLAR DISORDER (MANIC DEPRESSIVE ILLNESS) *Clinical Features* A cyclical mood disorder in which episodes of major depression are interspersed with episodes of mania or hypomania; 1% of the population is affected. Most pts initially present with a manic episode in adolescence or young adulthood, but 20% present with a major depression. Antidepressant therapy is usually contraindicated in pts with a cyclical mood disorder because it may provoke a manic episode. Pts with a major depressive episode and a prior history of "highs" (mania or hypomania—which can be pleasant/euphoric or irritable/impulsive) and/or a family history of bipolar disorder should not be treated with antidepressants but must be referred promptly to a psychiatrist.

With mania, an elevated, expansive mood, irritability, angry outbursts, and impulsivity are characteristic. Specific symptoms include: (1) increased motor activity and restlessness; (2) unusual talkativeness; (3) flight of ideas and racing thoughts; (4) inflated self-esteem that can become delusional; (5) decreased need for sleep (often the first feature of an incipient manic episode); (6) decreased appetite; (7) distractability; (8) excessive involvement in risky activities (buying sprees, sexual indiscretions). Pts with full-blown mania can become psychotic. Hypomania is characterized by attenuated manic symptoms and is greatly underdiagnosed, as are "mixed episodes," where both depressive and manic or hypomanic symptoms coexist simultaneously.

Untreated, a manic or depressive episode typically lasts for 1–3 months, with cycles of 1–2 episodes per year. Risk for manic episodes increases in the spring and fall. Variants of bipolar disorder include rapid and ultrarapid cycling (manic and depressed episodes occurring at cycles of weeks, days, or hours). In many pts, especially females, antidepressants trigger rapid cycling and worsen the course of illness. Pts with bipolar disorder are at risk for psychoactive substance use, especially alcohol abuse, and for medical consequences of risky sexual behavior (STDs).

Bipolar disorder has a strong genetic component. Pts with bipolar disorder are vulnerable to sleep deprivation, to changes in the photoperiod, and to the effects of jet lag.

℞ TREATMENT

Bipolar disorder is a serious, chronic illness that requires lifelong monitoring by a psychiatrist. Acutely manic pts often require hospitalization to reduce environmental stimulation and to protect themselves and others from the consequences of their reckless behavior. Mood stabilizers (lithium, valproic acid, carbamazepine, lamotrigine, topiramate) are effective for the resolution of acute episodes and for prophylaxis of future episodes. Antipsychotic medication, benzodiazepines, and antidepressants such as bupropion may be part of the treatment regimen. As in unipolar depression, rapid therapeutic intervention may decrease the risk of future relapse.

Schizophrenia and Other Psychotic Disorders

SCHIZOPHRENIA *Clinical Features* Occurs in 1% of the population worldwide; 30–40% of the homeless are affected. Characterized by a waxing and waning vulnerability to psychosis, i.e., an impaired ability to monitor reality, resulting in altered mood, thinking, language, perceptions, behavior, and interpersonal interactions. Pts usually present between late adolescence and the third decade, often after an insidious premorbid course of subtle psychosocial difficulties. Core psychotic features last ≥6 months and include: (1) delusions, which can be paranoid, jealous, somatic, grandiose, religious, nihilistic, or simply bizarre; (2) hallucinations, often auditory hallucinations of a voice or voices maintaining a running commentary; (3) disorders of language and thinking: incoherence, loosening of associations, tangentiality, illogical thinking; (4) inappropriate affect and bizarre, catatonic, or grossly disorganized behavior.

Prognosis depends not on symptom severity but on the response to antipsychotic medication. A permanent remission without recurrence does occasionally occur. About 10% of schizophrenic patients commit suicide. Comorbid substance abuse is common, especially of nicotine, alcohol, and stimulants.

 TREATMENT

Hospitalization is required for acutely psychotic pts, especially those with violent command hallucinations, who may be dangerous to themselves or others. Conventional antipsychotic medications are effective against hallucinations, agitation, and thought disorder (the so-called positive symptoms) in 60% of pts but are often less useful for apathy, blunted affect, social isolation, and anhedonia (negative symptoms). The novel antipsychotic medications— clozapine, risperidone, olanzapine, quetiapine, and others—have become the mainstay of treatment as they are helpful in pts unresponsive to conventional neuroleptics and may also be useful for negative and cognitive symptoms. Long-acting injectable forms of haloperidol and fluphenazine are ideal for noncompliant pts. Psychosocial intervention, rehabilitation, and family support are also essential.

OTHER PSYCHOTIC DISORDERS   These include schizoaffective disorder (where symptoms of chronic psychosis are interspersed with major mood episodes) and delusional disorders (in which a fixed, unshakable delusional belief is held in the absence of the other stigmata of schizophrenia). Pts with somatic delusions can be especially difficult to diagnose; they may become violent towards the physician if they feel misunderstood or thwarted and they almost always resist referral to a psychiatrist.

Anxiety Disorders

Characterized by severe, persistent anxiety or sense of dread in the absence of psychosis or a severe change in mood. Most prevalent psychiatric illness seen in the community; present in 15–20% of medical clinic patients.

PANIC DISORDER   Occurs in 1–3% of the population; female:male ratio of 2:1. Familial aggregation may occur. Onset in second or third decade. Initial presentation is almost always to a nonpsychiatric physician, frequently in the ER, as a possible heart attack or serious respiratory problem. The disorder is often initially unrecognized or misdiagnosed.

Clinical Features   Characterized by panic attacks, which are sudden, unexpected, overwhelming paroxysms of terror and apprehension with multiple associated somatic symptoms. Attacks usually reach a peak within 10 min, then slowly resolve spontaneously. Diagnostic criteria for panic disorder require four or more panic attacks within 4 weeks occurring in nonthreatening or nonexertional settings, and attacks must be accompanied by at least four of the following: dyspnea, palpitations, chest pain or discomfort, choking/smothering feelings, dizziness/vertigo/unsteady feelings, feelings of unreality, paresthesia, hot and cold flashes, sweating, faintness, trembling, and fear of dying, going crazy, or doing something uncontrolled during an attack. Panic disorder is often associated with a concomitant major depression.

When the disorder goes unrecognized and untreated, pts often experience significant morbidity: they become afraid of leaving home and may develop anticipatory anxiety, agoraphobia, and other spreading phobias; many turn to self-medication with alcohol or benzodiazepines.

Panic disorder must be differentiated from cardiovascular and respiratory disorders. Conditions that may mimic or worsen panic attacks include hyperthyroidism, pheochromocytoma, hypoglycemia, drug ingestions (amphetamines, cocaine, caffeine, sympathomimetic nasal decongestants), and drug withdrawal (alcohol, barbiturates, opiates, minor tranquilizers).

Rx TREATMENT

Cognitive-behavioral psychotherapy (identifying and aborting panic attacks through relaxation and breathing techniques)—either alone or combined with medication—can be effective. The cornerstone of drug therapy is antidepressant medication. The TCAs imipramine and clomipramine benefit 75–90% of panic disorder pts. Low doses (e.g., 10 to 25 mg/d) are given initially to avoid transient increased anxiety associated with heightened monoamine levels. SSRIs are equally effective; they should be started at one-third to one-half of their usual antidepressant dose (e.g., 5 to 10 mg fluoxetine, 25 to 50 mg sertraline, 10 mg paroxetine). Benzodiazepines (alprazolam 0.5–1 mg/qid or clonazepam 1–2 mg bid) may be used in the short term while waiting for antidepressants to take effect.

GENERALIZED ANXIETY DISORDER (GAD)   Characterized by persistent, chronic anxiety but without the specific symptoms of phobic, panic, or obsessive-compulsive disorders; occurs in 5–6% of the population.

Clinical Features   Pts experience persistent, excessive, and/or unrealistic worry associated with muscle tension, impaired concentration, autonomic arousal, feeling "on edge" or restless, and insomnia. Pts worry excessively over minor matters, with life-disrupting effects; unlike panic disorder, complaints of shortness of breath, palpitations, and tachycardia are relatively rare. Secondary depression is common, as is social phobia.

Rx TREATMENT

Benzodiazepines are the initial agents of choice when generalized anxiety is severe and acute enough to warrant drug therapy. A trial of an SSRI antidepressant should then be started as many pts will experience significant relief with this class of medications. Physicians must be alert to psychological and physical dependence on benzodiazepines. A subgroup of pts respond to buspirone, a nonbenzodiazepine anxiolytic. Anticonvulsants with GABA-ergic properties (gabapentin, oxcarbazepine, tiagabine) may also be effective against anxiety. Psychotherapy and relaxation training can be useful.

OBSESSIVE-COMPULSIVE DISORDER (OCD)   A severe disorder present in 2–3% of the population and characterized by recurrent obsessions (persistent intrusive thoughts) and compulsions (repetitive behaviors) that the pt experiences as involuntary, senseless, or repugnant. Pts are often ashamed of their symptoms and only seek help after they have become debilitated.

Clinical Features   Common obsessions include thoughts of violence (such as killing a loved one), obsessive slowness for fear of making a mistake, fears of germs or contamination, and excessive doubt or uncertainty. Examples of compulsions include repeated checking to be assured that something was done properly, hand washing, extreme neatness and ordering behavior, and counting rituals, such as numbering one's steps while walking.

Onset is usually in adolescence, with 65% of cases manifest before age 25. It is more common in males and in first-born children. In families of OCD patients, an increased incidence of both OCD and Tourette's syndrome is found. The course of OCD is usually episodic with periods of incomplete remission. Pts with severe disease may become completely housebound. Major depression, substance abuse, and social impairment are common.

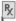 **TREATMENT**

Clomipramine and the SSRIs (fluoxetine, fluvoxamine) are highly effective. A combination of drug therapy and CBT is most effective for the majority of pts. Education and referral to a national support organization is also useful.

POSTTRAUMATIC STRESS DISORDER (PTSD)   Occurs in a subgroup of individuals exposed to a severe life-threatening trauma. Predisposing factors include a prior history of traumatization and/or a diathesis toward anxiety responses. Early psychological intervention following a traumatic event may reduce the risk for chronic PTSD.

Clinical Features   Three core sets of symptoms: (1) *reexperiencing*, where the pt unwillingly reexperiences the trauma through recurrent intrusive recollections, recurrent dreams, or by suddenly feeling as if the traumatic event is recurring; (2) *avoidance and numbing*, where the pt experiences reduced responsiveness to, and involvement with, the external world, a sense of a foreshortened future, and avoidance of activities that arouse recollection of the traumatic event; (3) *arousal*, characterized by hypervigilance, hyperalertness, an exaggerated startle response, sleep disturbance, guilt about having survived when others have not or about behavior required for survival, memory impairment or trouble concentrating, and intensification of symptoms by exposure to events that symbolize or resemble the traumatic event. Comorbid substance abuse and other mood and anxiety disorders are common. This disorder is extremely debilitating, particularly as it becomes chronic and affects psychosocial functioning. Most pts require referral to a psychiatrist for ongoing care.

 TREATMENT

Medications used with varying success include a combination of an SSRI and trazodone, 50–200 mg qhs for sleep; TCAs can also be effective. Group psychotherapy (with other trauma survivors), alone or with individual psychotherapy, is useful.

PHOBIC DISORDERS   *Clinical Features*   Recurring, irrational fears of specific objects, activities, or situations, with subsequent avoidance behavior of the phobic stimulus. Diagnosis is made only when the avoidance behavior is a significant source of distress or interferes with social or occupational functioning.

1.   *Agoraphobia*: Fear of being in public places. May occur in absence of panic disorder, but is almost invariably preceded by that condition.
2.   *Social phobia*: Persistent irrational fear of, and need to avoid, any situation where there is risk of scrutiny by others, with potential for embarassment or humiliation. Common examples include excessive fear of public speaking and excessive fear of social engagements.
3.   *Simple phobias*: Persistent irrational fears and avoidance of specific objects. Common examples include fear of heights (acrophobia), closed spaces (claustrophobia), and animals.

℞ TREATMENT

Agoraphobia is treated as for panic disorder. Beta blockers (e.g., propranolol, 20 to 40 mg orally 2 h before the event) are particularly effective in the treatment of "performance anxiety." SSRIs are very helpful in treating social phobias. Social and simple phobias respond well to CBT and relaxation techniques and to systematic desensitization and exposure treatment.

SOMATOFORM DISORDERS *Clinical Features* Pts with multiple somatic complaints that cannot be explained by a known medical condition or by the effects of substances; seen commonly in primary care practice (prevalence of 5%). In somatization disorder, the pt presents with multiple physical complaints referable to different organ systems. Onset is before age 30, and the disorder is persistent; pts with somatization disorder can be impulsive and demanding. In *conversion disorder*, the symptoms involve voluntary motor or sensory function. In *hypochondriasis*, the pt believes there is a serious medical illness, despite reassurance and appropriate medical evaluation. As with somatization disorder, these pts have a history of poor relationships with physicians due to their sense that they have not received adequate evaluation. Hypochondriasis can be disabling and show a waxing and waning course. In *factitious illnesses*, the pt consciously and voluntarily produces physical symptoms; the sick role is gratifying. *Munchausen's syndrome* refers to individuals with dramatic, chronic, or severe factitious illness. A variety of signs, symptoms, and diseases have been simulated in factitious illnesses; most common are chronic diarrhea, fever of unknown origin, intestinal bleeding, hematuria, seizures, hypoglycemia. In *malingering*, the fabrication of illness derives from a desire for an external gain (narcotics, disability).

℞ TREATMENT

Pts with somatoform disorders are usually subjected to multiple diagnostic tests and exploratory surgeries in an attempt to find their "real" illness. This approach is doomed to failure. Successful treatment is achieved through behavior modification, in which access to the physician is adjusted to provide a consistent, sustained, and predictable level of support that is not contingent on the pt's level of presenting symptoms or distress. Visits are brief, supportive, and structured and are not associated with a need for diagnostic or treatment action. Pts often benefit from antidepressant treatment. Consultation with a psychiatrist is essential.

PERSONALITY DISORDERS (AXIS II DIAGNOSES)

Defined as an inappropriate, stereotyped, maladaptive use of a certain set of psychological characteristics; affects 5–15% of the general population. The pattern of behavior is enduring and affects the person's relationships and ability to function satisfactorily in life.

Comorbid Axis I diagnosis is common, as is a psychoactive substance use disorder. In medical and surgical settings, pts with personality disorders often become engaged in hostile, manipulative, or unproductive relationships with their physicians. Long-term psychotherapy is beneficial for pts who are motivated to change. Antidepressants and low-dose antipsychotic medications can be helpful, particularly for episodes of decompensation, but should be prescribed in consultation with a psychiatrist as misdiagnosis is common.

DSM-IV describes three major categories of personality disorders; pts usually present with a combination of features.

Cluster A Personality Disorders

Affected pts are often characterized as "wild" or "mad." The *paranoid* personality is suspicious, hypersensitive, guarded, hostile, and can occasionally become threatening or dangerous. The *schizoid* personality is interpersonally isolated, cold, and indifferent, while the *schizotypal* personality is eccentric and superstitious, with magical thinking and unusual beliefs resembling schizophrenia.

Cluster B Personality Disorders

Patients with these disorders are often "wild" or "bad." The *borderline* personality is impulsive and manipulative, with unpredictable and fluctuating intense moods and unstable relationships, a fear of abandonment, and occasional rage episodes. The *histrionic* pt is dramatic, engaging, seductive, and attention-seeking. The *narcissistic* pt is self-centered and has an inflated sense of self-importance combined with a tendency to devalue or demean others, while pts with *antisocial* personality disorder use other people to achieve their own ends and engage in exploitative and manipulative behavior with no sense of remorse. Some aspects of the Cluster B personality disorders appear related to mood disorders.

Cluster C Personality Disorders

Patients with these disorders are often "whiny" or "sad." The *dependent* pt fears separation, tries to engage others to assume responsibility, and often has a help-rejecting style. Pts with *compulsive* personality disorder are meticulous and perfectionistic but also inflexible and indecisive, while those who are *passive-aggressive* request help, appear compliant on the surface, but undo or resist all efforts aimed at change. *Avoidant* pts are anxious about social contact and have difficulty assuming responsibility for their isolation. The personality disorders share some features with the anxiety disorders.

For a more detailed discussion, see Reus VI: Mental Disorders, Chap. 371, p. 2547, in HPIM-16.

PSYCHIATRIC MEDICATIONS

Four major classes are commonly used in adults: (1) antidepressants, (2) anxiolytics, (3) antipsychotics, and (4) mood stabilizing agents. Nonpsychiatric physicians should become familiar with one or two drugs in each of the first three classes so that the indications, dose range, efficacy, potential side effects, and interactions with other medications are well known.

GENERAL PRINCIPLES OF USE

1. Most treatment failures are due to undermedication and impatience. For a proper medication trial to take place, an effective dose must

be taken for an adequate amount of time. For antidepressants, antipsychotics, and mood stabilizers, full effects may take weeks or months to occur.

2. History of a positive response to a medication usually indicates that a response to the same drug will occur again. A family history of a positive response to a specific medication is also useful.

3. Pts who fail to respond to one drug will often respond to another in the same class; one should attempt another trial with a drug that has a different mechanism of action or a different chemical structure. Treatment failures should be referred to a psychiatrist, as should all pts with psychotic symptoms or who require mood stabilizers.

4. Avoid polypharmacy; a pt who is not responding to standard monotherapy requires referral to a psychiatrist.

5. Pharmacokinetics may be altered in the elderly, with smaller volumes of distribution, reduced renal and hepatic clearance, longer biologic half-lives, and greater potential for CNS toxicity. The rule with elderly pts is to "start low and go slow."

6. Never stop treatment abruptly; especially true for antidepressants and anxiolytics. In general, medications should be slowly tapered and discontinued over 2–4 weeks.

7. Review possible side effects each time a drug is prescribed; educate pts and family members about side effects and need for patience in awaiting a response.

ANTIDEPRESSANTS (ADS)

Useful to group according to known actions on CNS monoaminergic systems (Table 202-1). The selective serotonin reuptake inhibitors (SSRIs) have predominant effects on serotonergic neurotransmission, also reflected in side effect profile. The TCAs, or tricyclic antidepressants, affect noradrenergic and, to a lesser extent, serotonergic neurotransmission but also have anticholinergic and antihistaminic effects. Venlafaxine and mirtazapine have relatively "pure" noradrenergic and serotonergic effects. Bupropion is a novel antidepressant that enhances noradrenergic function. Trazodone and nefazodone have mixed effects on serotonin receptors and on other neurotransmitter systems. The MAOIs inhibit monoamine oxidase, the primary enzyme responsible for the degradation of monoamines in the synaptic cleft.

ADs are effective against major depression, particularly when neurovegetative symptoms and signs are present. In very severe depression with many endogenous features, TCAs or MAOIs are more efficacious than SSRIs. ADs are also useful in treatment of panic disorder, posttraumatic stress disorder, chronic pain syndromes, and generalized anxiety disorder. The TCA clomipramine and the SSRIs successfully treat obsessive-compulsive disorder.

All ADs require at least 2 weeks at a therapeutic dose before clinical improvement is observed. All ADs also have the potential to trigger a manic episode or rapid cycling when given to a pt with bipolar disorder. The MAOIs must not be prescribed concurrently with other ADs or with narcotics, as potentially fatal reactions may occur. "Withdrawal syndromes" usually consisting of malaise can occur when ADs are stopped abruptly.

ANXIOLYTICS

Benzodiazepines bind to sites on the γ-aminobutyric acid receptor and are cross-tolerant with alcohol and with barbiturates. Four clinical properties: (1) sedative, (2) anxiolytic, (3) skeletal muscle relaxant, and (4) antiepileptic. Individual drugs differ in terms of potency, onset of action, duration of action (related to

Table 202-1

Antidepressants

Name	Usual Daily Dose, mg	Side Effects	Comments
SSRIs			
Fluoxetine (Prozac)	10–80	Headache; nausea and other GI effects; jitteriness; insomnia; sexual dysfunction; can affect plasma levels of other meds (except sertraline); akathisia rare	Once daily dosing, usually in A.M.; fluoxetine has very long half-life; must not be combined with MAOIs
Sertraline (Zoloft)	50–200		
Paroxetine (Paxil)	20–60		
Fluvoxamine (Luvox)	100–300		
Citalopram (Celexa)	20–60		
Escitalopram (Lexapro)	10–30		
TCAs			
Amitriptyline (Elavil)	150–300	Anticholinergic (dry mouth, tachycardia, constipation, urinary retention, blurred vision); sweating; tremor; postural hypotension; cardiac conduction delay; sedation; weight gain	Once daily dosing, usually qhs; blood levels of most TCAs available; can be lethal in O.D. (lethal dose = 2 g); nortriptyline best tolerated, especially by elderly
Nortriptyline (Pamelor)	50–200		
Imipramine (Tofranil)	150–300		
Desipramine (Norpramin)	150–300		
Doxepin (Sinequan)	150–300		
Clomipramine (Anafranil)	150–300		

964

Drug	Dose (mg)	Side Effects	Comments
Mixed norepinephrine/serotonin reuptake inhibitors			
Venlafaxine (Effexor)	75–375	Nausea; dizziness; dry mouth; headaches; increased blood pressure; anxiety and insomnia	Bid-tid dosing (extended release available); lower potential for drug interactions than SSRIs; contraindicated with MAOIs
Mirtazapine (Remeron)	15–45	Somnolence; weight gain; neutropenia rare	Once daily dosing
Mixed-action drugs			
Bupropion (Wellbutrin)	250–450	Jitteriness; flushing; seizures in at-risk patients; anorexia; tachycardia; psychosis	Tid dosing, but sustained release also available; fewer sexual side effects than SSRIs or TCAs; may be useful for adult ADD
Trazodone (Desyrel)	200–600	Sedation; dry mouth; ventricular irritability; postural hypotension; priapism rare	Useful in low doses for sleep because of sedating effects with no anticholinergic side effects
Nefazodone (Serzone)	300–600	Sedation; headache; dry mouth; nausea; constipation	Once daily dosing; no effect on REM sleep unlike other antidepressants
Amoxapine (Asendin)	200–600	Sexual dysfunction	Lethality in overdose; EPSEs possible
MAOIs			
Phenelzine (Nardil)	45–90	Insomnia; hypotension; anorgasmia; weight gain; hypertensive crisis; tyramine cheese reaction; lethal reactions with SSRIs; serious reactions with narcotics	May be more effective in patients with atypical features or treatment-refractory depression
Tranylcypromine (Parnate)	20–50		
Isocarboxazid (Marplan)	20–60		

Note: ADD, attention deficit disorder; MAOI, monoamine oxidase inhibitor; REM, rapid eye movement; SSRI, selective serotonin reuptake inhibitor; TCA, tricyclic antidepressant; EPSEs, extrapyramidal side effects.

Table 202-2

Anxiolytics

Name	Equivalent PO dose, mg	Onset of Action	Half-life, h	Comments
Benzodiazepines				
Diazepam (Valium)	5	Fast	20–70	Active metabolites; quite sedating
Flurazepam (Dalmane)	15	Fast	30–100	Flurazepam is a pro-drug; metabolites are active; quite sedating
Triazolam (Halcion)	0.25	Intermediate	1.5–5	No active metabolites; can induce confusion and delirium, especially in elderly
Lorazepam (Ativan)	1	Intermediate	10–20	No active metabolites; direct hepatic glucuronide conjugation; quite sedating
Alprazolam (Xanax)	0.5	Intermediate	12–15	Active metabolites; not too sedating; may have specific antidepressant and antipanic activity; tolerance and dependence develop easily
Chlordiazepoxide (Librium)	10	Intermediate	5–30	Active metabolites; moderately sedating
Oxazepam (Serax)	15	Slow	5–15	No active metabolites; direct glucuronide conjugation; not too sedating
Temazepam (Restoril)	15	Slow	9–12	No active metabolites; moderately sedating
Clonazepam (Klonopin)	0.5	Slow	18–50	No active metabolites; moderately sedating
Non-benzodiazepines				
Buspirone (BuSpar)	7.5	2 weeks	2–3	Active metabolites; tid dosing—usual daily dose 10–20 mg tid; nonsedating; no additive effects with alcohol; useful for agitation in demented or brain-injured patients

Table 202-3

Antipsychotic Agents

Name	Usual PO Daily Dose, mg	Side Effects	Sedation	Comments
TYPICAL ANTIPSYCHOTICS				
Low-potency				
Chlorpromazine (Thorazine)	100–600	Anticholinergic effects; orthostasis; photosensitivity; QT prolongation	+ + +	EPSEs usually not prominent; can cause anticholinergic delirium in elderly patients
Thioridazine (Mellaril)	100–600	cholestasis; QT prolongation		
Mid-potency				
Trifluoperazine (Stelazine)	2–15	Fewer anticholinergic side effects; fewer EPSEs	+ +	Well tolerated by most patients
Perphenazine (Trilafon)	4–32	than with higher potency agents	+ +	
Loxapine (Loxitane)	20–250	Frequent EPSEs	+ +	Little weight gain
Molindone (Moban)	50–225	Frequent EPSEs	0	
High potency				
Haloperidol (Haldol)	0.5–10	No anticholinergic side effects; EPSEs often prominent	0/+	Often prescribed in doses that are too high; long-acting injectable forms of haloperidol and fluphenazine available
Fluphenazine (Prolixin)	1–10	Frequent EPSEs	0/+	
Thiothixene (Navane)	2–20	Frequent EPSEs	0/+	
NOVEL ANTIPSYCHOTICS				
Clozapine (Clozaril)	200–600	Agranulocytosis (1%); weight gain; seizures; drooling; hyperthermia	+ +	Requires weekly WBC
Risperidone (Risperdal)	2–6	Orthostasis	+	Requires slow titration; EPSEs observed with doses >6 mg qd
Olanzapine (Zyprexa)	10–20	Weight gain	+ +	Mild prolactin elevation
Quetiapine (Seroquel)	350–700	Sedation; weight gain; anxiety	+ + +	Bid dosing
Ziprasidone (Geodon)	40–60	Orthostatic hypotension	+/+ +	Mimimal weight gain; increases QT interval
Aripiprazole (Abilify)	10–30	Nausea, anxiety, insomnia	0/+	Mixed agonist/antagonist

Note: EPSEs, extrapyramidal side effects; WBC, white blood count.

967

half-life and presence of active metabolites), and metabolism (Table 202-2). Benzodiazepines have additive effects with alcohol; like alcohol, they can produce tolerance and physiologic dependence, with serious withdrawal syndromes (tremors, seizures, delirium, and autonomic hyperactivity) if discontinued too quickly, especially for those with short half-lives.

Buspirone is a nonbenzodiazepine anxiolytic that is nonsedating, is not cross-tolerant with alcohol, and does not induce tolerance or dependence. It requires at least 2 weeks at therapeutic doses to achieve full effects.

ANTIPSYCHOTIC MEDICATIONS

These include the typical (or conventional) neuroleptics, which act by blocking dopamine D_2 receptors, and the atypical (or novel) neuroleptics, which act on dopamine, serotonin, and other neurotransmitter systems. Some antipsychotic effect may occur within hours or days of initiating treatment, but full effects usually require 6 weeks to several months of daily, therapeutic dosing.

CONVENTIONAL ANTIPSYCHOTICS Useful to group into high-, mid-, and low-potency neuroleptics (Table 202-3). High-potency neuroleptics are least sedating, have almost no anticholinergic side effects, and have a strong tendency to induce extrapyramidal side effects (EPSEs). The EPSEs occur within several hours to several weeks of beginning treatment and include acute dystonias, akathisia, and pseudo-parkinsonism. Extrapyramidal symptoms re-

Table 202-4

Clinical Pharmacology of Mood Stabilizers

Agent and Dosing	Side Effects and Other Effects

Lithium
  Starting dose: 300 mg bid or tid
  Therapeutic blood level: 0.8–1.2 meq/L
	Common side effects: Nausea/anorexia/diarrhea, fine tremor, thirst, polyuria, fatigue, weight gain, acne, folliculitis, neutrophilia, hypothyroidism
	Blood level is increased by thiazides, tetracyclines, and NSAIDs
	Blood level is decreased by bronchodilators, verapamil, and carbonic anhydrase inhibitors
	Rare side effects: Neurotoxicity, renal toxicity, hypercalcemia, ECG changes

Valproic acid
  Starting dose: 250 mg tid
  Therapeutic blood level: 50–125 μg/mL
	Common side effects: Nausea/anorexia, weight gain, sedation, tremor, rash, alopecia
	Inhibits hepatic metabolism of other medications
	Rare side effects: Pancreatitis, hepatotoxicity, Stevens-Johnson syndrome

Carbamazepine/oxcarbazepine
  Starting dose: 200 mg bid for carbamazepine, 150 bid for oxcarbazepine
  Therapeutic blood level: 4–12 μg/mL for carbamazepine
	Common side effects: Nausea/anorexia, sedation, rash, dizziness/ataxia
	Carbamazepine, but not oxcarbazepine, induces hepatic metabolism of other medications
	Rare side effects: Hyponatremia, agranulocytosis, Stevens-Johnson syndrome

Lamotrigine Starting dose: 25 mg/d	*Common side effects*: Rash, dizziness, headache, tremor, sedation, nausea *Rare side effect*: Stevens-Johnson syndrome

spond well to trihexyphenidyl, 2 mg bid, or benztropine mesylate, 1 to 2 mg bid. Akathisia may respond to beta blockers. Low-potency neuroleptics are very sedating, may cause orthostastic hypotension, are anticholinergic, and tend not to induce EPSEs.

Up to 20% of pts treated with conventional antipsychotic agents for >1 year develop tardive dyskinesia (probably due to dopamine receptor supersensitivity), an abnormal involuntary movement disorder most often observed in the face and distal extremities. Treatment includes gradual withdrawal of the neuroleptic, with possible switch to a novel neuroleptic; anticholinergic agents can worsen the disorder.

1–2% of pts exposed to neuroleptics develop neuroleptic malignant syndrome (NMS), a life-threatening complication with a mortality rate as high as 25%; hyperpyrexia, autonomic hyperactivity, muscle rigidity, obtundation, and agitation are characteristic, associated with increased WBC, increased CPK, and myoglobinuria. Treatment involves immediate discontinuation of neuroleptics, supportive care, and use of dantrolene and bromocriptine.

NOVEL ANTIPSYCHOTICS   A new class of agents that has become the first line of treatment (Table 202-3); efficacious in treatment-resistant pts, tend not to induce EPSEs or tardive dyskinesia, and appear to have uniquely beneficial properties on negative symptoms and cognitive dysfunction. Main problem is side effect of weight gain (most prominent in clozapine and in olanzapine; can induce diabetes).

MOOD-STABILIZING AGENTS

Four mood stabilizers in common use: lithium, carbamazepine, valproic acid, and lamotrigine (Table 202-4). Lithium is the "gold standard" and the best studied, and along with carbamazepine and valproic acid, is used for treatment of acute manic episodes; 1–2 weeks to reach full effect. As prophylaxis, the mood stabilizers reduce frequency and severity of both manic and depressed episodes in cyclical mood disorders. In refractory bipolar disorder, combinations of mood stabilizers may be beneficial.

For a more detailed discussion, see Reus VI: Mental Disorders, Chap. 371, p. 2547, in HPIM-16.

EATING DISORDERS

Definitions

Anorexia nervosa is characterized by refusal to maintain normal body weight, resulting in a body weight < 85% of the expected weight for age and height. *Bulimia nervosa* is characterized by recurrent episodes of binge eating followed by abnormal compensatory behaviors, such as self-induced vomiting, laxative abuse, or excessive exercise. Weight is in the normal range or above.

Both anorexia nervosa and bulimia nervosa occur primarily among previously healthy young women who become overly concerned with body shape and weight. Binge eating and purging behavior may be present in both conditions, with the critical distinction between the two resting on the weight of the individual. The diagnostic criteria for each of these disorders are shown in Tables 203-1 and 203-2.

Clinical Features

ANOREXIA NERVOSA

* General: hypothermia
* Skin, hair, nails: alopecia, lanugo, acrocyanosis, edema
* Cardiovascular: bradycardia, hypotension
* Gastrointestinal: salivary gland enlargement, slow gastric emptying, constipation, elevated liver enzymes
* Hematopoietic: normochromic, normocytic anemia; leukopenia
* Fluid/electrolyte: increased BUN, increased creatinine, hyponatremia, hypokalemia
* Endocrine: low luteinizing hormone and follicle-stimulating hormone with secondary amenorrhea, hypoglycemia, normal thyroid-stimulating hormone with low normal thyroxine, increased plasma cortisol, osteopenia

BULIMIA NERVOSA

* Gastrointestinal: salivary gland enlargement, dental erosion
* Fluid/electrolyte: hypokalemia, hypochloremia, alkalosis (from vomiting) or acidosis (from laxative abuse)
* Other: loss of dental enamel, callus on dorsum of hand

℞ TREATMENT

Anorexia Nervosa   Weight restoration to 90% of predicted weight is the primary goal in the treatment of anorexia nervosa. The intensity of the initial treatment, including the need for hospitalization, is determined by the pt's current weight, the rapidity of recent weight loss, and the severity of medical and psychological complications (Fig. 203-1). Severe electrolyte imbalances should be identified and corrected. Nutritional restoration can almost always be successfully accomplished by oral feeding. For severely underweight pts, sufficient calories should be provided initially in divided meals as food or liquid supplements to maintain weight and to permit stabilization of fluid and electrolyte balance (1500–1800 kcal/d intake). Calories can be gradually increased to achieve a weight gain of 1 to 2 kg per week (3000–4000 kcal/d intake). Meals must be supervised. Intake of vitamin D (400 IU/d) and calcium (1500 mg/d) should be sufficient to minimize bone loss. The assistance of psychiatrists or psychologists experienced in the treatment of anorexia nervosa is usually necessary. No psychotropic medications are of established value in the treatment of anorexia nervosa. Medical complications occasionally occur during refeeding; most patients transiently retain excess fluid, occasionally resulting in peripheral edema. Congestive heart failure and acute gastric dilatation have been described when refeeding is rapid. Transient modest elevations in serum levels of liver enzymes occasionally occur. Low levels of magnesium and phosphate should be replaced. Mortality is 5% per decade, either from chronic starvation or suicide.

Bulimia Nervosa   Bulimia nervosa can usually be treated on an outpatient basis (Fig. 203-1). Cognitive behavioral therapy and fluoxetine (Prozac) are first-line therapies. The recommended treatment dose for fluoxetine (60 mg/d) is higher than that typically used to treat depression.

Table 203-1

Diagnostic Criteria for Anorexia Nervosa

1. Refusal to maintain body weight at or above a minimally normal weight for age and height (e.g., weight loss leading to maintenance of body weight <85% of that expected; or failure to make expected weight gain during period of growth, leading to body weight <85% of that expected).
2. Intense fear of gaining weight or becoming fat, even though underweight.
3. Disturbance in the way in which one's body weight or shape is experienced, undue influence of body weight or shape on self-evaluation, or denial of the seriousness of the current low body weight.
4. In postmenarchal females, amenorrhea, i.e., the absence of at least three consecutive menstrual cycles, (A woman is considered to have amenorrhea if her periods occur only following hormone, e.g., estrogen administration.)

Specify type:
Restricting type: During the episode of anorexia nervosa, the person has not regularly engaged in binge-eating or purging behavior (i.e., self-induced vomiting or the misuse of laxatives, diuretics or enemas).
Binge eating/purging type: During the episode of anorexia nervosa, the person has regularly engaged in binge-eating or purging behavior (i.e., self-induced vomiting or the misuse of laxatives, diuretics, or enemas).

Source: From the *Diagnostic and Statistical Manual of Mental Disorders*, 4th ed, Washington, DC, American Psychiatric Association, 1994.

Table 203-2

Diagnostic Criteria for Bulimia Nervosa

1. Recurrent episodes of binge eating. An episode of binge eating is characterized by both of the following:
   a. Eating, in a discrete period of time (e.g., within any 2-h period), an amount of food that is definitely larger than most people would eat during a similar period of time and under similar circumtances.
   b. A sense of lack of control over eating during the episode (e.g., a feeling that one cannot stop eating or control what or how much one is eating).
2. Recurrent inappropriate compensatory behavior in order to prevent weight gain, such as self-induced vomiting, misuse of laxatives or diuretics, enemas, or other medications; fasting; or excessive exercise.
3. The binge eating and inappropriate compensatory behaviors both occur, on average, at least twice a week for 3 months.
4. Self-evaluation is unduly influenced by body shape and weight.
5. The disturbance does not occur exclusively during episodes of anorexia nervosa.

Specify type:
Purging type: During the current episode of bulimia nervosa, the person has regularly engaged in self-induced vomiting or the misuse of laxatives, diuretics, or enemas.
Nonpurging type: During the current episode of bulimia nervosa, the person has used other inappropriate compensatory behaviors such as fasting or excessive exercise but has not regularly engaged in self-induced vomiting or the misuse of laxatives, diuretics, or enemas.

Source: From the *Diagnostic and Statistical Manual of Mental Disorders*, 4th ed, Washington, DC, American Psychiatric Association, 1994.

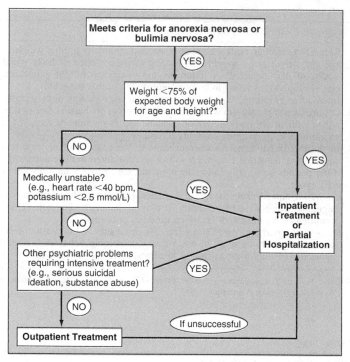

FIGURE 203-1

For a more detailed discussion, see Walsh TB: Eating Disorders, Chap. 65, p. 430, in HPIM-16.

204

ALCOHOLISM

Alcoholism and alcohol abuse are defined by the regular and excessive use of alcohol with concomitant social, occupational, and/or physical problems; alcohol is associated with half of all traffic fatalities and half of all homicides. In *alcohol dependence*, the regular use of alcohol has resulted in a state of physiologic tolerance and dependence. A pt may never suffer from withdrawal symptoms and still meet criteria for *alcohol abuse*.

Alcoholism is a multifactorial disorder in which genetic, biologic, and sociocultural factors interact. Typically, the first major life problem from excessive alcohol use appears in early adulthood, followed by periods of exacerbation and remission; the lifespan of the alcoholic is shortened by an average of 15 years due to increased risk of death from heart disease, cancer, accidents, or suicide.

Clinical Features

One out of five of the average physician's pts will suffer from alcoholism. Routine medical care requires attention to potential alcohol-related illness and to alcoholism itself:

1. Neurologic—blackouts, seizures, delirium tremens, cerebellar degeneration, neuropathy, myopathy
2. Gastrointestinal—esophagitis, gastritis, pancreatitis, hepatitis, cirrhosis, GI hemorrhage
3. Cardiovascular—hypertension, cardiomyopathy
4. Hematologic—macrocytosis, folate deficiency, thrombocytopenia, leukopenia
5. Endocrine—gynecomastia, testicular atrophy, amenorrhea, infertility
6. Skeletal—fractures, osteonecrosis
7. Cancer—breast cancer, oral and esophageal cancers, rectal cancers.

Most alcoholic pts do not have dramatic physical symptoms but instead present with psychosocial difficulties. Most common are marital difficulties, job problems (tardiness, absenteeism), and legal problems resulting from driving while intoxicated. A positive answer to any of the "CAGE questions" indicates a high probability of alcoholism: Are you . . . *C*utting down, or feel the need to? *A*nnoyed when people criticize your drinking? *G*uilty about your drinking? *E*ye-opening with a drink in the morning? Typically, pts will describe a host of difficulties but will then deny that they have a problem with alcohol abuse. Denial is a characteristic, if not the core, symptom of alcoholism.

Alcohol is a CNS depressant that acts on receptors for γ-aminobutyric acid (GABA), the major inhibitory neurotransmitter in the nervous system. Behavioral, cognitive, and psychomotor changes can occur at blood alcohol levels as low as 4–7 mmol/L (20–30 mg/dL), a level achieved after the ingestion of one or two typical drinks. Mild to moderate intoxication occurs at 17–43 mmol/L (80–200 mg/dL). Incoordination, tremor, ataxia, confusion, stupor, coma, and even death occur at progressively higher blood alcohol levels.

Chronic alcohol use produces CNS dependence. In such individuals, the earliest sign of alcohol withdrawal is tremulousness ("shakes" or "jitters"), which usually occurs 5–10 h after the last drink. This may be followed by generalized seizures ("rum fits") in the first 24–48 h; these do not require initiation of anti-seizure medications. With severe withdrawal, autonomic hyperactivity ensues (sweating, hypertension, tachycardia, tachypnea, fever), accompanied by insomnia, nightmares, anxiety, and GI symptoms.

Delirium tremens (DTs), which may begin 3–5 days after the last drink, is a very severe withdrawal syndrome characterized by profound autonomic hyperactivity, extreme confusion, agitation, vivid delusions, and hallucinations (often visual and tactile); mortality is 5–15%. Wernicke's encephalopathy is an alcohol-related syndrome characterized by ataxia, ophthalmoplegia, and confusion, often with associated nystagmus, peripheral neuropathy, cerebellar signs, and hypotension; there is impaired short-term memory, inattention, and emotional lability. Korsakoff's syndrome follows as the encephalopathy and ocular findings resolve; it is characterized by anterograde and retrograde amnesia and confabulation. Wernicke-Korsakoff's syndrome is caused by chronic thiamine deficiency, resulting in damage to thalamic nuclei, mamillary bodies, and brainstem and cerebellar structures.

Laboratory Findings

Clues to alcoholism include mild anemia with macrocytosis, folate deficiency, thrombocytopenia, granulocytopenia, abnormal liver function tests, hyperuricemia, and elevated triglycerides. Two blood tests with between 70% and 80% sensitivity and specificity are γ-glutamyl transferase (GGT) (>30 U) and carbohydrate-deficient transferrin (CDT) (>20 U/L); the combination of the two is likely to be more accurate than either alone when screening pts for high levels of alcohol intake. Decreases in serum K, Mg, Zn, and PO_4 levels are common. A variety of diagnostic studies may show evidence of alcohol-related organ dysfunction.

 TREATMENT

> *Acute Withdrawal*   Acute alcohol withdrawal is treated with multiple B vitamins including thiamine (50–100 mg IV or PO daily for 1 week or longer) to replenish depleted stores; if Wernicke-Korsakoff's syndrome is suspected, the IV route must be used, since intestinal absorption is unreliable in alcoholics. CNS depressant drugs are used when seizures or autonomic hyperactivity is present. These drugs halt the rapid state of withdrawal in the CNS and allow for a slower, more controlled reduction of the substance. Low-potency benzodiazepines with long half-lives are the medication of choice (e.g., diazepam, chlordiazepoxide), because they produce fairly steady blood levels of drug and there is a wide dose range within which to work. These benefits must be weighed against the risks of overmedication and oversedation, which occur less commonly with shorter-acting agents (e.g., oxazepam, lorazepam). Typical doses are diazepam 5–10 mg or chlordiazepoxide 25–50 mg PO every 1–4 h as needed for objective signs of alcohol withdrawal (such as pulse < 90).
>
> In severe withdrawal or DTs, high doses of benzodiazepines are usually required. The physician must also look for evidence of infection or trauma that may be masked by prominent withdrawal symptoms or that contribute to the pt's debilitated state. Fluid and electrolyte status and blood glucose levels should be closely followed as well. Cardiovascular and hemodynamic monitoring are crucial, as hemodynamic collapse and cardiac arrhythmia are not uncommon. Generalized withdrawal seizures rarely require aggressive pharmacologic intervention beyond that given to the usual patient undergoing withdrawal, i.e., adequate doses of benzodiazepines.
>
> *Recovery and Sobriety*   Maneuvers in rehabilitation fall into several general categories. First are attempts to help the alcoholic achieve and maintain a high level of motivation toward abstinence. These include education about alcoholism and instructing family and/or friends to stop protecting the person from the problems caused by alcohol. The second step is to help the pt to readjust to life without alcohol and to reestablish a functional life-style through counseling, vocational rehabilitation, and self-help groups such as Alcoholics Anonymous. The third component, called *relapse prevention*, helps the person to identify situations in which a return to drinking is likely, formulate ways of managing these risks, and develop coping strategies that increase the chances of a return to abstinence if a slip occurs. There is no convincing evidence that inpatient rehabilitation is more effective than outpatient care.
>
> Disulfiram (Antabuse; 250 mg/d), a drug that inhibits aldehyde dehydrogenase and results in toxic symptoms (nausea, vomiting, diarrhea, tremor) due to accumulation of acetaldehyde if the pt consumes alcohol, is used in some centers. Disulfiram has many side effects, and the reactions with alcohol can be dangerous. Preliminary studies suggest that the opiate antagonists naltrexone and acamprosate may reduce recidivism in abstinent alcoholics.

For a more detailed discussion, see Schuckit MA: Alcohol and Alcoholism, Chap. 372, p. 2562, in HPIM-16.

205

NARCOTIC ABUSE

Narcotics, or opiates, bind to specific opioid receptors in the CNS and elsewhere in the body. These receptors mediate the opiate effects of analgesia, euphoria, respiratory depression, and constipation. Endogenous opiate peptides (enkephalins and endorphins) are natural ligands for the opioid receptors and play a role in analgesia, memory, learning, reward, mood regulation, and stress tolerance.

The prototypic opiates, morphine and codeine, are derived from the juice of the opium poppy, *Papaver somniferum*. The semisynthetic drugs produced from morphine include hydromorphone (Dilaudid), diacetylmorphine (heroin), and oxycodone. The purely synthetic opioids and their cousins include meperidine, propoxyphene, diphenoxylate, fentanyl, buprenorphine, tramadol, methadone, and pentazocine. All of these substances produce analgesia and euphoria as well as physical dependence when taken in high enough doses for prolonged periods of time.

1% of the U.S. population meets criteria for narcotic abuse or dependence at some time in their lives. 70% of narcotic-addicted individuals have another psychiatric disorder (usually major depression, alcoholism, or a personality disorder). Three groups of abusers can be identified: (1) "medical" abusers—pts with chronic pain syndromes who misuse their prescribed analgesics; (2) physicians, nurses, dentists, and pharmacists with easy access to narcotics; and (3) "street" abusers. The street abuser is typically a higher functioning individual who began by using tobacco, alcohol, and marijuana and then moved on to opiates.

Clinical Features

Acutely, all opiates have the following CNS effects: sedation, euphoria, decreased pain perception, decreased respiratory drive, and vomiting. In larger doses, markedly decreased respirations, bradycardia, pupillary miosis, stupor, and coma ensue. Additionally, the adulterants used to "cut" street drugs (quinine, phenacetin, strychnine, antipyrine, caffeine, powdered milk) can produce permanent neurologic damage, including peripheral neuropathy, amblyopia, myelopathy, and leukoencephalopathy. The shared use of contaminated needles is a major cause of brain abscesses, acute endocarditis, hepatitis B, AIDS, septic arthritis, and soft tissue infections. At least 25% of street abusers die within 10–20 years of starting active opiate abuse.

Chronic use of opiates will result in tolerance (requiring higher doses to achieve psychotropic effects) and physical dependence. With shorter-acting opiates such as heroin, morphine, or oxycodone, withdrawal signs begin 8–12 h after the last dose, peak at 2–3 days, and subside over 7–10 days. With longer-acting opiates such as methadone, withdrawal begins 2–4 days after the last dose, peaks at 3–4 days, and lasts several weeks.

Withdrawal produces nausea and diarrhea, coughing, lacrimation, rhinorrhea, diaphoresis, twitching muscles, piloerection, fever, tachypnea, hypertension, diffuse body pain, insomnia, and yawning. Relief of these exceedingly unpleasant symptoms by narcotic administration leads to more frequent narcotic use. Eventually, all of the person's efforts are consumed by drug-seeking behavior.

℞ TREATMENT

Overdose High doses of opiates, whether taken in a suicide attempt or accidentally when the potency is misjudged, are frequently lethal. Toxicity occurs immediately after IV administration and with a variable delay after oral ingestion. Symptoms include miosis, shallow respirations, bradycardia, hypothermia, stupor or coma, and pulmonary edema. Treatment requires cardiorespiratory support and administration of the opiate antagonist naloxone (0.4 mg IV repeated in 3–10 min if no or only partial response). Because the effects of naloxone diminish in 2–3 h compared with longer-lasting effects of heroin (up to 24 h) or methadone (up to 72 h), pts must be observed for at least 1–3 days for reappearance of the toxic state.

Withdrawal One treatment of withdrawal requires administration of any opioid (e.g., 10 to 25 mg of methadone bid) on day 1 to decrease symptoms. After several days of a stabilized drug dose, the opioid is then decreased by 10 to 20% of the original day's dose each day. However, detoxification with opioids is proscribed or limited in most states. Thus, pharmacologic treatments often center on relief of symptoms of diarrhea with loperamide, of "sniffles" with decongestants, and pain with nonopioid analgesics (e.g., ibuprofen). Comfort can be enhanced with administration of the α_2-adrenergic agonist clonidine in doses up to 0.3 mg given two to four times a day to decrease sympathetic nervous system overactivity. Blood pressure must be closely monitored. Some clinicians augment this regimen with low to moderate doses of benzodiazepines for 2 to 5 days to decrease agitation.

Opioid Maintenance Methadone maintenance is a widely used treatment strategy in the management of opiate addiction. Methadone is a long-acting opioid optimally dosed at 80 to 120 mg/d (gradually increased over time). This level is optimally effective in blocking heroin-induced euphoria, decreasing craving, and maintaining abstinence from illegal oipoids. Over three-quarters of patients in well-supervised methadone clinics are likely to remain heroin-free for ≥6 months. Methadone is administered as an oral liquid given once a day at the program, with weekend doses taken at home. The longer-acting analogues, such as LAAM, can be given in doses up to 80 mg two or three times a week. After a period of maintenance (usually 6 months to ≥1 year), the clinician can work to slowly decrease the dose by about 5% per week. An additional medication that has been used for maintenance treatment involves the μ opioid agonist and κ antagonist buprenorphine.

Opiate Antagonists The opiate antagonists (e.g., naltrexone) compete with heroin and other opioids at receptors, reducing the effects of the opioid agonists. Administered over long periods with the intention of blocking the opioid "high," these drugs can be useful as part of an overall treatment approach that includes counseling and support. Naltrexone doses of 50 mg/d antagonize 15 mg of heroin for 24 h, and the possibly more effective higher doses (125 to 150 mg) block the effects of 25 mg of intravenous heroin for up to 3 days. To avoid precipitating a withdrawal syndrome, patients must be free of opioids for a minimum of 5 days before beginning treatment with naltrexone and should first be challenged with 0.4 or 0.8 mg of the shorter-acting agent naloxone to be certain they can tolerate the long-acting antagonist.

Drug-Free Programs Most opioid-dependent individuals enter treatment programs based primarily on the cognitive-behavioral approaches of enhancing commitment to abstinence, helping individuals to rebuild their lives without substances, and preventing relapse. Whether carried out in inpatient or outpatient settings, patients do not receive medications.

Prevention Except for the terminally ill, physicians should carefully monitor opioid drug use in their patients, keeping doses as low as is practical and administering them over as short a period as the level of pain would warrant in the average person. Physicians must be vigilant regarding their own risk for opioid abuse and dependence, never prescribing these drugs for themselves. For the nonmedical intravenous drug–dependent person, all possible efforts must be made to prevent AIDS, hepatitis, bacterial endocarditis, and other consequences of contaminated needles both through methadone maintenance and by considering needle-exchange programs.

For a more detailed discussion, see Shuckit MA, Segal DS: Opioid Drug Abuse and Dependence, Chap. 373, p. 2567, in HPIM-16.

SECTION 16

ADVERSE DRUG REACTIONS

206

ADVERSE DRUG REACTIONS

Adverse drug reactions are among the most frequent problems encountered clinically and represent a common cause for hospitalization. They occur most frequent in pts receiving multiple drugs and are caused by

- Errors in self-administration of prescribed drugs (quite common in the elderly).
- Exaggeration of intended pharmacologic effect (e.g., hypotension in a pt given antihypertensive drugs).
- Concomitant administration of drugs with synergistic effects (e.g., aspirin and warfarin).
- Cytotoxic reactions (e.g., hepatic necrosis due to acetaminophen).
- Immunologic mechanisms (e.g., quinidine-induced thrombocytopenia, hydralazine-induced SLE).
- Genetically determined enzymatic defects (e.g., primaquine-induced hemolytic anemia in G6PD deficiency).
- Idiosyncratic reactions (e.g., chloramphenicol-induced aplastic anemia).

RECOGNITION History is of prime importance. Consider the following:

- Nonprescription drugs and topical agents as potential offenders
- Previous reaction to identical drugs
- Temporal association between drug administration and development of clinical manifestations
- Subsidence of manifestations when the agent is discontinued or reduced in dose
- Recurrence of manifestations with cautious readministration (for less hazardous reactions)
- *Rare:* (1) biochemical abnormalities, e.g., red cell G6PD deficiency as cause of drug-induced hemolytic anemia; (2) abnormal serum antibody in pts with agranulocytosis, thrombocytopenia, hemolytic anemia.

Table 206-1 lists a number of clinical manifestations of adverse effects of drugs. It is not designed to be complete or exhaustive.

Table 206-1

Clinical Manifestations of Adverse Reactions to Drugs

MULTISYSTEM MANIFESTATIONS

Anaphylaxis	**Angioedema**
Cephalosporins	ACE inhibitors
Dextran	**Drug-induced lupus**
Insulin	**erythematosus**
Iodinated drugs or contrast media	Cephalosporins
	Hydralazine
Lidocaine	Iodides
Penicillins	Isoniazid
Procaine	Methyldopa

(continued)

Table 206-1 *(Continued)*

Clinical Manifestations of Adverse Reactions to Drugs

MULTISYSTEM MANIFESTATIONS *(Continued)*

Phenytoin	**Hyperpyrexia**
Procainamide	Antipsychotics
Quinidine	**Serum sickness**
Sulfonamides	Aspirin
Thiouracil	Penicillins
Fever	Propylthiouracil
Aminosalicylic acid	Sulfonamides
Amphotericin B	
Antihistamines	
Penicillins	

ENDOCRINE MANIFESTATIONS

Addisonian-like syndrome	Guanethidine
Busulfan	Lithium
Ketoconazole	Major tranquilizers
Galactorrhea (may also cause	Methyldopa
amenorrhea)	Oral contraceptives
Methyldopa	Sedatives
Phenothiazines	**Thyroid function tests, disorders**
Tricyclic antidepressants	**of**
Gynecomastia	Acetazolamide
Calcium channel antagonists	Amiodarone
Digitalis	Chlorpropamide
Estrogens	Clofibrate
Griseofulvin	Colestipol and nicotinic acid
Isoniazid	Gold salts
Methyldopa	Iodides
Phenytoin	Lithium
Spironolactone	Oral contraceptives
Testosterone	Phenothiazines
Sexual dysfunction	Phenylbutazone
Beta blockers	Phenytoin
Clonidine	Sulfonamides
Diuretics	Tolbutamide

METABOLIC MANIFESTATIONS

Hyperbilirubinemia	Oral contraceptives
Rifampin	Thiazides
Hypercalcemia	**Hypoglycemia**
Antacids with absorbable alkali	Insulin
Thiazides	Oral hypoglycemics
Vitamin D	Quinine
Hyperglycemia	**Hyperkalemia**
Chlorthalidone	ACE inhibitors
Diazoxide	Amiloride
Encainide	Cytotoxics
Ethacrynic acid	Digitalis overdose
Furosemide	Heparin
Glucocorticoids	Lithium
Growth hormone	

(continued)

METABOLIC MANIFESTATIONS *(Continued)*

Potassium preparations including salt substitute
Potassium salts of drugs
Spironolactone
Succinylcholine
Triamterene

Hypokalemia
Alkali-induced alkalosis
Amphotericin B
Diuretics
Gentamicin
Insulin
Laxative abuse
Mineralocorticoids, some glucocorticoids
Osmotic diuretics
Sympathomimetics
Tetracycline
Theophylline
Vitamin B_{12}

Hyperuricemia
Aspirin
Cytotoxics

Ethacrynic acid
Furosemide
Hyperalimentation
Thiazides

Hyponatremia
1. Dilutional
   Carbamazepine
   Chlorpropamide
   Cyclophosphamide
   Diuretics
   Vincristine
2. Salt wasting
   Diuretics
   Enemas
   Mannitol

Metabolic acidosis
Acetazolamide
Paraldehyde
Salicylates
Spironolactone

DERMATOLOGIC MANIFESTATIONS

Acne
Anabolic and androgenic steroids
Bromides
Glucocorticoids
Iodides
Isoniazid
Oral contraceptives

Alopecia
Cytotoxics
Ethionamide
Heparin
Oral contraceptives (withdrawal)

Eczema
Captopril
Cream and lotion perservatives
Lanolin
Topical antihistamines
Topical antimicrobials
Topical local anesthetics

Erythema multiforme or Stevens-Johnson syndrome
Barbiturates
Chlorpropamide
Codeine
Penicillins
Phenylbutazone

Phenytoin
Salicylates
Sulfonamides
Sulfones
Tetracyclines
Thiazides

Erythema nodosum
Oral contraceptives
Penicillins
Sulfonamides

Exfoliative dermatitis
Barbiturates
Gold salts
Penicillins
Phenylbutazone
Phenytoin
Quinidine
Sulfonamides

Fixed drug eruptions
Barbiturates
Captopril
Phenylbutazone
Quinine
Salicylates
Sulfonamides

Hyperpigmentation
Bleomycin
Busulfan

(continued)

Table 206-1 *(Continued)*

Clinical Manifestations of Adverse Reactions to Drugs

DERMATOLOGIC MANIFESTATIONS *(Continued)*

Chloroquine and other
  antimalarials
Corticotropin
Cyclophosphamide
Gold salts
Hypervitaminosis A
Oral contraceptives
Phenothiazines
Lichenoid eruptions
  Aminosalicylic acid
  Antimalarials
  Chlorpropamide
  Gold salts
  Methyldopa
  Phenothiazines
Photodermatitis
  Captopril
  Chlordiazepoxide
  Furosemide
  Griseofulvin
  Nalidixic acid
  Oral contraceptives
  Phenothiazines
  Sulfonamides
  Sulfonylureas
  Tetracyclines, particularly
    demeclocycline
  Thiazides
Purpura (see also
  Thrombocytopenia)
  Allopurinol
  Ampicillin

Aspirin
Glucocorticoids
Rashes (nonspecific)
  Allopurinol
  Ampicillin
  Barbiturates
  Indapamide
  Methyldopa
  Phenytoin
Skin necrosis
  Warfarin
**Toxic epidermal necrolysis
  (bullous)**
  Allopurinol
  Barbiturates
  Bromides
  Iodides
  Nalidixic acid
  Penicillins
  Phenylbutazone
  Phenytoin
  Sulfonamides
Urticaria
  Aspirin
  Barbiturates
  Captopril
  Enalapril
  Penicillins
  Sulfonamides

HEMATOLOGIC MANIFESTATIONS

Agranulocytosis (see also
  Pancytopenia)
  Captopril
  Carbimazole
  Chloramphenicol
  Cytotoxics
  Gold salts
  Indomethacin
  Methimazole
  Oxyphenbutazone
  Phenothiazines
  Phenylbutazone
  Propylthiouracil
  Sulfonamides
  Tolbutamide
  Tricyclic antidepressants

**Clotting abnormalities/hypo-
  thrombinemia**
  Cefamandole
  Cefoperazone
  Moxalactam
Eosinophilia
  Aminosalicylic acid
  Chlorpropamide
  Erythromycin estolate
  Imipramine
  L-Tryptophan
  Methotrexate
  Nitrofurantoin
  Procarbazine
  Sulfonamides

(continued)

HEMATOLOGIC MANIFESTATIONS *(Continued)*

Hemolytic anemia
Aminosalicylic acid
Cephalosporins
Chlorpromazine
Dapsone
Insulin
Isoniazid
Levodopa
Mefenamic acid
Melphalan
Methyldopa
Penicillins
Phenacetin
Procainamide
Quinidine
Rifampin
Sulfonamides
Hemolytic anemias in G6PD deficiency
See Table 64-3
Leukocytosis
Glucocorticoids
Lithium
Lymphadenopathy
Phenytoin
Primidone
Megaloblastic anemia
Folate antagonists
Nitrous oxide
Oral contraceptives
Phenobarbital
Phenytoin
Primidone
Triamterene
Trimethroprim
Pancytopenia (aplastic anemia)
Carbamazepine
Chloramphenicol

Cytotoxics
Gold salts
Mephenytoin
Phenylbutazone
Phenytoin
Quinacrine
Sulfonamides
Trimethadione
Zidovudine (AZT)
Pure red cell aplasia
Azathioprine
Chlorpropamide
Isoniazid
Phenytoin
Thrombocytopenia (see also **Pancytopenia**)
Acetazolamine
Aspirin
Carbamazepine
Carbenicillin
Chlorpropamide
Chlorthalidone
Furosemide
Gold salts
Heparin
Indomethacin
Isoniazid
Methyldopa
Moxalactam
Phenylbutazone
Phenytoin and other hydantoins
Quinidine
Quinine
Thiazides
Ticarcillin

CARDIOVASCULAR MANIFESTATIONS

Angina exacerbation
Alpha blockers
Beta blocker withdrawal
Ergotamine
Excessive thyroxine
Hydralazine
Methysergide
Minoxidil
Nifedipine
Oxytocin
Vasopressin

Arrhythmias
Adriamycin
Antiarrhythmic drugs
Atropine
Anticholinesterases
Beta blockers
Digitalis
Emetine
Lithium
Phenothiazines
Sympathomimetics

(continued)

Table 206-1 *(Continued)*

Clinical Manifestations of Adverse Reactions to Drugs

CARDIOVASCULAR MANIFESTATIONS *(Continued)*

Thyroid hormone
Tricyclic antidepressants
Verapamil
AV block
 Clonidine
 Methyldopa
 Verapamil
Cardiomyopathy
 Adriamycin
 Daunorubicin
 Emetine
 Lithium
 Phenothiazines
 Sulfonamides
 Sympathomimetics
**Fluid retention or congestive
 heart failure**
 Beta blockers
 Calcium antagonists
 Estrogens
 Indomethacin
 Mannitol
 Minoxidil
 Phenylbutazone
 Steroids
Hypotension
 Calcium antagonists
 Citrated blood

Diuretics
Levodopa
Morphine
Nitroglycerin
Phenothiazines
Protamine
Quinidine
Hypertension
 Clonidine withdrawal
 Corticotropin
 Cyclosporine
 Glucocorticoids
 Monoamine oxidase inhibitors
  with sympathomimetics
 NSAIDs
 Oral contraceptives
 Sympathomimetics
 Tricyclic antidepressants with
  sympathomimetics
Pericarditis
 Emetine
 Hydralazine
 Methysergide
 Procainamide
Thromboembolism
 Oral contraceptives

RESPIRATORY MANIFESTATIONS

Airway obstruction
 Beta blockers
 Cephalosporins
 Cholinergic drugs
 NSAIDs
 Penicillins
 Pentazocine
 Streptomycin
 Tartrazine (drugs with yellow
  dye)
Cough
 ACE inhibitors
Pulmonary edema
 Contrast media
 Heroin
 Methadone
 Propoxyphene

Pulmonary infiltrates
 Acyclovir
 Amiodarone
 Azathioprine
 Bleomycin
 Busulfan
 Carmustine (BCNU)
 Chlorambucil
 Cyclophosphamide
 Melphalan
 Methotrexate
 Methysergide
 Mitomycin C
 Nitrofurantoin
 Procarbazine
 Sulfonamides

(continued)

GASTROINTESTINAL MANIFESTATIONS

Cholestatic jaundice
  Anabolic steroids
  Androgens
  Chlorpropamide
  Erythromycin estolate
  Gold salts
  Methimazole
  Nitrofurantoin
  Oral contraceptives
  Phenothiazines
Constipation or ileus
  Aluminum hydroxide
  Barium sulfate
  Calcium carbonate
  Ferrous sulfate
  Ion exchange resins
  Opiates
  Phenothiazines
  Tricyclic antidepressants
  Verapamil
Diarrhea or colitis
  Antibiotics (broad-spectrum)
  Colchicine
  Digitalis
  Magnesium in antacids
  Methyldopa
Diffuse hepatocellular damage
  Acetaminophen (paracetamol)
  Allopurinol
  Aminosalicylic acid
  Dapsone
  Erythromycin estolate
  Ethionamide
  Glyburide
  Halothane
  Isoniazid
  Ketoconazole
  Methimazole
  Methotrexate
  Methoxyflurane
  Methyldopa
  Monoamine oxidase inhibitors
  Niacin
  Nifedipine
  Nitrofurantoin
  Phenytoin
  Propoxyphene
  Propylthiouracil
  Pyridium
  Rifampin
  Salicylates

Sodium valproate
Sulfonamides
Tetracyclines
Verapamil
Zidovudine (AZT)
Intestinal ulceration
  Solid KCl preparations
Malabsorption
  Aminosalicylic acid
  Antibiotics (broad-spectrum)
  Cholestyramine
  Colchicine
  Colestipol
  Cytotoxics
  Neomycin
  Phenobarbital
  Phenytoin
Nausea or vomiting
  Digitalis
  Estrogens
  Ferrous sulfate
  Levodopa
  Opiates
  Potassium chloride
  Tetracyclines
  Theophylline
Oral conditions
  1. Gingival hyperplasia
     Callcium antagonists
     Cyclosporine
     Phenytoin
  2. Salivary gland swelling
     Bretylium
     Clonidine
     Guanethidine
     Iodides
     Phenylbutazone
  3. Taste disturbances
     Biguanides
     Captopril
     Griseofulvin
     Lithium
     Metronidazole
     Penicillamine
     Rifampin
  4. Ulceration
     Aspirin
     Cytotoxics
     Gentian violet
     Isoproterenol (sublingual)
     Pancreatin

(continued)

Table 206-1 *(Continued)*

Clinical Manifestations of Adverse Reactions to Drugs

GASTROINTESTINAL MANIFESTATIONS *(Continued)*

Pancreatitis
Azathioprine
Ethacrynic acid
Furosemide
Glucocorticoids
Opiates
Oral contraceptives

Sulfonamides
Thiazides
Peptic ulceration or hemorrhage
Aspirin
Ethacrynic acid
Glucocoricoids
NSAIDs

RENAL/URINARY MANIFESTATIONS

Bladder dysfunction
Anticholinergics
Disopyramide
Monoamine oxidase inhibitors
Tricyclic antidepressants
Calculi
Acetazolamide
Vitamin D
Concentrating defect with polyuria (or nephrogenic diabetes insipidus)
Demeclocycline
Lithium
Methoxyflurane
Vitamin D
Hemorrhagic cystitis
Cyclophosphamide
Interstitial nephritis
Allopurinol
Furosemide
Penicillins, esp. methicillin
Phenindione
Sulfonamides
Thiazides
Nephropathies
Due to analgesics (e.g., phenacetin)

Nephrotic syndrome
Captopril
Gold salts
Penicillamine
Phenindione
Probenecid
Obstructive uropathy
Extrarenal: methysergide
Intrarenal: cytotoxics
Renal dysfunction
Cyclosporine
NSAIDS
Triamterene
Renal tubular acidosis
Acetazolamide
Amphotericin B
Degraded tetracycline
Tubular necrosis
Aminoglycosides
Amphotericin B
Colistin
Cyclosporine
Methoxyflurane
Polymyxins
Radioiodinated contrast medium
Sulfonamides
Tetracyclines

NEUROLOGIC MANIFESTATIONS

Exacerbation of myasthenia
Aminoglycosides
Polymyxins
Extrapyramidal effects
Butyrophenones, e.g., haloperidol
Levodopa
Methyldopa
Metoclopramide
Oral contraceptives
Phenothiazines
Tricyclic antidepressants

Headache
Ergotamine (withdrawal)
Glyceryl trinitrate
Hydralazine
Indomethacin
Peripheral neuropathy
Amiodarone
Chloramphenicol
Chloroquine
Chlorpropamide
Clofibrate
Demeclocycline

(continued)

NEUROLOGIC MANIFESTATIONS *(Continued)*

Disopyramide
Ethambutol
Ethionamide
Glutethimide
Hydralazine
Isoniazid
Methysergide
Metronidazole
Nalidixic acid
Nitrofurantoin
Phenytoin
Polymyxin, colistin
Procarbazine
Streptomycin
Tolbutamide
Tricyclic antidepressants
Vincristine

Pseudotumor cerebri (or intra-cranial hypertension)
Amiodarone
Glucocorticoids, mineralocorticoids

Hypervitaminosis A
Oral contraceptives
Tetracyclines

Seizures
Amphetamines
Analeptics
Isoniazid
Lidocaine
Lithium
Nalidixic acid
Penicillins
Phenothiazines
Physostigmine
Theophylline
Tricyclic antidepressants
Vincristine

Stroke
Oral contraceptives

OCULAR MANIFESTATIONS

Cataracts
Busulfan
Chlorambucil
Glucocorticoids
Phenothiazines

Color vision alteration
Barbiturates
Digitalis
Methaqualone
Streptomycin
Thiazides

Corneal edema
Oral contraceptives

Corneal opacities
Chloroquine
Indomethacin
Vitamin D

Glaucoma
Mydriatics
Sympathomimetics

Optic neuritis
Aminosalicylic acid
Chloramphenicol
Ethambutol
Isoniazid
Penicillamine
Phenothiazines
Phenylbutazone
Quinine
Streptomycin

Retinopathy
Chloroquine
Phenothiazines

EAR MANIFESTATIONS

Deafness
Aminoglycosides
Aspirin
Bleomycin
Chloroquine
Erythromycin
Ethacrynic acid

Furosemide
Nortriptyline
Quinine

Vestibular disorders
Aminoglycosides
Quinine

MUSCULOSKELETAL MANIFESTATIONS

Bone disorders
1. Osteoporosis
   Glucocorticoids
   Heparin

2. Osteomalacia
   Aluminum hydroxide
   Anticonvulsants
   Glutethimide

(continued)

Table 206-1 *(Continued)*

Clinical Manifestations of Adverse Reactions to Drugs

MUSCULOSKELETAL MANIFESTATIONS *(Continued)*

Myopathy or myalgia
  Amphotericin B
  Chloroquine
  Clofibrate
  Glucocorticoids
  Oral contraceptives

Myositis
  Gemfibrozil
  Lovastatin

PSYCHIATRIC MANIFESTATIONS

Delirious or confusional states
  Amantadine
  Aminophylline
  Anticholinergics
  Antidepressants
  Cimetidine
  Digitalis
  Glucocorticoids
  Isoniazid
  Levodopa
  Methyldopa
  Penicillins
  Phenothiazines
  Sedatives and hypnotics
Depression
  Amphetamine withdrawal
  Beta blockers
  Centrally acting antihyperten-
    sives (reserpine, methyldopa,
    clonidine)
  Glucocorticoids
  Levodopa
Drowsiness
  Antihistamines
  Anxiolytic drugs
  Clonidine
  Major tranquilizers
  Methyldopa
  Tricyclic antidepressants

Hallucinatory states
  Amantadine
  Beta blockers
  Levodopa
  Meperidine
  Narcotics
  Pentazocine
  Tricyclic antidepressants
**Hypomania, mania, or excited
  reactions**
  Glucocorticoids
  Levodopa
  Monoamine oxidase inhibitors
  Sympathomimetics
  Tricyclic antidepressants
**Schizophrenic-like or paranoid
  reactions**
  Amphetamines
  Bromides
  Glucocorticoids
  Levodopa
  Lysergic acid
  Monoamine oxidase inhibitors
  Tricyclic antidepressants
Sleep disturbances
  Anorexiants
  Levodopa
  Monoamine oxidase inhibitors
  Sympathomimetics

Source: Adapted from AJJ Wood: HPIM-15, pp. 432–436.

For a more detailed discussion, see Roden DM: Principles of Clinical Phar-
macology, Chap. 3, p. 13, in HPIM-16; Wood AJJ: Adverse Reactions to
Drugs, Chap. 71, p. 430, in HPIM-15.

207

WOMEN'S HEALTH

The most common causes of death in both men and women are (1) heart disease, (2) cancer, and (3) cerebrovascular disease, with lung cancer the top cause of cancer death, despite common misperceptions that breast cancer is the most common cause of death in women. These misconceptions perpetuate inadequate attention to modifiable risk factors in women, such as dyslipidemia, hypertension, and cigarette smoking. Furthermore, since women in the Unites States live on average 5.7 years longer than men, the majority of the disease burden for many age-related disorders rests in women. For a discussion of the menopause transition and postmenopausal hormone therapy, see Chap. 178.

SEX DIFFERENCES IN HEALTH AND DISEASE
Alzheimer's Disease   (See also Chap. 190)

Alzheimer's disease (AD) affects approximately twice as many women as men, due to larger numbers of women surviving to older ages and to sex differences in brain size, structure, and functional organization. Postmenopausal hormone therapy may worsen cognitive function and the development of AD.

Coronary Heart Disease   (See also Chap. 123)

Coronary heart disease (CHD) presents differently in women, who are usually 10–15 years older than men with CHD and are more likely to have comorbidities, such as hypertension, congestive heart failure, and diabetes. Women more often have atypical symptoms, such as nausea, vomiting, indigestion, and upper back pain. Physicians are less likely to suspect heart disease in women with chest pain and are less likely to perform diagnostic and therapeutic cardiac procedures in women. The conventional risk factors for CHD are the same in both men and women, though women receive fewer interventions for modifiable risk factors than do men.

Diabetes Mellitus   (See also Chap. 176)

The prevalence of type 2 diabetes mellitus (DM) is higher in women, in part related to the higher prevalence of obesity among women. Polycystic ovary syndrome and gestational diabetes mellitus are both common conditions in premenopausal women that carry an increased risk for type 2 DM. Premenopausal women with DM have identical rates of CHD to males.

Hypertension   (See also Chap. 122)

Hypertension, as an age-related disorder, is more common in women than in men after age 60. Antihypertensive drugs appear to be equally effective in women and men; however, women may experience more side effects.

Autoimmune Disorders   (See also Chap. 161)

Most autoimmune disorders occur more commonly in women than in men; these include autoimmune thyroid and liver diseases, lupus, rheumatoid arthritis, scleroderma, multiple sclerosis, and idiopathic thrombocytopenic purpura. The mechanism for these sex differences remains obscure.

HIV Infection (See also Chap. 91)

Heterosexual contact with an at-risk partner is the fastest-growing transmission category of HIV. Women with HIV have more rapid decreases in their CD4 cell counts than men do. Other sexually transmitted diseases, such as chlamydial infection and gonorrhea, are important causes of infertility in women, and papilloma virus infection predisposes to cervical cancer.

Osteoporosis (See also Chap. 180)

Osteoporosis is much more prevalent in postmenopausal women than in age-matched men, since men accumulate more bone mass and lose bone more slowly than do women. Calcium intake, vitamin D, and estrogen all play important roles in bone formation and bone loss.

Pharmacology

On average, women have lower body weights, smaller organs, higher percent body fat, and lower total-body water than men do. Gonadal steroids, menstrual cycle phase, and pregnancy can all affect drug action. Women also take more medications than men do, including over-the-counter formulations and supplements. The greater use of medications, combined with biologic differences, may account for the reported higher frequency of adverse drug reactions in women.

Psychological Disorders (See also Chaps. 201 & 203)

Depression, anxiety, and eating disorders (bulimia and anorexia nervosa) are more common in women than in men. Depression occurs in 10% of women during pregnancy and 10–15% of women during the postpartum period.

Substance Abuse and Tobacco (See also Chap. 204)

Substance abuse is more common in men than women. However, women alcoholics are less likely to be diagnosed than men and are less likely to seek help. When they do seek help, it is more likely to be from a physician than from a treatment facility. Alcoholic women drink less than alcoholic men but exhibit the same degree of impairment. More men than women smoke tobacco, but the prevalence of smoking is declining faster in men than women.

Violence Against Women

Domestic violence is the most common cause of physical injury in women. Women may present with symptoms of chronic abdominal pain, headaches, substance abuse, and eating disorders, in addition to obvious manifestations such as trauma. Sexual assault is one of the most common crimes against women and is more likely by a spouse, ex-spouse, or acquaintance than by a stranger.

For a more detailed discussion, see Dunaif A: Women's Health, Chap. 5, p. 28, HPIM-16.

208

HEALTH MAINTENANCE AND DISEASE PREVENTION

A primary goal of health care is to prevent disease or to detect it early enough that interventions will be more effective. In general, screening is most effective when applied to relatively common disorders that carry a large disease burden and have a long latency period. Early detection of disease has the potential to reduce both morbidity and mortality; however, screening asymptomatic individuals carries some risk. False-positive results can lead to unnecessary lab tests and invasive procedures and can increase pt anxiety. Several measurements have been derived to better assess the potential gain from screening and prevention interventions:

- Number of subjects needed to be screened to alter the outcome in one individual
- Absolute impact of screening on disease (e.g., lives saved per thousand screened)
- Relative impact of screening on disease outcome (e.g., the % reduction in deaths)
- The cost per year of life saved
- The increase in average life expectancy for a population

Current recommendations include performance of a routine health care examination every 1–3 years before age 50 and every year thereafter. History should include medication use, allergies, dietary history, use of alcohol and tobacco, sexual practices, safety practices (seat belt and helmet use, gun possession), and a thorough family history. Routine measurements should include assessments of height, weight, body-mass index, and blood pressure. Screening should also be considered for domestic violence and depression.

Counseling by health care providers should be performed at health care visits. Tobacco and alcohol use, diet, and exercise represent the vast majority of factors that influence preventable deaths. While behavioral changes are frequently difficult to achieve, it should be emphasized that studies show even brief (<5 min) tobacco counseling by physicians results in a significant rate of long-term smoking cessation. Instruction about self-examination (e.g., skin, breast, testicular) should also be provided during preventative visits.

The top causes of age-specific mortality and corresponding preventative strategies are listed in Table 208-1. Formal recommendations from the U.S. Preventive Services Task Force are listed in Table 208-2.

Table 208-1

Age-Specific Causes of Mortality and Corresponding Preventative Options

Age Group	Top Causes of Age-Specific Mortality	Screening/Prevention Interventions to Consider for Each Specific Population
<35	1. Accidents 2. Suicide 3. Homicide 4. Malignancy 5. Heart disease 6. HIV	• Counseling on routine seat belt use (1) • Discuss dangers of drinking and driving (1) • Ask about tetanus vaccination status, repeat every 10 years (1) • Ask about gun use and/or gun possession (2,3) • Assess for substance abuse history including alcohol (2,3) • Screen for domestic violence (2,3) • Screen for depression and/or suicidal/homicidal ideation (2,3) • Annual Pap smear for cervical cancer screening (4) • Recommend skin, breast, and testicular self-exams (4) • Recommend UV light avoidance and regular sun screen use (4) • Annual measurement of blood pressure, height, weight, and body-mass index (5) • Discuss health risks of tobacco use, consider emphasis of cosmetic and economic issues to improve quit rates for younger smokers (4,5) • *Chlamydia* screening and contraceptive counseling for sexually active females (6) • HIV, hepatitis B, and syphilis testing if high-risk sexual behavior(s) or any prior history of sexually transmitted disease (6)
35–44	1. Malignancy 2. Accidents 3. Heart disease 4. Suicide 5. HIV 6. Chronic liver disease	*As above plus consider the following . . .* • Readdress smoking status, encourage cessation at every visit (1,3) • Obtain detailed family history of malignancies and begin early screening/prevention program if patient is at a significant increased risk (1) • Assess all cardiac risk factors (including screening for diabetes and hyperlipidemia) and consider primary prevention with aspirin for pts at >10% 10-year risk of a vascular event (3) • Assess for chronic alcohol abuse, risk factors for viral hepatitis, or other risks for development of chronic liver disease (6)

(continued)

Table 208-1 *(Continued)*

Age-Specific Causes of Mortality and Corresponding Preventative Options

Age Group	Top Causes of Age-Specific Mortality	Screening/Prevention Interventions to Consider for Each Specific Population
45–54	1. Malignancy 2. Heart disease 3. Accidents 4. Chronic liver disease 5. Cerebrovascular diseases 6. Suicide	*As above plus consider the following . . .* • Readdress smoking status, encourage cessation at every visit (1,2) • Begin breast cancer screening with yearly mammography at age 40 or 50 (1) • Consider prostate cancer screening with annual PSA and digital rectal exam at age 50 (or possibly earlier in African Americans or pts with family history) (1) • Begin colorectal cancer screening with either: fecal occult blood testing, flexible sigmoidoscopy, contrast barium enema, or colonoscopy (1) • Reassess vaccination status at age 50 and give special consideration to vaccines against *S. pneumoniae*, influenza, tetanus, and viral hepatitis (10)
55–64	1. Malignancy 2. Heart disease 3. Chronic lower respiratory disease 4. Cerebrovascular disease 5. Diabetes 6. Accidents 7. Pneumonia/influenza	*As above plus consider the following . . .* • Readdress smoking status, encourage cessation at every visit (1,2,3) • Reassess cardiac functional status and risk factors (2,5) • Initiate 1° or 2° prevention for coronary disease (2,5) • Consider screening exercise treadmill to risk stratify for coronary disease (2,5) • Consider pulmonary function testing for all long-term smokers to assess for development of chronic obstructive airway disease (3,7) • Vaccinate all smokers against influenza and *S. pneumoniae* at age 50 (3,7) • Screen all postmenopausal women (and all men with risk factors) for osteoporosis (6)
65–74	(1–7 same as 55–64 age group)	*As above plus consider the following . . .* • Readdress smoking status, encourage cessation at every visit (1,2,3) • Reassess vaccination status at age 65, emphasis on influenza and *S. pneumoniae* (3,7) • Screen for dementia and depression (4,6) • Screen for visual and hearing problems, home safety issues, and elder abuse (4,6)

Table 208-2

Clinical Preventive Services for Normal-Risk Adults Recommended by the U.S. Preventive Services Task Force

Test or Disorder	Population,[a] years	Frequency
Blood pressure, height and weight	>18	Periodically
Cholesterol	Men > 35	Every 5 years
	Women > 45	Every 5 years
Diabetes	>45 or earlier, if there are additional risk factors	Every 3 years
Pap smear	Within 3 years of onset of sexual activity or 21–65	Every 1–3 years
Chlamydia	Women 18–25	Every 1–2 years
Mammography[a]	Women > 40	Every 1–2 years
Colorectal cancer[a]	>50	Every 1 year
Fecal occult blood and/or sigmoidoscopy or colonoscopy		Every 5 years
		Every 10 years
Osteoporosis	Women > 65; > 60 at risk	Periodically
Alcohol use	>18	Periodically
Vision, hearing	>65	Periodically
Adult immunization		
Tetanus-diptheria (Td)	>18	Every 10 years
Varicella (VZV)	Susceptibles only, >18	Two doses
Measles, mumps, rubella (MMR)	Women, childbearing age	One dose
Pneumococcal	>65	One dose
Influenza	>50	Yearly

[a] Screening is performed earlier and more frequently when there is a strong family history. Randomized, controlled trials have documented that fecal occult blood testing (FOBT) confers a 15 to 30% reduction in mortality. Although randomized trials have not been performed for sigmoidoscopy or colonoscopy, well-designed case-control studies suggest similar or greater efficacy relative to FOBT.

Note: Prostate-specific antigen (PSA) testing is capable of enhancing the detection of early-stage prostate cancer, but evidence is inconclusive that it improves health outcomes. PSA testing is recommended by several professional organizations and is widely used in clinical practice, but it is not currently recommended by the U.S. Preventive Services Task Force.

Source: Adapted from the U.S. Preventive Services Task Force: *Guide to Clinical Prevention Services*, 2d and 3d eds (www.ahrq.gov/clinic/uspstfix.htm).

For a more detailed discussion, see Martin GJ: Screening and Prevention of Disease, Chap. 4, p. 26, in HPIM-16.

209

APPENDIX: LABORATORY VALUES OF CLINICAL IMPORTANCE

In preparing the Appendix, the authors have taken into account the fact that the system of international units (SI, système international d'unités) is used in most countries and in some medical journals. However, clinical laboratories may continue to report values in conventional units. Therefore, both systems are provided in the Appendix.

Conversion from one system to another can be made as follows:

$$\text{mmol/L} = \frac{\text{mg/dL} \times 10}{\text{atomic weight (or molecular weight)}}$$

$$\text{mg/dL} = \frac{\text{mmol/L} \times \text{atomic weight (or molecular weight)}}{10}$$

For a more complete list of laboratory values, consult the Appendices of HPIM, 16e.[a]

REFERENCE VALUES FOR LABORATORY TESTS

Table 209-1

Hematology and Coagulation

Analyte	SI Units	Conventional Units
Antithrombin III		
Antigenic	220–390 mg/L	22–39 mg/dL
Functional	0.8–1.30 U/L	80–130%
Bleeding time (adult)	2–9.5 min	2–9.5 min
Carboxyhemoglobin		
Nonsmoker	0–0.023	0–2.3%
Smoker	0.021–0.042	2.1–4.2%
D-Dimer	<0.5 mg/L	<0.5 μg/mL
Differential blood count		
Neutrophils	0.40–0.70	40–70%
Bands	0.0–0.10	0–10%
Lymphocytes	0.22–0.44	22–44%
Monocytes	0.04–0.11	4–11%
Eosinophils	0.0–0.8	0–8%
Basophils	0.0–0.03	0–3%
Erythrocyte count		
Adult males	$4.50–5.90 \times 10^{12}$/L	$4.50–5.90 \times 10^{6}$/mm^3
Adult females	$4.00–5.20 \times 10^{12}$/L	$4.00–5.20 \times 10^{6}$/mm^3

(continued)

[a]A variety of factors can influence reference values. Values supplied in this Appendix reflect typical reference ranges in adults. Pediatric reference ranges may vary significantly from adult values. Whenever possible, reference values provided by the laboratory performing the testing should be utilized in the interpretation of laboratory data.

Table 209-1 *(Continued)*

Hematology and Coagulation

Analyte	SI Units	Conventional Units
Erythrocyte sedimentation rate		
Females	1–25 mm/h	1–25 mm/h
Males	0–17 mm/h	0–17 mm/h
Ferritin		
Male	30–300 μg/L	30–300 ng/mL
Female	10–200 μg/L	10–200 ng/mL
Fibrin(ogen) degradation products	<2.5 mg/L	<2.5 μg/mL
Fibrinogen	1.50–4.00 g/L	150–400 mg/dL
Folate (folic acid): Normal	7.0–39.7 nmol/L	3.1–17.5 ng/mL
Haptoglobin	0.16–1.99 g/L	16–199 mg/dL
Hematocrit		
Adult males	0.41–0.53	41.0–53.0
Adult females	0.36–0.46	36.0–46.0
Hemoglobin		
Plasma	0.01–0.05 g/L	1–5 mg/dL
Whole blood:		
Adult males	8.4–10.9 mmol/L	13.5–17.5 g/dL
Adult females	7.4–9.9 mmol/L	12.0–16.0 g/dL
Hemoglobin electrophoresis		
Hemoglobin A	0.95–0.98	95–98%
Hemoglobin A_2	0.015–0.035	1.5–3.5%
Hemoglobin F	0–0.02	0–2.0%
Homocysteine	0–12 μmol/L	0–12 μmol/L
Iron	5.4–28.7 μmol/L	30–160 μg/dL
Iron binding capacity	40.8–76.7 μmol/L	228–428 μg/dL
Mean corpuscular hemoglobin (MCH)	26.0–34.0 pg/cell	26.0–34.0 pg/cell
Mean corpuscular hemoglobin concentration (MCHC)	310–370 g/L	31.0–37.0 g/dL
Mean corpuscular volume (MCV)		
Male (adult)	78–100 fl	78–100 μm³
Female (adult)	78–102 fl	78–102 μm³
Methemoglobin		Up to 1% of total hemoglobin
Partial thromboplastin time, activated	22.1–35.1 s	22.1–35.1 s
Plasminogen		
Antigen	84–140 mg/L	8.4–14.0 mg/dL
Functional	0.80–1.30	80–130%
Plasminogen activator inhibitor 1	4–43 μg/L	4–43 ng/mL
Platelet count	150–350 × 10⁹/L	150–350 × 10³/mm³
Protein C	0.70–1.40	70–140%
Protein S	0.70–1.40	70–140%
Prothrombin time	11.1–13.1 s	11.1–13.1 s
Reticulocyte count	0.005–0.025 red cells	0.5–2.5% red cells
Thrombin time	16–24 s	16–24 s
Total eosinophils	70–140 × 10⁶/L	70–440/mm³
Vitamin B_{12}	185 pmol/L	>250 pg/mL

Table 209-2

Clinical Chemistry

Constituent	SI Units	Conventional Units
Albumin	35–55 g/L	3.5–5.5 g/dL
Aldolase	0–100 nkat/L	0–6 U/L
α_1 antitrypsin	0.8–2.1 g/L	85–213 mg/dL
Alpha fetoprotein (adult)	<15 μg/L	<15 ng/mL
Aminotransferases		
Aspartate (AST, SGOT)	0–0.58 μkat/L	0–35 U/L
Alanine (ALT, SGPT)	0–0.58 μkat/L	0–35 U/L
Ammonia, as NH_3	6–47 μmol/L	10–80 μg/dL
Amylase	0.8–3.2 μkat/L	60–180 U/L
Angiotensin-converting enzyme (ACE)	<670 nkat/L	<40 U/L
Anion gap	7–16 mmol/L	7–16 mmol/L
Arterial blood gases		
$[HCO_3^-]$	21–28 mmol/L	21–30 meq/L
P_{CO_2}	4.7–5.9 kPa	35–45 mmHg
pH	7.38–7.44	
P_{O_2}	11–13 kPa	80–100 mmHg
β-2-Microglobulin	1.2–2.8 mg/L	1.2–2.8 mg/L
	$\leqq$200 μg/L	$\leqq$200 μg/L
Bilirubin		
Total	5.1–17 μmol/L	0.3–1.0 mg/dL
Direct	1.7–5.1 μmol/L	0.1–0.3 mg/dL
Indirect	3.4–12 μmol/L	0.2–0.7 mg/dL
Brain type natriuetic peptide (BNP)	Age and gender specific: <167 ng/L	Age and gender specific: <167 pg/mL
Calcium, ionized	1.1–1.4 mmol/L	4.5–5.6 mg/dL
Calcium	2.2–2.6 mmol/L	9–10.5 mg/dL
CA-15-3	0–30 kU/L	0–30 U/mL
CA 19-9	0–37 kU/L	0–37 U/mL
CA 27-29	0–32 kU/L	0–32 U/mL
CA 125	0–35 kU/L	0–35 U/mL
Calcitonin		
Male	3–26 ng/L	3–26 pg/mL
Female	2–17 ng/L	2–7 pg/mL
Carbon dioxide tension (P_{CO_2})	4.7–5.9 kPa	35–45 mmHg
Carbon monoxide content	Symptoms with 20% saturation of hemoglobin	
Carcinoembryonic antigen (CEA)	0.0–3.4 ug/L	0.0–3.4 ng/mL
Chloride	98–106 mmol/L	98–106 meq/L
C-peptide		
Creatine kinase (CK) (total)		
Females	0.67–2.50 μkat/L	40–150 U/L
Males	1.00–6.67 μkat/L	60–400 U/L
Creatine kinase-MB	0–7 μg/L	0–7 ng/mL
Creatinine	<133 μmol/L	<1.5 mg/dL

(continued)

Table 209-2 *(Continued)*

Clinical Chemistry

Constituent	SI Units	Conventional Units
Erythropoietin	5–36 U/L	
Ferritin		
Female	10–200 μg/L	10–200 ng/mL
Male	15–400 μg/L	15–400 ng/mL
Gamma glutamyltrans- ferase	1–94 U/L	1–94 U/L
Glucose (fasting)		
Normal	4.2–6.4 mmol/L	75–115 mg/dL
Diabetes mellitus	>7.0 mmol/L	>125 mg/dL
Glucose, 2 h post- prandial	<6.7 mmol/L	<120 mg/dL
Hemoglobin A_{1c}	0.038–0.064 Hb fraction	3.8–6.4%
Homocysteine	4–12 μmol/L	4–12 μmol/L
Iron	9–27 μmol/L	50–150 μg/dL
Iron-binding capacity	45–66 μmol/L	250–370 μg/dL
Iron-binding capacity saturation	0.2–0.45	20–45%
Lactate dehydrogenase	1.7–3.2 μkat/L	100–190 U/L
Lactate	0.6–1.7 mmol/L	5–15 mg/dL
Lipase	0–2.66 μkat/L	0–160 U/L
Lipoprotein (a)	0–300 mg/L	0–30 mg/dL
Magnesium	0.8–1.2 mmol/L	1.8–3 mg/dL
Microalbumin urine		
24-h urine	<0.2 g/L or <0.031 g/24 h	<20 mg/L or <31 mg/24 h
Spot AM urine	<0.03 g albumin/ g creatinine	<0.03 mg albumin/ mg creatinine
Myoglobin		
Male	19–92 μg/L	
Female	12–76 μg/L	
Osmolality	285–295 mmol/kg serum water	285–295 mosmol/kg serum water
Osteocalcin	3.1–14 μg/L	3.1–14 ng/mL
Oxygen percent satur- ation (sea level)	0.97 mol/mol 0.60–0.85 mol/mol	97% 60–85%
Oxygen tension (P_{O_2})	11–13 kPa	80–100 mmHg
pH	7.38–7.44	
Parathyroid hormone– related peptide	<1.3 pmol/L	<1.3 pmol/L
Phosphatase, acid	0.90 nkat/L	0–5.5 U/L
Phosphatase, alkaline	0.5–2.0 nkat/L	30–120 U/L
Phosphorus, inorganic	1.0–1.4 mmol/L	3–4.5 mg/dL
Potassium	3.5–5.0 mmol/L	3.5–5.0 meq/L

(continued)

Table 209-2 (*Continued*)

Clinical Chemistry

Constituent	SI Units	Conventional Units
Prostate-specific antigen (PSA)		
Female	<0.5 μg/L	<0.5 ng/mL
Male		
<40 years	0.0–2.0 μg/L	0.0–2.0 ng/mL
>40 years	0.0–4.0 μg/L	0.0–4.0 ng/mL
PSA, free, in males 45–75 years, with PSA values between 4 and 20 μg/L	>0.25 associated with benign prostatic hyperplasia (BPH)	>25% associated with BPH
Protein, total	55–80 g/L	5.5–8.0 g/dL
Protein fractions:		
Albumin	35–55 g/L	3.5–5.5 g/dL (50–60%)
Globulin	20–35 g/L	2.0–3.5 g/dL (40–50%)
Alpha$_1$	2–4 g/L	0.2–0.4 g/dL (4.2–7.2%)
Alpha$_2$	5–9 g/L	0.5–0.9 g/dL (6.8–12%)
Beta	6–11 g/L	0.6–1.1 g/dL (9.3–15%)
Gamma	7–17 g/L	0.7–1.7 g/dL (13–23%)
Sodium	136–145 mmol/L	136–145 meq/L
Transferrin	2.3–3.9 g/L	230–390 mg/dL
Triglycerides	<1.8 mmol/L	<160 mg/dL
Troponin I	0–0.4 μg/L	0–0.4 ng/mL
Troponin T	0–0.1 μg/L	0–0.1 ng/mL
Urea nitrogen	3.6–7.1 mmol/L	10–20 mg/dL
Uric acid		
Males	150–480 μmol/L	2.5–8.0 mg/dL
Females	90–360 μmol/L	1.5–6.0 mg/dL

Table 209-3

Metabolic and Endocrine Tests

Analyte	SI Units	Conventional Units
Adrenocorticotropin (ACTH)	1.3–16.7 pmol/L	6.0–76.0 pg/mL
Aldosterone (adult)		
Supine, normal sodium diet	55–250 pmol/L	2–9 ng/dL
Upright, normal sodium diet		2- to 5-fold increase over supine value
Supine, low-sodium diet		2- to 5-fold increase over normal sodium diet level
Cortisol		
Fasting, 8 AM–Noon	138–690 nmol/L	5–25 μg/dL
Noon–8 PM	138–414 nmol/L	5–15 μg/dL
8 PM–8 AM	0–276 nmol/L	0–10 μg/dL
Cortisol, free (urine)	55–193 nmol/24 h	20–70 μg/24 h
Epinephrine (urine)	0–109 nmol/d	0–20 μg/d

(continued)

Table 209-3 *(Continued)*

Metabolic and Endocrine Tests

Analyte	SI Units	Conventional Units
Estradiol		
Female		
Menstruating		
Follicular phase	184–532 pmol/L	20–145 pg/mL
Midcycle peak	411–1626 pmol/L	112–443 pg/mL
Luteal phase	184–885 pmol/L	20–241 pg/mL
Postmenopausal	<217 pmol/L	<59 pg/mL
Male	<184 pmol/L	<20 pg/mL
Follicle-stimulating hormone (FSH)		
Female		
Menstruating		
Follicular phase	3.0–20.0 IU/L	3.0–20.0 U/L
Ovulatory phase	9.0–26.0 IU/L	9.0–26.0 U/L
Luteal phase	1.0–12.0 IU/L	1.0–12.0 U/L
Postmenopausal	18.0–153.0 IU/L	18.0–153.0 U/L
Male	1.0–12.0 IU/L	1.0–12.0 U/L
Gastrin	<100 ng/L	<100 pg/mL
Growth hormone (resting)	0.5–17.0 μg/L	0.5–17.0 ng/mL
Human chorionic gonadotropin (HCG) (nonpregnant)	<5 IU/L	<5 mIU/mL
17-Hydroxyprogesterone (adult)		
Male	0.15 nmol/L	5–250 ng/dL
Female		
Follicular phase	0.6–3.0 nmol/L	20–100 ng/dL
Midcycle peak	3–7.5 nmol/L	100–250 ng/dL
Luteal phase	3–15 nmol/L	100–500 ng/dL
Postmenopausal	≤2.1 nmol/L	≤70 ng/dL
5-Hydroindoleacetic Acid [5-HIAA] (urine)	10.5–36.6 μmol/d	2–7 mg/d
17 Ketosteroids (urine)	10–42 μmol/d	3–12 mg/d
Luteinizing hormone (LH)		
Female		
Menstruating		
Follicular phase	2.0–15.0 U/L	2.0–15.0 U/L
Ovulatory phase	22.0–105.0 U/L	22.0–105.0 U/L
Luteal phase	0.6–19.0 U/L	0.6–19.0 U/L
Postmenopausal	16.0–64.0 U/L	16.0–64.0 U/L
Male	2.0–12.0 U/L	2.0–12.0 U/L
Metanephrine (urine)	0.03–0.69 mmol/mol creatinine	0.05–1.20 μg/mg creatinine
Norepinephrine (urine)	89–473 nmol/d	15–80 μg/d
Parathyroid hormone (PTH)	10–60 ng/L	10–60 pg/mL

(continued)

Table 209-3 (*Continued*)

Metabolic and Endocrine Tests

Analyte	SI Units	Conventional Units
Progesterone		
Female		
Follicular	<3.18 nmol/L	<1.0 ng/mL
Midluteal	9.54–63.6 nmol/L	3–20 ng/mL
Male	<3.18 nmol/L	<1.0 ng/mL
Prolactin		
Female	0–20 μg/L	1.9–25.9 ng/mL
Male	0–15 μg/L	1.6–23.0 ng/mL
Renin (adult, normal sodium diet)		
Supine	0.08–0.83 ng/(L-s)	0.3–3.0 ng/(mL/h)
Upright	0.28–2.5 ng/(L-s)	1–9.0 ng/(mL/h)
Somatomedin-C (IGF-1) (adult)		
16–24 years	182–780 μg/L	182–780 ng/mL
25–39 years	114–492 μg/L	114–492 ng/mL
40–54 years	90–360 μg/L	90–360 ng/mL
>54 years	71–290 μg/L	71–290 ng/mL
Testosterone, total, morning sample		
Female	0.21–2.98 nmol/L	6–86 ng/dL
Male	9.36–37.10 nmol/L	270–1070 ng/dL
Thyroglobulin	0–60 μg/L	0–60 ng/mL
Thyroid hormone binding index (THBI or T_3RU)	0.83–1.17 mol ratio	0.83–1.17
(Free) thyroxine index	4.2–13	4.2–13
Thyroid stimulating hormone	0.5–4.7 mU/L	0.5–4.7 μU/mL
Thyroxine, total (T4)	58–140 nmol/L	4.5–10.9 μg/dL
Triiodothyronine, total (T3)	0.92–2.78 nmol/L	60–181 ng/dL
Thyroxine, free (fT4)	10.3–35 pmol/L	0.8–2.7 ng/dL
Triiodothyronine, free (fT3)	0.22–6.78 pmol/L	1.4–4.4 pg/mL
Vanillylmandelic Acid (VMA) (urine)	7.6–37.9 μmol/d	0.15–1.2 mg/d

Note: P, plasma; S, serum; U, urine; WB, whole blood.

Table 209-4

Toxicology and Therapeutic Drug Monitoring

Drug	Therapeutic Range		Toxic Level	
	Conventional Units	SI Units	Conventional Units	SI Units
Acetaminophen	10–30 µg/mL	66–199 µmol/L	>200 µg/mL	>1324 µmol/L
Amikacin				
Peak	25–35 µg/mL	43–60 µmol/L	>35 µg/mL	>60 µmol/L
Trough	4–8 µg/mL	6.8–13.7 µmol/L	>10 µg/mL	>17 µmol/L
Cocaine			>1000 ng/mL	>3300 nmol/L
Cyclosporine	Depends on timing after dose and transplant type with ranges of 100–400 ng/mL	Depends on timing after dose and transplant type with ranges of 83–333 nmol/L	Varies with time after dose and transplant type	Varies with time after dose and transplant type
Digoxin	0.8–2.0 ng/mL	1.0–2.6 nmol/L	>2.5 ng/mL	>3.2 µmol/L
Ethanol			>300 mg/dL	>65 mmol/L
Behavioral changes	>20 mg/dL	>4.3 mmol/L		
Clinical intoxication	>100 mg/dL	>1 g/L		
Gentamicin				
Peak	8–10 µg/mL	16.7–20.9 µmol/L	>10 µg/mL	>21 µmol/L
Trough	2–4 µg/mL	4.2–8.4 µmol/L	>4 µg/mL	>8.4 µmol/L
Ibuprofen	10–50 µg/mL	49–243 µmol/L	100–700 µg/mL	485–3395 µmol/L
Lithium	0.6–1.2 meq/L	0.6–1.2 nmol/L	>2 meq/L	>2 nmol/L

Drug				
Methadone	100–400 ng/mL	0.32–1.29 µmol/L	>2000 ng/mL	>6.46 µmol/L
Phenytoin	10–20 µg/mL	40–79 µmol/L	>20 µg/mL	>79 µmol/L
Procainamide	4–10 µg/mL	17–42 µmol/L	>10–12 µg/mL	>42–51 µmol/L
Quinidine	2–5 µg/mL	6–15 µmol/L	>6 µg/mL	>18 µmol/L
Salicylates	150–300 µg/mL	1086–2172 µmol/L	>300 µg/mL	>2172 µmol/L
Theophylline	8–20 µg/mL	44–111 µmol/L	>20 µg/mL	>110 µmol/L
Tobramycin				
Peak	8–10 µg/mL	17–21 µmol/L	>10 µg/mL	>21 µmol/L
Trough	<4 µg/mL	<9 µmol/L	>4 µg/mL	>9 µmol/L
Vancomycin				
Peak	18–26 µg/mL	12–18 µmol/L	>80–100 µg/mL	>55–69 µmol/L
Trough	5–10 µg/mL	3–7 µmol/L		

Table 209-5

Vitamins and Selected Trace Minerals

Specimen	SI Units	Conventional Units
Aluminum	<0.2 μmol/L	<5.41 μg/L
	5–30 μg/L	0.19–1.11 μmol/L
Arsenic	0.03–0.31 μmol/L	2–23 μg/L
	0.07–0.67 μmol/d	5–50 μg/d
Folic acid	7–36 nmol/L cells	3–16 ng/mL cells
Lead (adult)	<0.5–1 μmol/L	<10–20 μg/dL
Mercury	3.0–294 nmol/L	0.6–59 μg/L
Vitamin A	0.7–3.5 μmol/L	20–100 μg/dL
Vitamin B_1 (thiamine)	0–75 nmol/L	0–2 μg/dL
Vitamin B_2 (riboflavin)	106–638 nmol/L	4–24 μg/dL
Vitamin B_6	20–121 nmol/L	5–30 ng/mL
Vitamin B_{12}	148–590 pmol/L	200–800 pg/mL
Vitamin C (ascorbic acid)	23–57 μmol/L	0.4–1.0 mg/dL
Vitamin D_3, 1,25-dihydroxy	60–108 pmol/L	25–45 pg/mL
Summer	37.4–200 nmol/L	15–80 ng/mL
Winter	34.9–105 nmol/L	14–42 ng/mL
Vitamin E	12–42 μmol/L	5–18 μg/mL
Vitamin K	0.29–2.64 nmol/L	0.13–1.19 ng/mL
Zinc	11.5–18.5 μmol/L	75–120 μg/dL

Table 209-6

Classification of LDL, Total, and HDL Cholesterol

LDL cholesterol
<100	Optimal
100–129	Near or above normal
130–159	Borderline high
160–189	High
≥190	Very high

Total cholesterol
<200	Desirable
200–239	Borderline high
≥240	High

HDL cholesterol
<40	Low
≥60	High

Note: HDL, high-density lipoprotein; LDL, low-density lipoprotein.
Source: Executive summary of the third report of the national cholesterol education program (NCEP) expert panel on detection, evaluation, and treatment of high blood cholesterol in adults (adult treatment panel III): JAMA 285:2486, 2001.

REFERENCE VALUES FOR SPECIFIC ANALYTES

Table 209-7

Cerebrospinal Fluid[a]

Constituent	SI Units	Conventional Units
pH	7.31–7.34	
Glucose	2.22–3.89 mmol/L	40–70 mg/dL
Total protein, lumbar	0.15–0.5 g/L	15–50 mg/dL
IgG	0.009–0.057 g/L	0.9–5.7 mg/dL
IgG index[b]	0.29–0.59	
Oligoclonal bands (OGB)	<2 bands not present in matched serum sample	
CSF pressure		50–180 mmH$_2$O
Red blood cells	0	
Leukocytes		
Total	0–5 mononuclear cells per mm^3	
Differential		
Lymphocytes	60–70%	
Monocytes	30–50%	
Neutrophils	None	

[a] Since cerebrospinal fluid concentrations are equilibrium values, measurements of the same parameters in blood plasma obtained at the same time are recommended. However, there is a time lag in attainment of equilibrium, and cerebrospinal levels of plasma constituents that can fluctuate rapidly (such as plasma glucose) may not achieve stable values until after a significant lag phase.
[b] IgG index = CSF IgG(mg/dL) × serum albumin(g/dL)/Serum IgG(g/dL) × CSF albumin(mg/dL)

Table 209-8

Urine Analysis

	SI Units	Conventional Units
Amylase/creatinine clearance ratio [(Cl$_{am}$/Cl$_{cr}$) × 100]	1–5	1–5
Calcium (10 meq/d or 200 mg/d dietary calcium)	<7.5 mmol/d	<300 mg/d
Creatinine	8.8–14 mmol/d	1.0–1.6 g/d
Eosinophils	<100 eosinophils/mL	<100 eosinophils/mL
Glucose, true (oxidase method)	0.3–1.7 mmol/d	50–300 mg/d
5-Hydroxyindoleacetic acid (5-HIAA)	10–47 μmol/d	2–9 mg/d
"Microalbumin"	<0.02 g/L	<20 mg/L
Oxalate	228–684 μmol/d	20–60 mg/d
pH	5.0–9.0	5.0–9.0
Phosphate (phosphorus) (varies with intake)	12.9–42.0 mmol/d	400–1300 mg/d
Potassium (varies with intake)	25–100 mmol/d	25–100 meq/d
Protein	<0.15 g/d	<150 mg/d
Sodium (varies with intake)	100–260 mmol/d	100–260 meq/d
Specific gravity	1.001–1.035	
Uric acid (normal diet)	1.49–4.76 mmol/d	250–800 mg/d

SPECIAL FUNCTION TESTS

Table 209-9

Circulatory Function Tests

Test	SI Units (Range)	Conventional Units (Range)
Arteriovenous oxygen difference	30–50 mL/L	30–50 mL/L
Cardiac output (Fick)	2.5–3.6 L/m² of body surface area per minute	2.5–3.6 L/m² of body surface area per minute
Contractility indices		
Max. left ventricular dp/dt (dp/dt)/DP when DP = 5.3 kPa (40 mmHg)	220 kPa/s (176–250 kPa/s) (37.6 ± 12.2)/s	1650 mmHg/s (1320–1880 mmHg/s) (37.6 ± 12.2)/s
Mean normalized systolic ejection rate (angiography)	3.32 ± 0.84 end-diastolic volumes per second	3.32 ± 0.84 end-diastolic volumes per second
Mean velocity of circumferential fiber shortening (angiography)	1.83 ± 0.56 circumferences per second	1.83 ± 0.56 circumferences per second
Ejection fraction; stroke volume/end diastolic volume (SV/EDV)	0.67 ± 0.08 (0.55–0.78)	0.67 ± 0.08 (0.55–0.78)
End-diastolic volume	70 ± 20.0 mL/m² (60–88 mL/m²)	70 ± 20.0 mL/m² (60–88 mL/m²)
End-systolic volume	25 ± 5.0 mL/m² (20–33 mL/m²)	25 ± 5.0 mL/m² (20–33 mL/m²)
Pulmonary vascular resistance	2–12 (kPa·s)/L	20–130 (dyn·s)/cm⁵
Systemic vascular resistance	77–150 (kPa·s)/L	770–1600 (dyn·s)/cm⁵

Note: DP, diastolic pressure.
Source: E Braunwald et al, *Heart Disease,* 6th ed. Philadelphia, Saunders, 2001, with permission.

Table 209-10

Summary of Values Useful in Pulmonary Physiology

	Symbol	Typical Values	
		Man Age 40, 75 kg, 175 cm Tall	Woman Age 40, 60 kg, 160 cm Tall
PULMONARY MECHANICS			
Spirometry—volume-time curves			
Forced vital capacity	FVC	4.8 L	3.3 L
Forced expiratory volume in 1 s	FEV₁	3.8 L	2.8 L
FEV₁/FVC	FEV₁%	76%	77%
Maximal midexpiratory flow	MMF (FEF 25–27)	4.8 L/s	3.6 L/s
Maximal expiratory flow rate	MEFR (FEF 200–1200)	9.4 L/s	6.1 L/s
Spirometry—flow-volume curves			
Maximal expiratory flow at 50% of expired vital capacity	V$_{max}$ 50 (FEF 50%)	6.1 L/s	4.6 L/s
Maximal expiratory flow at 75% of expired vital capacity	V$_{max}$ 75 (FEF 75%)	3.1 L/s	2.5 L/s
LUNG VOLUMES			
Total lung capacity	TLC	6.4 L	4.9 L
Functional residual capacity	FRC	2.2 L	2.6 L
Residual volume	RV	1.5 L	1.2 L
Inspiratory capacity	IC	4.8 L	3.7 L
Expiratory reserve volume	ERV	3.2 L	2.3 L
Vital capacity	VC	1.7 L	1.4 L

(continued)

Table 209-10 (Continued)

Summary of Values Useful in Pulmonary Physiology

	Symbol	Typical Values	
		Man Age 40, 75 kg, 175 cm Tall	Woman Age 40, 60 kg, 160 cm Tall
GAS EXCHANGE (SEA LEVEL)			
Arterial O_2 tension	Pa_{O_2}	12.7 ± 0.7 kPa (95 ± 5 mmHg)	
Arterial CO_2 tension	Pa_{CO_2}	5.3 ± 0.3 kPa (40 ± 2 mmHg)	
Arterial O_2 saturation	Sa_{O_2}	0.97 ± 0.02 ($97 \pm 2\%$)	
Arterial blood pH	pH	7.40 ± 0.02	
Arterial bicarbonate	HCO_3^-	24 ± 2 meq/L	
Base excess	BE	0 ± 2 meq/L	
Diffusing capacity for carbon monoxide (single breath)	DL_{CO}	0.42 mLCO/s per mmHg (25 mL CO/min per mmHg)	
Dead space volume	V_D	2 mL/kg body wt	
Physiologic dead space; dead space-tidal volume ratio	V_D/V_T		
Rest		$\leq 35\%$ V_T	
Exercise		$\leq 20\%$ V_T	
Alveolar-arterial difference for O_2	$P(A - a)_{O_2}$	≤ 2.7 kPa ≤ 20 mmHg (≤ 20 mmHg)	

Table 209-11

Gastrointestinal Tests

Test	SI Units	Conventional Units
Absorption tests		
D-Xylose: after overnight fast, 25 g xylose given in oral aqueous solution		
Urine, collected for following 5 h	33–53 mmol (or >20% of ingested dose)	5–8 g (or >20% of ingested dose)
Serum, 1 h after dose	1.7–2.7 mmol/L	25–40 mg/dL >3.6 ($\pm$1.1) μg/mL at 90 min
	>50% recovered in 6 h	>50% recovered in 6 h
Gastric juice		
pH	1.6–1.8	1.6–1.8
Acid output		
Basal		
Females (mean $\pm$ 1 SD)	0.6 $\pm$ 0.5 μmol/s	2.0 $\pm$ 1.8 meq/h
Males (mean $\pm$ 1 SD)	0.8 $\pm$ 0.6 μmol/s	3.0 $\pm$ 2.0 meq/h
Maximal (after stimulation)		
Females (mean $\pm$ 1 SD)	4.4 $\pm$ 1.4 μmol/s	16 $\pm$ 5 meq/h
Males (mean $\pm$ 1 SD)	6.4 $\pm$ 1.4 μmol/s	23 $\pm$ 5 meq/h
Basal acid output/maximal acid output ratio	≤0.6	≤0.6
Gastrin, serum	40–200 μg/L	40–200 pg/mL

Table 209-12

Normal Values of Doppler Echocardiographic Measurements in Adults

	Range	Mean
RVD (cm), measured at the base in apical 4-chamber view	2.6 to 4.3	3.5 $\pm$ 0.4
LVID (cm), measured in the parasternal long axis view	3.6 to 5.4	4.7 $\pm$ 0.4
Posterior LV wall thickness (cm)	0.6 to 1.1	0.9 $\pm$ 0.4
IVS wall thickness (cm)	0.6 to 1.1	0.9 $\pm$ 0.4
Left atrial dimension (cm), anteroposterior dimension	2.3 to 3.8	3.0 $\pm$ 0.3
Aortic root dimension (cm)	2.0 to 3.5	2.4 $\pm$ 0.4
Aortic cusps separation (cm)	1.5 to 2.6	1.9 $\pm$ 0.4
Percentage of fractional shortening	34 to 44%	36%
Mitral flow (m/s)	0.6 to 1.3	0.9
Tricuspid flow (m/s)	0.3 to 0.7	0.5
Pulmonary artery (m/s)	0.6 to 0.9	0.75
Aorta (m/s)	1.0 to 1.7	1.35

Note: IVS, interventricular septum; LV, left ventricle; LVID, left ventircular internal dimension; RVD, right ventricular dimension.
Source: From A Weyman: *Principles and Practice of Echocardiography*, 2d ed, Philadelphia, Lea & Febiger, with permission.

INDEX

Bold number indicates the start of the main discussion of the topic; numbers with "f" and "t" refer to figure and table pages.

Abacavir, for HIV infections, 431t
Abdomen, rigid, 207
Abdominal angina, 748
Abdominal infection
    actinomycosis, 494
    Escherichia coli, 472
    Klebsiella, 472
Abdominal pain, **136**
    acute, catastrophic, **206**
        treatment of, 207
    approach to, 137–138, 207
    causes of, 137t
    characteristics of, 137–138
    laboratory and radiologic studies of,
        138–139
    physical examination in, 138, 206–207
    by quadrant, 207
    symptoms associated with, 138
Abdominal reflexes, 872
Abdominal wall disorders, pain in, 137t
Abdominal x-ray
    in aortic aneurysm, 653
    in biliary tract disease, 750t
    indications for, 32
    in pancreatitis, 754, 756
    utility of, 32
Abducens (VI) nerve palsy, 57
Abiotrophia infection, 460
Abscess. *See specific sites*
ABVD regime, for Hodgkin's disease,
    306
Acanthocytes, 265
Acarbose, for diabetes mellitus, 833t
Accelerated idioventricular rhythm, myo-
    cardial infarction and, 625
Accessory nerve (XI), 872
    disorders of, 924
Accidents, prevention of, 992t–993t
ACE inhibitors
    for acute coronary syndromes, 637
    for aortic regurgitation, 608
    for chronic renal failure, 709
    cough and, 189, 984t
    for diabetic nephropathy, 717
    for dilated cardiomyopathy, 609
    for glomerulonephritis, 720
    for heart failure, 649t, 650, 651t
    for hypertension, 618–620, 620t
    for mitral regurgitation, 605
    for myocardial infarction, 625
    for myocardial infarction prophylaxis,
        630
    for systemic sclerosis, 784
Acetaminophen
    for fever, 158
    for low back pain, 151

for migraine, 143t–144t
for osteoarthritis, 795
for pain, 25, 26t
poisoning, 74, 78, 761
for tension headache, 146t
Acetazolamide
    for glaucoma, 242–243
    for metabolic alkalosis, 13
N-Acetylcysteine, for acetaminophen poi-
        soning, 78, 761
Acetylsalicylic acid, for pain, 26t
Achalasia, 204
    treatment of, 204
Acid-base balance, **5**
Acid-base disorders, **9**
    metabolic acidosis, 11–12, 11f
    metabolic alkalosis, 11f, 12–13
    mixed, 14
    nomogram for, 11f
    respiratory acidosis, 11f, 13–14
    respiratory alkalosis, 11f, 14
Acid-fast stain, 351
Acid maltase deficiency, 948
Acid poisoning, 78
Acinetobacter infection, **473**
    nosocomial, 443
    treatment of, 473–474
Acitretin, for psoriasis, 259
Acne, 262–263
    drug-induced, 981t
Acne rosacea, 258f, 263
    treatment of, 263
Acne vulgaris, 256f, 258f, 262
    treatment of, 263
Acoustic neuroma, 922
Acquired immunodeficiency syndrome.
        See HIV/AIDS
Acrodermatitis chronica atrophicans, 506
Acromegaly, **810**
    paraneoplastic, 344t
    treatment of, 811
Acrophobia, 960
ACTH, 807, 809t
    deficiency of, 811–812
    hypersecretion of, 823
    replacement therapy, 812t
ACTH-secreting tumor, 807
ACTH syndrome, ectopic, 346
Actinobacillus actinomycetemcomitans.
        See HACEK organisms
Actinomycetoma, 492
Actinomycosis, **494**
    treatment of, 495
Activated protein C therapy
        for meningococcal infections, 463
        for septic shock, 51

Acute abdomen, **206**
Acute coronary syndromes, **635**
Acute lung injury, 39
Acute motor axonal neuropathy, 941
Acute respiratory distress syndrome
    (ARDS), 20, **39**
    clinical course and pathophysiology of,
        39–40
    disorders associated with, 39t
    treatment of, 40
Acute retroviral syndrome, 425–426, 437
Acute transverse myelopathy, 935
Acyclovir
    for Bell's palsy, 922
    for chickenpox, 527
    for genital herpes, 406
    for herpes simplex virus infections,
        242, 522–523, 524t–525t
    for herpes zoster, 410t, 527
    for viral encephalitis, 893
    for viral esophagitis, 205
    for viral meningitis, 892
Adalimumab, for rheumatoid arthritis, 783
Addisonian-like syndrome, drug-induced,
    980t
Addison's disease, 826
    treatment of, 826
Adefovir, for chronic hepatitis B, 763,
    764t
Adenoma
    pituitary. See Pituitary adenoma
    small bowel, 323
    thyroid, 821
Adenosine, for arrhythmias, 641t
Adenosine deaminase deficiency, 776
Adenovirus infection, **539**
    pneumonia, 679, 684
Adhesive capsulitis, **802**
    treatment of, 802
Admission orders, **1**
    checklist mnemonic, 1–2
ADMIT VITALS AND PHYSICAL
    EXAM (admissions mnemonic),
    1–2
Adrenal gland disorder
    Addison's disease, 826
    adrenal cortex, **823**
    adrenal mass, incidental, 827
    aldosteronism, 825–826
    congenital hyperplasia, 843
    Cushing's syndrome, 823–825
    hyperfunction, 823–826
    hypoaldosteronism, 827
    hypofunction, 826–827
    pheochromocytoma. See Pheochromo-
        cytoma
Adrenal insufficiency
    paraneoplastic, 103
    primary, 826
    secondary, 826
    treatment of, 103
Adrenal mass, incidental, **827**
Adult T cell leukemia/lymphoma, 303
    treatment of, 303

Advanced sleep phase syndrome, 185
Adverse drug reactions, **979.** *See also*
    Drug-induced illness
    causes of, 979
    drug monitoring, 1002t–1003t
    recognition of, 979
Aeromonas infection, **474**
    cellulitis, 409
    diagnosis of, 354t
    treatment of, 474
Agammaglobulinemia, X-linked, 777–
    778
Agglutination, 569
Agoraphobia, 960–961
Agranulocytosis, drug-induced, 982t
AIDS. *See* HIV/AIDS
Air pollution, 675
Airway obstruction
    drug-induced, 984t
    dyspnea in, 186
Albendazole
    for ascariasis, 582
    for echinococcosis, 589
    for enterobiasis, 584
    for hookworm, 582
    for larva migrans, 581
    for strongyloidiasis, 583
    for trichinellosis, 581
Albumin
    serum, 222, 222t
    serum-ascites gradient, 224–225, 226t
Albuterol
    for asthma, 669
    for COPD, 677
    for cough, 189
    for respiratory failure, 678
Alcohol abuse, 972
Alcohol dependence, 972
Alcoholic liver disease, **767**
    treatment of, 767–768
Alcoholic polyneuropathy, 928–930
Alcoholism, **972**
    alcohol withdrawal, 973
    chronic pancreatitis and, 756
    clinical features of, 973
    dementia in, 907
    laboratory evaluation of, 974
    screening for, 992t, 994t
    treatment of, 974
        acute withdrawal, 974
        recovery and sobriety, 974
        relapse prevention, 974
Aldosteronism, **825**
    hypertension in, 617–618
    primary, 825
    secondary, 825
    treatment of, 825–826
Alefacept, for psoriasis, 259
Alemtuzumab, for chronic lymphocytic
    leukemia/lymphoma, 300
Alendronate, for osteoporosis, 854
Alkaline diuresis, forced
    for drug overdose, 77
    for salicylate poisoning, 87

Alkaline phosphatase, blood, 221–222, 754
Alkali poisoning, 78
Alkali therapy, for nephrolithiasis, 733t
Alkylating agents, 287t
Allergic angiitis and granulomatosis, 786
Allergic disease, immediate type hypersensitivity, **773**
Allergy, to insect stings, 114
Allodynia, 24, 930, 938
Allopurinol
  for chronic myeloid leukemia, 293
  for gout, 798
  for nephrolithiasis, 733t
  for tumor lysis syndrome, 104
Alopecia, drug-induced, 981t
Alosetron, for irritable bowel syndrome, 746
Alpha fetoprotein, in testicular cancer, 333
α-Heavy chain disease, 323–324
Alpha radiation, 127
Alprazolam
  dosage and adverse effects of, 966t
  for panic disorder, 959
Alprostadil injection, for erectile dysfunction, 838
Aluminum phosphate binders, for hyperphosphatemia, 851
Alveolar hypoventilation, **695**
Alveolitis, extrinsic allergic, **672**
Alzheimer's disease, 904, 906t, 907, **907**
  treatment of, 908–909
  in women, 989
Amantadine
  for influenza, 535
  for influenza prophylaxis, 536
  for Parkinson's disease, 914
Amaurosis fugax, 58, 173
Amebiasis
  diagnosis of, 359t
  diarrhea, 391
  treatment of, 391–392
Amebic liver abscess, 382
Amenorrhea, **840**
  approach to, 840, 841f
  primary, 840
  secondary, 840
  treatment of, 842
Amikacin
  for *Klebsiella* infections, 473
  for nontuberculous mycobacterial infections, 505
  for *Pseudomonas aeruginosa* infections, 476t
Amiloride
  for diabetes insipidus, 814
  for edema, 196t
Aminoglycosides, mechanisms, indications, and adverse effects of, 362
Aminophylline
  for anaphylaxis, 105
  for asthma, 672
Aminosalicylates, for inflammatory bowel disease, 743, 744t–745t

Aminotransferases, blood, 220–221, 222t
Amiodarone
  for arrhythmias, 641t
  for cardiac arrest, 43f
  for dilated cardiomyopathy, 609
  for hypertrophic cardiomyopathy, 612
  thyroid disease caused by, 820
  for ventricular tachycardia, 625
Amitriptyline
  for ciguatera poisoning, 111
  dosage and adverse effects of, 964t
  for irritable bowel syndrome, 746
  for migraine prophylaxis, 142, 145t
  for multiple sclerosis, 903
  for pain, 27t
Ammonia, blood, 222
Amodiaquine, for malaria, 571t
Amoxapine, dosage and adverse effects of, 965t
Amoxicillin
  for anthrax, 120t
  for COPD, 678
  for endocarditis prophylaxis, 379t
  for *Helicobacter pylori* eradication, 739t
  for leptospirosis, 509
  for Lyme borreliosis, 507
  for otitis media, 251t, 253
  for pneumococcal infections, 447
  for pneumonia, 680t
  for sinusitis, 250t
  for urinary tract infections, 726t
Amoxicillin/clavulanate
  for animal bite infections, 107t, 410t
  for *Haemophilus influenzae* infections, 467
  for otitis media, 251t
  for pneumonia, 680t
  for sinusitis, 250t
Amphotericin B, 555–556
  for aspergillosis, 559
  for blastomycosis, 563
  for candidiasis, 206, 558
  for coccidioidomycosis, 563
  for cryptococcosis, 560
  for fusariosis, 564
  for histoplasmosis, 562
  for leishmaniasis, 573, 576
  for neutropenia, 274
  for paracoccidioidomycosis, 564
  for penicilliosis marneffei, 564
  for pseudoallescheriasis, 565
  for sporotrichosis, 565
Ampicillin
  for actinomycosis, 495
  for bacterial meningitis, 890t, 891t
  for *Bartonella* infections, 484t
  for diverticular disease, 747
  for endocarditis, 376t, 377t
  for endocarditis prophylaxis, 379t
  for enterococcal infections, 459
  for HACEK endocarditis, 469t
  for leptospirosis, 509
  for listeriosis, 466

Ampicillin (*Cont.*):
  mechanisms, indications, and adverse
    effects of, 361
  for necrotizing fasciitis, 410t
  for osteomyelitis, 416t
  for peritonitis, 381
  for pneumococcal infections, 447
  for shigellosis, 390
  for urinary tract infections, 726t
Ampicillin/sulbactam
  for acute cholecystitis, 751
  for animal bite infections, 107t, 108t,
    410t
  for epiglottitis, 254
  for HACEK endocarditis, 469t
  for osteomyelitis, 416t
  for pneumonia, 680t
Amprenavir, for HIV infections, 435t
Amrinone
  for heart failure, 651
  for myocardial infarction, 627t
Amylase, serum, 754
Amylase-creatinine clearance ratio, uri-
    nary, 754
Amyl citrate, for cyanide poisoning, 82
Amyloidosis, **804**
  Aβ_2M, 805
  amyloid A, 805
  autonomic dysfunction in, 928
  clinical features of, 805
  heredofamilial, 805
  interstitial lung disease and, 688t
  light chain, 805
  localized or organ-limited, 805
  renal disease in, 719t
  treatment of, 805–806
Amyotrophic lateral sclerosis (ALS), **917**
  familial, 917
  treatment of, 918–920
Anaerobic infection, **485**
  botulism, 486–487
  cellulitis, 409
  clostridial, 487–489
  diagnosis of, 356t
  mixed, **489**
    treatment of, 491, 491t
  osteomyelitis, 416t
  pneumonia, 679
  tetanus, 485–486
Anagrelide, for essential thrombocytosis,
    296
Anakinra, for rheumatoid arthritis, 783
Anal cancer, 328
Anal condyloma, **749**
Anal fissure, **749**
Analgesia (reduced pain perception), 23
Analgesic(s), 25, 26t–27t
Analgesic nephropathy, 722–723
Anal reflex, 872
Anaphylaxis, **105**
  drug-induced, 979t
  prevention of, 105
  treatment of, 105
Anaplasmosis, 513t, **514**

Anastrazole, for breast cancer, 318, 320
Ancylostoma braziliense infection, 581
Ancylostoma duodenale infection, 582
Androgen deficiency, **835**
  clinical features of, 836
  treatment of, 836
Androgen deprivation, for prostate cancer,
    339
Androgen excess, in women, 843
Anemia, **232, 267**. *See also specific types*
    of anemia
  chemotherapy-related, 287t–288t, 288–
    289
  classification of, 233, 233f
  hypoproliferative, 267–269
    diagnosis of, 268t
  in inflammation, 268t
  microcytic, 269
    diagnosis of, 269t
  in renal failure, 708
  treatment of, 271–272
Anemia of chronic disease, 267
  treatment of, 271
Aneurysm, aortic, **653**
Angina pectoris, 133, **631**
  drug-induced, 983t
  laboratory evaluation of, 631
  recurrent, post-MI, 630
  signs and symptoms of, 631
  stress testing in, 631, 632f, 633t
  treatment of, 632–635
    long-term suppression, 632–634
    mechanical revascularization, 634–
      635, 634t
  unstable, **635**
    high-risk features in, 637t
    treatment of, 278t, 635–637, 636f
Angiodysplasia, 217
  colonic, **748**
Angioedema, 194, **773**
  drug-induced, 979t
  treatment of, 774
Angiography, hepatobiliary, 223
Angioma, senile, 257f
Angiotensin receptor antagonists
  for chronic renal failure, 709
  for diabetic nephropathy, 717
  for dilated cardiomyopathy, 609
  for glomerulonephritis, 720
  for heart failure, 649t, 650
  for hypertension, 618, 620t
  for myocardial infarction, 625
Animal bite, treatment of, 107t–108t,
    109, 410t–411t
Animal-borne viral infection, **547**
Anion gap, 9, 14
  negative, 11
  normal, 11
Anisocytosis, 265
Ankylosing spondylitis, **788**
  diagnosis of, 789, 790f
  treatment of, 789–790
Annular skin lesion, 255
Anomic aphasia, 180t

Anorectal disease, **748**
Anorexia nervosa, **969**
  binge eating/purging type, 971t
  clinical features of, 970
  diagnostic criteria for, 971t
  restricting type, 971t
  treatment of, 970, 972f
Anosagnosia, 58
Anosmia, 910
Anovulation, 839–840
Antacids
  complications of, 214
  for erosive gastropathy, 740
  for gastroesophageal reflux disease, 200
Anthrax
  as bioweapon, 118–119
  cutaneous, 122
  gastrointestinal, 122
  inhalation, 101, 122
  microbiology and clinical features of, 119, 120t
  prevention of, 122
  treatment of, 120t, 122
Anthrax vaccine, 122
Anti-AChR antibodies, 942
Antiarrhythmics
  for pain, 25, 27t
  poisoning, 78–79
Antibacterial resistance, 361, 444
Antibacterial therapy, **360**
  cancer chemotherapy, 288t
  classes of antibacterial agents, 361–365
  mechanisms of drug action, 361
  principles of, 360–361
Anticholinergic agents, poisoning, 79
Anticoagulants, 278–279
  for mitral valve prolapse, 606
  for myocardial infarction, 625
  for stroke, 61, 65
Anticonvulsants
  for nerve agent exposure, 126
  for pain, 25, 27t
  poisoning, 79–80
  for subarachnoid hemorrhage, 66
Antidepressants, **963**
  for chronic fatigue syndrome, 953
  for pain, 25, 27t
  poisoning, 82
Antidiuretic hormone, 813
  abnormalities of, 813–814
Antifungal treatment
  systemic agents, 555–556
  topical agents, 555
Antigenic drift, influenza virus, 534
Antigenic shift, influenza virus, 534
Antihistamines
  for pityriasis rosea, 259
  for scombroid poisoning, 112
Antimetabolites, cancer chemotherapy, 287t
Antineuronal antibodies, paraneoplastic, 348t
Antiplatelet agents, 279
  for myocardial infarction, 625
  for stroke, 61
  for stroke prevention, 63–65

Antipsychotics, **968**
  dosage and adverse effects of, 967t
  novel, 967t, 969
  typical, 967t, 968–969
Antisocial personality, 962
Antithyroid drugs
  for thyrotoxicosis, 818–819
  for toxic multinodular goiter, 821
α_1-Antitrypsin deficiency, 676
Antivenom, 110–111, 113
Antrectomy, for peptic ulcer disease, 739t
Ant sting, 114
Anxiety disorder, **958**
Anxiolytics, **963**
  dosage and adverse effects of, 966t
Aorta
  abdominal, occlusive disease of, **655**
  arteritis of, **655**
  coarctation of, hypertension in, 617
  diseases of, **653**
    echocardiography in, 603
Aortic aneurysm, **653**
  abdominal, 653
  laboratory evaluation of, 653
  thoracic, 653
  treatment of, 653
Aortic dissection, **653**
  chest pain in, 133, 135f
  classification of, 654f
  laboratory evaluation of, 654
  treatment of, 654–655, 655t
Aortic regurgitation, **606**
  echocardiography in, 602f
  laboratory evaluation of, 607
  treatment of, 608
Aortic stenosis, **606**
  echocardiography in, 602f
  laboratory evaluation of, 606
  treatment of, 606, 607f
APACHE II, 20
Aphasia, **179**
  clinical features of, 180t
  treatment of, 181
Aplastic anemia
  monocytopenia in, 274
  treatment of, 272
Aplastic crisis, parvovirus, 543
Apo B100, familial defective, 856t, 857
Apo CII deficiency, familial, 856t, 860
Appetite-suppressing drugs, 829
Apraclonidine, for glaucoma, 242–243
Aprepitant, for nausea and vomiting, 198, 288
Arachnoiditis, lumbar, pain in, 150
Arbovirus infection, **548**
  encephalitis, 891t, 892, 893t
  meningitis, 890, 891t
Arcanobacterium haemolyticum infection, 462
Argatroban
  for heparin-induced thrombocytopenia, 277
  for thrombotic disorders, 279

Aripiprazole, dosage and adverse effects of, 967t
Aromatase inhibitors, for breast cancer, 318–319
Arrhythmia, **638**
  diagnosis of, 638
  drug-induced, 983t
  electrocardiography in, 638, 639f
  preoperative evaluation of, 36
  syncope and, 166t
  treatment of, 638–644, 646t–647t
Arsenic poisoning, 80
Arsenic trioxide, for acute myeloid leukemia, 292
Artemether, for malaria, 571t
Artemether-lumefantrine, for malaria, 572t
Arterial blood gases
  in alveolar hypoventilation, 695–696
  in ARDS, 39
  in asthma, 669
  in COPD, 677
  in cyanosis, 193
  in hypersensitivity pneumonitis, 672
  in pulmonary edema, 53
  in pulmonary hypertension, 660f
  in shock, 46
Arterial embolism, **656**
  treatment of, 656
Arteriosclerosis, of peripheral arteries, **655**
  treatment of, 656
Artesunate, for malaria, 571t
Arthritis. *See also specific types*
  arbovirus, 550
  gonococcal, 400, 412
  infectious, **412**
    diagnosis of, 413
    treatment of, 413
  meningococcal, 463
  pain in, 162f
  in systemic lupus erythematosus, 780
  in systemic sclerosis, 783
Arthritis mutilans, 791
Arthropathy, parvovirus, 543
Arthropod bites/stings, **112**
Arthropod-borne viral infection, **548**
Arthroscopic debridement and lavage, for osteoarthritis, 795
Asbestosis, 673–674
Ascariasis, **582**
  treatment of, 582
Ascites, 194, **224**
  in acute pancreatitis, 755
  in cirrhosis, 225, 226t
  classification by serum-ascites albumin gradient, 224–225, 226t
  in diseases not involving peritoneum, 224
  in diseases of peritoneum, 224
  fluid characteristics, 226t
L-Asparagine, for acute lymphoid leukemia/lymphoma, 302
Aspartame aminotransferase, 754
Aspergilloma, 558–559

Aspergillosis, **558**
  allergic bronchopulmonary, 558–559
  brain abscess, 894
  endobronchial saprophytic pulmonary, 558
  HIV and, 559
  invasive, 559
  meningitis, 897t
  nosocomial, 444
  sinusitis, 249, 559
  treatment of, 559
Aspirates, culture of, 355t
Aspirin
  for acute coronary syndromes, 635
  for acute pericarditis, 613
  for angina pectoris, 634
  for fever, 158
  for migraine, 143t
  for mitral valve prolapse, 606
  for myocardial infarction, 622, 624f, 625
  for myocardial infarction prophylaxis, 630
  for pain, 25
  for rheumatoid arthritis, 783
  for stroke, 61
  for stroke prevention, 63, 65, 65t
  for tension headache, 146t
  for thrombotic disorders, 279
Assisted reproductive technologies, 837, 846
Asterixis, 177
Asthma, **668**
  allergic, 668
  approach to, 668–669
  chronic, 672
  cough, 189
  diagnosis of, 664t
  idiosyncratic, 668
  insomnia in, 182
  laboratory evaluation of, 669
  occupational, 675
  treatment of, 669–672, 670t
    emergencies, 672
Astrocytoma, 883–884
Asystole, management of cardiac arrest, 44f
Ataxia-telangiectasia, 777
Ataxic disorder, **914**
  approach to, 915, 916t
  clinical features of, 914
  etiology of, 916t
  evaluation of, 915, 916t
  inherited, 915
  treatment of, 915–916
  unilateral, 915
Atazanavir, for HIV infections, 436t
Atelectasis, 20
  diagnosis of, 664t
Atenolol, for syncope, 167
Atheroembolism, renal, 728
Atherosclerosis
  of abdominal aorta, 655
  Chlamydia pneumoniae and, 519
  prevention of complications of, **861**

Athetosis, 178
Atorvastatin, for hyperlipidemia, 859t
Atovaquone
    for babesiosis, 96t, 573
    for *Pneumocystis* infections, 567, 567t
    for *Pneumocystis* prophylaxis, 568t
Atovaquone-proguanil
    for malaria, 571t, 575t
    for malaria prophylaxis, 572, 574t
Atrial fibrillation, 641t
    antithrombotic prophylaxis for, 65, 65t
    treatment of, 638, 644, 645f
Atrial flutter, 639f, 641t
Atrial premature beats, 640t
Atrial tachycardia, 639f
    with block, 640t
    multifocal, 641t
Atropine
    for arrhythmias, 626
    for asthma, 671
    for cardiac arrest, 44f
    for cardiac glycoside poisoning, 82
    for inflammatory bowel disease, 743
    for insecticide poisoning, 86
    for nerve agent exposure, 126, 128t
Audiologic assessment, 244
Audiometry, 244, 872
Auer rods, 266
Auricular cellulitis, 252
Auscultation, **594**
Autoantibody disorders, treatment of, 19
Autoimmune autonomic neuropathy, 930
Autoimmune disease
    neutropenia in, 274
    in women, 989
Autoimmune hemolysis, treatment of, 272
Autologous transfusion, 18
Autonomic nervous system (ANS)
    activation of, 927t
    features of, 925
    structure and function of, 925, 926f
    symptoms of dysfunction of, 926–927
Autonomic nervous system (ANS) disorder, **925**
    autonomic neuropathies, 930t
    with brain involvement, 929t
    diagnosis of, 928
    with spinal cord involvement, 929t
Avascular necrosis. See Osteonecrosis
AV block
    drug-induced, 984t
    myocardial infarction and, 626
Avoidance and numbing, 960
Avoidant personality, 962
5-Azacytidine, for myelodysplastic syndromes, 295
Azathioprine
    for autoimmune hepatitis, 766
    for chronic inflammatory demyelinating polyneuropathy, 941
    for inflammatory bowel disease, 744, 744t–745t

for inflammatory myopathies, 948
    for multiple sclerosis, 903
    for myasthenia gravis, 944
    for myocarditis, 612
    for reactive arthritis, 793
    for rheumatoid arthritis, 783
    for systemic lupus erythematosus, 781
    for vasculitis, 788
Azelastine, for allergic rhinitis, 775
Azithromycin
    for babesiosis, 96t, 573
    for *Bartonella* infections, 484t
    for chancroid, 407
    for *Chlamydia pneumoniae* infections, 519
    for diarrhea, 369
    for donovanosis, 407
    for gonococcal infections, 401t
    for HACEK endocarditis, 469t
    for *Haemophilus influenzae* infections, 467
    for *Legionella* infections, 478–479
    for meningococcal infection prophylaxis, 464t, 889
    for *Mycoplasma pneumoniae* infections, 517
    for nontuberculous mycobacterial infections, 504
    for pertussis, 468
    for pneumococcal infections, 447
    for pneumonia, 680t, 683t
    for shigellosis, 390
    for traveler's diarrhea, 384
    for urethritis in men, 396
Azotemia, **227**, 720
    intrinsic renal, 705t
    prerenal, 703, 705t
Aztreonam
    for pneumonia, 682t
    for *Pseudomonas aeruginosa* infections, 476t
    for sepsis, 52t
    for urinary tract infections, 726t

Babesiosis, 95, 96t, **572**
    diagnosis of, 359t
    treatment of, 573
Babinski sign, 872
Bacillary angiomatosis, **483**, 484t
    treatment of, 410t–411t
Bacille Calmette-Guérin, 500
    intravesical instillation of, 332
Bacillus anthracis infection, 118–119. See also Anthrax
Bacillus cereus infection, 384
Bacillus fragilis infection, 489–491
Back pain
    in ankylosing spondylitis, 789
    low. See Low back pain
Back school, 151
Baclofen
    for multiple sclerosis, 903
    for myoclonus, 177
    for trigeminal neuralgia, 921

Bacteremia
  anaerobic, 490
  clostridial, 488
  Escherichia coli, 472
  Pseudomonas aeruginosa, 474–475
  Staphylococcus aureus, 450
  streptococcal, 457–458
Bacterial disease, diagnosis of, **351**
Bacterial vaginosis, 394t–395t, 396–397,
  402
Bacteriuria, asymptomatic, 725
Bacteroides fragilis infection, 489–491
  from animal bite, 108t
  meningitis, 891t
Balanitis, circinate, 793
Balloon dilation, for achalasia, 204
Bamboo spine, 789
Bannwarth's syndrome, 897t
Barbiturate, 80
Barium enema, air-contrast, 327
Barium radiography, upper GI, 216
Barium swallow, 322
Bark scorpion, 113
Barrett's esophagus, 200
Bartonella infection, 106, **483**
  treatment of, 484t
Basal cell carcinoma, 258f
  of skin, **308**
    treatment of, 308
Basic life support (BLS), 41–42, 42f–44f
Basophilia, 273
Basophilic stippling, 265
Baylisascaris procyonis meningitis, 897t
Bechterew's disease, **788**
Becker dystrophy, 947
Beclomethasone
  for allergic rhinitis, 775
  for asthma, 671
Bee sting, 114
Behçet's syndrome, 786
Bell's palsy, 521, **922**
  treatment of, 922
Benzathine penicillin
  for endemic treponematoses, 508
  for pharyngitis, 250t
  for streptococcal infections, 456
Benznidazole, for Chagas' disease, 577
Benzodiazepines, dosage and adverse effects of, 966t
Benzoyl peroxide, for acne vulgaris, 263
Benztropine
  for extrapyramidal side effects, 969
  for neuroleptic poisoning, 86
  for Parkinson's disease, 914
Berger's disease, **720**
Berylliosis, 674
Beta blockers
  for angina pectoris, 633
  for aortic dissection, 654, 655t
  for asthma, 669
  for dilated cardiomyopathy, 609
  for heart failure, 649t, 650–651
  for hypertension, 618–619, 620t
  for hypertrophic cardiomyopathy, 611

  for mitral stenosis, 604
  for myocardial infarction, 623, 625
  for myocardial infarction prophylaxis,
    630
  poisoning, 80–81
  for supraventricular arrhythmias, 625–
    626
Beta-carotene
  for macular degeneration, 243
  for porphyria, 864
Beta radiation, 127
Betaxolol, for glaucoma, 243
Bethanecol, for bladder dysfunction, 903
BFM regime, for Burkitt's lymphoma, 303
Bicarbonate therapy, for metabolic acidosis, 12
Bichloroacetic acid, for human papillomavirus infections, 407
Biguanide, for diabetes mellitus, 833t
Bile acid sequestrants, for hyperlipidemia,
  859t
Bile salt deficiency, 213t
Biliary pain, 133f
Biliary sphincterotomy, endoscopic, 752
Biliary tract disease, **749**
  radiologic and imaging modalities for,
    750t
Bilirubin
  blood test, 220, 754
  conjugated, 218
  metabolism of, 218
  unconjugated, 218
Biologic agents, cancer chemotherapy,
  288t
Biopsy. *See also specific organs*
  culture of biopsy material, 355t
Bioterrorism, 444
  chemical, **125**
  microbial, **118**
  radiation, **127**
Bipolar disorder, **957**
  treatment of, 957
Bismuth citrate, for *Helicobacter pylori*
  eradication, 739t
Bismuth subsalicylate
  for diarrhea, 369
  for *Helicobacter pylori* eradication,
    739t
  for traveler's diarrhea, 384
Bisphosphonates
  for hypercalcemia, 345
  for osteoporosis, 854
Bite wound, HACEK organisms, 470
Blackwater fever, 570
Bladder cancer, **331**
  paraneoplastic syndromes, 344t
  treatment of, 332
Blakemore-Sengstaken balloon tamponade, for esophagogastric varices,
    771
Blastomycosis, **563**
  meningitis, 897t
  South American, 564
  treatment of, 563

Bleeding disorder, **275**
  blood vessel wall defects, 276
  coagulation disorders, 276–277
  gastrointestinal, **214**
  platelet disorders, 275–276
Bleomycin
  for extragonadal germ cell tumor, 343
  for testicular cancer, 333
Blepharoconjunctivitis, 242
  treatment of, 242
Blepharospasm, 922
Blindness, transient monocular, 173
Blood alcohol level, 973
Blood culture, 352t
  in endocarditis, 374
  for mycobacteria, 352t
Blood flukes, diagnosis of, 359t
Blood loss, symptoms of, 214
Blood pressure, monitoring of, 994t
Blood smear, **265**
  erythrocyte abnormalities, 265
  leukocyte abnormalities, 265–266
  platelet abnormalities, 265–266
Blood tests
  of liver function, 220–222, 222t
  toxicologic analysis, 75
Body fluids, culture of, 354t–355t
Body louse, 590–591
Body mass index, 828
Body temperature, 156
Boerhaave's syndrome, 198
Bone disease. *See also* Musculoskeletal
      disease; *specific diseases*
  anaerobic infections, 490
  drug-induced, 987t
  neck pain in, 154
  osteomalacia, 854–855
  osteoporosis, 852–854
  Pseudomonas aeruginosa infections,
      475
Bone marrow
  aspiration of, 266
  biopsy of, 266
  cellularity of, 266
  erythroid:granulocytic ratio, 266–267
  examination of, **266**
Bone marrow failure, 274
Bone marrow transplant
  for acute myeloid leukemia, 292
  for chronic myeloid leukemia, 293
  infections in transplant recipients, 421–
      422, 421t
  for myelodysplastic syndromes, 294
  for severe combined immunodeficiency,
      777
Bone mineral density, 852, 854t
Bone scan, in osteomyelitis, 415t
Borderline personality disorder, 962
Bordetella pertussis infection. *See* Pertus-
      sis
Bornholm disease, 545
Borrelia burgdorferi infection. *See* Lyme
      borreliosis

Borrelia infection, relapsing fever, **509**
Bortezomib, for multiple myeloma, 304
Bosentan
  for pulmonary hypertension, 661
  for systemic sclerosis, 784
Botulinum toxin
  for achalasia, 204
  for anal fissure, 749
  as bioweapon, 121t, 124, 487
  for dystonia, 178
Botulism, 124, **486**
  autoimmune dysfunction in, 930
  food-borne, 487
  intestinal, 487
  treatment of, 121t, 487
  wound, 487
Botulism antitoxin, 487
Botulism immune globulin, 487
Bounding pulse, 593
Bowen's disease, 308
Brachial neuritis, acute, 154
Brachial plexus, injury to, pain in, 154
Bradyarrhythmia
  management of cardiac arrest, 44f
  myocardial infarction and, 626
Bradykinesia, 175–176
Brain abscess, 99t, 101, **894**
  anaerobic, 490
  diagnosis of, 894
  nocardiosis, 492
  Pseudomonas aeruginosa, 475
  streptococcal, 460
  treatment of, 894–895
Brain death, 57–58
Brain herniation, 67
Brain natriuretic peptide (BNP)
  in cardiomyopathy, 609
  for heart failure, 648
Brainstem auditory evoked responses
      (BAER), 244
Brainstem disorders, 924
  stroke, 59t
  weakness in, 176t, 177t
Brain tumor, **883**
  approach to, 883
  headache in, 142t
  primary intracranial, **883**
  treatment of, 883
  tumors metastatic to nervous system,
      884–885, 885t
BRCA genes, 316, 334
Breast
  clinical examination of, 282t
  mass in
      approach to, 317, 317f
      biopsy of, 317
  self-examination of, 282t, 317
Breast cancer, **316**
  diagnosis of, 283, 317–318, 317f
  genetics of, 316–317
  incidence and epidemiology of, 316
  metastases to nervous system, 885t
  paraneoplastic syndromes, 344t, 348t
  pleural effusion in, 691

Breast cancer (*Cont.*):
  prevention of, 283
  prognosis for, 320t
  risk factors for, 281–283, 316
  screening for, 281, 282t, 993t
  staging of, 318, 319t
  treatment of, 318–320
Bretylium, for arrhythmias, 641t
Brill-Zinsser disease, 513
Brimonidine, for glaucoma, 243
Broca's aphasia, 179–180, 180t
Bromocriptine
  for hyperprolactinemia, 810
  for Parkinson's disease, 913t
Bronchial aspirate, culture of, 353t
Bronchiolitis, respiratory syncytial virus, 538
Bronchitis, chronic, **675**
Bronchoalveolar carcinoma, 311
  treatment of, 314t, 316
Bronchoalveolar lavage, 667
Bronchodilators, for COPD, 677, 677t
Bronchopneumonia, 679
Bronchoscopy, 667
Brown-Séquard hemicord syndrome, 933
Brucellosis, **479**
  osteomyelitis, 414
  treatment of, 480
  tuberculosis versus, 480t
Brugia infection, 584
Bruton's tyrosine kinase, 777
Budesonide, for asthma, 671
Buerger's disease, **656**
Bulimia nervosa, **969**
  clinical features of, 970
  diagnostic criteria for, 971t
  nonpurging type, 971t
  purging type, 971t
  treatment of, 970, 972f
Bullae, 255, 408
Bumetanide
  for edema, 196t
  for pulmonary edema, 54
Bundle branch block
  electrocardiography in, 597f
  left, 597f, 644t
  right, 597f, 639f, 644t
Buprenorphine
  abuse of, **975**
  for narcotic abuse, 976
Bupropion, 963
  for bipolar disorder, 957
  dosage and adverse effects of, 965t
  for smoking cessation, 676
  for syncope, 167
Burkholderia cepacia infection, **475**
  treatment of, 477
Burkholderia mallei infection, 477
Burkholderia pseudomallei infection, 477
Burkitt's lymphoma, 302–303, 532, 532t
  treatment of, 303
Bursitis, **801**
  pain in, 162f
  treatment of, 802

Buruli ulcer, 505
Buspirone, 968
  dosage and adverse effects of, 966t
  for generalized anxiety disorder, 959
Butalbital, for tension headache, 146t
Butorphanol, for pain, 27t
Butterfly rash, 780
Byssinosis, 674

Cabergoline, for hyperprolactinemia, 810
Cadmium poisoning, 81
Caffeine
  for migraine, 143t
  for tension headache, 146t
CAGE questions, 973
Calcipotriol, for psoriasis, 259
Calcitonin, for hypercalcemia, 849t
Calcitriol
  for hypocalcemia, 850
  for osteomalacia, 855
Calcium acetate, for hyperphosphatemia, 708
Calcium carbonate, for hyperphosphatemia, 708
Calcium channel blockers
  for angina pectoris, 633–634
  for hypertension, 618, 620t, 621
  poisoning, 81
  for Prinzmetal's variant angina, 637
  for pulmonary hypertension, 661
Calcium gluconate
  for hyperkalemia, 10t
  for hypocalcemia, 850
  for marine envenomations, 110
Calcium oxalate deposition disease, **799**
Calcium oxalate stones, 732, 733t
Calcium phosphate stones, 732, 733t
Calcium pyrophosphate deposition disease, **798**
  treatment of, 798
Calcium therapy
  for beta-blocker poisoning, 81
  for colorectal cancer prevention, 283
  for ethylene glycol poisoning, 83
  for GI bleeding, 217
  for hypermagnesemia, 852
  for hypocalcemia, 850
  for osteoporosis, 854
  for primary sclerosing cholangitis, 753
  for renal tubular acidosis, 723
Calicivirus infection, diarrhea, 385
California (La Crosse) encephalitis, 552t, 893t, 894
Caloric intake, 3
Calymmatobacterium granulomatis infection. *See* Donovanosis
Campylobacter infection, 389
  diagnosis of, 353t
  proctocolitis, 399
  reactive arthritis, 792
  treatment of, 389
Cancer. *See also specific types and sites*
  in alcoholism, 973
  dementia in, 905t

Cancer (*Cont.*):
  depression and, 956
  early detection of, **280**, 282t
  immunization of cancer patients, 423t
  infections in cancer patients, **417**
  life-style factors that reduce risk for, 281t
  lymphadenopathy in, 237t
  obesity and, 829
  oncologic emergencies, **101**
  osteoporosis and, 853t
  prevention of, **280**, 992t–993t
    in high-risk groups, 281–284
  screening for, **280**, 282t, **991**
  tumor growth, 284–285
  tumors metastatic to nervous system, 884–885, 885t
Cancer chemotherapy, **284**
  categories of agents, 285, 287t–288t
  complications of, 285–286
  curability of cancers with, 286t
  development of drug resistance, 285, 286t
  immunization of patients receiving, 423t
  toxicity of, 285, 287t–288t
    anemia, 287t–288t, 288–289
    nausea and vomiting, 286–288, 287t–288t
    neutropenia, 287t–288t, 288
Cancer of unknown primary site (CUPS), **341**
  clinical presentation in, 341
  pathologic evaluation of biopsy specimens, 342t–343t
  prognosis for, 341–343
Candesartan, for myocardial infarction, 625
Candidemia, 557
Candidiasis, 262, **557**
  cutaneous, 557
  deeply invasive, 558
  esophageal, 205, 557–558
    treatment of, 206
  etiology and pathogenesis of, 557
  mucocutaneous, 779
  nosocomial, 443
  prevention of, 558
  thrush, 557
  treatment of, 262, 558
  urinary tract, 557
  vulvovaginal, 394t–395t, 397, 557–558
Capecitabine, for breast cancer, 320
Capnocytophaga canimorsus infection, 100, 106, 107t
  cellulitis, 409
Capsaicin, for osteoarthritis, 795
Captopril
  for heart failure, 650, 651t
  for myocardial infarction, 625
  for myocardial infarction prophylaxis, 630
Carbamate poisoning, 86

Carbamazepine
  for bipolar disorder, 957
  for brain tumor, 883
  for glossopharyngeal neuralgia, 923
  for multiple sclerosis, 903
  for pain, 27t
  for seizures, 880t–881t, 882t
  for trigeminal neuralgia, 921
Carbamazepine/oxcarbazepine, dosage and adverse effects of, 968t
Carbidopa/levodopa, for Parkinson's disease, 911, 912t
Carbimazole, for thyrotoxicosis, 818
Carbon monoxide poisoning, 69, 71, 74, 81
Carboplatin
  for bladder cancer, 332
  for head and neck cancer, 310
  for ovarian cancer, 335
  for peritoneal carcinomatosis, 343
Carboxyhemoglobinemia, 193t
Carbuncle, 449
Carcinoid syndrome, 329, 330t
Carcinoid tumor, **329**, 344t
  treatment of, 329
Carcinomatosis, peritoneal, in women, 343
Cardiac arrest, **41**
  differential diagnosis of, 41t
  follow-up of, 43
  management of, 41–42, 42f–44f
Cardiac biomarkers
  in acute coronary syndromes, 635
  in myocardial infarction, 622
Cardiac catheterization
  in cardiac tamponade, 615
  in cardiomyopathy, 610t, 611
  in constrictive pericarditis, 616
  in pulmonary hypertension, 659, 660f
Cardiac glycoside poisoning, 82
Cardiac hypertrophy, electrocardiography in, 600–601, 600t
Cardiac ischemia, insomnia in, 182
Cardiac risk factors, 630, 992t–993t
  assessment of surgical patient, 34–37, 34t, 35f
Cardiac risk index, 34t
Cardiac tamponade, **615**
  laboratory evaluation of, 615
  treatment of, 615
Cardiobacterium hominis. See HACEK organisms
Cardiogenic shock, 45t, 46t, 49, **626**, 628t
  treatment of, 627
Cardiomyopathy
  dilated, **609**
    laboratory evaluation of, 609, 610t
    treatment of, 609
  drug-induced, 984t
  hypertrophic obstructive, **611**
    echocardiography in, 603
    laboratory evaluation of, 610t, 611
    treatment of, 611–612
  laboratory evaluation of, 610t

Cardiomyopathy (*Cont.*):
  restrictive, **609**
    laboratory evaluation of, 610t, 611
    treatment of, 611
Cardiopulmonary bypass, rewarming by, 116
Cardiopulmonary resuscitation (CPR), 41–42, 42f–44f
  for hypoxic-ischemic encephalopathy, 71
Cardiovascular collapse, **41**
  differential diagnosis of, 41t
Cardiovascular disease. *See also* Heart disease; *specific diseases*
  in alcoholism, 973
  aortic disease, 653–655
  arrhythmias, 638–648
  cardiomyopathy, 609–612
  circulatory function tests, 1006t
  constipation in, 213t
  coronary artery disease, 631–637
  cor pulmonale, 652
  echocardiography in, 596–603
  electrocardiography in, 596–603
  heart failure, 648–651
  hypertension, 616–621
  myocardial infarction, 621–630
  myocarditis, 612
  pericardial disease, 612–616
  peripheral vascular disease, 655–658
  physical examination of heart, 593–596
  pulmonary hypertension, 658–661
  renal disease and, 721t
  in rheumatoid arthritis, 781
  in sarcoidosis, 803
  syncope in, 166t
  syphilis, 404
  in systemic sclerosis, 783
  valvular heart disease, 603–608
  vasculitis, 785–788
Cardioversion, for atrial fibrillation, 639
Carnitine palmitoyltransferase deficiency, 950
Carotid artery pulse, 593, 593f
Carotid endarterectomy, 65
Carotid sinus hypersensitivity, 166t
Carotid stenosis
  asymptomatic, 65
  symptomatic, 65
Carotid tests, 61
Carpal tunnel syndrome, 941
Carteolol, for glaucoma, 243
Carvedilol, for heart failure, 650
Caspofungin, 556
  for aspergillosis, 559
  for candidiasis, 558
Castleman's disease, 527
Cataplexy, 183, 184t, 185
Cataract, 242
  drug-induced, 987t
Cat bite, 106
Catfish envenomations, 110–111
Catheter-related infection, 417–418
  urinary catheter, 442–443, 725
  vascular catheter, 444

Cat-scratch disease, 106, **483**, 484t
Cauda equina lesion, 934
Causalgia, 24
Cavernous sinus syndrome, 924f, 925
Cefadroxil, for endocarditis prophylaxis, 379t
Cefazolin
  for endocarditis, 377t
  for endocarditis prophylaxis, 379t
  indications for, 362
  for osteomyelitis, 416t
  for *Staphylococcus aureus* infections, 452t
  for streptococcal infections, 459
Cefdinir, for otitis media, 251t
Cefepime
  for bacterial meningitis, 890t
  indications for, 362
  for pneumococcal infections, 446
  for pneumonia, 683t
  for *Pseudomonas aeruginosa* infections, 476t
  for sepsis, 52t
Cefixime, for gonococcal infections, 401t
Cefoperazone, for *Pseudomonas aeruginosa* infections, 476t
Cefotaxime
  for bacterial meningitis, 890t, 891t
  for brain abscess, 894
  for gonococcal infections, 401t
  for nocardiosis, 493t
  for pneumococcal infections, 446
  for pneumonia, 680t
  for sepsis, 52t
  for spontaneous bacterial peritonitis, 225
Cefotetan
  for gonococcal infections, 401t
  indications for, 362
  for osteomyelitis, 416t
  for pelvic inflammatory disease, 398
Cefoxitin
  for animal bites, 107t
  for diverticular disease, 747
  for gonococcal infections, 401t
  for *Klebsiella* infections, 473
  for nontuberculous mycobacterial infections, 505
  for pelvic inflammatory disease, 398
Cefpodoxime
  for pneumococcal infections, 446
  for pneumonia, 680t
  for urinary tract infections, 726t
  for urethritis in men, 393
Ceftazidime
  for brain abscess, 894
  for gram-negative sepsis, 96t
  for neutropenia, 274
  for osteomyelitis, 416t
  for *Pseudomonas aeruginosa* infections, 476t
Ceftizoxime
  for gonococcal infections, 401t
  for nocardiosis, 493t

Ceftriaxone
for acute bacterial endocarditis, 99t
for animal bite, 108t
for bacterial meningitis, 98t, 890t, 891t
for *Bartonella* infections, 484t
for brain abscess, 894
for brucellosis, 480
for chancroid, 407
for endocarditis, 375, 376t–377t
for epididymitis, 396
for gonococcal infections, 401t
for gram-positive sepsis, 96t
for HACEK endocarditis, 469t
for *Haemophilus influenzae* infections, 467
indications for, 362
for infectious arthritis, 413
for Lyme borreliosis, 507
for meningococcal infections, 97t, 464t
for meningococcal infection prophylaxis, 464t
for meningococcal meningitis prophylaxis, 889
for *Mycoplasma pneumoniae* infections, 517
for nocardiosis, 493t
for osteomyelitis, 416t
for otitis media, 251t
for pelvic inflammatory disease, 398
for peritonitis, 381
for pneumococcal infections, 446–447
for pneumonia, 680t–681t, 682t–683t
for purpura fulminans, 97t
for sepsis, 52t
for typhoid fever, 388
for urethritis in men, 393
for urinary tract infections, 726t
Cefuroxime
indications for, 362
for pneumonia, 680t, 682t–683t
Celecoxib, for pain, 26t
Celiac arteriography, 770
Cellulitis, 409, **409**
anaerobic, 488
Escherichia coli, 472
Klebsiella, 472
nocardiosis, 492
streptococcal, 456
treatment of, 410t–411t
Central European encephalitis, 552t
Central nervous system, paraneoplastic syndromes, 346–348, 347t
Central venous pressure, in shock, 46, 47f
Cephalexin
for *Bartonella* infections, 484t
for endocarditis prophylaxis, 379t
for pharyngitis, 250t
Cephalosporins
for listeriosis, 466
mechanisms, indications, and adverse effects of, 362
Cerebellar ataxia, 915, 916t
Cerebellar degeneration, paraneoplastic, 347, 348t

Cerebral cortex, diseases of, weakness in, 176t, 177t
Cerebral hemisphere, stroke involving, 59t
Cerebrospinal fluid (CSF), ventricular drainage of, 67
Cerebrospinal fluid (CSF) analysis
in acute bacterial meningitis, 888–889, 887t
in chronic meningitis, 896
culture, 354t
in multiple sclerosis, 900
in progressive multifocal leukoencephalopathy, 895
reference values for specific analytes, 1005t
in viral encephalitis, 893
in viral meningitis, 892
Cerebrovascular disease
prevention of, 993t
syncope in, 166t
Cerumen, 244
Cervical angina syndrome, 154
Cervical cancer, **337**
prevention of, 284
risk factors for, 284
screening for, 337, 992t
staging and survival in, 336t, 337
treatment of, 337
Cervical intraepithelial neoplasia, 284
Cervical radiculopathy, 155t
nonprogressive, 156
Cervical spine
disk disease, pain in, 154, 156
trauma to, pain in, 154
Cervicitis
gonococcal, 399
mucopurulent, **397**
Cestode infection, **587**
cysticercosis, 587–588
diphyllobothriasis, 589–590
echinococcosis, 589
taeniasis saginata, 587
taeniasis solium, 587–588
Cetirizine, for allergic rhinitis, 775
Cetuximab, for head and neck cancer, 310
Cevimeline, for Sjögren's syndrome, 785
Chagas' disease, **576**
acute, 576–577
chronic, 577
treatment of, 577
Chancroid, **406**
treatment of, 407
Charcoal, activated, 77
for porphyria, 864
Charcot's joint, 162f, 800
Charcot's triad, 752
Chelating agents
binding radioactive materials, 131
for hemochromatosis, 862
Chemical bioterrorism, **125**
nerve agents, 126–127
vesicants, 125–126

Chest pain, **133**
   angina pectoris, 631–635
   in ankylosing spondylitis, 789
   approach to, 135f, 136
   differential diagnosis of, 134f, 135f, 136t
   less serious causes, 133–134
   in myocardial infarction, 622
   noncardiac, 204
   serious causes, 133
Chest wall disorders, dyspnea in, 186
Chest wall pain, 133, 134f
Chest x-ray
   in abdominal pain, 138
   in acute pericarditis, 613
   in aortic aneurysm, 653
   in aortic dissection, 654
   in aortic regurgitation, 607
   in aortic stenosis, 606
   in ARDS, 37
   in cardiac tamponade, 615
   in cardiomyopathy, 609, 610t, 611
   in constrictive pericarditis, 615
   in COPD, 676
   in cor pulmonale, 652
   in environmental lung disease, 673
   in heart failure, 648
   in hemoptysis, 191
   in hypersensitivity pneumonitis, 672
   indications for, 32
   in interstitial lung disease, 689
   in mitral stenosis, 603
   in myocarditis, 612
   in pneumonia, 684
   preoperative, 35
   in pulmonary edema, 53
   in pulmonary hypertension, 659, 660f
   in respiratory disease, 666
   in shock, 46
   in stroke, 61
   utility of, 32
Chickenpox, **512**
   complications of, 526
   nosocomial, 444
   prevention of, 527
   treatment of, 527
Chickenpox vaccine, 527
Chikungunya virus, 550
Chlamydial infection, **517**
Chlamydia pneumoniae infection, 517, **519**, 679, 684
   atherosclerosis and, 519
   treatment of, 519
Chlamydia psittaci infection, 517, **518**
Chlamydia trachomatis infection, **400**, 517, **518**
   adult inclusion conjunctivitis, 518
   epididymitis, 396
   mucopurulent cervicitis, 397
   pelvic inflammatory disease, 397
   proctitis, 399
   reactive arthritis, 792
   trachoma, 518
   treatment of, 402

   urethritis/urethral syndrome in women, 393–396
   urinary tract, 724
Chlorambucil, for inflammatory myopathies, 948
Chloramphenicol
   for *Bartonella* infections, 484t
   mechanisms, indications, and adverse effects of, 363
   for meningococcal infections, 464t
   for murine typhus, 512
   for plague, 483
   for relapsing fever, 510
   for rickettsialpox, 512
   for tularemia, 481
Chlordiazepoxide
   for alcohol withdrawal, 974
   dosage and adverse effects of, 966t
Chloroquine
   for malaria, 571t
   for malaria prophylaxis, 574t
   for porphyria, 864
Chlorphenid, for tularemia, 121t
Chlorpromazine
   dosage and adverse effects of, 967t
   for migraine, 144t
   for serotonin syndrome, 87
Chlorpropamide, for diabetes insipidus, 814
Chlorthalidone, for edema, 196t
Cholangiography, 223
Cholangitis, **752**
   primary sclerosing, **752**
      treatment of, 753
   treatment of, 752
Cholecystectomy
   for acute cholecystitis, 751
   for choledocholithiasis/cholangitis, 752
   for cholelithiasis, 750
Cholecystitis
   acute, **751**
      treatment of, 751
   chronic, **751**
Cholecystogram, 750t
Choledocholithiasis, **752**
   treatment of, 752
Cholelithiasis, **749**
   pancreatitis and, 753
   treatment of, 750–751
Cholera, **384**
   treatment of, 384–385
Cholera vaccine, 371t
Cholestatic jaundice, 221t
Cholesteatoma, 245
Cholesterol, blood, 855
   classification of, 1004t
   monitoring of, 994t
Cholestipol, for hyperlipidemia, 859t
Cholestyramine
   for hyperlipidemia, 859t
   for irritable bowel syndrome, 746
   for nephrolithiasis, 733t
   for *Pfiesteria* poisoning, 112
   for porphyria, 864

Cholestyramine (*Cont.*):
  for primary biliary cirrhosis, 768
  for primary sclerosing cholangitis, 753
  for viral hepatitis, 761
Cholinergic crisis, from nerve agents, 126
CHOP regimen
  for gastric cancer, 322
  for lymphoma, 301–302
Choreoathetosis, 178
Chorioretinitis, herpes simplex virus, 521
Chromosomal abnormalities
  in Burkitt's lymphoma, 302
  in cancer of unknown primary site,
    342t
  in head and neck cancer, 309
  in lung cancer, 311
  in lymphoid malignancies, 298
  in myeloid leukemia, 290
  in testicular cancer, 333
Chronic ambulatory peritoneal dialysis,
    peritonitis in, 381
Chronic fatigue syndrome, **952**
  depression and, 956
  diagnosis of, 953
    CDC criteria for, 953t
  symptoms of, 952–953, 952t
  treatment of, 953–954
Chronic inflammatory demyelinating
    polyneuropathy, 941
Chronic obstructive pulmonary disease
    (COPD), **675**
  clinical features of, 676
  diagnosis of, 664t
  insomnia in, 183
  treatment of, 676–678
Chronic progressive external ophthalmo-
    plegia, 950
Churg-Strauss syndrome, 786
Chylomicrons, 856t, 857
Ciclopirox olamine, 555
  for dermatophyte infections, 262
Cidofovir
  for adenovirus infections, 539
  for cytomegalovirus infections, 531
  for herpes simplex virus infections,
    525t
Cigarette smoking, 861
  cessation of, 676, 690, 991, 992t, 993t
    preoperative, 37
  lung cancer and, 311
  passive, 675
Ciguatera poisoning, 111
  treatment of, 111
Cilostazol, for arteriosclerosis, 656
Cimetidine
  for erosive gastropathy, 740
  for snakebite, 110
Ciprofloxacin
  for *Aeromonas* infections, 474
  for animal bites, 107t
  for anthrax, 120t, 122
  for *Bartonella* infections, 484t
  for campylobacteriosis, 389
  for chancroid, 407

for cyclosporiasis, 387
for gonococcal infections, 401t
for infectious arthritis, 413
for inflammatory bowel disease, 744t–
  745t
for intestinal pseudoobstruction, 748
for isosporiasis, 387
for meningococcal infection prophylaxis, 464t, 889
for necrotizing fasciitis, 410t
for osteomyelitis, 416t
for peritonitis prophylaxis, 381
for plague, 483
for plague prophylaxis, 483
for pneumonia, 680t, 683t
for *Pseudomonas aeruginosa* infections, 477t
for Q fever, 516
for rickettsialpox, 512
for sepsis, 52t
for shigellosis, 390
for spontaneous bacterial peritonitis,
  225
for *Staphylococcus aureus* infections,
  453t
for tuberculosis, 498
for typhoid fever, 388
for urethritis in men, 393
Circadian rhythmicity disorder, 185
Circinate lesion, 255
Circulatory function tests, reference values for, 1006t
Circulatory overload, transfusion-related,
  18
Cirrhosis, **766**
  ascites in, 225, 226t
    complications of, 225–226
  classification of Child and Turcotte,
    770t
  clinical features of, 766
  diagnosis of, 767
  edema in, 194, 195f, 197
  primary biliary, **768**
    treatment of, 768
Cisapride
  for gastroesophageal reflux disease, 200
  for gastroparesis, 198
Cisplatin
  for bladder cancer, 332
  for cervical cancer, 337
  for cervical node metastasis, 343
  for endometrial cancer, 337
  for esophageal cancer, 321
  for extragonadal germ cell tumor, 343
  for gastric cancer, 322
  for head and neck cancer, 310
  for lung cancer, 313–315
  for ovarian cancer, 335
  for peritoneal carcinomatosis, 343
  for testicular cancer, 333
Citalopram, dosage and adverse effects of,
  964t
Citrate supplements, for nephrolithiasis,
  733t

Citrobacter infection, **473**
  treatment of, 473–474
Clarithromycin
  for endocarditis prophylaxis, 379t
  for *Haemophilus influenzae* infections,
    467
  for *Helicobacter pylori* eradication,
    739t
  for *Mycoplasma pneumoniae* infections,
    517
  for nontuberculous mycobacterial infec-
    tions, 504–505
  for pertussis, 468
  for pneumococcal infections, 447
  for pneumonia, 680t
Claudication, intermittent, 655
Claustrophobia, 960
Clenched-fist injury, 107t, 109
Clindamycin
  for anaerobic infections, 491
  for animal bites, 107t, 108t
  for anthrax, 120t, 122
  for babesiosis, 96t, 573
  for bacterial vaginosis, 395t
  for clostridial infections, 98t, 489
  for diphtheria, 461
  for gas gangrene, 410t
  for HACEK endocarditis, 469t
  mechanisms, indications, and adverse
    effects of, 363
  for necrotizing fasciitis, 98t, 410t, 457
  for osteomyelitis, 416t
  for pelvic inflammatory disease, 398
  for pneumococcal infections, 447
  for *Pneumocystis* infections, 567, 567t
  for pneumonia, 682t
  for sepsis, 52t
  for streptococcal infections, 459
  for toxic shock syndrome, 97t, 455,
    458
Clinical chemistry, reference values for
  laboratory tests, 997t–999t
Clofazimine, for leprosy, 503
Clomiphene citrate, for female infertility,
  846
Clomipramine, 963
  dosage and adverse effects of, 964t
  for hypersomnia, 185
  for obsessive-compulsive disorder, 960
  for panic disorder, 959
Clonazepam
  dosage and adverse effects of, 966t
  for myoclonus, 71, 177
  for panic disorder, 959
  for seizures, 882t
  for vertigo, 170t
Clonidine
  for menopausal symptoms, 845
  for narcotic withdrawal, 976
Clonorchiasis, 586
Clopidogrel
  for acute coronary syndromes, 635
  for myocardial infarction prophylaxis,
    630

  for stroke prevention, 63
  for thrombotic disorders, 279
Clostridial infection, **487**
  from animal bite, 108t
  nosocomial, 443
  treatment of, 489
Clostridium botulinum infection. *See* Bot-
  ulism
Clostridium difficile-associated disease
  (CDAD), 392
  treatment of, 392
Clostridium novyi infection, 487–489
Clostridium perfringens infection, 487–
  489
  food poisoning, 384
Clostridium septicum infection, 487–489
Clostridium tetani infection. *See* Tetanus
Clotrimazole, 555
  for candidiasis, 206, 558
Clozapine, 969
  dosage and adverse effects of, 967t
  for schizophrenia, 958
Clubbing, 193
Cluster headache, 140t, 144–146
CMV regimen, for bladder cancer, 332
Coagulation disorders, 276–277
  drug-induced, 982t
  reference values for laboratory tests,
    995t–996t
  treatment of, 277
Coagulation studies, for stroke, 61
Coal worker's pneumoconiosis, 674
Coarctation of aorta, hypertension in, 617
Coccidioidomycosis, **562**
  chronic fibrocavitary pulmonary, 562
  disseminated, 562–563
  meningitis, 897t
  primary pulmonary, 562
  treatment of, 563
Codeine
  abuse of, **975**
  for cough, 189
  for hemoptysis, 191
  for pain, 26t
CODOX-M regime, for Burkitt's lymphoma, 303
Cogan's syndrome, 786
Colchicine
  for amyloidosis, 806
  for fever, 159f
  for gout, 797
  for primary biliary cirrhosis, 768
Colectomy, for inflammatory bowel disease, 745
Colesevelam, for hyperlipidemia, 859t
Colistin, for *Pseudomonas aeruginosa* infections, 477t
Collagen vascular disease
  eosinophilia in, 273
  interstitial lung disease and, 690
  monocytosis in, 273
  pleural effusion in, 692t
Colloid, for hyponatremia, 5
Colonic angiodysplasia, **748**

Colonic polyps, **324**
  hereditary polyposis syndromes, 324–325, 325t
  hyperplastic, 324
  tubular adenoma, 324
  villous adenoma, 324
Colonoscopy, 327, 993t
Colorectal cancer, **326**
  etiology of, 326
  prevention of, 283, 327–328
  prognosis for, 326, 326t
  risk factors for, 283, 326
  screening for, 281, 282t, 327, 993t, 994t
  staging of, 326, 326t
  treatment of, 327
Color vision abnormalities, drug-induced, 987t
Coma, **54**
  approach to, 55–56
  brain death, 57–58
  differential diagnosis of, 55t
  drug-induced, 54
  in head trauma, 69
  hyperosmolar, **89**
  in hypoxic ischemic encephalopathy, 70f
  neurologic evaluation of, 56–57
  radiologic examination for, 57
Common cold, 248, 536, 538
Common peroneal neuropathy, 940t
Common variable immunodeficiency, 779
Complex regional pain syndrome, **930**
Complicated parapneumonic effusion, 691
Compression stockings, 658
Compulsive personality, 962
Computed tomography (CT)
  in abdominal pain, 139
  in aortic aneurysm, 653
  in aortic dissection, 654
  in biliary tract disease, 750t
  in coma, 57
  in constrictive pericarditis, 616
  in head trauma, 69
  hepatobiliary, 223
  indications for, 33
  in interstitial lung disease, 689
  neuroimaging, 873–875, 874t
  in osteomyelitis, 415t
  in pancreatitis, 754, 756
  in pneumonia, 684
  in poisoning or drug overdose, 75
  in respiratory disease, 666
  in subarachnoid hemorrhage, 66
  utility of, 33
Concussion, 68
  post-concussion headache, 146
Conduction aphasia, 180, 180t
Conductive hearing loss, 245
Condylomata lata, 403
Confusion, **54**
  neurologic evaluation of, 56–57
  radiologic examination for, 57

Conjunctivitis
  adult inclusion, **518**
    treatment of, 518
  enteroviral, 546
Connective tissue disease, **779**
  interstitial lung disease and, 688t
  mixed, 784
  rheumatoid arthritis, 781–783
  Sjögren's syndrome, 784–785
  systemic lupus erythematosus, 781–782
  systemic sclerosis, 783–784
Consciousness, impaired, **54**
  approach to, 55–56
  head trauma, 68–69
  neurologic evaluation of, 56–57
  radiologic examination for, 57
Constipation, **213**
  causes of, 213
  drug-induced, 985t
  treatment of, 213–214
Contact dermatitis, 258f
  allergic, 260
  irritant, 260
Continuous renal replacement therapy, 706
Contraception, female, **845**
Contraceptive patch, 845
Conversion disorder, 961
Coordination, testing of, **873**
Copper, toxic accumulation of, 864
Corneal disorder
  drug-induced, 987t
  infection, 242
Coronary arteriography, 631, 637
Coronary artery bypass graft (CABG)
  for angina pectoris, 634t, 635
  indications for, 623f
Coronary artery disease (CAD), **631**. See also Angina pectoris
  laboratory evaluation of, 631
  preoperative evaluation of, 36
  in women, 989
Coronary artery spasm, **637**
Coronavirus infection, **537**
Cor pulmonale, **652**
  causes of, 652
  laboratory evaluation of, 652
  treatment of, 652
Cortisol, excess, 823
Cortisone acetate, for hypopituitarism, 812
Corynebacterium diphtheriae infection. *See also* Diphtheria
  pharyngitis, 253
Corynebacterium jeikeium infection, 461–462
Corynebacterium urealyticum infection, 462
Costochondral pain, 133, 134f
Cotton dust exposure, 674
Cough, **187**
  ACE inhibitor, 619, 984t
  approach to, 188–189, 188f

Cough (*Cont.*):
  causes of, 187–188
  drug-induced, 189, 984t
  smoker's, 189
  treatment of, 189
Cough headache, 147
Coxiella burnetii infection. *See also* Q fever
  pneumonia, 684
Coxsackievirus infection, **545**
Cranial nerves
  disorders of, **920**
    multiple cranial nerve palsies, **924**
  examination of, **868**
  I. *See* Olfactory nerve (I)
  II, 868
  III, 869–870
  IV, 869–870
  V. *See* Trigeminal nerve (V)
  VI, 869–870
  VII. *See* Facial nerve (VII)
  VIII, 871–872
  IX, 872
  X. *See* Vagus nerve (X)
  XI. *See* Accessory nerve (XI)
  XII. *See* Hypoglossal nerve (XII)
Creatine phosphokinase, in myocardial infarction, 622
Creatinine clearance, 227
CREST syndrome, 783
Critical care medicine, principles of, **19**
Critically ill patient
  approach to, 19–20
  monitoring in ICU, 21
  prevention of complications, 21
Crocodile tears, 922
Crohn's disease, **742**
  arthritis in, 799
  extraintestinal manifestations of, 743
  treatment of, 743–745, 744t–745t
Cromolyn sodium
  for allergic rhinitis, 775
  for asthma, 670t, 671
  for systemic mastocytosis, 776
Croup, 253
Crust, 256, 408
Cryoglobulinemia, 719t
  essential mixed, 786
Cryoprecipitate, 19
  for von Willebrand's disease, 277
Cryptococcosis, **559**
  brain abscess, 894
  HIV and, 560
  meningitis, 897t
  treatment of, 560
Cryptosporidiosis, 386
  diagnosis of, 359t
  treatment of, 386
Crystalloid
  for hyponatremia, 5
  for shock, 47f
Culture
  diagnosis of infectious disease, 351, 352t–357t, 358

specimen collection and transport, 352t–357t
Cunninghamella infection, 560–561
Cushing's syndrome, 823
  diagnosis of, 823–825, 824f
  drug-induced, 823
  hypertension in, 617–618
  paraneoplastic, 344–346, 344t
  treatment of, 825
Cyanide poisoning, 69, 82
Cyanosis, **192**
  approach to, 193
  causes of, 193t
  central, 192–193, 193t
  peripheral, 192–193, 193t
Cyclobenzaprine, for low back pain, 151
Cyclophosphamide
  for acute renal failure, 706
  for breast cancer, 318–319
  for chronic inflammatory demyelinating polyneuropathy, 941
  for glomerulonephritis, 716
  for inflammatory myopathies, 948
  for interstitial lung disease, 690
  for multiple sclerosis, 903
  for myasthenia gravis, 944
  for rheumatoid arthritis, 783
  for systemic lupus erythematosus, 781
  for systemic sclerosis, 784
  for vasculitis, 788
  for Wegener's granulomatosis, 715
Cyclosporiasis, 387
  treatment of, 387
Cyclosporine
  immunosuppression for renal transplant, 712
  for inflammatory bowel disease, 744t–745t, 745
  for inflammatory myopathies, 948
  for myasthenia gravis, 944
  for psoriasis, 259
  for rheumatoid arthritis, 783
Cyproheptadine
  for migraine prophylaxis, 145t
  for serotonin syndrome, 87
  for urticaria/angioedema, 774
Cyst
  breast, 317
  mediastinal, **693**
  skin lesion, 255
Cystectomy, for bladder cancer, 332
Cysticercosis, **587**
  diagnosis of, 588, 588t
  meningitis, 897t
  treatment of, 588
Cystine stones, 732, 733t
Cystitis, **724**
  clinical features of, 724
  treatment of, 726t
Cytarabine
  for acute lymphoid leukemia/lymphoma, 302
  for acute myeloid leukemia, 292
Cytoadherance, 569

Cytomegalovirus infection, 529–531
  in AIDS, 530
  congenital, 529
  in immunocompromised host, 529–530
  mononucleosis, 529
  perinatal, 529
  treatment of, 530–531

Dacarbazine, for melanoma, 308
Danazol, for idiopathic thrombocytopenic
    purpura, 277
Dantrolene, for malignant hyperthermia,
    160
Dapsone
  for leprosy, 503
  for *Pneumocystis* infections, 567
  for *Pneumocystis* prophylaxis, 568t
Daptomycin
  for osteomyelitis, 416t
  for *Staphylococcus aureus* infections,
    453t
Daunorubicin
  for acute lymphoid leukemia/lym-
    phoma, 302
  for acute myeloid leukemia, 292
Daytime sleepiness, excessive, **183**, 184t,
    988t
Deafferentation pain, 141t
Death, brain death, 57–58
DeBakey classification, of aortic dissec-
    tion, 654f
Debranching enzyme deficiency, 948
Decerebration, 56
Decortication, 56
Deep-brain stimulation, for Parkinson's
    disease, 914
Deep venous thrombosis (DVT), **657**, 686
  prevention of, 658
  risk factors for, 657t
  treatment of, 278t, 279, 657, 687
Defecation, 208
Deferoxamine
  for hemochromatosis, 862
  for iron poisoning, 83
Defibrillation, for ventricular fibrillation/
    tachycardia, 41, 43f
Delavirdine, for HIV/AIDS, 432t, 439
Delayed sleep phase syndrome, 185
Delirium, 904
  drug-induced, 988t
Delirium tremens, 973–974
Delta agent. *See* Hepatitis D
Delusion(s), 957
Delusional disorder, 958
Demeclocycline, for syndrome of inappro-
    priate ADH, 103, 815
Dementia, **904**
  Alzheimer's disease, 907–909
  approach to, 904–907, 908t
  diagnosis of, 904
  differential diagnosis of, 905t
  differentiation of major dementias, 906t
  frontotemporal, 904, 906t, 907, 909
  Huntington's disease, 909–910

with Lewy bodies, 904, 906t, 907, 909
  multi-infarct, 904
  treatment of, 908–909
  vascular, 906t, 909
Dementia pugilistica, 904–907
Dengue fever, **549**
Dengue hemorrhagic fever/dengue shock
    syndrome, **554**
Dental pain, 147
Dental procedures, endocarditis prophy-
    laxis for, 378t, 379t
Dependent personality, 962
Depo-Provera, 845
Depression
  in Alzheimer's disease, 909
  drug-induced, 956, 988t
  major, **955**
    treatment of, 956
  with medical illness, 956
  screening for, 992t
Dermatitis
  allergic contact, 260
  atopic, 256f, 257f, 260
    treatment of, 260
  contact, 258f
  drug-induced, 981t
  irritant contact, 260
  seborrheic, 258f, 260–261
    treatment of, 261
  stasis, 257f
Dermatofibroma, 257f
Dermatomes, 870f, 871f
Dermatomyositis, 948, 949t
  treatment of, 948
Dermatophyte infection, 262
  treatment of, 262
Desipramine
  dosage and adverse effects of, 964t
  for pain, 27t
Desloradine, for allergic rhinitis, 775
Desmopressin
  for diabetes insipidus, 814
  for hypernatremia, 6–7
  for hypopituitarism, 812
Devic's syndrome, 903
Dexamethasone
  for bacterial meningitis, 887
  for brain tumor, 883
  for *Haemophilus influenzae* infections,
    467
  for hirsutism in female, 843
  for increased intracranial pressure, 68t
  for multiple myeloma, 304
  for nausea and vomiting, 286
  for spinal cord compression, 102, 934
  for thyrotoxic crisis, 820
  for typhoid fever, 388
Dexamethasone androgen-suppression
    test, 843
Dexamethasone test, for Cushing's syn-
    drome, 823
Dextroamphetamine, for hypersomnia,
    185
Dextromethorphan, for cough, 189

Dextrose, for status epilepticus, 72
Diabetes insipidus, **813**
    central, 6–7, 229, 230f, 813
    clinical features of, 813
    diagnosis of, 813–814
    drug-induced, 986t
    nephrogenic, 6–7, 229, 230f, 813
    treatment of, 814
Diabetes mellitus, **830**
    autonomic dysfunction in, 928
    clinical features of, 831
    complications of, 831, 833
    depression and, 956
    diagnosis of, 830
    gestational, 830
    in hospitalized patient, 834–835
    hypertension in, 621
    maturity-onset diabetes of the young,
        830
    nephropathy in, **717,** 833
    retinopathy in, 243
    treatment of, 92, 93f, 832–835, 832t,
        834f, 834t
    type 1 (insulin-dependent), 830
    type 2 (insulin-independent), 830
        risk factors for, 831t
    in women, 989
Diabetic ketoacidosis, **89**
    laboratory feature of, 89t
    treatment of, 90t
Dialysis, **709**
    for acute renal failure, 706
    for chronic renal failure, 709
    hemodialysis, 709–710
    for hypercalcemia, 849t
    for hyperkalemia, 10t
    for hypermagnesemia, 852
    indications for, 706, 709
    for methanol poisoning, 85
    peritoneal, 710–711
    for poisoning/drug overdose, 78
    slow low efficiency, 706
    for theophylline poisoning, 88
    for tumor lysis syndrome, 104
Diaphragmatic paralysis, **695**
Diarrhea, **208**
    acute, treatment of, 211, 211f
    in AIDS, 210t
    from altered intestinal motility, 209
    amebiosis, 391
    calicivirus, 385
    campylobacteriosis, 389
    cholera, 384
    chronic, treatment of, 211, 212f
    Clostridium difficile-associated disease,
        392
    cryptosporidiosis, 386
    cyclosporiasis, 387
    drug-induced, 985t
    enterohemorrhagic *E. coli,* 390
    evaluation of, 209–210
    exudative, 209
    food poisoning, 384
    giardiasis, 385–386

    infectious, **383**
        approach to, 383
    inflammatory, 387–393
    isosporiasis, 387
    microsporidiosis, 387
    noninflammatory, 384–387
    Norwalk virus, 385
    osmotic, 208
    rotavirus, 385
    salmonellosis, 387–388
    secretory, 209
    shigellosis, 390
    stool examination, 210
    travel advice, 366, 369, 371–372
    traveler's, 384
    Vibrio parahaemolyticus, 385
    yersiniosis, 390–391
Diascopy, 258–259
Diastolic blood pressure, 618f–619f
Diazepam
    for alcohol withdrawal, 974
    dosage and adverse effects of, 966t
    for marine envenomations, 110
    for multiple sclerosis, 903
    for myocardial infarction, 623
    for nerve agent exposure, 126
    for tetanus, 486
    for vertigo, 170t
Dichloralphenazone, for migraine, 144t
Diclofenac, for tension headache, 146t
Dicyclomine
    for diverticular disease, 747
    for irritable bowel syndrome, 746
Didanosine, for HIV infections, 429t
Dietary reference intakes (DRI), 3
Diethylcarbamazine, for filariasis, 584
Diffusing capacity of lung, 666
DiGeorge's syndrome, 777
Digitalis
    for heart failure, 649t
    for mitral stenosis, 604
Digitalis toxicity, 650
Digital rectal examination, 282t, 993t
    in prostate disorders, 338–339, 340f
Digoxin
    for cor pulmonale, 652
    for heart failure, 650
    for mitral regurgitation, 605
    poisoning, 82
    for supraventricular arrhythmias, 625
Dihydroergotamine, for migraine, 143t–
        144t
Diltiazem
    for aortic dissection, 654
    for arrhythmias, 641t
    for hypertrophic cardiomyopathy, 611
    for mitral stenosis, 604
Dimenhydrinate
    for nausea and vomiting, 198
    for vertigo, 170t
Dimercaprol
    for arsenic poisoning, 80
    for mercury poisoning, 85
D-Dimer test, 657, 685

Dimorphic fungi, 555
Diphenhydramine
    for anaphylaxis, 105
    for neuroleptic poisoning, 86
    for snakebite, 110
    for urticaria/angioedema, 774
Diphenoxylate
    abuse of, **975**
    for diarrhea, 211
    for inflammatory bowel disease, 743
    for irritable bowel syndrome, 746
Diphtheria, **460**
    prevention of, 461
    respiratory, 460
    treatment of, 461
Diphtheria antitoxin, 461
Diphyllobothriasis, **589**
Dipivefrin, for glaucoma, 243
Diplopia. *See* Double vision
Dipyrimadole, for stroke prevention, 63
Disease-modifying antirheumatic drugs
        (DMARD), for rheumatoid arthri-
        tis, 783
Disease prevention, **991**
Disequilibrium syndrome (dialysis), 710
Disopyramide
    for arrhythmias, 646t
    for hypertrophic cardiomyopathy, 611
Disseminated intravascular coagulation (DIC)
    thrombocytopenia in, 275
    treatment of, 277
Distributive shock, 45, 45t, 46t
Disulfiram, for alcoholism, 974
Diuretics
    complications of, 197t
    for cor pulmonale, 652
    for diabetes insipidus, 814
    for edema, 196t
    for heart failure, 626, 649, 649t
    for hypertension, 618–619, 620t
    hypokalemia caused by, 8
    for increased intracranial pressure, 67
    loop, 196t
    for mitral regurgitation, 605
    for mitral stenosis, 604
    for myocardial infarction, 628t
    for nephrolithiasis, 733t
    osmotic, for increased intracranial pres-
        sure, 67
    potassium-losing, 196t
    for pulmonary hypertension, 661
    for restrictive cardiomyopathy, 611
    for tricuspid regurgitation, 608
    for vertigo, 170t
Diverticular disease, **747**
    treatment of, 747
Diverticulitis, 747
Diverticulosis, 217
Dizziness, **168**
Dobutamine
    for heart failure, 626, 651
    for myocardial infarction, 627t, 628t
    for pulmonary edema, 54
    for shock, 48, 48t

Docusate salts
    for constipation, 214
    for myocardial infarction, 623
Dofetilide, for arrhythmias, 641t
Dog bite, 100, 106, 107t
Döhle bodies, 265
Domestic violence, 990, 992t
Donepezil, for Alzheimer's disease, 908–
        909
Donovanosis, **407**
    treatment of, 407
Dopamine
    for heart failure, 651
    for increased intracranial pressure,
        68t
    for myocardial infarction, 627t
    for shock, 48, 48t
    for vasospasm in subarachnoid hemor-
        rhage, 66
Dopamine agonists
    for hyperprolactinemia, 810
    for Parkinson's disease, 911, 913t
Dorsal root ganglionopathy, paraneoplas-
        tic, 346–348, 347t
Double vision, **171,** 241
    causes of, 174–175, 174t
Doxepin
    dosage and adverse effects of, 964t
    for pain, 27t
Doxorubicin
    for breast cancer, 318–319
    for carcinoid tumor, 329
    for endometrial cancer, 337
    for multiple myeloma, 304
    for pancreatic islet-cell tumors, 331
    for Zollinger-Ellison syndrome, 741
Doxycycline
    for animal bite, 108t
    for anthrax, 120t, 122
    for *Bartonella* infections, 484t
    for brucellosis, 480
    for *Chlamydia* infections, 402
    for cholera, 384
    for COPD, 678
    for donovanosis, 407
    for endemic treponematoses, 508
    for epidemic typhus, 513
    for epididymitis, 396
    for gonococcal infections, 401t
    for *Legionella* infections, 479
    for leptospirosis, 509
    for Lyme borreliosis, 507
    for malaria prophylaxis, 574t
    mechanisms, indications, and adverse
        effects of, 363
    for murine typhus, 512
    for *Mycoplasma pneumoniae* infections,
        517
    for onchocerciasis, 585
    for pelvic inflammatory disease, 398
    for plague, 483
    for plague prophylaxis, 483
    for pneumococcal infections, 447
    for pneumonia, 680t

Doxycycline (*Cont.*):
    for Q fever, 516
    for relapsing fever, 510
    for rickettsialpox, 512
    for Rocky Mountain spotted fever, 97t, 511
    for tularemia, 121t
    for urethritis in men, 396
Drug-induced illness, **979**
    acne, 981t
    Addisonian-like syndrome, 980t
    agranulocytosis, 982t
    airway obstruction, 984t
    alopecia, 981t
    anaphylaxis, 979t
    angina, 983t
    angioedema, 979t
    arrhythmias, 983t
    AV block, 984t
    bladder dysfunction, 986t
    bone disorders, 987t
    cardiomyopathy, 984t
    cardiovascular disease, 983t–984t
    cataract, 987t
    clotting abnormalities, 982t
    color vision abnormalities, 987t
    coma/stupor, 54
    constipation, 985t
    corneal disorders, 987t
    cough, 189, 984t
    Cushing's syndrome, 823
    cutaneous reactions, 264
    cystitis, 986t
    delirium, 988t
    depression, 956, 988t
    dermatitis, 981t
    diabetes insipidus, 986t
    diarrhea, 985t
    drowsiness, 988t
    drug monitoring, 1002t–1003t
    ear disease, 987t
    eczema, 981t
    edema, 195
    eosinophilia, 982t
    erectile dysfunction, 837
    erythema multiforme, 981t
    erythema nodosum, 981t
    esophagitis, 206
    eye disease, 987t
    fever, 980t
    fixed drug eruption, 981t
    galactorrhea, 980t
    gastrointestinal disease, 985t–986t
    glaucoma, 987t
    glomerulonephritis, 715t
    hallucinations, 988t
    headache, 986t
    hearing loss, 245, 987t
    heart failure, 984t
    heat stroke, 160
    hematologic disease, 982t–983t
    hemolytic anemia, 983t
    hepatitis, 761–762
    hirsutism, 842

hyperbilirubinemia, 980t
hypercalcemia, 980t
hyperglycemia, 980t
hyperkalemia, 980t
hyperpigmentation, 981t
hyperpyrexia, 980t
hypertension, 984t
hyperuricemia, 981t
hypoglycemia, 980t
hypokalemia, 981t
hypomania, 988t
hyponatremia, 981t
hypotension, 927, 931, 984t
insomnias, 182
interstitial nephritis, 720–722, 986t
jaundice, 218t, 220, 985t
leukocytosis, 983t
lichenoid eruptions, 982t
liver disease, 985t
lupus, 780, 979t
lymphadenopathy, 983t
malabsorption, 985t
megaloblastic anemia, 983t
metabolic acidosis, 981t
musculoskeletal disease, 987t–988t
myasthenia, 986t
myopathy, 951, 951t, 988t
myositis/myalgia, 988t
nausea/vomiting, 985t
nephropathy, 986t
nephrotic syndrome, 986t
neurologic disease, 986t–987t
neutropenia, 274
obesity, 829
optic neuritis, 987t
oral conditions, 985t
orthostatic hypotension, 927, 931
osteoporosis, 852
pancreatitis, 986t
pancytopenia, 983t
peptic ulcers, 986t
pericarditis, 984t
peripheral neuropathy, 986t
photodermatitis, 982t
pleural effusion, 692t
potassium imbalance, 8
pseudotumor cerebri, 987t
psychiatric disorders, 988t
pulmonary edema, 984t
pulmonary infiltrates, 984t
pure red cell aplasia, 983t
purpura, 982t
rash, 982t
renal disease, 986t
renal tubular acidosis, 986t
respiratory disease, 984t
retinopathy, 987t
schizophrenic-like reaction, 988t
seizures, 877t, 987t
serum sickness, 980t
sexual dysfunction, 980t
skin disease, 981t–982t
skin necrosis, 982t
sleep disorders, 988t

Drug-induced illness (*Cont.*):
  stroke, 897t
  syndrome of inappropriate ADH, 814t
  thrombocytopenia, 275, 277, 983t
  thromboembolism, 984t
  thyroid disease, 980t
  toxic epidermal necrolysis, 982t
  tubular necrosis, 986t
  urinary disease, 986t
  uropathy, 986t
  urticaria, 982t
  vasculitis, 787
  vestibular disorders, 987t
  weight loss, 201t
  in women, 990
Drug monitoring, 1002t–1003t
Drug overdose, **74.** *See also* Poisoning
  treatment of, 75–78
Drusen, 243
DTaP (diphtheria, tetanus toxoid, acellular
    pertussis) vaccine, 461
DTP (diphtheria, tetanus, pertussis) vac-
    cine, 367f
  in immunocompromised patients, 423t
Dual-energy x-ray absorptiometry, 852
Duchenne dystrophy, **947**
Duke criteria, for infective endocarditis,
    374t
Dysautonomia, 925
  paraneoplastic, 930
Dysbetalipoproteinemia, 856t, 860–861
Dysesthesia, 24
Dyskinesia, 911
Dysmenorrhea, 839
  primary, 842
Dyspepsia, 198
  functional, 200
  nonulcer, 737
Dysphagia, **203, 923**
  approach to, 203
  esophageal, 204–206
  oropharyngeal, 203–204
Dysphonia, **923**
Dyspnea, **185**
  approach to, 186–187
  cardiac versus pulmonary, 187t
  causes of, 186–187
  paroxysmal nocturnal, 183
Dystonia, 178

Ear disease
  drug-induced, 987t
  external ear infections, 252
  hearing disorders, 244–248
  middle ear infections, 252–253
  Pseudomonas aeruginosa infections,
    475
  vertigo, **168**
Eastern equine encephalitis, 550, 552t,
    893t
Eating disorder, **969**
  clinical features of, 970
  treatment of, 970–971, 972f
Ebola virus infection, **554**

Echinocandins, 556
Echinococcosis, **589**
  treatment of, 589
Echinocytes, 265
Echocardiography, **596**
  in acute pericarditis, 613
  in aortic aneurysm, 653
  in aortic regurgitation, 607
  in aortic stenosis, 606
  in cardiac tamponade, 615
  in cardiomyopathy, 609, 610t, 611
  in constrictive pericarditis, 615
  in cor pulmonale, 652
  2-D, 600t, 601f
  Doppler, 600t
    normal values of, 1009t
  in endocarditis, 375
  in heart failure, 648
  indications for, 600t, 602–603
  in mitral regurgitation, 605
  in mitral stenosis, 603
  in mitral valve prolapse, 606
  in myocardial infarction, 622
  in myocarditis, 612
  in pulmonary hypertension, 659, 660f
  in shock, 46
  stress, 600t
  transesophageal, 600t
  in valvular disease, 602, 602f
Echolalia, 180t
Ecthyma gangrenosum, 100, 475
Ectoparasites, **590**
Ectopic atrial contractions, 639f
Ectopic ventricular contractions, 639f
Eczema, 260–261
  asteatotic, 257f
  drug-induced, 981t
  dyshidrotic, 256f
  hand, 256f
Eczema herpeticum, 521
Edema, **194**
  approach to, 195f
  drug-induced, 195
  generalized, 194
  idiopathic, 195
  localized, 194
  peripheral, 649
  pulmonary. *See* Pulmonary edema
  treatment of, 195–197
    diuretics, 196t
Edetate calcium disodium, for lead poi-
    soning, 84
Efalizumab, for psoriasis, 259
Efavirenz, for HIV/AIDS, 432t, 439
Eflornithine, for sleeping sickness, 578
Ehrlichiosis, human monocytotropic, **513,**
    514t
Ehrlichiosis ewingii, **514,** 514t
Eikenella corrodens. See HACEK orga-
    nisms
Elderly, joint pain in, 164
Electrocardiography (ECG)
  in abdominal pain, 138
  in acute coronary syndromes, 635

Electrocardiography (ECG) (*Cont.*):
  in acute pericarditis, 613, 613t, 614f
  in aortic regurgitation, 607
  in aortic stenosis, 606
  in arrhythmias, 638, 639f
  in AV block, 645
  in bundle branch block, 597f
  in cardiac hypertrophy, 600–601, 600t
  in cardiac tamponade, 615
  in cardiomyopathy, 609, 610t, 611
  in coma, 57
  in constrictive pericarditis, 615
  in coronary artery disease, 631
  in cor pulmonale, 652
  heart rate, 596
  in hyperkalemia, 9, 9f
  lead system, 597f
  mean axis in, 599
  in mitral stenosis, 603
  in myocardial infarction, 598f, 599f,
    599t, 601, 613t, 622
  in myocarditis, 612
  preoperative, 35
  PR interval, 599
  QRS interval, 600
  QT interval, 600
  rhythm, 599
  in shock, 46
  in stroke, 61
  ST-T waves, 601
  in subarachnoid hemorrhage, 66
  in ventricular tachycardia, 644t
  in Wolff-Parkinson-White syndrome,
    644–645
Electrocochleography, 244
Electroconvulsive therapy, for depression,
  956
Electroencephalography
  in coma, 57
  in seizure, 876–877
Electrolyte balance, **5.** *See also specific
    electrolytes*
Electromyography
  in inflammatory myopathies, 949t
  in polyneuropathy, 939
Elementary body, 517
Elliptocytes, 265
Embolism
  cardiac source of, 602
  pulmonary. *See* Pulmonary embolism
Emergencies, medical
  acute respiratory distress syndrome,
    39–40
  anaphylaxis, 105–106
  asthma, 672
  bioterrorism, 118–132
  cardiovascular collapse and sudden
    death, 41–44
  coma/stupor, 54–58
  diabetic ketoacidosis, 89–91
  drug overdose, 74–88
  frostbite, 116–117
  head injury, 67–69
  hyperosmolar coma, 89–91

  hypoglycemia, 91–94
  hypothermia, 115–116
  hypoxic-ischemic encephalopathy, 69–
    71
  increased intracranial pressure, 67–69
  infectious disease, 94–101
  mammalian bites, 106–108
  oncologic, 101–104
  poisoning, 74–88
  pulmonary edema, acute, 53–54
  septic shock, 49–53
  shock, 44–49
  status epilepticus, 72–73
  stroke, 58–65
  subarachnoid hemorrhage, 66–67
Emergency contraceptive pills, 845
Emotional disorders, chest pain in, 134
Emphysema, **675**
  mediastinal, chest pain in, 133
Empyema, 488, 490, 691–692
  nocardiosis, 492
  streptococcal, 457
  tuberculous, 497
Emtricitabine, for HIV infections, 431t
Enalapril, for heart failure, 651t
Encephalitis
  acute, **886**
    approach to, 886, 888f–889f
  arboviral, **550,** 552t
  coxsackievirus, 545
  herpes simplex virus, 521, 525t
  limbic, paraneoplastic, 346
  measles, 540
  viral, **892**
    diagnosis of, 893
    etiology of, 891t, 892, 893t
    treatment of, 893–894
Encephalomyelitis, acute disseminated,
  903
Encephalopathy
  hepatic, **772**
  hypoxic-ischemic, **69**
    prognosis in, 70f
    treatment of, 71
Endocarditis, infective, **372**
  acute, 373
  acute bacterial, 99t, 101
  clinical features of, 373
  coagulase-negative staphylococci,
    451
  culture-negative, 484t, 485
  diagnosis of, 374–375, 374t
  echocardiography in, 602–603
  enterococcal, 376t, 459
  epidemiology of, 372
  etiology of, 372–373
  HACEK organisms, 377t, 469t, 470
  in IV drug users, 372
  listerial, 465
  native valve, 372
  nosocomial, 372
  paravalvular, 373
  pneumococcal, 446
    treatment of, 447

Endocarditis, infective (*Cont.*):
  prophylaxis
    antimicrobial regimens, 379t, 380
    in cardiac disease, 379t
    indications for, 378t, 379t
  prosthetic valve, 372, 450
  Pseudomonas aeruginosa, 475
  staphylococcal, 376t–377t
  Staphylococcus aureus, 450, 454
  streptococcal, 376t, 460
  subacute, 373
  treatment of, 454
    antimicrobials, 375, 376t–377t
    surgical, 375, 378t, 380
  tricuspid valve, 373
Endocrine disease. *See also specific diseases*
  adrenal, 823–828
  in alcoholism, 973
  in amyloidosis, 805
  anterior pituitary, 807–813
  dementia in, 905t
  diabetes mellitus, 830–835
  drug-induced, 980t
  lymphadenopathy in, 237t
  muscle disease in, 950
  osteoporosis and, 853t
  posterior pituitary, 813–815
  reference values for laboratory tests, 999t–1001t
  reproductive system disorders
    female, 839–846
    male, 835–838
  thyroid, 815–823
  weight loss in, 201t
Endocrine paraneoplastic syndromes, **344**
Endocrine tumors
  of GI tract, **329,** 330t
  of pancreas, **329,** 330t
Endometrial cancer, **335**
  staging and survival in, 335, 336t
  treatment of, 335–337
Endometrial tissue sampling, 282t
Endometritis, 397
Endoscopic band ligation, for esophago-gastric varices, 771
Endoscopic retrograde cholangiopancrea-tography, 750t, 752
Endoscopy, for GI bleeding, 215, 215f, 216f
Enfuvirtide, for HIV/AIDS, 436t, 439
Enoxaparin
  for deep venous thrombosis, 657
  for heart failure, 649
  for myocardial infarction, 625
Entacapone, for Parkinson's disease, 914
Entamoeba histolytica infection, 391
Enteral nutrition, **14**
  decision tree for initiating, 15f
  formulas for, 16
Enteritis, **398**
  treatment of, 399
Enterobacter infection, **473**
  nosocomial, 443
  osteomyelitis, 416t

  treatment of, 473–474
  urinary tract, 724
Enterobiasis, **583**
  treatment of, 584
Enterococcal infection, **459**
  infective endocarditis, 376t
  nosocomial, 443
  treatment of, 459
  urinary tract, 724
Enterocolitis, **398**
  infectious, 743
  treatment of, 399
Enterocytozoon infection, 387
Enteropathic arthritis, **799**
  treatment of, 799
Enteroviral infection, **544**
  coxsackievirus, 545
  encephalitis, 891t, 892
  meningitis, 890, 891t
  poliovirus, 544–545
  treatment of, 546
Enthesitis, 792
Environmental lung disease, **673**
Enzyme immunoassay (EIA), 351
Eosinopenia, 274
Eosinophilia, 273
  drug-induced, 982t
Eosinophilic granuloma, **690**
Ependymoma, 884
Ephedrine, for vertigo, 170t
Epidemic typhus, **512**
  treatment of, 513
Epididymitis, **396**
  treatment of, 396
Epidural abscess
  spinal, 99t, 101, 935
  Staphylococcus aureus, 449
Epidural hematoma, spinal, 935
Epiglottitis, 253–254
  Haemophilus influenzae, 467
Epilepsy, **875.** *See also* Seizure
  status epilepticus, **72**
  temporal lobe, 882
Epinephrine
  for anaphylaxis, 105, 114
  for asthma, 669
  for cardiac arrest, 43f–44f
  for glaucoma, 243
Epirubicin, for gastric cancer, 322
Epley procedure, 171
Epoprostenol
  for pulmonary hypertension, 661
  for systemic sclerosis, 784
Epstein-Barr virus infection, **531,** 532t
  clinical features of, 531–532
  diagnosis of, 532
  encephalitis, 893
  in lymphoid malignancies, 298
  treatment of, 533
Eptifibatide, for acute coronary syndromes, 635
Erectile dysfunction, **837**
  approach to, 837–838, 838f
  causes of, 837

Erectile dysfunction (*Cont.*):
  clinical features of, 837–838
  drug-induced, 837
  treatment of, 838, 838f
Ergot alkaloids, for Parkinson's disease, 913t
Ergotamine
  for cluster headache prophylaxis, 145
  for migraine, 143t
Erosion, 256
Ertapenem, 362
Erysipelas, 261, 409, 456
Erythema infectiosum, 543
Erythema migrans, 506
Erythema multiforme, 263, 521, 525t
  drug-induced, 981t
  treatment of, 263
Erythema nodosum, 263
  drug-induced, 981t
  treatment of, 263
Erythema nodosum leproticum, 503
Erythrocytosis. *See* Polycythemia
Erythroderma, 100
Erythroid:granulocytic ratio, bone marrow, 266–267
Erythromycin
  for acne vulgaris, 263
  for adult inclusion conjunctivitis, 518
  for animal bites, 107t
  for bacillary angiomatosis, 410t
  for *Bartonella* infections, 484t
  for campylobacteriosis, 389
  for chancroid, 407
  for *Chlamydia* infections, 402, 519
  for cholera, 384
  for diphtheria, 461
  for gastroparesis, 198
  for leptospirosis, 509
  for Lyme borreliosis, 507
  for pertussis, 468
  for pharyngitis, 250t
  for psittacosis, 519
  for relapsing fever, 510
  for streptococcal infections, 456, 459
  for trachoma prophylaxis, 518
Erythropoiesis
  hypoproliferative, 233
  ineffective, 218, 233
Erythropoietin, 267, 708
  for anemia, 288–289
  serum, 295
Eschar, 409
Escherichia coli infection
  enteroaggregative and diffusely adhering (EAEC/DAEC), 471
  enterohemorrhagic (EHEC), 390, 471
  enteroinvasive (EIEC), 471
  enteropathogenic (EPEC), 471
  enterotoxigenic (ETEC), 384
  extraintestinal, 471–472
    treatment of, 472
  intestinal, 471
    treatment of, 471
  meningitis, 887t

  osteomyelitis, 416t
  pneumonia, 681
  prostatitis, 727
  Shiga-toxin (STEC), 471
  urinary tract, 724, 727
Escherichia coli O157:H7, 353t, 390
Escitalopram, dosage and adverse effects of, 964t
Esmolol, for aortic dissection, 655t
Esophageal cancer, **320**
  treatment of, 321
Esophageal disorders
  dysphagia in, 204–206
  inflammation, 205–206
  motility disorders, 204–205
Esophageal pain, 133, 134f
Esophageal rupture, 134f
Esophageal spasm
  dysphagia in, 204–205
  treatment of, 205
Esophagitis
  in AIDS, 206
  candidal, 205–206
  GI bleeding in, 215
  herpes simplex virus, 522
  pill-related, 206
  viral, 205
    treatment of, 205
Esophagogastric varices, 215, **770**
  treatment of, 217, 771
Esophagogastroscopy, 770
Esophagus
  Barrett's, 200
  nutcracker, 205
Estradiol
  for abnormal uterine bleeding, 839
  for hypopituitarism, 812
  for menopausal symptoms, 845
Estramustine, for prostate cancer, 339
Estrogens
  conjugated
    for abnormal uterine bleeding, 839
    for amenorrhea, 842
    for menopausal symptoms, 845
  for hyperprolactinemia, 810
  for hypopituitarism, 812
Etanercept
  for ankylosing spondylitis, 789
  for psoriasis, 259
  for psoriatic arthritis, 792
  for rheumatoid arthritis, 783
Ethacrynic acid, for edema, 196t
Ethambutol
  for nontuberculous mycobacterial infections, 504–505
  for tuberculosis, 498
Ethanol therapy
  for ethylene glycol poisoning, 83
  for methanol poisoning, 85
Ethinylestradiol, for GI telangiectases, 217
Ethosuximide, for seizures, 880t–881t, 882t
Ethylene glycol poisoning, 83

Etoposide
  for extragonadal germ cell tumor, 343
  for testicular cancer, 333
Eustachian tube dysfunction, 245
Exanthem subitum, 527
Exchange transfusion, 17
  for malaria, 570
Excoriation, 256
Exemestane, for breast cancer, 318
Exercise testing
  in coronary artery disease, 631
  after myocardial infarction, 630
Expiratory reserve volume, 663f
External otitis, 475
Extracorporeal shockwave lithotripsy, 750
Extrapyramidal side effects, 968–969,
    986t
Eye disease, **241**
  assessment of, 241
  double vision, **171,** 241
  drug-induced, 987t
  herpes simplex infections, 521
  infection, 242
  inflammation, 242
  in inflammatory bowel disease, 743
  larva migrans, 581
  in malnutrition, 4
  Pseudomonas aeruginosa infections,
    475
  in reactive arthritis, 792
  red/painful eye, 241–242
    causes of, 241t
    treatment of, 241
  in rheumatoid arthritis, 781
  in sarcoidosis, 803
  toxoplasmosis, 579
  visual loss
    acute, **171,** 241–242
    chronic, 242–244
Eye movements, in confusion and coma,
    57
Eye trauma, 241–242
Ezetimibe, for hyperlipidemia, 859t

Facial diplegia, 925
Facial myokymia, 922
Facial nerve (VII), 870–871
  disorders of, **921**
    Bell's palsy, 922
Facial numbness, 920
Facial pain, 141t, 147, 920
Facial weakness, **921**
  bilateral, 922
Facioscapulohumeral dystrophy, **947**
Factitious illness, 961
Factor VIII replacement, 277
Facultative anaerobes, 489
Faintness, **164,** 168
Famciclovir
  for genital herpes, 406
  for herpes simplex virus infections,
    523, 524t–525t
  for herpes zoster, 527
  for viral meningitis, 892

Familial polyposis coli (FPC), 324, 325t
Famotidine, for erosive gastropathy,
    740
Fanconi syndrome, 722t
Fanning, 872
Farmer's lung, 674
Fasciculations, 872
Fascioliasis, 587
Fatigue, 944
  chronic fatigue syndrome, 952–954
Fatty liver, 767
Fecal occult blood test, 214, 282t, 327,
    993t
Fecal specimen, parasite diagnosis, 358–
    360, 359t
Feeding tube, 14
Felbamate, for seizures, 882t
Female infertility, **845**
  causes of, 845, 846f
  treatment of, 846
Fenofibrate, for hyperlipidemia, 859t
Fenoprofen, for pain, 26t
Fenoterol, for asthma, 669
Fentanyl
  abuse of, **975**
  for pain, 25, 27t
Ferriman-Gallwey score, 842
Fever, **156**
  cancer treatment-related, 104
    treatment of, 104
  clinical features of, 157–158
  definitions, 156–157
  diagnosis and treatment of febrile neu-
    tropenia, 419–420, 420f
  drug-induced, 980t
  with rash, 158
  in returned traveler, 372
Fever of unknown origin (FUO), **156**
  approach to, 158, 159f
  classic, 156–157
  HIV-associated, 157
  neutropenic, 157, 419–420, 420f
  nosocomial, 156–157
  treatment of, 158
Fexofenadine, for allergic rhinitis, 775
Fiber, dietary, 213
  for diverticular disease, 747
  for irritable bowel syndrome, 746
Fibric acid derivatives, for hyperlipid-
    emia, 859t, 860–861
Fibrinolytic agents, 279
Fibrinolytic therapy
  for myocardial infarction, 622–623,
    623f
  for pulmonary embolism, 687
Fibromyalgia, **800**
  depression and, 956
  pain in, 162f
  treatment of, 801
Fifth disease, 543
Filariasis, **584**
  lymphatic, 584
    treatment of, 584
  nocturnally periodic forms, 584

Filariasis (*Cont.*):
  onchocerciasis, 585
  subperiodic forms, 584
Finasteride
  for prostate cancer prevention, 283
  for prostate hyperplasia, 338
Fire coral, 110
Fisher syndrome, 941
Fish oils, for hyperlipidemia, 859t
Fitz-Hugh-Curtis syndrome, 397
Fixed drug eruption, 981t
Flea-borne typhus fever, **512**
Flecainide, for arrhythmias, 646t
Floxuridine, for colorectal cancer, 327
Flu. *See* Influenza
Fluconazole, 555–556
  for blastomycosis, 563
  for candidiasis, 206, 395t, 558
  for coccidioidomycosis, 563
  for cryptococcosis, 560
Fludarabine, for chronic lymphocytic leukemia/lymphoma, 299
Fludrocortisone
  for Addison's disease, 826
  for adrenal insufficiency, 103
  distinguishing types of hyperkalemia, 9
  for hypoaldosteronism, 827
  for orthostatic hypotension, 931
  for septic shock, 51
Fluid restriction
  for ascites, 225
  for heart failure, 649
  for hyponatremia, 345
  for syndrome of inappropriate ADH, 815
Fluid therapy
  for ARDS, 40
  for cholera, 384
  for diabetic ketoacidosis, 90t
  for hyperglycemic hyperosmolar state, 91
  for nephrolithiasis, 733
  for septic shock, 51
Flumazenil
  for anticonvulsant poisoning, 79
  for benzodiazepine poisoning, 80
  for hepatic encephalopathy, 772
Flunisolide, for asthma, 671
Fluoroquinolones
  for animal bite, 107t, 108t
  for diarrhea, 369
  for HACEK endocarditis, 469t
  mechanisms, indications, and adverse effects of, 364
5-Fluorouracil (5-FU)
  for anal cancer, 328
  for carcinoid tumor, 329
  for cervical cancer, 337
  for cervical node metastasis, 343
  for esophageal cancer, 321
  for gastric cancer, 322
  for head and neck cancer, 310
  for hypersomnia, 185
  for Zollinger-Ellison syndrome, 741

Fluoxetine
  for bulimia nervosa, 970
  dosage and adverse effects of, 964t
  for hypersomnia, 185
  for obsessive-compulsive disorder, 960
  for panic disorder, 959
  for systemic sclerosis, 784
Fluphenazine
  dosage and adverse effects of, 967t
  for schizophrenia, 958
Flurazepam, dosage and adverse effects of, 966t
Flutamide, for prostate cancer, 339
Fluticasone, for allergic rhinitis, 775
Fluticasone/salmeterol, for asthma, 670t, 671
Fluvastatin, for hyperlipidemia, 859t
Fluvoxamine
  dosage and adverse effects of, 964t
  for obsessive-compulsive disorder, 960
Folate deficiency
  anemia and, 269
  treatment of, 271
Follicle-stimulating hormone, 807
Follicular center lymphoma, 300
  treatment of, 300
Folliculitis, 256f, 409
  hot-tub, 409, 475
  Staphylococcus aureus, 449
Fomepizole
  for ethylene glycol poisoning, 83
  for methanol poisoning, 85
Fondaparimax, for thrombotic disorders, 279
Food poisoning
  bacterial, 384
  staphylococcal, 451
Foot, muscles and innervation of, 868t–869t
Foramen magnum
  compressive lesions of, 918
  lesions near, 934
Forced expiratory volume in 1 s, 663, 665t
Forced vital capacity, 663, 665t
Forearm, muscles and innervation of, 868t–869t
Formoterol, for asthma, 670t
Fosamprenavir, for HIV infections, 435t
Foscarnet
  for cytomegalovirus infections, 531
  for herpes simplex virus infections, 525t
Fosphenytoin, for status epilepticus, 72, 73f
Fracture
  in osteoporosis, 852–854
  pain in, 162f
Francisella tularensis infection, 106, 124. *See also* Tularemia
Fresh-frozen plasma (FFP), 17, 19
  for thrombotic thrombocytopenic purpura, 277
Friedreich's ataxia, 915, 917

Frostbite, **116**
  treatment of, 117, 117t
Frozen shoulder, 802
Functional residual capacity, 663f
Fungal infection, **555**
  diagnosis of, **351**, 355t
  treatment of, **555**
Furazolidone, for giardiasis, 386
Furosemide
  for ascites, 225
  for edema, 196t
  for heart failure, 626, 649
  for hypercalcemia, 345, 849t
  for hyperkalemia, 10t
  for myocardial infarction, 628t
  for pulmonary edema, 54
  for syndrome of inappropriate ADH,
    103
Furuncle, 449
Fusariosis, **564**
  treatment of, 564
Fusion inhibitors, 436t
Fusobacterium infection, 489–491
  meningitis, 891t

Gabapentin
  for generalized anxiety disorder, 959
  for pain, 25
  for seizures, 882t
Gag reflex, 872
Gait analysis, **873**
Galactorrhea, drug-induced, 980t
Galantamine, for Alzheimer's disease,
    908–909
Gallbladder
  calcified, 750
  porcelain, 750
Gallstones, 749–751
Gametocyte, *Plasmodium*, 569
Gamma radiation, 129
Ganciclovir
  for cytomegalovirus infections, 530–
    531
  for viral esophagitis, 205
Gardner's syndrome, 324–325, 325t
Gas exchange, disturbances of, 665–666
Gas gangrene, 488
  treatment of, 410t–411t
Gastric atrophy, 740
Gastric bypass surgery, 830
Gastric cancer, **321**
  staging of, 323t
  treatment of, 322
Gastric lavage, 77
Gastric pain, 133f
Gastric tumors, benign, **322**
Gastrinoma, 329, **740**
Gastritis
  atrophic, 740
  chronic, **740**
  superficial, 740
  treatment of, 217
  type A, 740
  type B, 740

Gastroesophageal reflux disease (GERD),
    198
  insomnia and, 183
  treatment of, 200
Gastrointestinal bleeding, **214**
  in colonic angiodysplasia, 748
  in diverticular disease, 747
  esophagogastric varices, 215, 770–771
  lower, 216–217
    causes of, 216
    evaluation of, 216–217, 216f
    treatment of, 217
  of obscure origin, 217
  upper, 215–216
    causes of, 215
    evaluation of, 215–216, 215f
    treatment of, 217
Gastrointestinal cancer, **320**
  anal cancer, 328
  colorectal cancer, 326–327
  esophageal cancer, 320–321
  gastric cancer, 321–322
  hepatocellular carcinoma, 328
  pancreatic cancer, 328
Gastrointestinal decontamination, 77
Gastrointestinal disease. *See also specific*
    diseases
  alcoholic liver disease, 767–768, 973
  in amyloidosis, 805
  anorectal disease, 748–749
  cholecystitis
    acute, 751
    chronic, 751–752
  choledocholithiasis/cholangitis, 752
  cholelithiasis, 749–751
  cirrhosis, 766–768
  clostridial, 488
  colonic angiodysplasia, 748
  diverticular disease, 747
  drug-induced, 985t–986t
  endocrine tumors, 329–331, 330t
  gastropathies, 740
  hepatic failure, acute, 761–762
  hepatitis
    acute, 757–761
    chronic, 762–766
  infectious, in immunocompromised
    host, 419
  inflammatory bowel disease, 742–746
  intestinal pseudoobstruction, 747–748
  irritable bowel syndrome, 746–747
  listerial, 465
  measles, 540
  osteoporosis and, 853t
  pancreatitis, 753–756
  peptic ulcer, 737–739
  pleural effusion in, 692t
  portal hypertension, 769–772
  primary biliary cirrhosis, 768
  primary sclerosing cholangitis, 752–
    753
  reference values for laboratory tests,
    1009t
  in systemic sclerosis, 783

Gastrointestinal disease (*Cont.*):
    travel advice, 366, 369
    tuberculosis, 497
    vascular, 748
    weight loss in, 201t
    Zollinger-Ellison syndrome, 740–741
Gastrointestinal procedures, endocarditis
        prophylaxis for, 378t, 379t
Gastrointestinal tract, functions of, 208
Gastroparesis, 198
Gastropathy, **740**
    erosive, 740
        treatment of, 740
    GI bleeding in, 215
Gastroplasty, vertically banded, 830
Gatifloxacin
    for pneumococcal infections, 447
    for pneumonia, 680t–681t, 682t
    for tuberculosis, 498
Gefitinib, for bronchoalveolar carcinoma,
        314t, 316
Gemcitabine
    for bladder cancer, 332
    for breast cancer, 320
    for pancreatic cancer, 328
Gemfibrozil, for hyperlipidemia, 859t
Generalized anxiety disorder, **959**
    treatment of, 959
Generalized tonic-clonic status epilepti-
        cus, 72
Genital herpes, 396–397, **406,** 521, 524t
Genital warts, **749**
Genitourinary cancer, **331**
    bladder cancer, 331–332
    renal cancer, 332–333
    testicular cancer, 333–334
Genitourinary disease, infectious, in im-
        munocompromised host, 419
Genitourinary procedures, endocarditis
        prophylaxis for, 378t, 379t
Gentamicin
    for *Abiotrophia* infections, 460
    for bacterial meningitis, 890t, 891t
    for *Bartonella* infections, 484t
    for brucellosis, 480
    for endocarditis, 375, 376t–377t
    for endocarditis prophylaxis, 379t
    for enterococcal infections, 459
    for gram-positive sepsis, 96t
    for HACEK endocarditis, 469t
    for listeriosis, 466
    for necrotizing fasciitis, 98t
    for pelvic inflammatory disease, 398
    for plague, 120t, 483
    for *Pseudomonas aeruginosa* infec-
        tions, 476t
    for sepsis, 52t
    for septic arthritis, 458
    for tularemia, 121t, 481
    for urinary tract infections, 726t
German measles. *See* Rubella
Germ cell tumor, extragonadal, unrecog-
        nized, 343
Germinoma, 884

Giant cell arteritis, 786, 788
    headache in, 142t
    visual loss in, 173
Giardiasis, 385–386, 399
    diagnosis of, 359t
    treatment of, 386
Gilbert's syndrome, 220
Gingivitis
    anaerobic infection, 489
    necrotizing ulcerative, 489
Gingivostomatitis, herpes simplex virus,
        520
Ginkgo biloba, 909
Glanders, 477
Glatiramer acetate, for multiple sclerosis,
        901
Glaucoma, 172f, 243
    acute angle-closure, 242
        treatment of, 242
    drug-induced, 987t
    headache in, 142t
    treatment of, 243
Glimepiride, for diabetes mellitus, 833t
Glipizide, for diabetes mellitus, 833t
Global aphasia, 180, 180t
Globulin, blood test, 222
Globus pharyngeus, 203
Glomerular disease, **713**
Glomerular filtration rate (GFR), 227
    in tubulointerstitial disease, 722t
Glomerulonephritis
    acute, 699, **713**
        causes of, 714t
    azotemia in, 228f
    chronic, 720
    drug-induced, 715t
    membranoproliferative, **717**
    membranous, **716**
    postinfectious, **714**
    poststreptococcal, 455, **714**
    rapidly progressing, 699, **715**
        causes of, 715t
Glomerulosclerosis, focal, **717**
Glossopharyngeal neuralgia, 166t, **923**
    treatment of, 923
Glucagonoma, 329, 330t
Glucagon therapy, for beta-blocker poi-
        soning, 81
Glucocorticoids. *See also specific drugs*
    for acute renal failure, 706
    for adhesive capsulitis, 802
    adverse effects of, 827–828, 828t
    for anaphylaxis, 105
    for ankylosing spondylitis, 790
    for asthma, 670t, 671
    for atopic dermatitis, 260
    for chronic inflammatory demyelinating
        polyneuropathy, 941
    clinical uses of, 827–828, 828t
    for COPD, 677, 677t
    for cysticercosis, 588
    for Epstein-Barr virus infections, 533
    for fever, 158
    for glomerulonephritis, 716–717

Glucocorticoids (*Cont.*):
  for gout, 797
  for Hymenoptera stings, 114
  for hypercalcemia, 103
  for hypersensitivity pneumonitis, 673
  for inflammatory bowel disease, 744, 744t–745t
  for inflammatory myopathies, 948
  for leprosy, 503
  for lichen planus, 260
  for meningococcal infections, 463
  for osteoarthritis, 795
  for pityriasis rosea, 259
  for *Pneumocystis* infections, 567
  preparations, 827t
  for psoriasis, 259
  for reactive arthritis, 793
  for respiratory failure, 678
  for rheumatoid arthritis, 783
  for sarcoidosis, 804
  for SARS, 537
  for seborrheic dermatitis, 261
  for Sjögren's syndrome, 785
  for systemic lupus erythematosus, 781
  for systemic mastocytosis, 776
  for systemic sclerosis, 784
  for tendinitis, 802
  for toxoplasmosis, 579
  for trichinellosis, 581
  for urticaria/angioedema, 774
  for vertigo, 170t
Glucosamine and chondroitin, for osteoarthritis, 795
Glucose
  blood, 830
  for cardiac glycoside poisoning, 82
  for hypoglycemia, 94
Glucose-lowering agents, oral, for diabetes mellitus, 832, 833t
Glucose-6-phosphate dehydrogenase deficiency, 270
  drugs causing hemolysis in, 270t
γ-Glutamyltranspeptidase, 222
Glyburide, for diabetes mellitus, 833t
Glycogen storage disease, 948
Glycolytic defects, 948
Goiter, 811, 816
  nontoxic, **820**
  substernal, 820
  toxic nodular, **821**
Gold compounds, for rheumatoid arthritis, 783
Gonadotropin(s), 807, 809t
  deficiency of, 811–812
  for female infertility, 846
  hypersecretion of, 811
  replacement therapy, 812t
Gonadotropin-releasing hormone (GnRH) deficiency, 835
Gonadotropin-secreting tumor, **811**
Gonorrhea, **399**
  anorectal, 399
  ocular, 400
  pharyngeal, 253, 400

  in pregnancy, 400
  treatment of, 400, 401t
  urethritis in men, 393–396
Goodpasture's syndrome, **690, 714,** 719t
Goserelin, for prostate cancer, 339
Gout, **796**
  acute gouty arthritis, 796–797
  clinical features of, 796–797
  evaluation of, 797
  pain in, 162f
  treatment of, 797–798
Gouty arthritis, 796–797
Graft-versus-host disease, 688t
  transfusion-related, 18, 18t
Grain dust exposure, 674
Gram-negative enteric bacteria, infections caused by, **471**
Gram's stain, 351
Granulocyte colony-stimulating factor (G-CSF), indications for, 288, 289t
Granulocyte-macrophage colony-stimulating factor (GM-CSF), indications for, 288, 289t
Granuloma, eosinophilic, **690**
Granulomatous disease, monocytosis in, 273
Graphesthesia, 873
Graves' disease, 818
Graves' ophthalmopathy, 950
Griseofulvin, 555
  for dermatophyte infections, 262
Growth hormone, 807, 809t
  deficiency of, 811–812
  hypersecretion of, 810–811
  replacement therapy, 812t
Growth hormone-releasing hormone-secreting tumor, 810
Growth hormone-secreting tumor, 807, 809
Guillain-Barré syndrome, 925, 930, 939–941
Gumma, 404
Guttate lesion, 255
Gynecologic cancer, **334**
  cervical, 337
  endometrial, 335–337
  ovarian, 334–335
Gynecomastia
  drug-induced, 980t
  paraneoplastic, 344t

HAART regimen, 438–439
HACEK organisms, **470**
  infective endocarditis, 377t
  treatment of, 469t
Haemophilus. See HACEK organisms
Haemophilus ducreyi infection. *See* Chancroid
Haemophilus influenzae infection, **466**
  from animal bites, 107t
  epiglottitis, 253, 467
  meningitis, 466–467, 887t, 891t
  nosocomial, 443
  pneumonia, 467, 679

Haemophilus influenzae infection (*Cont.*):
　prevention of, 467
　sinusitis, 249
　treatment of, 467
Haemophilus influenzae type b vaccine,
　　367f, 467
　in immunocompromised patients, 423t
Haemophilus parainfluenzae infection,
　　epiglottitis, 254
Hair, in malnutrition, 4
Hallucinations, **957**
　drug-induced, 988t
　hypnogogic, 184t, 185
Hallucinogens, poisoning, 83
Haloperidol
　for Alzheimer's disease, 909
　dosage and adverse effects of, 967t
　for nausea and vomiting, 198
　for schizophrenia, 958
　for tics, 179
Haloprogin, for dermatophyte infections,
　　262
Hand, muscles and innervation of, 868t–
　　869t
Hand-foot-and-mouth disease, 545
Hand hygiene, 442
Hantaan virus, 551
Hantavirus pulmonary syndrome, **551**
HDL cholesterol, 855, 856t
　classification of, 1004t
　patient goals, 861
Headache, **139**
　classification of, 140t–141t
　cluster, 140t, 144–146
　cough, 147
　drug-induced, 986t
　lumbar puncture, 146–147
　migraine, 139–144, 173
　post-concussion, 146
　serious causes of, 142t
　symptoms that suggest underlying dis-
　　order, 142t
　tension, 140t, 144
Head and neck cancer, **309**
　local disease, 310
　locally advanced disease, 310
　paraneoplastic syndromes, 344t
　prevention of, 284
　recurrent or metastatic, 310
　risk factors for, 284
　treatment of, 310
Head and neck region infection
　actinomycosis, 494
　anaerobic, 489–490
Head louse, 590–591
Head trauma, **67**
　headache in, 140t
Health care workers
　HIV infection and, 441
　narcotic abuse in, 975, 977
Health maintenance, **991**
Hearing aid, 247–248
Hearing disorders, **244**
　approach to, 244, 246f
　audiologic assessment, 244

　imaging studies in, 245
　prevention of, 248
　treatment of, 247–248
Hearing loss
　causes of, 245–247
　conductive, 245
　drug-induced, 245, 987t
　noise-induced, 248
　sensorineural, 245–246
Heart, physical examination of, **593**
Heart block, **645**
　first degree, 639f, 645
　second degree, 639f
　　Mobitz I, 645
　　Mobitz II, 645
　third degree, 639f, 645–648
Heartburn, **198**
Heart disease. *See also* Cardiovascular
　　disease; *specific diseases*
　in amyloidosis, 805
　arrhythmias, 638–648
　cardiomyopathy, 609–612
　congenital, echocardiography in, 603
　coronary artery disease, 631–637
　cor pulmonale, 652
　depression and, 956
　dyspnea in, 186
　echocardiography in, 596–603
　electrocardiography in, 596–603
　endocarditis prophylaxis and, 379t
　heart failure, 648–651
　myocardial infarction. *See* Myocardial
　　infarction
　myocarditis, 612
　pericardial disease, 612–616
　physical examination of heart, 593–596
　prevention of, 992t–993t
　valvular, 603–608
　weight loss in, 201t
Heart failure, **648**
　ascites in, 226t
　conditions that mimic, 648–649
　drug-induced, 984t
　edema in, 194, 195f, 196
　laboratory evaluation of, 648
　precipitating factors, 648
　preoperative evaluation of, 36
　treatment of, 626, 649–651, 649t, 651t
Heart murmur, 595–596, 595t, 596f
　diastolic, 595–596, 595t
　systolic, 595, 595t
Heart sounds, 594–595, 594f
　ejection clicks, 595
　first, 594
　fourth, 595
　midsystolic clicks, 595
　opening snap, 595
　second, 594
　third, 595
Heart transplant, infections in transplant
　　recipients, 422
Heat stroke, 160
　drug-induced, 160
　exertional, 160
　nonexertional, 160

Heerfordt-Waldenström syndrome, 803
Height, ideal weight for, 3t
Heimlich maneuver, 41
Heinz bodies, 265
Helicobacter pylori infection
  detection of, 738, 738t
  eradication of, 738, 739t
  in lymphoid malignancies, 298
  peptic ulcer disease, 737
Helminthic infection, **580**
  cestodes, 587–590
  nematodes, 580–585
  trematodes, 585–587
Hemapheresis, therapeutic, **19**
Hematemesis, 214
Hematin, for porphyria, 863
Hematochezia, 214
Hematologic disease. *See also specific*
    diseases
  in alcoholism, 973
  in amyloidosis, 805
  blood smear, 265
  bone marrow examination, 266–267
  drug-induced, 982t–983t
  neutropenia in, 274
  osteoporosis and, 853t
  reference values for laboratory tests,
    995t–996t
  in rheumatoid arthritis, 781
  in systemic lupus erythematosus,
    780
Hematopoiesis, extramedullary, 238t
Hematopoietic cell transplant
  for chronic lymphocytic leukemia/
    lymphoma, 300
  for follicular center lymphoma, 300
Hematuria, 232, 701, 718t
  approach to, 231f
  causes of, 229t
  gross, 232
  microscopic, 232
Heme albumin, for porphyria, 863
Heme arginate, for porphyria, 863
Hemianopia
  bilateral, 172f
  right homonymous, 172f
Hemifacial spasm, 922
Hemiparesis, 58–59, 176t
Hemochromatosis, **861**
  approach to, 862, 863f
  hereditary, 861
  treatment of, 862
Hemodiafiltration, 706
Hemodialysis, 709–710
  for acute renal failure, 706
  complications of, 710, 710t
  intermittent, 706
  rewarming by, 116
Hemoglobin, abnormal, 192–193, 193t
Hemolytic anemia
  classification of, 269t
  drug-induced, 983t
  macroangiopathic, 271
  microangiopathic, 271

Hemolytic disorders, jaundice in, 218t
Hemolytic-uremic syndrome, **730**
Hemophilia A, 276
  treatment of, 277
Hemophilia B, 276
  treatment of, 277
Hemoptysis, **189**
  approach to, 190–191, 191f
  differential diagnosis of, 190t
  massive, 191
  treatment of, 191–192
Hemorrhage. *See specific types and sites*
Hemorrhagic fevers, viral, **550**
  as bioweapons, 121t, 124
  with renal syndrome, 551
  treatment of, 121t
Hemorrhoids, **748**
Hemosiderosis, idiopathic pulmonary,
  690
Hemothorax, 691
Henoch-Schönlein purpura, 786
  renal disease in, 715, 719t
Heparin
  for arterial embolism, 656
  for deep venous thrombosis, 657, 687
  for deep venous thrombosis prevention,
    658
  low-molecular-weight, 278t
    for acute coronary syndromes, 635
    for stroke, 61
  for myocardial infarction, 623, 624f,
    625
  for pulmonary embolism, 686–687
  for stroke, 61
  for thrombotic disorders, 278–279
  unfractionated, 278, 278t
    for acute coronary syndromes, 635
Heparin-induced thrombocytopenia, 275
  treatment of, 277
Hepatic encephalopathy, **772**
  treatment of, 772
Hepatic failure
  acute, **761**
    treatment of, 762
  fulminant, 67
Hepatitis
  acute, **757**
  alcoholic, 767
  autoimmune, **764**
    treatment of, 766
    type I, 764
    type II, 764
    type III, 764
  chronic, **762**
  toxic/drug-induced, **761**, 762
    treatment of, 761
  viral, **757**
    treatment of, 761
Hepatitis A
  acute, **757**, 758t
    clinical and laboratory features of,
    759f
  prevention of, 757

Hepatitis A vaccine, 367f, 368f, 370f,
 371t, 757, 766
 in immunocompromised patients, 423t
Hepatitis B, 788
 acute, **757,** 758t
  clinical and laboratory features of, 759f
 chronic, **762**
  treatment of, 763, 764t
 hepatocellular carcinoma and, 328
 prevention of, 759
Hepatitis B vaccine, 367f, 368f, 370f,
 371t, 759–760
 in immunocompromised patients, 423t
Hepatitis C, 788
 acute, 758t, **759**
  prevention of, 760
  serologic course of, 760f
 chronic, 762, **763,** 956
  treatment of, 764, 765t
 hepatocellular carcinoma and, 328
Hepatitis D
 acute, 758t, **760**
 chronic, 762
Hepatitis E, acute, 758t, **760**
Hepatobiliary imaging, **223**
Hepatocellular carcinoma, **328**
Hepatomegaly, **220**
Hepatorenal syndrome, 227
Herniated disc, 935
 cervical, 156
Heroin abuse, **975**
Herpangina, 545
Herpes B virus, 106
Herpes gladiatorum, 521
Herpes labialis, 258f
Herpes simplex, 261
Herpes simplex virus infection, **520**
 acyclovir-resistant, 525t
 diagnosis of, 522
 encephalitis, 891t, 894
 epidemiology of, 520
 genital, 396–397, **406,** 521, 524t
  treatment of, 406
 herpes gladiatorum, 521
 keratitis, 242
 meningitis, 891t
 neonatal, 522, 525t
 neurologic, 521–522, 525t
 ocular, 521
 oral-facial, 520–521, 524t
 prevention of, 523
 proctitis, 399
 treatment of, 522–523, 524t–525t
 urethritis, 393
 urethritis/urethral syndrome in women,
  396
 urinary tract, 724
 visceral, 522, 525t
 whitlow, 521, 524t
Herpesvirus infection, **520**
Herpes zoster, 256f, 261, **526**
 complications of, 526
 neck pain in, 154
 treatment of, 410t–411t, 527

Herpetiform lesion, 255
Heterophile test, 532
Hirsutism
 drug-induced, 842
 in female, **842**
  approach to, 843, 844f
  treatment of, 843
Histamine blockers, for carcinoid tumor,
 329
Histiocytosis X, **690**
Histoplasmosis, **561**
 acute pulmonary, 561
 chronic pulmonary, 561–562
 disseminated, 562
 mediastinal fibrosis, 561
 meningitis, 897t
 treatment of, 562
Histrionic personality, 962
HIV/AIDS, **424**
 advanced HIV disease, 426
 aspergillosis and, 559
 clinical features of, 425–426
  acute retroviral syndrome, 425–426,
   437
  asymptomatic infection, 437
  symptomatic disease, 437–438
 cryptococcosis and, 560
 cytomegalovirus infection and, 530
 definition of AIDS, 424
 depression and, 956
 diagnosis of HIV infection, 426–427,
  427f
 diarrhea in, 210t
 encephalitis in, 893
 epidemiology of, 425
 esophagitis in, 206
 establishment of chronic/persistent infection, 426
 etiology of, 424–425
 fever of unknown origin in, 157
 health care workers and, 441
 immune abnormalities in, 426
 immune response to HIV infection,
  426
 laboratory monitoring of, 427, 437
 lymphoma in, 302
 meningitis in, 891t, 898
 nontuberculous mycobacterial infections in, 504
 pathophysiology and immunopathoge-
  nesis of, 425–426
 penicilliosis marneffei and, 564
 Pneumocystis infection and, 566–568
 prevention of, 441, 992t
 primary infection, 425–426
 progressive multifocal leukoencephalopathy in, 895
 risk factors for, 425
 screening for HIV infection, 426
 sepsis in, treatment of, 52t
 toxoplasmosis and, 579–580
 travel advice for infected traveler, 369–
  371

HIV/AIDS (*Cont.*):
　treatment of
　　antiretroviral drugs, 428t–436t, 438–439
　　indications to change antiretroviral therapy, 440t
　　principles of, 440t
　　prophylaxis against secondary infections, 440–441
　　tuberculosis and, 497
　　in women, 990
HIV vaccine, 441
HMG-CoA reductase inhibitors
　for acute coronary syndromes, 637
　for hyperlipidemia, 859t, 860–861
Hodgkin's disease, 297t, **304**
　EBV-associated, 532
　paraneoplastic syndromes, 348t
　staging of, 305–306, 306t
　treatment of, 306
Homicide, 992t
Hookworm, **582**
　treatment of, 582
Hormone replacement therapy, for menopausal symptoms, 843
Hospital-acquired infection. *See* Nosocomial infections
Hospitalized patient, care of
　acid-base balance, 5–14
　admission orders, **1**
　critical care medicine, 19–22
　electrolyte balance, 5–14
　enteral nutrition, 14–17
　imaging, **32**
　nutritional assessment, 2–4
　pain and pain management, 23–27
　parenteral nutrition, 14–17
　procedures performed by internists, **28**
　respiratory failure, 21–23
　surgical patient, evaluation of, **34**
　transfusion and pheresis therapy, 17–19
Howell-Jolly bodies, 265
Human bite
　clenched-fist injury, 107t, 109
　occlusional, 107t, 109
Human chorionic gonadotropin
　for hypopituitarism, 812
　in testicular cancer, 333
Human herpesvirus 6, **527**
Human herpesvirus 7, **527**
Human herpesvirus 8, **527**
　in lymphoid malignancies, 298
Human immunodeficiency virus infection. *See* HIV/AIDS
Human papillomavirus (HPV) infection, 407
　treatment of, 407–408
Human T-lymphotropic virus type I, in lymphoid malignancies, 298
Huntington's disease, 907, **909**
Hydatid cyst, 589
Hydralazine
　for dilated cardiomyopathy, 609
　for heart failure, 650–651, 651t
　for mitral regurgitation, 605

Hydrocephalus
　normal-pressure, 904, 907, 909
　obstructive, 67
　in subarachnoid hemorrhage, 66
Hydrochloric acid, for metabolic alkalosis, 13
Hydrochlorothiazide, for edema, 196t
Hydrocodone, for hemoptysis, 191
Hydrocortisone
　for Addison's disease, 826
　for adrenal insufficiency, 103
　for chronic fatigue syndrome, 954
　for hypopituitarism, 812
　for inflammatory bowel disease, 744
　for meningococcal infections, 463
　for myxedema coma, 817
　for septic shock, 51
Hydrofludrocortisone, for syncope, 167
Hydroid envenomations, 110
Hydromorphone
　abuse of, **975**
　for pain, 26t
Hydronephrosis, 228f, 734
Hydrotherapy, for low back pain, 151
Hydroxyapatite arthropathy, **798**
Hydroxychloroquine
　for porphyria, 864
　for Q fever, 516
　for rheumatoid arthritis, 783
　for Sjögren's syndrome, 785
　for systemic lupus erythematosus, 781
Hydroxyprogesterone
　for abnormal uterine bleeding, 839
　for endometrial cancer, 337
Hydroxyurea
　for cervical cancer, 337
　for essential thrombocytosis, 296
　for sickle cell anemia, 271
Hydroxyzine
　for ciguatera poisoning, 111
　for urticaria/angioedema, 774
Hymenoptera sting, **114**
　treatment of, 114
Hyoscyamine, for irritable bowel syndrome, 746
Hyperalgesia, 24
Hyperbaric oxygen therapy
　for carbon monoxide poisoning, 71
　for clostridial infections, 489
Hyperbilirubinemia
　causes of, 218, 218t
　drug-induced, 980t
Hypercalcemia, **847**
　causes of, 847–848, 847t
　differential diagnosis of, 848t
　drug-induced, 980t
　familial hypocalciuric, 848, 850
　paraneoplastic, 103, 344t, 345, 847, 847t, 848t, 850
　treatment of, 103, 848–850, 849t
Hypercalciuria, 848
Hypercapnia, 666
Hyperchloremic acidosis, 722t

Hypercholesterolemia, **855**
  approach to, 857, 858f, 859t
  familial, 856t, 857
  with hypertriglyceridemia, 856t, **860**
  isolated, 856t, **857**
  polygenic, 856t, 857
  treatment of, 857, 858f, 859t
Hypercoagulable state, 277–280
  treatment of, 278–279, 278t, 280f
Hyperesthesia, 24
Hyperglycemia, drug-induced, 980t
Hyperglycemic hyperosmolar state, **90**
  laboratory feature of, 89t
  treatment of, 91
Hyperhidrosis, primary, 930
Hyper-IgE syndrome, 779
Hyperkalemia, 8–9
  causes of, 8t
  drug-induced, 980t
  electrocardiogram in, 9, 9f
  treatment of, 10t, 708
  in tubulointerstitial disease, 722t
Hyperlipidemia, **855**, 856t
  combined, 856t, **860**
Hyperlipoproteinemia, **855**
Hypermagnesemia, **852**
Hypernatremia, 6–7
  treatment of, 6–7, 6t
Hyperosmolar coma, **89**
Hyperoxaluria, 732
Hyperparathyroidism
  familial, 847
  primary, 847–848
  secondary, 848, 850, 855
  tertiary, 848, 850
Hyperpathia, 930, 938
Hyperphosphatemia, 850, **851**
  treatment of, 708
Hyperpigmentation, drug-induced, 981t
Hyperprolactinemia, **809**
  treatment of, 810
Hyperpyrexia, drug-induced, 980t
Hypersensitivity disorder, immediate type,
    773
  allergic rhinitis, 774–775
  angioedema, 773–774
  systemic mastocytosis, 775–776
  urticaria, 773–774
Hypersensitivity pneumonitis, **672**, 688t
  treatment of, 673
Hypersomnia, **183**, 184t
  treatment of, 183–185
Hypersplenism, 271, 274
Hypertension, **616**
  approach to, 617–618
  definition of, 616
  in diabetes mellitus, 621
  drug-induced, 984t
  essential, 616
  isolated systolic, 616
  malignant, 621
    visual loss in, 173
  portal. *See* Portal hypertension
  in pregnancy, 621

  preoperative evaluation of, 36–37
  pulmonary. *See* Pulmonary hyperten-
      sion
  in renal failure, 708–709
    approach to, 700t, 702
  renovascular, 729–730
  secondary, **616**
    approach to, 617
    treatment of, 618–621, 618f–619f,
        620t
  in women, 989
Hyperthermia, **160**
  malignant, 160
  treatment of, 160
Hyperthyroidism
  depression and, 956
  insomnia in, 183
  muscle disease in, 950
  subclinical, 821
  with TSH-secreting adenoma, 811
Hypertransfusion therapy, 17
Hypertriglyceridemia, **855**
  in acute pancreatitis, 754
  familial, 856t, 860
  with hypercholesterolemia, 856t, **860**
  isolated, 856t, **857**
  treatment of, 860
Hypertrophic osteoarthropathy, **800**
  treatment of, 800
Hyperuricemia
  asymptomatic, 797
  drug-induced, 981t
Hyperventilation, **698**
  for increased intracranial pressure, 68,
      68t
Hyperviscosity state, treatment of, 19
Hypoalbuminemia, 850
  in acute pancreatitis, 754
Hypoaldosteronism, **827**
  hyporeninemic, 827
Hypoalgesia, 24
Hypocalcemia, **850**, 851
  in acute pancreatitis, 754
  treatment of, 850
Hypochondriasis, 961
Hypogammaglobulinemia of infancy,
    transient, 778
Hypoglossal nerve (XII), 872
  disorders of, 924
Hypoglycemia, **91**
  autoimmune, 93f
  diagnosis of, 91–92, 93f, 94t
  drug-induced, 980t
  fasting, 92
  paraneoplastic, 344t
  postprandial, 92
  reactive, 93f
  treatment of, 93–94
Hypogonadism
  hypogonadotropic, 835–836
  osteoporosis and, 853t
  primary, 835, 837
  secondary, 835

Hypokalemia, 8
  causes of, 7t
  drug-induced, 981t
  treatment of, 8
Hypolipidemic drugs, 859t
Hypomagnesemia, 850, **851**
  treatment of, 851
Hypomania, drug-induced, 988t
Hyponatremia, 5–7
  dilutional, 649
  drug-induced, 981t
  euvolemic, 5–6
  hypervolemic, 5
  hypovolemic, 5
  paraneoplastic, 345–346
  treatment of, 5–6
Hypoparathyroidism, 850–851
Hypophosphatemia, **850**
  treatment of, 851
Hypopituitarism, **811**
  treatment of, 812, 812t
Hypopnea, 697
Hypotension
  drug-induced, 984t
  myocardial infarction and, 627, 629f
  orthostatic. *See* Orthostatic hypotension
Hypothalamus, 808f
Hypothermia, **115**
  for hypoxic-ischemic encephalopathy,
    71
  neuroprotection in stroke, 61
  risk factors for, 115t
  treatment of, 116
Hypothyroidism, 815–817
  causes of, 815–816, 816t
  clinical (overt), 816
  dementia in, 907
  depression in, 956
  edema in, 195
  evaluation of, 816–817, 817f
  muscle disease in, 950
  subclinical (mild), 816
  treatment of, 817
Hypoventilation syndromes, **696**, 696t
  neuromuscular, 696t, 697
  obesity-hypoventilation, 696t, 697
  primary alveolar, 20, **695**, 696
Hypoxemia
  in acute pancreatitis, 754
  approach to, 664f
  mechanisms of, 666
  nocturnal, 697
Hypoxia, 71
  histotoxic, 69
  nocturnal, 697
Hypoxic-ischemic encephalopathy, **69**
  prognosis in, 70f
  treatment of, 71
Hysterectomy, for cervical cancer, 337

Ibuprofen
  for pain, 26t
  for systemic lupus erythematosus, 781
  for tension headache, 146t

Ibutilide, for arrhythmias, 641t
Icterus. *See* Jaundice
Idarubicin, for acute myeloid leukemia,
    292
Idebenone, for ataxia, 917
Idiopathic thrombocytopenic purpura
    (ITP), 275
  treatment of, 277
Ifosfamide, for cervical cancer, 337
IgA nephropathy, **720**
IgG subclass deficiency, 778
Illness-severity scales, 20
Imaging, diagnostic, **32**
Imatinib
  for chronic myeloid leukemia, 293
  for gastric cancer, 322
Imidazoles, 555
Imipenem
  for anaerobic infections, 491t
  for animal bites, 107t
  for diverticular disease, 747
  for enterococcal infections, 459
  for nocardiosis, 493t
  for peritonitis, 381
  for pneumonia, 680t–681t, 683t
Imipenem-cilastin
  for acute pancreatitis, 754
  for *Pseudomonas aeruginosa* infec-
    tions, 476t
  for sepsis, 52t
  for urinary tract infections, 726t
Imipramine
  dosage and adverse effects of, 964t
  for noncardiac chest pain, 204
  for pain, 27t
  for panic disorder, 959
Imiquimod, for human papillomavirus in-
    fections, 408
Immune-complex disorders, treatment of,
    19
Immune disease
  back pain in, 150
  renal, 721t
Immune globulin, intravenous
  for chronic inflammatory demyelinating
    polyneuropathy, 941
  for chronic lymphocytic leukemia/lym-
    phoma, 299
  for Guillain-Barré syndrome, 941
  for immunoglobulin deficiency, 779
  for inflammatory myopathies, 948
  for myasthenia gravis, 944
  for streptococcal toxic shock syndrome,
    458
  for toxic shock syndrome, 455
Immune hyperplasia, 238t
Immunization, **365**
  active, 365
  of adults with medical conditions, 370f
  of immunocompromised patients, 423t
  passive, 365
  schedule
    for adults, 366, 368f–369f, 994t
    for children and adolescents, 366, 367f
  for travel, 366, 371t

Immunocompromised host
  cytomegalovirus infection in, 529–530
  immunizations in, 423t, 424
  infections in, **417**
  parvovirus infection in, 543
  toxoplasmosis in, 579
Immunodeficiency disease
  immunoglobulin deficiency syndromes, 777–779
  lymphopenia in, 274
  primary, **776**
    laboratory evaluation of, 778t
    severe combined immunodeficiency, 776–777
    T cell immunodeficiency, 777
    X-linked immunodeficiency with increased IgM, 779
Immunofluorescent stain, 351
Immunoglobulin deficiency syndrome, **777**
  treatment of, 779
Immunohemolytic anemia, 271
  cold antibody, 271
  warm antibody, 271
Immunoproliferative small-intestinal disease (IPSID), 323–324
Immunosuppressive therapy
  for liver transplant, 769
  for renal transplant, 711–713
Impetigo, 261, 456
  bullous, 261
  treatment of, 261
Implantable automatic defibrillator, for hypertrophic cardiomyopathy, 612
Inclusion body myositis, 948, 949t
  treatment of, 948
Inclusion cyst, epidermal, 256f
Indigestion, **198**
  treatment of, 200
Indinavir sulfate, for HIV infections, 434t
Indomethacin
  for acute pericarditis, 613
  for ankylosing spondylitis, 789
  for diabetes insipidus, 814
  for pain, 26t
  for reactive arthritis, 793
Infectious disease. *See also specific diseases*
  Acinetobacter, 473–474
  actinomycosis, 494–495
  adenovirus, 539
  Aeromonas, 474
  anaerobes. *See* Anaerobic infection
  anaplasmosis, 514–515
  arthritis, 412–413
  aspergillosis, 558
  Bartonella, 483–485, 484t
  blastomycosis, 563
  brain abscess, 894–895
  brucellosis, 479–480
  Burkholderia cepacia, 475–477
  in cancer patients, 417–421
  candidiasis, 557
  catheter-related, 417–418
  chlamydial, 517–520
  Citrobacter, 473–474
  coccidioidomycosis, 562–563
  coronavirus, 537
  Corynebacterium, 461–462
  cryptococcosis, 559–560
  cytomegalovirus, 529–531
  dementia in, 905t
  diagnosis of, 95, **351**
    antigen detection, 351
    culture, 351, 352t–357t, 358
    microscopy, 351
    nucleic acid probes, 358
    serology, 358
    susceptibility testing, 358
  diarrhea, 383–393
  diphtheria, 460–461
  ehrlichiosis, 513–514
  emergencies, **94**
  encephalitis, acute, 886–894
  endemic treponematoses, 507–508
  endocarditis, 372–380
  Enterobacter, 473–474
  enterococcal, **459**
  enteroviral, 544–546
  epidemic typhus, 512–513
  Epstein-Barr virus, 531–533
  focal infections with fulminant course, 99t, 101
  fungal, 555–565
  fusariosis, 564
  gram-negative enteric bacteria, **471**
  HACEK organisms, 470
  Haemophilus influenzae, 466–467
  helminthic, 580–591
  herpesvirus infection, 520–528
  histoplasmosis, 561–562
  HIV/AIDS. *See* HIV/AIDS
  hospital-acquired, 442–444
  human herpesvirus types 6, 7, and 8, 527–528
  immunization, 365–372
  in immunocompromised host, 417–424
  influenza, 533–536
  intraabdominal, 380–383
  Klebsiella, 472–473
  Legionella, 478–479
  leprosy, 500–503
  leptospirosis, 508–509
  listerial, 465–466
  Lyme borreliosis, 506–507
  lymphadenopathy in, 237t
  Malassezia, 564
  measles, 539–541
  meningitis
    acute, 886–894
    chronic, 896–898
  meningococcal, 462–465
  metapneumovirus, 538
  Moraxella catarrhalis, 468
  Morganella, 473–474
  mucormycosis, 560–561

Infectious disease (*Cont.*):
  mumps, 542
  murine typhus, 512
  Mycoplasma, 516–517
  myelopathy, 935
  neurologic infections, 98t, 100–101,
    419
  neutropenia in, 274
  nocardiosis, 492–494
  nontuberculous mycobacteria, 503–
    505
  normal barriers to, 418t
  osteomyelitis, 414–417
  paracoccidioidomycosis, 564
  parainfluenza virus, 538–539
  parvovirus B19, 542–543
  penicilliosis marneffei, 564
  pertussis, 467–468
  plague, 481–483
  pleural effusion in, 692t
  pneumococcal, 445–448
  Pneumocystis, 565–568
  Proteus, 473
  protozoal, 569–580
  Providencia, 473–474
  pseudoallescheriasis, 564–565
  Pseudomonas, 474–475
  Q fever, 515–516
  rabies, 547–548
  relapsing fever, 509–510
  of reproductive tract, 393–408
  respiratory syncytial virus, 537–538
  rhinovirus, 536
  rickettsial, 510–516
  rickettsialpox, 511–512
  Rocky Mountain spotted fever, 510–
    511
  rubella, 541–542
  scrub typhus, 513
  sepsis
    with obvious primary infection, 95,
      96t
    with skin manifestations, 95, 97t,
      100
    with soft tissue/muscle findings, 98t,
      100
  Serratia marcescens, 473–474
  sexually transmitted, 393–408
  of skin, 261–262, 417
  of skin and soft tissue, 408–412
  spirochetal, 506–510
  sporotrichosis, 565
  staphylococcal, 448–455
  Stenotrophomonas maltophilia, 475–
    477
  streptococcal, 455–460
  transfusion-related, 18, 18t
  in transplant recipients, **421**
  travel advice, 366–372
  treatment of, antibacterial therapy,
    360–365
  tuberculosis, 495–505
  tularemia, 480–481
  varicella-zoster virus, 523–527
  viral
    animal-borne, **547**
    insect-borne, **547**
    rodent-borne, **548**
  weight loss in, 201t
Inferior vena cava interruption, 687
Infertility
  female, **845**
  male, **836**
Inflammatory bowel disease, **742**
  Crohn's disease, 742–743
  extraintestinal manifestations of, 743
  treatment of, 743–745, 744t–745t
  ulcerative colitis, 742
Infliximab
  for ankylosing spondylitis, 789
  for inflammatory bowel disease, 744t–
    745t
  for psoriatic arthritis, 792
  for rheumatoid arthritis, 783
Influenza, **533**
  clinical features of, 534
  complications of, 534–535
  epidemiology of, 534
  pneumonia, 679, 684
  prevention of, 535-536
  treatment of, 535
Influenza vaccine, 367f, 368f, 370f, 535,
    536t, 993t, 994t
  in immunocompromised patients, 423t
Insect-borne viral infection, **547**
Insecticide poisoning, 86
Insect sting, 114
Insomnia, **181**, 184t
  drug-induced, 182
  extrinsic, 181
  long-term (chronic), 181
  in medical disorders, 182, 184t
  in movement disorders, 182
  in psychiatric disease, 182
  psychophysiologic, 182
  rebound, 182
  short-term, 181
  sleep-offset, 181
  sleep-onset, 181
  transient, 181
  transient situational, 182
  treatment of, 183
Inspiratory capacity, 663f
Insulin
  for cardiac glycoside poisoning, 82
  for diabetes mellitus, 832–833, 832t
  for diabetic ketoacidosis, 90t
  for hyperglycemic hyperosmolar state, 91
  for hyperkalemia, 10t
  pharmacokinetics of insulin prepara-
    tions, 832t
Insulinoma, 93f, 94t, 329, 330t
Insulin resistance syndrome, 831
Intensive care unit. *See* Critically ill pa-
    tient
Interferon-α therapy
  for anal condylomas, 749
  for carcinoid tumor, 329

Interferon-α therapy (*Cont.*):
  for chronic hepatitis B, 763, 764t
  for chronic hepatitis C, 764, 765t
  for chronic myeloid leukemia, 293
  for essential thrombocytosis, 296
  for melanoma, 307
  for renal cancer, 333
  for viral hepatitis, 761
  for Zollinger-Ellison syndrome, 741
Interferon-β therapy, for multiple sclerosis, 901, 903
Interferon therapy, for human papillomavirus infections, 407
Interleukin 2 therapy
  for melanoma, 308
  for renal cancer, 333
Interstitial lung disease, **687**
Intestinal motility, 208
  altered, 209
Intestinal pseudoobstruction, **747**
  treatment of, 748
Intraabdominal abscess, **381**
Intraabdominal infection, **380**
  abscess, 381–383
  clostridial, 488
  peritonitis, 380–381
Intraaortic balloon counterpulsation, 627, 628t
Intraaortic balloon pump, for myocardial infarction, 629
Intracerebral hemorrhage, 67
  treatment of, 61
Intracranial hemorrhage, 59–60
  headache in, 142t
Intracranial infection, suppurative, 98t
Intracranial pressure (ICP)
  increased, 57, **67**, 883, 886
    treatment of, 67–68, 68t
  monitoring of, 68
Intracranial tumor, primary, **883**
Intracytoplasmic sperm injection (ICSI), 837, 846
Intrauterine insemination, 846
Intravascular device infections, 443–444
  gram-negative enteric bacteria, 473
Intravenous drug user
  endocarditis in, 372
  sepsis in, treatment of, 52t
In vitro fertilization, 837
Involucrum, 414
Iodinated glycerol, for cough, 189
Iodine deficiency, 820
Iododoxyrubicin, for amyloidosis, 806
Iodoquinol, for amebiasis, 391
Ipratropium
  for asthma, 671
  for COPD, 677
  for cough, 189
Irinotecan
  for breast cancer, 320
  for cervical cancer, 337
  for colorectal cancer, 327
Iris/target lesion, 255
Iritis, 242

Iron
  oral, for anemia, 271
  poisoning, 83
Iron-deficiency anemia, 267, 268f, 268t, 269, 269t
  treatment of, 271
Iron overload, transfusion-related, 18
Irritable bowel disease, **746**
  diagnosis of, 746, 747t
  treatment of, 746–747
Ischemia, hypoxic-ischemic encephalopathy, **69**, 70f
Ischemic nephropathy, **730**
Ischemic stroke, 58, 60
  causes of, 63t
  treatment of, 61
Isocarboxazid, dosage and adverse effects of, 965t
Isoetharine, for asthma, 669
Isolated IgA deficiency, 778
Isolation aphasia, 180t
Isolation techniques, 442
Isometheptene, for migraine, 144t
Isoniazid
  for nontuberculous mycobacterial infections, 505
  poisoning, 83–84
  for tuberculosis, 498, 499t, 501t
Isopropyl alcohol poisoning, 84
Isoproterenol, for asthma, 669
Isosorbide dinitrate
  for achalasia, 204
  for angina pectoris, 633t
  for esophageal spasm, 205
  for heart failure, 650–651
Isosorbide mononitrate, for angina pectoris, 633t
Isosporiasis, 387
  treatment of, 387
Isotretinoin, for acne vulgaris, 263
Itraconazole, 555–556
  for aspergillosis, 559
  for blastomycosis, 563
  for candidiasis, 206, 558
  for coccidioidomycosis, 563
  for histoplasmosis, 562
  for paracoccidioidomycosis, 564
  for penicilliosis marneffei, 564
  for pseudoallescheriasis, 565
  for sporotrichosis, 565
Ivermectin
  for larva migrans, 581
  for onchocerciasis, 585
  for pediculosis, 591
  for scabies, 590
  for strongyloidiasis, 583

Japanese encephalitis, 550, 552t
Japanese encephalitis vaccine, 371t
Jarisch-Herxheimer reaction, 404
Jaundice, **218**
  causes of, 218, 218t
  cholestatic, 221t
  drug-induced, 218t, 220, 985t

Jaundice (*Cont.*):
   evaluation of, 218–219, 219f
   hepatocellular conditions that produce,
     220t
Jellyfish envenomations, 110
Jet-lag, 185
Joint disease
   anaerobic infections, 490
   in inflammatory bowel disease, 743
   Pseudomonas aeruginosa infections,
     475
   swelling in, **161**
Joint pain, **161**
   in elderly, 164
   history of, 161
   imaging in, 164
   initial assessment of, 161, 162f
   laboratory tests in, 162–163
   physical examination in, 161
   synovial fluid analysis, 163f, 164
Joint replacement, for osteoarthritis, 796
Jugular foramen syndrome, 924
Jugular venous pulsation, 593
Juvenile arthritis, pain in, 162f
Juvenile polyposis, 325, 325t

Kala-azar, 573
Kallmann's syndrome, 835
Kaolin-pectin, for diarrhea, 211
Kaposi's sarcoma, 437, 527
Katayama fever, 586
Kawasaki disease, 786
Kayexalate
   for cardiac glycoside poisoning, 82
   for hyperkalemia, 10t, 708
Keratitis, 242
   herpes simplex, 242, 521
   nocardiosis, 492
   treatment of, 242
Keratoderma blennorrhagica, 793
Keratosis
   actinic, 257f, 258f
   seborrheic, 257f
Keratosis pilaris, 257f
Ketanserin, for systemic sclerosis, 784
Ketoacidosis, diabetic, **89,** 89t, 90t
Ketoconazole, 555
   for candidal esophagitis, 206
   for Cushing's syndrome, 825
   for ectopic ACTH syndrome, 346
Ketolides, mechanisms, indications, and
    adverse effects of, 362–363
Ketorolac, for pain, 26t
Kidney disease. *See* Renal disease
Kingella kingae infection. *See also* HA-
    CEK organisms
   arthritis, 412
Klebsiella infection, **472**
   nosocomial, 443
   pneumonia, 681
   prostatitis, 727
   treatment of, 472–473
Klinefelter's syndrome, 835–836
Koplik's spots, 539–540

Korsakoff's syndrome, 973
K-phos, for hypophosphatemia, 851
Kwashiorkor, 4

Labetalol
   for aortic dissection, 655t
   for malignant hypertension, 621
Laboratory values, **995**
Labyrinthine dysfunction
   acute bilateral, 169
   acute unilateral, 169
   recurrent, 169
Labyrinthitis, acute, 169
La Crosse encephalitis, 552t, 893t, 894
β-Lactams
   for *Escherichia coli* infections, 472
   mechanisms, indications, and adverse
    effects of, 361–362
Lactic acidosis, 12
Lactic dehydrogenase, serum, 754
Lactilol, for hepatic encephalopathy, 772
Lactulose
   for constipation, 214
   for hepatic encephalopathy, 772
Lacunar syndromes, 58–59, 62
Lambert-Eaton syndrome, 348t, 942
Lamivudine
   for chronic hepatitis B, 763, 764t
   for HIV/AIDS, 430t, 439
Lamotrigine, 969
   for bipolar disorder, 957
   dosage and adverse effects of, 968t
   for seizures, 880t–881t, 882t
Langerhans cell pulmonary histiocytosis,
   690
Lansoprazole, for *Helicobacter pylori*
    eradication, 739t
Larva migrans
   cutaneous, **581**
   ocular, **581**
   treatment of, 581
   visceral, **581**
Laryngeal palsy, 923–924
Laryngitis, 253
Lassa fever, 551
Latanoprost, for glaucoma, 243
Latex agglutination assay, 351
Laxatives, for constipation, 214
LDL cholesterol, 855, 856t
   classification of, 1004t
   patient goals, 861
Lead poisoning, 84, 723
Lead-time bias, 281
Leech infestation, **591**
Leflunomide, for rheumatoid arthritis, 783
Legionella infection, **478**
   diagnosis of, 356t
   nosocomial, 444
   pneumonia, 679, 684
   treatment of, 478–479
Legionnaires' disease, 478
Leiomyosarcoma, gastric, 322
Leishmaniasis, **574**
   cutaneous, 576
   mucosal, 576

Leishmaniasis (*Cont.*):
  treatment of, 573–576
  visceral, 573–576
Lemierre syndrome, 490
Lennox-Gastaut syndrome, 880t–881t
Lepirudin
  for heparin-induced thrombocytopenia,
    277
  for thrombotic disorders, 279
Leprosy, **500**
  complications of, 503
  lepromatous, 502
  treatment of, 503
  tuberculous, 502
Leptomeningeal metastasis, 885, 885t
Leptospirosis, **508**
  anicteric, 508
  from animal bite, 108t
  icteric, 508
  treatment of, 509
Leriche syndrome, 655
Letrozole, for breast cancer, 318, 320
Leucovorin
  for gastric cancer, 322
  for *Pneumocystis* infections, 567t, 568t
Leukapheresis, 19
Leukemia
  monocytopenia in, 274
  myeloid, **290**
Leukemoid reaction, 273
Leukocytes
  inclusions and nuclear abnormalities,
    265–266
  normal values in blood, 272t
Leukocytosis, **272**
  in acute pancreatitis, 754
  drug-induced, 983t
Leukoerythroblastic reaction, 273
Leukopenia, **273**
Leukoplakia, 258f
  oral, 284
  oral hairy, 258f, 532
Leuprolide, for prostate cancer, 339
Levetiracetam, for seizures, 882t
Levobunolol, for glaucoma, 243
Levodopa, for Parkinson's disease, 911,
    912t
Levofloxacin
  for *Chlamydia pneumoniae* infections,
    519
  for epididymitis, 396
  for gonococcal infections, 401t
  for *Legionella* infections, 478
  for *Mycoplasma pneumoniae* infections,
    517
  for pelvic inflammatory disease, 398
  for pneumonia, 680t–681t, 682t
  for *Pseudomonas aeruginosa* infec-
    tions, 477t
  for sepsis, 52t
  for sinusitis, 250t
  for *Staphylococcus aureus* infections,
    453t
  for tuberculosis, 498

Levorphanol, for pain, 25, 26t
Levothyroxine
  for hypothyroidism, 817, 820
  for nontoxic goiter, 820
  for thyroid cancer, 822
Lewisite, 125–126
Lewy bodies, 909–910
Lhermitte's symptom, 899
Lichenification, 256
Lichenoid eruption, drug-induced, 982t
Lichen planus, 256f, 258f, 260
Lichen simplex chronicus, 257f
Lidocaine
  for arrhythmias, 646t
  for cardiac arrest, 43f
  for ventricular tachycardia, 625
Lightheadedness, 168
Limb-girdle dystrophy, **947**
Lincosamides, mechanisms, indications,
    and adverse effects of, 363
Linear skin lesion, 255
Linezolid
  for enterococcal infections, 459
  mechanisms, indications, and adverse
    effects of, 364–365
  for osteomyelitis, 416t
  for *Staphylococcus aureus* infections,
    453t
Liothyronine
  for myxedema coma, 817
  for thyroid cancer, 822
Lipase, serum, 754
Lipemia retinalis, 857
Lipid metabolism, disorders of, **855**
Lipid storage disease, lymphadenopathy
    in, 237t
Lipodystrophy syndrome, HAART-re-
    lated, 438
Lipoprotein analysis, 855
Lipoprotein lipase deficiency, familial,
    856t, 860
Liquid nitrogen, for anal condylomas, 749
Lisinopril, for heart failure, 651t
Listeriosis, **465**
  meningitis, 886, 887, 891t
  neonatal, 465–466
  in pregnancy, 465–466
  treatment of, 466
Lithium, 969
  for bipolar disorder, 957
  for cluster headache prophylaxis, 145
  dosage and adverse effects of, 968t
  poisoning, 84
Liver abscess
  amebic, 382
  streptococcal, 460
Liver biopsy, percutaneous, 223–224
Liver disease. *See also specific diseases*
  alcoholic, **767**
  in amyloidosis, 805
  benign tumors, **328**
  coagulation disorders in, 276
  drug-induced, 985t
  hepatobiliary imaging, **223**

Liver disease (*Cont.*):
  in inflammatory bowel disease, 743
  prevention of, 992t–993t
  in sarcoidosis, 803
Liver fluke, **586**
Liver function tests, 220–222, 222t
Liver transplant, **768**
  for acute hepatic failure, 762
  for alcoholic liver disease, 768
  contraindications, 769
  for hepatic encephalopathy, 772
  indications for, 769
  infections in transplant recipients, 422
  for primary biliary cirrhosis, 768
  for primary sclerosing cholangitis, 753
  for toxic/drug-induced hepatitis, 761
  for viral hepatitis, 761
Löffler's syndrome, 582
Lofgren's syndrome, 803
Looser's zones, 854
Lo/Ovral, 845
Loperamide
  for diarrhea, 211, 366
  for inflammatory bowel disease, 743
  for irritable bowel syndrome, 746
  for narcotic withdrawal, 976
  for traveler's diarrhea, 384
Lopinavir/ritonavir, for HIV infections, 436t
Loratadine, for allergic rhinitis, 775
Lorazepam
  dosage and adverse effects of, 966t
  for status epilepticus, 72, 73f
Losartan
  for heart failure, 650
  for systemic sclerosis, 784
Louse-borne relapsing fever, **509**
Louse-borne typhus fever, **512**
Lovastatin, for hyperlipidemia, 859t
Low back pain, **147**
  acute
    causes of, 150t
    treatment of, 150–151, 152f–153f
  causes of, 148–150, 150t
  chronic, treatment of, 151
  examination in, 147–148, 149t
  types of, 147
Low back strain/sprain, 148
Lower extremity, edema of, 194
Lower motor neuron dysfunction, 175
Loxapine, dosage and adverse effects of, 967t
Ludwig's angina, 489
Lumbar disk disease, pain in, 148
Lumbar puncture, **29**
Lumbar puncture headache, 146–147
Lumbosacral radiculopathy, 149t
Lumpectomy, 318
Lung abscess, 681–684
  anaerobic, 490
Lung cancer, **310**
  asbestosis and, 674
  classification of, 311
  clinical features of, 311

metastases to nervous system, 885t
metastatic, 311
non-small cell, 311, 314t, 315
paraneoplastic syndromes, 344t, 348t
pleural effusion in, 691
prevention of, 283
risk factors for, 283, 311
screening for, 281, 282t
small cell, 311, 314t, 315
staging of, 311–312, 312t–313t
treatment of, 313–316, 313t–314t
Lung disease. *See also specific diseases*
  diffuse parenchymal, dyspnea in, 186
  environmental, **673**
    approach to, 673
    inorganic dusts, 673–674
    management of, 675
    organic dusts, 674
    toxic chemicals, 674–675
    treatment of, 675
  interstitial, **687**
    approach to, 688–689
    categories of, 688t
    diagnosis of, 664t
    treatment of, 690
  in sarcoidosis, 803
Lung fluke, **587**
Lung injury, acute, 38
Lung transplant
  for COPD, 677
  infections in transplant recipients, 422
Lung volume(s), 663, 663f
Lung volume reduction surgery, 677
Lupus, drug-induced, 979t
Luteinizing hormone, 807
Lyme borreliosis, **506**
  arthritis, 506–507
  disseminated infection, 506
  localized infection, 506
  meningitis, 897t
  persistent infection, 506
  prevention of, 507
  treatment of, 507
Lymphadenitis, in tuberculosis, 496
Lymphadenopathy, **235**
  approach to, 236
  diseases associated with, 237t
  drug-induced, 983t
  due to hyperplasia, 236
  due to infiltration, 236
  in HIV/AIDS, 438
  treatment of, 236
Lymphangiectasia, intestinal, 274
Lymphedema, 194, **658**
  treatment of, 658
  unilateral, 658
Lymph nodes
  biopsy of, 236
  cervical, metastases to, 343
Lymphoblastic leukemia, acute, 302
  treatment of, 302
Lymphoblastic lymphoma, acute, 302
  treatment of, 302
Lymphocutaneous syndrome, nocardiosis, 492

Lymphocytic choriomeningitis, **548**
Lymphocytic leukemia, chronic, 298–300
  staging of, 299, 299t
  treatment of, 299–300
Lymphocytosis, 273
Lymphoepithelioma, 309
Lymphogranuloma venereum, 399
Lymphoid leukemia/lymphoma
  acute, 297t, **302**
  chronic, 297t, **298**
Lymphoid malignancy, **296**
  classification of, 296–297, 297t
  definition of, 296
  diagnosis and staging of, 298
  incidence and etiology of, 297–298
Lymphoma. *See also* Lymphoid leukemia/
    lymphoma
  aggressive, 297t, **301**
    approach to, 301
    prognosis for, 301t
    treatment of, 301–302
  EBV-associated, 532
  gastric, 322
  indolent, 297t, **300**
  intestinal, 323
  lymphopenia in, 274
  paraneoplastic syndromes, 348t
  pleural effusion in, 691
  primary CNS, 884
Lymphopenia, 274
Lymphoproliferative disease, Epstein-Barr
    virus, 532–533
Lymphoproliferative syndrome, X-linked,
    779
Lynch syndrome, 325, 325t

Maalox, for erosive gastropathy, 740
Machado-Joseph disease, 915
Macrolides, mechanisms, indications, and
    adverse effects of, 362–363
Macular degeneration, 172f, 173, 243
  dry, 243
  wet, 243
Macule, 255
Magnesium chloride, for hypomagnese-
    mia, 851
Magnesium sulfate
  for cardiac arrest, 43f
  for hypomagnesemia, 851
Magnetic resonance angiography, in renal
    artery stenosis, 729
Magnetic resonance cholangiography,
    750t
Magnetic resonance imaging (MRI)
  in aortic aneurysm, 653
  in aortic dissection, 654
  in coma, 57
  in constrictive pericarditis, 616
  FLAIR, 882
  in hearing disorders, 245
  hepatobiliary, 223
  indications for, 33–34
  neuroimaging, 873, 874t, 875
  in osteomyelitis, 415t
  in poisoning or drug overdose, 75
  in respiratory disease, 666
  in stroke, 61
  utility of, 33–34
Malabsorption syndromes, **213**
  causes of, 213t
  drug-induced, 985t
Malaria, **569**
  cerebral, 99t, 569
  chemoprophylaxis, 572, 574t
  clinical features of, 569–570
  diagnosis of, 359t
  in pregnancy, 570
  prevention of, 570–572
    in travelers, 366
  transfusion, 570
  treatment of, 570, 571t–572t
    self-treatment, 575t
Malassezia infection, **564**
Malathion, for pediculosis, 591
Maldigestion, 213
Male infertility, **836**
  treatment of, 837
Malignant hyperthermia, 160
Mallory-Weiss syndrome, 198
Mallory-Weiss tear, 215
Malnutrition, **3**
  clinical features of, 4
  severe, 4
Mammalian bites, **106**, 107t–108t
Mammography, screening, 282t, 317–
    318, 993t, 994t
Mandelamine, for nephrolithiasis, 733t
Mania, drug-induced, 988t
Manic depressive illness. *See* Bipolar dis-
    order
Mannitol, for increased intracranial pres-
    sure, 67, 68t
Marasmus, 4
Marburg virus infection, **554**
Marie-Strumpell disease, **788**
Marine envenomations, **110**
  invertebrates, 110
  treatment of, 110–111
  vertebrates, 110–111
Marine poisoning, **111**
Mastectomy, modified radical, 318
Mastitis, *Staphylococcus aureus*, 449
Mastocytosis, systemic, **775**
  diagnosis of, 775, 775t
  treatment of, 776
Mastoiditis, 253
Maturity-onset diabetes of the young, 830
McArdle's disease, 950
Measles, **539**
  atypical, 540
  clinical features of, 540
  complications of, 540
  prevention of, 541
  treatment of, 540–541
Measles vaccine, 539, 541
Mebendazole
  for ascariasis, 582
  for enterobiasis, 584

Mebendazole (*Cont.*):
  for hookworm, 582
  for trichinellosis, 581
Mechanical ventilation. *See* Ventilatory
    support
Meclizine, for vertigo, 170t
Median neuropathy, 940t, 941
Mediastinal disease, **693**
Mediastinal mass, 693, 695t
Mediastinitis, **693**
Mediastinoscopy, 667
Medroxyprogesterone
  for abnormal uterine bleeding, 840
  for amenorrhea, 842
  for menopausal symptoms, 845
Mefloquine
  for malaria, 571t
  for malaria prophylaxis, 574t
Megaloblastic anemia, drug-induced, 983t
Megaloblastic madness, 936
Megastrol, for endometrial cancer, 337
Meglitinide, for diabetes mellitus, 833t
Meglumine antimonate, for leishmaniasis,
    573
Melanoma, **307**
  acral lentiginous, 307
  lentigo maligna, 307
  metastases to nervous system, 885t
  nodular, 307
  paraneoplastic syndromes, 348t
  superficial spreading, 307
  treatment of, 307–308
Melarsoprol, for sleeping sickness, 578
Melasma, 258f
Melena, 214
Meleney's gangrene, 490
Melioidosis, 477
Melphalan, for multiple myeloma, 304
Memantine, for Alzheimer's disease, 909
Ménière's disease, 169, 245–246
  treatment of, 171
Meningeal biopsy, 898
Meningioma, 884
Meningitis
  acute, **886**
    approach to, 886, 888f–889f
  acute bacterial, **886**
    clinical features of, 886–887
    differential diagnosis of, 887
    treatment of, 887, 890t, 891t
  aseptic, 545
  bacterial, 98t, 100–101
  chronic, **896**
    approach to, 896–897
    bacterial, 897t
    causes of, 897t, 898t
    symptoms and signs of, 896t
    treatment of, 898
    viral, 897t
  Escherichia coli, 472
  Haemophilus influenzae, 466–467
  headache in, 142t
  herpes simplex virus, 522, 525t
  meningococcal, 462–465

mumps, 542
  pneumococcal, 446
    treatment of, 447
  Pseudomonas aeruginosa, 475
  streptococcal, 458
  tuberculous, 497
  viral, **890**
    chronic, 897t
    diagnosis of, 892
    etiology of, 890, 891t
    seasonal prevalence of viruses, 891t
    treatment of, 892
Meningococcal infection, **462**
  chemoprophylaxis, 464t
  meningitis, 886, 887, 887t, 891t
    prophylaxis for, 887
  prevention of, 464–465, 464t
  treatment of, 463–464, 464t
Meningococcal vaccine, 368f, 371t, 464–
    465, 464t
  in immunocompromised patients, 423t
Meningococcemia, 462–463
  treatment of, 97t
Meningoencephalitis, cryptococcosis, 560
Menometrorrhagia, 839
Menopausal gonadotropins, for hypopitui-
    tarism, 812
Menopause, **843**
  insomnia and, 183
  treatment of symptoms of, 843–845
Menorrhagia, 839
Menstrual disorders, 839–842
Mental status examination, **867,** 867t
Meperidine
  abuse of, **975**
  for acute cholecystitis, 751
  for acute pancreatitis, 754
  for pain, 27t
6-Mercaptopurine, for inflammatory
    bowel disease, 744, 744t–745t
Mercury poisoning, 84–85
Meropenem
  for anaerobic infections, 491t
  for bacterial meningitis, 890t
  for brain abscess, 894
  for meningococcal infections, 464t
  for pneumonia, 680t, 683t
  for *Pseudomonas aeruginosa* infec-
    tions, 476t
  for sepsis, 52t
Merozoite, 569
Mesenteric arteriography, 216, 770
Mesenteric insufficiency, chronic, **748**
Mesenteric ischemia
  acute, **748**
    mechanisms of, 748
Mesothelioma, 674
Metabolic acidosis, 11–12, 11f
  causes of, 12t
  drug-induced, 981t
  treatment of, 12
Metabolic alkalosis, 11f, 12–13
  causes of, 13, 13t
  treatment of, 13

Metabolic disease. *See also specific diseases*
  abdominal pain in, 137t
  drug-induced, 980t
  reference values for laboratory tests, 999t–1001t
  syncope in, 166t
Metabolic syndrome, 831
Metamucil, for irritable bowel syndrome, 746
Metapneumovirus infection, **538**
Metaproterenol, for asthma, 669
Metformin, for diabetes mellitus, 832, 833t
Methadone
  abuse of, **975**
  maintenance therapy, 976
  for narcotic withdrawal, 976
  for pain, 25, 26t
Methamphetamine, for hypersomnia, 185
Methanol poisoning, 85
Methemoglobinemia, 85–86, 192, 193t
Methimazole, for thyrotoxicosis, 818
Methocarbanol, for low back pain, 151
Methotrexate
  for acute lymphoid leukemia/lymphoma, 302
  for ankylosing spondylitis, 790
  for chronic inflammatory demyelinating polyneuropathy, 941
  for head and neck cancer, 310
  for inflammatory myopathies, 948
  for multiple sclerosis, 903
  for psoriasis, 259
  for psoriatic arthritis, 792
  for reactive arthritis, 793
  for rheumatoid arthritis, 783
  for sarcoidosis, 804
  for vasculitis, 788
Methylene blue, for methemoglobinemia, 85–86
Methylphenidate, for hypersomnia, 184t, 185
Methylprednisolone
  for acute transverse myelopathy, 935
  for asthma, 670t, 671
  for multiple sclerosis, 901–903
  for optic neuritis, 173
  for renal transplant rejection, 711
Methylsergide, for migraine prophylaxis, 145t
Metipranolol, for glaucoma, 243
Metoclopramide
  for migraine, 144t
  for nausea and vomiting, 198
  for systemic sclerosis, 784
Metolazone, 196
  for edema, 196t
  for heart failure, 649
Metoprolol
  for acute coronary syndromes, 636
  for myocardial infarction, 625
  for myocardial infarction prophylaxis, 630
  for syncope, 167

Metronidazole
  for acne rosacea, 263
  for amebiasis, 391
  for anaerobic infections, 491, 491t
  for bacterial meningitis, 890t, 891t
  for bacterial vaginosis, 395t
  for brain abscess, 99t, 894
  for *Clostridium difficile*-associated disease, 392
  for giardiasis, 386
  for *Helicobacter pylori* eradication, 739t
  for hepatic encephalopathy, 772
  for inflammatory bowel disease, 744, 744t–745t
  for intestinal pseudoobstruction, 748
  for intracranial infections, 98t
  mechanisms, indications, and adverse effects of, 364
  for pelvic inflammatory disease, 398
  for peritonitis, 381
  for pneumonia, 681t
  for tetanus, 486
  for trichomonal vaginitis, 395t
  for urethritis in men, 396
Metrorrhagia, 839
Metyrapone
  for Cushing's syndrome, 825
  for ectopic ACTH syndrome, 346
Mexiletine, for arrhythmias, 646t
Mezlocillin
  for HACEK endocarditis, 469t
  for *Pseudomonas aeruginosa* infections, 476t
MHC class II deficiency, 777
Miconazole, 555
  for vulvovaginal candidiasis, 395t
Microaerophilic bacteria, 489
Microalbuminuria, 230, 833
Microbial bioterrorism, **118**
  anthrax, 118–119
  botulinum toxin, 121t, 124, 487
  CDC category A, B, and C agents, 119t
  features of agents used as bioweapons, 118t
  plague, 121t, 122–123
  preparedness, 125
  prevention of, 125
  smallpox, 121t, 123–124
  tularemia, 121t, 124
  viral hemorrhagic fevers, 121t, 124
Micronutrient deficiency, 16t, 17
Microscopy, diagnostic, 351
Microsporidiosis, 387
  treatment of, 387
Midazolam
  for increased intracranial pressure, 68t
  for status epilepticus, 72, 73f
Midodrine, for orthostatic hypotension, 931
Miglitol, for diabetes mellitus, 833t
Migraine, **139**, 140t, 173
  classic, 139–140
  common, 140–141

Migraine (*Cont.*):
  prophylactic treatment of, 145t
  seizures versus, 877t
  treatment of, 141–142, 143t–144t
    staged approach, 145t
Milk of magnesia, for *Pfiesteria* poisoning, 112
Milrinone, for myocardial infarction, 627t
Miltefosine, for leishmaniasis, 576
Mineral oil, for constipation, 214
Minimal change disease, **716**
Mini-mental status examination, 867t
Mini-transplant
  for chronic lymphocytic leukemia/lymphoma, 300
  for follicular center lymphoma, 300
Minocycline
  for leprosy, 503
  for nocardiosis, 493t
  for *Staphylococcus aureus* infections, 453t, 454
Mirtazapine, 963
  dosage and adverse effects of, 965t
Misoprostol, for erosive gastropathy, 740
Mite borne spotted fever, **510**
Mitochondrial cytopathies, 950
Mitomycin, for anal cancer, 328
Mitotane, for Cushing's syndrome, 825
Mitoxantrone
  for multiple sclerosis, 903
  for prostate cancer, 339
Mitral regurgitation, **604**
  acute, 627–628
  echocardiography in, 602f
  treatment of, 605
Mitral stenosis, **603**
  echocardiography in, 602f
  laboratory evaluation of, 603
  treatment of, 604, 604f
Mitral valve prolapse, **605**
  echocardiography in, 603
  treatment of, 606
Mittelschmerz, 842
Mixed connective tissue disease, **784**
MMR (measles, mumps, rubella) vaccine, 367f, 368f, 370f, 994t
  in immunocompromised patients, 423t, 542
Modafinil, for hypersomnia, 183, 184t
Mold, 555
Molindone, dosage and adverse effects of, 967t
Mollaret's meningitis, 522
Monkey bite, 106, 108t
Monoamine oxidase inhibitors (MAOI), 963
  dosage and adverse effects of, 965t
Monocytopenia, 274
Monocytosis, 273
Mononeuropathy, 940t, 941
Mononeuropathy multiplex, 941
Mononucleosis
  cytomegalovirus, 529
  Epstein-Barr virus, 531–533, 532t

Montelukast, for asthma, 670t, 671
Mood disorder, **955**
Mood stabilizers, 968t, **969**
MOPP/ABV regimen, for Hodgkin's disease, 306
MOPP/ABVD regimen, for Hodgkin's disease, 306
Moraxella catarrhalis infection, 468
  otitis media, 252
  pneumonia, 679
  sinusitis, 249
  treatment of, 468
Morbilliform lesion, 255
Morganella infection, **473**
Morphine
  abuse of, **975**
  for acute coronary syndromes, 637
  for increased intracranial pressure, 68t
  for myocardial infarction, 623
  for pain, 25, 26t
  for pulmonary edema, 54
Mortality, age-specific causes, 992t–993t
Morulae, 513
Motor exam, 868t–869t, **872**
Motor fluctuations, 911
Motor impairment, in spinal cord disease, 933
Motor neuron disease, **917**
  acute, 917t, 941
  amyotrophic lateral sclerosis, 917–920
  chronic, 917t
  etiology and investigation of, 919t
Motor unit dysfunction, 175
  weakness in, 176t, 177t
Movement disorders, **175**
  insomnia in, 182
Moxifloxacin
  for *Legionella* infections, 478
  for pneumonia, 680t–681t, 682t
  for tuberculosis, 498
Mucormycosis, **560**
  nose and paranasal sinus, 561
  pulmonary, 561
  rhinocerebral, 101, 249
  treatment of, 561
Mucous membranes, in malnutrition, 4
Mucous patch, 403
Multifocal motor neuropathy with conduction block, 918
Multiorgan system failure, 21
Multiple cranial nerve palsies, **924**
Multiple endocrine neoplasia (MEN), MEN1, 740–741
Multiple myeloma, 303–304
  renal disease in, 719t
  staging of, 305t
  treatment of, 304
Multiple sclerosis (MS), **899**
  acute (Marburg's variant), 903
  clinical features of, 899
  clinical variants of, **903**
  diagnostic criteria for, 900t
  disorders that mimic, 901t
  facial nerve disorders in, 922

Multiple sclerosis (MS) (*Cont.*):
  laboratory findings in, 900
  primary progressive, 899
  progressive-relapsing, 899
  relapsing-remitting, 899
  secondary progressive, 899
  spinal cord involvement in, 936
  treatment of, 901–903, 902f
    acute relapses, 901–903
    progressive symptoms, 903
    prophylaxis against relapses, 901
Multiple system atrophy, 928
Mumps, 542
Mumps vaccine, 542
Munchausen's syndrome, 961
Mupirocin, mechanisms and indications
  for, 365
Murine typhus, endemic, **512**
  treatment of, 512
Murmur. *See* Heart murmur
Muscle atrophy, 872
Muscle contracture, 944
Muscle cramp, 944
Muscle disease, **944.** *See also specific dis-
    eases*
  in endocrine disease, 950
  inflammatory, 948–950
  metabolic, 948–950
  mitochondrial, 950
  muscular dystrophies, 944–948
  paraneoplastic, 347t, 348–349
  periodic paralysis, 950
  toxic, 950, 951t
  weakness in, 176t, 177t
Muscle relaxants, poisoning, 86
Muscle spasm, low back pain and, 147
Muscle strength testing, 872
Muscle weakness, 944
  approach to, 945f, 946f
  intermittent, 946f
  persistent, 945f
Muscular dystrophy, **944**
  Duchenne, 947–948
  facioscapulohumeral, 947
  limb-girdle, 947
  myotonic dystrophy, 944–947
  oculopharyngeal, 948
Musculoskeletal disease. *See also specific
    diseases*
  in alcoholism, 973
  in amyloidosis, 805
  drug-induced, 987t–988t
  Escherichia coli, 472
  in sarcoidosis, 803
  tuberculosis, 497
Musculoskeletal pain, **161**
  history of, 161
  imaging in, 164
  initial assessment of, 161, 162f
  laboratory tests in, 162–163
  physical examination in, 161
M-VAC regimen, for bladder cancer, 332
Myalgia, 944
  drug-induced, 988t

Myasthenia gravis, **942**
  clinical features of, 942
  differential diagnosis of, 942
  double vision in, 174
  laboratory findings in, 942–943
  paraneoplastic, 348t
  treatment of, 943–944, 943f
Myasthenic crisis, 944
Mycobacterial infection
  brain abscess, 894
  diagnosis of, 352t, 356t
  nontuberculous, **503**
    in HIV/AIDS, 504
    treatment of, 504–505
Mycobacterium abscessus infection, 505
Mycobacterium avium complex infection,
  504
Mycobacterium chelonae infection, 505
Mycobacterium fortuitum infection, 505
Mycobacterium kansasii infection, 504–
  505
Mycobacterium leprae infection. *See* Leprosy
Mycobacterium marinum infection, 505
Mycobacterium tuberculosis infection. *See*
  Tuberculosis
Mycobacterium ulcerans infection, 505
Mycophenolate mofetil
  immunosuppression for renal trans-
    plant, 713
  for inflammatory myopathies, 948
  for myasthenia gravis, 944
  for systemic lupus erythematosus, 781
Mycoplasma genitalium infection
  mucopurulent cervicitis, 397
  pelvic inflammatory disease, 397
  urethritis, 393
Mycoplasmal infection, **516**
  genital, **402**
    treatment of, 403
Mycoplasma pneumoniae infection, **516**
  pneumonia, 679, 684
  treatment of, 517
Mydriatic agents, 242
Myelodysplastic syndromes (MDS), **294**
  classification of, 294t
  prognostic scoring system for, 295t
  treatment of, 294–295
Myelofibrosis, 273
  idiopathic, 295
Myelography, 875
Myeloid leukemia, **290**
  acute, **290**
    classification of, 291t
    features of, 290–291
    incidence and etiology of, 290
    treatment of, 291–292
  chronic, **292**
    features of, 292–293
    incidence and etiology of, 292
    natural history of, 293
    treatment of, 293–294, 293t
Myelopathy
  acute transverse, 935
  infectious, 935

Myelopathy (*Cont.*):
  retrovirus-associated, 935
  spondylitic, 935
Myelophthisis, 273
Myeloproliferative syndromes, **295**
Myiasis, **591**
Myocardial infarction
  accelerated idioventricular rhythm and, 625
  acute pericarditis versus, 613t
  AV block and, 626
  bradyarrhythmias and, 626
  cardiogenic shock and, 626–627, 628t
  chest pain in, 622
  complications of, 625–628
  electrocardiography in, 598f, 599f, 599t, 601, 613t, 622
  heart failure and, 626
  hemodynamic complications of, 628t
  hypotension and, 627, 629f
  laboratory evaluation of, 622
  mechanical complications of, 627–628
  non-Q-wave, 601, 622
  non-ST-elevation, **635**
    high-risk features in, 637t
    treatment of, 635–637, 636f
  pain in, 133, 134f, 135f
  pericarditis and, 629
  Q wave, 598f, 600t, 601
  recurrent angina and, 630
  secondary prevention of, 630
  ST-segment elevation, **621**
  supraventricular arrhythmias and, 625–626
  treatment of, 278t, 279, 622–625, 623f, 624f, 627t
  ventricular aneurysm and, 630
  ventricular arrhythmias and, 625
Myocardial perfusion imaging, 622
Myocarditis, **612**
  coxsackievirus, 545
  in diphtheria, 460
  laboratory evaluation of, 612
  treatment of, 612
Myoclonus, 177
  posthypoxic, 71
Myonecrosis, 412, **412**
  clostridial, 98t, 100, 488
Myopathy
  drug-induced, 951, 951t, 988t
  inflammatory, **948**
    diagnosis of, 949t
  metabolic, **948**
  mitochondrial, **950**
  simulating muscular dystrophy, 950
  toxic, 950, 951t
Myophosphorylase deficiency, 948
Myositis, **412**
  drug-induced, 988t
Myotonia, 944, 950
Myotonic dystrophy, **944**
  treatment of, 947
Myxedema coma, 816
  treatment of, 817

Nadolol
  for syncope, 167
  for variceal bleeding, 217, 771
Nafcillin
  for bacterial meningitis, 890t, 891t
  for cellulitis, 410t
  for endocarditis, 376t–377t
  for osteomyelitis, 416t
  for sepsis, 52t
  for *Staphylococcus aureus* infections, 452t
Nails, in malnutrition, 4
Naloxone
  for narcotic overdose, 976
  for primary biliary cirrhosis, 768
  for status epilepticus, 72
Naltrexone, for narcotic abuse, 976
Naproxen
  for pain, 26t
  for tension headache, 146t
Naratriptan, for migraine, 143t
Narcissistic personality, 962
Narcolepsy, 183, 184t
  symptoms of, 185t
Narcotic(s)
  for acute abdomen, 207
  for migraine, 144t
  for pain, 26t
Narcotic abuse, **975**
  clinical features of, 975–976
  prevention of, 977
  treatment of
    drug-free programs, 977
    opiate antagonists, 976–977
    opioid maintenance, 976
    overdose, 976
    withdrawal, 976
Nasal swab, 353t
Nasogastric aspiration, for GI bleeding, 215
Nasopharyngeal cancer, 309, 532, 532t
Nausea and vomiting, **197**
  causes of, 199t
  chemotherapy-related, 286–288, 287t–288t
  complications of, 198
  drug-induced, 985t
  treatment of, 198
Necator americanus infection, 582
Neck pain, **154,** 155t
  causes of, 154
  treatment of, 156
Neck weakness, **924**
Necrotizing fasciitis, 98t, 100, **409**
  mixed anaerobic-aerobic infection, 490
  streptococcal, 457
  treatment of, 410t–411t
Nedocromil sodium, for asthma, 670t, 671
Nefazodone, 963
  dosage and adverse effects of, 965t
Negri bodies, 547
Neisseria gonorrhoeae infection. *See also* Gonorrhea
  arthritis, 412
  disseminated, 400, 401t

Neisseria gonorrhoeae infection (*Cont.*):
  epididymitis, 396
  mucopurulent cervicitis, 397
  pelvic inflammatory disease, 397
  proctitis, 399
  urethritis/urethral syndrome in women,
    396
  urinary tract, 724
Neisseria meningitidis infection. *See* Meningococcal infection
Nelfinavir mesylate, for HIV infections,
  434t
Nelson's syndrome, 825
Nematode infection, **580**
  ascariasis, 582
  enterobiasis, 583–584
  filariasis, 584–585
  hookworm, 582
  intestinal, 582–584
  larva migrans, 581
  onchocerciasis, 585
  strongyloidiasis, 582–583
  tissue, 580–581
  trichinellosis, 580–581
Neomycin, for hepatic encephalopathy,
  772
Neonate
  herpes simplex virus infection in, 522,
    525t
  listerial infection in, 465–466
  streptococcal infections in, group B,
    458–459
  tetanus in, 486
Nephrectomy, for renal cancer, 333
Nephritic syndrome, 232
Nephritis
  acute, approach to, 700t
  acute (allergic) interstitial, **720**
  chronic interstitial, **722**
  interstitial
    azotemia in, 228f
    drug-induced, 986t
Nephrolithiasis, **731**
  approach to, 700t, 702, 732, 732t
  signs and symptoms of, 731
  stone composition, 732, 733t
  treatment of, 733, 733t
Nephropathy
  diabetic, 717, 833
  drug-induced, 986t
  IgA, 720
  ischemic, **730**
  sickle cell, 731
Nephrosclerosis, arteriolar, **730**
Nephrotic syndrome, **716**
  approach to, 699, 700t
  causes of, 716t
  drug-induced, 986t
  edema in, 194, 195f
  evaluation of, 718t
Nerve agents
  bioweapons, 126–127
  treatment of exposure to, 127, 128t
Nerve conduction studies, in polyneuropathy, 939

Nerve trunk pain, 141t
Nervous system tumor, **883**
  approach to, 883
  treatment of, 883
Nesiritide
  for heart failure, 651, 651t
  for pulmonary edema, 54
Nateglinide, for diabetes mellitus, 833t
Neuralgia, 24
  cranial, 141t
  postherpetic, 526–527
Neurasthenia, 942
Neuroborreliosis, 506–507
Neurocysticercosis, 588, 894
Neuroendocrine small cell tumor, bladder,
  331
Neurogenic tumor, mediastinal, 693
Neuroimaging, **873**
  in brain abscess, 894
  in brain tumor, 883
  in chronic meningitis, 897–898
  in encephalitis, 893
  guidelines for, 874t
  in multiple sclerosis, 900
  in progressive multifocal leukoencepha-
    lopathy, 895
  in seizures, 882
Neuroleptic malignant syndrome, 160,
  969
Neuroleptic poisoning, 86
Neurologic disease. *See also specific diseases*
  in alcoholism, 973
  in amyloidosis, 805
  anaerobic infections, 490
  ataxic disorders, 914–917
  autonomic nervous system disorders,
    925–932
  brain abscess, 894–895
  cranial nerve disorders, 920–925
  dementias, 904–910
  depression and, 956
  diagnosis of, 867–873
    neuroimaging, 873–875
  drug-induced, 986t–987t
  encephalitis, acute, 886–894
  in HIV/AIDS, 437
  infectious, 98t, 100–101
    in immunocompromised host, 419
  insomnia in, 182
  in leprosy, 503
  in malnutrition, 4
  meningitis
    acute, 886–894
    chronic, 896–898
  motor neuron disease, 917–920
  multiple sclerosis, 899–904
  myasthenia gravis, 942–944
  nervous system tumors, 883–885
  Parkinson's disease, 910–914
  peripheral neuropathy, 936–941
  progressive multifocal leukoencepha-
    lopathy, 895
  radiation therapy-related, 885

Neurologic disease (*Cont.*):
    in rheumatoid arthritis, 781
    in sarcoidosis, 803
    seizures, 875–883
    spinal cord disease, 932–936
    in systemic lupus erythematosus, 780
    weight loss in, 201t
Neurologic examination, **867**
    for confusion and coma, 56–57
    coordination and gait analysis, 873
    cranial nerve exam, 868–872
    mental status exam, 867–868, 867t
    motor exam, 868t–869t, 872
    reflex testing, 872
    sensory exam, 870f, 871f, 873
Neurologic paraneoplastic syndrome, **346,**
        347t
    of CNS and dorsal root ganglia, 346–
        347, 347t
    of nerve and muscle, 347t, 348–349
Neuromuscular junction disorders, weak-
        ness in, 176t, 177t
Neuromyelitis optica, 903
Neuropathic joint disease, **800**
Neurosyphilis, 403–404, 405t, 897t
Neutraphos, for hypophosphatemia, 851
Neutron particles, 129
Neutropenia, 274
    cancer-treatment related, 104, 287t–
        288t, 288
        treatment of, 104
    diagnosis and treatment of febrile neu-
        tropenia, 419–420, 420f
    sepsis in, treatment of, 52t
    treatment of, 274
Neutrophilia, 272
Nevirapine, for HIV/AIDS, 432t, 439
Niacin, for hyperlipidemia, 859t, 860
Niacin deficiency, 16t
Nicotine replacement therapy, 676
Nifedipine
    for achalasia, 204
    for aortic regurgitation, 608
    for esophageal spasm, 205
    for pulmonary hypertension, 661
    for systemic sclerosis, 784
    for vasospastic disorders, 656
Nifurtimox, for Chagas' disease, 577
Nimodipine, for vasospasm in subarach-
        noid hemorrhage, 66
Nipah virus, 892
Nitazoxanide, for cryptosporidiosis, 386
Nitrates
    for angina pectoris, 632, 633t
    for dilated cardiomyopathy, 609
    for heart failure, 651t
    for Prinzmetal's variant angina, 637
Nitric oxide, inhaled, for cor pulmonale,
        652
Nitrofurantoin
    mechanisms and indications for, 365
    for urinary tract infections, 726t
    for urinary tract infection prophylaxis,
        727

Nitrogen mustard, 125–126
Nitroglycerin
    for acute coronary syndromes, 635
    for anal fissure, 749
    for angina pectoris, 632, 633t
    for esophagogastric varices, 771
    for heart failure, 626, 651t
    for malignant hypertension, 621
    for myocardial infarction, 623, 627t,
        628t
    for pulmonary edema, 54
Nitroprusside
    for heart failure, 626, 650, 651t
    for mitral regurgitation, 605
    for myocardial infarction, 627t, 629
Nocardiosis, **492**
    brain abscess, 894
    treatment of, 493–494, 493t
Nodular lesions, 409
Nodule, 255
Nonfluent transcortical aphasia, 180t
Nonpolyposis syndrome, 325, 325t
Nonsteroidal anti-inflammatory drugs
        (NSAID)
    for acute cholecystitis, 751
    for chronic fatigue syndrome, 953
    for fever, 158, 159f
    for gout, 797
    for low back pain, 151
    for migraine, 142, 143t
    for osteoarthritis, 795
    for pain, 25
    peptic ulcer disease and, 737
    for psoriatic arthritis, 792
    for rheumatoid arthritis, 783
    for tendinitis, 802
Norepinephrine
    for increased intracranial pressure, 68t
    for shock, 48, 48t
Norethisterone, for GI telangiectases, 217
Norfloxacin, for spontaneous bacterial
        peritonitis, 225
Norplant, 845
Nortriptyline
    dosage and adverse effects of, 964t
    for migraine prophylaxis, 145t
    for pain, 25, 27t
Norwalk virus infection, diarrhea, 385
Nosocomial infections, **442**
    epidemic and emerging problems, 444
    intravascular device infections, 443–444
    pneumonia, 443, 685
    prevention of, 1, 442
    surgical wound, 443
    urinary tract infections, 442–443
Nucleic acid probes, 358
Nucleoside analogues, 438
5′-Nucleotidase, blood, 222, 222t
Nude syndrome, 777
Nutrients, GI absorption of, 208
Nutritional status, assessment of, **2**
Nutritional support
    decision tree for initiating, 15f
    enteral nutrition, 14–17
    parenteral nutrition, 14–17

Nystagmus, 870
Nystatin, 555
  for candidiasis, 206, 558

Obesity, **828**
  causes of, 828–839
  central, 828
  clinical features of, 829
  defined, 828
  drug-induced, 829
  treatment of, 829–830
Obesity-hypoventilation, 696t, 697
Obsessive-compulsive disorder, **959**
  treatment of, 960
Obstructive shock, extracardiac, 45t, 46t
Octreotide
  for acromegaly, 811
  for carcinoid tumor, 329
  for esophagogastric varices, 771
  for pancreatic islet-cell tumors, 331
  for variceal bleeding, 217
Octreotide scan, 741
Ocular motor nerve palsy, 174
Oculopharyngeal dystrophy, **948**
Odynophagia, 203
Ofloxacin
  for epididymitis, 396
  for gonococcal infections, 401t
  for leprosy, 503
  for meningococcal infection prophy-
    laxis, 464t
  for pelvic inflammatory disease, 398
  for typhoid fever, 388
Olanzapine, 969
  dosage and adverse effects of, 967t
  for schizophrenia, 958
Olfactory dysfunction, **922**, 923t
Olfactory nerve (I), 868
  disorders of, **922**, 923t
Oligemic shock, 45, 45t, 46t
Oligoblastic leukemia, 294
Oligodendroglioma, 884
Oliguria, 228
Olivopontocerebellar degeneration,
  915
Omeprazole
  for gastroesophageal reflux disease,
    200
  for *Helicobacter pylori* eradication,
    739t
  for noncardiac chest pain, 204
  for systemic sclerosis, 784
  for Zollinger-Ellison syndrome, 741
Onchocerciasis, **585**
  treatment of, 585
Oncologic emergencies, **101**
  paraneoplastic syndromes, 103
  structural/obstructive, 101–102
  treatment complications, 104
Ondansetron, for nausea and vomiting,
  198
Ophthalmia neonatorum, 400, 401t
Ophthalmoplegia, 925
  chronic progressive external, 950

Opiate abuse, **975**
Opisthorchiasis, 586
Opsoclonus-myoclonus syndrome, parane-
    oplastic, 347
Optic chiasm, lesion of, 172, 172f, 243–
    244
Optic nerve disorders, 172f
  tumors, 243–244
Optic neuritis, 172f, 173
  drug-induced, 987t
Optic neuropathy, 172f
  anterior ischemic, 173
Optic radiations, lesions of, 172f
Optic tract lesions, 172f
Oral contraceptives
  for abnormal uterine bleeding, 839–
    840
  for amenorrhea, 842
  for hirsutism in female, 843
  for menopausal symptoms, 843
  for pelvic pain in women, 842
  for pregnancy prevention, 845
Orchiectomy, for testicular cancer, 333
Orchitis, mumps, 542
Organophosphate insecticide poisoning,
    86
Organophosphorus nerve agents, 126–127
Orientia tsutsugamushi infection. *See*
    Scrub typhus
Orlistat, for obesity, 829
Oropharyngeal dysphagia, 203–204
Oroya fever, **483**, 484t
Orthostatic hypotension, 165, 927
  approach to, 927–928
  drug-induced, 927, 931
  treatment of, 167–168, 931, 931t
Oseltamivir
  for influenza, 535
  for influenza prophylaxis, 536
Osteoarthritis, **794**
  back pain in, 148
  clinical features of, 794–795
  erosive, 794
  generalized, 794
  primary, 794
  secondary, 794
  treatment of, 795–796
Osteochondritis, 475
Osteomalacia, **854**
  treatment of, 855
Osteomyelitis, **414**
  acute hematogenous, 414–415
  chronic, 414, 417
  contiguous-focus, 414, 417
  HACEK organisms, 470
  imaging in, 414, 415t
  Pseudomonas aeruginosa, 475
  staphylococcal, 414
  Staphylococcus aureus, 449, 454
  treatment of, 415–417, 416t
  vertebral, 417
    brucellosis, 479
    pain in, 150

Osteonecrosis, **801**
  pain in, 162f
  treatment of, 801
Osteoporosis, **852**
  back pain in, 150
  diseases associated with, 853t
  drug-induced, 852
  risk factors for fracture, 853t
  screening for, 993t, 994t
  treatment of, 854
    in women, 990
Otitis externa, 252
  acute diffuse, 252
  acute localized, 252
  chronic, 252
  malignant or necrotizing, 252
Otitis media
  acute, 252
    diagnosis of, 251t
    treatment of, 251t
  chronic, 253
  measles, 540
  Moraxella catarrhalis, 468
  pneumococcal, 445
  serous, 253
Otoacoustic emissions, 244
Otosclerosis, 245
Ovarian ablation, for breast cancer, 318
Ovarian cancer, **334**
  paraneoplastic syndromes, 348t
  staging and survival in, 335, 336t
Ovarian failure, 840, 842
Overdiagnosis, 281
Overweight, 828
Ovral, 845
Oxacillin
  for brain abscess, 99t
  for cellulitis, 410t
  for endocarditis, 376t–377t
  for epidural abscess, 99t
  for infectious arthritis, 413
  for intracranial infections, 98t
  mechanisms, indications, and adverse
    effects of, 361
  for osteomyelitis, 416t
  for sepsis, 52t
  for *Staphylococcus aureus* infections,
    452t
  for toxic shock syndrome, 97t
Oxaliplatin, for colorectal cancer, 327
Oxalosis, 723
Oxazepam, dosage and adverse effects of,
  966t
Oxcarbazepine, for generalized anxiety
    disorder, 959
Oxcarbazine, for pain, 27t
Oxime therapy, for nerve agent exposure,
    126, 128t
Oxybutynin, for bladder dysfunction, 903
Oxycodone
  abuse of, **975**
  for pain, 26t
Oxygen therapy
  for carbon monoxide poisoning, 81
  in cardiogenic shock, 627
  for cluster headache, 146
  for COPD, 677
  for cor pulmonale, 652
  for heart failure, 626
  for interstitial lung disease, 690
  for myocardial infarction, 623
  for pulmonary edema, 54
  for pulmonary hypertension, 661
  for respiratory failure, 678
  for seizures, 882
  for shock, 48
Oxytocin, 813

Pacemaker, artificial
  for hypertrophic cardiomyopathy, 612
  indications for, 626
Paclitaxel
  for bladder cancer, 332
  for breast cancer, 318
  for head and neck cancer, 310
  for ovarian cancer, 335
  for peritoneal carcinomatosis, 343
Pain, **23**
  abdominal, **136**
  acute, treatment of, 25, 26t–27t
  acute abdomen, **206**
  chest, **133**, 204
  chest wall, 133, 134f
  chronic, 25
    treatment of, 25, 26t–27t
  costochondral, 133, 134f
  in diverticular disease, 747
  esophageal, 133, 134f
  evaluation of, 24–25, 24t
  eye, 241–242
  facial, 141t, 147, 920
  joint, **161**
  low back, **147**
  management of, **23**
  neck, **154**, 155t
  neuropathic, 24, 24t
  organization of pain pathways, 23–24
  in osteoarthritis, 794
  pelvic, 842
    chronic pelvic pain syndrome, 727–
      728
  referred, 25
  shoulder, **154**, 155t
  somatic, 24t
  in spinal cord disease, 933
  spontaneous, 930
  visceral, 24t
Pallidotomy, for Parkinson's disease, 914
Palosetron, for nausea and vomiting, 198
Palpation, precordial, 593–594, 594f
Pamidronate, for hypercalcemia, 103, 345,
    849t
Pancreatectomy, subtotal, 756
Pancreatic abscess, 755
Pancreatic cancer, 328
Pancreatic enzyme replacement, 756
Pancreatic islet-cell tumor, **329**, 344t
  treatment of, 331
Pancreatic necrosis, 755

Pancreatic pseudocyst, 755
Pancreatitis
  acute, **753**
    complications of, 754–755, 755t
    treatment of, 754
  ascites in, 226t
  chronic, **755**
    complications of, 756
    treatment of, 756
  drug-induced, 986t
  edematous, 753
  necrotizing, 753–754
  pleural effusion in, 691
Pancytopenia, drug-induced, 983t
Panic disorder, **958**
  treatment of, 959
Papillary necrosis, **727**
Papilledema, 173
Pappenheimer bodies, 265
Pap smear, 282t, 337, 992t, 994t
Papular lesions, 409
Papule, 255
Para-aminosalicylic acid, for tuberculosis,
  499t
Paracentesis, **30**
  for acute abdomen, 207
  diagnostic, 224
  large-volume, for ascites, 225
Paracoccidioidomycosis, **564**
  treatment of, 564
Paragonimus infection, 587
Parainfluenza virus infection, **538**
  pneumonia, 684
Paralysis, **175**
  diaphragmatic, 695
  periodic, 950
Paralytic shellfish poisoning, 111–112
Paramomycin
  for amebiasis, 391
  for cryptosporidiosis, 386
Paraneoplastic syndrome
  emergent, 103
  endocrine, **344**
  neurologic, **346,** 347t
  treatment of, 345
Paranoid personality, 962
Paraparesis, 176t
Paraplegia, 933
  familial spastic, 936
Parasites
  blood and tissue, diagnosis of, 359t,
    360
  diagnosis of, **358**
    antibody and antigen detection, 360
    direct diagnosis, 358–360, 359t
  intestinal, diagnosis of, 358–360, 359t
  in red blood cells, 265
Parathyroid hormone, for osteoporosis,
  854
Parenteral nutrition, **14**
  decision tree for initiating, 15f
Paresthesia, in spinal cord disease, 933
Parkinsonian syndrome, 907

Parkinson's disease, **910**
  clinical features of, 910
  differential diagnosis of, 911
  etiology of, 910
  treatment of, 911–914, 912t–913t
Parotitis, mumps, 542
Paroxetine
  dosage and adverse effects of, 964t
  for irritable bowel syndrome, 746
  for panic disorder, 959
  for syncope, 167
Paroxysmal nocturnal dyspnea, 183
Paroxysmal supraventricular tachycardia,
  639f, 640t
Parvovirus B19 infection, **542**
  treatment of, 543
Passive-aggressive personality, 962
Pasteurella multocida infection
  from animal bites, 106, 107t–108t
  cellulitis, 409
Patch test, 259
Pediculosis, **590**
  treatment of, 591
Pelvic abscess, clostridial, 488
Pelvic infection
  actinomycosis, 494
  anaerobic, 490
  Escherichia coli, 472
Pelvic inflammatory disease (PID), **397**
  treatment of, 398
Pelvic pain
  chronic, **727**
  in female, **842**
    treatment of, 842
Pemoline, for breast cancer, 320
Penicillamine
  for mercury poisoning, 85
  for nephrolithiasis, 733t
  for rheumatoid arthritis, 783
  for systemic sclerosis, 784
  for Wilson's disease, 865
Penicillin
  for actinomycosis, 495
  for anaerobic infections, 491
  for anthrax, 122
  for brain abscess, 99t
  for clostridial infections, 98t, 489
  for enterococcal infections, 459
  for HACEK endocarditis, 469t
  for listeriosis, 466
  mechanisms, indications, and adverse
    effects of, 361
  for meningococcemia, 97t
  for necrotizing fasciitis, 98t, 410t, 457
  for pneumococcal infections, 447
  for septic arthritis, 458
  for streptococcal toxic shock syndrome,
    458
  for toxic shock syndrome, 97t, 455
Penicillin G
  for bacterial meningitis, 890t, 891t
  for endocarditis, 376t
  for gas gangrene, 410t
  for leptospirosis, 509

Penicillin G (*Cont.*):
for meningococcal infections, 464t
for *Staphylococcus aureus* infections, 452t, 454
for streptococcal infections, 459
Penicillin V
for pharyngitis, 250t
for streptococcal carriage, 456
for streptococcal infections, 456
Penicillin VK, for animal bite, 108t
Penicilliosis marneffei, **564**
treatment of, 564
Pentamidine
for leishmaniasis, 576
for *Pneumocystis* infections, 567t
for *Pneumocystis* prophylaxis, 568t
for sleeping sickness, 578
Pentazocine abuse, **975**
Pentobarbital coma, 68t, 72, 73f
Pentoxifylline
for alcoholic liver disease, 768
for arteriosclerosis of peripheral arteries, 656
Peptic ulcer disease (PUD), 200, 329, **737**
approach to, 729
causes of, 737
diagnosis of, 738, 738t, 741t
drug-induced, 986t
duodenal, 737–739
gastric, 737–739
GI bleeding in, 215
treatment of
medical, 738, 739t
surgical, 738–739, 739t
Peptostreptococcus infection, 489–491
Percutaneous balloon valvuloplasty, for mitral stenosis, 604
Percutaneous coronary intervention (PCI)
for acute coronary syndromes, 637
for angina pectoris, 634, 634t
for cardiogenic shock, 627
for myocardial infarction, 622, 623f
Percutaneous electrical nerve stimulation, for low back pain, 151
Percutaneous needle aspiration, of lung, 667
Percutaneous transhepatic cholangiography, 750t
Percutaneous transluminal angioplasty, for angina pectoris, 634, 634t
Pergolide, for Parkinson's disease, 913t
Periappendicitis, 397
Periarticular disorder, **801**
Pericardial disease, **612**
acute pericarditis, 612–614
cardiac tamponade, 615
constrictive pericarditis, 615–616
Pericardial effusion
echocardiography in, 603
oncologic emergency, 102
symptomatic, approach to, 616
treatment of, 102
Pericardial tamponade, oncologic emergency, 102

Pericardiectomy, 615
Pericarditis
acute, **612**
causes of, 612, 613t
laboratory evaluation of, 613, 613t, 614f
pain in, 133, 135f
treatment of, 613t
constrictive, **615**
laboratory evaluation of, 615–616
treatment of, 616
coxsackievirus, 545
drug-induced, 984t
myocardial infarction and, 629
tuberculous, 497
Perichondritis, 252
Perihepatitis, 397
Perimenopause, 843
Perinephric abscess, 382–383
Periodic limb movement disorder, 182, 184t
Periodic paralysis, **950**
hyperkalemic, 950
hypokalemic, 950
Periodontal disease, anaerobic infection, 489
Peripherally inserted central catheter (PICC), for parenteral nutrition, 16
Peripheral nerves, cutaneous areas supplied by, 870f, 871f
Peripheral neuropathy
approach to, 937f
autonomic dysfunction in, 928
drug-induced, 986t
mononeuropathy, 940t, 941
polyneuropathy, 936–941
weakness in, 176t, 177t
Peripheral vascular disease, **655**
arterial, 655–657
venous, 657–658
Peritoneal dialysis, 710–711
complications of, 710t, 711
Peritoneal disease
ascites in, 224
pain in, 137t
Peritoneal lavage, for acute abdomen, 207
Peritonitis, **380**
in chronic ambulatory peritoneal dialysis, 381
secondary, 381
spontaneous bacterial, 225–227, 226t, 380–381
treatment of, 381
tuberculous, 226t
Perlèche, 258f
Permethrin, for pediculosis, 591
Personality disorder, **961**
cluster A, 962
cluster B, 962
cluster C, 962
Pertussis, **467**
catarrhal phase of, 467
convalescent phase of, 468
paroxysmal phase of, 467–468

Pertussis (*Cont.*):
  prevention of, 468
  treatment of, 468
Peutz-Jeghers syndrome, 325, 325t
Pfiesteria poisoning, 112
  treatment of, 112
Pharyngitis
  acute, 253
    diagnosis of, 250t
    treatment of, 250t
  bacterial, 253
  herpes simplex virus, 520
  streptococcus group A, 455–456
    treatment of, 456
  viral, 253
Pharyngoconjunctival fever, 539
Pharynx, necrotizing infections of, 489
Phenelzine
  dosage and adverse effects of, 965t
  for migraine prophylaxis, 145t
Phenobarbital
  for seizures, 882t
  for status epilepticus, 72, 73f
Phenothiazine, for nausea and vomiting, 198
Phentolamine, for sympathomimetic poisoning, 88
Phenylephrine
  for increased intracranial pressure, 68t
  for shock, 48, 48t
  for vasospasm in subarachnoid hemorrhage, 66
Phenytoin
  for brain tumor, 883
  for multiple sclerosis, 903
  for myotonic dystrophy, 947
  for pain, 27t
  for seizures, 880t–881t, 882t
  for status epilepticus, 72, 73f
  for trigeminal neuralgia, 920
Pheochromocytoma, 823
  hypertension in, 617–618
Phlebotomy
  for hemochromatosis, 862
  for polycythemia, 235
  for porphyria, 864
  for pulmonary edema, 54
Phobic disorder, **960**
  treatment of, 961
Phosphate therapy, for hypophosphatemia, 851
Phosphofructokinase deficiency, 950
Photodermatitis, drug-induced, 982t
Phototherapy, for primary biliary cirrhosis, 768
Physostigmine
  for anticholinergic poisoning, 79
  for cyclic antidepressant poisoning, 82
  for muscle relaxant poisoning, 86
Pilocarpine
  for glaucoma, 242–243
  for Sjögren's syndrome, 785
Pink eye, 242
Pinta, 507–508

Pinworm, **583**
Pioglitazone, for diabetes mellitus, 833t
Piperacillin
  mechanisms, indications, and adverse
    effects of, 361
  for osteomyelitis, 416t
  for pneumonia, 683t
  for *Pseudomonas aeruginosa* infections, 476t
Piperacillin/tazobactam
  for anaerobic infections, 491t
  for gram-negative sepsis, 96t
  for osteomyelitis, 416t
  for peritonitis, 381
  for pneumonia, 680t–681t, 682t–683t
  for *Pseudomonas aeruginosa* infections, 476t
  for sepsis, 52t
Pitting, 239
Pitting edema, 658
Pituitary adenoma, **807**
  diagnosis of, 807, 809t
  gonadotropin-producing, **811**
  nonfunctioning, **811**
  treatment of, 809
  TSH-producing, 811
Pituitary apoplexy, 807, 809
Pituitary disorder
  anterior, **807**
  posterior, **813**
Pituitary hormone hypersecretion syndromes, **809**
Pituitary tumor, 244, **807**
Pityriasis rosea, 256f, 259
  treatment of, 259
Plague, **481**
  as bioweapon, 121t, 122–123
  bubonic, 482
  pneumonic, 122, 482
  septicemic, 482
  treatment of, 121t, 482–483
Plantar reflex, 872
Plaque, skin lesions, 255
Plaques, lesions of multiple sclerosis, 899
Plasma cell disorders, 297t, **303**
Plasmacytoma, 304
Plasma exchange
  for acute renal failure, 706
  for glomerulonephritis, 716
  for multiple sclerosis, 903
Plasmapheresis, 19
  for acute renal failure, 706
  for chronic inflammatory demyelinating
    polyneuropathy, 941
  for myasthenia gravis, 944
  for primary biliary cirrhosis, 768
  for thrombotic thrombocytopenic purpura, 277
  for vasculitis, 788
Plasmodium infection, **569**. *See also* Malaria
Platelet clumping, 266
Platelet count, 275

Platelet disorders, 275–276
  platelet function disorders, 276–277
  thrombocytopenia, 275
Plateletpheresis, 19
Platelet transfusion, 18
Platinum agents
  for breast cancer, 320
  cancer chemotherapy, 287t
Pleconaril, for enterovirus infections, 546
Plesiomonas infection, 354t
Pleural biopsy, 667
Pleural disease, **691**
  tuberculous, 496–497
Pleural effusion, **691**
  in acute pancreatitis, 755
  approach to, 694f
  drug-induced, 692t
  eosinophilic, 691
  exudative, 692t
  parapneumonic, 691–692
  in pneumonia, 681
  tests for, 693t
  transudative, 692t
Pleural plaques, 674
Pleurisy, **691**
  pain in, 133
Pleurodynia, coxsackievirus, 545
Pneumatic compression boots, 658
Pneumococcal infection, 95, **445**
  endocarditis, 446–447
  epiglottitis, 254
  meningitis, 446, 886, 887t, 890t
  nosocomial, 443
  otitis media, 252, 445
  penicillin-resistant, 446
  pneumonia, 445–447, 679, 681, 684
  prevention of, 447
  sinusitis, 249, 445
  treatment of, 446–447
Pneumococcal vaccine, 367f, 368f, 370f,
    447, 993t, 994t
  in immunocompromised patients, 423t
Pneumocystis infection, 437, 565–568,
    684
  HIV and, 566–568
  prevention of, 568, 568t
  treatment of, 567–568, 567t
Pneumonia, **679**
  aspiration, 490, 679, 681t, 684
  bronchopneumonia, 679
  Chlamydia pneumoniae, 519
  community-acquired, 679–685
    clinical features of, 679–681
    complications of, 681–684
    diagnosis of, 684
    in long-term care facilities, 684
    treatment of, 680t, 684–685
  desquamative interstitial, **689**
  diagnosis of, 664t
  diphtheria, 461
  eosinophilic, 688t, **690**
  Escherichia coli, 472
  gram-negative enteric bacteria, 473
  Haemophilus influenzae, 467

  hospital-acquired, 685
    treatment of, 680t, 682t–683t
  influenza virus, 534
  interstitial, 679, 688t
  Klebsiella, 472
  lobar, 679
  miliary, 679
  Moraxella catarrhalis, 468
  Mycoplasma pneumoniae, 516–517
  nocardiosis, 492
  nosocomial, 443
  pneumococcal, 445–447
    treatment of, 447
  Pneumocystis, 437, 565–568, 684
  Pseudomonas aeruginosa, 474
  respiratory syncytial virus, 538
  routes of infection, 679
  Staphylococcus aureus, 450
  streptococcal, 457
  Toxoplasma, 579
  usual interstitial, **689**
  varicella, 526
  ventilator-associated, 474
Pneumonitis
  herpes simplex virus, 522
  hypersensitivity. *See* Hypersensitivity
    pneumonitis
  necrotizing, 490
Pneumothorax, **692**
  pain in, 135f
Podofilox, for human papillomavirus in-
    fections, 408
Podophyllin
  for human papillomavirus infections,
    407
  for warts, 262
Podophyllotoxin, for anal condylomas,
    749
Poikilocytosis, 265
Poisoning, **74**
  acetaminophen, 74, 78, 761
  alkali and acid, 78
  antiarrhythmic drugs, 78–79
  anticholinergic agents, 79
  anticonvulsants, 79–80
  antidepressants, cyclic, 82
  arsenic, 80
  barbiturates, 80
  beta-blockers, 80–81
  cadmium, 81
  calcium channel blockers, 81
  carbon monoxide, 69, 71, 74, 81
  cardiac glycosides, 82
  cyanide, 69, 82
  digoxin, 82
  enhancement of poison elimination,
    76t, 77–78
  ethylene glycol, 83
  hallucinogens, 83
  insecticides, 86
  iron, 83
  isoniazid, 83–84
  isopropyl alcohol, 84
  lead, 84, 723

Poisoning (*Cont.*):
  lithium, 84
  marine, **111**
  mercury, 84–85
  methanol, 85
  muscle relaxants, 86
  neuroleptics, 86
  prevention of absorption, 76t, 77
  salicylates, 86–87
  sympathomimetics, 87–88
  thallium, 88
  theophylline, 88
  treatment of, 75–78
Polio vaccine, 367f, 544, 546
  in immunocompromised patients, 423t
Poliovirus infection, **544**
  paralytic disease, 544
  postpolio syndrome, 545
  prevention of, 546
Polyangiitis, microscopic, 786
Polyangiitis overlap syndrome, 786
Polyarteritis, renal disease in, 719t
Polyarteritis nodosa, 715, 786
Polychondritis, relapsing, **800**
  treatment of, 800
Polycystic kidney disease, **722**
Polycystic ovarian syndrome, 839–840
Polycythemia, **234**
  approach to, 234f
  secondary, 235
  treatment of, 235
Polycythemia vera, 235, 295
Polydipsia, 230f, 813
Polyene macrolide, 555
Polyethylene glycol, for constipation, 214
Polymyalgia rheumatica, **801**
  pain in, 162f
  treatment of, 801
Polymyositis, 948, 949t
  pain in, 162f
  treatment of, 948
Polymyxin B, for *Pseudomonas aeruginosa* infections, 477t
Polyneuropathy, **936**
  acute inflammatory demyelinating, 939–941
  alcoholic, 928–930
  axonal, 937–938, 938t
  chronic inflammatory demyelinating, 941
  clinical features of, 936–937
  demyelinative, 937–938, 938t
  diagnosis of, 938–939, 939t
  in diphtheria, 461
  electrodiagnosis of, 939
  time course of, 939t
Polyps
  colonic, **324**
  gastric, 322–323
Polythiol resins, for mercury poisoning, 85
Polyuria, 228–229, 722t
  approach to, 230f
  causes of, 229t

Pontiac fever, 478
Porphyria, **862**
  acute intermittent, 862
    autoimmune dysfunction in, 930
  erythropoietic, 862, 864
  hepatic, 862
  treatment of, 863–864
Porphyria cutanea tarda, 863
  treatment of, 864
Porphyromonas infection, 489–491
Portal hypertension, **769**
  classification of, 769, 770t
Portuguese man-of-war, 110
Posaconazole, 555
Postcoital contraception, 845
Posterior fossa mass, 67
Postherpetic neuralgia, 526–527
Postpolio syndrome, 545
Postradiation fibrosis, 154
Posttraumatic stress disorder (PTSD), **960**
  treatment of, 960
Postural orthostatic tachycardia syndrome, 930
Potassium, disorders of, **7**
Potassium acetate, for hypokalemia, 8
Potassium bicarbonate, for hypokalemia, 8
Potassium chloride
  for hypokalemia, 8
  for metabolic alkalosis, 13
Potassium hydroxide preparation, 257–258
Potassium iodide, for sporotrichosis, 565
Potassium therapy, for diabetic ketoacidosis, 90t
Pott's disease, 497
Powassan encephalitis, 552t
PPD skin test, 498
Pralidoxime
  for insecticide poisoning, 86
  for nerve agent exposure, 126, 128t
Pramipexole
  for Parkinson's disease, 913t
  for periodic limb movements of sleep, 184t
  for restless legs syndrome, 182
Pravastatin, for hyperlipidemia, 859t
Praziquantel
  for diphyllobothriasis, 590
  for echinococcosis, 589
  for liver flukes, 587
  for lung flukes, 587
  for schistosomiasis, 586
  for taeniasis, 588
  for taeniasis saginata, 587
Prazocin, for vasospastic disorders, 656
Prednisolone
  for alcoholic liver disease, 768
  for asthma, 670t, 671
  for autoimmune hepatitis, 766
  for respiratory failure, 678
Prednisone
  for acute lymphoid leukemia/lymphoma, 302
  for acute pericarditis, 613

Prednisone (*Cont.*):
for alcoholic liver disease, 768
for amyloidosis, 805
for asthma, 670t, 671
for autoimmune hepatitis, 766
for Bell's palsy, 922
for cluster headache prophylaxis, 145
for COPD, 678
for hypercalcemia, 849t
for hypersensitivity pneumonitis, 673
for hypopituitarism, 812
for idiopathic thrombocytopenic purpura, 277
immunosuppression for renal transplant, 712–713
for inflammatory bowel disease, 744
for interstitial lung disease, 690
for multiple myeloma, 304
for multiple sclerosis, 903
for myasthenia gravis, 944
for optic neuritis, 173
for *Pneumocystis* infections, 567t
for polymyalgia rheumatica, 801
for reflex sympathetic dystrophy, 801
for relapsing polychondritis, 800
for thyrotoxicosis, 819
for vasculitis, 788
Preeclampsia, 731
Preexcitation syndrome, **644**
Pregnancy
gonorrhea in, 400
hypertension in, 621
listeriosis in, 465–466
malaria in, 570
streptococcal infection in, group B, 459
syphilis in, 405t
toxemias of, 731
travel advice, 369
Preleukemia, 294
Premenstrual syndrome, 842
Presbycusis, 245
Preventive services, **991**, 994t
Prevotella infection, 489–491
pelvic inflammatory disease, 397
Primaquine
for malaria, 570
for malaria prophylaxis, 572, 574t
for *Pneumocystis* infections, 567, 567t
Primidone, for seizures, 882t
Primitive neuro-ectodermal tumor (PNET), 884
Prinzmetal's variant angina, **637**
Prion disease, 904, 906t
Probenecid, for gout, 798
Procainamide
for arrhythmias, 646t
for cardiac arrest, 43f
for malignant hyperthermia, 160
for myotonic dystrophy, 947
for ventricular tachycardia, 625
Procaine penicillin G, for diphtheria, 461
Prochlorperazine
for migraine, 144t
for nausea and vomiting, 198, 286
for vertigo, 170t

Proctitis, **398**
herpes simplex virus, 524t
treatment of, 399
Proctocolitis, **398**
treatment of, 399
Progesterone, for hypopituitarism, 812
Progressive external ophthalmoplegia, **948**
Progressive multifocal leukoencephalopathy, **895**
Progressive supranuclear palsy, 906t, 907
Proguanil, for malaria prophylaxis, 574t
Prolactin, 807, 809t
hypersecretion of, 809–810
Prolactin-secreting tumor, 807, 809
Promethazine
for nausea and vomiting, 198
for vertigo, 170t
Propafenone, for arrhythmias, 646t
Propionibacterium acnes infection, 489–491
Propofol
for increased intracranial pressure, 68t
for status epilepticus, 72, 73f
Propoxyphene abuse, **975**
Propranolol
for aortic dissection, 655t
for esophagogastric varices, 771
for migraine prophylaxis, 145t
for phobias, 961
for thyrotoxicosis, 818, 820
for variceal bleeding, 217
Propylthiouracil, for thyrotoxicosis, 818–820
Prostacyclin, for cor pulmonale, 652
Prostascint scanning, for prostate cancer, 339
Prostate cancer, **338**
biopsy in, 339, 340f
bone metastasis, 343
diagnosis of, 339, 340f
prevention of, 283
risk factors for, 283
screening for, 281, 282t, 993t
treatment of, 339–341
Prostatectomy, radical retropubic, 339
Prostate hyperplasia, **338**
treatment of, 338
Prostate-specific antigen (PSA), 282t
bound and free, 339
in prostate cancer, 338–339, 340f
in prostate hyperplasia, 338
PSA density, 339
Prostatitis, **727**
acute bacterial, 727
chronic bacterial, 727
Prosthetic joint infection, 412–413, 454
Protease inhibitors, 433t–436t
Protein-calorie malnutrition, 4
Protein-losing enteropathy, 213
Protein restriction, for chronic renal failure, 709
Proteinuria, 230–232, 701, 718t, 722t
nephrotic range, 231

Proteus infection, **473**
  from animal bite, 108t
  prostatitis, 727
  treatment of, 473
  urinary tract, 724
Prothrombin time, 222, 222t
Proto-oncogenes, 285
Protozoal infection, **569**
  babesiosis, 572–573
  blood and tissue, diagnosis of, 359t
  intestinal, diagnosis of, 359t
  leishmaniasis, 574–576
  malaria, 569–572
  toxoplasmosis, 578–580
  trypanosomiasis, 576–578
Protriptyline
  for hypersomnia, 185
  for sleep apnea, 184t
Providencia infection, **473**
Prussian blue, for thallium poisoning, 88
Pseudoallescheriasis, **564**
  treatment of, 565
Pseudocyst, pancreatic, 755
Pseudoephedrine, for allergic rhinitis, 775
Pseudogout, **798**
  pain in, 162f
Pseudohypoparathyroidism, 850
Pseudomelena, 214
Pseudomonas aeruginosa infection, **474**
  from animal bite, 108t
  cellulitis, 409
  clinical features of, 474–475
  meningitis, 891t
  nosocomial, 443
  osteomyelitis, 416t
  otitis externa, 252
  pneumonia, 681, 685
  sinusitis, 249
  treatment of, 475, 476t–477t
  urinary tract, 724
Pseudoseizure, 876
Pseudothrombocytopenia, 276
Pseudotumor cerebri
  drug-induced, 987t
  visual loss in, 173
Psittacosis, **518**
  treatment of, 519
Psoas abscess, 383
Psoriasis, 256f, 257f, 259
  treatment of, 259
Psoriatic arthritis, 259, **791**
  pattern of joint involvement, 791
  pain in, 162f
  treatment of, 791–792
Psychiatric disorder, **955**. *See also specific diseases*
  anxiety disorders, 958–961
  bipolar disorder, 957
  dementia in, 905t
  depression, 955–957
  drug-induced, 988t
  eating disorders, 969–972
  generalized anxiety disorder, 959
  insomnia in, 182

  mood disorders, **955**
  obsessive-compulsive disorder, 959–960
  panic disorder, 958–959
  personality disorders, 961–962
  phobic disorders, 960–961
  posttraumatic stress disorder, 960
  schizophrenia, 957–958
  seizures in, 877t
  somatoform disorder, 961
  syncope in, 166t
  weight loss in, 201t
  in women, 990
Psychiatric medications, **962**
  antidepressants, 963, 964t–965t
  antipsychotics, 968–969
  anxiolytics, 963
  mood stabilizers, 968t, 969
  principles of use of, 962–963
Psyllium extract
  for constipation, 213
  for diverticular disease, 747
  for irritable bowel syndrome, 746
Pubic louse, 590–591
Puerperal sepsis, streptococcal, 457
Pulmonary alveolar proteinosis, 688t
Pulmonary angiography, 660f, 667
Pulmonary capillary wedge (PCW) pressure, in shock, 46, 47f
Pulmonary circulation, disturbances of, 665
Pulmonary disease. *See also* Respiratory disease; *specific diseases*
  anaerobic infections, 490
  coccidioidomycosis, 562–563
  cor pulmonale, 652
  cryptococcosis, 560
  cyanosis in, 192, 193t
  histoplasmosis, 561–562
  mucormycosis, 561
  nocardiosis, 492
  nontuberculous mycobacteria, 504–505
  postoperative, risk factors for, 36t
  pulmonary hypertension, 659t
  in rheumatoid arthritis, 781
  in systemic sclerosis, 783
Pulmonary edema
  acute, **53**
    precipitants of, 53t
    treatment of, 54
  diagnosis of, 664t
  drug-induced, 984t
Pulmonary embolism, **685**
  approach to, 686f
  chest pain in, 133, 135f
  dyspnea in, 186
  pleural effusion in, 692t
  pulmonary hypertension in, 659t
  treatment of, 278t, 279, 686–687, 687f
Pulmonary fibrosis, 688t
  idiopathic, **689**
Pulmonary function tests, 667
  in asthma, 669
  in COPD, 675–676

Pulmonary function tests (*Cont.*):
  in environmental lung disease, 673
  in hypersensitivity pneumonitis, 672
  preoperative, 36t, 37
  in pulmonary hypertension, 659, 660f
  reference values for, 1007t–1008t
Pulmonary hemorrhage syndrome, 688t
Pulmonary hypertension, **658**
  arterial, 659t
  causes of, 659t
  laboratory evaluation of, 659
  primary, **659**
    approach to, 660f
    differential diagnosis of, 659–661
    laboratory evaluation of, 659
    treatment of, 661
  venous, 659t
Pulmonary infiltrate, drug-induced, 984t
Pulmonary scintigraphy, 667
Pulmonary thromboembolic disease, 659t
Pulmonary vascular disease, diagnosis of,
    664t
Pulseless disease, **655**
Pulseless electrical activity, management
    of cardiac arrest, 43f
Pulse oximeter, 666
Pulsus alternans, 593, 593f
Pulsus bisferiens, 593, 593f
Pulsus paradoxus, 593
Pulsus parvus, 593, 593f
Pulsus tardus, 593, 593f
Pupils, in confusion and coma, 56–57
Pure alexia, 180t
Pure red cell aplasia, drug-induced, 983t
Pure tone audiometry, 244
Pure word deafness, 180t
Purine nucleoside phosphorylase defi-
    ciency, 777
Purpura. *See also specific types*
  drug-induced, 982t
  thrombotic thrombocytopenic, 276–277
Purpura fulminans, 97t, 100
Pustule, 255
Puumala virus, 551
PUVA therapy, for psoriasis, 259
Pyelonephritis, **724**
  azotemia in, 228f
  clinical features of, 724
  emphysematous, **727**
  treatment of, 726t
Pyloroplasty, for peptic ulcer disease,
    739t
Pyomyositis, 412
  Staphylococcus aureus, 450
Pyrantel pamoate
  for ascariasis, 582
  for enterobiasis, 584
  for hookworm, 582
Pyrazinamide, for tuberculosis, 498, 499t,
    502t
Pyridostigmine
  for myasthenia gravis, 943–944
  for orthostatic hypotension, 931
Pyridoxine, for isoniazid poisoning, 84

Pyridoxine deficiency, 16t
Pyrimethamine
  for isosporiasis, 387
  for malaria, 571t
  for *Pneumocystis* prophylaxis, 568t
  for toxoplasmosis, 579
Pyuria, 232, 701
  sterile, 232

Q fever, **515**
  acute, 515
  chronic, 515
  treatment of, 516
Quadrantopia, 172f
Quadriparesis, 176t
Quadriplegia, 933
Quantitative sudomotor axon reflex test,
    928
Quetiapine
  dosage and adverse effects of, 967t
  for schizophrenia, 958
Quinacrine, for giardiasis, 386
Quincke's sign, 607
Quinidine
  for arrhythmias, 646t
  for malaria, 570, 571t
Quinine
  for babesiosis, 96t, 573
  for malaria, 99t, 570, 571t
  for myotonic dystrophy, 947
Quinolone, for urinary tract infections,
    726t
Quinupristin/dalfopristin
  for enterococcal infections, 459
  for *Staphylococcus aureus* infections,
    453t, 454

Rabies, 106, **547**
  brainstem dysfunction period, 547
  coma and death, 547
  encephalitis phase of, 547
  postexposure prophylaxis, 548, 549t
  preexposure prophylaxis, 548
  prodromal period, 547
  sylvatic, 547
  treatment of, 548
  urban, 547
Rabies vaccine, 371t
Radiation bioterrorism, **127**
  acute radiation sickness, 129–131
  exposure
    external contamination, 129
    internal contamination, 129
    localized, 129
    whole-body, 129
  types of radiation, 127–129
Radiation sickness, acute, **129**
  stages of, 130
  treatment of, 130–131, 131f
Radiation therapy
  for breast cancer, 320
  for cancer, 288t
  for cervical cancer, 337
  for colorectal cancer, 327

Radiation therapy (*Cont.*):
  complications of CNS radiation, 885
  for endometrial cancer, 335
  for esophageal cancer, 321
  for gastric cancer, 322
  for head and neck cancer, 310
  for Hodgkin's disease, 306
  for lung cancer, 313t–314t, 315
  for prostate cancer, 339
  for spinal cord compression, 102
  for testicular cancer, 333
Radioiodine
  for thyroid cancer, 822
  for thyrotoxicosis, 818–820
  for toxic multinodular goiter, 821
Radionuclide ingestion, treatment of, 130
Radionuclide scan
  in cardiomyopathy, 610t
  hepatobiliary, 223
  in osteomyelitis, 415t
Radon exposure, 675
Ragged red fibers, 950
Raloxifene
  for breast cancer prevention, 283
  for osteoporosis, 854
Ramsay Hunt syndrome, 526, 922
Ranitidine
  for gastroesophageal reflux disease, 200
  for *Helicobacter pylori* eradication,
    739t
  for urticaria/angioedema, 774
Rapid shallow breathing index (RSBI), 21
Rasburicase, for tumor lysis syndrome,
    104
Rash
  classification of, 158
  drug-induced, 982t
Rat-bite fever, 106
Rattlesnake bite, 109
Ravuconazole, 555
Raynaud's phenomenon, 656
Reactive arthritis, **792**
  treatment of, 793
Rebleeding, in subarachnoid hemorrhage,
    66
Recluse spider bite, 112
  treatment of, 113
Recommended dietary allowances (RDA),
    3
Rectal cancer. *See* Colorectal cancer
Red blood cell(s)
  inclusions, 265
  intracellular abnormalities, 270
  membrane abnormalities, 271
  morphology of, 233f, 234, 265
  packed, 17
Red blood cell disorders, **267**
  anemia due to RBC destruction or
    blood loss, 270–271
  hypoproliferative anemias, 267–269,
    268t
  maturation disorders, 269–270
Red blood cell indices, 233
Red blood cell transfusion, 17–18

Red eye, 241–242, 241t
  treatment of, 241
Reexperiencing, 960
Reference values, laboratory tests, **995**
Referred pain, abdominal, 137t
Reflexes
  in confusion and coma, 57
  testing of, **872**
Reflex sympathetic dystrophy syndrome,
    801, 930
  treatment of, 801
Regurgitation, 197–198
Reiter's syndrome, 388, 413, **792**
  pain in, 162f
Relapsing fever, **509**
  chill phase of, 509
  flush phase of, 509
  louse-borne, 509
  tick-borne, 509
  treatment of, 510
Renal abscess, 382–383
Renal artery
  occlusion of
    acute, **728**
    azotemia in, 228f
  stenosis of, **729**
    clinical features of, 729t
    hypertension in, 616–618
  thrombosis of, 728
Renal atheroembolism, 728
Renal cancer, **332**
  paraneoplastic syndromes, 344t
  treatment of, 333
Renal disease. *See also specific diseases*
  in amyloidosis, 805
  anemia in, 268t
  approach to, **699, 700t**
  dialysis, 709–711
  drug-induced, 986t
  glomerular, 713–720
    in multisystem diseases, 719t
  hypertension in, 621
  nephrolithiasis, 702, 731–733
  nephrotic syndrome, 699
  parenchymal, hypertension in, 617–618
  renal failure. *See* Renal failure
  renal transplant, 711–713
  renal tubular disease, 701, 720–723
  renovascular disease, 728–731
  in sarcoidosis, 803
  in systemic sclerosis, 783
  urinary tract infections, 701, 724–728
  urinary tract obstruction, 702, 734–735
  weight loss in, 201t
Renal failure
  acute, **702**
    approach to, 699, 700t
    causes of, 704t
    definition of, 702
    differential diagnosis of, 703
    findings and diagnostic workup,
      703–705, 705t
    intrinsic, 703, 704t, 705
    postrenal, 703, 704t, 705

Renal failure (*Cont.*):
  prerenal, 703, 704t, 705
    treatment of, 705–706
  chronic, **707**
    approach to, 699
    causes of, 707t
    differential diagnosis of, 707–708
    laboratory evaluation of, 708
    renovascular disease and, 730
    slowing progression of, 709
    treatment of, 708–709
  edema in, 194, 195f
Renal stones, **731**
Renal transplant, **711**
  complications of, 713
  contraindications to, 712t
  factors influencing graft survival, 712t
  immunosuppressive therapy for, 711–713
  infections in transplant recipients, 422
  rejection of, 711
Renal tubular acidosis, **723**
  distal (type I), 723
  drug-induced, 986t
  proximal (type II), 723
  treatment of, 723
  type IV, 723
Renal tubular disease, **720**
  approach to, 700t, 701
  causes of, 721t
  transport dysfunction in, 722t
Renal vein occlusion, azotemia in, 228f
Renal vein thrombosis, **728**
Renovascular disease, **728**
  arteriolar nephrosclerosis, 730
  hemolytic-uremic syndrome, 730
  ischemic nephropathy, 730
  renal artery occlusion, 728
  renal artery stenosis, 729–730
  renal vein occlusion, 228f
  renal vein thrombosis, 728
  scleroderma, 730
  sickle cell nephropathy, 731
  toxemia of pregnancy, 731
  vasculitis, 731
Repaglinide, for diabetes mellitus, 833t
Reproductive system disorder, **393**
  female, **839**
  male, **835**
Residual volume, 663, 663f, 665t
Respiratory acidosis, 11f, 13–14
  treatment of, 13–14
Respiratory alkalosis, 11f, 14
  treatment of, 14
Respiratory disease. *See also* Pulmonary
    disease; *specific diseases*
  in amyloidosis, 805
  ARDS, 39–40
  asthma, 668–672
  Chlamydia pneumoniae, 519
  COPD, 675–678
  diagnosis of, **666**
  drug-induced, 984t
  environmental, 673–675

  hypersensitivity pneumonitis, 672–673
  infectious, in immunocompromised
    host, 419
  interstitial lung disease, 687–690
  meningococcal, 463
  obstructive, 664t, 665t
  pneumonia, 679–685
  prevention of, 993t
  Pseudomonas aeruginosa, 474
  pulmonary embolism, 685–687
  respiratory failure, 678
  restrictive
    extraparenchymal, 664t, 665t
    parenchymal, 664t, 665t
  in sarcoidosis, 803
  sleep apnea, 697–698
  specimens for culture, 353t
  Staphylococcus aureus, 450
  upper respiratory infections, **248**
  ventilatory disorders, 695–697
  viral, **533**
  weight loss in, 201t
Respiratory failure, **20, 22, 678**
  acute, 22
  acute or chronic, 22
  chronic, 22
  clinical evaluation of, 22–23
  mechanism of
    alveolar network dysfunction, 22–23
    controller dysfunction, 22–23
    pulmonary vascular dysfunction, 22–23
    pump dysfunction, 22–23
  treatment of, 21, 23
  type I (acute hypoxemic), 20
  type II, 20
  type III, 20
  type IV, 21
Respiratory function, disturbances of
  aspiration of lung in, 667
  bronchoalveolar lavage in, 667
  bronchoscopy in, 667
  gas exchange, 665–666
  imaging in, 666
  mechanisms of, 666
  mediastinoscopy in, 667
  pleural biopsy in, 667
  pulmonary angiography in, 667
  pulmonary circulation, 665
  pulmonary function tests in, 667
  scintigraphy in, 667
  skin tests for, 666
  sputum exam in, 666
  thoracentesis in, 667
  ventilatory, 663–665, 663f, 664f, 664t,
    665t
  video-assisted thoracic surgery in, 667
Respiratory muscle dysfunction, 186
Respiratory pattern, in confusion and
    coma, 57
Respiratory procedures, endocarditis pro-
    phylaxis for, 378t, 379t
Respiratory quotient, 665

Respiratory support, for nerve agent exposure, 127
Respiratory syncytial virus immune globulin, 538
Respiratory syncytial virus infection, **537**
  pneumonia, 679
  treatment of, 538
Responsiveness, assessment of impaired consciousness, 56
Restless legs syndrome, 182, 184t
Retching, 197
Reticulate body, 517
Reticulated lesion, 255
Reticulocyte(s), 265
Reticulocyte index, 233–234, 233f
Reticuloendothelial system hyperplasia, 238t
Retinal artery occlusion, 172f
Retinal vein occlusion, 172f, 173
Retinitis, herpes simplex virus, 521
Retinitis pigmentosa, 172f
Retinoic acid
  for acne vulgaris, 263
  for acute myeloid leukemia, 292
  for head and neck cancer prevention, 310
  for oral leukoplakia, 284
Retinopathy
  diabetic, 243
    treatment of, 243
  drug-induced, 987t
Retrochiasmal lesion, 172, 172f
Retroperitoneal abscess, 382
Reverse transcriptase inhibitors, 428t–432t
  nonnucleoside, 439
Rewarming
  active, 116
  passive, 116
Reye's syndrome, 535
Rheumatic fever, acute, 455
Rheumatoid arthritis, **781**
  interstitial lung disease in, 690
  neck pain in, 154
  pain in, 162f
  pleural effusion in, 691
  treatment of, 782–783, 782f
Rhinitis, allergic, **774**
  treatment of, 774–775
Rhinovirus infection, **536**
Rhizomucor infection, 560–561
Rhizopus infection, 560–561
Ribavirin
  for adenovirus infections, 539
  for chronic hepatitis C, 764, 765t
  for hemorrhagic fever, 551
  for Lassa fever, 551
  for measles, 541
  for respiratory syncytial virus infections, 538
  for SARS, 537
  for viral encephalitis, 893
  for viral hemorrhagic fevers, 121t
Rickettsia akari infection. *See* Rickettsialpox

Rickettsial disease, **510**
Rickettsialpox, **511**
  treatment of, 512
Rickettsia rickettsii infection. *See* Rocky Mountain spotted fever
Rifabutin, for mycobacterial infections, 504–505
Rifampin
  for anthrax, 122
  for *Bartonella* infections, 484t
  for brucellosis, 480
  for *Clostridium difficile*-associated disease, 392
  for diphtheria, 461
  for endocarditis, 375, 377t
  for *Haemophilus influenzae* prophylaxis, 467
  for *Legionella* infections, 479
  for leprosy, 503
  mechanisms, indications, and adverse effects of, 364
  for meningococcal infection prophylaxis, 464t, 887
  for nontuberculous mycobacterial infections, 505
  for primary biliary cirrhosis, 768
  for Q fever, 516
  for streptococcal carriage, 456
  for tuberculosis, 498, 499t, 501t
Rift Valley fever, 551
Riluzole, for amyotrophic lateral sclerosis, 918
Rimantadine
  for influenza, 535
  for influenza prophylaxis, 536
Ringworm, 262
Rinne test, 244, 871
Risedronate, for osteoporosis, 854
Risperidone
  dosage and adverse effects of, 967t
  for schizophrenia, 958
Ritonavir, for HIV infections, 433t
Rituximab
  for chronic lymphocytic leukemia/lymphoma, 300
  for gastric cancer, 322
  for idiopathic thrombocytopenic purpura, 277
Rivastigmine, for Alzheimer's disease, 908–909
River blindness, 585
Rizatriptan, for migraine, 143t
Rocky Mountain spotted fever, 97t, 100, **510**
  treatment of, 511
Rodent bite, 106, 108t
Rodent-borne viral infection, **548**
Romaña's sign, 576–577
Romberg sign, 914
Romberg test, 873
Ropinirole
  for Parkinson's disease, 913t
  for restless legs syndrome, 182
Roseola infantum, 527

Rosetting, 569
Rosiglitazone, for diabetes mellitus, 833t
Ross River virus, 550
Rosuvastatin, for hyperlipidemia, 859t
Rotavirus infection, diarrhea, 385
Rouleaux formation, 265
Rubella, **541**
  congenital rubella syndrome, 541
Rubella vaccine, 541
Rubeola. *See* Measles
Rumination, 197
Russian spring-summer encephalitis, 552t

Saccades, 870
St. Louis encephalitis, 552t, 893t
Salicylates
  for osteoarthritis, 795
  poisoning, 86–87
Salicylic acid, for scabies, 590
Saline diuresis, for poisoning/drug overdose, 77
Saline therapy
  for hypercalcemia, 103, 849t
  for hyponatremia, 6
  for metabolic alkalosis, 13
  for syndrome of inappropriate ADH, 815
Salmeterol
  for asthma, 669, 670t
  for COPD, 677
Salmonella infection, 387
  diagnosis of, 353t
  reactive arthritis, 792
Salmonellosis, **387**
  nontyphoidal, 388–389
  treatment of, 388–389
Salpingitis, 397
Salt wasting, 722t
Saquinavir mesylate, for HIV infections, 433t
Sarcoidosis, **802**
  acute, 803
  clinical features of, 803
  insidious onset, 803
  treatment of, 804
Sarcoma
  Kaposi's, 437, 527
  paraneoplastic syndromes, 344t
Sarcoptes scabiei. See Scabies
Scabies, **590**
  treatment of, 590
Scalded-skin syndrome, staphylococcal, 451
Scale, 256
Scar, 256
Scar carcinoma, 308
Scarlet fever, 456
Schistocytes, 265
Schistosomiasis, **585**
  acute, 586
  cercarial invasion, 586
  chronic, 586
  diagnosis of, 359t
  treatment of, 586

Schizoaffective disorder, 958
Schizoid personality, 962
Schizont, 569
Schizophrenia, **957**
  treatment of, 958
Schizophrenic-like reaction, drug-induced, 988t
Schizotypal personality, 962
Schwannoma, 884
  vestibular, 246
Scintigraphy, for biliary tract disease, 750t
Scleroderma, **783**. *See also* Systemic sclerosis
  diffuse cutaneous, 783
  dysphagia in, 205
  limited cutaneous, 783
  pain in, 162f
  renovascular disease in, 730
Sclerotherapy, for esophagogastric varices, 771
Scombroid poisoning, 112
Scopolamine
  for nausea and vomiting, 198
  for vertigo, 170t
Scorpionfish, 110–111
Scorpion sting, **113**
  treatment of, 113
Scotoma, 172f
Screening recommendations, **991**
Scrofula, 496
Scrub typhus, **513**
Sea anemone envenomations, 110
Segmental signs, in spinal cord disease, 933
Seizure, **875**. *See also* Epilepsy
  absence (petit mal), 875, 880t, 882t
  causes of, 875, 876t, 877t
  classification of, 875
  clinical evaluation of, 876, 878f–879f
  complex-partial, 875
  differential diagnosis of, 877t
  drug-induced, 877t, 987t
  electroencephalography in, 876–877
  generalized, 875
  neuroimaging in, 882
  partial (focal), 875, 880t, 882t
  from poisoning/drug overdose, 76–77
  simple-partial, 875
  syncope versus, 165, 877t
  tonic-clonic (grand mal), 875, 880t, 882t
  treatment of, 880t–881t, 882, 882t
Selection bias, 281
Selective serotonin reuptake inhibitors (SSRI), 963
  dosage and adverse effects of, 964t
Selegiline
  for Alzheimer's disease, 909
  for Parkinson's disease, 911
Seminoma, 333
Sensitization, 24
Sensorineural hearing loss, 245–246
Sensory exam, 870f, 871f, **873**

Sensory level, 102
Sensory neuronopathy, paraneoplastic, 348t
Sepsis
 clostridial, 488
 gram-negative, 96t
 gram-positive, 96t
 listerial, 465
 without obvious primary infection, 95, 96t
 puerperal, 475
 severe, **49.** *See also* Septic shock
  antimicrobial therapy for, 52t
  infectious disease emergencies, **94**
  with skin manifestations, 95, 97t, 100
  with soft tissue/muscle findings, 98t, 100
 Staphylococcus aureus, 450
Septic arthritis
 brucellosis, 479
 HACEK organisms, 470
 Staphylococcus aureus, 450, 454
 streptococcal, 458
Septic shock, 45, **49**
 clinical features of, 50–51
 epidemiology and risk factors for, 49–50
 treatment of, 51–53, 52t
Sequestra, 414
Serologic diagnosis, 358
Serotonin syndrome, 87
Serratia marcescens infection, **473**
 urinary tract, 724
Sertraline
 dosage and adverse effects of, 964t
 for panic disorder, 959
Serum sickness, 787
 drug-induced, 980t
Sevelamer, for hyperphosphatemia, 708
Severe acute respiratory syndrome (SARS), **537**
 epidemiology of, 537
 treatment of, 537
Severe combined immunodeficiency (SCID), **776**
 adenosine deaminase deficiency, 776
 Swiss-type, 776
 treatment of, 777
 X-linked, 776–777
Sexual dysfunction, drug-induced, 980t
Sexually transmitted disease (STD), **393**
 chancroid, 406–407
 Chlamydia infections, 400–402
 donovanosis, 407
 enteritis, 398–399
 enterocolitis, 398–399
 epididymitis, 396
 gonorrhea, 399–400
 herpes simplex virus infections, 406
 human papillomavirus infections, 407–408
 mucopurulent cervicitis, 397
 mycoplasmal infections, 402–403
 pelvic inflammatory disease, 397–398

 proctitis, 398–399
 proctocolitis, 398–399
 syphilis, 403–406
 ulcerative genital lesions, 398
 urethral syndrome in women, 396
 urethritis
  in men, 393–396
  in women, 396
 vulvovaginal infections, 396–397
Shigella infection, 390
 diagnosis of, 353t
 proctocolitis, 399
 reactive arthritis, 792
 treatment of, 390
Shingles. *See* Herpes zoster
Shock, 20, **44.** *See also specific types of shock*
 approach to, 45
 forms of, 45t
 in GI bleeding, 214
 hemodynamic profiles in, 46t
 laboratory evaluation of, 46
 oligemic, 45, 45t, 46t
 physical examination for, 45–46
 treatment of, 46–49, 47f
  vasopressors, 48t
Shoulder
 adhesive capsulitis of, 802
 muscles and innervation of, 868t–869t
Shoulder pain, **154,** 155t
Sibutramine, for obesity, 829
Sicca symptoms, 784
Sick euthyroid syndrome, **820**
Sickle cell anemia, 270
 clinical manifestations of, 270, 270t
 nephropathy in, **731**
 treatment of, 271–272
Sickled cells, 265
Sideroblastic anemia, 269, 269t
Sigmoidoscopy, 282t, 327
Sildenafil
 adverse effects of, 623, 636
 for erectile dysfunction, 838
 for systemic sclerosis, 784
Silent ischemia, 631
Silicosis, 674
Simple phobia, 960–961
Simvastatin, for hyperlipidemia, 859t
Sindbis virus, 550
Sinusitis, 248–252
 acute, 249
  diagnosis of, 250t
  treatment of, 249, 250t
 anaerobic infection, 490
 Aspergillus, 559
 chronic, 249–250
  bacterial, 249
  fungal, 249–250
 pneumococcal, 445
 streptococcal, 460
Sinus rhythm, 599
Sinus tachycardia, 639f, 640t
 myocardial infarction and, 625
Sirolimus, immunosuppression for renal transplant, 713

Sister Mary Joseph's nodule, 224
Sjögren's syndrome, **784**
  treatment of, 785
Skeletal disease. *See* Bone disease; Musculoskeletal disease
Skeletal muscle-central nervous system syndrome, 950
Skin
  biopsy of, 258
  examination of, **255**
Skin cancer, **307**
  basal cell carcinoma, 308
  melanoma, 307
  prevention of, 309
  screening for, 282t
  squamous cell carcinoma, 308–309
Skin disease. *See also specific diseases*
  acne, 262–263
  in amyloidosis, 805
  anaerobic infections, 490
  clostridial, 488
  common, **259**
  diagnosis of, 257–259
  drug-induced, 264, 981t–982t
  eczematous, 260–261
  history in, 257
  infectious, 261–262, 408–412
    in immunocompromised host, 417
  in inflammatory bowel disease, 743
  larva migrans, 581
  lesion characteristics
    arrangement and shape, 255
    distribution, 255, 256f–258f
  in malnutrition, 4
  papulosquamous, 259–260
  primary lesions, 255
  Pseudomonas aeruginosa infections, 475
  in returned traveler, 372
  in rheumatoid arthritis, 781
  in sarcoidosis, 803
  secondary lesions, 256
  staphylococcal, 449
  streptococcal, 456–457
  in systemic lupus erythematosus, 780
  in systemic sclerosis, 783
  vascular disorders, 263–264
Skin necrosis, drug-induced, 982t
Skin tag, 257f, 258f
Skin test, in respiratory disease, 666
Sleep, nonrestorative, 181
Sleep apnea, **697**
  central, 183, 697
  mixed, 183
  obstructive, 183, 184t, 697, 698t
  treatment of, 697–698, 698t
Sleep disorder, **181**
  approach to, **181**
  drug-induced, 988t
  seizures in, 877t
Sleep hygiene, 183
  inadequate, 182
Sleeping sickness, **577**
  treatment of, 578

Sleep paralysis, 184t, 185
Slow-reacting substance of anaphylaxis, 773
Small-bowel tumor, **323**
  treatment of, 324
Smallpox
  as bioweapon, 121t, 123–124
  hemorrhagic, 123
  malignant, 123
  microbiology and clinical features of, 122
  treatment of, 121t, 123
  vaccination and prevention of, 121t, 123–124
Smell, disorders of sense of, **922, 923t**
Smoke inhalation, 674
Smoking cessation, 37, 676, 690, 991, 992t, 993t
Snakebite, venomous, 108t, **109**
  treatment of, 109–110
Social phobia, 960–961
Sodium, disorders of, **5**
Sodium bicarbonate
  for cardiac arrest, 42, 43f–44f
  for hyperkalemia, 10t
  for iron poisoning, 83
  for metabolic acidosis, 12
  for shock, 49
Sodium nitrite, for cyanide poisoning, 82
Sodium nitroprusside, for aortic dissection, 654, 655t
Sodium restriction
  for aldosteronism, 825
  for ascites, 225
  for cor pulmonale, 652
  for heart failure, 649, 651
  for hyponatremia, 5
  for mitral stenosis, 604
  for restrictive cardiomyopathy, 611
Sodium stibogluconate, for leishmaniasis, 573–576
Sodium thiosulfate, for cyanide poisoning, 82
Sodium valproate
  for migraine prophylaxis, 145t
  for posthypoxic myoclonus, 71
Soft tissue infection, 408–412
  anaerobic, 490
  clostridial, 488
  Klebsiella, 472
  Pseudomonas aeruginosa, 475
  streptococcal, 456–457
Solid organ transplant, infections in transplant recipients, 422
Solitary pulmonary nodule, 314
  approach to, 315f
Solute diuresis, 230f
Somatization disorder, 961
Somatoform disorder, **961**
  treatment of, 961
Somatostatin, for esophagogastric varices, 771
Somatostatinoma, 329, 330t
Somatotropin, for hypopituitarism, 81

Sotalol, for arrhythmias, 641t
South American hemorrhagic fever syn-
    drome, 551
Soy products, for menopausal symptoms,
    845
Spastic paraplegia, familial, 936
Spectinomycin, for gonococcal infections,
    401t
Speech audiometry, 244
Speech therapy, 181
Spherocytes, 265
Sphincteric reflex, 872
Spider bite, **112**
Spinal cord, anatomy of, 933f
Spinal cord compression
    neoplastic compression, 885, 885t, 934
        oncologic emergency, 102
        treatment of, 102
Spinal cord disease, **932**
    acute, 934–935
    approach to, 934
    cervical cord, 934
    chronic myelopathy, 935–936
    complications of, 936
    lumbar cord, 934
    sacral cord, 934
    specific signs by cord level, 934
    symptoms and signs of, 932–933
    thoracic cord, 934
    trauma, autonomic dysfunction in, 928
    treatable, 932t
    weakness in, 176t, 177t
Spinal cord infarction, 935
Spinal epidural abscess, 935
Spinal epidural hematoma, 935
Spinal shock, 933
Spinal stenosis, pain in, 148
Spinocerebellar ataxia, 915
Spirillum minor infection, 106
Spirochetal infection, **506**
Spironolactone
    for aldosteronism, 825
    for ascites, 225
    for dilated cardiomyopathy, 609
    for edema, 196t
    for heart failure, 649t, 650
    for hirsutism in female, 843
Splenectomy, 240
    for esophagogastric varices, 771
    postsplenectomy infection, 95
        treatment of, 52t
Splenic abscess, 382
Splenomegaly, **236**
    diseases associated with, 238t–239t
    mechanisms of, 238t–239t, 239
    tropical, 570
Spondylitic myelopathy, 935
Spondylolisthesis, pain in, 148
Spondylosis, cervical, pain in, 154, 156
Spondylotic myelopathy, 156
Sporotrichosis, **565**
    extracutaneous, 565
    lymphangitis, 565
    meningitis, 897t

plaque, 565
    treatment of, 565
Sporozoite, 569
Spotted fever, tick- and mite-born, **510**
Sputum culture, 353t
Sputum examination, 666, 684
Squamous cell carcinoma, 258f
    of esophagus, 321
    of skin, **308**
        treatment of, 308–309
Staghorn calculi, 731
Standard precautions, 442
Stanford classification, of aortic dissec-
    tion, 654f
Staphylococcal infection, **448**
    arthritis, 412
    coagulase-negative, **451**
        endocarditis, 451
        meningitis, 886, 891t
        prosthetic device-related, 451
        treatment of, 454
    endocarditis, 376t–377t
    urinary tract, 724
Staphylococcus aureus infection, **448**
    from animal bites, 107t
    bacteremia, 450
    colonization of humans, 448
    diagnosis of, 449
    endocarditis, 450, 454
    epidemiology of, 448
    epiglottitis, 254
    food poisoning, 384, 451
    impetigo, 261
    invasive disease, 448–449
    meningitis, 886
    methicillin-resistant, 448
    musculoskeletal, 449, 454
    nosocomial, 443
    osteomyelitis, 414, 416t
    pneumonia, 679, 684
    prevention of, 451
    prosthetic-device related, 450, 454
    respiratory, 450
    risk factors for, 449
    scalded-skin syndrome, 451
    sepsis, 450
    sinusitis, 249
    skin and soft tissue, 449
    toxic shock syndrome, 100, 451, 455
    toxin-mediated disease, 449, 451
    treatment of, 452t–453t, 454–455
    urinary tract, 450
Stasis ulcer, 257f
Stat DRIP (medications mnemonic), 2
Statins, 859t
Stat medications, 2
Status epilepticus, **72**
    treatment of, 72, 73f
Stauffers' syndrome, 332
Stavudine, for HIV infections, 430t
Stenotrophomonas maltophilia infection,
    475
    treatment of, 477
Stent, vascular, for angina pectoris, 634,
    634t

Stereognosis, 873
Sternoclavicular pyarthrosis, 475
Steroid injection, for psoriatic arthritis, 792
Stevens-Johnson syndrome, 263
Stiff neck, 886
Stingrays, 110–111
Stomatitis, aphthous, 258f
Stool examination
    diagnosis of infectious disease, 353t–354t
    in diarrhea, 210
Straight-leg raising sign, 147
    crossed, 147
    reverse, 147–148
Streptobacillus moniliformis infection, from animal bite, 106, 108t
Streptococcal infection, **455**
    cellulitis, 409
    dog bite, 107t
    group A, 455
        bacteremia, 457
        cellulitis, 456
        epiglottitis, 254
        erysipelas, 456–457
        impetigo, 456
        necrotizing fasciitis, 457
        nosocomial, 443–444
        pharyngitis, 253, 455–456
        pneumonia, 457, 681
        poststreptococcal glomerulonephritis, 714
        puerperal sepsis, 457
        toxic shock syndrome, 457–458, 457t
    group B
        meningitis, 886, 887t
        neonatal infection, 458–459
        pelvic inflammatory disease, 397
        treatment of, 458
    group C, 458
    group D, 459
    group G, 458
    hemolytic patterns, 455
    infective endocarditis, 376t
    nutritionally variant streptococci, 460
    osteomyelitis, 415t
    scarlet fever, 456
    skin and soft tissue, 456–457
    toxic shock syndrome, 100
    viridans streptococci, 459–460
Streptogramins, mechanisms, indications, and adverse effects of, 365
Streptokinase
    for myocardial infarction, 623
    for thrombotic disorders, 279
Streptomycin
    for brucellosis, 480
    for enterococcal infections, 459
    for nontuberculous mycobacterial infections, 504
    for plague, 121t, 483
    for tuberculosis, 498, 499t
    for tularemia, 121t, 481

Streptozotocin
    for carcinoid tumor, 329
    for pancreatic islet-cell tumors, 331
    for Zollinger-Ellison syndrome, 741
Stress testing, in coronary artery disease, 631, 632f, 633t
Stroke, **58**
    anatomic localization in, 59t
    causes of, 63t
        determination of, 61–62
    clinical presentation of, 58–60
    drug-induced, 987t
    embolic, 65
    hemorrhagic, 60
    ischemic, 58, 60–61, 63t
    prevention of, 62–65
    risk factors for, 62, 64t
    treatment of, 60–61, 60t
Strongyloidiasis, **582**
    diagnosis of, 359t
    treatment of, 583
Struvite stones, 732, 733t
Stupor, **54**
Subacute sclerosing panencephalitis, 540
Subarachnoid hemorrhage (SAH), **66**
    with hydrocephalus, 67
    laboratory evaluation of, 66
    rebleeding, 66
    treatment of, 66
Subdural hematoma, 904
Substance abuse
    alcoholism, 972–975
    narcotic abuse, 975–977
    in women, 990
Succimer
    for arsenic poisoning, 80
    for lead poisoning, 84
    for mercury poisoning, 85
Sucralfate, for erosive gastropathy, 740
Sudden death, **41**
Suicide, 955–956, 958, 992t–993t
Sulfadiazine, for toxoplasmosis, 579
Sulfadoxine, for malaria, 571t
Sulfadoxine/pyrimethamine, for malaria, 575t
Sulfasalazine
    for ankylosing spondylitis, 790
    for inflammatory bowel disease, 743
    for psoriatic arthritis, 792
    for reactive arthritis, 793
    for rheumatoid arthritis, 783
Sulfhemoglobinemia, 192, 193t
Sulfinpyrazone, for gout, 798
Sulfonamides
    mechanisms, indications, and adverse effects of, 363–364
    for nocardiosis, 493, 493t
Sulfonylurea
    for diabetes mellitus, 832, 832t
    hypoglycemia from, 93f, 94, 94t
Sulfur granules, 494
Sulfur mustard, 125–126
    treatment of exposure to, 126

Sumatriptan
  for cluster headache, 146
  for migraine, 143t, 144t
Summer grippe, 545
Superior vena cava syndrome, **693**
  oncologic emergency, 101–102
  treatment of, 102
Supraventricular arrhythmia, myocardial
    infarction and, 625–626
Supraventricular tachycardia, 643t
  from poisoning/drug overdose, 75–76
Suramin, for sleeping sickness, 578
Surgical patient, evaluation of, **34**
  cardiac risk assessment, 34–37, 34t,
    35f
  pulmonary evaluation, 36t, 37
Susceptibility testing, diagnostic, 358
Swallowing disorder, **203**
Swimmer's ear, 252, 475
Swimmer's itch, 586
Sympathomimetics
  for heart failure, 651
  poisoning, 87–88
Symphysis pubis infection, 475
Syncope, **164**
  approach to, 165, 167f
  causes of, 165, 166t
  seizure versus, 165, 877t
  treatment of, 167–168
  vasodepressor, 165
  vasovagal, 165, 166t, 167
Syndrome of inappropriate ADH
    (SIADH), **814**
  causes of, 814, 814t
  drug-induced, 814t
  paraneoplastic, 103, 344t, 345–346,
    814t
  treatment of, 103, 815
Syndrome X, 831
Synkinesis, 922
Synovial fluid analysis, 163f, 164
  in gout, 797
Syphilis, **403**
  cardiovascular, 404
  congenital, 404
  diagnosis of, 404
  endemic, 507–508
  late, 403–404
  late benign, 404
  latent, 403, 405t
  in pregnancy, 405t
  primary, 403, 405t
  secondary, 403, 405t
  tertiary, 936
  treatment of, 404–406, 405t
Syringomyelia, 935–936
Syrup of ipecac, 77, 88
Systemic inflammatory response syn-
    drome (SIRS), 49
Systemic lupus erythematosus (SLE), **781**
  interstitial lung disease in, 690
  pain in, 162f
  renal disease in, 714, 719t
  treatment of, 780–781

Systemic sclerosis, **783**
  interstitial lung disease in, 690
  treatment of, 784
Systolic blood pressure, 618f–619f

Tabes dorsalis, 936
Tachyarrhythmia
  electrocardiography in, 639f
  syncope and, 166t
  treatment of, 638
Tacrine, for Alzheimer's disease, 908–909
Tacrolimus, immunosuppression for renal
    transplant, 712
Tadalafil, adverse effects of, 623, 636
Taeniasis saginata, **587**
  treatment of, 587
Taeniasis solium, **587**
  treatment of, 588
Takayasu's arteritis, **655,** 786, 788
Tamoxifen
  for breast cancer, 318–319
  for breast cancer prevention, 283
  for endometrial cancer, 337
  for melanoma, 308
Tandem walk test, 873
Tapeworm. *See* Cestode infection
Tardive dyskinesia, 969
Target cells, 265
T cell immunodeficiency, **777**
  treatment of, 777
T cell receptor complex deficiency, 777
Td (tetanus, diphtheria) vaccine, 368f,
    370f, 994t
Teardrop cells, 265
Tegaserod, for irritable bowel syndrome,
    747
Telangiectasia, GI tract, 217
Telithromycin, for pneumonia, 680t
Temazepam, dosage and adverse effects
    of, 966t
Temozolamide, for melanoma, 308
Temporal arteritis. *See* Giant cell arteritis
Tendinitis, **802**
  calcific, **802**
  pain in, 162f
  treatment of, 802
Tendon xanthoma, 857
Tenofovir, for HIV infections, 431t
Tenosynovitis, in gout, 796
Tensilon (edrophonium) test, 942
Tension headache, 140t, 144
  treatment of, 146t
Teratodermoid, 693
Terazosin, for prostate hyperplasia, 338
Terbinafine, 555
Terbutaline, for asthma, 669
Testicular cancer, **333**
  paraneoplastic syndromes, 344t
  treatment of, 333–334
Testicular failure, 835
Testosterone
  for androgen deficiency, 836
  deficiency of, 835–836
  for hypopituitarism, 812

Tetanus, 106, **485**
  generalized, 485–486
  local, 486
  neonatal, 486
  prevention of, 486
  treatment of, 486
Tetanus booster, 109
Tetanus immune globulin, 486
Tetanus vaccine, 486, 992t, 993t, 994t
Tetracycline
  for acne rosacea, 263
  for acne vulgaris, 263
  for adult inclusion conjunctivitis, 518
  for cerebral malaria, 99t
  for *Chlamydia pneumoniae* infections, 519
  for diverticular disease, 747
  for *Helicobacter pylori* eradication, 739t
  for intestinal pseudoobstruction, 748
  mechanisms, indications, and adverse effects of, 363
  for *Moraxella catarrhalis* infections, 468
  for psittacosis, 519
  for trachoma prophylaxis, 518
  for tularemia, 481
Tetrathiomolybdate, for Wilson's disease, 865
Thalamotomy, for Parkinson's disease, 914
Thalassemia, 269, 269t
  treatment of, 272
Thalidomide
  for leprosy, 503
  for multiple myeloma, 304
Thallium 201 imaging, in coronary artery disease, 631
Thallium poisoning, 88
Theophylline
  for asthma, 670t, 671
  for COPD, 677, 677t
  poisoning, 88
Thermoregulatory sweat test, 928
Thiabendazole, for strongyloidiasis, 583
Thiamine
  for alcoholism, 974
  deficiency of, 16t
  for status epilepticus, 72
Thigh, muscles and innervation of, 868t–869t
Thioridazine, dosage and adverse effects of, 967t
Thiothixene, dosage and adverse effects of, 967t
Thoracentesis, **28,** 667
Thoracic disease, actinomycosis, 494
Thoracic outlet syndrome
  arterial, 154
  disputed, 154
  true neurogenic, 154
Thoracic surgery, video-assisted, 667
Throat culture, 353t, 456
Thromboangiitis obliterans, **656**

Thrombocytopenia, 275
  drug-induced, 275, 983t
  treatment of, 277
Thrombocytosis, 276
  essential, 296
Thromboembolism, drug-induced, 984t
Thrombolytic therapy
  for arterial embolism, 656
  for myocardial infarction, 624f
  for stroke, 61, 62t
Thrombophlebitis, superficial, **657**
Thrombotic disorders, **277**
Thrombotic thrombocytopenic purpura (TTP), 276
  treatment of, 277
Thrush, oral, 557
Thumb, muscles and innervation of, 868t–869t
Thymectomy, for myasthenia gravis, 944
Thymoma, 348t, 693, 779, 942
Thyroid adenoma, **821**
  toxic, **821**
Thyroid cancer, 815, **821**
  treatment of, 822
Thyroid disease, **815**
  amiodarone-related, 820
  drug-induced, 980t
  goiter
    nontoxic, 820–821
    toxic multinodular, 821
  hypothyroidism, 815–817
  neoplastic, 815
  sick euthyroid syndrome, 820
  thyrotoxicosis, 818–820
  toxic adenoma, 821
Thyroid nodule, solitary, 821
  approach to, 822f
Thyroid-stimulating hormone (TSH), 807, 809t, 815
  deficiency of, 811–812
  replacement therapy, 812t
Thyroid-stimulating hormone-secreting tumor, 809, 811
Thyroid storm. *See* Thyrotoxic crisis
Thyrotoxic crisis, 818
  treatment of, 819–820
Thyrotoxicosis, 815, **818,** 821
  causes of, 818
  evaluation of, 818, 819f
  treatment of, 818–820
Thyrotropin-releasing hormone (TRH), 815
Thyroxine, 815–823
  for hypopituitarism, 812
Tiagabine
  for generalized anxiety disorder, 959
  for seizures, 882t
Tic(s), 178–179
Ticarcillin, for *Pseudomonas aeruginosa* infections, 476t
Ticarcillin/clavulanate
  for anaerobic infections, 491t
  for *Pseudomonas aeruginosa* infections, 476t

Ticarcillin/clavulanate (*Cont.*):
  for sepsis, 52t
  for urinary tract infections, 726t
Tic douloureux. *See* Trigeminal neuralgia
Tick bite, **114**
  treatment of, 114–115
Tick-borne relapsing fever, **509**
Tick-borne spotted fever, **510**
Tick paralysis, **114**
Tidal irrigation, for osteoarthritis, 795
Tidal volume, 663f
Tilt-table testing, 928
Timolol
  for glaucoma, 242–243
  for migraine prophylaxis, 145t
  for myocardial infarction prophylaxis,
    630
Tinea capitis, 262
Tinea cruris, 257f, 262
Tinea pedis, 256f, 257f, 262
Tinea unguium, 262
Tinnitus, 247
  treatment of, 248
Tirofiban, for acute coronary syndromes,
    635
Tissue plasminogen activator (tPA)
  for myocardial infarction, 624f
  for stroke, 61, 62t
  for thrombotic disorders, 279
Tobramycin
  for gram-negative sepsis, 96t
  for osteomyelitis, 416t
  for *Pseudomonas aeruginosa* infec-
    tions, 476t
  for sepsis, 52t
Toes, muscles and innervation of, 868t–
    869t
Tolcapone, for Parkinson's disease, 914
Tolnaftate, for dermatophyte infections,
    262
Tolosa-Hunt syndrome, 925
Tongue, geographic, 258f
Tongue paralysis, **924**
Tophi, 796
Topiramate
  for bipolar disorder, 957
  for seizures, 882t
Topoisomerase inhibitors, 287t
Torsades de pointes, 643t
Total lung capacity, 663, 663f, 665t
Toxemia of pregnancy, **731**
Toxic epidermal necrolysis, drug-induced,
    982t
Toxic granulations, 265
Toxicologic analysis, for poisoning or
    drug overdose, 75
Toxic shock syndrome, 97t
  staphylococcal, 100, 451
    treatment of, 455
  streptococcal, 100, 457–458, 457t
Toxins, renal disease and, 721t
Toxoplasmosis, **578**
  brain abscess, 894
  congenital, 579

diagnosis of, 359t
  HIV and, 579–580
  meningitis, 897t
  ocular, 579
  prevention of, 580
  treatment of, 579
Trace minerals, reference values for labo-
    ratory tests, 1004t
Tracheobronchitis
  Moraxella catarrhalis, 468
  respiratory syncytial virus, 538
Trachoma, **518**
  treatment of, 518
Tramadol
  abuse of, **975**
  for osteoarthritis, 795
  for pain, 27t
Transaminases, blood, 220–221, 222t
Transfusion, **17**
  autologous, 18
  complications of, 18, 18t
  exchange, 17, 570
  for GI bleeding, 217
  of plasma components, 19
  platelet, 18
  red blood cell, 17–18
  for shock, 47f
  whole blood, 17
Transient hypogammaglobulinemia of in-
    fancy, 778
Transient ischemic attack (TIA), 58
Transjugular intrahepatic portosystemic
    shunt (TIPS), 771
  for ascites, 225
Transplant recipient
  cytomegalovirus infection in, 530
  infections in, **421**
Transurethral microwave thermotherapy
    (TUMT), for prostate hyperplasia,
    338
Transurethral resection of prostate
    (TURP), 338
Tranylcypromine, dosage and adverse ef-
    fects of, 965t
Trastuzumab, for breast cancer, 320
Travel advice, **366**
  gastrointestinal illness, 366, 369
  for HIV-infected traveler, 369–371
  immunization, 366, 371t
  malaria prevention, 366
  in pregnancy, 369
  problems after return, 371–372
Traveler's diarrhea, 384
Trazodone, 963
  dosage and adverse effects of, 965t
  for insomnia, 183
  for posttraumatic stress disorder, 960
Trematode infection, **585**
  liver flukes, 586–587
  lung flukes, **587**
  schistosomiasis, 585–586
Tremor, 177
  in Parkinson's disease, 910
Trench fever, **483**, 484t

Trench mouth, 489
Treponema pallidum infection. *See* Syphilis
Treponematosis, endemic, **507**
    treatment of, 508
Treprostinil, for pulmonary hypertension, 661
Triamcinolone
    for asthma, 671
    for cough, 189
Triamterene, for edema, 196t
Triazolam
    dosage and adverse effects of, 966t
    for insomnia, 183
Triazoles, 555
Trichinellosis, **580**
    meningitis, 897t
    treatment of, 581
Trichloroacetic acid, for human papillomavirus infections, 407
Trichomoniasis, 396–397
    urethritis, 393
Triclabendazole, for liver flukes, 587
Tricuspid regurgitation, **608**
    treatment of, 608
Tricuspid stenosis, **608**
    treatment of, 608
Tricuspid valve endocarditis, 373
Tricyclic antidepressants, 963
    dosage and adverse effects of, 964t
Trientene, for Wilson's disease, 864–865
Trifluoperazine, dosage and adverse effects of, 967t
Trifluorothymidine, for herpes simplex virus infections, 525t
Trigeminal nerve (V), 870
    disorders of, **920,** 921t
    sensory divisions of, 921f
Trigeminal neuralgia, 147, **920**
    treatment of, 920
Trigeminal neuropathy, **920**
    causes of, 920–921, 921t
Trihexyphenidyl
    for extrapyramidal side effects, 969
    for Parkinson's disease, 914
Triiodothyronine, 815–823
Trimethoprim
    mechanisms, indications, and adverse effects of, 363–364
    for *Pneumocystis* infections, 567t
    for urinary tract infection prophylaxis, 727
Trimethoprim-sulfamethoxazole (TMP-SMX)
    for animal bites, 107t, 108t
    for *Aeromonas* infections, 474
    for brucellosis, 480
    for *Burkholderia cepacia* infections, 477
    for COPD, 677–678
    for cyclosporiasis, 387
    for HACEK endocarditis, 469t
    for *Haemophilus influenzae* infections, 467

for isosporiasis, 387
for *Legionella* infections, 479
for listeriosis, 466
for *Moraxella catarrhalis* infections, 468
for nephrolithiasis, 733t
for nocardiosis, 493, 493t
for otitis media, 251t
for peritonitis prophylaxis, 381
for pertussis, 468
for *Pneumocystis* infections, 567, 567t
for *Pneumocystis* prophylaxis, 568t
for salmonellosis, 389
for shigellosis, 390
for sinusitis, 250t
for spontaneous bacterial peritonitis, 225
for *Staphylococcus aureus* infections, 453t, 454
for *Stenotrophomonas maltophilia* infections, 477
for toxoplasmosis prophylaxis, 580
for urinary tract infection prophylaxis, 727
for urinary tract infections, 726t
Trimetrexate, for *Pneumocystis* infections, 567t
Trophozoite, 569
Troponins, cardiac-specific, 622
Trypanosomiasis, **576**
Tuberculosis, **495**
    AIDS and, 497
    brucellosis versus, 480t
    diagnosis of, 497–498
    epidemiology of, 495–496
    extrapulmonary, 496–497
    latent, 500, 501t–502t
    miliary, 497
    multidrug-resistant, 495, 499
    nosocomial, 444
    osteomyelitis, 414
    pathogenesis of, 496
    pleural effusion in, 691
    prevention of, 500
    pulmonary
        postprimary disease, 496
        primary disease, 496
    treatment of, 498–500, 499t, 501t–502t
Tubular necrosis
    acute, azotemia in, 228f
    drug-induced, 986t
Tubulin poisons, 287t
Tubulointerstitial disease, **720**
Tularemia, 95, 106, **480**
    as bioweapon, 121t, 124
    oculoglandular, 481
    oropharyngeal, 481
    pulmonary, 481
    treatment of, 121t, 481
    typhoidal, 481
    ulceroglandular, 481
Tumor lysis syndrome, 104
    treatment of, 104

Turcot's syndrome, 325, 325t
Two-point discrimination, 873
Tympanometry, 244
Typhoid fever, 388
treatment of, 388
Typhoid vaccine, 371t
Typhus fever
flea-borne, 512–513
louse-borne, 512–513
Tzanck preparation, 258, 522

Ulcer
peptic. *See* Peptic ulcer disease
skin, 256, 409
Ulcerative colitis, **742**
arthritis in, 799
extraintestinal manifestations of, 743
treatment of, 743–745, 744t–745t
Ulcerative genital lesions, **398**
Ulnar neuropathy, 940t, 941
Ultrasonography
in abdominal pain, 139
in acute abdomen, 207
in aortic aneurysm, 653
in aortic dissection, 654
in biliary tract disease, 750t
Doppler, in peripheral vascular disease, 656–657
endoscopic, 741
in biliary tract disease, 750t
hepatobiliary, 223
indications for, 32–33
neuroimaging, 874t
in osteomyelitis, 415t
in pancreatitis, 754, 756
renal, 707
utility of, 32–33
Undecylenic acid, for dermatophyte infections, 262
Upper motor neuron dysfunction, 175
weakness in, 176t, 177t
Upper respiratory infection, **248**
ear infections, 252–253
larynx and epiglottis, 253–254
nonspecific, 248
pharyngitis, 253
sinusitis, 248–252
Urate nephrosis, 797
Urea breath test, 738t
Ureaplasma urealyticum infection, 402
urethritis, 393
Ureidopenicillin, for acute cholecystitis, 751
Uremic syndrome, **708**
Ureteral obstruction, 734
Urethral syndrome, in women, **396**
Urethritis, **724**
clinical features of, 724
gonococcal, 393–396, 399
in men, **393**
treatment of, 393–396
nongonococcal, 393–396, 402
in women, **396**
acid nephropathy, 797

Uric acid stones, 732, 733t, 797
Urinalysis
in acute renal failure, 703–705, 705t
in chronic renal failure, 708
reference values for specific analytes, 1005t
toxicologic analysis, 75
in urinary tract infections, 725
urine culture, 354t
Urinary abnormalities
approach to, 700t, 701
asymptomatic, 701, **718**, 718t
glomerular causes of, 718t
urine composition, **230**
urine volume, **228**
Urinary tract infection (UTI), **724**
acute, 724
approach to, 700t, 701
clinical features of, 724
complicated, 726t
device-related, 442–443
emphysematous pyelonephritis, 727
enterococcal, 459
Escherichia coli, 471
gram-negative enteric bacteria, 473
Klebsiella, 472
nephrolithiasis and, 731
nosocomial, 442–443
papillary necrosis, 727
prevention of, 727
prostatitis, 727
Proteus, 473
Pseudomonas aeruginosa, 475
Staphylococcus aureus, 450
treatment of, 725, 726t
Urinary tract obstruction, **734**
approach to, 701t, 702, 735f
clinical features of, 734, 735f
treatment of, 706, 734–735
Urogenital secretions, culture of, 354t
Urokinase, for thrombotic disorders, 279
Ursodeoxycholic acid
for cholelithiasis, 750
for primary biliary cirrhosis, 768
for primary sclerosing cholangitis, 753
Urticaria, 263–264, **773**
drug-induced, 982t
treatment of, 774
Uterine bleeding
abnormal, **839**
treatment of, 839–840
dysfunctional (anovulatory), 839

Vaginal infection
diagnosis of, 394t
treatment of, 394t
Vaginitis, trichomonal, 394t–395t
Vaginosis, bacterial, 394t–395t, 396–397, 402
Vagotomy, for peptic ulcer disease, 739t
Vagus nerve (X), 872
disorders of, 923

Valacyclovir
  for genital herpes, 406
  for herpes simplex virus infections, 523, 524t–525t
  for herpes zoster, 527
  for viral meningitis, 892
Valganciclovir
  for cytomegalovirus infections, 530
  for viral esophagitis, 205
Valproic acid, 969
  for bipolar disorder, 957
  for brain tumor, 883
  dosage and adverse effects of, 968t
  for myoclonus, 177
  for seizures, 880t–881t, 882t
Valsalva maneuver, 928
Valsartan, for myocardial infarction, 625
Valvular heart disease, **603**. See also specific valves
  echocardiography in, 602, 602f
  preoperative evaluation of, 36
Vancomycin
  for acute bacterial endocarditis, 99t
  for bacterial meningitis, 890t, 891t
  for brain abscess, 894
  for Clostridium difficile-associated disease, 392
  for endocarditis, 375, 376t–377t
  for endocarditis prophylaxis, 379t
  for enterococcal infections, 459
  for gram-positive sepsis, 96t
  for HACEK endocarditis, 469t
  for hepatic encephalopathy, 772
  for infectious arthritis, 413
  mechanisms, indications, and adverse effects of, 362
  for osteomyelitis, 416t
  for pneumococcal infections, 447
  for pneumonia, 681t, 682t–683t
  for sepsis, 52t
  for Staphylococcus aureus infections, 452t–453t, 454
  for streptococcal infections, 459
Varicella vaccine, 367f, 368f, 370f, 994t
  in immunocompromised patients, 423t
Varicella-zoster immune globulin, 528t
Varicella-zoster virus infection, **523**
  diagnosis of, 526–527
  encephalitis, 892–893
Vascular disorders. See also Cardiovascular disease
  abdominal pain in, 137t
  gastrointestinal, **748**
  headache with, 140t
  skin conditions, 263–264
  syncope in, 166t
Vascular malformation, chronic myelopathy and, 935
Vascular shunting, anatomic, cyanosis in, 192, 193t
Vasculitis, 264, **785**
  approach to, 787, 787f
  azotemia in, 228f
  cutaneous, 786

definition and pathogenesis of, 785–786
  isolated, of CNS, 786
  primary vasculitis syndromes, **786**
  renal disease and, 715, 731
  secondary vasculitis syndromes, **787**
  treatment of, 264, 788
Vasodilators, for heart failure, 626, 650–651, 651t
Vasopressin, 813
  for cardiac arrest, 43f
  for diverticulosis, 217
  for esophagogastric varices, 771
  replacement therapy, 812t
  for shock, 48, 48t
Vasopressors, for shock, 48t
Vasospasm, in subarachnoid hemorrhage, 66
Vasospastic disorders, **656**
  treatment of, 656
Venezuelan equine encephalitis, 552t, 893t
Venlafaxine, 963
  dosage and adverse effects of, 965t
  for pain, 27t
Venous obstruction, edema in, 194, 195f
Ventilatory function, disturbances in, **663**, 663f, 664f, 664t, 665t, **695**
  extraparenchymal, 663
  obstructive, 663, 664t
  parenchymal, 663
  restrictive, 663, 664t
Ventilatory support
  for amyotrophic lateral sclerosis, 920
  for ARDS, 40
  care of ventilated patient, 21
  indications in critically ill patient, 20
  for respiratory failure, 23, 678
  weaning from mechanical ventilation, 21
Ventricular aneurysm
  myocardial infarction and, 630
  pseudoaneurysm, 630
  true, 630
Ventricular arrhythmia, myocardial infarction and, 625
Ventricular fibrillation, 639f, 642t
  management of cardiac arrest, 41, 43f
  myocardial infarction and, 625
Ventricular hypertrophy, 602
Ventricular premature beats, 642t
Ventricular septal rupture, 627–628
Ventricular tachycardia, 639f, 642t
  electrocardiography in, 644t
  management of cardiac arrest, 43f
  myocardial infarction and, 625
  from poisoning/drug overdose, 76
Verapamil
  for aortic dissection, 654
  for arrhythmias, 641t
  for hypertrophic cardiomyopathy, 611
  for migraine prophylaxis, 142, 145t
  for mitral stenosis, 604
  for supraventricular arrhythmias, 626

Verruca peruana, **483,** 484t
Verruca plana, 256f
Verruca vulgaris, 257f
Verrucous carcinoma, 308
Vertebral fracture, 148, 852
Vertebral metastasis, back pain in, 148–150
Vertebrobasilar insufficiency, visual loss in, 173
Vertigo, **168**
  approach to, 171
  benign paroxysmal positional, 169t, 170
  benign positional, 171
  central, 168, 169t, 170
  central positional, 169t
  pathologic, 168
  peripheral, 168, 169t
  physiologic, 168
  psychogenic, 170
  treatment of, 170t, 171
Vesicants, 125–126
Vesicle, 255, 409
Vestibular disorder, drug-induced, 987t
Vestibular neuronitis, 169
Vestibular schwannoma, 246
Vibrio cholerae infection. *See* Cholera
Vibrio cholerae non-O1 infection, 385
Vibrio parahaemolyticus infection, diarrhea, 385
Vibrio vulnificus infection, 100
Vinblastine, for lung cancer, 313
Vincent's angina, 489
Vincristine
  for acute lymphoid leukemia/lymphoma, 302
  for multiple myeloma, 304
Vindesine, for lung cancer, 313
Vinorelban, for lung cancer, 313
Vinorelbine, for breast cancer, 320
Violence, against women, 990, 992t
VIPoma, 329, 330t
Viral disease, diagnosis of, **351,** 357t
Virilization, 843
Visceral abscess, 382–383
Visceral disease, back pain in, 150, 151t
Visceral distention, pain in, 137t
Visceral spasm, pain in, 137t
Vision testing, 868–869
Visual cortex lesions, 172f
Visual field mapping, 172, 172f
Visual loss
  acute, **171,** 241–242
  chronic, 242–244
    causes of, 243t
  transient or sudden, 173
Vital capacity, 663f, 665t
Vitamin(s)
  reference values for laboratory tests, 1004t
  therapy for vitamin deficiencies, 16t
Vitamin A, for measles, 540–541
Vitamin A deficiency, 16t

Vitamin B$_{12}$ deficiency, 907, 936
  anemia and, 269
  treatment of, 271
Vitamin C
  for macular degeneration, 243
  for nephrolithiasis, 733t
Vitamin C deficiency, 16t
Vitamin D
  for osteomalacia, 855
  for osteoporosis, 854
  for primary biliary cirrhosis, 768
  for primary sclerosing cholangitis, 753
  for psoriasis, 259
Vitamin D deficiency, 854–855
Vitamin E
  for Alzheimer's disease, 909
  for macular degeneration, 243
  for menopausal symptoms, 845
Vitamin E deficiency, 16t, 915
Vitamin K, for primary biliary cirrhosis, 768
Vitamin K deficiency, 16t, 276–277
Vitreous detachment, 173
Vitreous hemorrhage, 173
Vomiting, **197.** *See also* Nausea and vomiting
von Hippel-Lindau disease, 332
von Willebrand's disease, 276
  treatment of, 277
Voriconazole, 555–556
  for aspergillosis, 559
  for fusariosis, 564
  for pseudoallescheriasis, 565
V/Q nuclear scan, in pulmonary hypertension, 659, 660f
Vulvovaginal infection, **396**

Waldenström's macroglobulinemia, 719t
Warfarin
  for cor pulmonale, 652
  for deep venous thrombosis, 657
  for deep venous thrombosis prevention, 658
  for dilated cardiomyopathy, 609
  for heparin-induced thrombocytopenia, 277
  for mitral stenosis, 604
  for renal vein thrombosis, 728
  for stroke prevention, 65, 65t
  for thrombotic disorders, 278t, 279
  for thyrotoxicosis, 819
Warts, 262
  anal, **749**
  treatment of, 262
Wasp sting, 114
Water restriction
  for hyponatremia, 5–6
  for syndrome of inappropriate ADH, 103
Weakness, 175. *See also* Muscle weakness
  approach to, 178f
  causes of, 177t

Weakness (*Cont.*):
from different areas of nervous system, 176t
Weaning, for mechanical ventilation, 21
Weaponization, 118
Weber test, 244, 872
Wegener's granulomatosis, 715, 786, 788
Weight, ideal weight for height, 3t
Weight loss, **201**
causes of, 201, 201t
drug-induced, 201t
laboratory evaluation of, 202t
Weil's syndrome, 508
Wernicke-Korsakoff's syndrome, 973–974
Wernicke's aphasia, 179, 180t
Western equine encephalitis, 552t, 893t
West Nile virus encephalitis, 550, 552t, 892, 893t, 894
Wet mount, 351
Wheal, 255
Whiplash injury, 154
Whipple's disease, **799**
Whipple's triad, 92, 93f
Whitlow, herpetic, 521, 524t
Whole blood transfusion, 17
Whole-bowel irrigation, 77
Widow spider bite, 113
treatment of, 113
Wilson's disease, **864**
treatment of, 864–865
Winking owl sign, 102
Winterbottom's sign, 577
Wiskott-Aldrich syndrome, 779
Withdrawal of care, 21–22
Wolff-Parkinson-White syndrome, 639f, **644**
Women's health, **989**
Alzheimer's disease, 989
autoimmune disease, 989
coronary artery disease, 989
diabetes mellitus, 989
drug-induced illness, 990
HIV infection, 990
hypertension, 989
osteoporosis, 990
psychiatric disorders, 990
substance abuse, 990
violence, 990
Wood's light examination, 259
Work hardening, 151

Wound infection
culture of wound material, 355t
nosocomial, 443
Wrist, muscles and innervation of, 868t–869t
Wuchereria bancrofti infection, 584

Xanthelasma, 258f, 857
Xanthoma
eruptive, 857
tendon, 857
tuberous, 857
X-rays. *See also* Abdominal x-ray; Chest x-ray
bioterrorism, 129
in osteomyelitis, 415t

Yaws, 507–508
Yeast, 555
Yellow fever, **553**
Yellow fever vaccine, 371t
Yersinia pestis infection, 122–123. *See also* Plague
Yersiniosis, 390–391
diagnosis of, 353t
reactive arthritis, 792
treatment of, 391

Zafirlukast, for asthma, 670t, 671
Zalcitabine, for HIV infections, 429t
Zaleplon, for insomnia, 183
Zanamivir
for influenza, 535
for influenza prophylaxis, 536
Zap70 kinase deficiency, 777
Zidovudine, for HIV infections, 428t, 438
Zileuton, for asthma, 670t, 671
Zinc deficiency, 16t
Zinc therapy
for macular degeneration, 243
for Wilson's disease, 864–865
Ziprasidone, dosage and adverse effects of, 967t
Zoledronate, for hypercalcemia, 103, 345, 849t
Zollinger-Ellison syndrome, 329, 330t, **740**
diagnosis of, 741, 741t
treatment of, 741
Zolmitriptan, for migraine, 143t
Zolpidem, for insomnia, 183, 184t
Zonisamide, for seizures, 882t
Zoster ophthalmicus, 526–527